PARAMEDIC PRINCIPLES AND PRACTICE ANZ

A clinical reasoning approach 2E

PARAMEDIC PRINCIPLES AND PRACTICE ANZ

A clinical reasoning approach 2E

Brett Williams

BAVocEd, Grad Cert IntensiveCarePara,
Grad Dip EmergHlth, MHlthSc, PhD, FACP,
Registered Paramedic

Linda Ross

BTeach, GradDipPhysEd, DipHlth(Amb),
BParaStud, MHlthProfEd, PhD

ELSEVIER

ELSEVIER

Elsevier Australia. ACN 001 002 357
(a division of Reed International Books Australia Pty Ltd)
Tower 1, 475 Victoria Avenue, Chatswood, NSW 2067

ISBN: 978-0-7295-4306-4

National Library of Australia Cataloguing-in-Publication Data

A catalogue record for this book is available from the National Library of Australia

Content Strategist: Rachel Simone Ford
Content Project Manager: Fariha Nadeem
Copy edited by Leanne Peters
Proofread by Tim Learner
Cover by Georgette Hall
Index by Innodata Indexing
Typeset by New Best-Set, China
Printed in China

Last digit is the print number: 9 8 7 6 5 4 3

Contents

Foreword

Professor Brett Williams, Dr Linda Ross and the contributing authors are some of Australia and New Zealand's most experienced paramedics, educators, researchers and emergency physicians. So it was with great pleasure that I accepted the invitation to write this foreword for *Paramedic Principles and Practice ANZ 2nd ed*, a unique and valuable resource that integrates knowledge and decision-making in the Australian and New Zealand context that they know and understand so well.

Paramedics are required to adapt and improve their range of clinical capabilities to provide care. This brings increased responsibility as professional clinicians to be aware of the potential impact they have on the lives of others. This impact cannot be underestimated.

As paramedics adapt and change, the authors saw the need to adapt and change this edition. They have added further chapters:

- Pharmacokinetics and pharmacodynamics
- Evidence-based practice in paramedicine
- Interpersonal communication and patient-focused care
- Mass casualty
- Tropical medicine
- Older patients
- Family violence
- Paediatric patients.

These chapters have added to the book's practical approach and continue to bring art and science together.

The shift of paramedic education from vocational to a university model has resulted in clinicians who enter the workforce with a complex understanding of anatomy, physiology, pathology and pharmacology. There is little doubt that this science has been an important step in the development of the paramedic profession. However, new graduate paramedics now have much less clinical exposure where they can learn the art of being a paramedic. I am impressed with the way this text lays out the pathway for graduates to develop and grow to be expert clinicians by bringing together the art and science of paramedicine. The inclusion of real-life stories reinforces this message and brings to life important theoretical models related to developing as an expert clinician and lifelong learner.

This text goes beyond the technical aspects of emergency care: it drives and reinforces the importance of professional attitudes, behaviours, clinical competence, teamwork, communication skills and the humanitarian approach required of paramedics. It is a refreshing approach to the complex challenges paramedics face in the context of an ageing population, high instances of chronic health problems, a health system that offers limited access to community-based clinicians and limited technological assistance for paramedic decision making. This book will be a valuable tool for those wanting to provide high-quality, patient-focused care in this challenging healthcare environment.

Healthcare starts at the patient, not at the emergency department or at a hospital or clinic door. In this context it is notable that decisions and clinical interventions performed by paramedics often keep patients alive until they can receive more definitive care.

Paramedic assessments, decisions and interventions have the capacity to keep patients out of the hospital system entirely, reduce morbidity and reduce the length of hospital stay, all of which have the potential to reduce the social and economic burden on the health system.

I recommend this edition to you as a resource that will assist you to contribute confidently to the care of your community and further develop your professional practice and career.

Success depends upon previous preparation, and without such preparation there is sure to be failure.

Confucius

Adjunct Associate Professor Ian Patrick

ASM, FPA, LMPA

Preface

Nothing in life is to be feared, it is only to be understood. Now is the time to understand more, so that we may fear less.

Marie Curie (1867–1934)

The best paramedic clinicians combine their knowledge, experience and non-technical behaviours and skills to form reasoned decisions in the best interest of patients. We cannot teach experience; that comes with time. Non-technical skills and behaviours are many, varied and can be innate to individuals; however, they can be enhanced through reflection and practice. This book aims to arm you with knowledge that underpins paramedic practice and decision-making based on the experience of the authors and best available evidence. It also endeavours to contextualise this knowledge and consider the human factors at play realising that paramedic practice is both multidimensional and unpredictable. Every case you attend as a paramedic will require you to call upon this knowledge, but to practise effectively you also need to be able to interpret people and situations.

To be a safe paramedic you need to elicit accurate information from patients, family members and bystanders who will differ from you in gender, generation, culture, social situation and health. You then have to determine what information is relevant and finally draw together all of these knowledge sets, skills, behaviours and attitudes to determine a diagnosis and treatment plan.

The process of clinical reasoning is probably the most difficult for students of any medical discipline to learn. Anatomy, physiology and pharmacology will come easily to those blessed with a good memory but will also eventually sink into the minds of the rest of us. Similarly, guidelines and clinical skills can be learned with practice. But how do you take all of this knowledge and use it when you are confronted with a patient?

An alternative method is to apply the clinical reasoning approach to conditions as you learn them. This text is not a substitute for content-specific texts that describe the anatomy, pathophysiology and pharmacology in far more detail. What the editors hope to offer is a text that allows you to see the links between the pathophysiology of a disease, how this creates the signs and symptoms perceived by the patient and how these need to be managed in the out-of-hospital environment.

Clinical reasoning is a real-time, living mystery. Traditional teaching methods offer you the clues that allow you to solve the clinical puzzle. But in real life, paramedics have to extract and sort the clues by importance before they must decide on an answer. To help you to develop this skill, this book is structured in two parts.

Part 1, Paramedic Principles, articulates the principles that support good paramedic practice: the ability to communicate effectively, gather essential clinical information in difficult environments and use this information to make safe and effective clinical decisions. Part 2, Paramedic Practice, presents the various conditions that paramedics can expect to encounter. Each chapter outlines the relevant background information and knowledge used to inform the clinical reasoning process. A series of case studies step you through each scenario to link the clues and, importantly, reveal the process of reaching a safe and effective management plan.

About the editors

Brett Williams

Professor Brett Williams is the current Head of the Department of Paramedicine at Monash University. Brett has won numerous national teaching awards and has published over 270 peer-reviewed publications, 11 book chapters and recently co-edited a book. Brett is committed to developing and finding the next generation of paramedic PhD scholars, professionalising paramedic care and building capacity for paramedics domestically and internationally. He currently supervises 16 paramedic PhD students and has supervised to timely completion eight doctoral and numerous master's and honours research projects.

Linda Ross

Linda is Deputy Head of Paramedicine at Monash University and leads the Postgraduate Programs. She practised as an advanced life support paramedic with Ambulance Victoria for 15 years before becoming a full-time academic in 2012. Since that time she has completed a Master of Health Professional Education investigating establishing rapport with patients and a PhD investigating the psychosocial needs of older people and developing paramedic awareness of these issues. She continues to explore research endeavours that enhance paramedic education and improve patient outcomes. She is well published in these areas with over 30 peer-reviewed publications and many national and international conference presentations, winning the 2015 Mary Lawson prize for best presentation at the 6th International Clinical Skills Conference in Prato, Italy. Linda is a passionate paramedic educator and believes in challenging, motivating and encouraging students to become lifelong learners who are able to use creativity and critical thinking to problem-solve, draw conclusions and make decisions.

Contributing authors

Tim Andrews GradDipEmergHlth

Intensive Care Paramedic, Ambulance Victoria, Victoria, Australia; Teaching Associate, Monash University, Victoria, Australia

Jason C Bendall AdvDipHlth (Amb), BMedSc (Hons), MBBS, MM (ClinEpi), PhD, FANZCA

Clinical Dean (Manning Clinical School), Department of Rural Health, University of Newcastle, New South Wales, Australia; Specialist Anaesthetist, Department of Anaesthesia, John Hunter Hospital, New South Wales, Australia

Andrew Bishop BHlthSci (Pre-Hospital Care), GradDipEmergHlth (MICA Paramedic), GradCert EmergHlth (Aeromedical & Retrieval)

Intensive Care (MICA) Flight Paramedic, Ambulance Victoria, Victoria, Australia; Teaching Associate, Monash University, Victoria, Australia

Rosemarie Boland RN, RM, MN, PhD

NETS Educator/NeoResus Web Content Developer and PIPER (Neonatal/Perinatal); Postdoctoral Research Fellow: Murdoch Children's Research Institute, Victoria, Australia; Honorary Clinical Senior Lecturer, University of Melbourne, Victoria, Australia

Kelly-Ann Bowles BSc (HumMoveSci), PhD

Director of Research, Department of Paramedicine, and Director of Research, School of Primary and Allied Health Care, Monash University, Victoria, Australia

Kate Carroll PhD, BBiolSci

Lecturer, School of Biomedical Sciences, Monash University, Victoria, Australia

John Craven BSc (Hons), BMBS, FRACP, FACEM

Head of Unit, SA Ambulance Service (SAAS) MedSTAR Kids Paediatric Retrieval Service, South Australia, Australia; Emergency Consultant, Flinders Medical Service, South Australia, Australia; Paediatric Emergency Consultant, Women's and Children's Hospital, South Australia; Senior Lecturer, Flinders University, South Australia, Australia

Daniel Cudini BExSci, BEmergHlth (Paramedic), GradDipEmergHlth (ICP)

Clinical Support Officer/Intensive Care Paramedic, Ambulance Victoria, Victoria, Australia; Teaching Associate, Monash University, Victoria, Australia

Ashley Denham BHlthSc (Paramedic), GradCertTEd

Lecturer, Bachelor of Paramedic Science, Central Queensland University, South Australia, Australia

Haydn Drake BA, BHSc (Paramedicine), GradDipHlthSci

Lecturer in Paramedicine, Auckland University of Technology, Auckland, New Zealand

Rosamond Dwyer MBBS, BMedSci, FACEM

Consultant Emergency Physician, Peninsula Health, Victoria, Australia; Retrieval Consultant, Adult Retrieval Victoria, Victoria, Australia

Sharon Flecknoe BSc (Biomed), BSc (Honours), PhD, GradDipEd (Secondary)

Director of Biomedicine Education Team in Allied Health and Director of Outreach Education, Monash University, Victoria, Australia

Boyd Furmston BNurs, GradDipNurs (Intensive Care), GradDipPara

Teaching Associate, Department of Paramedicine, Monash University, Victoria, Australia; Advanced Life Support Paramedic, Ambulance Victoria, Victoria, Australia

Hugh Grantham ASM, MBBS, FRACGP

Adjunct Professor, Curtin University, CQU University; Senior Medical Practitioner SAAS; Senior Medical Officer, Flinders Medical Centre Emergency Department, South Australia, Australia

Cameron Gosling BAppSc (HM), GradDip (ExRehab), MAppSc, PhD

Head of Undergraduate Paramedic Programs, Department of Paramedicine, Monash University, Victoria, Australia

Joelene Gott BParaSc, GradDipParaSc (Critical Care)

Lecturer, Bachelor of Paramedic Science, CQUniversity, Queensland, Australia

Shaun Greene MBChB, MSc (Medical Toxicology), FACEM, FACMT

Medical Director, Victorian Poisons information Centre, Victoria, Australia; Clinical Toxicologist and Emergency Physician, Victoria, Australia

Brian Haskins BHlthSc (Highest Honours), GradCertLearn&TeachHigherEd, GradDipOutdoorEd, GradDipEMS, MHlthServMgt

Lecturer and Pre Hospital Trauma Life Support (PHTLS) Program Director, Department of Paramedicine, Monash University, Victoria, Australia; Department of Epidemiology and Preventive Medicine, Monash University, Victoria, Australia

Dianne Inglis BN, AdvDip MICA, AssDip HlthSci (Paramedic), CertIV TAE

Intensive Care Paramedic; Clinical Education Manager (ret.), Victoria, Australia

Paul A. Jennings BNur, GradCertAdvNur, AdvDipMICAStud, GCHPE, GradCertBiostats, MClinEpi, PhD, FPA

Regional Improvement Lead, Barwon South West Region, Operational Improvement, Ambulance Victoria, Victoria, Australia; Adjunct Associate Professor, Department of Epidemiology and Preventive Medicine and Department of Paramedicine, Monash University, Victoria, Australia

Jeff Kenneally ASM, BBus, GradCert MICA, AssDip HlthSci (Paramedic), CertIV TAE

Intensive Care Paramedic; MICA team manager (ret.); Lecturer, College of Health and Biomedicine, Victoria University, Victoria, Australia

Jessica Lacey BEmergHealth (Pmed), BSc

Teaching Associate, Department of Paramedicine, Monash University, Victoria, Australia; Advanced Life Support Paramedic, Ambulance Victoria, Victoria, Australia

Peter A. Leggat AM, ADC, MD, PhD, DrPH, FAFPHM, FFPH RCP (UK), FPHAA, FACTM, FFTM ACTM, FFTM RCPS (Glasg), FISTM, FACRRM, FACAsM, Hon.FFPM RCP (UK), Hon.FACTM, Hon.FFTM ACTM

Professor and Co-Director, World Health Organization Collaborating Centre for Vector-borne and Neglected Tropical Diseases, College of Public Health, Medical and Veterinary Sciences, James Cook University, Queensland, Australia; Adjunct Professor, School of Public Health and Social Work, Queensland University of Technology, Queensland, Australia

Judy Lowthian PhD, MPH, BAppSc (SpPath)

Principal Research Fellow and Head of Research, Bolton Clarke Research Institute, Victoria, Australia; Adjunct Professor, Faculty of Health and Behavioural Sciences, University of Queensland, Queensland, Australia; Adjunct Associate Professor, School of Public Health and Preventive Medicine, Monash University, Victoria, Australia; Adjunct Associate Professor, Institute of Future Environments, Queensland University of Technology, Queensland, Australia

Andrew McDonell PA, NP, MICA-P, BAppSc, GradDipE&Train, GradDipEmergHlth, MBus, MPAS, FACN, MACRRM

Intensive Care (MICA) Paramedic, Ambulance Victoria, Victoria, Australia

Gayle McLelland PhD, MEd (ICT), GradCertHlthInformatics, BEdStudies

Associate Professor, Southern Cross University, Lismore, New South Wales, Australia; Adjunct, Monash University, Victoria, Australia

Tegwyn McManamny BEmergHealth (Hons), GradDipEmergHlth (ICP)

Teaching Associate, Monash University, Victoria, Australia; Intensive Care Paramedic, Ambulance Victoria, Victoria, Australia

Ben Meadley BAppSc (Human Movement), DipParamediSc (Prehospital Care), GradDipIntensiveCareParamed, GradDipEmergHlth (MICA), GradCertEmergHlth (Aeromed Retrieval)

Adjunct Lecturer, Department of Paramedicine, Monash University, Victoria, Australia; Intensive Care (MICA) Flight Paramedic, Ambulance Victoria, Victoria, Australia

Kim Murphy BSc (Hons), PhD, GradDipEd, MPH

Senior Lecturer, Immunology, Monash University, Victoria, Australia

Ziad Nehme BEmergHlth(Paramedic) (Hons), PhD

Paramedic and Senior Research Fellow, Ambulance Victoria, Victoria, Australia; Research Fellow & Adjunct Senior Lecturer, Monash University, Victoria, Australia.

Alexander Olaussen BEmergHlth (Paramedic), BMedSc (Hons), MBBS (Hons)

Adjunct Senior Lecturer, Department of Paramedicine, Monash University, Victoria, Australia; Research Fellow, National Trauma Research Institute, The Alfred Hospital, Victoria, Australia; Emergency Doctor, Northeast Health Wangaratta, Victoria, Australia

Robin Pap NDipEmergMedCare, HDipHigherEd&Trng, BTechEmergMedCare, MScMed (Emerg Med)

Lecturer in Paramedicine, Western Sydney University, New South Wales, Australia

Ravina Ravi BSc(Hons), PhD

Clinical Research Associate, Novotech, Melbourne, Australia

David Reid MHM(Hons), GradCert HSM, BSci (Paramedical Science), DipHlthSci (Prehospital Care), GAICD, MACPara

Director Paramedical Science, Edith Cowan University, Western Australia, Australia; Paramedic St John Ambulance (NT) Inc., Northern Territory, Australia

Louise Roberts BN, BHSc (Paramedics) (Hons), PhD

Lecturer, Paramedic Unit, College of Medicine and Public Health, Flinders University, South Australia, Australia

Joe-Anthony Rotella MBBS, BSc, MMedTox, FACEM

Toxicology Fellow and Emergency Physician, Austin Health, Victoria, Australia; Honorary Clinical Senior Lecturer, Austin Clinical School, University of Melbourne, Victoria, Australia

Auston Rotheram MEd, GradDipEmergHlth (MICA),GradCertMgt, GradCertRes

Senior Lecturer, University of Tasmania, Tasmania, Australia

Simon Sawyer BPsychMgtMktg, BEmergHealth (Pmed), PhD

Lecturer, Department of Paramedicine, Monash University, Victoria, Australia; Advanced Life Support Paramedic, Ambulance Victoria, Victoria, Australia

Brendan Shannon BEmergHlth (Paramedic) (Hons)

Lecturer, Department of Paramedicine, Monash University, Victoria, Australia; Registered Advanced Life Support Paramedic, Ambulance Victoria, Victoria, Australia

Paul Simpson AdvDip (ParamedScience), BEd (PDHPE), BHSc (PrehospCare), GradCertPaeds, GradCertClinEd, MScM (ClinEpi), PhD

Registered Paramedic (Intensive Care), NSW Ambulance, New South Wales, Australia; Senior Lecturer and Director of Academic Program (Paramedicine), Western Sydney University, New South Wales, Australia

Erin Smith PhD, MPH, MClinEpi

Associate Professor, School of Medical and Health Sciences, Edith Cowan University, Western Australia, Australia; Adjunct Senior Lecturer, Medical and Veterinary Sciences, Division of Tropical Health and Medicine, College of Public Health, James Cook University, Queensland, Australia

Yvonne Singer RN, DSc, BSc, GDipClinNur, CF

Program Coordinator, Victorian Adult Burn Service, Victoria, Australia; Burn Registry of Australia & New Zealand Associate; Monash University, Victoria, Australia

Toby St. Clair DipAmbParaStudies, GradDipEmerHlth(MP), GradCertEmAeroMedRet, MSpecParamed

Teaching Associate, Monash University, Victoria, Australia; Mobile Intensive Care Paramedic, Ambulance Victoria, Victoria, Australia

Brian Stoffell BA (Hons 1), LLB (Hons 1), PhD

Course Coordinator, Bachelor of Letters (Health), Flinders University, South Australia, Australia

Liz Thyer PhD (Melb), BSc (Hons), DipAmbParaStudies, GCTE

Director of Learning and Teaching, Senior Lecturer, School of Science and Health, Western Sydney University, New South Wales, Australia

Abigail Trewin BHlthSt (Paramedic), ADipAmb Studies, GradCertIntPara, GradCertHumLdshp, MPHTM

Director Disaster Preparedness and Response, National Critical Care and Trauma Response Centre, Northern Territory, Australia

Jarrod Wakeling BHlthSc (Paramed), GDEmergHlth (Intensive Care Paramed), MEmergHlth

Intensive Care Paramedic, Ambulance Victoria, Victoria, Australia; Teaching Associate, Monash University, Victoria, Australia

Helen Webb BEd, TeachCert, MHlthSc (Hons), PhD

Associate Professor in Paramedicine, Australian Catholic University, Victoria, Australia

Julian White AM, MB, BS, MD, FACTM

Head of Toxinology, Women's and Children's Hospital, Adelaide, Australia

Denise Wilson BA(SocSc), MA(Hons), PhD

Professor, Māori Health; Associate Dean, Māori Advancement, Faculty of Health & Environmental Sciences, Auckland University of Technology, Auckland, New Zealand; Co-Director, Taupua Waiora Māori Health Research Centre, Auckland University of Technology, Auckland, New Zealand

Shaun Whitmore RN, AssocDipHealthSci, AdvDipMICA (Paramedic), GradCertAeromedicalRetrieval

Intensive Care Flight Paramedic Air Ambulance Victoria, Australia

Reviewers

Malcolm Boyle ADipHlthSci(AmbOff), MICA Cert, BInfoTech(InfoSys), MClinEpi, GCertAcadPrac, PhD, RP, FACPara

Associate Professor/Academic Lead, School of Medicine—Paramedicine, Griffith University, Queensland, Australia

Daniel DeGoey BClinicalPrac (Paramedic), BSc (Chiropractic), FHEA

Advanced Care Paramedic II, Queensland Ambulance Service, Australia; Lecturer of Paramedical Sciences, Queensland University of Technology, Queensland, Australia

Sonja Maria BClinPrac(Paramedic) PhD(c)

Senior Lecturer in Paramedicine, Strategic Liasion Officer, Masters of Paramedicine coordinator, School of Biomedical Science, Charles Sturt University, New South Wales, Australia

David McLeod AdDipPubSafty (Emerg Man), BHlthSc (Paramedicine), GDipStratLeadership, MACPara

Clinical Educator, New South Wales Ambulance, New South Wales, Australia

Roshan Raja DipHSci (Paramedicine), BApSci (OHS), BHSci (Paramedicine), GCTE, MEd

Advanced Life Support Paramedic and Clinical Instructor, Ambulance Victoria, Victoria, Australia; Lecturer, Paramedicine, Victoria University, Victoria, Australia

James Thompson BHSc Hons, GCHE, BNsg, DipAppSc (Ambulance Studies)

Teaching Specialist/Senior Lecturer, Paramedic Unit, School of Medicine, Flinders Southern Adelaide Clinical School, Flinders University, Adelaide, Australia

The key to improving your clinical practice

The ability to reach safe and accurate clinical decisions is not solely influenced by the paramedic's knowledge of disease and clinical practice guidelines. Clinical decision-making can be influenced by numerous factors including patient demographics and expectations, paramedic experience and fatigue levels, resourcing and the environment in which patient care occurs.

This text therefore aims to not only link pathology with signs and symptoms, but also to contextualise paramedic practice and reveal the unique strategies experienced paramedics use to practise effectively in the out-of-hospital environment. Under internal and external pressures, the best paramedics are often unaware of the decision-making process they use to devise treatment plans. This book will explore some of the processes involved and provide students with a guide to making safe and effective clinical decisions for a wide variety of clinical presentations.

Each chapter in Part 2, Paramedic Practice, presents case studies based on genuine cases. In practice, paramedics begin the problem-solving process the moment the case is dispatched. They begin to consider potential diagnoses; things to consider given age, location and other factors; and potential treatment options. The initial case study in each chapter describes the typical presentation for a particular condition and the signs and symptoms that should not be missed. It identifies a particular pathology and how this links to the patient's signs and symptoms, and outlines how the condition commonly presents, the clinical decision-making challenges often associated with it and how it can be managed. As each chapter progresses, the presentation becomes less 'classic' and the chapter describes how to reach a clinical decision when faced with increasing uncertainty. The subsequent case studies in each chapter thus present less-typical examples, enabling novice practitioners to examine the decision-making processes of more experienced clinicians and to explore how safe and effective clinical decisions can be made.

Understanding how you make clinical decisions is the key to improving your skills, and learning why clinicians make errors in collecting or processing information allows you to identify these behaviours in yourself and correct them. Even for experienced clinicians, there is value in understanding the process: when experts are faced with a condition they have not encountered before, they may switch to the form of clinical reasoning more often used by novices. This meta-cognition (analysing how you think) is what separates expert paramedics from those with simply a good memory.

Key features

CASE STUDY

Case 14519, 0947 hrs.

Dispatch details: A 74-year-old female with chest pain. The patient has a cardiac history.

Initial presentation: The patient is sitting in a chair on the front verandah as the crew arrive. As they approach she coughs vigorously and produces a large volume of purulent mucus that she spits delicately into a tissue. She tells the paramedics she has had a chest cold with thick spit for about a week but today when she stands up her chest hurts, and it hurts more when she coughs.

Case study
Each case study is based on a genuine case and reflects the experience of the chapter author(s). The introduction section to each case outlines the dispatch number and call-out time, the dispatch details as noted by the call-taker and the patient's initial presentation when the paramedics arrive on the scene.

Clinical reasoning steps

For every case study we take you through the four-step clinical reasoning process of **assess**, **confirm**, **treat** and **evaluate**. This process is critical to improving your clinical decision-making: it is an internal process used by most clinicians and therefore rarely visible in practice.

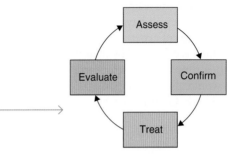

1 Assess

Assessment of patients in the out-of-hospital setting is limited by time and equipment. An accurate history and a structured approach are therefore the two most important elements in this environment. Each case study identifies the most pertinent signs and symptoms associated with a particular condition.

2 Confirm

In addition to linking the pathophysiology of a condition with the symptoms, each case study details the various differential diagnoses that should be considered when you are presented with a particular case history. This reflects the way experienced clinicians think: exploring a range of potential causes for a patient's condition and systematically eliminating them until the best management plan is reached.

3 Treat

Each case study outlines the principles of managing the condition with special consideration for the out-of-hospital environment. The treatments are not based around a particular skill set, but start with the most basic elements and extend through to an intensive care level.

4 Evaluate

The evaluation phase is important as the patient's response to treatment can indicate the accuracy of the initial diagnosis. Not all treatments available to paramedics will demonstrate an effect in the timeframes associated with emergency care. In some cases the treatment may be instantaneous but inevitably some will take longer or may not be effective at all.

Ongoing management

We conclude the case studies with an outline of what happens once the patient arrives at hospital, because understanding where out-of-hospital and in-hospital treatments align and differ can assist in determining how aggressive out-of-hospital management should be and where transport should be considered as treatment.

Acknowledgements

The editors would like to acknowledge and thank the chapter authors. They all have genuine passion for their respective areas of expertise and the paramedic profession, which is evidenced by their willingness to contribute their time in the development of this text. The editors would also like to thank the first edition editors and Hugh Grantham who was consulted in the early stages of this new 2nd edition. The editors would also like to thank all those willing to support and progress the paramedic profession and in particular paramedic education. Finally, the editors would like to acknowledge their colleagues, friends and families for their patience and support during the editing of this text.

PART ONE
PARAMEDIC PRINCIPLES

SECTION 1:
Introduction to Paramedic Principles and Practice

In this section:

CHAPTER 1

Introduction

By Linda Ross and Brett Williams

The paramedic profession is ever evolving. This evolution is based on a multitude of connected factors including advances in medicine, patient demographics, government policy and health system structure, and education. The public's perception of paramedics and their role is often garnered from news bulletins and reality television shows highlighting emergency situations. The day-to-day reality can be very different, with paramedics attending to a wide variety of patients who may be suffering from chronic and non-life-threatening conditions. Regardless of the perception and the reality, what is a constant—and at the heart of paramedic practice—is patient care.

Paramedics are required to possess advanced clinical skills and be able to manage a range of conditions under pressure. They have to solve complex clinical problems in public environments, often surrounded by the patient's family, friends and bystanders. In addition, they can be operating in extreme environments and be subject to external distractions and complications such as traffic. Furthermore, they are subject to time pressures imposed by their service and the patient's condition, and have limited diagnostic tools at their disposal. Paramedics must therefore possess not only clinical knowledge and skill but also traits that allow them to operate effectively under pressure. This text will not only explore clinical concepts and patient presentations but will discuss the human factors influencing paramedic practice.

This text is designed to be used in conjunction with a quality educational program to assist both undergraduate and graduate paramedics to link theory to practice. Experienced clinicians and experts in their field have written each chapter. They have been able to draw upon their knowledge and years of experience to add context and provide the most up-to-date and relevant information possible. This text will act as a valuable resource for any paramedics aiming to provide quality patient care in the out-of-hospital environment.

Professionalism

A profession is a disciplined group of individuals who adhere to ethical standards and who hold themselves out as, and are accepted by the public as, possessing special knowledge and skills in a widely recognised body of learning derived from research, education and training at a high level, and who are prepared to apply this knowledge and exercise these skills in the interest of others.

(Australian Council of Professions, 2019)

It is incumbent on paramedics to uphold the principles, laws, ethics and conventions of the paramedic profession.

National Registration

In 2018, the Australian Healthcare Practitioner Regulation Authority (AHPRA) added the discipline of paramedicine to its list of nationally registered health professionals (Paramedicine Board of Australia, 2018a). This development recognised the complexity of contemporary paramedic practice, and illustrates how far paramedicine has moved from its traditional roots as a transport service. With national registration comes the standards that paramedics must meet in order to be become registered and maintain that status. These include continuing professional development, criminal history checks, English-language skills, recency of practice and insurance standards. Once registered, paramedics have a professional and ethical obligation to protect and promote public health and safe healthcare.

Code of Conduct

In 2018, the Paramedic Board of Australia released a code of conduct for paramedics (Paramedicine Board of Australia, 2018b). This code is designed to support individual practitioners in the challenging task of providing good healthcare and fulfilling their professional roles and to provide a framework to guide professional judgment. In addition, it assists the Board in their role of protecting the public by setting and maintaining standards of good practice, and is a guide to the public and consumers of health services about what good practice is and the standard of behaviour they should expect from paramedics. Standards covered by the paramedic code of conduct are listed in Box 1.1.

Professional development

Professionalism goes beyond the scope and boundaries set by AHPRA registration. While minimum professional development standards are mandated, it is incumbent on individual paramedics to seek their own development opportunities beyond this.

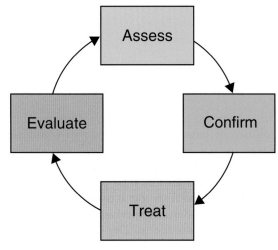

Figure 1.1
The clinical reasoning model.

This may take the form of formal education in postgraduate programs, membership and participation in national discipline-specific bodies, reading contemporary research, profession networks with other healthcare providers, or combinations of these.

Reflective practice

Paramedics of all experience levels are encouraged to incorporate reflective practice into their daily routines. There are numerous models describing the steps involved in reflection; however, the purpose remains the same regardless of the process. In order to become better clinicians paramedics need to be able to reflect on their own performance in order to continue learning. Reflection does not have to be a formal process and may be as simple as taking a moment or two to reflect on what you did well in a particular case and what you could improve on. Taking the time to reflect on these aspects always helps you to then form strategies for maintenance or improvement.

Paramedic Principles and Practice 2nd edition

Paramedic Principles and Practice 2nd edition is divided into two parts: paramedic principles and paramedic practice. Each part consists of multiple sections incorporating chapters related to each section's theme. It also contains some new chapters based on the current paramedic profession climate and reader feedback. New chapters include:
- Pharmacokinetics and pharmacodynamics
- Evidence-based practice in paramedicine
- Interpersonal communication and patient-focused care
- Mass casualty

- Tropical medicine
- Older patients
- Family violence
- Paediatric patients.

Part 1—Paramedic principles

Part 1, Paramedic principles, explores foundation knowledge and concepts that underpin patient conditions and care. It begins with some key physiological processes that are common to a wide range of diseases and injuries. A thorough understanding of perfusion and of autonomic and inflammatory responses is vital as these processes serve to inform paramedic understanding of patient presentations and the effects of pharmaceutical and non-pharmaceutical interventions. We also look at the role of the paramedic and how that has evolved over time along with education standards, scopes of practice and patient demographics. Part 1 also talks about errors, mitigating legal and ethical factors, and looking after your own health and wellbeing.

Clinical reasoning is also introduced in this part of the text. It is an intriguing and complex process that is essential for the generally autonomous paramedic in the out-of-hospital environment. This chapter will help you to understand the clinical reasoning process and then explore how your perspective, attitude, communication, preconceptions and philosophy can influence your ability to make safe and effective decisions (Figure 1.1).

Part 1 contains three new chapters: *Pharmacokinetics and pharmacodynamics*, which explores the key underlying principles of drug actions and interactions within the physiological system; *Evidence-based practice in paramedicine*, which looks at the origins and importance of research to the profession; and *Interpersonal communication and patient-focused care*, which highlights the significance of this aspect of paramedic practice.

Part 2—Paramedic practice

Part 2, Paramedic practice, begins with the structured clinical approach and patient-centred interview. These processes are integral to patient care and outcomes as they set the scene and provide the information from which decisions are made. The ensuing sections take the reader through various patient presentations encountered in the out-of-hospital environment. These include cardiac, respiratory, medical, environmental and mental health conditions. We also look at trauma presentations and unique population groups such as Indigenous, paediatric and older patients. The chapters within this part of the text not only provide detailed background knowledge of conditions but also explore contextual implications pertinent to paramedic practice. The expert authors have provided case studies that guide the reader through the clinical reasoning process and elaborate on considerations at each step.

Part 2 contains five new chapters: *Mass casualty*, which explores the role and responsibilities of paramedics in multi-casualty or major incidents; *Tropical medicine*, which explores tropical disease transmission and treatment; *Older patients*, which discusses the unique biopsychosocial issues applicable to older patients and how to recognise and manage these; *Family violence*, which discusses the prevalence of family violence and the role of paramedics when they encounter it; and *Paediatric patients*, which discusses the differences between paediatric patients and some common conditions.

Summary

This text examines the complex cognitive processes involved in reaching effective clinical decisions in the high-pressure, time-poor environments in which paramedics have to operate. As a paramedic, you will accumulate knowledge, skills, experience and attitudes that will allow you to perform your work safely and efficiently. Chapters have been written by content specialists who are able to share some of their knowledge and experience with you. Use their expertise to supplement your learning and practice. Finally, never lose sight of who is at the centre of your practice as a paramedic: the patient.

References

Australian Council of Professions. (2019). *What is a Profession?* Retrieved from: http://www.professions.com.au/about-us/what-is-a-professional.

Paramedicine Board of Australia. (2018a). *Paramedicine Board of Australia.* Retrieved from: http://www.paramedicineboard.gov.au/.

Paramedicine Board of Australia. (2018b). *Codes, guidelines and policies.* Retrieved from: https://www.paramedicineboard.gov.au/Professional-standards/Codes-guidelines-and-policies.aspx.

SECTION 2:
Foundation Knowledge

In this section:

A number of essential physiological concepts underpin paramedic practice and are common to a wide range of diseases and injuries. Perfusion, the autonomic nervous system and inflammation are concepts that all paramedics must understand in order to make safe and effective clinical decisions. These homeostatic responses are common across nearly all conditions that paramedics confront, and the importance of understanding how they integrate into the disease process cannot be over-emphasised. In addition, this section will explore the key underlying principles of drug actions and interactions within the physiological system. As paramedics, it is vital to understand pharmacological interventions and their therapeutic and potential adverse effects.

This foundation section does not attempt to cover these concepts to their full breadth and depth. It is designed as a quick reference to aid in understanding of concepts which are fundamental to other sections within this text. More detailed concepts and explanations can be found in content-specific pathophysiology and pharmacology texts. The reference and suggested reading lists at the end of each chapter will provide you with a range of further texts.

CHAPTER 2

Perfusion

By Sharon Flecknoe and Kate Carroll

Introduction

One of the consequences of working in an environment subject to time pressures and few diagnostic tools is paramedics' propensity to summarise complex physiological responses into axioms that can be used as rules to assist in decision-making. For example: 'The first two rules of paramedic practice are: (1) the air must go in and out; and (2) the blood must go around and around'. Simplistic certainly, but these sayings are not only reinforced by the primary survey (A, B, C) but are also the basis of sustaining life: no cell can survive without an adequate supply of oxygen and nutrients. In order to provide continuous supply of these essential factors, tissues must be adequately perfused with oxygen- and nutrient-rich blood. Perfusion is the focus of this chapter because it is not only central to homeostasis but will also determine how you, as a clinician, correct disturbances caused by illness or injury. Without an understanding of the concept of perfusion, you risk simply treating the patient's symptoms rather than managing the underlying cause.

What is perfusion?

In simple terms, perfusion is the flow of blood through a particular capillary bed within an organ or tissue. Therefore, tissues can be adequately perfused or inadequately perfused, depending on the amount of blood flowing to them. However, in practice, it is not this simple. Given that the role of the circulatory system is to deliver oxygen and nutrients (at the same time as removing waste products), it becomes evident that cells receiving adequate circulation but blood which is depleted of oxygen or nutrients (e.g. due to hypoxaemia or hypoglycaemia) would not function effectively. Consequently, in this chapter we will discuss the interplay that exists between the circulatory, respiratory and digestive systems to allow adequate perfusion with quality blood, as well as provide examples of how inadequacies in these systems can lead to adverse outcomes (see Table 2.1). Let's start by considering the factors that lead to normal perfusion.

Factors leading to normal perfusion

The continuous circulation of oxygen and nutrient-rich blood in a healthy individual requires a series of well-orchestrated events across multiple organ systems as explained in Figure 2.1. Let's commence our discussions by considering the blood returning to the right side of the heart from the body (systemic circulation). This blood is oxygen-poor (deoxygenated) and must be pumped to the lungs.

The lungs

With each breath we take, air is drawn into the alveoli of the lungs, allowing diffusion of oxygen into the red blood cells (RBC) that are concurrently passing through the adjacent alveolar capillaries. It takes an RBC approximately 0.75 seconds to pass through the alveolar capillary at rest, but only 0.25 seconds for diffusion of gases to occur (West & Luks, 2016). As you can see, in a healthy individual, gas exchange is efficient!

The blood

Once oxygen diffuses into the blood it passes into RBCs and binds with haemoglobin (Hb). The amount of oxygen capable of being transported by the cardiovascular system is dependent on the amount of Hb present in the blood (Marieb & Hoehn, 2016). Oxygenated blood is returned to the left side of the heart for subsequent delivery to the systemic circulation.

The heart

The left ventricle of the heart pumps oxygenated blood to the tissues via the systemic circulation. Blood flow through this system is dependent on the difference in pressure within vessels across two points (i.e. the pressure in the arteries is greater than the veins, therefore driving blood flow). However, pressure itself is dependent on the resistance to blood flow as well as the amount of blood carried in the vessels. As a result, the left ventricle must generate large amounts of pressure in the arteries to promote efficient circulation of blood. In order to do this, the heart can beat faster (increasing heart rate) or stronger (via increasing the force of contraction which increases the volume of blood ejected with each contraction; this is known as stroke volume). Alterations in either heart rate or stroke volume lead to changes in the volume of blood pumped from the left ventricle in each minute (known as cardiac output): cardiac output (CO) = heart rate (HR) × stroke volume (SV).

The blood vessels

Oxygenated blood leaving the heart travels via arteries and arterioles to reach the capillaries: the

Table 2.1: Factors affecting delivery of oxygen and nutrients to cells

Organs/tissues involved	Normal function	Common factors leading to decreased oxygen/nutrient delivery to cells
Lungs	Uptake of oxygen, removal of carbon dioxide	• Inability to get oxygen to alveoli (via airways) • Decreased diffusion of oxygen at alveoli
Blood	Haemoglobin binds with oxygen for transport	• Decreased blood volume (hypovolaemia) • Decreased haemoglobin (anaemia)

Heart	Left ventricle contracts to establish pressure gradient for blood flow through systemic circulation
	Heart rate and contractility (stroke volume) vary leading to alterations in cardiac output
		• Altered heart rate:
		  › tachycardia (increased heart rate—too little time for ventricular filling)
		  › bradycardia (decreased heart rate—too little cardiac output)
		• Decrease stroke volume caused by:
		  › alteration in rhythm
		  › injury to myocardium
		  › decreased preload
		  › decreased contractility
		  › increased afterload

Blood vessels	Directs blood flow to different organs Allows gas and nutrient exchange	• Redirection of blood flow via sympathetic innervation and adrenaline • Blood diverted from skin to essential organs • Damaged blood vessels/blood loss leading to hypovolaemia
Liver (with help of pancreas)	Stores and secretes glucose in response to pancreatic hormones	• Altered release of glucose into blood during times of need (or inability for cells to use glucose) due to pancreatic hormones

site of gas and nutrient exchange at the level of the tissues. Once nutrients have been offloaded and waste collected, deoxygenated blood travels back to the heart via the veins. The level of perfusion for each organ is tightly regulated to maintain homeostasis. Smooth muscle in the walls of the arterioles can constrict or dilate the vessel, increasing or decreasing resistance and thereby directing the flow of blood to areas in need.

The liver

Although we have spoken about blood flow to different organs for the purposes of maintaining homeostasis, some tissues also contribute to blood via the release of hormones or nutrients (in addition to waste). For example, the liver receives oxygenated blood from the systemic arterial circulation but also receives nutrient-rich blood directly from the gastrointestinal tract (Marieb & Hoehn, 2016). Depending on the demands of the body, the liver responds to pancreatic hormones by either extracting glucose from the blood and subsequently storing it for later use, or alternatively, releasing stored glucose back into the bloodstream to provide energy for cellular processes.

The cells

At the level of the tissues, oxygen diffuses across the capillary walls, through the interstitial space and into the cells. With the help of insulin (released by the pancreas), glucose also enters the cells, allowing metabolic processes to continue. Without oxygen and glucose, cells are unable to function, therefore demonstrating the critical need for adequate tissue perfusion.

Disturbances of perfusion

Owing to the complexity of the cardiovascular, respiratory and digestive systems, multiple factors must align to allow for adequate perfusion of tissues. Disturbances in any of these factors will result in decreased supply of oxygen and glucose to the tissue, as well as poor removal of waste (see Table 2.1).

The lungs

The ability of the lungs to provide a continuous supply of oxygen to the blood is an essential component of maintaining normal cell function. A

> **REFLECTIVE BOX**
>
> Exercise represents a physiological stress to your body. Consider how your body responds when you exercise. What happens to your heart rate, rate and depth of breathing, and blood flow to the skin? How do these changes maintain blood flow and oxygenation? How would your glucose levels be maintained in the absence of additional food sources?

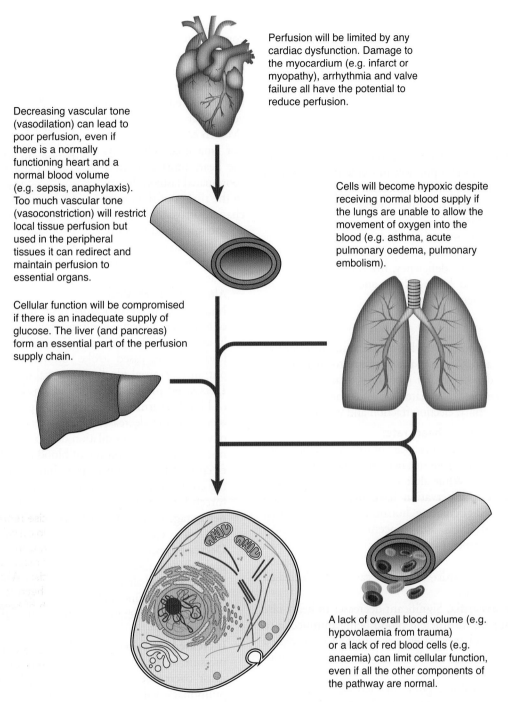

Perfusion will be limited by any cardiac dysfunction. Damage to the myocardium (e.g. infarct or myopathy), arrhythmia and valve failure all have the potential to reduce perfusion.

Decreasing vascular tone (vasodilation) can lead to poor perfusion, even if there is a normally functioning heart and a normal blood volume (e.g. sepsis, anaphylaxis). Too much vascular tone (vasoconstriction) will restrict local tissue perfusion but used in the peripheral tissues it can redirect and maintain perfusion to essential organs.

Cells will become hypoxic despite receiving normal blood supply if the lungs are unable to allow the movement of oxygen into the blood (e.g. asthma, acute pulmonary oedema, pulmonary embolism).

Cellular function will be compromised if there is an inadequate supply of glucose. The liver (and pancreas) form an essential part of the perfusion supply chain.

A lack of overall blood volume (e.g. hypovolaemia from trauma) or a lack of red blood cells (e.g. anaemia) can limit cellular function, even if all the other components of the pathway are normal.

Figure 2.1
Factors affecting perfusion quality.

decreased ability to oxygenate the blood can occur because of problems with ventilation (the ability to move gas in and out of the alveoli), external respiration (the ability of oxygen to diffuse from the alveoli to the blood) or both.

Issues with ventilation include:
- choking and airway obstruction
- narrowed airways due to asthma, croup and anaphylaxis

- an inability to inspire due to spinal cord injury or physical damage of the chest wall or diaphragm.

Issues with external respiration include:
- decreased surface area for gas exchange (e.g. chronic obstructive pulmonary disease)
- increased distance for oxygen diffusion (e.g. acute pulmonary oedema)
- altered pulmonary blood supply (e.g. pulmonary embolism)

changes to atmospheric pressure that occur with diving and aviation (i.e. altitude).

The blood

Decreases in blood volume (hypovolaemia) or haemoglobin content (anaemia) result in inadequately perfused tissue.

Causes of hypovolaemia include:

- injuries that cause significant bleeding (burns, musculoskeletal injuries, postpartum haemorrhage)
- conditions that promote movement of fluid from blood vessels to the interstitial space, thereby decreasing circulating blood volume (burns, anaphylaxis).

Causes of anaemia include:

- diseases that cause a decrease in RBCs (kidney disease, B12 deficiency, iron deficiency)
- undetected haemorrhage such as a persistent bowel bleed.

The heart

The critical role of the heart in maintaining cardiac output, and therefore the pressure to drive blood flow, is dependent on its ability to regulate heart rate and achieve adequate stroke volume (determined by contractility, ejection fraction and venous return).

Disturbances to heart rate

Under normal circumstances, heart rate is tightly controlled via the autonomic nervous system to maintain homeostasis. While alterations in parasympathetic/sympathetic innervation have marked effects on heart rate, circulating hormone (e.g. adrenaline, thyroxine) levels, ion concentrations (e.g. Ca^{2+}, K^+) and temperature (e.g. fever) also play a role in determining heart rate. Abnormally fast (tachycardia) or slow (bradycardia) heart rates can lead to decreased cardiac output.

- **Bradycardia.** Significant decreases in heart rate result in insufficient blood being pumped into the circulatory system per minute (i.e. decreased cardiac output), thereby decreasing delivery of oxygen and glucose.
- **Tachycardia.** Significant increases in heart rate (e.g. 200 bpm) reduce the time for the ventricles to fill, thereby reducing the volume of blood available for ejection with each contraction. Consequently, stroke volume is decreased, and despite the high heart rate, cardiac output can be compromised. In the absence of compensatory mechanisms, reductions in cardiac output ultimately lead to decreased perfusion.

Disturbances in stroke volume

Stroke volume is determined by subtracting the volume of blood within the ventricle at the end of ventricular systole (contraction) from the volume of blood present prior to contraction (i.e. at the end of diastole when maximal filling has occurred); this represents the volume of blood ejected with each ventricular contraction (Marieb & Hoehn, 2016). For maximal efficiency, the heart must beat in a coordinated fashion. Injury to the tissues of the heart, changes in venous return or systemic blood pressure can all lead to decreases in the efficiency of ventricular contraction.

- **Alterations in rhythm.** Injury to the heart myocardial tissue or pacemaker cells can alter its regular rate and rhythm, as well as its ability to contract in a coordinated fashion, thus leading to decreased stroke volume and cardiac output (e.g. atrial fibrillation, atrial flutter).
- **Decreased preload.** Reductions in the volume of blood returning to the heart (e.g. decreased blood volume; decreased filling time; obstruction of venous return; vasodilation due to anaphylaxis) not only alter the volume of blood available for ejection with each contraction, but also decrease the contractility of the heart, resulting in a less forceful ventricular contraction and a lower percentage of ventricular volume being ejected (known as ejection fraction).
- **Decreased contractility.** In addition to a decreased preload (described above), decreased sympathetic innervation and altered ion (K^+, Ca^{2+}) or hormone levels (e.g. thyroxine, adrenalin) can all have effects on the force generated by the heart with each contraction.
- **Increased afterload.** Afterload refers to the pressure in the great arteries which the ventricle must overcome in order to open the aortic/pulmonary valve to eject blood. In cases of hypertension, afterload increases, leading to decreased ejection fractions.

The blood vessels

The layer of smooth muscle present in the walls of blood vessels (in particular arteries and arterioles) provides a mechanism by which the diameter of the blood vessels can be altered (Marieb & Hoehn, 2016). Contracting the smooth muscle allows the vessel to constrict, increasing resistance to blood flow and maintaining pressure in the case of fluid (blood) loss. In contrast, relaxation of the smooth

> ## REFLECTIVE BOX
>
> Approximately 30% of Australians over the age of 25 have hypertension (McCance & Huether, 2015). Consider what would happen to afterload in the case of high blood pressure. How would this affect stroke volume? What compensatory mechanisms might be required to maintain cardiac output in these patients?

muscle layer allows the vessel to dilate. Both vaso-constriction and vasodilation are regulated by the autonomic nervous system. However, the smooth muscle layer is also responsive to hormones such as adrenaline and substances released during the inflammatory process.

Causes of **vasoconstriction** include:

- sympathetic nervous system innervation
- adrenaline, noradrenaline release.

Causes of **vasodilation** include:

- decreased sympathetic innervation
- inflammatory substances such as histamine (anaphylaxis) and nitric oxide
- drugs such as glyceryl trinitrate and morphine
- low levels of oxygen and/or high levels of CO_2 in the systemic system, and high levels of oxygen in the pulmonary system.

The liver

In combination with the pancreas and the gastro-intestinal (GI) system, the liver plays a vital role in determining blood glucose levels. Consequently, injury or disease affecting any one of these three organs can result in disturbances of glucose levels. The pancreatic hormones insulin and glucagon determine the uptake or release of glucose by the liver respectively. Diabetes and pancreatitis affect the amount of insulin and/or glucagon released from the pancreas but can also affect tissue sensitivity to these hormones. Intentional or accidental misman-agement of diabetic medications can cause hypo-glycaemia. Chronic liver and GI diseases do not commonly present as health emergencies but they may complicate the diagnosis and management of other health emergencies.

Assessment of perfusion

The body's ability to compensate for inadequate perfusion poses a number of problems for the paramedic. At the extreme end of the scale—no perfusion—the clinical picture is clear: the patient will be unconscious, pulseless and cool to touch. However, the speed at which this state develops, and the range of symptoms that present as the patient passes from adequate perfusion to no perfusion, are less clear.

Nearly all perfusion assessment tools use a combination of blood pressure, heart rate, skin and conscious state to categorise the severity of the condition. Of all of these, blood pressure can be the least reliable indicator of perfusion status. For example, patients who are normally hypertensive can suffer inadequate perfusion even when their systolic and diastolic pressures are within normal range. Without a pre-event measure of blood pressure,

it can be difficult to evaluate the significance of a reading during a health crisis (however, an initial recording is useful in setting a baseline with which subsequent measurements can be compared). The body's response of raising the heart rate and diverting blood flow to essential organs also 'protects' the blood pressure until there is no more capacity for compensation. Hypotension is therefore generally considered a late sign of inadequate perfusion.

An early sign of inadequate perfusion is often an increased heart rate (Craft et al., 2015). In response to sympathetic innervation, the increase in heart rate can support cardiac output in the presence of decreased blood volume (and therefore, decreased stroke volume). In the field, this tachy-cardia needs to be distinguished from anxiety and a response to pain; consequently, matching the tachycardia with the broader clinical picture is important. Assessing the skin provides additional information; cool, pale and clammy skin indicates shunting of the blood from non-essential organs (due to sympathetic vasoconstriction) and is a reliable indicator that the tachycardia is not simply a response to pain but more likely to be due inadequate perfusion.

Conscious state is the last of the four perfusion indicators that are usually assessed. In the setting of hypovolaemia, an altered conscious state is a late indicator, as the brain preferentially receives blood as the body responds to blood loss. However, the brain is sensitive to hypoxia and hypoglycaemia. Changes in these parameters often alter the conscious state long before changes occur to the skin. Remem-ber, though, that the body is adept at maintaining its perfusion and the progression from normal to extremely ill may not be apparent in a single assess-ment. It will, however, become obvious if a series of accurate assessments are performed over time. This highlights the importance of undertaking regular observations for any patient you suspect could develop perfusion problems.

Principles of medical management of perfusion

With an understanding of the causes of inadequate perfusion, combined with an accurate patient assessment, paramedics should be able to effectively identify and manage patients with perfusion issues.

Ventilate

As per rule 1 (air must go in and out) and the primary survey, always ensure the patient is ventilat-ing adequately before you start looking for other issues. For example, hypoxia will initially raise the heart rate but, if prolonged, the heart rate may slow and concurrently reduce perfusion. Ensuring adequate ventilation can be as simple as positioning the patient or providing jaw support. Alternatively, it can be as complex as decompressing a tension pneumothorax. Do not move to the circulation (C) until you have resolved any issues with airway (A) and breathing (B).

The heart

Disturbances of heart rate and rhythm should be identified during the vital signs survey and, if associated with inadequate perfusion, managed as a priority. Intensive care paramedics across Australia and New Zealand carry a range of antiarrhythmic medications such as atropine, adrenaline, verapamil, amiodarone and adenosine. The use of external defibrillators to electrically revert dangerous arrhythmias and conduct external pacing is also common practice. In addition, intensive care paramedics administer a range of medications to improve ventricular contractility. This group of medications (known as inotropes) can increase the ejection fraction and improve cardiac output.

The liver

The brain has a high metabolic demand and no mechanism for storing significant amounts of glucose or oxygen (McCance & Huether, 2015). As a result, the conscious state decreases rapidly if supplies of either glucose or oxygen are compromised. It is unusual for inadequate blood supply to be the cause of the problem when a patient is unconscious but has palpable distal pulses. If you have resolved any ventilation issues and have an unconscious patient with distal pulses, consider whether the blood being delivered to the brain is carrying sufficient glucose.

Volume, inotrope, pressor (VIP)

Restoring lost blood volume with intravenous fluids is widely supported by ambulance guidelines across Australia and New Zealand. If other causes of inadequate perfusion have been eliminated or treated and the patient remains poorly perfused, replacing lost volume is the first step in managing the patient. In most settings an initial dose of 20 mL/kg of isotonic crystalloid is recommended, followed by a repeat if the patient remains inadequately perfused. The aim is to increase preload back to an optimum level, thus ensuring that the heart receives optimum filling and stretch pressures, thereby restoring contractility and stroke volume.

If the patient remains inadequately perfused despite improved filling and pressures, the standard treatment is to commence inotrope therapy. Adrenaline, noradrenaline or dopamine all promote varying degrees of vasoconstriction and increase circulatory pressures but should not be commenced until normal intravascular volumes have been restored.

In patients with low or absent vascular tone, normal preload will not be restored by volume alone and vasopressors (adrenaline, noradrenaline or even metaraminol) have to be used to improve venous return. This 'fill then squeeze' approach aims to ensure there is sufficient circulating volume before vasoconstriction restricts blood flow to some organs. Paramedics in Australia and New Zealand do not commonly use selective pressors such as metaraminol. Unlike the inotrope family of drugs, which have effects on both the heart and the blood vessels, the pressors produce only potent vasoconstriction.

There are a number of controversies surrounding the best fluid to use to restore perfusion (isotonic, hypertonic, crystalloid, colloid), how much should be administered and even whether it should be administered if there is a suspicion the patient may still be bleeding. This area is likely to see significant changes in guidelines over the next decade as data is collected and assessed.

Summary

The term 'perfusion' describes the ability of the cardiovascular system to supply the body's cells with adequate oxygenation and nutrition, while also removing wastes. Perfusion is often used synonymously with the terms 'pressure' or 'blood flow', but it is important to keep in mind that neither of these terms is adequate in describing the critical requirements of the body's cells for oxygen and glucose.

Assessing perfusion involves a number of factors including heart rate, blood pressure, conscious state and circulation to the skin.

Regardless of the cause, inadequate perfusion usually triggers a sympathetic nervous system response. However, there is no heart rate or blood pressure that is exclusively indicative of adequate/inadequate perfusion; individual anatomy and physiology can alter the delivery of nutrients to cells as pressures fluctuate. Consequently, rates and pressures outside the normal range should always be considered pathological until proven otherwise.

Suggested reading

Marieb, E. N., & Hoehn, K. (2016). *Human anatomy & physiology* (10th ed.). Pearson Education.

References

Craft, J., Gordon, C., Huether, S. E., McCance, K. L., & Brashers, V. L. (2015). *Understanding pathophysiology*. Elsevier Health Sciences.

Marieb, E. N., & Hoehn, K. (2016). *Human anatomy & physiology* (10th ed.). Pearson Education.

McCance, K. L., & Huether, S. E. (2015). *Pathophysiology-E-Book: the biologic basis for disease in adults and children*. Elsevier Health Sciences.

West, J. B., & Luks, A. (2016). *West's respiratory physiology: the essentials* (10th ed.). Wolters Kluwer.

CHAPTER 3

The Autonomic Response

By Kate Carroll and Sharon Flecknoe

Introduction

The nervous system is one of two major control systems within the body (the other being the endocrine system). Therefore, it is important for paramedics to have an understanding of the fundamentals of how the nervous system works to control, regulate and coordinate all of the body's systems. Neurons (also called nerve cells) predominantly use electrical signals to communicate and control the body's functions. Electrical messages are transported along the axons of neurons until they reach the axon terminal; at this point, neurotransmitters (chemical messengers) are released to relay messages across synapses (the gap between two neurons or a neuron and its target cell) permitting messages to be transferred from one neuron to another, or from the neuron to a target cell.

The nervous system is the master control system of the body, consisting of a number of subdivisions, as illustrated in Figure 3.1. The system contains two main divisions: the central nervous system (CNS), which consists of the brain and the spinal cord; and the peripheral nervous system (PNS), which lies outside of the CNS and consists of both sensory and motor divisions. Communication between the two main divisions is made possible by cranial and spinal nerves which send and receive electrical signals between the CNS and PNS. While all elements of the nervous system are important, the autonomic nervous system has a significant impact on paramedic practice and is therefore the focus of this chapter.

The autonomic nervous system

The autonomic nervous system (ANS) contains two divisions: the parasympathetic nervous system and the sympathetic nervous system. The ANS is also referred to as the involuntary nervous system as it innervates and controls the involuntary functions of cardiac and smooth muscle and glands (Marieb & Hoehn, 2016). The parasympathetic nervous system is most active during periods of rest and recovery ('rest and digest'), allowing the body to conserve and restore energy, while the sympathetic nervous system mobilises energy stores and prepares the body for action, particularly in moments of acute stress ('fight or flight'). Under normal conditions, there is a balance between parasympathetic and sympathetic activity within the body's tissues and organs. The background activity created by these divisions is the autonomic tone, whereby one division is responsible for the predominant tone (background activity) of a tissue or organ (see Table 3.1). Together, the parasympathetic and sympathetic divisions of the ANS function to maintain homeostasis. Figure 3.2 summarises the effects of the parasympathetic and sympathetic divisions of the ANS on various tissues and organs. An understanding of each division of the ANS is important for paramedics, as both can negatively impact patient outcomes if the innervation of one division dominates inappropriately over the other.

In order to exert an effect on target tissues and organs, the ANS utilises a chain of two neurons to relay messages from the CNS to an effector. The cell body of the first neuron in the chain, the *preganglionic neuron*, is located in the CNS (brain stem or spinal cord) and its axon is located in the PNS. The preganglionic neuron synapses with the cell body of a second neuron, the *postganglionic* neuron, in a region known as the autonomic ganglia, in the PNS. The postganglionic neuron will eventually synapse with its effector (target cells). When comparing the parasympathetic and sympathetic divisions, each contains pre- and postganglionic neurons, but they differ in their site of exit from the CNS, relative lengths of pre- and postganglionic axons and the type of neurotransmitters released at their synapses (see Fig 3.3).

The parasympathetic nervous system

The parasympathetic nervous system is also referred to as the craniosacral division due to the location from which its preganglionic neurons exit the CNS. Preganglionic neurons arise from nuclei (cell bodies in the CNS) within the brain stem via cranial nerves and sacral segments (S2–S4) of the spinal cord (see Fig 3.2A). The preganglionic neurons arising from the brainstem travel within cranial nerves, such as the oculomotor (III), facial (VII), glossopharyngeal (IX) and vagus (X) nerves, towards the viscera of the head, thorax and abdomen where they synapse with a postganglionic neuron. The postganglionic neuron then travels to and innervates its target, causing an effect; for example, innervation of the

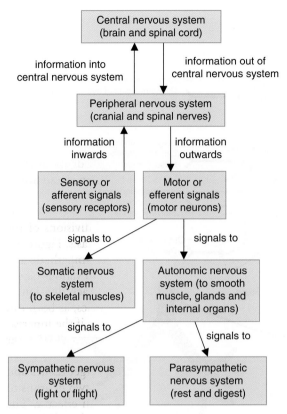

Figure 3.1
Subdivisions of the nervous system.
Source: Craft et al. (2015).

Table 3.1: Autonomic tone

Site	Predominant tone
Ciliary muscle	Parasympathetic
Iris	Parasympathetic
Sinoatrial node	Parasympathetic
Arterioles	Sympathetic
Veins	Sympathetic
Gastrointestinal tract	Parasympathetic
Uterus	Parasympathetic
Urinary bladder	Parasympathetic
Salivary glands	Parasympathetic
Sweat glands	Sympathetic

small intestine by a parasympathetic postganglionic neuron will increase intestinal motility (i.e. to assist in the 'rest and DIGEST'). The preganglionic neurons of the parasympathetic division are long and the postganglionic neurons are short (see Fig 3.3), with their autonomic ganglia located in or near the structures they innervate (Marieb & Hoehn, 2016).

The sympathetic nervous system

The sympathetic nervous system is also referred to as the thoracolumbar division as the preganglionic neurons arise from cell bodies located in the thoracic (T1–T12) and lumbar (L1–L2) regions of the spinal cord (see Fig 3.2B). The preganglionic neurons of the sympathetic division are short, forming synapses with their postganglionic neurons close to the spinal cord in a region known as the sympathetic trunk ganglia (see Figs 3.2B and 3.3). Postganglionic neurons then travel to and innervate their target cells to regulate certain activities in the body associated with the 'fight or flight' response; for example, innervation of cardiac muscle tissue of the heart increases force of contraction during times of acute stress. Unlike the parasympathetic division, some preganglionic sympathetic neurons can pass through ganglia without synapsing with a postganglionic neuron. Instead, the preganglionic neuron can synapse directly with cells of the adrenal medulla (see Fig 3.3), causing the release of the hormones adrenaline and noradrenaline which help mobilise energy stores during the 'fight or flight' response.

Neurotransmitters of the ANS

The communication between pre- and postganglionic neurons and target cells in both the sympathetic and the parasympathetic divisions relies on the release of neurotransmitters from the one neuron and their subsequent binding to appropriate receptors on the next neuron or target cell. It is the binding of these neurotransmitters to their appropriate receptors that eventually leads to a response within target cells. Two major neurotransmitters of the ANS are acetylcholine and noradrenaline.

Parasympathetic neurotransmitters and receptors

Both pre- and postganglionic neurons in the parasympathetic nervous system release the neurotransmitter acetylcholine, and are therefore collectively known as cholinergic neurons (see Fig 3.3). Acetylcholine exerts its effect by binding to cholinergic receptors, which are broadly categorised as either nicotinic or muscarinic receptors (both of which

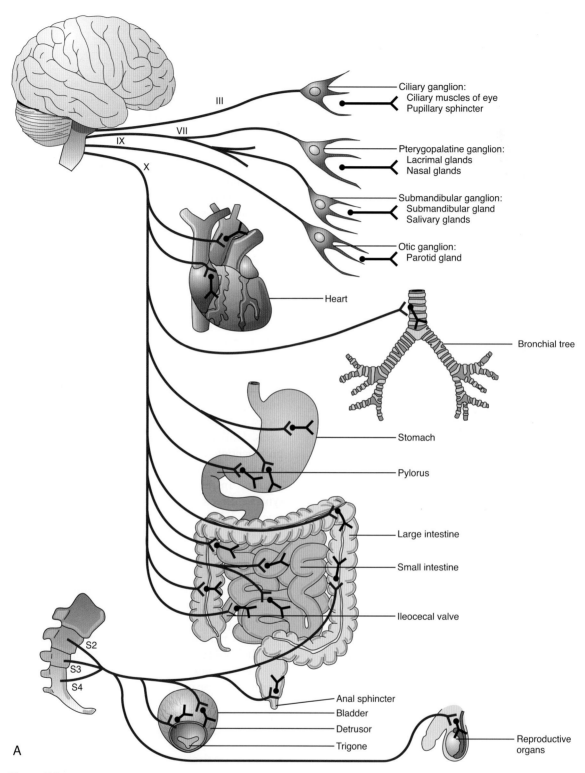

Figure 3.2
Summary of the effects of the **A** parasympathetic and **B** sympathetic nervous systems.
Source: Copstead & Banasik (2010).

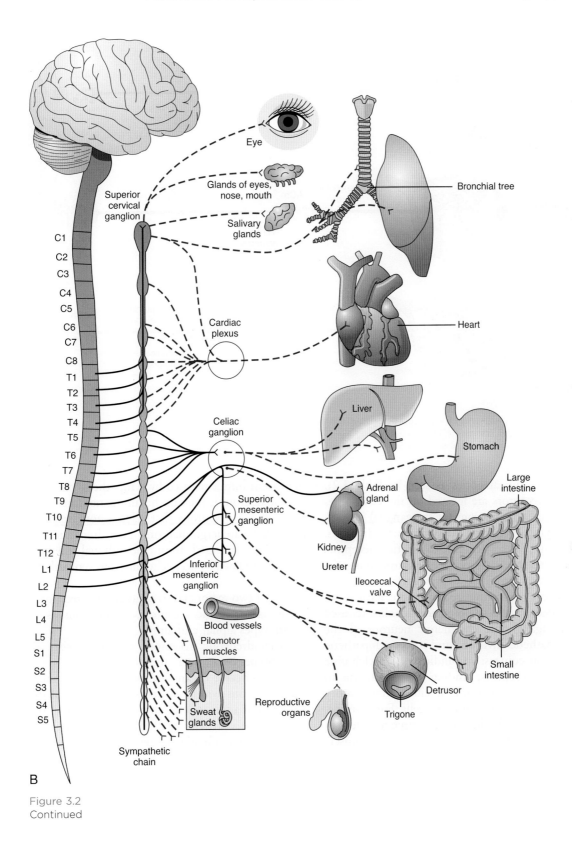

C1
C2
C3
C4
C5
C6
C7
C8
T1
T2
T3
T4
T5
T6
T7
T8
T9
T10
T11
T12
L1
L2
L3
L4
L5
S1
S2
S3
S4
S5

B

Superior
cervical
ganglion

Cardiac
plexus

Celiac
ganglion

Superior
mesenteric
ganglion

Inferior
mesenteric
ganglion

Blood vessels

Pilomotor
muscles

Sweat
glands

Reproductive
organs

Sympathetic
chain

Eye

Glands of eyes,
nose, mouth

Salivary
glands

Bronchial tree

Heart

Liver

Stomach

Large
intestine

Adrenal
gland

Kidney

Ureter

Ileocecal
valve

Small
intestine

Detrusor

Trigone

Figure 3.2
Continued

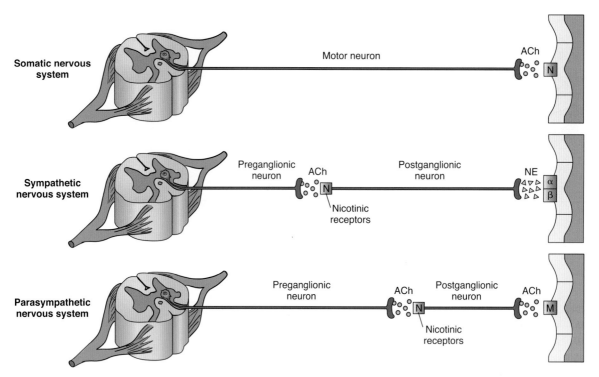

Figure 3.3
Sympathetic and parasympathetic neurotransmitters and receptors.
Source: Copstead & Banasik (2010).

have further subcategories as seen in Table 3.2). Nicotinic receptors are located on the cell bodies of postganglionic neurons (at the ganglia) in both the parasympathetic and the sympathetic divisions. The binding of acetylcholine to nicotinic receptors always exerts an excitatory effect, ensuring transmission of messages from pre- to postganglionic neurons. In contrast, muscarinic receptors are located on target (effector) cells and bind acetylcholine released from postganglionic cholinergic neurons of the parasympathetic division (and a few sympathetic neurons). In contrast to binding of acetylcholine to nicotinic receptors, binding of acetylcholine to muscarinic receptors can have either an excitatory or an inhibitory effect on target cells. For example, binding of acetylcholine to muscarinic receptors in the gastrointestinal tract increases smooth muscle activity associated with digestion. However, binding of acetylcholine to muscarinic receptors in the smooth muscle of anal sphincters allows muscle relaxation, and hence defecation. The effects of acetylcholine binding to muscarinic receptors on target organs are summarised in Table 3.2.

Sympathetic neurotransmitters and receptors

Although preganglionic neurons of the sympathetic nervous system release acetylcholine, the main neurotransmitter released by sympathetic postganglionic neurons is the catecholamine noradrenaline (see Fig 3.3). Neurons that release noradrenaline are called adrenergic neurons. Noradrenaline and adrenaline (released from the adrenal medulla when stimulated by acetylcholine from sympathetic preganglionic neurons) exert their effect by binding to one of two major classes of adrenergic receptors:
- alpha-adrenergic receptors, which consists of subtypes $alpha_1$ and $alpha_2$
- beta-adrenergic receptors which consists of subtypes $beta_1$, $beta_2$ and $beta_3$.

Each effector organ innervated by the sympathetic nervous system contains at least one of the subtypes of adrenergic receptors. For example, the cells of the ventricles of the heart contain $beta_1$ receptors that can bind noradrenaline and adrenaline, resulting in an increase in the force of contraction of the heart. The effects of noradrenaline and adrenaline binding to various types of adrenergic receptors on target organs are summarised in Table 3.2 and Box 3.1.

Intracellular second messengers

Neurotransmitters cannot enter a target cell but instead act as the first messenger by binding to and activating their receptors, leading to the eventual activation of second messengers that have an

Table 3.2: Effect of parasympathetic and sympathetic nervous system on various tissues and organs

Effector organ	Sympathetic nervous system		Parasympathetic nervous system	
	Adrenergic receptor	Effect of stimulation	Muscarinic receptor	Effect of stimulation
Blood vessels	Alpha$_1$	Vasoconstriction	–	–
Heart				
Sinoatrial node	Beta$_1$	Increased heart rate	M2	Decreased heart rate
Ventricles	Beta$_1$	Increased force of contraction	–	–
Lung smooth muscle	Beta$_2$	Bronchodilation	M3	Bronchoconstriction
Digestive system				
Smooth muscle	Beta$_2$	Decreased activity	M3	Increased activity
Sphincters	Beta$_2$	Constriction (sphincters closed)	M3	Relaxation (sphincters open)
Gastric glands	–	–	M3	Increased secretions
Eyes	Alpha$_1$	Pupil dilation	M3	Pupil constriction
Kidneys	Beta$_1$	Renin secretion	–	–
Adipose	Beta$_3$	Breakdown of fat stores	–	–
Pancreas	Alpha$_2$	Inhibition of insulin secretion	M3	Stimulation of insulin secretion
Urinary bladder sphincter	Alpha$_1$	Constriction (sphincter closed)	M3	Relaxation (sphincter open)

Note: Nicotinic receptors have been omitted from the table as activation of these receptors always results in an excitatory effect.
Source: Craft et al. (2015).

BOX 3.1 Noradrenaline: neurotransmitter or hormone?

When noradrenaline is released by neurons into a synapse, it acts as a neurotransmitter and its effects are short lived. In contrast, when noradrenaline is released into the bloodstream, it acts as a hormone and its effects are longer lasting (Craft et al., 2015).

intracellular effect. Activation of second messengers can have a long-lasting effect. Changes within target cells brought about by second messengers include alterations in gene expression, activation of enzymes and the opening and closing of ion channels (Marieb & Hoehn, 2016). An awareness of some of the intracellular second messengers, particularly those associated with the sympathetic nervous system, is relevant to paramedic practice. Some relevant examples are discussed in the following paragraphs.

Example 1: When beta$_1$ receptors bind noradrenaline released via the sympathetic nervous system (e.g. from postganglionic cells), the now active receptors stimulate the activation of the enzyme adenylyl cyclase, resulting in the production of the intracellular second messenger cyclic adenosine monophosphate (cAMP). When this occurs in cells in the ventricles of the heart, the increased levels of cAMP cause changes to free intracellular calcium that increase the force of contraction and decrease membrane stability, both resulting in an increased heart rate. If cAMP is synthesised in excess, ectopic beats and eventual ventricular tachycardia/ventricular fibrillation can occur (Bryant & Knights, 2014).

Example 2: Similarly, in the lungs, stimulation of beta$_2$ receptors by noradrenaline released via the sympathetic nervous system results in an increase in cAMP causing bronchodilation. In contrast, stimulation of muscarinic receptors in the lungs by acetylcholine released via the parasympathetic nervous system results in an increase in cyclic guanine monophosphate (cGMP), which has the opposite effect of cAMP, causing bronchoconstriction. A balance between the levels of cAMP and cGMP determines many cellular responses to signals from the ANS.

Example 3: Sympathetic stimulation of alpha$_1$ receptors in peripheral blood vessels activates the intracellular second messenger inositol triphosphate which acts on smooth muscle cells causing vasoconstriction. The effect of inositol triphosphate is opposed by increasing levels of intracellular cGMP, which is formed in response to nitric oxide within blood vessels. The relevance of this to paramedic practice is that glyceryl trinitrate (GTN), a drug used to treat angina pectoris, acts by stimulating the production of cGMP which causes vasodilation. A potentially hazardous drug interaction exists between GTN and the erectile dysfunction drugs that work by blocking the breakdown of cGMP: this is the reason behind the relative contraindication of GTN in the presence of these drugs (Bryant & Knights, 2014).

Example 4: During the fight or flight response, there is an increase in the breakdown of glycogen (our stored energy) into glucose for energy production. Under normal conditions, the hormone glucagon increases cAMP levels which eventually causes the breakdown of glycogen to glucose. During sympathetic activation, an increase in adrenaline also causes an increase in cAMP levels resulting in further breakdown of glycogen to glucose. The importance of cAMP in the breakdown of glycogen explains how adrenaline is able to increase blood glucose levels and how glucagon is able to indirectly increase the heart rate. Glucagon's ability to indirectly increase heart rate means it can be used as an alternative treatment when a patient is suffering from an overdose of beta-blockers (Bryant & Knights, 2014).

> ### REFLECTIVE BOX
>
> Considering the role of cAMP, what would be the consequences for the body if a drug unexpectedly interfered with the production of the enzyme adenylyl cyclase? Which division of the ANS would most likely be affected?

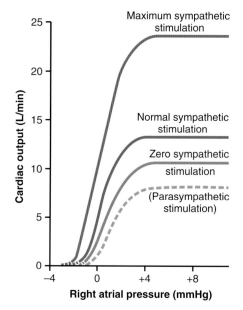

Figure 3.4
The effect of sympathetic and parasympathetic stimulation on cardiac output.
Source: Hall (2011).

significantly, reducing systemic blood pressure and thus reducing blood flow (Marieb & Hoehn, 2016). Furthermore, parasympathetic innervation of the heart becomes dominant, resulting in bradycardia.

Assessment of ANS function

Parasympathetic division

The effects of parasympathetic stimulation are seen in everyday life and ordinary circumstances. The parasympathetic system is the 'rest and digest' division. Given this, it does not normally present a problem in patient assessment for paramedics (reflex responses are rarely evaluated in the out-of-hospital setting). However, some abnormal responses are easily observed and they may indicate autonomic nerve injury. These responses include loss of temperature control, hypotension (in the absence of volume loss), bradycardia (in the absence of hypoxia) and priapism (Sanders, 2012) and they are often found in patients with a relatively high-level spinal cord injury. Normally, sympathetic stimulation maintains the muscle tone that keeps blood vessels at their usual diameter. If sympathetic stimulation is disrupted by an injury to the spinal cord or medulla, neurodepressive drugs, emotional stress or some other factor, the blood vessels dilate

Sympathetic division

Most of the patients paramedics encounter will be experiencing some level of heightened sympathetic nervous system response. Paramedics are usually called when an adverse health event exceeds the coping mechanisms or resources of the patient or their family. This indicates that there is a high likelihood that the sympathetic 'fight or flight' response is in effect. This is most likely to affect the patient's physiological parameters and it is almost impossible to distinguish whether the vital signs you are recording are purely related to a pathophysiological state or are augmented by sympathetic stimulation. The effect of sympathetic innervation on cardiac output is illustrated in Figure 3.4.

To illustrate this complexity, imagine that a patient has cut his finger with a butcher's knife and lost a significant amount of blood. He presents as tachycardic, cool, pale and clammy. The injury will result in sympathetic innervation, which will increase his heart rate. This increase in heart rate will support cardiac output for a period of time despite the decreased blood volume from the bleed (cardiac output = heart rate × stroke volume). The paramedic must determine whether the tachycardia is purely an expected sympathetic response or because of pain or other pathophysiology. The vasoconstrictor effect of the sympathetic response on the vessels leading to non-essential organs is a strong indication that the tachycardia is not simply a response to pain and is reliably measured by assessing the skin. Cool, pale and clammy skin indicates shunting of the blood and a state of inadequate perfusion. This simplistic case demonstrates the interconnectedness between the sympathetic response and the patient's presentation.

Critical illness is a potent stimulus of the sympathetic nervous system and, if prolonged, can have increasingly detrimental effects. Several organ systems may be affected. The heart seems to be most susceptible to sympathetic overstimulation. Detrimental effects include impaired diastolic function, tachycardia, tachyarrhythmia and myocardial ischaemia. Adverse effects have also been observed in other organs such as the lungs (pulmonary oedema, elevated pulmonary arterial pressures), the coagulation system (hypercoagulability, thrombus formation), the gastrointestinal system (hypoperfusion, inhibition of peristalsis), the endocrine system (decreased prolactin, thyroid and growth hormone secretion), the immune system (immunomodulation, stimulation of bacterial growth), metabolism (increase in cell energy expenditure, hyperglycaemia and electrolyte changes), bone marrow (anaemia) and skeletal muscles (apoptosis) (Dünser & Hasibeder, 2009).

Principles of management

Potential therapeutic options to manage excessive sympathetic reactions comprise temperature control, adequate use of sedative/analgesic drugs, aiming for reasonable cardiovascular targets, adequate fluid therapy and use of medications such as steroids and antibiotics to reduce underlying inflammatory or infective responses (Dünser & Hasibeder, 2009). Potential therapeutic options to manage inadequate sympathetic response comprise administration of IV fluids and adrenergic agonists. The patient with a spinal cord injury will also need to be monitored for hypothermia due to hypothalamic dysfunction (Brown & Edwards, 2014).

Summary

The autonomic nervous system has two divisions: the parasympathetic nervous system and the sympathetic nervous system. These systems govern involuntary functions of cardiac and smooth (involuntary) muscle and glands. The sympathetic nervous system responds to stress and prepares the body for action ('fight or flight'), while the parasympathetic nervous system dominates during periods of rest and recovery ('rest and digest').

A number of illnesses or injuries can trigger a widespread sympathetic response, and recognising this 'pattern' can assist in determining the cause. Poor perfusion, hypoglycaemia, pain and other noxious stimuli can all trigger the sympathetic nervous system, and the signs of sympathetic innervation can help identify the underlying illness or injury.

References

Brown, D., & Edwards, H. (2014). *Lewis's Medical–Surgical nursing* (3rd ed.). Sydney: Elsevier.

Bryant, B., & Knights, K. (2014). *Pharmacology for health professionals* (4th ed.). Sydney: Elsevier.

Copstead, L. C., & Banasik, J. L. (2010). *Pathophysiology* (4th ed.). Missouri: Saunders.

Craft, J., Gordon, C., & Tiziani, A. (2015). *Understanding pathophysiology*. Sydney: Elsevier.

Dünser, M., & Hasibeder, W. (2009). Sympathetic overstimulation during critical illness: adverse effects of adrenergic stress. *Journal of Intensive Care Medicine, 24*(5), 293–316.

Hall, J. E. (2011). *Guyton and Hall textbook of medical physiology* (12th ed.). Philadelphia: Saunders.

Marieb, E. N., & Hoehn, K. (2016). *Human anatomy and physiology* (10th ed.). Pearson Education Limited.

Sanders, M. (2012). *Mosby's paramedic textbook* (3rd ed.). St Louis: Mosby.

CHAPTER 4

The Inflammatory Response

By Kim Murphy

Introduction

Chapter 2 established how a constant supply of nutrients to cells is essential to homeostasis. But accidental exposure to pressure, heat, cold, microbes, chemicals and radiation will quickly injure and kill the cells that make up human tissue. In fact, when you consider the number of potential diseases and accidents that can befall any one of us, the body's ability to locate and heal damaged tissue is as essential to health as its more immediate needs for oxygen or glucose. Despite the vast number of different causes of cell damage, the methods by which the body responds are remarkably consistent. This **inflammatory response** is extremely sensitive and finely balanced, but in some circumstances the complex interactions between the numerous chemicals and compounds that drive the inflammatory response can spread beyond the area of damaged tissue. Ironically, when this occurs the inflammatory response can harm healthy tissue, particularly if the response is inappropriate or prolonged.

The detrimental effects of an uncontrolled or misdirected inflammatory response is recognised as the cause of many chronic diseases including rheumatoid arthritis, diabetes, coeliac disease and multiple sclerosis. It is also responsible for many acute events such as asthma, anaphylaxis, sepsis, burn shock and even cardiovascular disease. The notion that the process for injury response and healing can cause harm is somewhat counterintuitive, but it is something that paramedics must understand because it impacts on the chronic and acute conditions they are required to recognise and treat. Thankfully, as complex as the inflammatory response can be when examined in detail, the underlying principles behind inflammation are relatively easy to understand, predictable and can often be managed in the emergency setting.

This chapter provides an introduction to the inflammatory process but does not go into the level of detail needed to understand many of the complex interactions surrounding the inflammatory response. The reader is strongly encouraged to study this important area in more depth using specific immunology and pathophysiology textbooks on the subject.

What is inflammation?

Inflammation is the immune response to tissue injury, due to either pathogenic microbes or physical injury. It results from a cascade of chemical and biological immune reactions that drive further chemical reactions. The inflammatory response is triggered in response to infection in order to control and eliminate harm, minimise further injury to the body and promote healing. Generally, inflammation is tightly controlled and is restricted to the site of infected or damaged tissue. However, occasionally this response can cascade out of control and begin to affect tissues distant to the site of infection or injury and can even evolve into a life-threatening condition. Inflammation is characterised by heat, pain, redness, swelling and loss of function. In addition to the classic instigators of infection and tissue injury, there is a range of adverse conditions that initiate the inflammatory response (see Box 4.1). These include ischaemia, genetic defects, immune defects, temperature extremes, chemical agents, nutrient deprivation and radiation (McCance & Huether, 2014).

The basics of normal inflammation

The key to understanding the inflammatory response is to remember that it is designed to minimise further injury, clean the area of damaged tissues and promote new cell growth. Accordingly, the primary action of the inflammatory process can be summarised as increasing blood flow to the area of injury. This allows large numbers of specialised white blood cells (leukocytes) to migrate to the site of injury, remove dead tissue and fight infection. Of course, open wounds can result in large amounts of blood loss, so the inflammatory response also plays a role in blood clotting.

When the body receives a minor injury, inflammation provides increased blood supply to the site of injury and is the first stage of the healing process. Tissue damage is detected by macrophages in the tissue; macrophages are specialised immune cells which have the ability to phagocytose (devour) infectious microbes and damaged cells. Upon detection and phagocytosis, macrophages release chemical mediators known as chemokines and cytokines which trigger vasodilation, increased vascular permeability (where the blood vessel walls become 'leaky', allowing more leukocytes to access the injured tissue) and chemotaxis (the movement of leukocytes into the

BOX 4.1 Causes of acute inflammation

- Trauma: pressure, abrasion, laceration
- Thermal injury: burns, frostbite
- Tissue necrosis from hypoxia or poor perfusion
- Infections: bacterial, viral, parasitic
- Microbial toxins (e.g. tetanus toxin)
- Immune reactions (e.g. allergy)
- Irradiation and chemical agents

BOX 4.2 The inflammatory response

The process of the inflammatory response involves three key processes:
1. vasodilation, resulting in increased blood flow, and reduced blood velocity, to the injured or damaged tissue (causing warmth and redness)
2. increased vascular permeability, as plasma leaks from blood vessels into the damaged tissue (causing swelling)
3. chemotaxis, the emigration of leukocytes and plasma proteins into the damaged tissue.

tissues) (see Box 4.2). Collectively, this allows inflammatory cells to move to the site of damage and stimulates the release of other biological pathways (complement cascade, kinin and clotting) that limits the effect of the foreign substance, allowing time for an effective immune response (see Fig 4.1).

Mast cells are another important cell involved in inflammation; mast cells are found lining the tissues that interact with the environment (such as the skin). Mast cells also release potent inflammatory mediators including cytokines and chemokines, and others such as histamine. Mast cell degranulation is of greatest clinical importance in allergy; exposure to a trigger allergen can cause mast cells to release their cellular contents resulting in early and late stages of allergic inflammation. This can range from relatively mild symptoms, such as hives, to more severe symptoms such as anaphylactic shock. In physiological inflammation mast cells have overlapping functions with macrophages, producing inflammatory mediators that cause vasodilation, chemotaxis and pain.

In more detail, the inflammatory process can be viewed as occurring over four stages as described in the following example.

Stage 1: Injury

A fit, healthy male has fallen from his bicycle and has a deep abrasion to his forearm. As his arm was compressed against the concrete gutter and his momentum forced it to slide across the rough surface, the skin was scoured away and the softer connective tissue underneath suffered a mix of compression, abrasion and heat. As a result, individual cell membranes were damaged and substances usually only found inside cells were released into the interstitial space.

Stage 2: Detection

The release of intracellular contents (particularly K^+ ions, proteins and uric acid) into the extracellular space is the usual trigger for the inflammatory response that occurs after trauma. These damage-associated molecular patterns (DAMPs) are detected by macrophages which reside under the skin. Macrophages are potent activators of the inflammatory immune response and are commonly found in tissues that are subject to injury or exposed to infectious agents (e.g. the skin, the lining of the lungs, the gastrointestinal system), along with other immune cells. Precursors to macrophages, known as monocytes, can also be found in the blood. Inflammatory mediator release can also be triggered by hypoxia or cell damage or, alternatively, in response to inflammatory mediators from other cells elsewhere in the body.

Stage 3: Response and recruitment

As immunologists explore the inflammatory response in increasing detail, they are unravelling what appears to be a never-ending string of precursor chemicals that trigger subsequent reactions that drive the inflammatory response forwards. For this chapter we deal with just the primary drivers involved in the process: if you are interested in learning more about the structure and function of the immune system, see Chapter 12 in Craft et al. (2015).

Macrophages become activated when they recognise DAMPs and release a range of inflammatory mediators; these mediators attract cells that further drive the inflammatory response. In particular macrophages secrete a number of different cytokines and chemokines (small chemical mediators that have effects on immune and other cells) that cause vascular changes including increased vascular permeability, thereby allowing more plasma proteins into the tissue. These chemical mediators also attract neutrophils and, subsequently, monocytes to the tissue; later, if required, lymphocytes are also recruited.

Inflammatory mediators can be divided into several groups, but the primary and most immediate effect of most of them is to alter blood flow in the

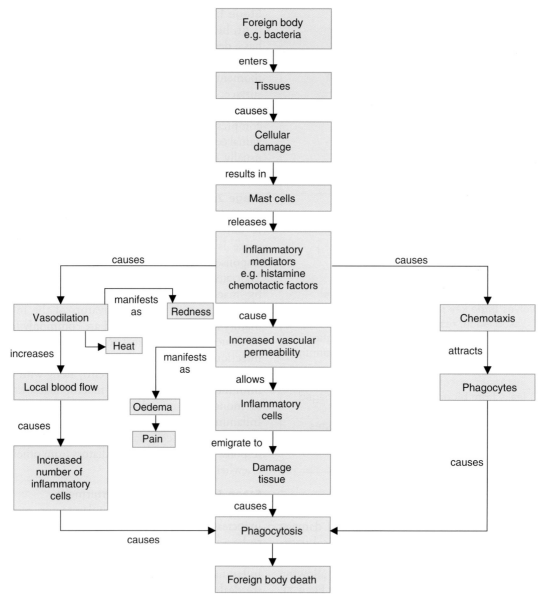

Figure 4.1
The inflammatory response to minor injury.
Source: Modified from McCance & Huether (2014).

area of the injury. They cause this change through two mechanisms: vasodilation and increased vessel permeability. Inflammatory mediators are very vasoactive (meaning they act on blood vessels): they increase blood flow to the area and allow plasma proteins and leucocytes (mainly neutrophils) that are normally trapped within the circulatory system to escape into the extracellular space (Netea et al., 2017). Neutrophils recognise DAMPs (or pathogen-associated molecular patterns [PAMPs] found on microbes) and these phagocytose-injured cells that release powerful inflammatory mediators or release nets of DNA to capture and destroy microbes, while

the plasma proteins prolong vasodilation and also act to destroy foreign cells and promote clotting (see below). In addition, the presence of the plasma proteins in the interstitial space creates an osmotic pressure that draws plasma from the intravascular space. This increase in blood flow and fluid leakage from vessels triggers two of the classic signs of inflammation: redness and swelling (see Fig 4.2). Pro-inflammatory cytokines cause rapid dilation of the post-capillary venules, which results in increased blood flow into the microcirculation. Cytokines also cause increased vascular permeability resulting from retraction of endothelial cells lining the capillaries.

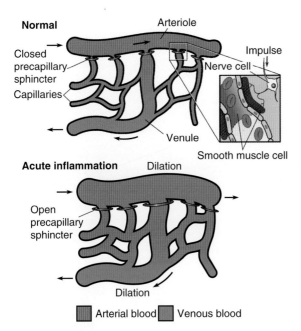

Normal

Closed precapillary sphincter

Capillaries

Arteriole

Impulse

Nerve cell

Venule

Smooth muscle cell

Acute inflammation

Dilation

Open precapillary sphincter

Dilation

Arterial blood   Venous blood

Figure 4.2
Capillary changes due to inflammation.
Source: Craft et al. (2015).

BOX 4.3 The lymphatic system and inflammation

The role of lymphatic vessels is to drain interstitial fluid and return it to the main circulatory system. The fluid in the lymph system passes through lymph nodes where immune cells (particularly B lymphocytes) produce antibodies specific to the bacteria that is detected. One function of antibodies is to bind to the bacteria and identify them to macrophages and neutrophils. A second function is to activate the complement system. Lymph nodes that drain injured or infected limbs will become swollen and painful in response to activation and proliferation of lymphocytes.

The movement of fluid from the intravascular to the interstitial space challenges the lymphatic system, which may not be capable of draining all the exudate from the area (see Box 4.3).

The role of plasma proteins in inflammation

The relationship between inflammation and healing is demonstrated by the activation of various plasma proteins. The tissue damage and subsequent vasodilation and increased vessel permeability triggered by the release of the inflammatory cytokines attracts plasma proteins from three interrelated systems to the site of injury. These proteins are integral to the

inflammatory response and are classified as belonging to the complement system, the clotting system or the kinin system (see Fig 4.3).

- The complement system. Of the more than 30 proteins in the complement system, all are inactive in the plasma until injury or infection occurs. In reality, many of the group's proteins simply form enzymes that cleave a further protein within the complement system. This promotes inflammation, recruits neutrophils and macrophages to the site of inflammation, coats pathogens to make them more visible to neutrophils and macrophages, and can also form a pore in the foreign cell leading to the destruction of the cell.
- The clotting system. The clotting system is activated by a group of plasma proteins when they are exposed to damaged tissue. This can occur when connective tissue and vessels are damaged by trauma; once activated, the plasma proteins in this system promote coagulation through fibrin, which both prevents bleeding and limits the spread of potential pathogens. The clotting system also releases pro-inflammatory cytokines; in this way inflammation and clotting are intrinsically connected.
- The kinin system. The kinin and coagulation systems are intertwined with one of the plasma proteins involved in coagulation (the Hageman factor or factor XII), converting the inactive kinin protein (prekallikrein) into its active form (bradykinin). Once activated through the factor XII, most of the potent kinin proteins cause vasodilation and increased vessel permeability, and also convert one of the complement plasma proteins to its active form.

Stage 4: Resolution and repair
The numerous cytokines and chemokines that drive the inflammatory pathways are part of a finely balanced cascade: many of these chemicals stimulate the production of some inflammatory cytokines while suppressing the production of others. When it works perfectly, the process initially drives the inflammatory response forwards, but eventually the change in the affected tissue, such as the removal of microbes, starts to retard inflammation. At a cellular level, neutrophils with their potent effects are replaced by alternatively activated (anti-inflammatory) macrophages which remove dead cells and initiate wound repair.

Alternative trigger: infection
Apart from direct injury by trauma, the introduction of pathogens into the interstitial space also triggers the inflammatory process. In some cases the pathogen is recognised directly by inflammatory cells sensing PAMPs, while in other instances the activity of the

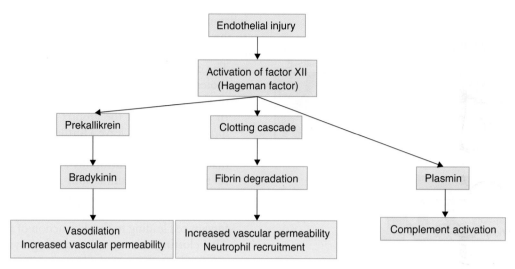

Figure 4.3
Plasma proteins in the inflammatory response.

pathogen triggers the inflammatory response (e.g. the release of toxins). Some foreign substances, such as silica, are not necessarily infective but are known to produce an aggressive inflammatory response.

Abnormal inflammation

There are a number of conditions where the delicate balance between pro- and anti-inflammatory mediators that normally promote healing leads to more tissue damage. At their most severe, these abnormal reactions can lead to acute life-threatening episodes of anaphylaxis and asthma (see Fig 4.4), although there are conditions where the effects are less acute but they are persistent and cause structural changes to the tissues (e.g. autoimmune conditions such as rheumatoid arthritis).

The effects of abnormal inflammation depend on the degree of insult and the organs affected, but the process is consistent with that of physiological (normal) inflammation, starting with cellular or tissue damage and leading to various degrees of a local or systemic response. In many conditions the acute phase will not completely resolve and instead becomes chronic.

Step 1: Tissue damage or infection

The introduction of particular types of antigens (e.g. *S. aureus*) or the destruction of a large amount of tissue (e.g. from burns) can cause the release of a massive amount of pro-inflammatory cytokines that can cascade out of control, spreading away from the initial site of injury and causing systemic effects. In addition to causing vasodilation and increased vessel permeability, most inflammatory mediators can cause small muscle constriction, which is of particular concern when they affect the bronchioles of the lungs or the walls of the gastrointestinal system.

Step 2: Systemic manifestations

Hypotension

Widespread small vessel dilation allows blood to pool and decreases venous return to the heart. Combined with a shift of plasma from the intravascular space to the interstitial space this can rapidly reduce cardiac output (see Chapter 2). As cellular perfusion deteriorates, cells start to die, releasing their contents into the interstitial space and driving the inflammatory process further forwards.

Signs: Hypotension, tachycardia, warm red skin (due to blood pooling in the capillaries), *oedema* (due to plasma pooling in the interstitial space).

Hypoxia

If a severe inflammatory response is triggered in the lungs, spasm of the smooth muscle in the bronchioles reduces the airway diameter and impedes ventilation. This can be further complicated by the stimulation of mucus-producing cells. In extreme cases, the change in vessel permeability can cause airway swelling that leads to further airway occlusion.

Signs: Wheeze (bronchoconstriction), *cough* (mucus production), *stridor* (laryngeal oedema).

Fever

Elevations in body temperature are commonly associated with the inflammatory process, especially in response to inflammatory cytokines produced during infections. Pro-inflammatory cytokines act on the hypothalamus to produce prostaglandins that cause fever. Fever is an important part of the immune response and many cytokines have the ability to cause fever; fever has the potential to both inhibit

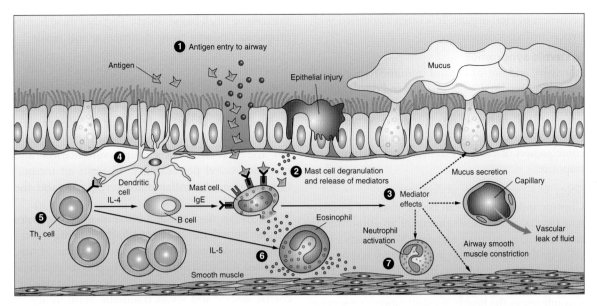

Figure 4.4
Inflammatory effects in asthma.
Asthma is a disease driven by the inflammatory response in both the acute and the chronic phases. Inhaled antigens (1) bind to immunoglobulin E (IgE) on mast cells and trigger the mast cells to degranulate (2) and release mediators such as histamine, leukotrienes, prostaglandin D_2, interleukins and platelet-activating factor. Combined, these mediators (3) induce bronchospasm and oedema from increased capillary permeability and trigger goblet cells to secrete mucus. The antigens are also detected by dendritic cells (4) that process and present them to Th_2 cells (5). This produces interleukin-4 (IL-4), which promotes B cells to form more IgE. Th_2 cells also produce interleukin-5 (IL-5) (6), which activates eosinophils. Eosinophil products damage the respiratory epithelium, leading to more inflammation and damage. Other inflammatory cells, including neutrophils (7), also contribute to the inflammatory process.
Source: McCance & Huether (2014).

BOX 4.4 Playing with prostaglandins

Derived from arachidonic acid, prostaglandins are important mediators in the inflammatory process and cause increased vascular permeability, neutrophil chemotaxis and pain by direct effects on nerves. Activation of phospholipase A_2 by hypoxia, cell damage and the inflammatory cascade is the first step in the cellular response. Phospholipase A_2 breaks down phospholipids to release arachidonic acid, the raw material for the production of prostaglandins (via the enzyme cyclooxygenase, COX) and leukotrienes (via the enzyme lipoxygenase). A number of anti-inflammatory drugs (aspirin and NSAIDs) are specifically aimed at inhibiting prostaglandin production acting on the COX enzymes to reduce pain and fever. The intrinsic link between inflammation and coagulation (the COX system also produces thromboxanes that are involved in platelet aggregation) is evidenced by the increased bleeding times caused by these drugs. Certain anti-inflammatory drugs have been shown to cause increased coagulability and have led to an increased risk of heart attack or stroke (Bryant & Knights, 2014), although the risk is dose dependent.

microbial growth and also improve the immune response to microbes. Medications that inhibit prostaglandin synthesis (aspirin, ibuprofen) are effective in reducing fever (see Box 4.4).

Signs: Temperature > 38°C or < 36°C. Although a temperature above 37°C can be considered febrile, significant fevers will generate a temperature greater than 38°C. The shunting of blood to the skin in the inflammatory response can ultimately cause a significant temperature loss and patients with sepsis will not be able to sustain a fever over long periods; this can lead to the late sign of 'cold sepsis'.

Organ dysfunction
Typically a late sign of a severe, prolonged inflammatory response, this reflects widespread inadequate

perfusion of vital organs. It is often associated with hyper- or hypocoagulation.

Systemic syndromes

A massive and out-of-control immune response will result in generalised inflammation and organ failure. Two terms—systemic inflammatory response syndrome (SIRS) and multi-organ dysfunction syndrome (MODS)—are used to describe the overwhelming consequences of a severely dysregulated inflammatory response.

Step 3: Chronic inflammation

Chronic inflammation can be the result of a persistent infection, the development of an autoimmune condition (an immune response to the body's own cells) or the failure of the inflammatory response to transition to the resolution phase. Regardless of the cause, this condition represents a debilitating process that influences the health of many patients presenting to paramedics. Tissue that has become chronically inflamed is typically infiltrated with large numbers of macrophages, lymphocytes and plasma cells, as well as excessive small blood vessels. Together these factors propagate ongoing tissue destruction and repair.

Summary

Inflammation is a homeostatic response to injury or infection that protects the body from further damage and promotes healing. The complex cascade of chemicals involved in the inflammatory response has the net effect of causing vasodilation and increased vessel permeability. There is an integral link between the inflammatory response and the clotting system.

Excessive, uncontrolled inflammatory responses are the underlying cause of life-threatening conditions such as anaphylaxis, sepsis and burns shock. Localised abnormal inflammatory responses contribute to conditions such as asthma, cardiovascular disease, coeliac disease and severe traumatic brain injury.

Chronic inflammation results when the inflammatory response does not resolve and causes further tissue damage.

References

Bryant, B., & Knights, K. (2014). *Pharmacology for health professionals* (4th ed.). Chatswood: Mosby.

Craft, J., Gordon, C., & Tiziani, A. (2015). *Understanding pathophysiology* (2nd ed.). Sydney: Elsevier.

McCance, K., & Huether, S. (2014). *Pathophysiology: the biologic basis for disease in adults and children* (7th ed.). St Louis: Mosby.

Netea, G. M., Balkwill, F., Chonchol, M., Cominelli, F., Donath, M. Y., Giamarellos-Bourboulis, E. J., Golenbock, D., Gresnigt, M. S., Heneka, M. T., Hoffman, H. M., Hotchkiss, R., Joosten, L. A. B., Kastner, D. L., Korte, M., Latz, E., Libby, P., Mandrup-Poulsen, T., Mantovani, A., Mills, K. H. G., Nowak, K. L., O'Neill, L. A., Pickkers, P., van der Poll, T., Ridker, P. M., Schalkwijk, J., Schwartz, D. A., Siegmund, B., Steer, C. J., Tilg, H., van der Meer, J. W. M., van de Veerdonk, F. L., & Dinarello, C. A. (2017). A guiding map for inflammation. *Nature Immunology*, *18*(8), 826–831.

CHAPTER 5

Pharmacokinetics and Pharmacodynamics

By Ravina Ravi and Boyd Furmston

Introduction

Pharmacology is a scientific discipline concerned with the action, purpose, physiological effects and toxicology of chemical substances (i.e. drugs, hormones, neurotransmitters etc.) on living systems. The origin of the word 'pharmacology' traces back to the ancient Greek word *pharmakon*, which translates as 'drug' meaning both 'remedy' and 'poison' (Derrida, 1981).

In this foundations chapter, we explore the key underlying principles of drug actions and interactions within the physiological system. The basic concepts of pharmacology can be divided broadly into two sections, pharmacodynamics (things that affect the action of drugs) and pharmacokinetics (things that affect the concentration of drugs in the system), both of which will be covered in this chapter. As paramedics, it is vital to understand the pharmacological interventions that are administered and their application to the dynamic and potentially deteriorating patient. Knowledge of these concepts is essential in understanding and predicting the therapeutic effects of treatment as well as anticipating potential drug interactions and adverse reactions to facilitate better patient outcomes.

Definitions

Key terms used within this chapter are defined in Table 5.1.

Pharmacodynamics (what the drug does to the body)

Targets of drug action

'*Corpora non agunt nisi fixate*' ('drugs will not work unless they are bound') is a famous phrase coined by the German researcher, Paul Ehrlich (1854–1915), who is best known for his contributions to the advancement of a number of scientific disciplines including pharmacology (Bosch & Rosich, 2008). While there are of course exceptions to the rules (e.g. activated charcoal, osmotic diuretics, antacids, antimicrobials), Ehrlich's theory holds true for the majority of drugs. Molecules (i.e. drugs, hormones, neurotransmitters etc.) which bind to molecular targets on cells are referred to as **ligands**. Ligands have the ability to bind reversibly or irreversibly, activate or inactivate their target, thereby consequently increasing or decreasing the function of that cell. Once bound to their relevant molecular target, a complex series of sequential events is initiated in order to produce a physiological response. Indeed, drugs are simply **exogenous** ligands mimicking and/or modifying our normal physiological processes and therefore utilise the same molecular targets as the body's own **endogenous** ligands.

In order to understand how a drug works, we need to first understand how and where drugs bind, in addition to the associated signalling and intracellular pathways involved in eliciting a physiological response. With few exceptions as outlined previously, the four main types of regulatory proteins commonly involved as molecular drug targets are:

- receptors
- ion channels
- enzymes
- carrier molecules (transporters) (Lambert, 2004).

Receptors

Receptors are protein molecules typically located on the cell membrane or within cells and are activated by endogenous ligands such as neurotransmitters, hormones or inflammatory mediators. Receptors exhibit a level of chemical exclusivity such that they will only interact with ligands which display compatible properties based on their shape, size and charge. The 'lock and key' analogy is a popular way in which to describe this level of compatibility, whereby, if the key (ligand) has the wrong properties, then it is unable to engage with the lock (receptor) (see Fig 5.1).

Receptors are further subdivided into four families, based on their molecular structure and the nature of the sequence of events following receptor occupation to the relevant physiological response (see Table 5.2 and Fig 5.2).

Ion channels

Ions are charged molecules (common examples include potassium [K^+], sodium [Na^+] and chloride [Cl^-]). Ion channels are in essence gateways located in the cell membrane which regulate the passage of selected ions. There are two types of ion channels: ligand gated and voltage gated. As the names suggest, ion movement across ligand-gated channels is triggered by the relevant ligand binding and are more suitably classified as receptors (see Table 5.2 and

Table 5.1: Key definitions

Term	Definition
Absorption	Process relating to the movement of unchanged drug from the administration site to the systemic circulation
Affinity	Describes the attraction and tendency of a ligand to bind to its target
Agonist	Ligand which binds to and activates the receptor to elicit a physiological response
Allosteric modulation	Ligand which binds to a receptor's allosteric site (distinct from the activate site) to modulate the response
Antagonist	Ligand which binds to the receptor and blocks the response (by preventing agonist binding)
Bioavailability	Describes the proportion of drug which enters the systemic circulation unchanged and is available to interact at its site of activity
Clearance	Describes the rate at which a drug is removed from the plasma
Distribution	Process relating to the reversible transfer of a drug from the circulation into other compartments in the body (i.e. fluid, cells or tissues)
EC_{50}	Describes the concentration of drug required to produce 50% of the maximum response
Efficacy	Describes the ability of the drug, once bound, to elicit a response
Endogenous	Describes a substance that has originated or been produced internally (within the organism or system)
Excretion	Process relating to the irreversible loss of drug from the body
Exogenous	Describes a substance that has originated or been produced externally (outside the organism or system)
First-order (normal) kinetics	When the amount of drug in the plasma is eliminated at a constant proportion per unit time
Half-life	Describes the time taken for a drug to be eliminated to half its original concentration in the plasma
Ligands	Molecules which bind to protein targets; drugs, hormones and neurotransmitters that bind to their targets are referred to as ligands
Metabolism	Process relating to the breakdown or transformation of a drug, through a number of mechanisms, to a form which is easily excreted by the body
Potency	Defined as how much drug is required to produce the desired/required response
Selectivity	A drug's target
Specificity	A drug's effects
Steady state	Describes the point at which the rate of drug input is equal to the rate of drug elimination
Tachyphylaxis and desensitisation	Describes the diminished effects (rapid and gradual) of a drug over time following repeated administration
Therapeutic window	Describes the therapeutic dosage/concentration range of a drug (between the minimum effective concentration [MEC] and the minimum toxic concentration [MTC])
Zero-order (saturation) kinetics	When a constant proportion of drug is eliminated per unit time irrespective of the amount of drug in the plasma

Source: Raffa et al. (2014); Rang et al. (2012); Bryant & Knights (2011).

Fig 5.2), while voltage-gated channels are mediated by changes in the membrane potential. Local anaesthetics are examples of commonly utilised drugs which act by blocking voltage-gated sodium channels (Camerino et al., 2007), thereby preventing depolarisation and signal transmission.

Enzymes
Enzymes are biological catalysts which control the rate of biochemical reactions in a cell. Some examples of enzymes include 3-hydroxy-3-methyl-glutaryl-coenzyme A reductase (HMG-CoA), which is involved in cholesterol synthesis and angiotensin II (Ang II) which is involved in blood pressure regulation.

Drugs can act by interfering with the active site of the enzymes by:
- acting as a substrate analogue—competitively (e.g. perindopril, acts on angiotensin-converting enzyme [ACE]) or non-competitively (e.g. aspirin, acts on cyclo-oxygenase [COX]), or

Table 5.2: An overview of the four main types of receptors and examples of drugs that act at these sites

Types	Type 1: Ligand-gated ion channels	Type 2: G protein-coupled receptors (GPCRs)	Type 3: Kinase-linked receptors	Type 4: Nuclear receptors
Features	• Receptors are linked to ion channels	• Constitute the largest family of receptors • Membrane receptors coupled to intracellular effectors via G protein • Mechanism involves second messenger systems (i.e. cAMP and cGMP)	• Respond mainly to protein mediators (i.e. cytokines, growth factors, insulin) • Predominantly involved in the control of cell growth and differentiation	• Generally located in the cytosol but migrates to the nucleus following activation • Regulate gene transcription and protein synthesis
Location	Cell membrane	Cell membrane	Cell membrane	Intracellular
Receptor examples	nAChR; GABA$_A$ receptors	Adrenoceptors; opioid receptors	Insulin, growth factors	Steroid receptors
Drug examples	Suxamethonium Benzodiazepine	Adrenaline Morphine	Insulin	Thyroxine Oestrogen

Source: Adapted from Rang et al. (2012) (Table 3.2).

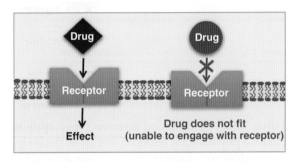

Figure 5.1
Graphical representation of the 'lock and key' concept as it relates to pharmacology.

• acting as false substrates to produce a non-functional product (e.g. anticancer drug fluorouracil, replaces uracil inhibiting DNA synthesis and cell division) (Rang et al., 2012).

Carrier/transporter molecules

Due to the lipid bilayer of the cell membrane, only ions and small molecules with sufficient lipid solubility are able to diffuse across. Those lacking in this property require transportation via carrier proteins located within the membrane, a process which requires metabolic energy as molecules are transported against their concentration gradient.

There are three different types of carrier molecules: symporters (move molecules in the same direction; e.g. loop diuretics; renal), antiporters (move molecules in opposite directions; e.g. digoxin; heart) and uptake carriers (stop uptake and consequently the breakdown of chemicals at the nerve terminal, prolonging their effects; e.g. cocaine) (Alexander et al., 2017).

Specificity versus selectivity

Specificity is a term used to describe the number of effects a drug produces or the number of mechanisms involved. Ideally, in order to avoid any unwanted side effects (i.e. adverse reactions), a given drug will act on one target, at one site and produce one physiological response; unfortunately, no drugs possess this property. Most drugs, however, will exhibit **selectivity**, thereby showing preference for a particular molecular target. Thus, selectivity describes the number of targets a drug will interact with. It is important to note, however, that while the majority of drugs will exhibit some degree of selectivity within a particular dose range, in most instances, increasing the dose may invariably generate off-target effects, resulting in adverse reactions.

Drug–target interactions

Now that we have covered the basics of drug targets, we can delve into drug–target interactions including the relationship between drug concentration and the associated response.

Following the administration of a drug, the ensuing response usually increases as more drug is given until a point where increasing the dose does not contribute to a higher response (response plateaus). The relationship between drug concentration and resultant effect is often represented as a concentration-response (C-R) curve whereby the concentration of the drug is plotted against a semi-logarithmic scale. The sigmoidal shape of the

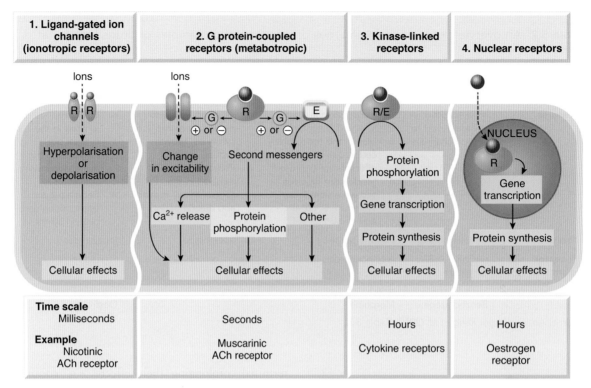

Figure 5.2
Overview of the four main receptor types and their associated signalling pathways, ACh-acetylcholine.
E = enzyme; G = G protein; R = receptor.
Source: Rang et al. (2012) (Fig 3.2).

resultant curves against this scale includes a linear segment, generally between 20% and 80% of the maximal response and often reflects the therapeutic concentrations of that drug (**therapeutic window**). Below this section reflects the subtherapeutic effects while increasing the drug concentration above 80% of the maximal response generally enhances the risk of adverse reactions without the additional therapeutic benefits (see Fig 5.3). Indeed, understanding the fundamental concepts relating to C-R curves allows us to compare the effects of drugs which act on the same molecular target. Because the response is proportional to the log drug concentration for the middle section of the C-R curve we would not expect a doubling of the concentration to produce a doubling of the response. An example of a practical application of this is when giving intravenous opiate analgesia it is necessary to more than double the dose to achieve double the effect. Continuing to repeat the same small dose that did not achieve analgesia is not going to control our patient's pain.

It should be noted that with respect to drug-receptor interactions, occupation by a drug does not always result in the activation of that receptor. Therefore, drugs can be defined into two broad categories, agonists and antagonists. An **agonist** is a drug which binds to and activates the receptor to induce a physiological response, similar to the body's own endogenous ligands. When a drug activates its receptor, but produces less than the maximal effect despite all targets being occupied, then that drug is often referred to as a *partial agonist*. Fentanyl and morphine are examples of *full agonists* (able to produce a maximal response) while buprenorphine is an example of a partial agonist which targets the same opioid receptors (Lambert, 2004) (see Box 5.1).

Affinity, potency and efficacy
Now that we understand the basis of the concentration-response relationship, we can discuss several parameters which play a role in this relationship. **Affinity** describes the tendency of a ligand/drug to interact and bind with its target. In other words, it is a measure of how well the drug binds—the higher the affinity the more likely the drug is to bind and the greater the time spent bound to that receptor. The **potency** of a drug is therefore linked to its affinity—the higher the attraction between the drug and its receptor, the more likely it is to interact to produce a physiological response, even at low concentrations (see Fig 5.4). It should be noted, however, that this is not always a proportional relationship.

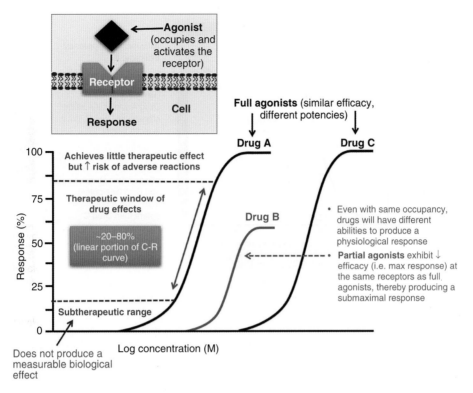

Figure 5.3
Illustrative depiction of the concept of an agonist and the concentration-response relationship.
Source: Adapted from Raffa et al. (2014) (Fig 1.8) and Bryant & Knights (2011) (Fig 5.5).

BOX 5.1 Spare receptor theory

- The spare receptor theory relates to the notion that not all receptors associated with a particular physiological response need to be occupied in order to facilitate a maximal response.
- Due to their reduced efficacy, partial agonists are only able to elicit a submaximal physiological response, even when all receptors are occupied, compared to full agonists.
- Partial agonists can actually compete with full agonists for receptor occupancy and impede the overall physiological response.

Source: Stephenson (1956).

BOX 5.2 Affinity, potency and efficacy summary

It is important to remember the following.
- High affinity binding can be achieved at low drug concentrations. As such we cannot make inferences about affinity based on the C-R curves.
- The concepts of potency and efficacy are not interchangeable such that displaying high potency does not necessarily confer high efficacy and vice versa.
- Agonists exhibit both affinity and efficacy (i.e. attracted to, occupies and activates the receptor).
- Antagonists, described opposite, exhibit affinity but no efficacy (i.e. attracted to and occupies the receptor but prevents it from being activated = blocks response).

Source: Lambert (2004).

Once bound to the target, **efficacy** is a measure of the drug's ability to activate that target (e.g. receptor) and elicit a response. Utilising the C-R curves, we are able to determine the maximum response a drug can produce (E_{max}) as well as the concentration of the drug required to produce 50% of the maximum response (**EC_{50}**), parameters which are useful when trying to compare drug efficacy and potency respectively. It

should be noted that drugs which act on the same target can exhibit similar potency (EC_{50}) but differ in their efficacy (E_{max}) or conversely have differing potencies but similar efficacies. This concept is depicted in Figure 5.4 and Box 5.2.

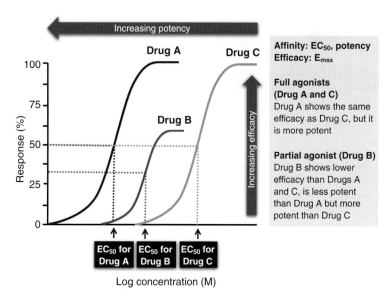

Figure 5.4
Diagrammatic overview of the basic concepts of potency and efficacy as well as the associated effects on the C-R curve. It should be noted that affinity cannot be compared using C-R curves.
Source: Adapted from Raffa et al. (2014) (Figs 1.20 and 1.21) and Bryant & Knights (2011) (Figs 5.5 and 5.6).

Antagonists, commonly referred to as 'blockers' or 'inhibitors', occupy the receptor, impeding the access and binding of the endogenous ligand to the active site, thereby preventing the ensuing physiological response. Antagonism can either be reversible or irreversible and we can exploit this feature therapeutically to block any unwanted physiological effects. Atropine is an example of a competitive, reversible antagonist which will compete with an agonist (i.e. ACh) for binding at muscarinic receptor sites, thereby decreasing parasympathetic stimulation (Raffa et al., 2014).

Thus, using the 'lock and key analogy', both agonists and antagonists act as keys and are able to fit into the lock (receptor); however, only the agonist is able to turn and open the lock. Refer to Table 5.3 and Figure 5.5 for an overview of the three main types of antagonism and the resultant effects these have on the C-R curve.

In addition to the active (orthosteric) site, receptors may also possess an alternative (allosteric) binding site. Indeed, another way in which a drug can modify the activity of a receptor is by binding to its allosteric site (Abdel-Magid, 2015; Christopoulos et al., 2014). These drugs are termed **allosteric modulators** and can act to either augment (positive allosteric modulator [PAMs]) or inhibit (negative allosteric modulators [NAMs]) the activity of that receptor and the relevant ligand (Abdel-Magid, 2015). Benzodiazepines are allosteric modulators of the $GABA_A$ receptor (ligand-gated ion channel), inducing a structural change in

the receptor such that the effect of the endogenous inhibitory neurotransmitter, GABA, is increased (Sigel & Steinmann, 2012).

Tachyphylaxis and desensitisation

The repeated administration of a drug can sometimes result in its diminished effects over time. The terms **tachyphylaxis** and **desensitisation** have been used synonymously to describe this phenomenon although, depending on the source, these definitions may differ slightly. The main difference between the two terms is time, with tachyphylaxis often used to describe the rapid onset of this phenomenon. Another term which is commonly utilised is *tolerance*, which describes the gradual decrease in the body's responsiveness to the drug (days or weeks). While the distinction between these terms is not always clear, some of the mechanisms thought to be involved include:

- conformational change of the receptors such that normal signalling processes are impeded
- loss or translocation of the receptors
- depletion of mediators
- augmented metabolism of the drug, and/or
- physiological adaptation whereby the body compensates by opposing the effects of the drug (Rang et al., 2012; Gainetdinov et al., 2004; Neubig et al., 2003).

In essence, tolerance mechanisms are geared towards opposing the effectiveness of the drug such that more drug is required to achieve the same response.

Table 5.3: Summary of the main types of antagonists

Types	Competitive reversible antagonists	Irreversible antagonists	Non-competitive antagonists
Features	Binds reversibly to the active site of the receptor (agonist and antagonist compete for the **same site**) Antagonism can be overcome by increasing agonist dose (i.e. the inhibition is surmountable)	Binds irreversibly to the active site of the receptor (agonist and antagonist compete for the **same site**) Antagonism cannot be overcome with increasing agonist dose	Binds to an alternative site to the active site (agonist and antagonist bind to **different sites**) Antagonism cannot be overcome with increasing agonist dose
Effect on the C-R curves	Parallel rightward shift with no effect on maximum response	Decrease in maximum response	Decrease in maximum response
Drug examples	Atropine (mAChR antagonist) Naloxone (opioid receptor antagonist)	Phenoxybenzamine (alpha-adrenoceptor antagonist)	Ketamine (NMDA receptor antagonist)

Source: Rang et al. (2012); Lambert (2004); Neubig et al. (2003).

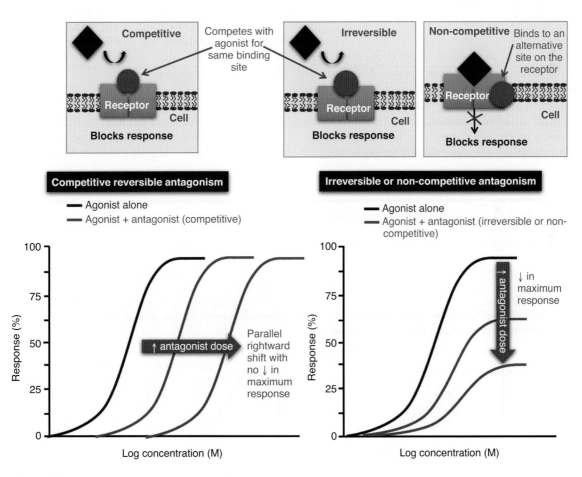

Figure 5.5
Illustrative overview of the main forms of antagonism and the associated effects on the concentration-response relationship.
Source: Adapted from Raffa et al. (2014) (Figs 1.9 and 1.23) and Bryant & Knights (2011) (Fig 5.7).

Pharmacokinetics (what the body does to the drug)

Pharmacokinetics is the branch of pharmacology concerned with the way drugs move throughout the body and how this concentration is modified as it travels through the different parts of the body. As mentioned in the previous section, in order to elicit an effect, the drug needs to reach and bind to its molecular target. The subsequent effect is often influenced by the concentration of the drug at its site of action, which is determined by a series of complex processes collectively denoted by the acronym **ADME** (absorption, distribution, metabolism and excretion). For all these processes, the movement of drug molecules across biological membranes predominantly occurs via passive diffusion; however, where drugs are required to be transported against their concentration gradient, carrier-mediated transport (active transport) is employed.

Absorption

The process of **absorption** relates to the movement of the unchanged drug from the site of administration into the systemic circulation, where it is then transported to its site of action. In addition to its route of administration, factors such as composition of the cell membrane, blood flow to the administration site, drug solubility, ionisation and formulation can all influence the rate and quantity of drug absorbed.

Oral administration is the most common route due to its high patient compliance, convenience and relatively fewer delivery complications. For orally ingested drugs, the major site of absorption is the small intestine; however, prior to entering the systemic circulation, the drug is first metabolised by the liver via a process known as *first-pass* **metabolism** (see Fig 5.6). Indeed, only drugs that enter the gastrointestinal tract, which is then transported into the hepatic portal system, are subject to first-pass metabolism.

The term **bioavailability** is used to describe the proportion of drug which reaches the circulation unchanged and is usually expressed as a percentage. The bioavailability of a drug is therefore influenced by its absorption and first-pass metabolism (i.e. oral administration). In contrast to oral administration, the intravenous (IV) route is the fastest with the highest bioavailability (i.e. 100%) as it is directly administered into the circulation, bypassing all absorption barriers (see Box 5.3).

Distribution

Upon entering the systemic circulation, a drug can then be transferred reversibly from one location in the body to another (e.g. tissue, muscle, fat) via a

BOX 5.3 Route of administration summary

The route of administration influences the:
- onset time (arrival at therapeutic range)
- peak plasma concentration
- duration of action (time spent in therapeutic range).

Theoretical illustration of the plasma concentration-time profile of a drug administered following a single oral dose and the interplay between the pharmacokinetic processes. It is important to note that factors such as the route of administration, disease state, genetics and environmental factors may influence the pharmacokinetic profile of a drug.

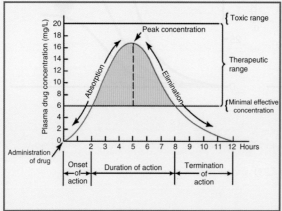
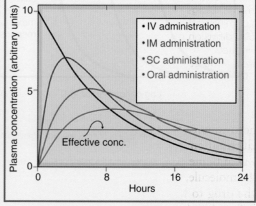

Source: Bryant & Knights (2011) (Fig 8.1).

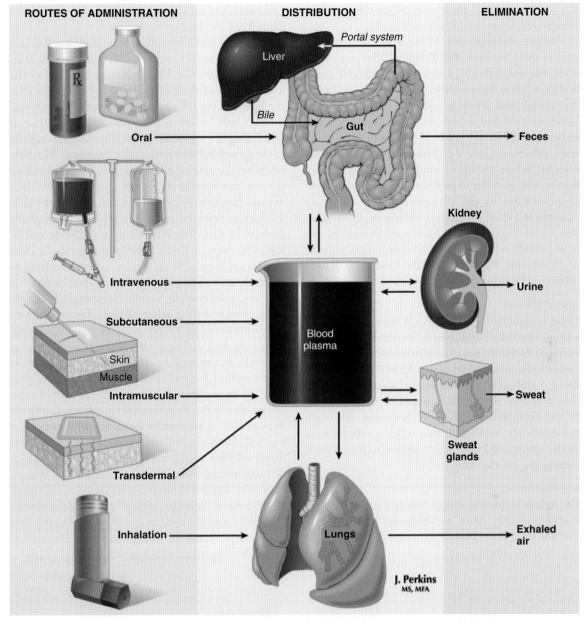

Figure 5.6
Overview of the main routes of administration and their associated absorption, distribution and elimination pathways. Drugs administered orally are predominantly absorbed in the gastrointestinal tract (GI). Intravenous (IV) administration enters the circulation directly while the intramuscular (IM) and subcutaneous (SC) routes require diffusion into the bloodstream. Other routes include, but are not limited to, inhalation, topical and sublingual.
Source: Raffa et al. (2014) (Fig 1.24).

process referred to as **distribution**. Drug distribution is mostly uneven with the location, extent and degree of distribution being dependent on capillary and cell membrane permeability, tissue perfusion, size of the molecule, regional pH as well as the tendency of the drug to bind to plasma proteins and tissue (i.e. lipophilic/lipid-soluble drugs). Furthermore, specialised barriers such as the blood–brain barrier (BBB) and placental barrier restrict the passage of certain drugs. As such, while some drugs will remain almost entirely in the plasma, others will have the propensity to diffuse to well-perfused organs or move to areas of poorer perfusion such as skeletal muscle or fat. It is important to note that only free drug (i.e. unbound) can interact with receptors, while drug bound to tissue or plasma proteins act like repositories and are released when the free drug is removed from the circulation.

Volume of distribution (Vd) indicates the distribution of drug between the blood and the rest of the body. Put simplistically, drugs which are highly tissue bound tend to have smaller amounts remaining in the circulation thereby equating to low plasma concentration but a high Vd. The opposite tends to be observed in drugs which remain in the circulation, exhibiting low Vd. This process is clinically relevant when trying to establish an appropriate *loading dose* in order to promptly achieve the desired concentration in the plasma. Amiodarone is an example of a drug with a large volume of distribution due to its highly lipophilic nature (Goldschlager et al., 2000), while warfarin exhibits a small volume of distribution due to its extensive binding to plasma proteins (Holford & Yim, 2016).

Metabolism

Drug metabolism is the physical transformation of a drug, normally conducted by enzymes, to an easily excreted form. In some instances, metabolism can convert the drug to an active form (i.e. prodrug). Drug metabolism predominantly occurs within the liver and typically involves functionalisation (Phase I) and conjugation (Phase II) reactions, although not explicitly with numerous other locations such as the lungs and kidneys also shown to play a part, depending on the drug.

Excretion

Excretion is the irreversible loss of a drug from the body, primarily from the kidneys, although the pulmonary system, breastmilk, tears, saliva and sweat may also contribute to this process. Both metabolism and excretion contribute to the elimination of the drug from the body.

The time taken for a drug to be eliminated to half its original plasma concentration is referred to as its *plasma half-life (t$_{1/2}$)*. The time taken for half of the total amount of drug in the body to be eliminated is the **half-life (t$_{1/2}$)**. The key factors which determine a drug's half-life are the Vd and **clearance** (rate at which drug is removed from the plasma). The majority of drugs will exhibit **first-order (normal) kinetics**, whereby the rate of elimination is proportional to the concentration of the free drug and in accordance with its half-life. For example, if a drug's half-life is 4 hours as depicted in Figure 5.7, then half of the amount of that drug remaining in the body will be removed every 4 hours. The point at which drug absorption is equal to drug elimination is referred to as **steady state**, whereby plasma drug concentration is constant, and hopefully, within the desired therapeutic range. Steady state is achieved either via continuous administration (i.e. IV infusion) or repeated dosing. Assuming drug dosing is fixed and repeated at regular intervals, as a general rule, steady state is reached in approximately 3–5 half-lives (see Fig 5.7). Where drug elimination occurs at a constant rate per unit of time, irrespective of the drug concentration, this is referred to as exhibiting **zero-order (saturation) kinetics** (see Fig 5.8). Both alcohol and warfarin are examples of drugs relevant to the out-of-hospital setting which demonstrate zero-order kinetics and in cases of toxicity, they may require extended periods of monitoring. As a general concept, drugs which demonstrate first-order kinetics tend to be more predictable and therefore preferred for therapeutic use compared to those showing zero-order kinetics.

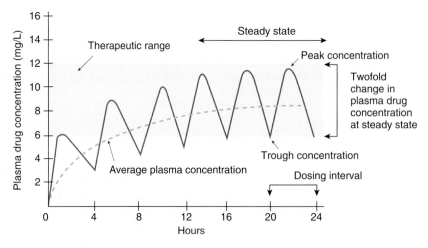

Figure 5.7
Graphical depiction of the concepts of half-life and steady state. In this example, a fixed dose of the drug is administered every 4 hours with a half-life of 4 hours and steady state being achieved after 3–5 half-lives. *Source: Bryant & Knights (2011) (Fig 8.6).*

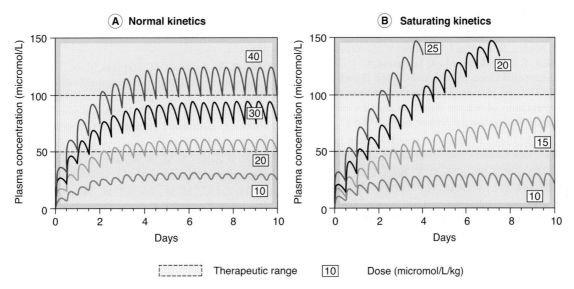

Figure 5.8
Comparison of normal versus saturation kinetics of an orally administered medication every 12 hours. As depicted in the figure on the right, if the amount of drug administered exceeds the set rate of elimination, the resultant effects may be disproportionate and unpredictable.
Source: Rang et al. (2012) (Fig 10.9).

The effects of population variance on pharmacokinetics

Elderly

A common expression used is to 'start low, go slow'. Factors such as a reduction in renal and hepatic capabilities with decreased drug clearance, in addition to changes in body composition (i.e. decrease in adipose tissue and muscle mass), should be considered in this population.

Paediatrics

It is important to note that paediatric patients are not just little adults. Paediatric patients may oxidise some drugs more rapidly or conjugation reactions may develop more slowly, and as such an altered metabolism should be considered in this population.

Pregnancy

Differences in blood volume and cardiac output during pregnancy along with increased renal and hepatic perfusion as well as function needs to be considered. Fetal risk assessment should be considered with drug administration due to its ability to cross the placental barrier.

Other

Considerations such as co-morbidities, genetic predisposition and the associated drug-to-drug interactions, in addition to how this relates to organ dysfunction with all patients, should be considered.

Summary

By understanding the pharmacological processes involved, drug dosing and formulations can be manipulated in order to achieve the desired pharmacodynamic or pharmacokinetic profile. Detailed study of a clinical pharmacological text in support of this chapter is strongly recommended.

References

Abdel-Magid, A. F. (2015). Allosteric modulators: an emerging concept in drug discovery. *American Chemical Society Medicinal Chemistry Letters, 6*(2), 104–107.

Alexander, S. P. H., Kelly, E., Marrion, N. V., Peters, J. A., Faccenda, E., Harding, S. D., Pawson, A. J., Sharman, J. L., Southan, C., Davies, J. A., & CGTP Collaborators. (2017). The concise guide to pharmacology 2017/18: transporters. *British Journal of Pharmacology, 174*(S1), S360–S446.

Bosch, F., & Rosich, L. (2008). The contributions of Paul Ehrlich to pharmacology: a tribute on the occasion of the centenary of his Nobel Prize. *Pharmacology, 82,* 171–179.

Bryant, B., & Knights, K. (2011). *Pharmacology for health professionals* (3rd ed.). Sydney: Mosby.

Camerino, D. C., Tricarico, D., & Desaphy, J. (2007). Ion channel pharmacology. *Neurotherapeutics: The Journal of the American Society for Experimental NeuroTherapeutics, 4,* 184–198.

Christopoulos, A., Changeux, J. P., Catterall, W. A., Fabbro, D., Burris, T. P., Cidlowski, J. A., Olsen, R. W., Peters, J. A., Neubig, R. R., Pin, J. P., Sexton, P. M., Kenakin, T., Ehlert, F. J., Spedding, M., & Langmead, C. J. (2014). International Union of Basic and Clinical Pharmacology. XC. Multisite pharmacology: recommendations of the nomenclature of receptor allosterism and allosteric ligands. *Pharmacological Reviews, 66*(4), 918–947.

Derrida, J. (1981). *Dissemination* trans B Johnson (pp. 63–171). Chicago: University of Chicago Press.

Gainetdinov, R. R., Premont, R. T., Bohn, L. M., Lefkowitz, R. J., & Caron, M. G. (2004). Desensitisation of G protein-coupled receptors and neuronal functions. *Annual Review of Neuroscience, 27*, 107–144.

Goldschlager, N., Epstein, A. E., Naccarelli, G., Olshansky, B., & Singh, B. (2000). Practical guidelines for clinicians who treat patients with amiodarone. *Archives of Internal Medicine, 160*, 1741–1748.

Holford, N., & Yim, D.-S. (2016). Volume of distribution. *Translational and Clinical Pharmacology, 24*(2), 74–77.

Lambert, D. G. (2004). Drugs and receptors. *Continuing Education on Anaesthesia, Critical Care & Pain, 4*(6), 181–184.

Neubig, R. R., Spedding, M., Kenakin, T., & Christopoulos, A. (2003). International Union of Pharmacology Committee on receptor nomenclature and drug classification. XXXVIII. Update on terms and symbols in quantitative pharmacology. *Pharmacological Reviews, 55*(4), 597–606.

Raffa, R. B., Rawls, S. M., & Beyzarov, E. P. (2014). *Netter's illustrated pharmacology* (2nd ed.). Philadelphia: Elsevier.

Rang, H. P., Dale, M. M., Ritter, J. M., Flower, R. J., & Henderson, G. (2012). *Rang and Dale's pharmacology* (7th ed.). Edinburgh: Churchill Livingstone.

Sigel, E., & Steinmann, M. E. (2012). Structure, function and modulation of $GABA_A$ receptors. *The Journal of Biological Chemistry, 287*(48), 40224–40231.

Stephenson, R. P. (1956). A modification of receptor theory. *British Journal of Pharmacology and Chemotherapy, 11*(4), 379–393.

SECTION 3:
Foundation Concepts

In this section:

Evidence-based practice and clinical reasoning may seem like an odd pairing; however, they are both concepts that underpin paramedic practice. Evidence-based practice serves to advance and inform the paramedic profession and clinical practice. Paramedics must take responsibility for clinical practice and guidelines that are not only based on best evidence, but evidence produced by the profession and for the out-of-hospital context. While evidence-based practice informs service- and profession-wide clinical guidelines, the clinical reasoning process is referring to the individual paramedic's ability to gather and process information in order to make informed decisions about patient treatment. The clinical reasoning chapter discusses the factors that contribute to decision-making and describes a four-step process to guide clinical reasoning, which is utilised throughout this text.

CHAPTER 6

Evidence-Based Practice in Paramedicine

By Kelly-Ann Bowles and Cameron Gosling

OVERVIEW

- Continuous improvement in patient outcomes is reliant on the engagement of ambulance services in research and the development of practice guidelines based on the latest evidence.
- To effectively treat patients, paramedics need to be able to interpret clinical practice guidelines using their clinical knowledge and experience, while considering the needs and values of the patient.
- Evidence-based practice is the combination of research evidence, clinical experience and the patient values and circumstances.

- Effective evidence-based practice in paramedicine is reliant on translation of appropriate research findings to ambulance services and clinical guidelines.
- The more paramedics engage in research, the more relevant the research evidence will be for their clinical role and the easier it will be for them to actively engage in evidence-based practice.

Case 1

An ambulance service has identified that their graduate paramedics are reporting issues with their sleep patterns since starting shift work. Older colleagues suggest that they start a structured exercise program as this helped them with sleep when they were new to the job. As the service would like to put an evidence-based suggestion out to all graduates, they work with researchers to find the latest, relevant evidence. As the graduates are saying that they just prefer to sit on the couch during their down time, the service wants to demonstrate to the graduates that exercise may be more beneficial than sedentary behaviour when it comes to establishing sleep patterns with shift work.

Introduction

The role of a paramedic has changed drastically over the last 30 to 40 years. What was traditionally a service that saw an 'ambulance driver' go to a patient and then take them to hospital, current practice has dictated that the paramedic take a more clinical role in patient care. The increase in academic education and the introduction of a diverse range of skills and practice has led to the recognition of paramedics as registered health professionals in some countries, similar to nurses and other allied health clinicians. As with other registered professions, paramedics are now responsible to consistently update their own clinician professional development, which can be viewed as an important part of the evidence-based practice framework.

Evidence-based practice (EBP) was developed from the idea that decisions made in regards to the treatment of patients, and the development of guidelines or policies behind these treatments, need to be based on best evidence. The initial development in the area of evidence-based practice focused on research that discussed the perceived success or failure of a drug or treatment. It originated from the area of evidence-based medicine, classically defined by Sackett and colleagues stating that 'evidence-based medicine (EBM) is the conscientious, explicit and judicious use of current best evidence in making decisions about the care of individual patients. The practice of evidence-based medicine means integrating individual clinical expertise with the best available external clinical evidence from systematic research' (Sackett et al., 1996). However, evidence-based practice takes the theories of evidence-based medicine a further step, by integrating the best evidence with the clinician's experience and the values and circumstances of the patient.

To help with the understanding of evidence-based practice, the diagram in Figure 6.1 is often used. The principle gives equal emphasis to the three components of evidence-based practice that lead to the final treatment decision. Although some versions of this image may differ slightly in the terminology used, the key idea is that the practice used to treat the patient is individualised based on each component. What may work well for one patient or one clinician in one setting may not be suitable for the next. As each health profession has their own 'experience' to add to the development of the evidence-based

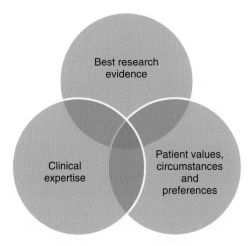

Figure 6.1
Components of evidence-based practice.

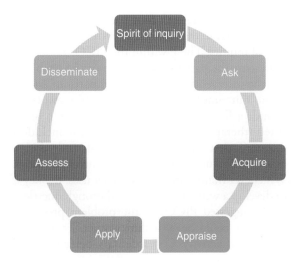

Figure 6.2
The seven steps in an evidence-based practice framework.

practice model, it is important that the unique working conditions that paramedics see themselves in are paramount in deciding the optimal practice for their own profession. It is not surprising, then, that many health professional organisations view evidence-based practice as a key part of patient care.

Introduction to evidence-based practice

Steps of evidence-based practice

With the three components of evidence-based practice discussed, we need to determine the different research findings we should use to help us decide on the best treatment for our patients. The individual clinical experience and patients' needs will vary from case to case, but ambulance services frequently revisit and review their clinical practice guidelines based on the latest evidence. This then allows the services to provide their clinicians with the latest relevant research findings to guide their clinical practice.

The best practice implementation of research findings into an evidence-based practice guideline utilises a well-established five-step framework (Sackett et al., 1996). These steps focus on the themes of *ask, acquire, appraise, apply and assess*. Over the years this five-step process has been modified and expanded to add a final step of dissemination so that all clinicians understand the importance of sharing their experiences with their peers. Some resources have gone further to suggest that evidence-based practice is actually a seven-step process, with an additional step described as developing the spirit of inquiry (Melnyk et al., 2010) (see Fig 6.2).

Spirit of inquiry

The first step is to develop an ethos that encourages members to question the way things are currently done and to strive to do things better. These questions may focus on clinical practices, education processes or the way in which a service functions. By exposing paramedic students to research subjects and giving students and clinicians the opportunity to be actively involved in research, the spirit of inquiry becomes the accepted norm.

A survey of paramedics in Australia found that paramedics generally agree that research and evidence-based practice is important to their practice (Simpson et al., 2012). Simpson and colleagues also reported that tertiary-qualified clinicians regarded evidence-based practice as more important than vocationally trained clinicians. Clinicians who had been paramedics for a longer period of time and senior-level clinicians (such as intensive care paramedics) did view evidence-based practice as important, but to a lesser extent than newly qualified paramedics. The authors suggested that more needs to be done to engage the senior clinicians in paramedic services, as they provide role modelling. The authors stated that this need to engage senior clinicians has been identified as an important factor in European services as well. So to truly ensure that evidence-based practice can flourish in the paramedic setting, it is important that leaders encourage their services to develop a spirit of inquiry.

Ask

Once a clinician has developed a spirit of inquiry, it is important they have the requisite skills required to then ask a quality question. Within tertiary-level research subjects, students are generally taught frameworks to increase their chances of developing a good research question. The most commonly used one is the PICO framework (Schardt et al., 2007).

Within this framework four parts of the question are identified so that the question truly matches the area of inquiry. The P within the PICO framework represents the patient, population or the problem; I is the intervention; C is the comparison; and O is the outcome. Some expand the framework to include a T to represent the type of question being asked (therapy, diagnosis etc.) and some include a second T that represents the type of study design (e.g. cohort study or randomised controlled study). Whichever framework the researcher uses, the key is to develop a well-structured and thorough question.

A suggested PICO for the problem presented in Case 1 could be: P = shift worker, I = exercise or physical activity, C = sedentary behaviour and O = sleep.

Acquire

Once the question is developed it is important to acquire all the research outputs published to date. For most researchers this will happen using a database repository such as Medline, CINAHL (Cumulative Index of Nursing and Allied Health Literature) or PubMed. Once a research question is developed using a PICO framework, researchers spend time making a list of synonyms for the words within each PICO element. Different databases also use subject headings or MeSH (Medical Subject Headings) terms, which are a way for the databases to group research on the same topic. It is important to identify which research database is suitable for the set question as databases include citations linked to different areas, with Medline often used for medical research and databases like ERIC (Educational Resources Information Centre) often used to search educational research. Within the database, the research then needs to use Boolean operators (terms such as AND, OR and NOT) to expand or limit the search. By using the OR function between the synonyms, the search is expanded within each element of the PICO. Elements are then combined by applying the AND operator to limit our final search to only include research that addresses all four aspects of the research question. Librarians are trained to help researchers use these databases and gather all the relevant publications so that the researcher can confidently answer their research question.

Revisiting the problem presented in Case 1, the following search may be used to find the relevant research.

1. Shift work schedule (as a subject heading) OR 'shift work' (as a keyword)

2. Exercise (as a subject heading) OR exercise OR 'physical activity'

3. Sedentary behaviour (as a subject heading) OR sedentary OR rest

4. Sleep (as a subject heading) OR sleep OR fatigue

5. Combine 1 AND 2 AND 3 AND 4

Appraise

With all the relevant research outputs found, the next step is to appraise the quality of the research and to think about the results specific to the clinical area. Researchers often use quality or risk of bias tools to help them systematically identify the strengths and weakness of each research output found. This is not so much about giving a research publication a score; it is more about establishing how valid the results of the research are when we take into account weakness that may greatly affect the results (like patients knowing that they have been given a placebo). It is important to understand the study type that we are appraising (e.g. randomised controlled trial or cohort study), as it is important to use a quality appraisal tool suitable for the included study. While appraising the research it is still important to consider all components of the evidence-based practice components of clinical experience and patient values and beliefs. Finally, we need to look at all of the research publications to really determine if there is a consistent finding that could be used in the evidence-based practice recommendation.

Apply

It is important then to apply, or translate, best-evidence findings to the relevant clinical setting. The concept of translational research for many traditionalists has been based on the notion of 'bench to bedside' (Woolf, 2008). However, the pathway to changes in clinical practice for paramedics is often not as easily defined. Woolf (2008) and Westfall and colleagues (2007) describe three translational stages that must be navigated for research to lead to changes to clinical guidelines, policies and practices. These three translational steps (or blocks) are: T1—can the research discoveries positively impact change in humans; T2—can the same positive effects be observed in patients; and finally T3—can the efficacy established in patient trials demonstrate similar results across the whole of practice (see Fig 6.3). The focus for paramedic research in making real-world changes is the translation to patients and practice.

It is great that the current research may find that a new lifting device reduces musculoskeletal injuries in hospital staff, but if this equipment cannot be used in an out-of-hospital setting, this research may not be applicable for paramedics. Ideally, we need to implement the findings in the area where

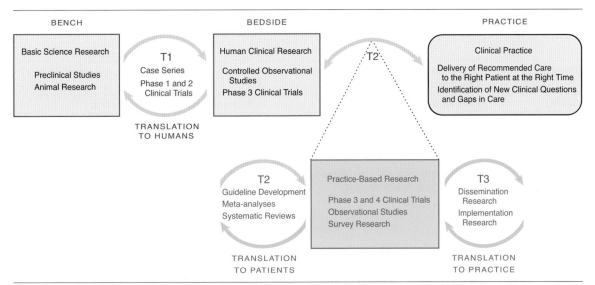

The current National Institutes of Health (NIH) Roadmap for Medical Research includes 2 major research laboratories (bench and bedside) and 2 translational steps (T1 and T2). Historically, moving new medical discoveries into clinical practice (T2) has been haphazard, occurring largely through continuing medical education programs, pharmaceutical detailing and guideline development. Proposed expansion of the NIH Roadmap (blue) includes an additional research laboratory (Practice-based Research) and translational step (T3) to improve incorporation of research discoveries into day-to-day clinical care. The research roadmap is a continuum, with overlap between sites of research and translational steps. The figure includes examples of the types of research common in each research laboratory and translational step. This map is not exhaustive; other important types of research that might be included are community-based participatory research, public health research and health policy analysis.

Figure 6.3
The 'Blue Highways' on the National Institutes of Health (NIH) Roadmap.
Source: Westfall, Mold & Fagnan, 2007.

the future recommendation will be made. This may occur through efficacy trials and/or effectiveness trials. Although there is not the scope to greatly detail these types of trials in this chapter, it is important to understand the difference.

Efficacy trails are primarily designed to see if the new intervention is successful in a controlled environment. It will often assess both the benefit and the harm of the potential intervention. This could be a randomised controlled trial against a placebo condition. To truly understand if the new intervention works, the trial is very 'controlled' with strict inclusion and exclusion criteria. Patients included in the trial would ideally all have the same disease and stage, and may not have any other comorbidities. Likewise, the clinicians providing the treatment are usually a select, well-trained team to ensure that the intervention is provided in exactly the same way for each patient. To ensure compliance, research assistants may telephone participants on a regular basis to ensure that they are adhering to the requirements of the trial. The overall aim of these trials is to determine if the new intervention does actually work. As these trials will be completed in such a controlled environment, the results are often an overestimate of the effect of the new intervention and may not be generalisable to the wider population. Efficacy trials are an important step in ensuring

patient safety and the genuine ability of the intervention to be successful. However, without an effectiveness trial we cannot truly understand if the intervention would be successful in the real world.

When we then want to see if this new treatment can work in a 'real-world' setting, next we would complete an effectiveness trial. This type of trial is more related to the real health setting and often less controlled in the way the intervention is delivered. We could still use a randomised controlled trial but now we might test against current practice or another common treatment approach. The aim of an effectiveness trial is to take the results from the efficacy trial and see if they are still relevant in a real-world setting. For an effectiveness trial the participants would be a better representation of the patient population. It is all well and good to show that a new spinal immobilisation protocol can decrease secondary damage when moving a patient, but if the clinicians cannot carry the new board to the patient or the protocol requires more people than is usually available, the effectiveness of the intervention will not be as great. Table 6.1 describes the differences between efficacy and effectiveness trials.

Assess

Once the evidence has been applied to the clinical setting, it is very important to assess the outcomes

Table 6.1: Differences between efficacy and effectiveness studies

	Efficacy study	Effectiveness study
Question	Does the intervention work under ideal circumstances?	Does the intervention work in real-world practice?
Setting	Resource-intensive 'ideal setting'	Real-world everyday clinical setting
Study population	Highly selected, homogenous population	Heterogeneous population Few to no exclusion criteria
Providers	Highly experienced and trained	Representative usual providers
Intervention	Strictly enforced and standardised No concurrent interventions	Applied with flexibility Concurrent interventions and cross-over permitted

Source: Singal, Higgins & Waljee, 2014.

of your setting. We need to quantify the benefits or cost to the patients or the service. At this stage, engagement of a health economist will help quantify the benefits to the service, the health system and/ or the patients and society. We also need to see if our results differ from those in the previous research. If our findings were very different, could there have been an error in the way we applied our research (i.e. were the clinicians not very good at giving the treatment)? We should also think very practically about our new finding, especially in the health setting. Will our recommendation be suitable within the health service or are we asking our clinicians to do something they cannot be equipped to do? Additionally, how do our results sit with your patient's values and preferences?

Disseminate

Perhaps the most important step in the evidence-based practice framework is that of dissemination. There is no point finding good results that could potentially greatly improve patient outcomes if we do not disseminate the findings. In fact, researchers have an ethical obligation to report their findings regardless of the outcome (Alley et al., 2015). Dissemination can be done through peer-reviewed publications and research conference presentations; however, to ensure change in clinical practice, findings need to filter through directly to the clinicians. Australian paramedics are now required to complete 30 hours of continuing professional development (CPD) each year as part of their ongoing registration as health professionals. To accommodate this requirement, professional bodies are offering CPD sessions to clinicians, as are most ambulance services. These sessions are an optimal way to disseminate research findings and changes in clinical practice to clinicians.

What must be remembered is the fact that the cycle of evidence-based practice is a continuous one. As one research question is answered, new questions will continue to develop. The process of evidence-based practice is ever developing to integrate new treatments or approaches to clinical care.

Strengths of evidence-based practice

Evidence-based practice has been used across different health settings and within different research contexts. Positive results have been seen regarding patient outcomes, staff satisfaction, higher quality healthcare and sustainable health service delivery (Melnyk et al., 2010). Utilising an evidence-based practice model facilitates the clinician to incorporate their own experience within decision-making processes, thus allowing for individualised treatment. The importance of evidence-based practice has been well proven in nursing, and it is perhaps even more important in paramedic settings where clinicians may not have large teams to consult with prior to providing treatment. Paramedics also attend to diverse members of the community at different stages of their lives. This may include patients in the later stages of life. The evidence-based practice model allows the paramedic to incorporate the patients' values and needs with equal emphasis as the research. This may prevent patients from receiving treatment they did not wish to receive or that is against their ethical or cultural beliefs.

Barriers and weaknesses of evidence-based practice

One major barrier to evidence-based medicine in emerging areas such as paramedicine is the general lack of current research in the area. This does make it difficult for researchers to confidently acquire and appraise relevant research. There may then be barriers to applying a finding in their own research, as without strong evidence health services or ethics boards may be hesitant to approve new or novel research approaches to clinical practice. Additionally, the current scope of practice for paramedics throughout the world and the very distinct differences between services, may make it difficult for research results to be generalisable across systems (Youngquist et al., 2010).

Some research has also reported hesitation to adopt an evidence-based practice approach, as clinicians feel that the strict process may negatively affect the autonomy of their practice (Watson et al., 2012). In these instances it is important to stress to clinicians the three distinct components to the evidence-based practice model and that the clinician experience is as important as the current research.

So what does this all mean for paramedics?

Over the years there has been a large transformation in the paramedic profession, from in-house unstructured training models to vocational training and now university degrees. Although clinical practice has also changed over this time, some of the practice guidelines may not have necessarily been led by evidence, although they may have been defensible and logical based on other health service areas. The profession of paramedicine does have its challenges. Research in this clinical setting is still in its infancy

and the transferability of research findings from other settings, which do not have the unpredictable environment that paramedics work in on a daily basis, may be questionable. However, as paramedics are often the first health professional to attend to patients, they are instrumental in starting the treatment plan for the patient and therefore require understanding of evidence-based practice, to ensure the best possible outcomes for the patients in their care (FitzGerald, 2015).

As research output directly related to paramedic practice increases in volume and quality, it will be easier for the profession to set its own evidence-based guidelines to determine optimal patient care in the out-of-hospital setting.

Case 1 conclusion

Although there is no research directly related to paramedics and this situation, there is some work looking at the effect of exercise on sleep. No work has completed the full framework of evidence-based practice so we are not yet at a stage where we can make a confident recommendation. Some of the research has suggested that physical activity may have a positive effect on sleep for shift workers but the research tends to be of low quality (Slanger et al., 2016). It is probably a good time to have an efficacy and effectiveness trial to help with the next stages of the evidence-based practice framework.

References

Alley, A. B., Seo, J.-W., & Hong, S.-T. (2015). Reporting results of research involving human subjects: an ethical obligation. *Journal of Korean Medical Science*, 30(6), 673–675.

FitzGerald, G. J. (2015). Paramedics and scope of practice. *The Medical Journal of Australia*, 203(6), 240–241.

Melnyk, B. M., Fineout-Overholt, E., Stillwell, S. B., & Williamson, K. M. (2010). Evidence-based practice: step by step: the seven steps of evidence-based practice. *The American Journal of Nursing*, 110(1), 51–53.

Sackett, D. L., Rosenberg, W. M., Gray, J. A., Haynes, R. B., & Richardson, W. S. (1996). *Evidence based medicine: what it is and what it isn't*. British Medical Journal Publishing Group.

Schardt, C., Adams, M. B., Owens, T., Keitz, S., & Fontelo, P. (2007). Utilization of the PICO framework to improve searching PubMed for clinical questions. *BMC Medical Informatics and Decision Making*, 7(1), 16.

Simpson, P. M., Bendall, J. C., Patterson, J., & Middleton, P. M. (2012). Beliefs and expectations of paramedics towards evidence-based practice and research. *International Journal of Evidence-Based Healthcare*, 10(3), 197–203.

Singal, A. G., Higgins, P. D., & Waljee, A. K. (2014). A primer on effectiveness and efficacy trials. *Clinical and Translational Gastroenterology*, 5(1), e45.

Slanger, T. E., Gross, J. V., Pinger, A., Morfeld, P., Bellinger, M., Duhme, A. L., Reichardt Ortega, R. A., Costa, G., Driscoll, T. R., Foster, R. G., Fritschi, L., Sallinen, M., Liira, J., & Erren, T. C. (2016). Person-directed, non-pharmacological interventions for sleepiness at work and sleep disturbances caused by shift work. *The Cochrane Database of Systematic Reviews*, (8), CD010641.

Watson, D. L. B., Burges Watson, D. L., Sanoff, R., Mackintosh, J. E., Saver, J. L., Ford, G. A., Price, C., Starkman, S., Eckstein, M., Conwit, R., Grace, A., & Murtagh, M. J. (2012). Evidence from the scene: paramedic perspectives on involvement in out-of-hospital research. *Annals of Emergency Medicine*, 60(5), 641–650.

Westfall, J. M., Mold, J., & Fagnan, L. (2007). Practice-based research—'Blue Highways' on the NIH roadmap. *JAMA*, 297(4), 403–406.

Woolf, S. H. (2008). The meaning of translational research and why it matters. *JAMA*, 299(2), 211–213.

Youngquist, S. T., Gausche-Hill, M., Squire, B. T., & Koenig, W. J. (2010). Barriers to adoption of evidence-based prehospital airway management practices in California. *Prehospital Emergency Care*, 14(4), 505–509.

CHAPTER 7

The Clinical Reasoning Process

By Paul Simpson and Liz Thyer

OVERVIEW

- Paramedics and other clinicians working in emergency medicine must be able to accurately assess a wide range of conditions using limited diagnostic tools, time and resources.
- The process of paramedic clinical decision-making has not been well researched.
- Traditional analytical models of clinical decision-making do not fully describe how expert clinicians solve clinical problems with more accuracy than novices.
- Expert clinicians are generally unaware of the cognitive processes that drive their decision-making (Geary & Kennedy, 2010).
- Two distinct models or systems of clinical reasoning exist: one is rapid, instinctive and unconscious; the other is slow, analytical and controlled.

- Neither the rapid/instinctive system nor the slow/analytical system is suited to every circumstance. Both have inherent errors and the most effective method is to recruit the strengths of each in reaching a clinical decision.
- Cognitive disposition to respond, emotion and human factors can all influence a clinician's ability to make informed unbiased decisions.
- Metacognition should enhance a paramedic's ability not only to progress towards expert reasoning but also to detect when errors occur and to maintain patient safety in the face of diagnostic uncertainty.

Introduction

In 2018, the Australian Healthcare Practitioner Regulation Authority (AHPRA) added the discipline of paramedicine to its list of nationally registered health professionals (Paramedicine Board of Australia, 2018). This development recognised the complexity of contemporary paramedic practice and illustrates how far paramedicine has moved away from its traditional roots as a transport service. If you were training to be a paramedic 30 years ago, you would most probably have undertaken a diploma course with a strong focus on management of trauma and transport of patients to hospital. All your patients would have gone to hospital, your scope of practice was comparatively narrow and the need to make complex clinical decisions was negated by a heavy reliance on step-by-step protocols.

Over the last decade, paramedic scope of practice has rapidly expanded as the role of paramedics in health systems has undergone dramatic transformation (Lord & Simpson, 2018). While paramedics traditionally functioned in an 'assess, treat, stabilise and transport' paradigm, they are now required to perform advanced patient examination and treatment with a view to determining a clinically appropriate disposition that is as likely to involve referral of the patient to an integrated community-based care pathway as it is transport to an emergency department (Williams et al., 2009).

This transformation in role and practice has led to a greater demand for enhanced clinical decision-making among paramedics (Lord & Simpson, 2018). Decision-making is underpinned by reasoning; in this context, clinical reasoning. This chapter aims to inform the novice (or experienced) paramedic how reasoning is performed, how decisions are made, how reasoning can be disrupted and how the impacts of these disruptions can potentially be mitigated.

How do paramedics make decisions?

How do paramedics make decisions? The truth currently is that we don't know. There is very little evidence describing how paramedics engage in clinical reasoning or critical thinking more broadly (Lord & Simpson, 2018). We do know that paramedics make their decisions in complicated, dynamic and unpredictable settings and that multiple operational, logistical, situational and cultural factors exert influence on the reasoning process (Simpson et al., 2017; O'Hara et al., 2015). This does not make paramedicine unique: all health disciplines have their own particular contexts and confounders to good reasoning, highlighted wonderfully in the medical context by Groopman in the well-known book entitled *How Doctors Think* (Groopman & Prichard, 2007). What it suggests is that an assumption that a 'one size fits all' approach to explaining how decisions are made 'on the road' or 'on the ward' would most likely be flawed. In the context of a lack of paramedicine-specific evidence, most of what is known about models of clinical reasoning arises from neighbouring disciplines, most notably emergency medicine. While the two are distinctly different, there are many commonalities between them that make emergency medicine the most appropriate discipline from which to extrapolate information (Lord & Simpson, 2018). While other medical and health disciplines have amassed substantial bodies of research exploring models of reasoning within their own practice, paramedicine as a discipline is yet to achieve this. It will be important for the discipline to gain a better understanding of how paramedics make decisions, as this will lead to improvement in patient safety and clinical quality (Croskerry, 2000, 2002).

Theoretical and conceptual foundations of clinical reasoning

Key to developing an effective clinical reasoning approach is a sound understanding of the theories and concepts that seek to explain how decisions are made (Croskerry, 2000). A novice paramedic without a theoretical and conceptual understanding may develop a flawed approach to reasoning that will increase risk of error and may compromise patient safety. Flawed reasoning may sit latent within a paramedic's practice, only to emerge and exert an effect when demands on the reasoning process increase, particularly when faced with complex situations. At this point, it must be emphasised that complexity in patient care may be found in any patient regardless of the perceived or actual acuity of presentation (Nagree et al., 2013). High-acuity cases can actually be low in complexity, and low-acuity cases high in complexity (see Box 7.1). The perceived acuity of a case has been reported in an Australian study to strongly impact on the decision-making process engaged in by paramedics under the belief that low-acuity presentations require low levels of reasoning (Simpson et al., 2017). The authors identified what they called 'low-acuity bias', a form of cognitive bias not previously discussed that may lead to flawed or erroneous decisions (see Box 7.1). Cognitive bias in clinical reasoning will be discussed in more detail later in this chapter, and the impact of 'low-acuity bias' is illustrated in the case at the start of the chapter.

> ## BOX 7.1 Key points regarding clinical reasoning in the context of paramedicine
>
> - There is always time to stop and think. A high-acuity emergency patient does not benefit from defaulting, consciously or unconsciously, to intuitive thinking as this may expose the patient, and you, to a higher risk of error.
> - When making decisions in high-acuity situations, remember that 'slow can be fast'. Taking a minute in the present to pause, check and confirm prior to acting might save 10 minutes in the future by actually increasing your efficiency and accuracy.
> - Low-acuity less-urgent cases require the same reasoning process as high-acuity cases. Be aware of 'low-acuity bias' that might promote intuitive, shortcut thinking and increase risk of error.

Dual-process theory—a framework for reasoning

The predominant theory attempting to explain how humans make decisions is dual-process theory (DPT) (Evans, 2003; Stanovich & West, 2000). The original work by psychologists on this theory was not specific to clinical settings, and its origins lie in non-clinical research. The use of DPT to explain clinical reasoning began to emerge in the late 1990s in the context of how doctors make decisions.

DPT states that decisions can be reached by either a fast, intuitive pathway or a slower, analytic pathway. In the simplest form, when faced with something familiar, we employ the fast, intuitive thinking pathway, or the 'System 1' pathway (Shaban, 2015). When faced with something unfamiliar, we employ the slower, analytic thinking pathway, or the 'System 2' pathway. To illustrate this, consider your experiences when you started learning to drive a car. In the initial period of learning, you had to think hard about each thing you had to do: activating the indicator to change lanes, while checking other traffic, while concentrating on what the driving instructor was telling you. Your actions were slow, cumbersome and methodical, consuming a huge amount of your cognitive capacity and concentration. You were primarily using your type 2 pathway, as the task was unfamiliar or unrecognised by your brain. Now, some years later,

CASE STUDY 1

Case 4321, 1600 hrs

Dispatch details: A 20-year-old female with ankle injury.

You are in your third month on the road as a graduate intern. Your normal partner is on sick leave and you are working with Tim, a paramedic of 15 years' experience who is starting leave at the end of the shift.

It is 1600 on a Saturday in June and you are attending your fourth sports-related injury of the day. You and Tim arrive at the sports complex and are directed to the sidelines of a local netball match where the team's trainer is treating a 20-year-old female who has twisted her ankle; the match has just finished. The patient says she is normally fit and healthy, but after colliding with another player and falling to the ground, there is deformation of her right ankle and it hurts to weight-bear. Tim briefly assesses the patient noting HR 120, BP 120/80 mmHg, RR 20. He advises her to keep it elevated and if she wants to, get a friend to take her to a clinic; he then starts to pack up the gear.

You have noticed that the patient did not feel you touching the sole of her foot while Tim was talking to her, you couldn't find a pedal pulse and her foot felt a lot colder compared to the other foot, even though they hadn't used ice. You want to bring this up with Tim, but he is already walking towards the ambulance, mumbling about people wasting the paramedics' time.

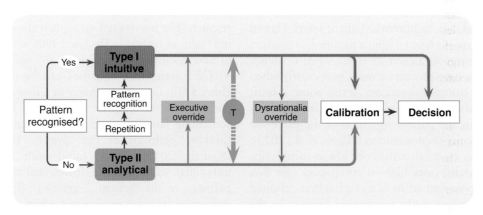

Figure 7.1
Type 1 and 2 systems within the dual-process theory of decision-making. T = toggle.
Source: Stiegler & Tung (2014).

you perform all the same functions with seemingly minimal concentration or effort. Your decisions to change lanes, or to accelerate or slow down when a traffic light turns amber, happen quickly without deliberation or delay. Figure 7.1 illustrates DPT in the context of clinical decision-making, including how repeated exposure to a situation (or a clinical situation) can lead to a switch in processing pathway over time. The green 'T' refers to 'toggling' back and forth between systems, as it is not 'one or the other' process. In the process of a task, depending on a range of variables, our mind might 'toggle' consciously or unconsciously from one system to the other as the reasoning process unfolds (Croskerry et al., 2013a).

In the context of clinical reasoning, the same dual pathway of thinking is in operation. A novice or 'early career' paramedic will have much the same experience as when they learned to drive. The gathering of data through patient assessment and the subsequent analysis and interpretation will be slow and methodical and consume a large amount of cognitive capacity: it will be a predominantly System 2 meditated process. Most of the patients and presentations encountered early on will not be familiar and won't represent a recognised 'pattern' of patient presentation. The more experienced paramedic, faced with the same situation and assuming they have seen similar presentations previously, will tend to arrive at a decision more quickly having utilised reasoning processes dominated by the System 1 pathway. This suggests that 'recognition' or 'familiarity' is important in determining which processing pathway dominates and assumes that these would come with 'experience' given that the experienced paramedic is more likely to have seen the same or similar presentations many times before. The general properties of System 1 and System 2 pathways within DPT are illustrated in Table 7.1.

As can be seen when comparing properties of the two systems, each has strengths and weaknesses. System 1 is fast, economical, efficient, and because it consumes less cognitive effort, facilitates greater capacity to perform multiple tasks simultaneously. It is however more susceptible to error, is less reliable and is associated with low scientific rigour. System 1 involves the use of 'heuristics', or thinking 'short cuts' (Gigerenzer & Gaissmaier, 2011). As we will discuss later in the chapter, another weakness of System 1 is that it is quite susceptible to compromise by a paramedic's emotions, beliefs and behaviour. On the other hand, System 2 has high reliability, results in fewer errors and has high scientific rigour. It is less susceptible to emotional compromise, but demands much higher cognitive effort therefore decreasing overall efficiency by limiting ability to perform concurrent tasks. System 1 is the 'natural state' for our minds and is where we spend most of our time under normal circumstances (Evans, 2003).

A key point to remember is that your mind has a preference for System 1 thinking because it consumes less cognitive effort, even though it may result in a lower level of accuracy. This has been labelled the 'accuracy-effort trade-off' (Gigerenzer

Table 7.1: General properties of System 1 and System 2 pathways in dual-processing theory

Property	System 1: Intuitive	System 2: Analytical
Reasoning style	Heuristic Associative Concrete	Normative Deductive Abstract
Awareness	Low	High
Prototypical	Yes	No, based on sets
Action	Reflexive, skilled	Deliberate, rule based
Automaticity	High	Low
Speed	Fast	Slow
Channels	Multiple, parallel	Single, linear
Propensities	Causal	Statistical
Effort	Minimal	Considerable
Cost	Low	High
Vulnerability to bias	Yes	Less so
Reliability	Low, variable	High, consistent
Errors	Common	Few
Affective valence	Often	Rarely
Predictive power	Low	High
Hard-wired	May be	No
Scientific rigour	Low	High
Context importance	High	Low

Source: Croskerry (2009).

& Gaissmaier, 2011; Shah & Oppenheimer, 2008). As mentioned earlier, heuristics are the 'shortcuts, rules of thumb, maxims, or any strategy that achieves abbreviation and avoids the laborious working through of all known options in the course of problem-solving' (Croskerry, 2000, p. 1226). Heuristic thinking is the default position for our brain, making it easy to slip into this type of thinking without being aware of it. The unrecognised use of heuristics in a context-demanding System 2 analysis can increase the risk of flawed reasoning and subsequent error.

On first thought, System 1 could be perceived as being 'bad' and that clinical reasoning should be consciously channelled through System 2 pathways of thinking. This is certainly not the case; in fact, System 1 is critically important and appears to play a pivotal role in what has been called the 'flesh and blood' reasoning engaged in by physicians in the emergency department setting (Croskerry, 2000; Sandhu et al., 2006). Not all clinical decisions require System 2 thinking, and one's cognitive capacity would be easily overwhelmed if System 2 was required for each. Paramedic clinical practice occurs in a 'decision-dense' environment: within the course of a single patient encounter, paramedics make a myriad of decisions in a short time, often based on incomplete or limited information and frequently in a resource-poor context (Jensen et al., 2011). There are small decisions that won't require much reasoning at all (e.g. at what point in the flow of the case should a blood pressure be performed or which route of administration is most appropriate to administer a required medication). Conversely, there are other larger decisions that demand a System 2-dominated reasoning approach (e.g. formulating a clinical impression upon which to initiate patient care, when determining how best to extricate a patient from a difficult location, or when determining whether non-transport and referral is appropriate following assessment and/or treatment). The great difficulty for clinicians is to find the balance between System 1 and System 2 in a given situation. This requires you to develop a 'real-time' awareness as to which system you are operating, and the ability to consciously 'override' a system if the context requires it (refer Box 7.1). This is extremely difficult to do, and it doesn't happen by accident, but it represents an advanced end point that early-career and experienced paramedics should aim to achieve.

Approaches to decision-making 'on the ground'

Earlier in the chapter, we discussed the 'neat and tidy' concept of DPT, but this does not always play out in such clear definition in practice. Therefore, it can be helpful to conceptualise System 1 and System 2 thinking (or intuitive and analytical thinking, respectively) as existing at either ends of a continuum of reasoning, rather than as a one-or-the-other structure. Along this continuum, there are various decision-making approaches that have elements of analytical and intuitive thinking, but none represents the exclusive use of System 1 or 2 thinking. Each approach has shortcomings and advantages, so none is preferred to the other, but should be selected for optimal use based on a given situation and various converging factors.

Table 7.2 details several common approaches to decision-making identified by psychologists in research exploring how doctors make decisions in emergency departments; these have been referred to as 'flesh and blood' decision-making processes (Sandhu et al., 2006).

Factors affecting the clinical reasoning process

Clinical reasoning by paramedics or any other health professional does not happen in a vacuum: it cannot therefore be isolated from the context in which it occurs. As important as it is to know the underpinning theory of how your mind functions, it is as important to be aware of, and understand, how you mind dysfunctions (Croskerry, 2000). In short, a paramedic at any point on the continuum from novice to expert must develop metacognition: the ability to 'think about how you think' (Flavell, 1979; Croskerry, 2000). Being metacognitive means that you are developing a reflective capacity in which you are thinking not only about how your mind works, but also of the tricks your brain may play on you, the pitfalls that exist in reasoning processes, and the situations and contexts in which these are most likely to exert an effect (Croskerry et al., 2013a). Being aware of how your mind is working as it is working (e.g. being aware of whether you are engaging in intuitive or analytical reasoning) will allow you to engage in more efficient clinical reasoning resulting in safer clinical decisions (Schull et al., 2001; Croskerry, 2003; Sandhu et al., 2006). While the factors that may muddy the waters of the clinical reasoning process are many, we'll focus on a select few that will be of most relevance to the novice or early-career paramedic: cognitive bias, affective bias, cognitive load and human factors.

Cognitive bias or 'cognitive dispositions to respond'

Cognitive bias refers to failed heuristic thinking, or System 1 thinking, that when unchecked has failed and is strongly associated with faulty reasoning

Table 7.2: 'Flesh and blood' approaches to decision-making in emergency medicine

Cognitive strategy	Key features	Key shortcomings	Key advantages
Hypotheticodeductive	Inference based on preliminary findings Idea modification based on subsequent findings, response to therapy and exclusion of competing possibilities	Faulty hypothesis can precipitate dangerous actions Premature closure can result in erroneous conclusions Heterogenous pathway and conclusions: difficult to teach	Flexible
Algorithmic	Preset diagnostic or therapeutic pathway based on preestablished criteria	Inflexible Removes independent thinking	Pre-physician initiation Standardised case Easy to teach
Pattern recognition	Combination of salient features establish likely diagnosis with corresponding evaluation, management and disposition plan	Anchoring bias Confirmation bias	Rapid assessment and clinical plan
Rule out worst-case scenario	Consideration of preexisting mental list of 'cannot miss' diagnoses for a given presenting complaint	Incomplete differential diagnosis list missing less common disease entities Overtesting Anecdotal practice Value-induced bias	Increased probability of considering/recognising presentations of critical illness
Exhaustive	Accumulate facts indiscriminately and then sift through them for the diagnosis	Excessive resource use Time consumption	Thorough evaluations
Event driven	Treat symptoms and then re-evaluate with further evaluation, depending on response to therapy	Dangerous actions possible if faulty hypotheses Potentially inefficient	Flexible Accommodates ED environment

Source: Sandhu et al. (2006).

and clinical error. More recently, cognitive bias as a term has been rephrased to avoid the negative connotations associated with the term 'bias': they are now known as 'cognitive dispositions to respond' (CDR). CDRs are predictable heuristic decisions that paramedics (or any healthcare worker) fall victim to in particular situations under particular circumstances. In simple terms, you could consider them 'mind tricks': tricks our mind plays on us without us generally realising it has done so. While as many as 50 specific CDRs have been identified in the medical literature (Croskerry, 2003), we'll limit our discussion here to several of the most common that are applicable to paramedic practice.

'Anchoring' and 'confirmation bias' are among the most prevalent CDRs and they frequently occur together. Anchoring bias occurs when the paramedic 'locks' onto salient features of a case early on, but fails to adjust their clinical impression when other information later becomes known. An example could be when you are called to a person with breathing difficulties, and the dispatch information includes that the patient has a history of asthma. After

arriving at the case, the paramedic may inadvertently 'anchor' on the asthma information, and ignore signs or symptoms suggesting an alternative respiratory problem. Anchoring is illustrated in Case study 2 at the end of the chapter, where the paramedics maintain a diagnosis of drug overdose despite signs and symptoms indicating otherwise. Anchoring can lead to another CDR called 'premature diagnostic closure', in which the provisional diagnosis is finalised too early without due investigation or consideration of other possible diagnoses. This if often compounded by 'overconfidence bias', or the 'universal tendency to think we know more than we know' and therefore rely on intuition or hunches rather than objective information arising from a comprehensive assessment (Croskerry, 2003). Linked to this, 'confirmation bias' occurs when the paramedic selectively looks for signs and symptoms to support their initial clinical impression rather than challenge it.

With the increasing volume of patient presentations arising from mental illness, it is worth mentioning that such cases are high-risk for CDR. 'Psyche-out error' is a bias occurring frequently in the context of mental health patients, in which the patient's mental illness dominates the encounter and alters the paramedic's perception of the legitimacy or seriousness of the patient's complaint. 'Diagnostic overshadowing' occurs when the physical complaint of a patient with mental illness is incorrectly attributed to their mental illness rather than a true underlying pathology (Shefer et al., 2014; Jones et al., 2008). It is not necessary to be aware of all CDRs identified in the literature; however, extensive lists and explanations of the plethora of CDRs can be found in the detailed works of Croskerry (Croskerry, 2002, 2003).

Affective bias or 'affective dispositions to respond' (ADR)

While the awareness of CDR has increased markedly in the past 20 years, the powerful effect of emotion, or affect, has received less attention. There is strong evidence that the emotional state of the paramedic profoundly influences the clinical reasoning process, and if we cast our mind back to Figure 7.1 illustrating DPT, we see that it is on System 1 that this phenomenon, known as the 'affect heuristic', will most likely augment or compromise reasoning (Croskerry, 2007; Slovic et al., 2002). It is therefore vital for paramedics to develop an approach to clinical reasoning and decision-making that includes an ability to recognise their emotional state and regulate it in real time. This may sound easy, but emotional regulation at the point of care, while providing care, is difficult and requires a high level of self-awareness.

Clinicians and healthcare providers frequently encounter patients or situations that trigger overt or subtle emotional responses within themselves, leading to biased reasoning. In a clinical sense this was first recognised in 1978, when Groves published a seminal article 'Taking care of the hateful patient' in which the challenge of controlling one's emotions when dealing with various types of patients was first discussed (Groves, 1978). More recently, Croskerry identified three key areas of emotional influence on clinical reasoning: ambient, clinical and endogenous (Box 7.2).

Ambient influences may include workplace issues or frustrations, organisational or operational issues, interpersonal conflicts at home or work, stress,

fatigue due to long shifts or shift work, or any other variable that temporarily impacts mood and emotions. Recent Australian research by Simpson and colleagues investigating decision-making by paramedics when caring for older people who had fallen found that 'organisational confidence' and 'cultural norms' were powerful influencers of emotion, and that these emotions led to changes in reasoning that undermined System 2 thinking and promoted 'affect heuristics' (Simpson et al., 2017). Similarly, O'Hara and colleagues reported 'systems' factors within the workplace to exert profound influence on paramedics working within a British ambulance service (O'Hara et al., 2015).

Endogenous factors include clinically significant mental health or resilience issues within the paramedic such as anxiety or mood disorders, posttraumatic stress disorder (PTSD), depression, or other states of emotional dysregulation (Croskerry, 2007).

Of particular relevance to newer paramedic practitioners are the 'clinical situation induced' influences, or situational influences, where specific features of a patient or clinical task create bias that compromises reasoning. The most discussed of these influences is a phenomenon called 'counter-transference', the development of positive or negative feelings towards a patient (or situation) or patient group that impact on reasoning without the clinician being aware (Park et al., 2014; Croskerry, 2007; Croskerry et al., 2008). These feelings could be based on previous exposure to an individual patient or patient population that evokes emotions within the paramedic, and may result in labelling or categorisation of patients ('frequent flyers', 'drug seekers', 'psyches', 'fallers'). Subsequent patients are then categorised or labelled based on past experience, leading to biased reasoning towards the current patient and greater risk of misdiagnosis or error (Park et al., 2014; Simpson et al., 2017; Croskerry et al., 2010). Case study 2 at the end of this chapter illustrates how this can occur in practice.

Human factors

'Human factors' refers to an area of applied science with origins in the civil aviation industry that investigates the interplay between humans, machines and their work environments (Wachter, 2012). The contemporary paradigm of patient safety acknowledges that human factors play a substantial role in error in clinical settings, with systems errors relating to human factors commonly identified during analyses of patient safety incidents (Bleetman et al., 2012). While a detailed discussion of the science of human factors is beyond the scope of this chapter, a brief overview of human factors and their relationship to clinical reasoning is essential. Human factors can serve to compromise the clinical reasoning process in paramedic practice (Keebler et al., 2017). Based on data derived from aircraft maintenance studies, Gordon Dupont put forward the 12 most common human factors affecting people in their workplace that contribute to mistakes being made (Dupont, 1997). These have become known as 'Dupont's Dirty Dozen' (Table 7.3), and while their origins are not clinical, their application to human factors education in clinical settings is widespread (Marquardt et al., 2015).

Many of the factors listed above are relevant to the paramedic context. Think about an average day at work or on a recent practicum or supervised shift: how many of these factors might have been present at one time across the duration of the shift, potentially impacting negatively on your reasoning? While many of these are well known and are frequently referred to, 'lack of assertiveness' and 'norms' are less commonly discussed. These two factors have strong ties

to workplace culture, and have been identified as being powerful influences on paramedic decision-making (Simpson et al., 2017): they can lead to erroneous thinking dominated by heuristics, prone to cognitive and affective bias, and unchallenged by team members. They may also disproportionately impact on the novice practitioner or those new to an organisation who for a variety of reasons feel less empowered to be assertive or less willing to challenge organisational culture. Case study 1 at the beginning of the chapter illustrates how a lack of assertiveness can affect decision-making, in that instance compounded by a lack of communication and a strong element of complacency.

Decision density and cognitive load

'Cognitive load' refers to the amount of processing your mind is capable of dealing with effectively at any one time. Cognitive load theory (CLT) was proposed in the 1980s, when psychology research identified that we have a limited capacity for cognitive processing of sensory inputs (van Merriënboer & Sweller, 2010). CLT builds on Miller's seminal work that our minds can only manage 'seven plus or minus two' elements at once and can only actively process between two and four of these elements concurrently (Sweller, 1988; Miller, 1956). Once processed, information lasts for only 20 seconds unless there is reinforcement of that information in the short term; this is particularly the case when the cognitive activities involve unfamiliar or new information. Given the limited resources available to a paramedic crew in relation to the number of actions they need to perform in a relatively short, often pressured timeframe, a state of 'cognitive overload' may often be reached (Burgess, 2010). The result can be an unconscious shift to System 1 thinking as a strategy to keep up with sensory demand and processing needs.

Strategies to enhance quality of clinical reasoning

While not definitive, there is some evidence describing strategies that may help to optimise clinical reasoning (Croskerry, 2002). Embedding these approaches into your early-career practice may help develop a more robust model of reasoning that will have greater chance of withstanding the many challenges to effective reasoning that you will face.

- *Accept that you are susceptible to flawed reasoning.* Probably the most important initial strategy is to accept that you are susceptible to flawed reasoning, regardless of how good you believe yourself to be. The paramedic who is open to the fact that their reasoning can be flawed will

Table 7.3: The 'Dirty Dozen' of human factors contributing to error

Lack of communication	Lack of teamwork	Lack of resources	Stress
Lack of knowledge	Distraction	Pressure	Lack of awareness
Complacency	Fatigue	Lack of assertiveness	Norms

Source: Adapted from Dupont (1997).

Table 7.4: High-risk situations for cognitive and affective bias

High-risk situation	Potential biases
1. Was this patient handed off to me from a previous shift?	Diagnosis momentum, framing
2. Was the diagnosis suggested to me by the patient, nurse or another physician?	Premature closure, framing bias
3. Did I just accept the first diagnosis that came to mind?	Anchoring, availability, search satisficing, premature closure
4. Did I consider other organ systems besides the obvious one?	Anchoring, search satisficing, premature closure
5. Is this a patient I don't like, or like too much, for some reason?	Affective bias
6. Have I been interrupted or distracted while evaluation this patient?	All biases
7. Am I feeling fatigued right now?	All biases
8. Did I sleep poorly last night?	All biases
9. Am I cognitively overloaded or overextended right now?	All biases
10. Am I stereotyping this patient?	Representative bias, affective bias, anchoring, fundamental attribution error, psych out error
11. Have I effectively ruled out must-not-miss diagnoses?	Overconfidence, anchoring, confirmation bias

Note: A description of specific biases can be found in Croskerry.
Source: Adapted from Graber et al. (2012).

more likely be able to successfully implement approaches to adapt and overcome.

- *Develop metacognitive practice.* Start thinking about how you think. Studying this chapter has been a first step in developing metacognition, so continue to learn more about how reasoning occurs. Importantly, learn more about how your own mind works, and what cognitive or affective strengths and weaknesses you bring to the patient encounter.
- *Recognise and detect CDR and ADR.* Increasing your awareness of CDR and ADR is critical. Importantly, increase your awareness of 'high-risk situations' in which you might be most susceptible to bias. Table 7.4 provides an excellent overview of commonly encountered 'high-risk' situations for bias (Croskerry et al., 2013b). Recognition and detection should occur ideally before and during the patient encounter, allowing for real-time mitigation and self-regulation. A useful quick self-assessment to gauge your emotional temperature leading into a patient encounter can be framed around the mnemonic **HALT** (i.e. are you Hungry, Angry, Late or Tired?), these being factors may cause emotional dysregulation during the case (Adams & Murray, 1998).
- *Implement cognitive forcing strategies.* A forcing strategy is a conscious 'metacognitive step' built into a paramedic's practice that forces the paramedic to consider alternatives and/or conduct a self-check (Croskerry et al., 2013b;

Graber et al., 2012; Ely et al., 2011). A simple cognitive forcing strategy easily applied to paramedic contexts is the 'clinical pause'. At or around the same time point in each case, after forming a provisional diagnosis but before you act and treat, embed a conscious 'pause' in your routine. During this stop, 'force' yourself to think about the reasoning process you have engaged in and the presence of any influences or biases that could be impacting your process. A cognitive check can also be embedded in your preparatory routine on your way to a case. After considering the dispatch details, develop a habit of conducting a 'risk of bias' using the information available to you from the call and a quick self-check of your own emotional state. This may then increase your awareness of potential biases as you commence the case, bookended by a time-out later on.

- *Reduce cognitive load.* If working with a partner, actively reduce your cognitive load by off-loading manual tasks and activities to your partner. This may free up your processing capacity and enhance your capacity for clearer reasoning and System 2 thinking. Look to distribute responsibilities among your team members should there be others around.
- *Embrace cognitive aids and decision-assistance rules.* Decision rules are becoming more common in clinical practice, and there is good evidence to support their superiority over human reasoning

(Bandiera et al., 2003; Grove & Meehl, 1996; McGinn et al., 2008). An increasingly common example would be the adoption of spinal clearance rules such as the Canadian C-Spine or NEXUS by ambulance services rather than relying on paramedic judgment alone (Hoffman et al., 1992; Stiell et al., 2001; Vaillancourt et al., 2009). Cognitive aids such as the humble checklist also act to reduce reliance on memory and reduce your overall cognitive load (Ely et al., 2011).

A step-by-step guide to clinical decision-making

In order to structure the clinical reasoning process, we use the four-step model of assess, confirm, treat and evaluate (see Fig 7.2).

① ### Step 1: Assess

Chapter 4 described using a standardised assessment process to reduce the cognitive workload in the high-stimulus environments in which paramedics find themselves working. This is equally important for novices and experts. Regardless of whether you have well-formed 'illness scripts' or not, you will inevitably find yourself creating hypotheses about the cause of a patient's condition during the assessment process. These judgments may occur before you even meet the patient, based on dispatch details, the patient's age, their appearance or the way they meet you at the door. Using all this information to create possible causes for a patient's presentation is advisable but be sure not to 'anchor' on these initial impressions. Regardless of your evolving impression of the patient or the case, always finish the assessment

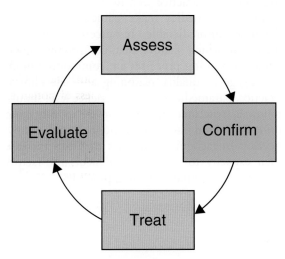

Figure 7.2
The clinical reasoning model.
Source: Johnson, M. et al. (2015). Paramedic principles and practice ANZ. A clinical reasoning approach. Sydney: Elsevier.

process. Never make a decision based on incomplete information; this would result in premature diagnostic closure, a very common form of cognitive bias. A decision can only be as good as the information used to make it: poor assessment results in poor information and subsequently a flawed reasoning process.

② ### Step 2: Confirm

Following a thorough assessment and determination of a provisional diagnosis, you must work to confirm your suspicion by considering a short-list of differential diagnoses and eliminating these where safe to do so. It is as important to rule out what it can't be as to rule in what it could be. For every case presented in this text, we suggest alternatives or 'differentials' for each presentation. In cases where the omission of a particular differential diagnosis could endanger the patient, we include a 'red flag' as a warning. Most of the differential diagnoses offered should be able to be eliminated quickly, but a few may require you to return to the assessment stage and conduct further assessment. This 'backward step' should be considered a success, not a failing of your reasoning process.

A vital action at this time, before determining and then implementing a treatment plan, is to enact a 'clinical pause' (Croskerry et al., 2013b). The momentum of a case, particularly in a higher-acuity context, can lead to a tendency to rush forward without considering all aspects of the case. This clinical pause represents a 'cognitive check', or a review of the reasoning process that has led you to your provisional diagnosis.

A final key process in confirming your decision is to consult when possible. Consultation takes many forms, but most commonly will involve your shift partner. In most ambulance service models, paramedics function as a two-person team. It would be uncommon for an early-career paramedic in Australasia to practise without a qualified partner and discussing your decision with them does not convey uncertainty or indecisiveness, but rather a high level of self-awareness and commitment to patient safety. This is not only relevant to early-career paramedics; practitioners at any level will often have opportunities to consult with a partner or another health professional who may be present, regardless of self-perception of expertise and experience. In simple terms, 'two heads are better than one', and the likelihood of safe practice will increase with twice the cognitive power.

③ ### Step 3: Treat

Clinical decision-making must extend into the treatment phase (remember, treatment doesn't necessarily

CASE STUDY 2

Case 1205, 0120 hrs.

Dispatch details: An 18-year-old female patient classified by dispatch as a 'drug overdose'.

Initial presentation: You are called to assess an 18-year-old female patient at a dance party. The case is classified by the dispatch system as 'drug overdose'. You are escorted to her by the security guards, who tell you that seven people have been transported to hospital from the event so far, all due to drug overdoses. The 18-year-old appears sweaty and in an altered conscious state and her breath smells of alcohol.

mean treating with medications or procedures; it can include transport, advice or referral). You need to determine whether the treatment is safe and acceptable to the patient, and whether benefits from treatment outweigh the risks of not providing a treatment.

 Step 4: Evaluate

Although the effectiveness of medical treatments can vary, most conditions will respond to appropriate treatment. How a patient responds to your treatment plan is invaluable information about the accuracy of your initial assessment and the results should feed back into the decision-making loop (Geary & Kennedy, 2010). When a patient fails to respond to treatment, it might indicate that your initial assessment was incorrect: take this new information and reassess your patient and your decision-making. This text should provide you with a guide as to how responsive each condition is to correct treatment.

Anchoring bias occurs when the paramedics use external information, in this case the information about the drugs from the security guards, to presume a diagnosis without assessing all the information from the patient. Irrespective of what new information becomes available the paramedic with an anchoring bias will not change their initial position, leading to **premature diagnostic closure**.

Fundamental attribution error is when the patient is considered to be at least partly responsible for their presentation. In this case, the 18-year-old may have taken drugs at the dance party and this may affect the way the paramedics assess or treat her.

Having completed the chapter, let's revisit Case study 1.

Summary

Modern paramedic practice demands a high level of clinical reasoning commensurate to the expanding models of practice seen in Australasian health services. Paramedics make clinical decisions in dynamic, unpredictable, resource-poor environments in which factors that compromise good clinical reasoning processes are commonly found. To engage in quality reasoning and safe clinical practice, paramedics of any experience level should follow a structured approach to decision-making using theoretical frameworks, and most importantly, develop metacognitive abilities that will increase their capacity to recognise and neutralise factors that threaten sound reasoning processes.

CASE STUDY 1 REVISITED

Case 4321, 1600 hrs

You are in your third month on the road as a graduate intern. Your normal partner is on sick leave and you are working with Tim, a paramedic of 15 years' experience who is starting leave at the end of the shift.

It is 1600 on a Saturday in June and you are attending your fourth sports-related injury of the day. As you and Tim arrive at the sports complex, he complains about 'another sporting job' and suggests that you assess the patient as he is feeling tired and wants to start holidays. You are directed to the sidelines of a local netball match where the team's trainer is treating a 20-year-old female who has twisted her ankle; the match has just finished.

You start a systematic assessment of the patient who says she is normally fit and healthy, but after colliding with another player and falling to the ground, there is deformation of her right ankle and it hurts to weight-bear. The patient is fully conscious, with HR 120, BP 120/80 mmHg and RR 20. She has no other injuries apart from swelling to the right ankle. You notice that you cannot locate a pedal pulse and the foot appears very cold; there also appears to be decreased sensation. You ask Tim to assess the foot and he confirms this identifying that this is a more serious injury than expected.

You and Tim take a moment to discuss the presentation and determine a course of action. You outline to Tim your thoughts on clinical management and map out a treatment plan, to which he agrees. You then advise the patient that she should attend hospital with you and she agrees.

1. What was done differently in this case compared to the case at the start of the chapter?

2. What potential influences on clinical reasoning were present, and how did the paramedic team work to mitigate them?

References

Adams, J., & Murray, R., III. (1998). The general approach to the difficult patient. *Emergency Medicine Clinics of North America, 16*, 689–700.

Bandiera, G., Stiell, I. G., Wells, G. A., Clement, C., De Maio, V., Vandemheen, K. L., Greenberg, G. H., Lesiuk, H., Brison, R., & Cass, D. (2003). The Canadian C-spine rule performs better than unstructured physician judgment. *Annals of Emergency Medicine, 42*, 395–402.

Bleetman, A., Sanusi, S., Dale, T., & Brace, S. (2012). Human factors and error prevention in emergency medicine. *Emergency Medicine Journal, 29*, 389–393.

Burgess, D. J. (2010). Are providers more likely to contribute to healthcare disparities under high levels of cognitive load? How features of the healthcare setting may lead to biases in medical decision making. *Medical Decision Making, 30*, 246–257.

Croskerry, P. (2000). The cognitive imperative thinking about how we think. *Academic Emergency Medicine: Official Journal of the Society for Academic Emergency Medicine, 7*, 1223–1231.

Croskerry, P. (2002). Achieving quality in clinical decision making: cognitive strategies and detection of bias. *Academic Emergency Medicine: Official Journal of the Society for Academic Emergency Medicine, 9*, 1184–1204.

Croskerry, P. (2003). The importance of cognitive errors in diagnosis and strategies to minimize them. *Academic Medicine: Journal of the Association of American Medical Colleges, 78*, 775–780.

Croskerry, P. (2007). Commentary: the affective imperative: coming to terms with our emotions. *Academic Emergency Medicine: Official Journal of the Society for Academic Emergency Medicine, 14*, 184–186.

Croskerry, P. (2009). Context is everything or how could I have been that stupid. *Healthcare Quarterly, 12,* e171–e176.

Croskerry, P., Abbass, A., & Wu, A. W. (2010). Emotional influences in patient safety. *Journal of Patient Safety, 6,* 199–205.

Croskerry, P., Abbass, A. A., & Wu, A. W. (2008). How doctors feel: affective issues in patients' safety. *The Lancet, 372,* 1205–1206.

Croskerry, P., Singhal, G., & Mamede, S. (2013a). Cognitive debiasing 1: origins of bias and theory of debiasing. *BMJ Quality & Safety,* bmjqs-2012-001712.

Croskerry, P., Singhal, G., & Mamede, S. (2013b). Cognitive debiasing 2: impediments to and strategies for change. *BMJ Quality & Safety, 22,* ii65–ii72.

Dupont, G. (1997). *The Dirty Dozen Errors in Maintenance.* Human Error in Aviation Maintenance. Federal Aviation Administration.

Ely, J. W., Graber, M. L., & Croskerry, P. (2011). Checklists to reduce diagnostic errors. *Academic Medicine: Journal of the Association of American Medical Colleges, 86,* 307–313.

Evans, J. S. B. (2003). In two minds: dual-process accounts of reasoning. *Trends in Cognitive Sciences, 7,* 454–459.

Flavell, J. H. (1979). Metacognition and cognitive monitoring: a new area of cognitive–developmental inquiry. *American Psychologist, 34,* 906.

Geary, U., & Kennedy, U. (2010). Clinical decision-making in emergency medicine. *Emergencias, 22,* 56–60.

Gigerenzer, G., & Gaissmaier, W. (2011). Heuristic decision making. *Annual Review of Psychology, 62,* 451–482.

Graber, M. L., Kissam, S., Payne, V. L., Meyer, A. N., Sorensen, A., Lenfestey, N., Tant, E., Henriksen, K., Labresh, K., & Singh, H. (2012). Cognitive interventions to reduce diagnostic error: a narrative review. *BMJ Quality & Safety,* bmjqs-2011-000149.

Groopman, J. E., & Prichard, M. (2007). *How doctors Think.* Boston: Houghton Mifflin.

Grove, W. M., & Meehl, P. E. (1996). Comparative efficiency of informal (subjective, impressionistic) and formal (mechanical, algorithmic) prediction procedures: the clinical–statistical controversy. *Psychology, Public Policy, and Law, 2,* 293.

Groves, J. (1978). Taking care of the hateful patient. *The New England Journal of Medicine, 298,* 883–887.

Hoffman, J. R., Schriger, D. L., Mower, W., Luo, J. S., & Zucker, M. (1992). Low-risk criteria for cervical-spine radiography in blunt trauma: a prospective study. *Annals of Emergency Medicine, 21,* 1454–1460.

Jensen, J. L., Croskerry, P., & Travers, A. H. (2011). Consensus on paramedic clinical decisions during high-acuity emergency calls: results of a Canadian Delphi study. *CJEM, 13,* 310–318.

Jones, S., Howard, L., & Thornicroft, G. (2008). 'Diagnostic overshadowing': worse physical health care for people with mental illness. *Acta Psychiatrica Scandinavica, 118,* 169–171.

Keebler, J. R., Lazzara, E. H., & Misasi, P. (2017). *Human factors and ergonomics of prehospital emergency care.* CRC Press.

Lord, B., & Simpson, P. (2018). Clinical reasoning in paramedicine. In J. Higgs, G. Jensen, S. Loftus & N. Christensen (Eds.), *Clinical reasoning in the health professions* (4th ed.). London, United Kingdom: Elsevier.

Marquardt, N., Treffenstadt, C., Gerstmeyer, K., & Gades-Buettrich, R. (2015). Mental workload and cognitive performance in operating rooms. *International Journal of Psychology Research, 10,* 209.

McGinn, T., Jervis, R., Wisnivesky, J., Keitz, S., & Wyer, P. C., GROUP, E.-B. M. T. T. W. (2008). Tips for teachers of evidence-based medicine: clinical prediction rules (CPRs) and estimating pretest probability. *Journal of General Internal Medicine, 23,* 1261–1268.

Miller, G. A. (1956). The magical number seven, plus or minus two: some limits on our capacity for processing information. *Psychological Review, 63,* 81.

Nagree, Y., Camarda, V. J., Fatovich, D. M., Cameron, P. A., Dey, I., Gosbell, A. D., McCarthy, S. M., & Mountain, D. (2013). Quantifying the proportion of general practice and low-acuity patients in the emergency department. *The Medical Journal of Australia, 198,* 612–615.

O'Hara, R., Johnson, M., Siriwardena, A. N., Weyman, A., Turner, J., Shaw, D., Mortimer, P., Newman, C., Hirst, E., & Storey, M. (2015). A qualitative study of systemic influences on paramedic decision making: care transitions and patient safety. *Journal of Health Services Research & Policy, 20,* 45–53.

Paramedicine Board of Australia. (2018). Retrieved from: https://www.paramedicineboard.gov.au/About.aspx.

Park, D. B., Berkwitt, A. K., Tuuri, R. E., & Russell, W. S. (2014). The hateful physician: the role of affect bias in the care of the psychiatric patient in the ED. *The American Journal of Emergency Medicine, 32,* 483–485.

Sandhu, H., Carpenter, C., Freeman, K., Nabors, S. G., & Olson, A. (2006). Clinical decisionmaking: opening the black box of cognitive reasoning. *Annals of Emergency Medicine, 48,* 713–719.

Schull, M. J., Ferris, L. E., Tu, J. V., Hux, J. E., & Redelmeier, D. A. (2001). Problems for clinical judgement: 3. Thinking clearly in an emergency. *CMAJ: Canadian Medical Association Journal = Journal de l'Association Medicale Canadienne, 164,* 1170–1175.

Shaban, R. (2015). Theories of clinical judgment and decision-making: a review of the theoretical literature. *Australasian Journal of Paramedicine, 3.*

Shah, A. K., & Oppenheimer, D. M. (2008). Heuristics made easy: an effort-reduction framework. *Psychological Bulletin, 134,* 207.

Shefer, G., Henderson, C., Howard, L. M., Murray, J., & Thornicroft, G. (2014). Diagnostic overshadowing and other challenges involved in the diagnostic process of patients with mental illness who present in emergency departments with physical symptoms–a qualitative study. *PLoS ONE, 9,* e111682.

Simpson, P., Thomas, R., Bendall, J., Lord, B., Lord, S., & Close, J. (2017). 'Popping nana back into bed'—a qualitative exploration of paramedic decision making when caring for older people who have fallen. *BMC Health Services Research, 17,* 299.

Slovic, P., Finucane, M., & Peters, E. (2002). The affect heuristic. In T. Gilovich, D. Griffin & D. Kahneman (Eds.), *Heuristics and biases: the psychology of intuitive judgment.* Cambridge, MA: University Press.

Stanovich, K. E., & West, R. F. (2000). Individual differences in reasoning: implications for the rationality debate? *The Behavioral and Brain Sciences, 23,* 645–665.

Stiegler, M. P., & Tung, A. (2014). Cognitive processes in anesthesiology decision making. *Anesthesiology, 120,* 204–217.

Stiell, I. G., Wells, G. A., Vandemheen, K. L., Clement, C. M., Lesiuk, H., De Maio, V. J., Laupacis, A., Schull, M.,

McKnight, R. D., & Verbeek, R. (2001). The Canadian C-spine rule for radiography in alert and stable trauma patients. *JAMA, 286,* 1841–1848.

Sweller, J. (1988). Cognitive load during problem solving: effects on learning. *Cognitive Science, 12,* 257–285.

Vaillancourt, C., Stiell, I. G., Beaudoin, T., Maloney, J., Anton, A. R., Bradford, P., Cain, E., Travers, A., Stempien, M., & Lees, M. (2009). The out-of-hospital validation of the Canadian C-Spine Rule by paramedics. *Annals of Emergency Medicine, 54,* 663–671.e1.

van Merriënboer, J. J., & Sweller, J. (2010). Cognitive load theory in health professional education: design principles and strategies. *Medical Education, 44,* 85–93.

Wachter, R. (2012). *Understanding patient safety. 2.* New York, NY: McGraw-Hill Medical.

Williams, B., Onsman, A., & Brown, T. (2009). From stretcher-bearer to paramedic: the Australian paramedics' move towards professionalisation. *Australasian Journal of Paramedicine, 7.*

SECTION 4:
Communication and Non-technical Skills

In this section:

Interpersonal communication and patient-focused care are pivotal skills in paramedic practice. Gaining the patient's trust, support and cooperation is essential to the effective management of a patient's condition. This section discuss communication types and strategies, and the impact interpersonal skills can have on the quality of patient care. Patient-focused, or holistic, care is also paramount in order to appreciate and treat all the intertwined aspects of a patient's condition. A paramedic's awareness of their own strengths and weaknesses in this area encourages reflection, growth and development in their ability to establish and maintain good paramedic–patient relationships in a wide variety of situations.

CHAPTER 8

Interpersonal Communication and Patient-Focused Care

By Robin Pap and Paul Simpson

OVERVIEW

- Communication plays a critical part in the everyday work of a paramedic. The best way to facilitate effective communication is to have a thorough understanding of the underlying principles.
- Effective paramedic–patient communication is fundamental to collecting sufficient information to determine an accurate diagnosis and gaining the support of the patient for the preferred treatment.
- In the diagnostically limited setting of emergency healthcare, the paramedic's ability to communicate effectively is often the primary tool to gather information that will assist in developing a treatment plan.

- Patient-focused care is care that goes beyond merely forming a provisional diagnosis and medical treatment; it aims to understand the patient holistically, and in that way enables improved patient satisfaction and outcomes; patient-centred communication forms a vital part of this.
- The ability to communicate effectively is not a personality trait. There is evidence suggesting that effective medical communication can be taught and improved.

Introduction

Throughout a shift and other professional activities, paramedics interact with a variety of people from diverse backgrounds and for multiple reasons. These interactions demand the ability to communicate with and relate to other people, most importantly patients. Effective communication is a major premise for patient-centredness. Patient-focused care therefore requires interpersonal communication skills as much as it does clinical skills.

A recent literature review of ambulance service complaints in the United Kingdom (UK) listed 'attitude/conduct/behaviour' as one of the top three themes of complaints received by UK National Health Service/Public Ambulance Services (Brady, 2017). Poor communication was a recurring contributing factor to this and other themes. Studies have also shown that miscommunication places patient safety at significant risk (Wilk et al., 2018). Effective communication, on the other hand, is linked to improved patient outcomes (Stewart, 1995; Stewart et al., 1999), fewer malpractice claims (Levinson et al., 1997) and fewer medication errors (Kohn et al., 2000). Research has also shown that paramedics are cognisant of how vital providing emotional support and effective communication is for delivering patient-focused care (Ayub et al., 2017). Specifically, interpersonal communication skills are critical in establishing rapport with patients, and are therefore recognised in the Paramedicine Board of Australia's *Professional Capabilities for Registered Paramedics* (2018) (see Box 8.1).

Effective communication entails more than simply sending and receiving words. It occurs in many forms, including vocalising without words (e.g. laughing or crying), non-verbal cues (e.g. eye contact and facial expressions) and material forms (e.g. pictures or written words); multiple factors should be considered (O'Toole, 2016). Patient-focused care is an approach to the planning, delivery and evaluation of healthcare that is grounded in mutually beneficial partnerships among healthcare providers and patients (Institute for Patient- and Family-Centred Care, 2018). This chapter outlines the principles of interpersonal communication skills and the foundations of patient-focused care. Chapter 15 will deal with how these principles are applied in the setting of a patient interview.

Fundamental concepts of communication

Paramedics communicate with a variety of individuals for multiple reasons. Besides communicating with patients, paramedics are required to routinely interact with family members, members of the public, other health professionals, emergency service personnel and other paramedics. As healthcare professionals, paramedics should aim to provide safe and effective patient-focused care interactions with persons other than the patient. Paramedics should also aim to use interpersonal communication skills to gather and share information while including the patient. This requires developing rapport, a mutual understanding and a therapeutic relationship (O'Toole, 2016).

BOX 8.1 Professional capabilities for registered paramedics

Domain 2: Professional communication and collaboration

This domain covers registered paramedics' responsibility to utilise appropriate, clear and effective communication. It also addresses their responsibility to ensure that they function effectively with other healthcare team members at all times.

What registered paramedics must be able to do	Evidence of this capability for the paramedicine profession
1. **Communicate clearly, sensitively and effectively with patient/service user and their family or carers**	• Establish rapport with patient/service user to gain understanding of their issues and perspectives, and to encourage their active participation in care and treatment • communicate with the patient/service user and/or carers to collect and convey information and reach agreement about the purpose of any care and treatment • convey knowledge and procedural information in ways that engender trust and confidence and respects patient/service user confidentiality, privacy and dignity • respond appropriately to patient/service user queries or issues • use appropriate communication skills to effectively manage avoidance, confusion and confrontation • identify and effectively manage likely communication barriers, including anxiety and stress, specific to individual patients/service users and/or carers • make appropriate adjustments to communication style to suit the particular needs of the patient/service user including those from culturally and linguistically diverse backgrounds and Aboriginal and Torres Strait Islander people, and • make provisions to engage third parties, including interpreters, to facilitate effective communication with patients/service users whose first language is not English, wherever possible. **Communication needs** may be influenced by English language skills, health literacy, age, health status, culture. **Appropriate adjustments** may include the paramedic demonstrating an awareness of the ways that their own culture and experience affect their interpersonal style, and having an awareness of strategies to ensure this does not present an impediment. **Communication techniques** must include active listening, use of appropriate language and detail, use of appropriate verbal and non-verbal cues and language, and confirming that the other person has understood.
2. **Collaborate with other health practitioners**	• Establish and maintain effective and respectful collaborative working relationships as a member of a healthcare team • demonstrate understanding of professional roles and responsibilities of healthcare team members and other service providers and how they interact with the role of a paramedic • follow accepted protocols and procedures to provide relevant and timely verbal and written communication • effectively supervise tasks delegated to other healthcare team members • consult effectively with relevant healthcare team members and other service providers to facilitate continuity of care, and • make appropriate referrals to other healthcare team members and other service providers. **Healthcare team members** may include registered health practitioners, accredited health professionals, and licensed or unlicensed healthcare workers.

Source: Paramedicine Board of Australia (2018).

The scientific principles of exchanging information can be explained using models of communication. Originally developed by Claude E. Shannon and Warren Weaver in 1949 as a mathematical model of communication, the linear model of communication (see Fig 8.1) has been adapted for the social sciences and is frequently applied to the healthcare setting. It describes communication starting with a source which has a message intended for a destination. To do so, a transmitter encodes the message into a signal,

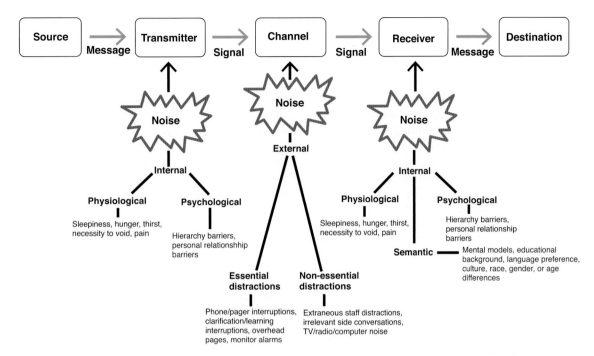

Figure 8.1
The linear model of communication.
Source: Mohorek & Webb (2015).

which is then conveyed through a channel; a receiver then decodes the signal back into a message for the destination (Mohorek & Webb, 2015). Throughout this process, 'noise' (synonymous with barriers) may be present which can corrupt the message.

The concept of signal versus noise in terms of information gathering is probably best described using the analogy of an old AM radio. In between the stations only static can be heard (noise), but when the radio is tuned in to the correct frequency the broadcast is clear (signal). If a station isn't quite tuned in, the mix of signal and noise makes it hard to discern what the announcer is saying. In fact, the amount of data we receive is exactly the same whether the station is correctly tuned in or not: the difference is that we can only understand the information if the signal is clear and there is no static. Internal noise (including physiological, psychological and semantic noise) corrupts the encoding/decoding of messages/signals whereas external noise corrupts signals present in channels.

Some examples of noise are more obvious than others. Feeling tired and fatigued towards the end of a busy night shift is a bodily barrier within the paramedic and thus poses a risk of producing physiological internal noise during communication. A language barrier often causes semantic internal noise in the receiver. An authoritarian paramedic approach may create psychological internal noise.

But some noise is much more complex to sense and mitigate. Culture, for example, is not limited by ethnicity, language or birthplace. It can be described as a system of shared values, beliefs and behaviours that shape how we contextualise our world (Carrillo et al., 1999). Religion, age, education, gender and sexual preference all contribute to culture and, if not appreciated, can create barriers to effective clinical communication (Carrillo et al., 1999). Of course, it simply isn't practical to learn all the cultural nuances that could affect patient care (who to address, how to address them, whether to shake hands or not etc.), and such a notion fails to recognise that individuals within a culture are unique and respond differently to illness. Beyond recognising that cultural barriers exist, the key is to ask (directly but politely) about the patient's beliefs and preferences (Carrillo et al., 1999). Paramedics, in fact, form a very strong cultural group described by a common understanding of disease processes, hierarchy, responsibility and processes. Historically, the paramedic culture consisted entirely of middle-aged males, and today young female paramedics can be subjected to cultural biases from patients. As unfair as cultural stereotyping is (regardless of the direction it flows), it does exist and the key to mollifying its effects are to first recognise the bias and then to seek or provide information to reduce its impact.

Verbal and non-verbal communication

Verbal communication is the sharing of information between individuals using words. The words we choose when we talk are important, but when we communicate with someone, we use much more than only words. Non-verbal communication (i.e. those parts of a communication other than words) contributes significantly to the meaning of the message we intentionally or unintentionally convey. In fact, up to 65% of a message's meaning may be conveyed non-verbally (Esposito et al., 2007). Non-verbal communication may be divided into body language and suprasegmental features. Body language refers to non-verbal cues such as posture, facial expression, proximity and appearance. Suprasegmental features, which includes prosodic and paralinguistic attributes, are non-verbal characteristics of the voice such as tone, volume, emphasis and timely pauses.

It is critical for paramedics to be aware of non-verbal communication, in both the messages they give and the ones they receive. Paramedics must be self-aware of their non-verbal communication and how it influences the way they are being perceived and heard. Paramedics need to ensure that in an effort to build an effective paramedic–patient relationship, non-verbal messages support rather than contradict the verbal messages (O'Toole, 2016). Apart from helping build rapport, non-verbal communication may affect patients' wellbeing. A recent hospital-based study investigating seriously ill patients' experiences of health professionals' non-verbal communication suggested that body language and tone of speech are essential in terms of promoting and protecting patients' positive thoughts and emotions, and therefore represent a significant ethical component in the communication encounter (Timmermann et al., 2017). At the same time, paramedics must gain skills and experience in sensing their patients' presentation and non-verbal communication and understand how this influences their overall patient assessment.

The science and art of patient communication

If we were all identical in beliefs, experiences and physiology, clinicians would not need to focus so closely on communicating with patients. They would simply need to ask a series of standard questions, perform the necessary tests and process the data, and it would always lead to a logical conclusion. But while medicine is based in science, it is a human undertaking that is practised in a world mired with beliefs, values, opinions and inconsistent levels of knowledge (Saunders, 2000; Tolana, 2007). Clinical decisions are

Table 8.1: Traditional clinician–patient role relationship

Patient	Clinician
Passive	Active
Seeks help	Provides help
Needs medical knowledge	Holder of medical knowledge
Information supply (answers)	Information collection (asks)
Complies with advice (cooperation)	Provides advice (guidance)

rarely based on scientific values alone: the variability of human bodies and disease presentations does not allow that degree of certainty. We need the rich details of the patient's story to help us reach a diagnosis.

How we express ourselves (verbally and non-verbally) is very dependent on the role we perceive we have in the circumstance: this is especially true when we communicate with people we have never met. Historically, the roles of patient and clinician are strongly 'socially legitimised' and were first described by American sociologist Talcott Parsons (Parsons, 1951). According to Parsons, the clinician is the holder of medical knowledge while the patient is the seeker of that knowledge. The clinician asks the questions; the patient answers them honestly. The clinician dispenses advice; the patient should accept and adhere to that advice (see Table 8.1). This active–passive divide attributed well-defined rights and obligations to both parties and characterised the interaction between them for much of the second half of the last century. But because it attributed complete control of the interaction to the doctor, it was rarely a construct that allowed the clinician to fully understand the patient's presentation and perspective. That it survived (and in some places grew) as a model of communication was probably due to its alignment with the social norms of the era and the aspirations of the medical profession in maintaining a distinct professional separation and control.

Key to this traditional role structure was that the clinician had to remain neutral to the patient's personal or social attributes and focus only on the disease (Lipkin et al., 1995). The model also suggested that any failure in the consultation was a result of either party failing to adhere to their roles and responsibilities. It was quickly noted, however, that the distinct role division was actually a cause of conflict between the two parties. Patients were not completely unaware of their illness; they formed ideas as to the cause, possible investigations and treatment (Katon & Kleinman, 1980). When their ideas of their illness were not addressed, they felt the clinician was either uncaring or incompetent (DiMatteo & Hays, 1980; Valentine, 1991). In such cases they were less likely to follow the clinician's advice, regardless of how appropriate it may have been. The concept of the patient as the unknowing seeker of medical advice was probably never entirely true but it is now rapidly decaying. Patients' ability to access medical information has rapidly accelerated over the past decade, with one study finding that 41% of participants were influenced by the internet about seeking medical care, treating an illness or questioning the advice they received from their doctor (Forkner-Dunn, 2003).

While the social distinction and power imbalance between patient and clinician described by Parsons is still evident today (and still actively pursued by some clinicians), the asymmetrical model describing the relationship between clinician and patient fails to accurately describe the actual encounter or act as a tool to build effective communication.

The explanatory model

Just as Parsons' model was published, other attempts were made to describe the clinician–patient relationship. Less authoritarian than the active–passive relationship described by Parsons, the explanatory model acknowledges not only the value of the patient's input into the interview but also how it can lead to conflict. The explanatory model recognises that nearly all patients have an understanding of the cause, severity and expected treatment for their illness (Carrillo et al., 1999; Kleinman et al., 1978). This explanation may be based on culture, beliefs and past experience more than scientific evidence, but unless it is recognised and addressed there is no means of developing a satisfying and effective management plan (Baer et al., 2008; Haidet et al., 2008). While Parsons' model bestowed professional expertise and authority on every clinician by virtue of their role, patients are actually reluctant to trust those who they consider have not listened to or understood their description of their illness (Roter & Hall, 2006).

The vital distinction that the explanatory model makes is between illness and disease (see Table 8.2). Patients are primarily concerned with illness—why they are ill, how the condition affects their lives, what it doesn't allow them to do—and they may create a narrative that explains all of these aspects. Paramedics are primarily focused on the biological dimensions of disease: linking the pathology to the abnormal function of tissues and extending this to the creation of specific symptoms (Stewart, 1995). Paramedics use this 'narrative' to create a coherent and logical story in their minds that identifies the underlying disease. As a result, there is enormous potential for

Table 8.2: Explanatory clinician–patient relationship

Patient	Clinician
Expert on illness	Expert on disease
Has concept of cause	Yet to form concept of cause
Needs concerns addressed	Needs to develop a management plan

BOX 8.2 Shared values

Although we communicate with people every day, the encounter between clinician and patient is not a typical social encounter. In addition to the stresses of pain and illness, any exchange between clinician and patient is framed by specified roles and responsibilities: the clinician as the caregiver and the patient as the care receiver. When we communicate, we constantly send and receive messages, encode and decode, and respond consciously and subconsciously in what can be described as a 'transactional' model (Buckman, 2002). This communication occurs in a fluid state: neither party is certain where it will go, and both parties are constantly trying to read and respond to the messages they are receiving. All this happens against background noise and requires perception, interpretation, filtering and modification, all contextualised by biases and prejudices, values and beliefs. To be an effective communicator you therefore need to analyse the other person's frame of reference. You also need to develop an awareness of the other person's perceptions, biases and preferred techniques—and become aware of your own. Finally, you need to become fluent in a range of communication strategies (see Chapter 15).

conflict between the two explanations if they are not explored and expressed appropriately (Kleinman et al., 1978). In reality, neither explanation has to be the sole focus of the interview and to ignore one or the other will leave one party unsatisfied. It shouldn't belittle the clinician to allow the patient to express their understanding of the illness as it is the only tool the paramedic has to develop a shared understanding of the disease and to negotiate a successful resolution of the health problem (see Box 8.2; Baer et al., 2008; Haidet et al., 2008). It may be difficult for some novice clinicians to accept that their role is not simply to diagnose the disease, nor is it the patient's role to accept that diagnosis with blind faith. To ensure that the patient believes their illness is being appropriately managed, paramedics may have to not only implement the correct treatment, but also convince the patient that their diagnosis is in fact correct.

The notion of the patient interview as a negotiation challenges many clinicians who instinctively feel patients should comply with expert opinion. However, the interview is not a negotiation in the commercial sense whereby, for example, two parties seek ownership of property, but is rather a negotiation to resolve the conflict between the clinician's and the patient's explanatory models. The result allows the paramedic to provide optimal clinical care, while the patient feels what they have received is in their best medical and personal interests (Buckman, 2002; Haidet et al., 2008; Lipkin et al., 1995). The ability to reach a negotiated 'truth' becomes the purpose of the interview.

Effective listening

Not being listened to is a major source of patient dissatisfaction (Boudreau et al., 2009). Just like sending messages (speaking), receiving messages (listening) requires skill. This is true in general life and essential for healthcare professionals (Stein-Parbury, 2014; Harms & Pierce, 2015). Effective listening means that the message is not just heard but understood and that both parties are assured that this process has taken place successfully. O'Toole (2016) defines effectives listening well and explains that it requires attention, reflection, clarification and validation. Attention means that the paramedic consciously focuses completely on the patient (Stein-Parbury, 2014; Berger, 2014; Egan, 2010). Reflecting back messages in both a verbal and a non-verbal way indicates to the patient that the paramedic understands not only what has been said but also the individual's thoughts and feelings about the complaint or illness (Devito, 2009). It's important that this takes place utilising lay language because medical terminology may cause confusion, escalation or unnecessary anxiety (Ayub et al., 2017). If uncertainty exists, the paramedic needs to ask questions to clarify (O'Toole, 2016). Finally, validating involves demonstrating that the patient's message and emotions have been understood accurately (O'Toole, 2016).

Considering these elements, it becomes clear that effective listening forms a key component of patient communication using the explanatory model and patient-focused care. Effective listening is not only about understanding the clinical presentation but understanding the patient and his/her pertinent background and perspective. Paramedics who listen

BOX 8.3 Reflective questions—non-verbal communication

Think about a time when you had an important conversation with someone.
1. Did you use non-verbal communication to support what you were saying?
2. Do you think it supported or contradicted your verbal messages?
3. What non-verbal communication do you think you use regularly and which aspects could develop to enhance your patient-focused care?

effectively are more successful in establishing a therapeutic relationship in which the patient feels valued and confident in the care they receive (see Box 8.3).

Patient-centred communication

The Australian Commission on Safety and Quality in Healthcare (ACSQHC) defines patient-centred care as 'healthcare that is respectful of, and responsive to, the needs and values of patients and consumers' (ACSQHC, 2011). Key to the provision of patient-centred care is patient-centred communication, which has been consistently associated with positive health outcomes and improved patient satisfaction (King & Hoppe, 2013). Epstein and Street define patient-centred communication as:

> (1) eliciting and understanding patient perspectives (concerns, ideas, expectations, needs, feelings and functioning), (2) understanding the patient within his or her unique psychosocial and cultural contexts, and (3) reaching a shared understanding of patient problems and the treatments that are concordant with patient values.
> (Epstein & Street, 2007)

This definition highlights that patient communication must involve more than objective elicitation of a structured and completed history; it focuses on terms such as 'understanding the patient', 'patient perspective' and 'shared understanding'. It is not enough, however, to achieve the three points described above; effective patient-centred communication requires the paramedic to demonstrate these points in such a way that the patient recognises that nature of the paramedic–patient relationship they are entering into. Due to the stress, fear, anxiety, worry or concern that a patient may be experiencing as a result of

BOX 8.4 Reflective questions—patient-centred communication

Think of a time when you have sought healthcare from a health practitioner of some kind.
1. What is your recollection of the nature of the relationship formed between you and the healthcare practitioner?
2. Did you feel included in the decision-making process?
3. Do you feel the care provided would have met the three key points of 'patient-centred care' detailed in the definition above?

BOX 8.5 Reflection questions—self-awareness

1. What would you consider your strengths and weaknesses with regard to your interpersonal communication skills?
2. Identify an academic, a student peer and a work-colleague or supervisor whose opinion you respect. Ask them each the same question about your strengths and weaknesses regarding interpersonal communication. How do their perceptions compare to your own self-assessment?

their complaint, they may not be well attuned to the communication being put forward by the paramedic (Fortin et al., 2012). It is important, then, that the paramedic maintains an acute awareness of themselves while developing an awareness of the patient as more than simply a 'chief complaint' (see Box 8.4).

Emotional and behavioural components of effective communication

Key aspects of paramedic communication that may influence the effectiveness of patient-centred communication are discussed in the following sections. Frequently in communication training for health professionals, the focus is solely on 'interviewing techniques' including verbal and non-verbal concepts such as body language, proxemics and listening techniques, with little focus on the emotional and behavioural contributors to effective communication. Self-awareness, bias and prejudice, sympathy and empathy, paramedic expectations and compassion are emotional and behavioural factors that play a critical role in patient-centred communication and may sit within the paramedic's sphere of control or regulation. An understanding of and appreciation for the role each plays in the paramedic–patient relationship is essential to developing a successful patient-centred approach to care.

Self-awareness

In order to engage in effective patient-centred communication, paramedics must develop a high level of awareness not just of the patient, but of themselves and what they bring knowingly or otherwise into the paramedic–patient relationship (O'Toole, 2016). Self-awareness offers many benefits to both the paramedic and the patient. For the paramedic, self-awareness may increase their understanding of themself, enhance their capacity for self-regulation of thoughts and behaviours (Devito, 2009) and improve their ability to recognise and respond appropriately to the needs of others (Schore, 2005). Importantly, self-awareness has been posited as being 'essential for developing a therapeutic relationship and for promoting open, honest and genuine health professionals who are not afraid to be caring human beings' (Stein-Parbury, 2009). Reflection and peer-observation are tools through which self-awareness can be heightened, providing a vehicle to explore the paramedic's own values, needs, implicit biases and personality characteristics, and to assess the impact of these values and needs on personal communication (O'Toole, 2016) (see Box 8.5).

Bias and prejudice

The presence of paramedic bias or prejudice during communication may have a negative impact on paramedic–patient relationships, leading to conflict, misunderstandings and communication breakdown (O'Toole, 2016).

Bias and prejudice may lead to a paramedic making stereotyped judgments about a patient and their presenting condition, taking the focus of care away from the patient. This has the capacity to reduce communication and cloud clinical reasoning, resulting in poor clinical judgment and less than optimal patient outcomes (see Fig 8.2).

It is essential that paramedics, novice or experienced, engage in communication that is free of bias and prejudice; however, this appears to be more easily said than done. This is because in most instances bias and prejudice are implicit in nature, occurring and impacting without the paramedic being aware of their presence or their effect on their clinical judgment (Fitzgerald & Hurst, 2017). Implicit biases have been extensively researched in healthcare; gender-, racial- and sexuality-based implicit bias have been demonstrated in numerous contexts across multiple professions (Wyatt et al., 2016).

The key challenge for novice or experienced paramedics is to recognise and accept that they, like the majority of health professionals, are susceptible to implicit bias and making stereotypical and moral judgments about patients. In a systematic review including 42 studies, Fitzgerald and Hurst found that 35 of those studies reported evidence of implicit bias among a broad cross-section of health professionals, and consistent evidence of a positive correlation between the presence of implicit bias and worse patient outcomes (Fitzgerald & Hurst, 2017). While none of the studies in the review included participants who were paramedics, the results can be generalised to paramedics as there is no valid

reason to suggest the paramedic workforce would behave differently.

It is important to recognise that it is not only the paramedic who may compromise communication in the clinical setting. A patient may also bring his or her own bias and prejudice into the clinical encounter (O'Toole, 2016). For example, a young paramedic may be perceived by a patient to be too inexperienced to competently manage their condition so the patient may without intention defer to an older-looking paramedic who is present. This may interfere with the younger paramedic's attempts to develop rapport and gather a concise and complete history (see Fig 8.3). A paramedic must therefore develop an awareness of their own bias and prejudice and implement strategies to mitigate them, but also an awareness of patient bias and prejudice and strategies to mitigate those. Strategies that may help a paramedic reduce their implicit bias or mitigate their impact are detailed in Box 8.6.

Paramedic expectations

A paramedic's expectations of the nature of the patients and presentations they are attending has the potential to negatively affect the quality of care a patient receives (Simpson et al., 2017). In a qualitative study of Australian paramedics, Simpson and colleagues reported the presence of a 'low acuity bias' in the attitudes and perceptions of paramedics towards their work. This bias arose from the paramedics' perception as to whether or not the patient and their presentation fit into the cultural definition of what 'real paramedic work' was. Work classified as 'non-emergency' or 'non-life-threatening' can be negatively perceived and may be viewed as work that did not 'need' a paramedic to attend. As a result, the affective and behavioural aspects of a paramedic's interaction with a patient may change, shifting the nature of the paramedic–patient relationship away from one that is patient-centred to one that is paramedic-centred (Simpson et al., 2017). Though uncommonly referred to in the paramedicine

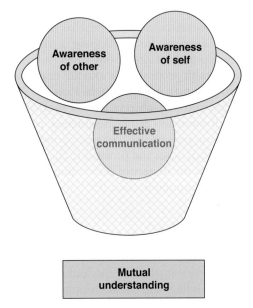

Figure 8.2
Mutual understanding.

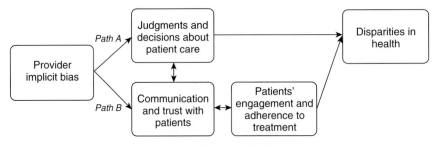

Figure 8.3
Model of paths through which provider-implicit bias may contribute to health disparities.
Source: Zestcott et al. (2016)

BOX 8.6 Evidence-based strategies to reduce implicit bias

- Stereotype replacement: recognising that a response is based on stereotype and consciously adjusting the response
- Counter-stereotypic imaging: imagining the individual as the opposite of the stereotype
- Individuation: seeing the person as an individual rather than a stereotype (e.g. learning about their personal history and the context that brought them to the doctor's office or health centre)
- Perspective taking: 'putting yourself in the other person's shoes'
- Increasing opportunities for contact with individuals from different groups: expanding one's network of friends and colleagues or attending events where people of other racial and ethnic groups, gender identities, sexual orientation and other groups may be present
- Partnership building: reframing the interaction with the patient as one between collaborating equals, rather than between a high-status person and a low-status person

Source: Devine et al. (2012).

literature, affective dispositions to respond (ADR), or emotional biases, have been described in detail in the medical literature (Croskerry, 2005) and should be considered by paramedics to be highly relevant in determining the effectiveness of communication with patients (Croskerry, 2007).

Empathy and sympathy

In the context of healthcare, empathy has been defined as 'a predominantly cognitive attribute that involves an understanding of the patient's experiences, concerns and perspective, combined with a capacity to communicate this understanding and an intention to help' (Hojat, 2016). Put simply, empathy is the ability to share and understand the feelings of others. Empathic communication by healthcare professionals may be associated with positive healthcare outcomes (Steinhausen et al., 2014; Lelorain et al., 2012). When health professionals demonstrate empathic behaviour, a more 'humanistic' relationship emerges between the professional and patient which may result in increased patient compliance and greater patient satisfaction (Kim et al., 2004). Potentially helpful verbal techniques for expressing empathy towards patients are summarised in Table 8.3 using the NURSE pneumonic (Hashim, 2017; Back et al., 2005).

While most health professionals would consider themselves to be empathetic in their communication with and behaviour towards patients, a vast body of research suggests developing and maintaining empathy may be more difficult than it appears. Cross-disciplinary research using validated survey tools to measure self-reported empathy levels has identified low levels of empathy in undergraduate students studying midwifery, nursing, paramedicine, occupational therapy, physiotherapy, medicine and nutrition (Williams et al., 2014; Williams et al., 2015). Across several studies, paramedicine students typically reported lower levels of empathy compared to their interprofessional colleagues (Boyle et al., 2010; Williams et al., 2012; Williams et al., 2016). Multidisciplinary research has tended to suggest that empathy levels decline as undergraduate study progresses (Chen et al., 2007; Hojat et al., 2004; Ward et al., 2012; Nunes et al., 2011; Sherman & Cramer, 2005). The formative years of a paramedic's development therefore appear to be important in establishing a baseline for empathetic communication and behaviour into the future.

Let's now revisit the definition of empathy described previously and pay particular attention to the part suggesting that empathy is 'predominantly cognitive' in nature. Cognitive refers to understanding of the patient's feelings, implying an objectivity that rarely exists. It is important to recognise that empathy has an 'affective' component interplaying with what we have said is a predominantly cognitive process. The affective component of empathy refers to a paramedic sharing the patient's emotions, in essence 'feeling what the patient is feeling'. The affective domain of empathy is an important component contributing the 'humanistic' interaction between paramedic and patient; however, an excessive amount of emotional involvement may cloud professional objectivity, resulting in flawed reasoning and reduced diagnostic accuracy. An affective over-investment in a patient or their situation may lead to strong feelings of sympathy, which if not regulated may be deleterious to the patient and the paramedic. Unregulated emotional investment or sympathy may lead to professional burnout and compassion fatigue (Figley, 1995), personal exhaustion and vicarious traumatisation (Linley & Joseph, 2007). In order to achieve optimal patient outcomes, empathy in communication should be maximised, while sympathy should be optimised but closely regulated (Hojat, 2016). Self-regulation is difficult to achieve, particularly at the novice practitioner level;

Table 8.3: Techniques for expressing empathy to patients: the NURSE mnemonic.

Technique	Examples (may overlap)
Naming	'It seems like you are feeling …' 'I wonder if you are feeling …' 'Some people would feel … in this situation.' 'I can see that this makes you feel …'
Understanding	'I can understand how that might upset you.' 'I can understand why you would be … given what you are going through.' 'I can imagine what that would feel like.' 'I can't imagine what that would feel like!' 'I know someone who had a similar experience. It is not easy.' 'This has been a hard time for you.' 'That makes sense to me.'
Respecting	'It must be a lot of stress to deal with …' 'I respect your courage to keep a positive attitude in spite of your difficulties.' 'You are a brave person.' 'I am impressed by how well you handled this.' 'It sounds like a lot to deal with.' 'You have been through a lot.' 'You did the right thing by coming in.'
Supporting	'I want to help in any way I can.' 'Please let me know if there is anything I can do to help.' 'I am here to help you in any way I can.' 'I will be with you in this difficult time.' 'I will be with you all the way.'
Exploring	'Tell me more about what you were feeling when you were sick.' 'How are you coping with this?' 'What has happened since we last met?'

Sources: Hashim (2017); Back et al. (2005).

however, ongoing engagement in reflective practice together with participation in mentoring and clinical supervision opportunities may enhance a paramedic's ability to first develop emotional regulation, then decrease erosion of empathy in subsequent years.

Compassion

Compassion is an important element of patient-centred care and communication (Frampton et al., 2013). Peters and colleagues describe compassion as 'a deep feeling of connectedness with the experience of human suffering that requires personal knowing of the suffering of others, evokes a moral response to the recognised suffering and that results in caring that brings comfort to the sufferer' (Peters et al., 2006). While there are no studies exploring compassion that are specific to paramedicine, there is a strong body of evidence from allied health disciplines, particularly nursing, suggesting compassion on the part of the health provider enhances communication and overall patient experience. However, Lown and colleagues reported a gap between health provider and patient perception of the prevalence of compassion in the healthcare they provided and received, respectively (Lown et al., 2011). In this survey, 78% of physicians believed most health professionals provided compassionate care, compared to 53% reported by patients.

Research has identified barriers to compassionate care and communication such as lack of time, support and resources, each of which resonates in the context in which paramedics work (Sinclair et al., 2016). Researchers have proposed that operational and workload pressures are a barrier to paramedics providing the quality of care they believe they should (Simpson et al., 2017). An ever-increasing technical and diagnostic aspect of healthcare provision has also been argued to be non-conducive to provision of compassionate care, with a decrease in 'soft skills' (Frampton et al., 2013). Maintaining an awareness of compassion as an essential ingredient for quality paramedical care may enhance communication between paramedic and patient and help keep the patient at the centre of the paramedic–patient relationship.

Summary

Communication is a critical component of safe and patient-focused care. The knowledge and skills required to communicate effectively can be learned. Communication entails sending, receiving and, most importantly, understanding messages. Messages are sent by much more than just words. Non-verbal communication and effective listening play an important role. Paramedics need to be self-aware and perceptive to internal and external factors that influence information exchange. Ultimately communication aims to gather, provide and relay information to build a therapeutic relationship and facilitate patient-focused care. Patient-focused care is care that goes beyond merely eliciting a medical history; it aims to understand the patient holistically, and in that way enables improved patient satisfaction and outcomes. Paramedics must develop self-awareness about their own biases and learn to mitigate these while at the same time learn to observe and interpret their patients' biases and prejudice. Empathy and sympathy are essential components of high-quality out-of-hospital care.

References

Australian Commission on Safety and Quality in Health Care. (2011). Patient centred care: improving quality and safety through partnerships with patients and consumers. ACSQHC, Sydney.

Ayub, E. M., Sampayo, E. M., Shah, M. I., & Doughty, C. B. (2017). Prehospital providers' perceptions on providing patient and family centred care. *Prehospital Emergency Care, 21*(2), 233–241.

Back, A. L., Arnold, R. M., Baile, W. F., Tulsky, J. A., & Fryer-Edwards, K. (2005). Approaching difficult communication tasks in oncology. *CA: A Cancer Journal for Clinicians, 55*, 164–177.

Baer, R. D., Weller, S. C., Garcia, J. G., & Rocha, A. L. (2008). Cross-cultural perspectives on physician and lay models of the common cold. *Medical Anthropology Quarterly, 22*(2), 146–148.

Berger, C. R. (Ed.), (2014). *Interpersonal communication*. Berlin/Boston: Walter de Gruyter GmbH.

Boudreau, J. D., Cassell, E., & Fuks, A. (2009). Preparing medical students to become attentive listeners. *Medical Teacher, 31*(1), 22–29.

Boyle, M., Williams, B., Brown, T., Molloy, A., McKenna, L., Molloy, L., & Lewis, B. (2010). Levels of empathy in undergraduate health science students. *The Internet Journal of Medical Education, 1*, 1–7.

Brady, M. (2017). UK ambulance service complaints: a review of the literature. *International Journal of Emergency Services, 6*(2), 104–121.

Buckman, R. (2002). Communications and emotions. *British Medical Journal, 325*(7366), 678–682.

Carrillo, J. E., Green, A. R., & Betancourt, J. R. (1999). Cross-cultural primary care: a patient-based approach. *Annals of Internal Medicine, 130*, 829–834.

Chen, D., Lew, R., Hershman, W., & Orlander, J. (2007). A cross-sectional measurement of medical student empathy. *Journal of General Internal Medicine, 22*, 1434–1438.

Croskerry, P. (2005). *Diagnostic failure: a cognitive and affective approach. Advances in patient safety: from research to implementation*. Rockville, MD: Agency for Health Care Research and Quality.

Croskerry, P. (2007). The affective imperative: Coming to terms with our emotions. *Academic Emergency Medicine: Official Journal of the Society for Academic Emergency Medicine, 14*, 184–186.

Devine, P. G., Forscher, P. S., Austin, A. J., & Cox, W. T. L. (2012). Long-term reduction in implicit race bias: a prejudice habit-breaking intervention. *Journal of Experimental Social Psychology, 48*, 1267–1278.

Devito, J. A. (2009). *The interpersonal communication book*. Boston: Pearson.

DiMatteo, M. R., & Hays, R. (1980). The significance of patients' perspectives of physician conduct. *Journal of Community Health, 6*, 18–34.

Egan, G. (2010). *The skilled helper* (10th ed.). Thomson: Belmont, CA.

Epstein, R. M., & Street, R. L. (2007). *Patient-Centered communication in cancer care: promoting healing and reducing suffering*. National Institutes of Health Publication Bethesda, MD: National Cancer Institute.

Esposito, A., Bratanić, M., Keller, E., & Marinaro, M. 2007. *Fundamentals of Verbal and Nonverbal Communication and the Biometric Issue*. NATO Security through Science Series E: Human and Social Dynamics, vol. 18.

Figley, C. R. (1995). *Compassion Fatigue: coping with secondary post-traumatic stress disorder in those who treat the traumatised*. New York, NY: Brunner/Mazel.

Fitzgerald, C., & Hurst, S. (2017). Implicit bias in healthcare professionals: a systematic review. *BMC Medical Ethics, 18*, 19.

Forkner-Dunn, J. (2003). Internet-based patient self-care: the next generation of health care delivery. *Journal of Medical Internet Research, 5*(2).

Fortin, A. H., Dwamena, F. C., Frankel, R. M., & Smith, R. C. (2012). *Smith's Patient-Centered interviewing: an Evidence-Based method*. New York, NY: McGraw-Hill.

Frampton, S. B., Guastello, S., & Lepore, M. (2013). Compassion as the foundation of patient-centered care: the importance of compassion in action. *Journal of Comparative Effectiveness Research, 2*, 443–455.

Haidet, P., O'Malley, K., Sharf, B., Gladney, A., Gresinger, A., & Street, R. (2008). Characterizing explanatory models of illness in healthcare: development and validation of the CONNECT instrument. *Patient Education and Counseling, 73*, 232–239.

Harms, L., & Pierce, J. (2015). *Working with people: communication skills for reflective practice*. Don Mills, Ontario: Oxford University Press.

Hashim, M. J. (2017). Patient-Centered communication: basic skills. *American Family Physician, 95*, 29–34.

Hojat, M. (2016). *Empathy in health professions education and patient care*. New York, NY: Springer.

Hojat, M., Mangione, S., Nasca, T. J., Rattner, S., Erdmann, J. B., Gonnella, J. S., & Magee, M. (2004). An empirical study of decline in empathy in medical school. *Medical Education, 38*, 934–941.

Institute for Patient- and Family-Centred Care (2018), *Patient- and Family-Centred Care. The Institute for Patient- and Family-Centred Care*, viewed 20 May 2018, <http://www.ipfcc.org/about/pfcc.html>.

Katon, W., & Kleinman, A. (1980). Doctor–patient negotiation and other social science strategies in patient care. In L. Eisenberg & A. Kleinman (Eds.), *The relevance of social science for medicine*. Boston: Reidel.

Kim, S. S., Kaplowitz, S., & Johnston, M. V. (2004). The effects of physician empathy on patient satisfaction and compliance. *Evaluation and the Health Professions, 27*(3), 237–251.

King, A., & Hoppe, R. (2013). 'Best Practice' for Patient-Centered communication: a narrative review. *Journal of Graduate Medical Education, 5*, 385–393.

Kleinman, A., Eisenberg, L., & Good, B. (1978). Culture, illness, and care: clinical lessons from anthropologic and cross-cultural research. *Annals of Internal Medicine, 88*, 251–258.

Kohn, L. T., Corrigan, J., & Donaldson, M. S. (2000). *To err is human: building a safer health system*. Washington, DC: National Academy Press.

Lelorain, S., Brédart, A., Dolbeault, S., & Sultan, S. (2012). A systematic review of the associations between empathy measures and patient outcomes in cancer care. *Psycho-Oncology, 21*(12), 1255–1264.

Levinson, W., Roter, D., Mullooly, J. P., Dull, V. T., & Frankel, R. M. (1997). Physician-patient communication. *Journal of American Medical Association, 277*(7), 553–559.

Linley, P. A., & Joseph, S. (2007). Therapy work and therapists' positive and negative well-being. *Journal of Social and Clinical Psychology, 26*, 385–403.

Lipkin, M., Putnam, S. M., & Lazare, A. (1995). *The medical interview*. New York: Springer.

Lown, B. A., Rosen, J., & Marttila, J. (2011). An agenda for improving compassionate care: a survey shows about half of patients say such care is missing. *Health Affairs, 30*, 1772–1778.

Mohorek, M., & Webb, T. P. (2015). Establishing a conceptual framework for handoffs using communication theory. *Journal of Surgical Education, 72*(3), 402–409.

Nunes, P., Williams, S., Sa, B., & Stevenson, K. (2011). A study of empathy decline in students from five health disciplines during their first year of training. *International Journal of Medical Education, 2*, 12.

O'Toole, G. (2016). *Communication: core interpersonal skills for health professionals* (2nd ed.). Chatswood: Elsevier.

Paramedicine Board of Australia. (2018). *Professional Capabilities for Registered Paramedics*, 29 June, <https://www.paramedicineboard.gov.au/Professional-standards/Professional-capabilities-for-registered-paramedics.aspx>.

Parsons, T. (1951). *The social system.*. Glencoe, IL: The Free Press.

Peters, M. A. (2006). Compassion: an investigation into the experience of nursing faculty. *International Journal for Human Caring, 10*.

Roter, D., & Hall, J. A. (2006). *Doctors talking with Patients/Patients talking with doctors*. Westport: Praeger.

Saunders, J. (2000). The practice of clinical medicine as an art and as a science. *Medical Humanities, 26*, 18–22.

Schore, A. N. (2005). Attachment, affect regulation and the developing right brain: linking developmental neuroscience to paediatrics. *Pediatrics in Review, 26*, 204–217.

Sherman, J. J., & Cramer, A. (2005). Measurement of changes in empathy during dental school. *Journal of Dental Education, 69*, 338–345.

Simpson, P., Thomas, R., Bendall, J., Lord, B., Lord, S., & Close, J. (2017). 'Popping nana back into bed'—a qualitative exploration of paramedic decision making when caring for older people who have fallen. *BMC Health Services Research, 17*, 299.

Sinclair, S., Norris, J. M., McConnell, S. J., Chochinov, H. M., Hack, T. F., Hagen, N. A., McClement, S., & Bouchal, S. R. (2016). Compassion: a scoping review of the healthcare literature. *BMC Palliative Care, 15*, 6.

Steinhausen, S., Ommen, O., Thüm, S., Lefering, R., Koehler, T., Neugebauer, E., & Pfaff, H. (2014). Physician empathy and subjective evaluation of medical treatment outcome in trauma surgery patients. *Patient Education and Counseling, 95*(1), 53–60.

Stein-Parbury, J. (2009). *Patient and person: interpersonal skills in nursing* (4th ed.). Sydney: Churchill Livingstone Elsevier.

Stein-Parbury, J. (2014). *Patient and person: interpersonal skills in nursing* (5th ed.). Sydney: Churchill Livingstone Elsevier.

Stewart, M. (1995). Effective physician–patient communication and health outcomes: a review. *CMAJ: Canadian Medical Association Journal = Journal de l'Association Medicale Canadienne, 152*(9), 1423–1433.

Stewart, M., Brown, J. B., Boon, H., Galajda, J., Meredith, L., & Sangster, M. (1999). Evidence of patient–doctor communication. *Cancer Prevention Control, 3*(1), 25–30.

Timmermann, C., Uhrenfeldt, L., & Birkelund, R. (2017). Ethics in the communicative encounter: seriously ill patients' experiences of health professionals' nonverbal communication. *Scandinavian Journal of Caring Sciences, 31*(1), 62–73.

Tolana, P. C. 2007. *Decision making in medicine and health*. New York: Nova Biomedical Books.

Valentine, K. L. (1991). Comprehensive assessment of caring and its relationship to outcome measures. *JAMA, 266*, 1831–1832.

Ward, J., Cody, J., Schaal, M., & Hojat, M. (2012). The empathy enigma: an empirical study of decline in empathy among undergraduate nursing students. *Journal of Professional Nursing, 28*, 34–40.

Wilk, S., Siegl, L., Siegl, K., & Hohenstein, C. (2018). Miscommunication as a risk focus in patient safety: work process analysis in prehospital emergency care. *Anaesthetist, 67*(4), 255–263.

Williams, B., Boyle, M., Brightwell, R., Devenish, S., Hartley, P., McCall, M., McMullen, P., Munro, G., O'Meara, P., & Webb, V. (2012). An assessment of undergraduate paramedic students' empathy levels. *International Journal of Medical Education, 3*, 98–102.

Williams, B., Brown, T., McKenna, L., Boyle, M. J., Palermo, C., Nestel, D., Brightwell, R., McCall, L., & Russo, V. (2014). Empathy levels among health professional students: a cross-sectional study at two universities in Australia. *Advances in medical education and practice, 5*.

Williams, B., Brown, T., McKenna, L., Palermo, C., Morgan, P., Nestel, D., Brightwell, R., Gilbert-Hunt, S., Stagnitti, K., Olaussen, A., & Wright, C. (2015). Student empathy levels across 12 medical and health professions: an interventional study. *Journal of Compassionate Health Care, 2*.

Williams, B., Boyle, M., & Howard, S. (2016). Empathy levels in undergraduate paramedic students: a three-year longitudinal study. *Nurse Education in Practice, 16*, 86–90.

Wyatt, R., Laderman, M., Botwinick, L., Mate, K., & Whittington, J. (2016). *Achieving health equity: a guide for health care Organizations—IHI white paper.* Cambridge, Massachusetts: Institute for Health Improvement.

Zestcott, C. A., Blair, I. V., & Stone, J. (2016). Examining the presence, consequences, and reduction of implicit bias in health care: a narrative review. *Group Processes & Intergroup Relations, 19*, 528–542.

SECTION 5:
The Australian and New Zealand Healthcare Systems

In this section:

Paramedics are a vital link in the healthcare system and often the first contact for patients in a health episode. It is therefore important for paramedics to understand where they fit within the complex healthcare system. The first chapter in the section explores how the paramedic profession evolved and discusses the variety of roles currently available to paramedics. The second chapter looks more specifically at patient demographics and ambulance service utilisation rates. This chapter also delves into the steps or stages a patient or caller goes through before calling for help and the reasoning behind it. Finally, it explains the triage and dispatch system and describes a fictitious ambulance call.

CHAPTER 9

The Paramedic Role in Healthcare

By Andrew McDonell

OVERVIEW

- Ambulance services are widely recognised as providing an emergency service to patients with life-threatening conditions.
- Providing safe transport to hospital in addition to providing emergency out-of-hospital care defines the paramedic role and distinguishes the role from that of other health professionals.
- Historically, the clinical emphasis of paramedic care has been on stabilising patients for rapid transport to hospital for definitive care.
- Ambulances staffed with two crew members are the primary method of service delivery in Australia and New Zealand, but this model is slowly changing.
- Paramedic scope of practice has increased significantly since 2000, but this is not as widely recognised among the public or other health professions.
- Ambulance workloads are increasing between 10% and 25% plus per annum. This growth is fuelled by patients suffering chronic conditions rather than the life-threatening emergencies traditionally associated with ambulance calls.
- New models of education, equipment and dispatch are being introduced by some ambulance services and governments to deal with the new caseload.
- Paramedics are state registered (Australia), educated in universities and graduating with qualifications equivalent to other health professionals.
- The traditional 'Respond, treat and transport' model of ambulance care is being replaced with 'Treat and leave' models.
- There is a rapidly growing emphasis on keeping patients out of hospital. This requires paramedics to engage in treatment pathways other than transport to the emergency department (ED).
- The complex interactions created when patients have multiple chronic conditions and need to be directed to the safest treatment pathway is increasing the complexity of paramedic clinical decision-making.
- Paramedics are under pressure to integrate with other healthcare providers and provide patient care in non-emergency community settings.
- Paramedics are undertaking advanced clinical programs such as paramedic practitioner, community paramedicine and physician associate to meet the needs of low-acuity patients and fill gaps in remote/rural locations that have poor or no medical coverage.
- First responders from the community, volunteer organisations and fire services are now engaging with the traditional ambulance role of responding to health emergencies.

 CASE STUDY

Case 14519, 0947 hrs.

Dispatch details: A 74-year-old female with chest pain. The patient has a cardiac history.

Initial presentation: The patient is sitting in a chair on the front verandah as the crew arrive. As they approach she coughs vigorously and produces a large volume of purulent mucus that she spits delicately into a tissue. She tells the paramedics she has had a chest cold with thick spit for about a week but today when she stands up her chest hurts, and it hurts more when she coughs.

Introduction

Paramedicine has come a long way from the ambulance services of the 19th and 20th century providing basic first aid and patient transport services to that of being a recognised profession and essential member of the healthcare community. The role of the paramedic is dynamic and roles are continually evolving to meet the needs of an ageing population and modernisation of the health workforce. The demand for the expertise of paramedics is on the rise and positions for paramedics have risen by 81.6% between 2011 and 2016 (Health and Community Services Workforce Council, 2017).

Paramedics are required to make decisions under intense time pressures, with incomplete (and often misleading) information, and with strong emotional and social input from the patient's family and friends (Shields & Flin, 2012; Wyatt, 2003). To the untrained observer, making clinical decisions probably does not appear to be all that difficult: collect all the information you need, compare it to the known causes of diseases, match it to an appropriate protocol/guideline that is based on good scientific evidence and follow the steps described in the protocol. In reality, however, there is well-documented evidence that novice clinicians across a number of medical professions struggle to integrate their knowledge into an effective decision-making strategy (Hoben et al., 2007; Patel & Groen, 1986; Rikers et al., 2004). For paramedic students the challenge is even greater: working with limited diagnostic tools and in a public setting, paramedics are rarely presented with a structured and linear form of clinical information (Shaban et al., 2004).

The value of the paramedic in the ongoing care of patients and the ability of the paramedic to contribute to patient outcomes are becoming well recognised. Gone are the days of paramedics 'dropping' a patient off at the hospital ED and just leaving. Paramedics are providing comprehensive clinical handovers, now staying longer and continuing patient treatment within the hospital setting. Changes to guidelines have resulted in direct admissions of patients to stroke units, cardiac catheter labs and trauma centres based on clinical diagnosis and treatment by paramedics (Flynn et al., 2017).

While decision-making is essential within an emergency out-of-hospital environment, the recognition of paramedics to make solid evidence-based patient assessment resulting in considered patient management delivery has resulted in the expansion of paramedicine into a wide range of health areas, particularly, general practice, community health and rural healthcare (Wankhade, 2016).

This chapter is going to explore how ambulance services, paramedics and paramedicine have evolved over time. The practice of paramedicine is changing as the profession becomes more holistic and integrates into the ever-changing health system. This is an exciting time, particularly for student and graduate paramedics.

The roles of ambulance services and paramedics in Australia and New Zealand

Traditional role—emergency response and transport to hospital

Like police and fire services, ambulances are a conspicuous part of nearly every community across the globe. Although the levels of skill, training and equipment may vary, the common public perception of ambulance services regardless of where they are based is that ambulances respond to medical emergencies (Lowthian et al., 2011a; Sheather, 2009). Tied intrinsically to this is the notion that ambulances provide rapid transport to hospital for definitive care. For paramedics managing and working in ambulance services it is becoming increasingly obvious that the role of the modern ambulance service will need to extend beyond this paradigm, but for those outside the profession the transport role of ambulance services remains firmly entrenched (see Box 9.1).

Development of ambulance services

Ambulance services in Commonwealth countries share a remarkably similar history. Most started after the 1880s and were established by the early 1900s as small teams of mostly volunteers (there were some paid staff by the early 20th century) trained and coordinated by charitable organisations

> **PRACTICE TIP**
>
> 'They put wheels on ambulances for a reason'. This is an axiom reminding paramedic students that transport is an integral part of 'ambulance care', but is it a part of paramedic care? This is changing with more advanced treatment and changes to scope of practice—paramedic practitioners! One day, paramedics might be presenting patients not only to doctors but to a range of advanced providers such as paramedic practitioners, nurse practitioners or physician associates.

> **PRACTICE TIP**
>
> 'Diesel with the foot flat down is a great paramedic drug'. This is often quoted by senior paramedics and indicative of an era when the only response to a patient's clinical deterioration was to transport them to the hospital faster. Is it appropriate in modern paramedicine?

BOX 9.1 Respond, treat and transport

The traditional 'Respond, treat and transport' model of ambulance services is not as universally applicable to the modern paramedic role as it once was. As ambulance services engage other treatment pathways, the pressure on decision-making increases: paramedics now need to decide which pathway other than transport to ED is most suitable for the patient. This may include arranging appointments in a general practice or referral to extended care paramedics (ECPs)/prescribing paramedic practitioner (PPPs).

or local community groups. The Order of St John established the St John Ambulance Association (training branch) and St John Ambulance Brigade (uniformed branch) which formed the majority of early ambulance services. There were exceptions to the St John domination such as the Civil Ambulance and Transport Brigade in New South Wales (which later amalgamated with St John to form the Ambulance Transport Corps) (Ambulance Service of NSW, 2015), City Ambulance Transport Brigade later to become the Queensland Ambulance Transport Brigade (Queensland Ambulance Service, 2017a) and Wellington Free Ambulance in New Zealand (Wellington Free Ambulance, 2014).

Australia

Based in the major cities, these early ambulance transport services did not lack work—traumatic and environmental injuries caused by increasing industrialisation were all too common—and the services quickly grew in size (Howie-Willis, 2009). With only rudimentary first-aid skills and virtually no medical equipment, the role of these early ambulance services was solely response and transport. In fact, an ability to operate the horse or vehicle that carried the patient was often the only essential qualification considered for the role. With most ambulance services structured along military command models (members of the Army Medical Corps often contributed to staffing), the progression from volunteers to paid employees saw the term 'Ambulance driver' evolve into 'Ambulance officer' and then to 'Paramedic', the common descriptor of the 'professional' role today.

The fundamental responsibility of providing an emergency response and transport function remains the most obvious and distinctive role of ambulance services worldwide. In Australia and New Zealand, this transport function has not only shaped public perception of the paramedic role, but also influenced the way governments have chosen to develop, fund and use ambulance services. In the early days, it was not uncommon for more than one organisation to offer ambulance services within a major city and support volunteer services in outlying areas. The various ambulance services were eventually incorporated into single statewide systems under government control (Howie-Willis, 2009). This process of consolidation occurred as early as 1919 in New South Wales and the 1950s in South Australia. Over the succeeding decades the states gradually absorbed within their borders any autonomous regions that delivered independent ambulance services and by the 1980s all Australian states and territories operated statewide ambulance services that recruited and trained their own staff, selected their own equipment and developed their own practice guidelines; largely in isolation from the other states. The model varies slightly in Western Australia and the Northern Territory, where the government contracts the delivery of ambulance services to St John Ambulance Australia. Overall state ambulance services represent a single organisation staffed by paramedics in the major cities, large rural centres and towns, with volunteer support in smaller regional locations.

New Zealand

The New Zealand ambulance services, much like Australia, started as local volunteer organisations but from 1957 the Hospital Act required hospitals to provide an ambulance service to their catchment area. Hospitals gradually contracted the role to the Order of St John, which now provides services to nearly 90% of the New Zealand population. In the Greater Wellington and Wairarapa regions, the Wellington Free Ambulance Service provides coverage.

Significant advancement

In the late 1960s and 1970s a number of research studies suggested that more advanced out-of-hospital emergency care of cardiac and trauma patients could dramatically improve patient outcomes (Boyd & Cowley, 1983; Pantridge & Geddes, 1967). In some countries this led to an increase in the level of patient care, with medical practitioners placed in ambulances, and this remains a standard in many parts of Europe including Germany and France (Dick, 2003). However, in Australia and New Zealand the system remained mostly one of taking the patient to the doctor at the hospital. Yet there were gradual changes in the education and scope of practice of the then ambulance officers, and over the past two decades the emergence of the term 'paramedic' (meaning: alongside medicine) reflects a shift from simply transporting the injured and acutely ill to treating them. In addition, faced with growing demand, a number of ambulance services have contracted the routine transport of low-acuity patients (e.g. transfers between hospitals) to private ambulance services in an attempt to quarantine their own resources for emergency responses.

Regardless of these changes, the emergency response and transport function remain the most visible and defined role provided by the various ambulance services operating in Australia and New Zealand. When patients phone for an ambulance their expectation is that a crew of two paramedics will attend, treat them to varying degrees and then transport them to hospital (see Box 9.1).

Terminology and title

In the past, there were no standards of practice, which resulted in a lack of consistency in the terms used to describe ambulance personnel and their level of training. During 2018, Australia established the Paramedicine Registration Board of Australia to nationally regulate paramedics and clinical practice. Registration of paramedics in New Zealand followed shortly after in 2020.

Stretcher bearers and ambulance drivers

These terms are hopefully well and truly defunct! Originally, the terms evolved from the military to describe the soldiers who collected and carried injured soldiers to aid posts. 'Ambulance driver' was used to describe the driver of the horse-drawn ambulances used in the military (Wallis & Boyle, 2014). The terminology transferred into civilian usage.

In New South Wales the term 'stretcher bearer' was used until the early 1900s and was replaced with 'ambulance driver' after the introduction of the horse-drawn ambulance fleet (Ambulance Service of NSW, 2015). Queensland used the term 'bearer' to describe rank. A person commenced as a bearer, progressed to a senior bearer, with the highest rank being a senior bearer driver. This terminology was phased out in the 1990s with the formation of the Queensland Ambulance Service (Queensland Ambulance Service, 2017b) (see Fig 9.1).

The term ambulance driver appears to be an accepted term worldwide for a person who works in an ambulance. Within Australasia, ambulance driver appears to have been used in all ambulance services well into the 1970s. The phasing out of the term seemed to come out of a report written

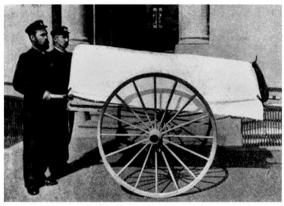

Figure 9.1
Brisbane's first paid stretcher bearers, employed by the City Ambulance Transport Brigade. Stretcher bearers rode to casualties on ponies, provided first aid and transported patients in a covered litter to hospital. Today paramedics respond in ambulances, have university education and advanced medical equipment and treatment protocols.
Source: State Library of Queensland and John Oxley Library.

by a Victorian Surgeon Gordon Trinca reviewing traumatic road accidents. Within the text the terms 'ambulance driver' and, for the first time, 'ambulance officer' were used interchangeably. This was the first time that ambulance drivers were recognised as providing patient care. It is not clear when ambulance officer became common usage, but it seems to have happened after industrial action resulting in a strike by ambulance drivers in 1972 by the Ambulance Employees Association of Victoria which won the establishment of an 'Ambulance Officers' Training Centre—'The AOTC' (Wilde, 1999) in Melbourne.

Unfortunately, the curse of the term of 'ambulance driver' continues to haunt modern-day paramedics!

First responder

The term 'first responder' generally refers to first-aid–trained or medically trained personnel (often volunteers) sent to emergency medical cases as part of a coordinated response. In some areas this includes fire crews trained in first aid, while in outlying areas it can include volunteer first-aiders registered with their local ambulance service. The term is sometimes used to include first-aid–trained bystanders. There is no agreed-upon definition of the role or scope of practice for first responders, but it is generally limited to basic care of the unconscious patient (oropharyngeal airway, bag-valve-mask ventilation and CPR) and basic assessment of the conscious patient (conscious state, pulse and blood pressure), although in some areas it includes application of automated external defibrillators (AEDs). Participants in volunteer first-responder programs come from a range of backgrounds and occupational groups. Traditionally, programs using community volunteers were more common in rural and remote areas.

Dispatch methods for first responders are evolving along with paramedic practice, aided by the use of technology. Through the use of app technology on mobile phones, the organisation and availability of first responders is significantly changing. No longer do first-responder teams need to be systematically organised into teams or groups. This technology allows individuals, who are registered as 'trusted responders', to be sent to a location to provide immediate first aid, CPR and/or defibrillation at the same time as an ambulance is being dispatched. This voluntary system of individual dispatch was first implemented in Europe and the United Kingdom (UK) with great success. This model is presently being rolled out across Australia and New Zealand (Ambulance Victoria, 2018).

Ambulance officer

As touched on earlier in 'Stretcher bearers and ambulance drivers', the term ambulance officer appears to have evolved in the quest for professionalism and through industrial action. In some parts of Australia and New Zealand, ambulance officer is used depending on the person's clinical skills and education, as well their role and legal responsibilities.

For a while, in Australian states and New Zealand regions the terms ambulance officer and paramedic were completely synonymous. Over time, the term ambulance officer has been passed down to volunteers who perform ambulance duties. The term paramedic has become the practice level of university graduates with a bachelor or higher academic degree. With the introduction of professional registration in Australia, the term paramedic is protected and can only be used by registered practitioners. This is presently not yet the case in New Zealand, although the profession is actively working towards paramedic registration.

The notation ambulance officer is still widely used, particularly in Australian and New Zealand ambulance services which use a large number of volunteers to provide direct response or support paramedics.

Paramedic

National registration in Australia protects the use of the name 'paramedic' for use by registered practitioners only (Paramedicine Registration Board of Australia, 2018a). In New Zealand, all paramedic positions are essentially based on ambulance services and unregulated. Agreement between the two major New Zealand ambulance services (Order of St John and Wellington Free Ambulance) has led to the development of a standardised professional role description. In North America the term denotes a higher level of training than the term 'emergency medical technician (EMT)'.

Generally, in Australia, the term paramedic describes a person who has completed a bachelor degree or higher qualification in paramedicine or equivalent approved academic qualification, registered with the Paramedicine Registration Board and practises paramedicine within the context of clinical, administration, academic and/or research communities.

Advanced life support (ALS) or advanced paramedic

Introduced during the early 2000s, this level of practice recognises a higher level of skills (e.g. intravenous [IV] access, use of adrenaline in cardiac arrest, IV analgesia, thrombolysis, 12-lead ECG, insertion of subglottic airways). The term was introduced to differentiate between basic life support (BLS) ambulance officers/paramedics and ALS paramedics.

ALS has become a clumsy term and largely redundant as university-based training has made ALS skills the basic level of care provided by paramedics. When we refer to paramedics in this text we infer that they are university qualified and accredited with ALS skills, although in some areas the descriptor BLS is still in place for paramedics with less training.

Critical care paramedic (CCP), intensive care paramedic (ICP) and mobile intensive care ambulance (MICA) paramedic

These terms generally refer to paramedics who have undergone additional postgraduate education after practising as a paramedic for a period of time. The selection and training of CCPs, ICPs and MICA paramedics was traditionally conducted by the various ambulance services. Training has mainly moved into a postgraduate model provided by universities, with standards determined by the services (see Fig 9.2).

These paramedics practise at an advanced clinical level and provide management techniques underpinned by advanced pharmacology (including a range of IV infusions), advanced airway skills often with anaesthetic skills, fluid resuscitation including blood transfusions in an out-of-hospital setting. The difference between an ALS paramedic and CCP/ ICP/MICA paramedic is in the depth of knowledge

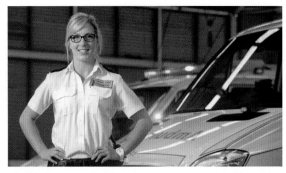

Figure 9.2
Intensive care and critical care paramedics provide advanced clinical skills such as inducing coma for endotracheal intubation, gastric intubation, thoracotomy, advanced drug therapy and administering blood transfusions in time-critical patients, enhancing care given by ambulance paramedics.
Source: https://www.examiner.com.au/story/2191567/ hard-work-study-key-intensive-care-paramedic/

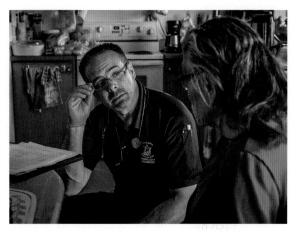

Figure 9.3
Are extended care paramedics and paramedic practitioners the future of response or preventing emergency ambulance response? Research now acknowledges that many patients who receive a fully equipped, double-crewed ambulance response do not need one.
Source: Courtesy of BC Emergency Health Services.

and associated problem-solving, clinical judgment and application of advanced clinical practice.

Extended care paramedic (ECP)

This term refers to paramedics who respond to cases of low acuity where there is a strong possibility that the patient can be treated and left at home or referred to other healthcare providers. Based on a UK model, this role is unique in that it does not intrinsically link ambulance response with patient transport, but aims to treat people in their home and avoid transfer to hospital.

ECP models vary from those providing direct patient care within a community setting, providing an alternative patient care pathway for well-defined predictable conditions to those collaborating in a multidisciplinary team, to providing out-of-hospital care to complex patients who have opted not to go to hospital (see Fig 9.3). This area of work sees paramedics forming close working relationships with a range of health providers including general practitioners, medical specialists, district nurses and palliative care teams providing high-quality care without hospitalisation (Hoyle et al., 2012).

Most ambulance services in Australia and New Zealand are now using this model. The qualifications to operate as an ECP vary considerably between services with some requiring an ICP qualification, while others do not. The scope of practice also varies widely. Within the Australasian context, success of the ECP programs is usually measured by the number of patients not transported to the ED, rather than patient outcomes (Boyle, 2017).

Internationally, roles such as ECP have evolved into more autonomous providers such as paramedic

practitioners in the UK and community paramedics in North America. These practitioner roles have given paramedics a career structure that allows public and private practice, with advanced legal authority to issue prescriptions, order tests and delegate treatment (Andalo, 2018). It will be interesting to see what happens in the next few years within the Australian and New Zealand context.

Funding of ambulance services and public health

Although ambulance services in Australia and New Zealand are based in the public health system (see Box 9.2) and funded almost entirely by government (see Box 9.3), the phrase 'public health' as it is used here refers to the concept of promoting and protecting (in addition to treating) the health of the community. The effectiveness of public health programs can be seen by the reductions in the number of cases of lung cancer and heart disease; for instance, due to research and education into factors such as smoking and diet (see Box 9.4).

Given the perceived role of ambulance services in responding to health emergencies, it is not difficult to see the disconnect that exists between the role the ambulance service can provide and the aims of public health to improve the social, political and economic factors that cause illness (Rothstein, 2002). The relationship could be described as one of reactivity, in which ambulance services respond to patients for whom public health initiatives have failed to prevent illness, injury or disability. Yet the role the ambulance service and paramedics plays

BOX 9.2 The public-sector ambulance model in Australia

- Health is a state responsibility.
- Ambulance services are organised at a state/territory level.
  - Each state/territory has an ambulance authority (a public agency).
  - Most have an Ambulance Act.
  - Registration of paramedics is a Commonwealth role, but impacts on state operations.
  - Each has a government department that sets standards, monitors ambulance performance and provides the bulk of service funding.
  - Public hospitals are also organised at a state level. All states/territories have a government department that sets standards, monitors hospital performance and provides the bulk of hospital funding.
- Paramedics in Australia are registered by the Paramedicine Registration Board of Australia, and the determination of practice of a paramedic is regulated under this body, authorised by national law ensuring the community is protected.
- The various state/territory ambulance authorities meet collaboratively under the banner of the Council of Ambulance Authorities to progress their mutual objectives.
- Paramedics Australasia is the professional organisation for paramedics.
- Paramedics are industrially represented by a range of unions such as the Ambulance Employees of Australia, United Voice Union, Health Services Union and Transport Workers Union of Australia and come under the banner of the National Council of Ambulance Unions.

BOX 9.3 Ambulance funding in Australasia

How the funds for the various Australian and New Zealand ambulance services are collected varies slightly (taxes, levies, subscription), but the services are essentially funded from the public purse. Interestingly, with the exception of Queensland and Tasmania there is still an expectation to recover fees from patients or insurers to a much greater extent than in public hospitals or other emergency services. Combined with a governance model that links the services directly back to the responsible minister, this has ambulance services competing with other health and emergency services for funding. It also makes them subject to political pressures and policies that may not reflect the best direction for the individual ambulance services. As an example of the funding base provided to Australian ambulance services, in the 2016/17 financial year, Ambulance Victoria obtained its revenue as follows: government contribution, $676 million; transport fees, $185 million; membership, $93.6 million; a total operating cost of over $955 million or $153 per citizen (Productivity Commission, 2018).

early administration of an external defibrillator. Increases in paramedic knowledge and education have resulted in increased skills expanding the paramedic's role to include treatments ranging from early post-resuscitation care to the use of advanced airway care such as rapid sequence intubation and the use of intensive-care-level drug therapy such as inotropes. During 2016/2017, there was a significant increase in out-of-hospital cardiac arrest survival in Australia, with up to 80% of patients who had a ventricular fibrillation cardiac arrest in the presence of a paramedic being discharged from hospital (Andrew et al., 2017).

The increased prevalence of chronic diseases across the community raises new challenges in both diagnosis and management (see Fig 9.4). Identifying patients who can be managed in the community is a clinical decision that many paramedics struggle with: as a profession, paramedicine has not traditionally engaged in chronic disease management and it remains underrepresented in many vocational and tertiary courses. Changes in paramedic practice is occurring with the introduction of ECP practice and consideration of introducing a prescribing paramedic practitioner model.

in the public health system is far more significant than simply transport and could be described as proactive: for example, ambulance services have been instrumental in initiatives such as the chain of survival, which has dramatically improved rates of survival from cardiac arrest (Victorian Ambulance Cardiac Arrest Registry, 2017; Nolan et al., 2006). Developed in the mid-1980s, the first chain of survival concept saw the role of the ambulance paramedics as providing a quick response and the

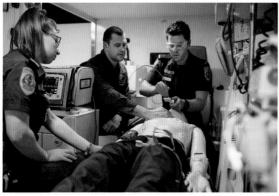

Figure 9.4
While the education and equipping of paramedics focuses on critical events such as cardiac arrests, car accidents and terrorist attacks, the vast majority of paramedic work involves responding to patients suffering from the complications of chronic diseases. *Source: Courtesy of Monash University.*

Community education

Although early ambulance services grew out of organisations offering first-aid education, very few retain significant public education programs. The emphasis on the emergency response and transport role has seen most modern ambulance services focus their resources in this area and move away from providing first-aid education to the public. This is despite the experience and credibility that paramedics could provide in first-aid training. The approach to providing community education as a public health service (e.g. road accident education), a means of improving emergency care (e.g. CPR and AED programs) or a funding stream is inconsistent across the ambulance services in Australia and New Zealand.

Workplace culture

The focus on transport has literally shaped the paramedic workforce: the historical need to load patients onto manually operated stretchers saw ambulance services initially employ an all-male workforce. This contrasted with the long-term recruitment of female nursing staff in hospitals and further differentiated the role of ambulance services until the early 1990s, when female paramedics began to be recruited in significant numbers. Up to 64% of undergraduate enrolments in paramedic courses were female in 2009 (Williams, 2009). For the first time, during 2016/2017, the number of females recruited into Ambulance Victoria was at 56.7%, and government policy required Ambulance Victoria to recruit a 50/50 gender split during the 2017/2018 period. Presently, Ambulance Victoria has more female paramedics than male (Hennessy, 2017). This is significant, as traditionally women were completely excluded from the ambulance workforce and only 10 years previously in 2008, the ambulance workforce was 80.3% male (Australian Bureau of Statistics [ABS], 2008). It is unfortunate that only data from Ambulance Victoria was available, as it would have been interesting to look at the changes in gender ratios in the ambulance workforce across Australia and New Zealand.

The shift to university-based education has affected workplace culture. Given that a large number of senior paramedics have been educated within the vocational model (usually a diploma), new university-trained paramedics holding a bachelor's degree are educated to a 'higher' level. However, the current university model is struggling to provide students with the necessary quality and amount of clinical placement experience, and this has implications for ambulance service planning and delivery. New graduates tend to need clinical support for longer periods, so graduate programs and 'on-road' clinical supervision have become a priority. Paramedics generally work in teams of two, and effective communication and consultation are essential. The disparate nature of the old and new staff often means that team members use different knowledge bases, communication styles and decision-making tools.

Ambulance services have been slow to embrace postgraduate education, with most failing to link career progression with formal qualifications. The result is a workplace where the majority of senior clinical staff are vocationally trained males over the age of 50 with extensive clinical experience, while the majority of new staff are university-trained females under the age of 35 with a mix of clinical experience (Williams et al., 2010).

In recent years growth of paramedic employment opportunities outside of government-sponsored ambulance services have been slow but it is steadily increasing. Companies that provide medical services to industrial sites, sporting events and festivals, as well as private patient transport operators, are offering paramedic employment and these new operators are likely to create their own workplace cultures that may not be consistent with those in the larger ambulance services. Some paramedics are already working for a number of different employers, both public and private.

Professionalism, regulation and professional standards

The notion of a 'profession' grew from occupational guilds and early universities and was the recognition that those in a particular profession possessed a unique body of knowledge and a defined role (Cruess et al., 2002). Since then, the term has grown to include the concepts of a code of conduct, membership of a professional body and regulation of practice (Sheather, 2009).

While it may appear pedantic to some observers, the argument over professionalism in paramedic practice actually has significant implications for how paramedics reach clinical decisions. The increasing complexity of paramedic practice over the past decade has inspired a number of discussions that suggest paramedicine should be considered as a profession (Grantham, 2004; Wyatt, 1998). This has been supported by the shift to university-based education, which has standardised the level of knowledge within paramedic practice, and the development of a professional body of knowledge through research. In other health professions, the professional organisation defines the necessary training, code of conduct, professional behaviours and required body of knowledge.

Within Australia during 2018, a significant step forward in professionalism of paramedics was made. Paramedics became nationally registered and a Paramedicine Registration Board of Australia added to Australian Health Professional Registration Authority (AHPRA) (Paramedicine Registration Board of Australia, 2018b). As a result, only a person who appears on the national register of practitioners will be able to call themselves a 'paramedic' as per national law. The code of conduct of registered paramedics will define the professional behaviours expected of paramedics, what education standard is required and the expectations of the development of a specific body of knowledge (Paramedicine Registration Board of Australia, 2018b). At this stage, paramedics in New Zealand remain subject to the regulation of the various employers of the industry.

Paramedic education

The past two decades have seen a significant shift in the way paramedics themselves are educated. Until the early 2000s paramedics were recruited and trained by their local ambulance service. This vocational model involved as few as 4 weeks' training and rarely more than 20 weeks' training, and recruited workers mainly from outside the health sector. It provided each ambulance service with a workforce that identified strongly with local guidelines and was especially reliant on protocols to guide decision-making. The shift to undergraduate and postgraduate paramedic degrees has substantially increased the knowledge base upon which paramedics can draw to solve clinical problems based on evidence-based research (see Box 9.5).

The future paramedic role

Over the past 30 years, although paramedic practice has embraced significantly higher standards of education and practice to move far beyond the traditional role (Brown, 2017), the underlying responsibilities of responding to health emergencies and providing transport to hospital have remained

> ### BOX 9.5 Evidence-based practice
>
> The clinical practice guidelines used by ambulance services are increasingly being scrutinised to ensure they are supported by scientific evidence. As a result, a number of long-held ambulance guidelines have been questioned and either modified or discontinued. Reporting of incidents under a patient-safety framework is designed to reduce the allocation of blame onto individuals and determine whether systematic errors were the cause. This proactive management of adverse incidents and the desire to maximise learning from incidents contrast with the clinical auditing methods traditionally used by some ambulance services.

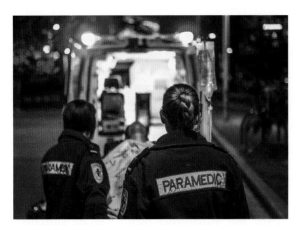

Figure 9.5
The media portrays paramedic work as a constant parade of acutely ill patients trapped in precarious situations requiring the crew to intervene immediately. However, most patients are suffering from a combination of chronic illnesses, which alone or in combination may be the cause of the current health emergency. To determine a safe treatment plan requires careful collection and sorting of symptoms, vital signs, medical history and the patient's own description of their condition.
Source: Courtesy of Ambulance Victoria.

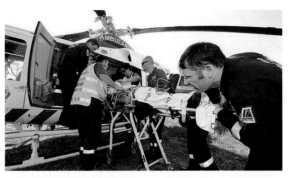

Figure 9.6
The demand for ambulance services in Australia is increasing between 8% and 12.5% per annum and in New Zealand by up to 25% between 2016 and 2017. This seems to affect response times.
Source: Courtesy of Ambulance Victoria.

largely intact. However, this narrow definition of the paramedic role is significantly changing as the profession has gained national registration and postgraduate education expands. How the role of the paramedic will actually change will depend on responses to pressures both within the profession and externally.

Internal pressures

Ambulance services are being forced to react to two dominant changes: increasing workloads and decreasing patient acuity (see Fig 9.5). In Australia, demand for services has increased by between 8% and 12.5% per year since the early 2000s (Productivity Commission, 2018). This is similar to changes faced overseas: demand increased by 10.4% in the UK in 2015/2016 (Comptroller and Auditor General, 2017) and by 25% in New Zealand in 2016/2017 (Order of St John, 2017).

The increase in workload is placing pressure on the politically important performance measure of response times. Although there is no scientific data to support a specific target figure for response times (see Fig 9.6) the public highly values reporting of the percentage of cases attended within the nominated target time and this is therefore a significant performance indicator for ambulance services. Increasing workloads invariably lead to longer response times unless more ambulances or first responders are introduced into service (Campbell & Elington, 2016).

This rise in demand is commonly attributed to the demands of an ageing population and escalating rates of diseases such as obesity and diabetes (Comptroller and Auditor General, 2017). The proportion of Australians aged 65 years or older rose from just 4% in 1901 to 13.5% by 2010 and is estimated to reach 21% by 2041 (ABS, 2011). With a strong correlation between age and disability (88% of Australians aged 90 have a disability compared with 40% aged 65–69) this is certainly one factor in increasing workloads, but it is not the only reason. The increasing workload is actually multifactorial, with decreasing out-of-hours access to GPs, well-publicised delays at EDs, public awareness campaigns into the dangers of stroke (Bray et al., 2011) and chest pain as well as changes to pricing for ambulance attendance all contributing to some degree (Lowthian et al., 2011a).

Simultaneously, improvements in public health strategies, medications and motor vehicle safety have reduced the frequency of life-threatening emergencies that have traditionally been identified as core ambulance cases. For example, male death rates from all diseases of the circulatory system decreased from 1020 deaths per 100,000 in 1968 to 234 deaths per 100,000 in 2008, while standardised death rates from motor vehicle crashes fell from 14.8% in 2000 to 9.6% in 2009 (ABS, 2011). A proportion of these decreases are almost certainly attributable to improvements in the out-of-hospital care provided by paramedics: for example, the survival rate for out-of-hospital cardiac arrest has improved significantly (Victorian Ambulance Cardiac Arrest Registry, 2017).

Clearly, the improvements in some areas of public health are shifting the bulk of paramedic cases from acute to chronic care (Lowthian et al., 2011b). This is further reflected in the evolution of dispatch codes used by some modern ambulance services. Whereas every call for an ambulance was once considered to be an emergency, most ambulance services now recognise that even using a highly risk-adverse triage tool, up to one-third of those who call for an ambulance can be immediately classified as not needing one so urgently that lights and sirens are used in the response. In 2017, the Queensland Ambulance Service responded to 593,206 incidents that were considered to need a lights-and-sirens response and 236,240 cases that were considered to be non-urgent (Department of Health, Queensland, 2017). Over the years it has been recognised that in reality, fewer than 10% of patients are suffering the life-threatening medical events for which the ambulance has been strongly identified (National Health Service [NHS], 2006).

External pressures

The wider public healthcare system is facing demographic and financial challenges. Designed for a past generation, the system is a complex and fragmented collection of services and sectors that lie across multiple layers of government and too often fail to integrate and coordinate effectively (Australian Institute of Health and Welfare [AIHW], 2016; Bray et al., 2011; National Health and Hospitals Reform Commission [NHHRC], 2009). Similar to the ambulance service, the system is effective for those suffering acute or emergency problems that can be resolved quickly, but it was not structured to meet the needs of people suffering multiple complex health and social problems (AIHW, 2016; NHHRC, 2009). Unlike the ambulance system, however, the hospital system has passed saturation point and the lack of beds and staff is forcing changes beyond simply trying to increase hospital capacity.

The most significant of these changes is the attempt to manage chronic illness in the community rather than in hospitals (AIHW, 2016; NHHRC, 2009). This community-based reform is challenging ambulance services to integrate with the wider healthcare system and is changing the fundamental nature of some ambulance responses.

Australian and New Zealand governments are seeking to reduce stresses on the hospital system. During 2014 Health Workforce Australia (HWA) commissioned a report evaluating an extended care paramedic trial which was funded by the Commonwealth of Australia and took part in all states and territories of Australia except Victoria (Centre for Health Service Development [CHSD], 2014).

The report demonstrated that paramedics could provide assessment and management of people with minor illness/injury and chronic illness across a range of diverse communities' settings, resulting in people staying in their community and not being unnecessarily transferred to hospital (CHSD, 2014).

In New Zealand, in an effort to avoid transport to hospital, two versions of the ECP concept were evaluated for their effectiveness and safety, while St John in Horowhenua and the Wellington Free Ambulance Service adopted similar models after effective trials (Hoyle et al., 2012). Both St John and Wellington Free Ambulance use ECPs as part of their normal dispatch process.

The Victorian and Queensland Ambulance Services are using a modified version of the call-taking process to refer patients identified as low-acuity to other services without dispatching an ambulance at all. Queensland Ambulance Service introduced a Secondary Triage and Referral (STAR) system during 2011. STAR prevented, on average, 46 ambulance transports per week in the Brisbane region, a 53% improvement compared to when the system was first implemented (Toloo et al., 2012), while the Victorian Triage Referral Service has reduced ambulance dispatches by 11.9% (Eastwood et al., 2017).

Alternative paramedic roles

Before 2018, in both Australia and New Zealand the lack of a national standard for training and a scope of practice had largely limited the ability of other industries to engage in the skill set offered by paramedics. The national registration of paramedics in Australia is resolving many of the regulatory barriers and in the future paramedics are likely to find roles and employment outside of the ambulance service. The emphasis that paramedic training and experience places on trauma and acute illness will make paramedics ideally suited to many of these roles. However, the need to assess and manage chronic conditions, as well as to engage with other health providers, will require additional education to augment the current paramedic skill set. Evolving roles include the following.

Industrial paramedic

A number of companies in the mining sector and other industries employ paramedics on worksites, ships and offshore drilling platforms. This rapidly growing sector lacks consistent regulatory guidelines regarding what services it must provide and what skill sets and qualification are required.

Community paramedic

The role of community paramedic is generally targeted at remote and rural communities that cannot attract a higher level of permanent medical care. In many ways the role is similar to that of an ECP, but not quite a paramedic practitioner. The role includes primary assessment of acute and chronic conditions, and ongoing management where possible or referral to higher levels of care where required. In reality, the close-knit nature of many rural communities means paramedics already perform these roles, as well as assisting staff at local hospitals in times of need (Mulholland et al., 2009).

The evolution of the community paramedic appears to be similar to that of the paramedic practitioner in the UK (see below), but from a North American perspective. Between 2014 and 2016 an international curriculum was developed and based on the National Curriculum and Career Pathway—Community Paramedic, which provided a framework for paramedics to advance to high levels of medical education similar to or higher than that of 'nurse practitioners and physician assistants' via tertiary education qualifications progressing through bachelor, master and doctorate levels (O'Meara et al., 2014; Paramedic Health Solutions, 2016).

Paramedic practitioners

Initially known as emergency care practitioners, paramedic practitioners evolved in the UK against a background of change in primary care provision to avoid the apparent increased utilisation of emergency ambulance services, particularly in the after-hours settings during the early 2000s. These opportunities in primary care allowed for a change and extended scope of paramedic practitioners to provided medical care within the community and general practice. The paramedic practitioner meets the NHS aim of 'treating the right patients in the right place at the right time' (Woollard, 2016). It was quickly realised that in-service training within ambulance services could not meet the educational needs of an autonomous healthcare practitioner, and the education of paramedic practitioners was transferred to universities, initially at an honours level (paramedic practitioner), being expanded to a masters (advanced paramedic practitioner) and doctorate (consultant paramedic practitioner) (NHS, 2004; Woollard, 2016).

Paramedic practitioners in the UK work in a range of settings including ambulance services, private practice, GP surgeries, critical care, urgent care centres and for medical specialists (Brown, 2017). On 1 April 2018, paramedic practitioners in the UK were given prescribing rights as independent prescribers (Andalo, 2018). This means that paramedic practitioners no longer follow Ambulance service guidelines. Paramedic practitioners can also

order imaging and pathology to aid them in diagnosis, then can either treat or delegate treatment to other health providers.

Within Australia and New Zealand, little work has been done in implementing a paramedic practitioner model. In January 2015, the Victorian Government announced the formation of a committee to investigate a range of issues. One of the initiatives included providing advice on the potential introduction of paramedic practitioners in Victoria (Victorian Labor, 2015). As a member of the new committee, the Ambulance Employees Australia—Victoria (AEAV) set up a working party to investigate the introduction of a prescribing paramedic practitioner (PPP) and reported back to the Minister for Ambulance Services (Victoria) (McGhie, 2017).

The AEAV working party produced two reports which were submitted to the Victorian Government in December 2017 and January 2018 (Rafael & Ousley, 2017; McDonell, 2018). The reports defined a PPP as follows:

A paramedic practitioner is a paramedic who has undergone top up education to be able to: order and interpret tests (pathology/imaging), perform physical examination, prescribe medications (including restricted drugs), refer to specialists, allied health and provide or delegate treatment in any health environment.

(Rafael & Ousley, 2017).

Scope of practice for the PPPs would include practising in a range of clinical environments similar to that of the UK and undertaking master (prescribing paramedic practitioner) and doctorate (consultant paramedic practitioner) academic programs.

Physician associate (PA)/rural paramedic practitioner (PA/RPP)

This physician assistant/associate is a role that frees up medical practitioners by allowing physicians to delegate a range of care, patient groups and medical/surgical procedures to PAs. PAs are members of the medical profession and conduct patient assessments, prescribe medications, order tests, diagnose and conduct or delegate patient care to other health providers (such as junior doctors, nurses or nursing assistants). Traditional professional roles are strongly guarded in medicine and, despite the success of the role of physician assistant (North American terminology) or physician associate (New Zealand and UK terminology) in other countries, Australia and New Zealand have struggled to introduce this role into their healthcare systems. In Australia, PAs practise mainly in Queensland, with a scattering practising within the private sector in a variety of locations around Australia (Murray & O'Kane, 2014). In New Zealand, a trial in three sites across the North Island commenced in 2012. As there were no domestic academic programs in New Zealand, the trial was restricted to PAs trained in the United States. The trial appears to have been successful; however, integration of a PA model into healthcare has not occurred on a large scale (Gammelin, 2014).

Within Australia, a number of paramedics have completed PA training. Reaburn and colleagues (2017) proposed a future model of care where experienced paramedics undertake postgraduate PA education to qualify as a rural paramedic practitioner (RPP). Based in rural and remote locations with low emergency workload, the RPP would always be able to be dispatched to emergency care and but in their downtime would be able to provide in-hospital/health service/general practice patient care and visit patients within their community. Three key treatment pathways for an RPP would be:

1. treat and leave
2. treat and refer
3. treat/retrieve and admit.

It is argued that the RPP model instead of a non-paramedic PA model could be built upon existing paramedic services that already exist in rural and remote locations, rather than recruiting health professions to that location. The RPP builds on existing paramedic knowledge and the addition of PA medical education, producing a provider that would straddle medical and paramedical domains: traditional dispatch with community, primary care and hospital patient care services (Reaburn et al., 2017).

Emergency management/humanitarian aid/disaster paramedic

The use of paramedics in responses to humanitarian disasters and providing emergency management is increasing. This probably reflects the usefulness of the paramedic skill set, but since some of the required knowledge and skills lie outside the traditional paramedic role, additional training in areas such as wound care, infection control and public health will be required if paramedics are to operate effectively in this role. However, with paramedics expanding their practice into roles such as extended care paramedic, paramedic practitioner, physician associate and rural paramedic practitioner, these positions would place paramedics in an ideal place to become more involved in emergency management and humanitarian roles.

Summary

The history of paramedic care has impacted strongly on the way governments are developing paramedic resources. The inherent link between emergency response and transport has also shaped the public's expectations of paramedic services. In addition, the way ambulance services have operated in the past has defined what paramedics expect their role to be in the future.

International and national health reforms are ongoing and are integrating ambulance services into the healthcare system in ways that were not perceived as little as a decade ago. The 'Respond, treat, leave or refer' reforms, and advanced paramedic practice (paramedic practitioner etc.) pose questions about not only education and equipment but also professional practice boundaries, accreditation and how paramedics interact with other health professionals. Paramedic registration will no doubt solve some of these perceived issues. None of these issues are insurmountable and whatever form the future paramedic role may take, it is almost certain that the need to make safe clinical decisions through effective reasoning is likely to increase as paramedics are faced with more complex patient problems and multiple treatment pathways. It is an exciting time.

References

Ambulance Victoria. (2018). *Life saving app set for 2018 release*. Press Release. Melbourne: Ambulance Victoria.

Ambulance Service of NSW. (2015). Celebrating 120 years. Sirens. April.

Andalo, D. (2018). Paramedics are now independent prescribers. *The Pharmaceutical Journal*, doi:10.1211/PJ.2018.20204628. April 3.

Andrew, E., Nehme, Z., Wolfe, R., Bernard, S., & Smith, K. (2017). Long-term survival following out-of-hospital cardiac arrest. *Heart (British Cardiac Society)*, *103*(14), 1104.

Australian Bureau of Statistics (ABS). (2008). *Health Care Delivery and Financing*. Year Book Australia. http://www.abs.gov.au/AUSSTATS/abs@.nsf/bb8db737e2af84b8ca2571780015701e/A50BD9743BF2733ACA2573D2001078D8?opendocument.

Australian Bureau of Statistics (ABS). (2011). *Life Expectancy Trends—Australia*. Canberra: Commonwealth of Australia. Retrieved from www.ausstats.abs.gov.au/ausstats/subscriber.nsf/LookupAttach/4102.0Publication23.03.112/$File/41020_Lifeexpectancy_Mar2011.pdf.

Australian Institute of Health and Welfare (AIHW). (2016). *Australian Health 2016. Australian Government*: https://www.aihw.gov.au/reports/australias-health/australias-health-2016/contents/summary.

Boyd, D. R., & Cowley, R. A. (1983). Comprehensive regional trauma/emergency medical services (EMS) delivery systems: the United States experience. *World Journal of Surgery, 7*(1), 149–157.

Boyle, M. (2017). Do we need extended care paramedics? *Australasian Journal of Paramedicine, 14*(1), Editorial.

Bray, J., Mosley, I., Barger, B., & Bladin, C. (2011). Stroke public awareness campaigns have increased ambulance dispatches for stroke in Melbourne, Australia. *Stroke; a Journal of Cerebral Circulation, 42*(11), 2154–2157.

Brown, P. (2017). A day in the life of a paramedic advanced clinical practitioner in primary care. *Journal of Paramedic Practice*, https://doi.org/10.12968/jpar.2017.9.9.378. September.

Campbell, A., & Elington, M. (2016). Reducing time to first on scene: an ambulance community first responder scheme. *Emergency Medicine International, 2016*, 1915895. doi:10.1155/2016/1915895. Published online 31 March.

Centre for Health Service Development (CHSD). 2014. HWA Expanded Scopes of practice program evaluation: extending the role of paramedics. *Final Report*. Australian Health Services Institute, University of Wollongong.

Comptroller and Auditor General (2017). NHS ambulance services. *National Audit Service: 11407 01/17 NAO*.

Cruess, S. R., Johnston, S., & Cruess, R. L. (2002). Professionalism for medicine: opportunities and obligations. *The Medical Journal of Australia, 177*(4), 208–211.

Department of Health (Queensland Health), (2017). *Queensland Ambulance Service Public Performance Indications*. www.ambulance.qld.gov.au.

Dick, W. F. (2003). Anglo-American vs. Franco-German emergency medical services system. *Prehospital Disaster Medicine, 18*(1), 29–35.

Eastwood, K., Smith, K., Morgans, A., & Stoelwinder, J. (2017). Appropriateness of cases presenting in the emergency department following ambulance service secondary telephone triage: a retrospective cohort study. *BMJ Open, 7*(10), http://bmjopen.bmj.com/content/7/10/e016845.

Flynn, D., Francis, R., Robalino, S., Lally, J., Snooks, H., Rodgers, H., McClelland, G., Ford, G., & Price, C. (2017). A review of enhanced paramedic roles during and after hospital handover of stroke, myocardial infarction and trauma patients. *BMC Emergency Medicine*, doi:10.1186/s12873-017-0118-5.

Gammelin, E. (2014). Physician assistants in New Zealand. *Journal of the American Academy of Physician Assistants: November 2014*, 10–11. doi:10.1097/01.JAA.0000455651.96800.6a.

Grantham, H. (2004). Prehospital care as a profession—are we there yet? *Journal of Emergency Primary Health Care, 2*(2–1).

Health and Community Services Workforce Council. (2017). *Paramedic*. Information Pamphlet, Give a health career a go.

Hennessy, J. (2017). Questions taken on notice—ambulance service portfolio. *Public Accounts and Estimates Committee, Parliament of Victoria*; 17 May.

Hoben, K., Varley, R., & Cox, R. (2007). Clinical reasoning skills of speech and language therapy students. *International Journal of Language, Communication and Communication Disorders, 42*(S1), 123–135.

Howie-Willis, I. (2009). The Australian ambulance system: a historical perspective. In P. O'Meara & C. Grbich (Eds.), *Paramedics in Australia: contemporary challenges of practice*. Frenchs Forest: Pearson Education Australia.

Hoyle, S., Swain, A., Fake, P., & Larsen, P. (2012). Introduction of an extended care paramedic model in New Zealand. *Emergency Medicine Australasia: EMA, 24*, 652–656.

Lowthian, J., Jolley, D., Curtis, A., Currell, A., Cameron, P., Stoelwinder, J., & McNeil, J. (2011b). The challenges of population ageing: accelerating demand for emergency ambulance services by older patients, 1995–2015. *The Medical Journal of Australia, 194*(11).

Lowthian, J. A., Cameron, P. A., Stoelwinder, J. U., Curtis, A. J., Currell, A., Cooke, M., & McNeil, J. J. (2011a). Increasing utilisation of emergency ambulances. *Australian Health Review, 35*, 63–69.

McDonell, A. (2018). *Prescribing Paramedic Practitioners*. Short Submission to Department of Health and Human Services Victoria. Melbourne.

McGhie, S. (2017). Prescribing paramedic practitioner forum. Bulletin. 25 May. Ambulance Employees Australia—Victoria (AEAV).

Mulholland, P., O'Meara, P., Walker, J., Stirling, C., & Tourle, V. (2009). Multidisciplinary practice in action: the rural paramedic—it's not only lights and sirens. *Journal of Emergency Primary Health Care, 7*(2).

Murray, R., & O'Kane, D. (2014). Physician assistants in Australia. *JAAPA, 27*(7), 9–10.

National Health and Hospitals Reform Commission (NHHRC). (2009). *National Health and Hospitals Reform Commission Report*. Canberra: NHHRC.

National Health Service (NHS). (2004). *A career framework for the NHS*. London: MHS Modernisation Agency.

National Health Service (NHS). (2006). *NHS ambulance services … More than just patient transport*. London: NHS Confederation.

Nolan, J., Soar, J., & Eikeland, H. (2006). The chain of survival. *Resuscitation, 71*, 270–271.

O'Meara, P., Ruest, M., & Stirling, C. (2014). Community paramedicine: higher education as an enabling factor. *Australasian Journal of Paramedicine*, https://ajp.paramedics.org/index.php/ajp/article/viewFile/22/29.

Order of St John (2017). *Annual Report 2017—Purongo-a-tau o Hato Hone*. Order of St John. Auckland.

Paramedic Health Solutions. (2016). *Community Paramedicine—National Curriculum & Career Pathways*. Mobile CE Inc. Partnership Program USA.

Paramedicine Registration Board of Australia. (2018a). *Professional Standards*. http://www.paramedicineboard.gov.au/Professional-standards.aspx.

Paramedicine Registration Board of Australia. (2018b). *Registration*. http://www.paramedicineboard.gov.au/Registration.aspx.

Pantridge, J. F., & Geddes, J. S. (1967). A mobile intensive-care unit in the management of myocardial infarction. *The Lancet, 2*, 271–273.

Patel, V. L., & Groen, G. J. (1986). Knowledge-based solution strategies in medical reasoning. *Cognitive Science, 10*, 91–116.

Productivity Commission. (2018). *Report on Government Services, 2018*. Canberra: Australian Government. http://www.pc.gov.au/research/ongoing/report-on-government-services. Chapter: 11.

Queensland Ambulance Service (2017a). *Pioneers and Ponies: The Early Years*. QAS Insight Magazine—Autumn Edition.

Queensland Ambulance Service (2017b). *QAS history and heritage*. https://www.ambulance.qld.gov.au/history.html Downloaded 26/4/2018.

Rafael, B., & Ousley, B. (2017). *Prescribing Paramedic Practitioner—Tapping into paramedic potential to contribute to primary care in Victoria. Ambulance Employees Australia (Victoria)—Report of Prescribing paramedic practitioner working group*. North Melbourne.

Reaburn, G., Zolcinski, R., & Fyfe, S. (2017). Rural paramedic practitioner—a future model of care. *Australasian Journal of Paramedicine, 14*(1).

Rikers, R. M., Loyens, S. M., & Schmidt, H. G. (2004). The role of encapsulated knowledge in clinical case representations of medical students and family doctors. *Medical Education, 38*, 1035–1043.

Rothstein, M. A. (2002). Rethinking the meaning of public health. *The Journal of Law, Medicine and Ethics, 30*(2), 144–149.

Shaban, R., Wyatt-Smith, C. M., & Cuming, J. J. (2004). Uncertainty, error and risk in human clinical judgment: introductory theoretical frameworks in paramedic practice. *Journal of Emergency Primary Health Care, 2*(1).

Sheather, R. (2009). Professionalism. In P. O'Meara & C. Grbich (Eds.), *Paramedics in Australia: contemporary*

challenges of practice. Frenchs Forest: Pearson Education Australia.

Shields, A., & Flin, R. (2012). Paramedics' non-technical skills: a literature review. *Journal of Emergency Medicine, 30*.

Toloo, S., Rego, J., FitzGerald, G., Aitken, P., Ting, J., Quinn, J., & Enraght-Moony, E. (2012). Emergency Health Services (EHS): demand and service delivery models. Monograph 2: Queensland EHS users' profile. QUT, Brisbane, Queensland.

Wallis, J., & Boyle, M. (2014). From Stretcher Bearer to paramedic. *Australasian Journal of Paramedicine, 11*, 3. Editorial.

Wankhade, P. (2016). Staff perceptions and changing role of pre-hospital profession in the UK ambulance services: an exploratory study. *International Journal of Emergency Services, 5*(Issue: 2), 126–144. https://doi.org/10.1108/IJES-02-2016-0004.

Wellington Free Ambulance (2014). *Our History*. http://www.wfa.org.nz/our-history Downloaded 27/4/2018.

Wilde, S. (1999). *From driver to paramedic: a history of training ambulance officers in Victoria*. Melbourne: AOTC.

Williams, B. (2009). Do undergraduate paramedic students embrace case-based learning using a blended teaching approach? A 3-year review. *Australasian Journal of Educational Technology, 25*(3).

Williams, B., Onsman, A., & Brown, T. (2010). Professionalism. Is the Australian paramedic discipline a full profession? *Journal of Emergency Primary Health Care, 8*(1).

Woollard, M. (2016). The role of the paramedic practitioner in the UK. *Journal of Primary Health Care, 4*(1), Article 990156.

World Health Organization (WHO). (2009). *Report on the global tobacco epidemic*. Geneva: WHO.

Wyatt, A. (1998). Toward professionalism—an analysis of ambulance practice. *Australasian Journal of Emergency Care, 5*(1), 16–20.

Wyatt, A. (2003). Paramedic practice—knowledge invested in action. *Journal of Emergency Primary Health Care, 1*(3–4).

Victorian Ambulance Cardiac Arrest Registry (2017) *2016/2017 Annual Report*. Ambulance Victoria, Melbourne.

Victorian Labor (2015). Working with paramedics to address the ambulance crisis. *Media Release*: https://www.viclabor.com.au/media-releases/working-with-paramedics-to-address-the-ambulance-crisis/.

CHAPTER 10

Characteristics of Ambulance Patients

By Brendan Shannon

OVERVIEW

- Knowing who your patients are and understanding how and why they come to be in your care will help you understand why they present with their illness and what they expect you to do about it.
- Understanding the characteristics of patients who choose to engage ambulance services can be a key step in assessing, understanding and managing patients.
- Understanding the characteristics and intent of the call-taking systems that dispatch ambulance services can also be an important step in assessing, diagnosing and managing patients, and in reducing stress on paramedics.
- Being aware of what patients experience before and after the ambulance service was called and appreciating their expectations of what the paramedic will do are essential in gaining an accurate history and clinical picture.

Introduction

At first, the characteristics of ambulance patients can appear variable and random. As experience is gained, a paramedic may start to see trends in the patients they attend. It is important for paramedics to understand what leads people to call an ambulance so that they can better empathise with them. A simple exploration of the process undertaken by those who call for an ambulance can highlight the disparity between the paramedic's and the patient's expectations. Paramedics can be frustrated by patients who they perceive to have conditions far from a medical emergency. However, paramedics need to understand and appreciate why patients call in order to assess and treat them appropriately. To achieve such an understanding, this chapter will examine four main themes related to the characteristics of patients and use of paramedic resources.

- *Who is using ambulance services?* Current utilisation, trends in utilisation, types of patients being attended.
- *What factors can lead to people calling an ambulance?* Factors increasing the likelihood of calling an ambulance, those who call but shouldn't, those who should call but don't.
- *From problem onset to the decision to call an ambulance.* How do patients recognise a health emergency and how do they decide what to do about it?
- *The process of calling for an ambulance.* How do patients interact with the ambulance service? What events can occur between when paramedics are dispatched to a case and when they arrive? How are patients allocated an ambulance resource and do all patients receive the traditional response of getting an ambulance attendance? Can we educate the public to call when necessary?

Who is using ambulance services?

Current utilisation

Over the past decade the steady increase in demand for ambulance resources has been driven by multiple factors and includes, but is not limited to, an ageing population and an increase in the incidence of chronic disease (Aminzadeh & Dalziel, 2002; Lowthian et al., 2011b). The increasing demand for ambulance services has led to the need for innovative responses to manage this demand. One such example is the introduction of secondary phone triage systems to refer patients to alternative service providers (Eastwood et al., 2018).

Within Australia 3.2 million patients were assessed, treated or transported by ambulance services in 2017. Of these patients 40.3% were triggered by call dispatch systems as an emergency requiring a lights and sirens response (Australian Government Productivity Commission [AGPC], 2017a).

Table 10.1 shows that of the 7.7 million people who presented to an emergency department (ED) in Australia in 2017, only 1.9 million actually arrived via ambulance, which means that more than 5.8 million made their way by some other means (Australian Institute of Health and

Table 10.1: Triage level and arrival mode selected hospitals, 2016–2017

Arrival mode	Triage level					
	Resuscitation	Emergency	Urgent	Semi-urgent	Non-urgent	Total
Ambulance, air ambulance or helicopter rescue service	46,882 (2.5%)	429,350 (22.5%)	946,031 (49.7%)	454,879 (23.9%)	26,139 (1.4%)	1,903,538 (24.5%)
Other means	9,661 (0.2%)	541,533 (9.3%)	1,905,946 (32.6%)	2,698,504 (46.2%)	692,880 (11.7%)	5,852,068 (75.5%)
Total	56,543 (0.8%)	970,883 (12.5%)	2,851,977 (36.8%)	3,153,383 (40.6%)	719,019 (9.3%)	7,755,606 (100%)

Source: Australian Government Productivity Commission (AGPC). 2017a. Report on Government Services 2017.

Welfare [AIHW], 2017). Further exploration of the data in Table 10.1 reveals the breakdown in triage levels differentiated into those who arrived via an ambulance vehicle and those who did not, and can be referred to at your leisure. However, this table reveals data that tells a fascinating story about who uses ambulance services and how sick they are. Less than half (44.2%) of emergency cases arrived by ambulance; only one-third (33.2%) of urgent cases arrived by ambulance; and just 14.4% of semi-urgent cases arrived by ambulance, with only a small proportion (3.6%) of non-urgent cases arriving by ambulance. While we would expect to see a decreasing utilisation of ambulance services as urgency decreases, the alarming rates of urgent and emergency patients not utilising out-of-hospital care via ambulance is of concern and raises questions as to why this is occurring.

Trends in utilisation

The utilisation of ambulance services can also be broken down by case type and time of day. While there is a higher proportion overall of medical case types, this demand changes with time of day and week (Cantwell et al., 2015). A study of an Australian ambulance service showed that peak demand occurred at two separate times of the day, namely at 12 pm and again at 7 pm. Medical cases were the cause of most demand with the mean age of patients suffering medical complaints being significantly different to and older than trauma cases. Trauma cases most often had peaks during the weekends, with trauma patients of a younger age being likely to coincide with recreational activities. Patients suffering medical complaints had a mean age of 57 years and cases usually occurred during working hours. This was significantly different for trauma cases, with patients having a mean age of 49 years. Further literature reflects the above statistics, showing that older people (aged 65+) are more likely to access ambulance services for a medical

condition than they are a traumatic injury (Lowthian et al., 2011a).

Types of patients being attended

Epidemiological research has shown that less than half of emergency patients actually access ambulance services as a method of arrival to definitive care at the ED. Even with the steady rise of demand for ambulance services the question must be asked why are more than half of emergency patients not using ambulance services? While there is a preconceived idea that ambulances services are predominantly utilised by the highest of acuity patients, data does not support this. Australian research has shown that most ambulance cases are medical in nature with 44% of patients aged over 65 years (Cantwell et al., 2015), and those aged 85 years or over were eight times more likely to be transported than any other age group (Lowthian et al., 2011b). Figure 10.1 highlights the distribution of utilisation by age.

This highlights the ageing population shift and bucks the trends so often perceived by the public (Crowe et al., 2016) that the cases attended by paramedics are predominantly time-critical emergencies such as cardiac arrest. Further to this, the most common triage categories patients are given on arriving to ED via ambulance are urgent and semi-urgent, and not solely distributed around resuscitation and emergency categories. While this information is unlikely to be surprising to paramedics or health professionals working in the emergency setting, it may come as an interesting statistic to the public or those new to the profession.

By and large, paramedics are not treating and transporting all emergency patients entering into the hospital system and are not always transporting only the sickest of patients from the community. In light of this information it is pertinent we now explore the factors that cause people to call (or not call) an ambulance.

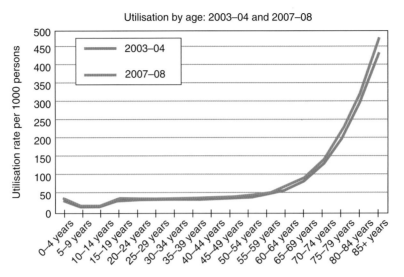

Figure 10.1
Ambulance utilisation per 1000 persons by age.
Source: Cantwell et al. (2015); data from Ambulance Victoria.

What factors can lead to people calling for an ambulance?

When a patient decides whether or not to use an ambulance service, there are really four main categories a patient will fall into, as Table 10.2 highlights. With these categories in mind, an Australian study (Morgans et al., 2015) identified a combination of factors that distinguish those people who are more likely to call an ambulance for a health problem from those who use alternative methods of transport to hospital.

Ambulance users are more likely to: possess a pension card; score higher on the 'powerful others' subscale of the health locus of control scale (indicating that they attribute a significant amount of control over their health to powerful others, such as health professionals); and use 'maladaptive' avoidance coping skills, particularly emotional discharge techniques like crying, to deal with the situation. This suggests that ambulance users are people who cope poorly when experiencing a health emergency. Rather than using thoughtful approaches to find a solution, they respond to their emotions related to the situation and defer responsibility to the available emergency healthcare resources (Morgans et al., 2015).

A study of ambulance patients in Queensland, Australia (Toloo et al., 2013) found that patients considered the urgency or severity of their conditions as reasons for calling an ambulance. Other factors that lead to calling included patients who:

- knew or felt they required special care
- believed they would get a higher priority at the ED

Table 10.2: Possible outcomes for patients deciding whether to use an ambulance service

	Patient requires medical care and transport to hospital	Patient doesn't require medical care or transport to hospital
Used ambulance	True emergency patient	'Inappropriate' ambulance service user
Didn't use ambulance	Delay/failure to use when appropriate	Non-urgent patient

- did not have a car
- had financial concerns.

We should not be surprised that users of ambulance services are more likely to have a pension card or suffer financial concerns. People who are socio-economically disadvantaged generally live shorter lives and suffer more illness and reduced quality of life than those who are well-off (AIHW, 2017). Someone holding a pension card is more likely to be older, and as we age we experience increasing health problems. So it stands to reason that, as a group, pensioners of all types (age, disability, veteran, etc.) will have greater health needs and will be more likely to need emergency healthcare (Ross et al., 2017). As previously discussed, this also has implications for why ambulance use is highest in our ageing population.

Conversely, people who use alternative means of transport to hospital are also more likely to combine the coping styles of cognitive avoidance and positive reappraisal (Morgans et al., 2015). This means that they avoid thinking about the current situation and its potential implications (like death or disability) and instead frame the situation in a more positive manner, expressing the view that the situation could be worse, and their situation is not that bad. The interesting thing about this group is that while they actively cope with their health emergency by self-medicating, seeking alternatives to ambulance care and contacting family and friends for advice and support, they waited a dangerously long time to arrive at a source of healthcare and in some cases had poorer health outcomes as a result. So an emotional coping style of crying, or panicking and calling an ambulance, can be more beneficial for some patients than trying to deal with the situation by relying on their own resources.

Those who shouldn't call

There are various reasons why patients call an ambulance. The disconnect between health professional and patient perspectives of what warrants a health emergency has been well established (Morgans & Burgess, 2011, 2012) and most ED attendance has been found to be for fever, chest pain and abdominal pain. While these conditions can be medical emergencies, it also indicates that patients perceive these conditions as emergencies (MacLean et al., 1999). There is evidence that health professionals (including paramedics) will rely more on physiological symptoms whereas patients will rely on how the health emergency makes them feel (Morgans & Burgess, 2012).

This is an important point to make as it has implications for paramedics treating patients in the community. The patient (or bystander) has been at a point of crisis and has called seeking assistance which, regardless of acuity and the disconnect between emergency perceptions, can be provided by paramedics (Ahl et al., 2006).

Both locally and internationally there is currently a steady increase in demand for ambulance services for low-acuity clinical problems (Eastwood et al., 2016). The straightforward process of dispatching an ambulance to all patients is clearly unsustainable. This is not to suggest that patients with low-acuity needs should be refused or be limited in accessing an appropriate level of care. While transporting low-acuity patients to EDs may actually delay the patient getting primary care promptly, it also creates unnecessary cost and strain on acute medical services such as ambulance services and EDs (Drummond, 2002; Gill, 1994). There are currently many novel ways being trialled and implemented across the globe

to deal with the growing demand of low-acuity patients. Services include extended-care paramedics, secondary phone triage and referral to alternative service providers, increasing community care services to high-risk patients recently discharged from hospitals, linking of primary care services for patients who frequently attend EDs, referral guidelines for use by paramedics, and government-funded educational media campaigns.

The use of ambulance services by patients with low-acuity complaints can lead to paramedics believing that these patients are inappropriately using their services. However, the use of terminology such as 'inappropriate patients' can have a negative connotation and lead to preconceived judgment unnecessarily. It's not that these patients shouldn't call; it's more that our traditional response model of sending every patient an ambulance needs to be adapted to refer patients to the most appropriate level of care in an appropriate timeframe for their complaint/condition (Eastwood et al., 2018).

Those that need to call but don't

Another population group of patients that warrants discussion are patients who should seek or require emergency healthcare but choose not to. Some people actively avoid seeking ambulance services. Table 10.3 shows the results of a survey of patients who attended EDs in Melbourne (Morgans et al., 2015).

There are many reasons given for not calling an ambulance, but the most common may be classified as social or perceptual barriers: lack of knowledge (not sure if it was an emergency); ambulance is just for transport (could be driven by others); and

Table 10.3: Reasons patient did not call an ambulance

Reason	% of responses
Unsure if it was an emergency	27.0
Could be driven to hospital by others	22.0
Did not want to cause a fuss	14.7
Too embarrassed to call an ambulance	7.0
Don't want to go to hospital	7.0
Other	5.8
Ambulance would take too long to arrive	4.5
Rather call local doctor	4.0
Costs: not an ambulance subscriber	4.0
Rather drive myself	3.0
Costs: not sure if covered	1.0

Source: Morgans et al. (2015).

embarrassment (didn't want to make a fuss). To make things even more complex, as previously discussed a health emergency is difficult to define, as changes in health conditions are dynamic and may vary in urgency over time. Interestingly, most researchers agree that there are no demographic factors that directly predict patterns of health service use (Lowthian et al., 2011a).

With this in mind, let's now explore the process a patient will go through prior to calling (or choosing not to call) an ambulance.

From problem onset to the decision to call for an ambulance

Making the decision to call

Research has revealed that patients report making health decisions based on the level of discomfort or pain they feel and on the advice of fellow laypeople, such as family and friends (Morgans et al., 2015). Patients can classify symptoms as an emergency not based on physiological criteria, but rather on when the symptoms were beyond their inherent ability to cope. Patients do not recognise medically significant symptoms as prompting them to seek emergency help, instead focusing on the nature of the presenting symptoms. Symptom onset that was sudden and severe can be interpreted as urgent, whereas slow-onset or mild and intermittent symptoms are interpreted as less urgent. This tendency to focus on rapid development rather than medically significant symptoms is a key difference between the medical and nonmedical categorisations of urgency. This may explain why patients report non-life-threatening symptoms as potentially serious and present 'unnecessarily' with symptoms that are of little medical urgency, or alternatively neglect to seek help for slow-onset or intermittent symptoms of a potentially serious nature, such as chest pain, shortness of breath or prodromal symptoms of significant aetiologies (Morgans & Burgess, 2011). A study investigating the patient decision-making process when calling for medical help has found that there are four distinct steps.

Step 1: Recognition

Patients use the following strategies to determine whether they have something to be worried about.

- Compare current health situation to 'normal' status.
- Identify symptoms: identification of symptoms is harder for people with chronic illnesses such as angina and asthma as these patients experience frequent exacerbation of symptoms.
- Mild symptoms are perceived as less serious.

- Intermittent symptoms can be confusing for patients.
- Identification of important symptoms depends on layperson knowledge of important symptoms, which varies greatly among patients and illnesses.
- Identify any pain: experiencing pain or discomfort tells a patient that things are not normal. Some patients may self-medicate, which can have an impact on the symptoms.
- Identify any traumatic mechanism of injury (e.g. fall, accident).

Once patients have decided that they are experiencing something abnormal, they then decide whether or not to do something about it.

Step 2: Identify the situation as an urgent health issue

Defining an event as a health emergency is difficult for patients and often involves consultation with another layperson for advice and reassurance. An emergency is often deemed to have occurred when patients felt that the situation was beyond their ability to control and manage. The outcome at this stage depends mostly on coping style and is affected by whether the illness is acute, chronic or an exacerbation of a chronic condition. Key factors that impact on whether a patient classifies their symptoms as urgent include the following.

- Sudden-onset symptoms are deemed as more urgent than those of gradual onset.
- If there is a traumatic mechanism of injury, the situation is quickly identified as urgent, even when the injury is minor.
- In chronic illnesses such as chest pain, abdominal pain, diabetes, asthma and chronic obstructive pulmonary disease (COPD), symptoms can fluctuate and patients find it harder to evaluate the urgency of their symptoms.

Patient perceptions of urgency have absolutely no correlation with in-hospital measures of medical urgency (Morgans & Burgess, 2011). Patients in this study did not generally consider medical issues when defining a health event as an emergency, instead focusing on social, personal and psychological responses to illness. When seeking healthcare for a perceived emergency condition, patients reported a belief that they were seriously unwell, required emergency medical care and expected to be admitted to hospital for medical assessment and treatment. Once patients have determined that a situation is urgent, they then have to decide what to do about it.

Step 3: Decide to get help

In the study by Morgans and Burgess, one in five people contacted an ambulance as soon as they identified an event as an emergency—meaning that four out of five called someone else first. In fact, the study showed that contacting a layperson (family and/or friends) was usually the first action taken by patients. This was followed by consideration of the healthcare services available at the time and seeking permission to use those services. Contrary to the beliefs of paramedics and hospital-based health professionals, seeking a source of medical healthcare was usually achieved only after arduous personal and social considerations by the patient. The types of actions taken by patients in the study once they had decided to seek help included the following.

- Calling a friend or relative. Fifty-five per cent of callers to ambulance services had called a friend or relative first to seek health advice and 'permission' to use emergency health resources.
- Self-medicating to try to relieve the symptoms. This included taking pain relief such as paracetamol or ibuprofen, anginine/GTN spray for chest pain or salbutamol for asthma. Self-medicating was particularly common in exacerbations of chronic illnesses, including cardiac and respiratory problems, and significantly contributed to the delay in seeking ambulance care.
- Seeking permission to use emergency health resources. In Australian studies it was presented that there was an increased delay to call associated with being with a primary healthcare provider (Coventry et al., 2015; Ingarfield et al., 2005).

Once patients decided to seek healthcare, they need to decide whether to call an ambulance, self-present to an ED or attend their GP or other primary healthcare.

Step 4: Decide where to get emergency medical help

The reality is that patient decision-making in out-of-hospital health emergencies is a layperson's decision-making process. It is affected by psychosocial factors rather than demographic or medical factors. Patients who seek emergency healthcare generally believe that what they are experiencing is a genuine emergency and that they are seeking the most appropriate source of care, which directly relates to their perception of the roles and responsibilities of the providers of emergency healthcare services. In the study by Morgans and colleagues (2008), patients and their carers reported that they found the emergency health experience frightening and worried about the experience and its outcomes for a long time after the event. Such fears were also evident in the proportion of people who tried to avoid hospital attendance because they feared a forced hospital admission. This helps to explain why it took patients on average 4.6 hours to identify their symptoms, define them as an emergency, seek help and advice, and then make the decision to pick up the phone to call the ambulance service.

Understanding the process a patient undergoes before they request help provides an understanding of why patients do or don't call. The question should be asked if we can better educate patients and the public now that we understand the decision-making process occurring. Can education alone help to better guide patients and bystanders to call when necessary in order reduce rates of unnecessary and/or delayed calls? While this is explored later in the chapter, at a minimum we can now understand why patients do or do not call, identify some factors that increase likelihood of using ambulance services and the decision-making process undertaken. This understanding can influence practice and empathy with patients.

The process of calling for an ambulance

Knowing the process of calling for an ambulance undertaken by patients enables paramedics to fully understand the early part of the patient journey towards care. For example, paramedics may take for granted the fact that animals and pets are usually kept secured prior to arrival, that medications are easily at hand and that the front house lights are on prior to arrival. These actions are requests which are usually asked of callers as a part of the call-taking process and is often not a logical foresight undertaken by the patients or requester of the ambulance.

So, what happens first? First, in Australia a call to 000, or in New Zealand a call to 111, is made (ESTA, 2018; St John Ambulance Services, 2017). The caller will be asked to decide whether they require ambulance, police or fire and the state or territory the caller is calling from. This is the first of many decisions to be made by the caller and is often not always straightforward. Once an ambulance is requested, the initial Telstra call-taker will then transfer the caller to an Emergency Services Telecommunications Authority (ESTA) ambulance call-taker and the caller's request will be triaged. Callers will initially be asked the following questions (ESTA, 2018).

- What is the exact location of the emergency?
- What is the phone number you are calling from?
- What is the problem? What exactly happened?
- How many people are hurt?
- How old is the person?
- Is the person conscious (awake)?
- Is the person breathing?

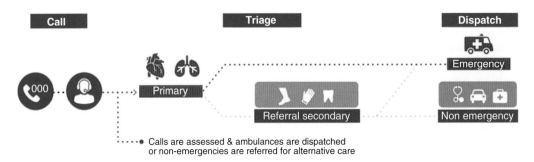

Figure 10.2
Ambulance Victoria's triage process.
Source: Ambulance Victoria (n.d.).

These questions rapidly determine the level of health response required and the location to which it should proceed. The call-taker will continue to ask more questions about the patient and is structured on the Medical Priority Dispatch System (MPDS).

MPDS triage

Medical triage of ambulance calls is generally governed by a structured process such as MPDS and involves identifying the primary problem and determining its severity (Cantwell et al., 2014). The triage depends on what the caller reports to the call-taker and hence the information, level and timeliness of response can only be influenced by the caller themselves. This is an important point for health professionals responding to the request to recall when the response is deemed as either over or under resourced. The aim of medical triage is to determine what resources the patient needs, and the level of clinical urgency compared to other patients. For example, if there are two cases and one ambulance, triage is used to determine which case the ambulance is sent to first. Automated triage systems like MPDS are designed to ensure a consistent level of resource allocation and prioritisation simultaneously.

Once the primary symptom has been identified, the call-taker can provide pre-arrival instructions to help the caller or the patient before the ambulance arrives. Instructions are commonly given for the following:
- scene safety and preparation
- CPR
- control of bleeding
- airway management
- childbirth.

Secondary triage

Once triage is complete, either an ambulance is sent to the requester or the caller may be referred to secondary phone triage. Through secondary triage, for ambulance services which have it in place, an appropriately qualified health professional will talk to the caller to further determine the appropriate level of response required. At this point the patient's request may be upgraded, downgraded or referred to other primary healthcare or self-care and an ambulance may not be sent (Eastwood et al., 2015). Figure 10.2 provides a diagram of the revised triage process including secondary phone triage used by Ambulance Victoria.

Cases 1 and 2 are examples of transcripts of ambulance calls and illustrate the call-taking process.

Can we educate patients to call when appropriate?

We have identified that ambulance utilisation for low-acuity complaints is increasing and that novel approaches to dealing with this issue are currently being implemented. Conversely, there is also the issue of patients who don't call but should, placing their health at great risk. Public education of when to call for an ambulance or seek emergency healthcare has been a point of discussion, with some research highlighting mass media campaigns as effective (Hickey et al., 2018; Nehme et al., 2017b; Nehme et al., 2017a) while other research questions its effectiveness (Bett et al., 2005). Education of the public must be considered if we are to improve the effective utilisation of ambulance services. While it's no surprise that most laypeople have inadequate health literacy, surprisingly approximately 40% of health professionals also have inadequate health literacy (AGPC, 2017b). Local campaigns that have been shown to be effective in educating laypeople of when they should and shouldn't call for an ambulance include informing them when to call for cardiac complaints (Nehme et al., 2017b), the improvement in early identification of stroke symptoms (Hickey et al., 2018) and (internationally) a program to reduce unnecessary calls (Ohshige, 2008). While educating the public of the need to

Case 1—Example ambulance call 1

John, a 39-year-old man, develops some chest pain while driving a forklift at a large manufacturing company. He goes to the first-aid room and the receptionist in administration decides to call an ambulance when the chest pain gets worse.

Emergency operator: 'Police, fire, or ambulance: which service do you require?'

Receptionist: 'Hello? We need an ambulance; he's got chest pain.'

Emergency operator: 'Which state or territory are you in?'

Receptionist: 'What? I'm in Deer Park and I need an ambulance please.'

Emergency operator: 'Is that Deer Park, Victoria?'

Receptionist: 'Yes. YES! Victoria! That's what I said!'

Ambulance call-taker: 'Ambulance. Where is your emergency?'

Receptionist: 'I already told them this. We need an ambulance please; there is a man here with chest pain.'

Ambulance call-taker: 'What address do you want the ambulance to come to?'

Receptionist: 'Plasticmakers Manufacturing, 59 Jones Street, Deer Park.'

Ambulance call-taker: 'Plasticmakers Manufacturing, 59 Jones Street, Deer Park. Is that near the intersection of Westall Road?

Receptionist: 'Yes, entrance B is just off Westall Road. Tell them to come in through entrance B … and hurry, I think he is getting worse, he looks terrible.'

Ambulance call-taker: 'What is the problem? Tell me exactly what has happened.'

Receptionist: 'He's been here in the office; he has chest pain and he needs an ambulance.'

Ambulance call-taker: 'How old is he?'

Receptionist: 'About 35, I think.'

Ambulance call-taker: 'Is he conscious?'

Receptionist: 'Yes.'

Ambulance call-taker: 'Is he breathing?'

Receptionist: 'Yes, but he's sort of gasping now, he's really struggling. Are they on their way?'

Ambulance call-taker: 'Is he completely awake and able to talk?'

Receptionist: 'Yes, he's struggling to talk, but he's awake.'

Ambulance call-taker: 'And you said he wasn't breathing normally, is that right?'

Receptionist: 'Yes, he's breathing hard.'

Ambulance call-taker: 'I have an ambulance organised for you coming to Plasticmakers Manufacturing, 59 Jones Street, Deer Park, entrance B off Westall Road. I have a couple more quick questions to help the ambulance, okay?'

Receptionist: 'Okay.'

Ambulance call-taker: 'Okay. Is he changing in colour?'

Receptionist: 'Well, he looks pale, almost a bit grey, and he's sweaty.'

Ambulance call-taker: 'Does he have any history of heart problems?'

Receptionist: 'Have you got heart problems, John? … He said he hasn't, no.'

Ambulance call-taker: 'Is he on any medications?'

Receptionist: 'Are you on medication, John? … He says he is on blood pressure medication but he can't remember what it's called.'

Ambulance call-taker: 'Okay, we have an ambulance organised; will someone be out the front to direct the ambulance to the right place?'

Receptionist: 'Yes, I can make them do that.'

Ambulance call-taker: 'That's good. Now you need to keep a careful eye on John, make sure he keeps breathing regularly and is awake and talking to you. If anything changes, you need to call me back immediately on 000. The ambulance is on its way to you now. Okay?'

Receptionist: 'Okay, thanks.'

request an ambulance is important, there also needs to be a balance between providing information that suggests patients should call and when they shouldn't to avoid confusion through conflicting messages.

Summary

The characteristics of ambulance patients is as variable as the day-to-day business of paramedics. Despite this variability, there are trends in utilisation we have now explored. We have identified patient factors that increase their likelihood of requesting ambulance care, and finally we covered the decision-making process patients undergo prior to deciding to call for an ambulance. In understanding the call-taking process we have an insight rarely gained by paramedics, who are likely to have had little exposure to the call-taking process. With the information we have learned from this chapter we can have an overall understanding of who ambulance patients are and the process they undertake to finally get a paramedic at their side. Understanding that patients call for many reasons and not just solely due to physiological complaints, paramedics can better empathise with patients, ultimately creating better satisfaction and health outcomes.

Case 2—Example ambulance call 2

Gail, a 56-year-old female, has suffered a fall.

Emergency operator: 'Police, fire, or ambulance: which service do you require?'

Patient: 'Ambulance, in Melbourne please.'

Ambulance call-taker: 'Ambulance. Where is your emergency?'

Patient: 'I've fallen out of my wheelchair and I am unable to get up.'

Ambulance call-taker: 'What address are you at?'

Patient: 'I've fallen from my wheelchair. I'm not hurt, but I can't get up!'

Ambulance call-taker: 'What is the address you are at?'

Patient: 'Oh sorry, I'm in Melbourne, I'm staying at the Inter-Continental in Melbourne.'

Ambulance call-taker: 'So you are at the Inter-Continental in Melbourne?'

Patient: 'Yes, that's the one!'

Ambulance call-taker: 'Does the address 495 Collins St, Melbourne, sound right, it's the address I'm getting for the motel.'

Patient: 'Yes, that the one, oh I'm so sorry I'm just so stuck and I have no help as I'm away on a trip.'

Ambulance call-taker: 'So you have fallen, is that right?'

Patient: 'Yes, that's right.'

Ambulance call-taker: 'How old are you?'

Patient: 'I'm 56.'

Ambulance call-taker: 'So you are breathing and conscious?'

Patient: 'Yes.'

Ambulance call-taker 'And you have fallen. Have you hurt yourself?'

Patient: 'Yes, I was just trying to move to the toilet from my wheelchair and I've slipped down onto the floor.'

Ambulance call-taker: 'And you are definitely not hurt?'

Patient: 'Yes, I'm definitely not hurt. My name is Gail.'

Ambulance call-taker: 'Okay, you poor thing Gail. Let's see if we can get you some help! We need to ask you some more questions.'

Patient: 'Okay.'

Ambulance call-taker: 'So that we can get you the help you need, I'm going to transfer you to one of our referral staff in a moment.'

Patient: 'Yes, that sounds fine.'

Ambulance call-taker: 'Okay, I'm transferring you now.'

Patient: 'Thank you.'

Line conference call …

Ambulance call-taker: 'Hello referral service. I have a patient by the name of Gail on the line who has fallen while transferring from her wheelchair. She is uninjured. Can you take the call?'

Referral service practitioner: 'Yes, of course I'll take the call.'

Ambulance call-taker: 'Great, transferring now.'

Referral service practitioner: 'Hello, Gail. It's Roger from referral service. I hear you have suffered a fall?'

Patient: 'Yes, unfortunately that's correct, I'm uninjured but I just can't get up. I'm away from home at the moment and have no one available locally who can help me. I'm so sorry for wasting your time, I really didn't want to call but I have no other option.'

Referral service practitioner: 'No stress at all, Gail, this is what we are here for. Now let's find out exactly what's happened and see if we can help.'

The patient was eventually triaged as a non-urgent call by the referral service practitioner and was sent a non-emergency ambulance. This resource could assist the patient who did not wish to be transported to ED after she was assisted back to her wheelchair.

References

Ahl, C., Nyström, M., & Jansson, L. (2006). Making up one's mind: Patients' experiences of calling an ambulance. *Accident and Emergency Nursing, 14*, 11–19.

Ambulance Victoria. (n.d.). *Delivering our patients the right care at the right time at the right place.* https://www.ambulance.vic.gov.au/wp-content/uploads/2017/07/delivering-our-patients-the-right-care-brochure-rev2.pdf.

Aminzadeh, F., & Dalziel, W. B. (2002). Older adults in the emergency department: a systematic review of patterns of use, adverse outcomes, and effectiveness of interventions. *Annals of Emergency Medicine, 39*, 238–247.

Australian Government Productivity Commission (AGPC). (2017a). *Report on Government Services 2017.*

Australian Government Productivity Commission (AGPC). (2017b). *Shifting the Dial: 5 year productivity review.*

Australian Institute of Health and Welfare (AIHW). (2017). *Emergency department care 2016–17: Australian hospital statistics.*

Bett, J., Tonkin, A., Thompson, P., & Aroney, C. (2005). Failure of current public educational campaigns to impact on the initial response of patients with possible heart attack. *Internal Medicine Journal, 35*, 279–282.

Cantwell, K., Morgans, A., Smith, K., Livingston, M., & Dietze, P. (2014). Improving the coding and classification of ambulance data through the application of International Classification of Disease 10th revision. *Australian Health Review, 38*, 70–79.

Cantwell, K., Morgans, A., Smith, K., Livingston, M., Spelman, T., & Dietze, P. (2015). Time of day and day of week trends in EMS demand. *Prehospital Emergency Care, 19*, 425–431.

Coventry, L. L., Bremner, A. P., Williams, T. A., & Celenza, A. (2015). The effect of presenting symptoms and patient characteristics on prehospital delay in MI patients presenting to emergency department by ambulance: a cohort study. *Heart, Lung and Circulation, 24*, 943–950.

Crowe, R. P., Levine, R., Rodriguez, S., Larrimore, A. D., & Pirrallo, R. G. (2016). Public perception of emergency medical services in the United States. *Prehospital and Disaster Medicine, 31*, S112–S117.

Drummond, A. J. (2002). No room at the inn: overcrowding in Ontario's emergency departments. *CJEM: Canadian Journal of Emergency Medical Care, 4*, 91–97.

Eastwood, K., Morgans, A., Smith, K., Hodgkinson, A., Becker, G., & Stoelwinder, J. (2016). A novel approach for managing the growing demand for ambulance services by low-acuity patients. *Australian Health Review, 40*, 378–384.

Eastwood, K., Morgans, A., Smith, K., & Stoelwinder, J. (2015). Secondary triage in prehospital emergency ambulance services: a systematic review. *Emergency Medicine Journal, 32*, 486–492.

Eastwood, K., Morgans, A., Stoelwinder, J., & Smith, K. (2018). Patient and case characteristics associated with 'no paramedic treatment' for low-acuity cases referred for emergency ambulance dispatch following a secondary telephone triage: a retrospective cohort study. *Scandinavian Journal of Trauma, Resuscitation and Emergency Medicine, 26*, 8.

ESTA. (2018). *Emergency Services Telecommunication Authority—our role*. Retrieved from: https://www.esta.vic.gov.au/our-role.

Gill, J. M. (1994). Nonurgent use of the emergency department: appropriate or not? *Annals of Emergency Medicine, 24*, 953–957.

Hickey, A., Mellon, L., Williams, D., Shelley, E., & Conroy, R. M. (2018). Does stroke health promotion increase awareness of appropriate behavioural response? Impact of the face, arm, speech and time (FAST) campaign on population knowledge of stroke risk factors, warning signs and emergency response. *European Stroke Journal, 3*, 117–125.

Ingarfield, S. L., Jacobs, I. G., Jelinek, G. A., & Mountain, D. (2005). Patient delay and use of ambulance by patients with chest pain. *Emergency Medicine Australasia: EMA, 17*, 218–223.

Lowthian, J. A., Cameron, P. A., Stoelwinder, J. U., Curtis, A., Currell, A., Cooke, M. W., & McNeil, J. J. (2011a).

Increasing utilisation of emergency ambulances. *Australian Health Review, 35*, 63–69.

Lowthian, J. A., Jolley, D. J., Curtis, A. J., Currell, A., Cameron, P. A., Stoelwinder, J. U., & McNeil, J. J. (2011b). The challenges of population ageing: accelerating demand for emergency ambulance services by older patients, 1995-2015. *The Medical Journal of Australia, 194*, 574.

MaClean, S. L., Bayley, E. W., Cole, F. L., Bernardo, L., Lenaghan, P., & Manton, A. (1999). The LUNAR project: a description of the population of individuals who seek health care at emergency departments. *Journal of Emergency Nursing, 25*, 269–282.

Morgans, A. E., Archer, F., & Allen, F. C. L. (2008). Patient decision making processes and outcomes when deciding to call an ambulance: what are patients thinking? *Journal of Emergency Primary Health Care.*

Morgans, A., Archer, F., & Allen, F. (2015). Patient decision making in prehospital health emergencies: determinants and predictors of patient delay. *Australasian Journal of Paramedicine, 6.*

Morgans, A., & Burgess, S. (2012). Judging a patient's decision to seek emergency healthcare: clues for managing increasing patient demand. *Australian Health Review, 36*, 110–114.

Morgans, A., & Burgess, S. J. (2011). What is a health emergency? The difference in definition and understanding between patients and health professionals. *Australian Health Review, 35*, 284–289.

Nehme, Z., Andrew, E., Bernard, S., Patsamanis, H., Cameron, P., Bray, J. E., Meredith, I. T., & Smith, K. (2017a). Impact of a public awareness campaign on out-of-hospital cardiac arrest incidence and mortality rates. *European Heart Journal, 38*, 1666–1673.

Nehme, Z., Cameron, P. A., Akram, M., Patsamanis, H., Bray, J. E., Meredith, I. T., & Smith, K. (2017b). Effect of a mass media campaign on ambulance use for chest pain. *The Medical Journal of Australia, 206*, 30–35.

Ohshige, K. (2008). Reduction in ambulance transports during a public awareness campaign for appropriate ambulance use. *Academic Emergency Medicine: Official Journal of the Society for Academic Emergency Medicine, 15*, 289–293.

Ross, L., Jennings, P. A., Smith, K., & Williams, B. (2017). Paramedic attendance to older patients in Australia, and the prevalence and implications of psychosocial issues. *Prehospital Emergency Care, 21*, 32–38.

St John Ambulance Services. (2017). *Annual Report 2017.*

Toloo, G., Fitzgerald, G. J., Aitken, P. J., Ting, J. Y. S., McKenzie, K., Rego, J., & Enraght-Moony, E. (2013). Ambulance use is associated with higher self-rated illness seriousness: user attitudes and perceptions. *Academic Emergency Medicine: Official Journal of the Society for Academic Emergency Medicine, 20*, 576–583.

SECTION 6:
Patient and Paramedic Safety

Patient safety and paramedic wellbeing have never been more topical than they are now, and with good reason. The first chapter in this section explores common errors in clinical practice, how and why they occur, and how they are mitigated and managed. The second chapter discusses paramedic health and safety. Paramedicine can be a stressful profession so being informed about the impact it can have on emotional and mental health is important. This chapter also discusses the challenges of shift work, and the roles of sleep, exercise and nutrition. Finally, the chapter talks about developing resilience and seeking support when needed.

CHAPTER 11

Patient Safety and Paramedicine

By Paul Jennings

OVERVIEW

- Patients deserve to receive high-quality healthcare and healthcare providers generally go to extreme lengths to provide it.
- Despite diligence and competence, all clinicians are subject to error.
- Medical errors are pervasive, substantial and affect all types of people, in all settings, receiving all types of treatment. Medical errors are not uncommon.
- Cultural issues such as blame and avoidance affect the number of medical incidents and near-misses that are reported.

- Disclosure of adverse events should be made easier and less punitive in order to identify and correct errors.
- The science of patient safety describes the extent of medical error and examines means to reduce risk and alter personal and organisational culture.
- Patient safety is intrinsically linked to evidence-based practice and the formation of clinical decision aids and guidelines that support clinical practice, but will always require effective clinical reasoning.

Introduction

It is often surprising to new medical, nursing and paramedic students that there is a discipline within healthcare known as patient safety. After all, the notion of healthcare is that it helps patients to recover from illness or injury. Indeed, the Hippocratic Oath (Collier & Son, 1910) states: 'Never do harm to anyone'. It is perhaps this disconnect—that caring for patients could actually harm them—that allowed a culture to develop whereby medical errors went largely unreported until the 1990s, when a series of disturbing studies discovered that medical errors were both more common and more serious than people had ever anticipated (Brennan et al., 1991; Thomas et al., 2000; Kohn et al., 1999). Far from being rare, one American study found that if medical errors were classified as a disease, they would be the sixth most common cause of death in the United States (National Center for Health Care Statistics at the Centers for Disease Control, 2005). In Australia, medical errors result in as many as 18,000 unnecessary deaths and more than 50,000 people becoming disabled each year (Weingart et al., 2000). As a result, the process of identifying why medical errors occur and what can be done to prevent them has developed into a specific discipline and a specialised form of risk management concerned with monitoring, analysing and preventing these errors.

Consumers of healthcare have the right to expect that they will receive high-quality and safe care regardless of the setting in which it is delivered: hospital, GP or out-of-hospital setting. Errors occur because those who are responsible for the provision of healthcare are human. Every day, competent, careful and conscientious people commit errors as a result of systemic or individual failures. For paramedics providing healthcare in the diagnostically limited and often chaotic environment of out-of-hospital emergency care, understanding the factors that contribute to errors and threaten patient safety is essential if such errors are to be avoided. This chapter examines the common causes of medical errors and how effective clinical reasoning is one tool that can be used to reduce both the frequency and the severity of errors.

The harm caused by healthcare errors

Until relatively recently, the notion of 'patient safety' was inseparable from 'patient care': it was assumed that by looking after their patients, clinicians were intrinsically making them safe. Patient safety is generally defined as 'the avoidance or reduction to acceptable levels of actual or potential harm from healthcare or the environment in which healthcare is delivered' (Australian Institute of Health and Welfare [AIHW], 2009). This definition is equally applicable to all healthcare settings and disciplines.

The cornerstone of patient safety is the systematic identification and monitoring of adverse events, or medical errors, and the improvement of healthcare through redesigning education and processes. The Harvard Medical Practice Study in the mid-1980s was one of the earliest studies reporting on adverse events (Brennan et al., 1991). The study screened a random sample of patient notes from 51 acute care facilities in New York State in order to identify records that contained an adverse event. The researchers found that some 13.6% of patients died as a result of an adverse or negligent event in hospital (Brennan et al., 1991; Leape et al., 1991; Localio et al., 1991). In a similar study conducted in Utah and Colorado in the early 1990s (Thomas et al., 2000) the authors found that 15.4% of adverse or negligent events caused death. This study also identified that the ED had a much higher error rate than other areas within hospitals due to the type and volume of work, and the staff involved. The Quality in Australian Health Care Study in the mid-1990s was the first Australian study to examine medical errors. The authors examined the incidence of adverse events, the likelihood these events might have led to death and the possibility that the events might have been prevented using patient records from 28 Australian hospitals across two states. The authors found that 4.9% of adverse events caused death and 51% of adverse events could have been prevented (Wilson et al., 1995).

The out-of-hospital environment is probably the health setting most analogous to the ED (see Fig 11.1) and the most recent study aiming to detect and reduce adverse events in the ED was reported in 2002. In this Victorian study, 2.85% of patient attendances were screened positive for one or more adverse events, and an adverse event was later confirmed in 1.24% of patient attendances, with 32.4% of these events being deemed severe. After

implementing various quality improvement activities (mostly changes to hospital policy and work practices), the number of adverse events fell dramatically (Wolff & Bourke, 2002).

Even though the magnitude of errors and adverse events has now been recognised, the degree to which they are acknowledged varies between settings. While there is considerable literature examining incident monitoring and adverse event tracking in the hospital environment (i.e. anaesthesia, operating theatres and intensive care units), there is scant literature relating to adverse events and incident reporting in the out-of-hospital environment. The findings of a systematic literature review conducted in 2009 found 88 papers covering seven themes of patient safety in paramedic practice (Bigham et al., 2012; see Table 11.1).

Types of medical error

While the factors that lead to medical errors are rarely simple or singular, medical errors can be classified into four categories: diagnostic, treatment, failure and preventive (Assaf et al., 2003).

- **Diagnostic errors** include a delay in making the correct diagnosis, missing a diagnosis and making an incorrect diagnosis that leads to patient harm (Singh et al., 2012). The rate of diagnostic errors is estimated to be between 10 and 15% (Graber et al., 2005; Shojania et al., 2003). It is this category of error that our text primarily seeks to address (see Fig 11.2).
- **Treatment errors** result in harm because of mistakes in a procedure such as a biopsy, suturing or intubation, but they also include medication errors. Because medication administration is so common, giving an incorrect drug dose, via the wrong route or even the wrong medication, is the most likely cause of medical error and subsequent patient harm (Assaf et al., 2003).

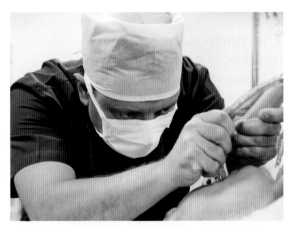

Figure 11.1
The concept of separating the process of treating patients from exposing them to risks has not been an easy transition for hospitals, but it is now a well-established practice that supports clinical care.
Source: Shutterstock/beerkoff.

Table 11.1: Patient safety themes emerging from the literature

Theme	Number of articles
Adverse events and medication error	22
Clinical judgment	13
Communication	6
Ground vehicle safety	9
Aircraft safety	6
Interfacility transport	16
Field intubation	16

Source: Bigham et al. (2012).

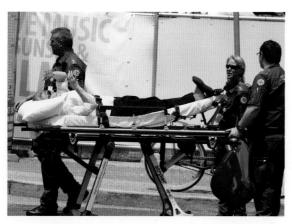

Figure 11.2
Working in the community setting, surrounded by distractions, it is likely that paramedics are at greater risk of making diagnostic and treatment errors than medical professionals working in controlled environments. Being aware that errors will pervade their clinical management at some point is the first step paramedics must make in reducing the potential consequences of any error.
Source: Shutterstock/paintings.

- **Failure errors** occur when a process or piece of equipment fails to function as designed. Instinctively this suggests the failure of equipment such as ventilators or monitors, but poor communication at handover, erroneous record keeping and patient misidentification are all typical failure errors in which people contribute to an error.
- **Preventive errors** are the instances when patients are harmed by a failure to deliver drugs or procedures that are known to reduce complications. Wound infection due to delayed changing of surgical dressings or omission of postoperative antibiotics are common examples of preventive errors.

Models of error

That errors occur frequently and patients are harmed have strongly motivated researchers to develop error mitigation strategies and a number of authors divide errors into two main models of causation: errors of the person and errors of the system (Graber et al., 2002; Nolan, 2000; Reason, 2000).

The person approach examines errors as a result of aberrant behaviour: care providers being forgetful, careless or even negligent. This model attributes blame to the person, and mitigation strategies introduced by organisations to address this type of error include educational programs, newsletters and posters aimed at coercing individuals to conform to newly devised procedures or protocols. Viewing

errors solely by this model can see organisations create an environment of fear to promote adherence to policy and, where errors are identified, implementing a program of naming, blaming, shaming and retraining (Nieva & Sorra, 2003; Reason, 2000).

The systems approach, on the other hand, accepts that individuals are not infallible and that errors will inevitably occur, irrespective of the will of organisations and clinicians. Humans will make mistakes, especially when the culture or system in which they are operating does not recognise the risk (Nieva & Sorra, 2003). In this approach, errors are seen as 'consequences rather than causes' (Reason, 2000), most often resulting from failures in systems or processes rather than individual inattention. Countermeasures are based on developing safety measures and processes that reduce the likelihood of clinicians making an error: engineering the risk out of risky situations and tasks. When errors do occur, the focus is not on who made the error, but rather why the defences failed (Reason, 2000).

Reducing diagnostic errors

This text is primarily focused on reducing diagnostic errors by improving information collection and clinical reasoning skills. Chapters 7, 14 and 15 identify specific areas, concepts and skills that can be developed to limit the perceptual and thought processes that lead to human error. However, it is important to realise that in addition to the personal and systemic factors that contribute to diagnostic error, there is also a category of 'no-fault' errors (Graber et al., 2002) that must be considered. These errors occur because no diagnostic test is infallible, diseases can present atypically and patients are (very) occasionally non-compliant in providing an accurate description of their condition.

Most ambulance services implement a system-level protection by ensuring that novices work with experienced paramedics. This is an example of a layered approach to error mitigation and it reduces, but does not completely mitigate, the chances of error.

Error defence

Reason (2000) is probably best known for his Swiss cheese model of system accidents (see Fig 11.3).

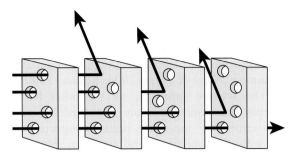

Figure 11.3
The Swiss cheese model of system accidents. Some holes can be thought of as active failures of systems or individuals, while others exist across the whole organisation.
Source: Adapted from Reason (2000).

> ## PRACTICE TIP
>
> Sodium and potassium chloride are harmless and dangerous medications, respectively, but they are often prepared in identical ampoules distinguished only by tiny type. Paramedics often wrap potassium chloride ampoules in tape when they stock them in their kit so that they can easily be identified in poor light or when crew are tired or distracted.

This model shows how most systems offer a series of defences, barriers or safeguards that block an error from progressing too far. However, despite a process, task or situation having a number of layers of defence (or cheese), errors can still occur. The defence layers (or countermeasures) may be engineered (physical barriers or alarms), may rely on people (paramedics, doctors, nurses) or may consist of procedures, protocols or administrative controls. The model illustrates that often the various layers of defence function independently of each other, with varying degrees (or indeed opportunities) for communication. Furthermore, despite the best intentions of each of the countermeasures, they may not be 100% infallible. While the countermeasures are generally effective in preventing hazards (or errors or incidents) from occurring, it is possible that some errors could slip through the holes, resulting in an adverse event. In the medical setting some holes in the cheese can be thought of as active failures of systems or individuals (e.g. distraction), while others are latent and exist across the whole organisation.

Error management

The inception of patient safety as a discipline has seen the introduction of a structured approach to reducing errors but, because it recognises that errors can never be totally avoided, it also demands that systems can tolerate and learn from any errors that do slip through. One of the most significant changes as a result has been the shift from a person approach to a systems view of errors. This enables individuals involved in errors to report the error into a constructive rather than a punitive environment and allows the organisation to respond by adapting the system rather than punishing the individual (Nieva & Sorra, 2003).

It is now widely accepted that in addition to having a responsibility to be vigilant in the provision of patient care, all healthcare practitioners have an equal responsibility to report any errors through the appropriate channel. Work is currently underway to integrate curriculum directly related to patient safety in paramedic undergraduate programs internationally (Batt et al., 2018), which should go some way to reinforcing the role of patient safety principles and providing tools to improve patient safety. Unfortunately today, many errors go unreported, often resulting in lost opportunities for process or training improvements. A study undertaken in the out-of-hospital environment identified six main reasons why clinicians are reluctant to report errors:

- the burden of reporting
- fear of disciplinary action
- fear of potential litigation
- fear of embarrassment
- fear of breaches of anonymity or confidentiality
- concern that 'nothing would change' even if the incident was reported (Jennings & Stella, 2011).

For the safety of our patients it is vital that these barriers are overcome to ensure complete and timely notification of errors, adverse events and near-misses. In some ambulance services support for reporting errors and near-misses, and building them into a continuous quality improvement link, is well-established, but in others it remains bound by a culture of blame.

Open disclosure

The culture of safety that has developed in some organisations that have embraced error management has extended beyond staff to include patients and their families. In healthcare systems that have a fully evolved culture of safety, the identification of hazards, adverse and sentinel events is rewarded and staff are shielded from punishment, while weaknesses in the system are rectified (Nieva & Sorra, 2003). However, the notion that patients should be informed openly and honestly about adverse events as soon as possible after they occur is alarming to clinicians working in organisations where error disclosure is primarily linked to disciplinary action (Hebert, 2001).

Sentinel events

Sentinel events are the most severe healthcare-related errors and must be notified to a health service

BOX 11.1 Australian sentinel events list

- Procedures involving the wrong patient or body part resulting in death or major permanent loss of function
- Suicide of a patient in an inpatient unit
- Retained instruments or other material after surgery requiring re-operation or further surgical procedure
- Intravascular gas embolism resulting in death or neurological damage
- Haemolytic blood transfusion reaction resulting from ABO incompatibility
- Medication error leading to the death of a patient reasonably believed to be due to incorrect administration of drugs
- Maternal death associated with pregnancy, birth and the puerperium
- Infant discharged to the wrong family

Source: Australian Commission on Safety and Quality in Health Care (2018).

BOX 11.2 Guiding principles of ambulance organisations focused on improving patient safety

- Clinicians are empowered to improve clinical care delivery.
- Clinicians actively involve consumers as partners in their care.
- Clinicians participate in designing systems and processes.
- Quality improvement activities are planned, prioritised and have sustainability strategies in place.
- Clinical care delivery is evidence based.
- Standards of clinical care are clearly articulated and communicated.
- Performance of clinical care processes and clinical outcomes are measured.
- Clinical performance measures, peer review and clinical audit are used to evaluate and improve performance.
- New procedures and therapies assuring quality and safety issues are considered.

Source: Department of Health, Victoria (2010).

provider's governing body, often the state Department of Health. In Australia a sentinel event is defined as 'a relatively infrequent, clear cut event that occurs independently of a patient's condition; it commonly reflects hospital system and process deficiencies, and results in unnecessary outcomes for the patient' (Department of Health, Victoria, 2010). Box 11.1 lists the eight Australian sentinel event classifications. These classifications are clearly more relevant to hospital and inpatient health settings, but ambulance services must be aware of their statutory responsibilities of reporting such incidents. Some health departments add an additional classification, such as 'other catastrophic event', to capture additional cases that meet the classification of a sentinel event (Department of Health [Victoria], 2010). It is into this classification that the majority of paramedic sentinel events fall.

Monitoring patient safety

Responsibility for ensuring patient safety must be shared between clinicians, health administrators, clinical leads and healthcare consumers (patients). There are a number of guiding principles around patient safety that ambulance organisations should focus on (see Box 11.2). As a minimum, ambulance managers should ensure that clinicians are involved in the development of clinical guidelines, designing systems and processes and monitoring the clinical effectiveness of their organisation. Clinicians should also actively participate in quality improvement

activities and embrace error reporting, peer review and clinical audit. The historical nature of ambulance services offering low-level clinical care saw many develop without a strong culture of clinical auditing. The self-contained nature of many services also resulted in auditing processes that were entirely internal and failed to seek broader clinical expertise. This was not that different from what most hospitals experienced when they started to embrace the notion of a patient safety system, and most of the patient safety auditing tools introduced by progressive ambulance services have come from the hospitals. Nonetheless, the move to such a system usually represents a cultural shift that is often difficult for both management and operational staff.

Patient safety and organisational culture

The development of a patient safety culture is critical to reducing patient risk (Nieva & Sorra, 2003). One effective way to inspire cultural change is through case reviews: recounting actual or realistic stories where clinicians were involved in an incident that resulted in actual or potential harm. The case study is an example of a vignette that can be posed, followed by questions to focus discussion. Clinicians are often able to relate to such events and help raise awareness of the learning principles. Organisations that have a culture of blame or avoidance of error

CASE STUDY

Case 1807, 2250 hrs.

Dispatch details: An advanced life support crew are dispatched to a 22-year-old female suffering from respiratory distress. The address is a nightclub and the call has come from club staff who state that she appears to be hyperventilating.

Initial presentation: On arrival the crew find a young woman with a raised respiratory rate who appears to be confused and is not able to answer questions. Her pulse is 110 bpm, BP 110/80 mmHg and RR 30; and the pulse oximetry reads 100%.

No-one at the club can give any details about her previous medical history or the events leading up to the ambulance being called. Apart from hyperventilation there is no other obvious abnormality. It seems that she has psychogenic hyperventilation so the crew try to slow her breathing down. The crew attempt to reassure her and slow her respiratory rate. Her blood glucose isn't checked at the scene as it is not deemed to be relevant. As she doesn't seem to be responding, the crew decide to transport her a short distance to the local ED. On arrival at the ED a routine blood glucose reveals her blood sugar to be 35 and the hospital staff comment on the strong smell of ketones.

No long-term harm seems to have been done and luckily the crew decided to transport the patient; however, they misdiagnosed ketoacidosis as psychogenic hyperventilation.

may benefit most from honest, open discussion of realistic stories that describe the fallibility of humans and systems.

Case study reflection
The patient's diabetic ketoacidosis was missed by the ambulance crew at the scene. If they had taken a blood sugar reading as routine for a patient in an altered conscious state, the diagnosis would have been clear. Similarly, if they had picked up the smell of ketones at the scene it would have raised the suspicion of diabetic ketoacidosis. Although no harm occurred on this occasion, the possibility exists that this could have been an error with significant consequences.

The paramedics were dispatched to a case labelled as 'hyperventilation' in a nightclub and it is possible that this created a preconceived idea. Preconceptions can lead to premature diagnostic closure (discussed in Ch 7), biases and ultimately missing the clinical diagnoses. The environment, with its extraneous odours and variable light, did not lend itself to obtaining good-quality observations and might account for why the smell of ketones was missed. Interestingly, the sensitivity to detect ketones in exhaled breath is variable and may have a genetic component (Forrai et al., 1981; Laska & Hubener, 2001), so both members of the crew might have been unable to detect ketones by smell.

As detailed in Reason's model, such factors aligned like the holes in Swiss cheese to enable this error to slide through. Luckily this was a near-miss situation rather than an error with major consequences, but it should nevertheless be followed up. Reviewing the case will suggest controls to prevent the situation occurring again for other patients or crew.

Risk management controls
The strongest controls to prevent a risk situation being repeated are mechanical controls, which

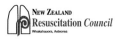

Advanced Life Support for Adults

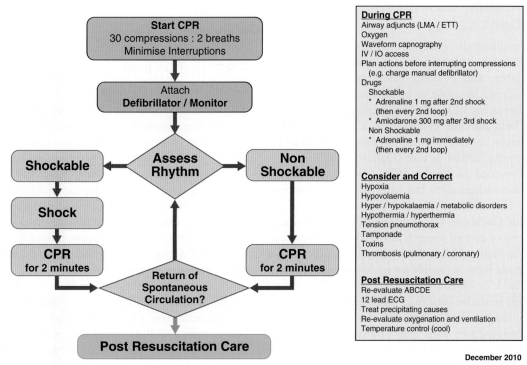

Start CPR
30 compressions : 2 breaths
Minimise Interruptions

Attach
Defibrillator / Monitor

Assess Rhythm

Shockable

Non Shockable

Shock

CPR for 2 minutes

CPR for 2 minutes

Return of Spontaneous Circulation?

Post Resuscitation Care

During CPR
Airway adjuncts (LMA / ETT)
Oxygen
Waveform capnography
IV / IO access
Plan actions before interrupting compressions
    (e.g. charge manual defibrillator)
Drugs
    Shockable
    * Adrenaline 1 mg after 2nd shock
        (then every 2nd loop)
    * Amiodarone 300 mg after 3rd shock
    Non Shockable
    * Adrenaline 1 mg immediately
        (then every 2nd loop)

Consider and Correct
Hypoxia
Hypovolaemia
Hyper / hypokalaemia / metabolic disorders
Hypothermia / hyperthermia
Tension pneumothorax
Tamponade
Toxins
Thrombosis (pulmonary / coronary)

Post Resuscitation Care
Re-evaluate ABCDE
12 lead ECG
Treat precipitating causes
Re-evaluate oxygenation and ventilation
Temperature control (cool)

December 2010

Figure 11.4
The NZRC/ARC guidelines for managing adult cardiac arrest are a good example of a guideline created on the basis of evidence that provides clinicians with a 'scaffold' to support them in a high-stimulus, high-workload environment.
Source: © 2014 Australian Resuscitation Council.

remove human behaviour completely from the process. An example of this is a safety handle on a piece of heavy machinery that automatically shuts the machine down if the handle is not pressed continually. However, mechanical controls are difficult to engineer in a clinical environment.

Procedural controls are also strong. Occasions when procedures or protocols create a safer environment than relying on paramedic reasoning and understanding include the first stages of a cardiac arrest (e.g. the New Zealand Resuscitation Council [NZRC]/Australian Resuscitation Council [ARC] cardiac arrest guidelines; see Fig 11.4) and high-intensity, low-frequency roles like neonatal resuscitation. Similarly, many ambulance services have a protocol that requires a blood glucose to be taken for all patients with an altered conscious state. In order for this control to work the behaviour needs to be driven by the protocol rather than relying on paramedic reasoning and understanding.

However, a procedure is useless unless it is followed and that is the function of education and clinical governance. Organisations must ensure adequate education of staff and auditing of procedures to identify individual or system weaknesses. Education can help us to make a strong link between the clinical experience we have just had (or hopefully somebody else had and told us about) and the reasons why we need to modify our behaviour in future: we now know why we should always remember the blood glucose.

The weakest controls are individually focused disciplinary approaches in which the individual is left in no doubt that they have made an error but no supporting education or system is put in place. Unfortunately, this disciplinary approach to risk management has been a feature of health service culture in the past.

Clinical practice for all professions is, in reality, a mixture of procedures or protocols and guidelines that are supported by clinical reasoning. In high-stress circumstances, a well-constructed guideline is an important element to patient safety and provides a scaffold for our clinical reasoning. In this sense guidelines are a function of evidence-based practice and risk management control.

Evidence-based practice and patient safety

Throughout the whole of medicine there is a move to base clinical guidelines on the best evidence available, and evidence-based practice (EBP) is considered by some to be an essential element of patient safety. EBP is the systematic process by which the best available evidence on a topic is used to underpin the decision-making process for a relevant treatment, action or task (Doherty, 2005).

Founded during the 1970s, EBP was influenced by two independent but intertwined movements. The first of these was led by epidemiologist Dr Archie Cochrane. Dr Cochrane called for systematic reviews of current research across all medical specialities so that evidence from scientific studies could be made more accessible for healthcare practitioners (Melnyk & Fineout-Overholt, 2005). The success of this initiative continues today and the results are published in the Cochrane Collaboration. Second, in conjunction with this production of clinical reviews, a new approach to medical practice was developed, known as evidence-based medicine (Guyett & Drummond, 2002). Initiated by clinical epidemiologists David Sackett, Brian Haynes, Peter Tugwell and Victor Neufeld at McMaster University in Canada, this new philosophy brought scientific decision-making to the bedside and by the early 1990s it had spread to other areas including allied health and nursing (Guyett & Drummond, 2002).

EBP includes data from a wide variety of evidential levels. Although some evidential levels are considered more reputable than others, EBP is selective—not exclusionary—between different types, recognising the diversity of evidence available. Practitioners gathering evidence incorporate data from sources such as randomised control trials (RCTs), systematic reviews, documented experiences, theories, documented patient reviews, role models, policy directives and expert opinion (le May, 1999). As a minimum, practitioners need to refer to more than one paper in order to refer to their practice as evidence based (Birnbaum, 1999; Doherty, 2005; Melnyk & Fineout-Overholt, 2005). Relying on only one paper does not recognise research differences and runs the risk of making recommendations on evidence that is not reputable, reliable or reproducible.

EBP, individual patients and clinical reasoning

The relationship between EBP and patient safety appears fundamental; patients will be diagnosed and receive treatment based on the results of large studies where the tests and interventions have been proven to be safe and effective (Savage & Williams, 2008). In terms of developing guidelines and protocols, this can be extremely useful to paramedics working in information- and time-poor settings: they can rely on the guidelines to reduce the cognitive load of decision-making and ensure the management plan is generally beneficial.

However, guidelines—even those developed by strong studies—should never completely negate clinical reasoning. One of the weaknesses of EBP is that even a well-designed trial is a summary of the 'net' effect of the test or drug: how did the majority of patients respond to the intervention? For interventions that are standard or routine this uniformity is undoubtedly beneficial; for example, the guideline that all patients in an altered conscious state should have their blood glucose level tested will ensure any episodes of hypo- or hyperglycaemia are identified. In routine procedures the essential element is including reliable interventions that provide a distinct treatment path; that is, for an altered conscious state test for hypoglycaemia: if hypoglycaemia is present, treat with IV glucose.

Where EBP cannot replace clinical reasoning is in acknowledging that the design of clinical trials aims to both reduce variables and identify a common response. In practice, clinicians will see cases that present or respond abnormally, and they will also be confronted by patients with multiple (acute and chronic) comorbidities that may influence their presentation or reaction to treatment (Savage & Williams, 2008). For paramedics, guidelines developed by EBP provide a simple solution for routine cases, but it remains the paramedic's responsibility to determine whether a patient can be described as 'routine'.

Rather than criticise EBP for its inability to deal with 'special cases', perhaps a better view is to embrace its utility to reduce the cognitive workload and decision-making in the majority of cases, and allow the clinician to detect the 'special cases'

PRACTICE TIP

Old clinical guidelines can be used to identify where EBP has been employed in paramedicine. For example, aminophylline for asthma, isoprenaline for bradycardia and atropine for cardiac arrest are all medications that were once routinely used in out-of-hospital medicine but have been replaced or simply excluded as either ineffective or harmful.

through effective reasoning and then integrate their knowledge of physiology and treatment to select the best management plan for that patient.

Summary

Medical practice is inherently complex. While it is the intent of all clinicians to protect their patients, this complexity can lead to errors. Medical errors are not usually caused by clinicians initiating the wrong treatment through a lack of knowledge; threats to patient safety are more often the result of clinicians working within flawed systems. The process of recognising and improving systems in healthcare is proving challenging as it can conflict with traditional clinical governance models that do not recognise error and tend to attribute blame to individuals rather than the system.

Nonetheless, over the past few decades there has been a significant change in the way some hospitals identify medical errors and seek to prevent them recurring. This should lead to much safer patient care in the longer term and has already been adopted by some ambulance services.

Consumers of healthcare have the right to expect the care they receive to be safe, regardless of the setting in which it is delivered. The current generation of clinicians being educated are the first to have concepts of human factors, error wisdom and patient safety embedded into their curriculums and, provided they are supported in the workplace, they should be the safest clinicians yet to enter practice.

References

Assaf, A. A. F., Bumpus, L. J., Carter, D., & Dixon, S. B. (2003). Preventing errors in healthcare: a call for action. *Hospital Topics, 81*(3), 5–12.

Australian Commission on Safety and Quality in Health Care. (2018). *Australian Sentinel Events List*. Retrieved 20 November 2018. Retrieved from https://www.safetyand quality.gov.au/our-work/indicators/australian-sentinel -events-list/.

Australian Institute of Health and Welfare [AIHW]. (2009). *Towards national indicators of safety and quality in health care. Cat. no. HSE 75.* Canberra: AIHW.

Batt, A. M., Henderson, L., Duncliffe, T. H., Robb, S., Jones, J. C., Crosetta, R., Smith, P., & Steary, D. (2018). Strategies for incorporating patient safety education in paramedic education using the IHI Open School. *Irish Journal of Paramedicine, 3*, 2. DOI: http://dx.doi.org/ 10.32378/ijp.v3i2.119.

Bigham, B. L., Buick, J. E., Brooks, S. C., Morrison, M., Shojania, K. G., & Morrison, L. J. (2012). Patient safety in emergency medical services: a systematic review of the literature. *Prehospital Emergency Care, 16*(1), 20–35. DOI: http://doi.org/10.3109/10903127.2011.621045.

Birnbaum, M. L. (1999). Guidelines, algorithms, critical pathways, templates, and evidence-based medicine [comment]. *Prehospital & Disaster Medicine, 14*(3), 114–115.

Brennan, T., Leape, L., Laird, N., Hebert, L., Localio, A. R., Lawthers, A. G., Newhouse, J. P., Weiler, P. C., & Hiatt, H. H. (1991). Incidence of adverse events and negligence in hospitalised patients: results of the Harvard Medical Practice Study I. *The New England Journal of Medicine, 324*(6), 370–376.

Collier, P. F., & Son (Eds.), (1910). *Oath of Hippocrates. Harvard classics* (Vol. 38). Boston: Harvard Press.

Department of Health, Victoria. (2010). Building foundations to support patient safety. *Sentinel event program annual report, 2009–2010. State of Victoria.*

Doherty, S. (2005). Evidence-based medicine: arguments for and against. *Emergency Medicine Australasia: EMA, 17*(4), 307–313.

Forrai, G., Bánkövi, G., Szabados, T., & Papp, E. S. (1981). Ketone compound smelling ability: study in Hungarian twins. *Acta Medica Academiae Scientiarum Hungaricae, 38*(2), 153–158.

Graber, M. L., Franklin, N., & Gordon, R. (2005). Diagnostic error in internal medicine. *Archives of Internal Medicine, 165*(13), 1493–1499.

Graber, M. L., Gordon, R., & Franklin, N. (2002). Reducing diagnostic errors in medicine: what's the goal? *Academic Medicine: Journal of the Association of American Medical Colleges, 77*(10), 981–987.

Guyett, G., & Drummond, R. (Eds.), (2002). *User's guide to the medical literature.* Chicago: AMA Press.

Hebert, P. C. (2001). Disclosure of adverse events and errors in healthcare. *Drug Safety, 24*(15), 1095–1104.

Jennings, P. A., & Stella, J. (2011). Barriers to incident notification in a regional prehospital setting. [comparative study research support, Non-U.S. Gov't.]. *Emergency Medicine Journal, 28*(6), 526–529.

Kohn, L. T., Corrigan, J. M., & Molla, S. (1999). *To err is human: building a safer health system.* Medicine. Washington, DC: National Academies Press.

Laska, M., & Hubener, F. (2001). Olfactory discrimination ability for homologous series of aliphatic ketones and acetic esters. *Behavioural Brain Research, 119*, 193–201.

le May, A. (1999). *Evidence-based practice nursing times monographs.* London: Emap Healthcare.

Leape, L., Brennan, T., Laird, N., Lawthers, A. G., Localio, A. R., Barnes, B. A., Hebert, L., Newhouse, J. P., Weiler, P. C., & Hiatt, H. (1991). The nature of adverse events in hospitalised patients: results of the Harvard Medical Study II. *The New England Journal of Medicine, 324*(6), 377–384.

Localio, A. R., Lawthers, A. G., Brennan, T. A., Laird, N. M., Hebert, L. E., Peterson, L. M., Newhouse, J. P., Weiler, P. C., & Hiatt, H. H. (1991). Relation between malpractice claims and adverse events due to negligence: results of the Harvard Medical Practice Study III. *The New England Journal of Medicine, 325*(4), 245–251.

Melnyk, B., & Fineout-Overholt, E. (2005). *Evidence-Based practice in nursing & healthcare: a guide to best practice.* Philadelphia: Lippincott Williams & Wilkins.

National Center for Health Care Statistics at the Centers for Disease Control. (2005). *Deaths/Mortality.* Retrieved March 2013 from www.cdc.gov/nchs/fastats/deaths.htm.

Nieva, V. F., & Sorra, J. (2003). Safety culture assessment: a tool for improving patient safety in healthcare organizations. *Quality and Safety in Health Care, 12*(Suppl.II), ii17–ii23.

Nolan, T. W. (2000). System changes to improve patient safety. *British Medical Journal, 18*(320), 771–773.

Reason, J. (2000). Human error: models and management. *British Medical Journal, 320*(7237), 768–770.

Savage, G. T., & Williams, E. S. (2008). Evidence-based medicine and patient safety: limitations and implications. In G. T. Savage & E. W. Ford (Eds.), *Advances in health care management: patient safety and health care management* (Vol. 7). Bingley, UK: Emerald Group.

Shojania, K. G., Burton, E., McDonald, M., & Goldman, L. (2003). Changes in rates of autopsy-detected diagnostic errors over time. *JAMA, 289,* 2849–2856.

Singh, H., Graber, M. L., Kissam, S. M., Sorensen, A. V., Lenfestey, N. F., Tant, E. M., Henriksen, K., & LaBresh, K. A. (2012). System-related interventions to reduce diagnostic errors: a narrative review. *BMJ Quality and Safety, 21,* 160–170.

Thomas, E. J., Stoddert, D. M., Burstin, H. R., Orav, E. J., Zeena, T., Williams, E. J., Howard, K. M., Weiler, P. C., & Brennan, T. A. (2000). Incidence and types of adverse events and negligent care in Utah and Colorado. *Medical Care, 38*(3), 261–271.

Weingart, S. N., Wilson, R. M., Gibberd, R. W., & Harrison, B. (2000). Epidemiology of medical error. *British Medical Journal, 320*(7237), 774–777.

Wilson, R. M., Runciman, W. B., Gibberd, R. W., Harrison, B. T., Newby, L., & Hamilton, J. D. (1995). The quality in Australian health care study. *The Medical Journal of Australia, 163*(9), 458–471.

Wolff, A. M., & Bourke, J. (2002). Detecting and reducing adverse events in an Australian rural base hospital emergency department using medical record screening and review. *Emergency Medicine Journal, 19,* 35–40.

CHAPTER 12

Paramedic Health and Wellbeing

By Ben Meadley and Tegwyn McManamny

OVERVIEW

- Working as a paramedic can be physically and emotionally demanding, and the role requires significant lifestyle adjustments.
- Paramedics can be exposed to highly stressful situations on a frequent basis.
- The unpredictable nature of the paramedic workplace can require crews to operate for long hours in uncomfortable environments with limited access to high-quality nutrition or rest breaks.

- Paramedics are at a high risk of suffering poor mental health due to the nature of their work, and are at a risk of misuse of alcohol and other drugs to cope with the demands of the profession.
- Poor physical, metabolic and mental health can arise from long-term exposure to shiftwork and complex patient situations.
- Many resources and strategies are available to enhance the health and wellbeing of paramedics.

Introduction

Paramedics work in a dynamic, often uncontrolled environment. Paramedics are required to care for people with varying states of physical and mental illness, and it is reasonable to suggest that this environment has physical or psychological impact on the paramedics themselves (Reynolds & O'Donnell, 2016). A paramedic's state of 'wellness', the decisions they make and the clinical care they deliver can have a significant bearing on the health outcomes of patients. Paramedics practise on a premise of a structured, systematic approach to patient assessment and clinical care. However, many other factors affect the way in which paramedics perform their role.

In this chapter we examine issues such as mental and physical health, nutrition, occupational stressors and what influence they may have on a paramedic's ability to provide high-quality clinical care, while maintaining a life balance. We also look at the paramedic's 'emotional capacity' and how it impacts on both the patient and the paramedic. Unlike some of the other factors involved in clinical decision-making, paramedic wellness as a whole can be difficult to quantify. Gaining an awareness of how the occupation of paramedicine affects one physically and emotionally can contribute to greater paramedic health, promote career longevity, reduce the risk of mental or physical injury, and ultimately lead to enhanced patient care.

Paramedic health and safety

Paramedics are exposed to a range of health and safety concerns that may affect their wellbeing, such as:

- exposure to contagious and infectious diseases from patients
- exposure to contagious or infectious diseases by sharps such as needles
- exposure to chemicals used in medical procedures such as methoxyflurane, nitrous oxide and industrial cleaning products
- physical tasks that involve awkward postures, repetition, force or overexertion
- exposure to extreme temperatures and inclement weather
- risk of injury from fire, explosions, unstable structures and surfaces, falling objects, traffic and occupational violence
- slips, trips and falls, often compounded by the fact that the paramedic is carrying a patient on a stretcher or in another extrication device
- transport dangers including driving at high speeds, often in difficult traffic or weather conditions
- shiftwork and extended workdays
- periods of intense psychological stress or trauma (Roberts et al., 2015).

These issues can present significant challenges for paramedics, who have to balance such welfare concerns with managing the health and wellbeing of their patients. Making good decisions that have positive impacts on patient wellbeing requires physically, mentally and emotionally healthy paramedics.

Definitions

Wellbeing

Wellbeing or wellness goes beyond feeling physically healthy; it is a multidimensional concept involving every part of a person: emotional/psychological, spiritual, intellectual and physical (Oades et al., 2017). This implies that many factors influence wellbeing, and that difficulties in one area may cause overall imbalance.

Attending to each individual component that makes up holistic 'wellbeing' is vital. For example:

- an *emotionally* well person is resilient to change and can make grounded decisions and adapt to circumstances rapidly.
- a *physically* well person can resist illness and maximise their physical capacity
- a *spiritually* well person is secure in their existence and purpose
- an *intellectually* well person is able to exercise their mental capacity to the fullest.

Stress

A paramedic's health and wellbeing can be significantly influenced by stress. A stressor is any condition or event (physiological, psychological or environmental) that causes a stress response (Ruotsalainen et al., 2014). A stress response occurs when a person is confronted by a perceivably threatening situation, leading to the sympathetic arousal of the autonomic nervous system; the 'fight or flight' response. It causes the release of the catecholamines adrenaline and noradrenaline from the adrenal medulla, preparing the body to stay and defend or to run away. The 'threat' message is conveyed initially through the autonomic nervous system but is sustained by a hormonal response that involves the release of adrenocorticotrophic hormone (ACTH) and glucocorticoids such as cortisol. Although stress is generally considered to be a psychological response, it has significant physiological components.

Long-term effects of stress

The health impacts of stress in the long term can be significant. Increased cortisol levels over a prolonged period of time lower the efficiency of the immune system, making the body more susceptible to infection and slowing the rate of wound healing (Martini, 2006). Chronically high levels of stress hormones trigger remodelling in cardiac and vascular tissue and can result in hypertension. Tiredness,

BOX 12.1 Signs and symptoms of acute stress

- Increased heart rate
- Increased blood pressure
- Pupil dilation
- Sweating
- Increased blood sugar levels
- Inhibition of digestive secretions
- Peripheral vasoconstriction
- Bronchodilation

sleep disorders, headaches, chronic pain and psychological difficulties such as anxiety, depression and panic attacks are also attributable to chronic exposure to stress hormones, as are changes in the brain structures involved in cognition and mental health (Lupien et al., 2009).

Acute and chronic stress

Much has been written about stressors and the effects of stress on healthcare workers. Stress is often divided into two categories: acute stress, usually related to exposure to critical incidents and traumatic events; and chronic stress, which is often linked to cumulative stress, burnout and everyday job-intrinsic stress (Hamilton, 2009).

Acute stress

Exposure to acute stressors such as critical incidents and traumatic events is often an integral part of the job for paramedics and other emergency workers (see Box 12.1 for signs of acute stress). A *critical incident* is defined as any event or circumstance that caused or could have caused (a 'near miss') unplanned harm, suffering, loss or damage (The Intensive Care Society, 2005). It can be extended to include any incident that overwhelms/threatens to overwhelm the individual's usual method of coping (Alexander & Klein, 2001).

The highest levels of critical incident stress appear to come from exposure to 'chaotic, tragic or gruesome circumstances' (Donnelly & Siebert, 2009). For paramedics, incidents involving children, suicides and grotesque mutilation are cited as being the most distressing (Gallagher & McGilloway, 2007). Paramedics may attend tragic and poignant scenes where they are confronted with deceased and dying patients, multi-casualty accidents and injured children. The effects of such exposure are unique to the person experiencing them. Emotional reactions may occur initially, but later effects can include nightmares, flashbacks and changes in mood. It is important to recognise the significant impact that critical incidents and traumatic events can have, and to be alert for signs of critical incident stress in yourself and your colleagues.

Chronic stress

While exposure to critical incidents and traumatic events can have a tremendous impact on the physical and mental wellbeing of paramedics, everyday operational duties can be just as stressful. Chronic stress, the 'enduring problems, conflicts and threats that many people face in their daily lives' (Pearlin, 1989), can be an ever-present background noise that paramedics must manage in addition to the provision of emergency healthcare. Causes of chronic stress in paramedics include:

- operational concerns such as organisational mismanagement
- inadequate operational support and dispatch errors (Alexander & Klein, 2001)
- lack of support from or conflict with colleagues (Donnelly & Siebert, 2009)
- shiftwork and sleep disruption
- working in hazardous conditions
- exposure to violence
- constant physiological arousal (when responding to or anticipating an incident) (Hegg-Deloye et al., 2014)
- high workloads.

The stress of not being stressed

It is commonly perceived that paramedics spend their days managing one acutely unwell patient after the other. The changing nature of the paramedic role (Reynolds & O'Donnell, 2016) has shown that they are primary healthcare providers rather than critical care experts. This can be a challenge for paramedics, who may feel that they are not contributing to patient healthcare in the way they anticipated. Paradoxically, this lack of exposure to critically ill patients can be stressful for paramedics, who feel their training and skills are being wasted. In reality, the primary healthcare role of paramedics can generate its own form of stress.

The cumulative effect of exposure to both acute and chronic stressors has been associated with negative outcomes for paramedics. These include ill health, burnout, premature mortality and high levels of workforce absenteeism (Clompus & Albarran, 2016). Paramedics are inadvertently affected by the chronic stressors around them, and it is important to recognise the impacts of this chronic exposure on their moods, decision-making and clinical practice.

Managing emotion

Several authors discuss the concept of an emotional bank account, cup or emotional pie (Covey, 1992).

According to this concept, our feelings of stress and wellbeing are rarely constant: the world and the people we interact with are constantly making deposits or withdrawals on our sense of wellbeing, filling or emptying our cup, or consuming parts of our 'pie'. When your emotional wellbeing is high, you have a deep reserve to draw on before you are affected. But if the people and situations around you all demand an emotional investment from you, your reserve will run down. Your reserves can be replenished by positive experiences and interactions, boosting your emotional wellbeing.

Running on empty

For paramedics facing a long shift full of emotionally charged situations, maintaining a degree of self-awareness and monitoring their stress and emotion levels throughout the shift become essential in avoiding triggers. Paramedics should recognise early which situations may deplete their reserves. Examples include not having a meal break on time, interacting with traumatised relatives of patients, communicating poorly with your work partner and facing busy nightshifts.

Replenish your reserves

Early in a paramedic's career, when the role is novel, it is difficult to imagine being unenthusiastic. But after a few years the break between shifts can seem too short to fully recharge before returning to work. Recognising this and using your downtime to positively recharge yourself are essential to wellness.

Protect yourself

The paramedic role by its nature involves a series of small stressors punctuated by the occasional large stressor. One of the keys to managing these stresses is to recognise the unique nature of the job, and to actively protect yourself at the start of every shift. Unlike other jobs where commercial or creative successes can actually make a day entirely positive, paramedics (like a number of healthcare roles) are often subject to a series of patients suffering crises.

Prepare yourself. Be well nourished, rested and physically well. If you are experiencing personal difficulties, ensure you let your work colleagues know so that they can keep an eye out for you at work, and consider other options for getting your wellbeing back on track, such as counselling or other support. All ambulance services will provide ample personal leave entitlements. If you need a break, take it. As such, consider personal leave as an important part of your wellness plan, and be wary of frivolous wastage of this entitlement.

It is important to realise that some situations may affect you more than others owing to past experiences or encounters and your current state of wellness. For example, a paramedic who is a keen cyclist may feel more empathy for cases involving bicycle crashes at work. Paramedics with young children are likely to find scenes with patients the same age as their children more challenging. If you are aware that some situations will challenge you more than others, it is important to remember the 'emotional reserve' concept and endeavour to keep your balance topped up. Recognise your emotions, speak to your work colleagues about any potential difficulties and consider addressing the root cause of your distress through counselling or other support services.

It is natural for paramedics to have an emotional reaction to the incidents they encounter. However, crossing the boundary between sympathy and empathy can result in a risky emotional attachment, leaving the paramedic's emotional state vulnerable. It is important to maintain a professional relationship with patients, understanding their needs without becoming too emotionally involved.

Fatigue

Fatigue has been defined as 'a state of tiredness, affecting both mind and body; where an individual is unable to function at their normal level of abilities' (Sofianopoulos et al., 2011). It is more than just being tired after a poor night's sleep and can be caused by a variety of influences including sleep disturbances, shiftwork, poor lifestyle and occupational stress. Fatigue is a reality for paramedics due to the nature of the job and shiftwork. It can significantly affect physical and psychological wellbeing, which can impact patient care. The symptoms of fatigue vary for each individual, and it is important to understand how fatigue affects you and the people around you. Reading the signs will help you know when to take action and make positive changes to ensure your health and safety, and that of your colleagues.

If you recognise the signs of fatigue in yourself or a colleague, act on this (see Box 12.2). Take a break wherever possible, ensure you are well nourished and hydrated, and monitor your condition. Studies indicate that judgment, alertness and concentration are all affected by fatigue (Dowson & Zee, 2005). Additionally, work performance is decreased due to changes in problem-solving and decision-making skills (Jansen et al., 2003); this has significant ramifications for patient care in the out-of-hospital setting.

How to manage fatigue

Paramedics can help reduce their fatigue, and recover more effectively from shiftwork, by remaining

> ## BOX 12.2 General signs of fatigue
>
> - Constant yawning
> - Heavy or sore eyes, rubbing your eyes
> - Trouble keeping your head upright
> - Delayed reactions
> - Irritability
> - Daydreaming
> - Taking longer than usual to perform simple tasks

self-aware and monitoring themselves. Key factors in the management of fatigue include:

- practising good sleep hygiene (leave adequate time for sleep, and set up the room for sleep during daylight with heavy curtains and noise insulation, put smart devices away)
- maintaining a healthy diet
- maintaining good physical fitness through regular exercise
- restricting your caffeine and alcohol intake, and avoiding using tobacco
- ensuring that your family and friends understand the demands of the paramedic lifestyle and can provide a supportive home environment.

Shiftwork

Paramedics work a variety of shifts. This results in a combination of long hours, overnight duties, rotating schedules, early starts and broken (or absent) nocturnal sleep. Shiftwork has been identified as having detrimental consequences on the health and wellbeing of workers (James et al., 2017), potentially resulting in compromised patient care. The discordant sleep patterns that result from rotations between day, afternoon and night shifts make it difficult to maintain consistently high sleep quality and natural circadian rhythms (James et al., 2017).

A novice paramedic may not feel the impact of shiftwork immediately. As a career of shiftwork progresses these effects become more pronounced. To reduce these, it is important to establish good work/rest habits by prioritising sleep, a healthy diet and exercise.

Self-care

There are some simple things you can do to positively contribute to your health and wellbeing and ensure longevity in the career you have chosen.

- *Catch up on sleep.* Ensure you are well rested both before and after your shifts. Hang heavy curtains in your bedroom to block out light and noise and use earplugs for afternoon naps.

- *Watch your diet.* Large meals and foods rich in fat and carbohydrates can make you feel drowsy as your body attempts to process them. Choose plenty of fresh vegetables with lean protein for your meals and have snacks such as nuts and fruits within easy access. Research has suggested that avoiding eating in the middle of nightshift can improve health outcomes (Bonnell et al., 2017).
- *Nap.* Studies have found that strategic napping during downtime on shifts (particularly night shifts) can reduce fatigue and the adverse effects on physiological functions (Davy & Göbel, 2018). Use your downtime to rest and regain some energy.
- *Seek help.* Having social supports and relationships are vital to wellbeing and discussing your experiences can be a valuable debriefing tool. Ambulance services also provide psychological support, counselling and critical incident debriefing for their staff. If your physical or psychological health deteriorates, seeking professional assistance can be difficult; however, a good first step is discussing any concerns with your local doctor, who can point you in the direction of further assistance where required.

Occupational violence

Occupational violence is a stark reality of paramedicine. Paramedic exposure to occupational violence is a growing concern, with data indicating significant rises in assaults against paramedics over the past decade (Maguire, 2018). In one study, 87% of paramedics reported exposure to occupational violence (Maguire et al., 2014). Violence may take many forms, including physical assault and injury, verbal threats, verbal assault and intimidation.

Paramedics are required to care for patients in a range of situations. This may include those affected by alcohol or other drugs, patients suffering mental illness where perceptions are distorted, relatives who are affected by the circumstances and bystanders who may have witnessed the event or provided assistance.

Most ambulance services recognise that occupational violence is a reality and have acted to protect the wellbeing of their staff. Specialised occupational training programs are compulsory in many ambulance services. These programs assist paramedics to recognise high-risk situations, develop strategies to manage and prevent episodes of actual or threatened violence (e.g. verbal de-escalation strategies) and as

a last resort, physically defend themselves (Spelten et al., 2017).

In addition to these specialised training programs, paramedics need to be constantly vigilant to ensure they are safe. In a manner similar to preventing manual-handling injury or poor nutrition, for example, paramedics should entertain the risk of occupational violence every time they come to work. Some strategies for managing this risk are listed below.

- Danger to you means STOP and make yourself safe, irrespective of patient condition.
- Assume any and every case could result in a threat to you or your colleagues.
- Be aware of your own mood and temperament. This may be affected by fatigue, hunger and workload among other factors.
- Manage your demeanour and confer with your colleagues if you need confirmation of how you may be perceived.
- Treat people humanely, and they will almost always reciprocate.
- Learn to recognise the signs of those affected by alcohol or other drugs.
- Retreat from situations if you have a bad feeling.
- Maintain a situational awareness of the scene.
- Always have an escape route.
- Know how to use your communication devices/ electronic distress alarms; use them when needed.
- Watch out for your colleagues.

Many occupational violence incidents in paramedicine can be avoided, but some cannot. As your experience grows, ensure you too evolve to gain a sense for high-risk situations. Learn to appreciate the dynamic nature of out-of-hospital care and protect the wellbeing of yourself and your colleagues.

Getting help

Extensive literature points to the psychological effects of accident and emergency work, with a strong indication that paramedics are at greater risk of developing physical and mental stress-related disorders (Asbury et al., 2018). Exposure to occupational violence can have serious emotional and mental health consequences for operational paramedics, with studies finding that negative impacts accumulate with repeated exposure to workplace violence (Mayhew & Chappell, 2009). Recognising changes in mental and physical health will help ensure that problems can be addressed early, which is vital for long-term wellbeing.

Out-of-hospital organisations have a responsibility to their employees in terms of preparing them for traumatic incidents as well as providing support post-incident. Paramedics suffering burnout, depression, anxiety or posttraumatic stress disorder (PTSD) require access to support and interventions to decrease stress, promote posttraumatic growth and increase resilience. Programs that address the stressful nature of the job at an organisational level may focus on support after critical incidents as well as management of chronic stress and burnout.

Critical incident stress management

In an acknowledgment of the distress experienced by paramedics and fire-fighters responding to traumatic incidents, a debriefing tool was created to facilitate their recovery (Mitchell, 1983). While controversy exists as to its effectiveness, many organisations use it worldwide. Critical incident stress debriefing (CISD) is conducted by trained facilitators. The process involves participants sharing their experiences of the event and reporting any symptoms, with the facilitator working to normalise stress responses and link participants to further aid if required (Halpern & Maunder, 2011).

Organisational help

Out-of-hospital organisations offer a wide array of other support services to their staff, including peer support, follow-up and referral services (to trained psychologists and counsellors), as well as education regarding emotional and mental health and how to obtain help. Educational programs may encourage self-awareness and monitoring of self and others, increasing awareness of stress and psychological health. It is important that such management tools are easily accessible for staff, and that emotional and psychological wellbeing is prioritised.

Personal strategies

It is important to remember the potential for positive experiences post-stress and the increased resilience and growth that may result. You need to monitor yourself for signs of stress, recognising when it is present and what has contributed to it. Identifying stress early allows you to seek help as soon as possible, creating the potential for growth and promoting psychological health. In addition, seeking assistance early helps you to learn effective coping strategies, rather than relying on poor mechanisms like denial, substance abuse and withdrawal (Clohessy & Ehlers, 1999).

The value of support services in the form of colleagues, friends and family can never be underrated. The people you know, trust and who know you well can be a wonderful source of support. Spending time with family and friends and engaging in activities you enjoy is a form of stress management that many find effective. Look for opportunities to improve your coping and stress management strategies, and never be afraid to seek help when you feel overwhelmed.

Physical injury, physical employment standards and physical activity

Physical injury

Paramedicine can be a physically demanding profession. This makes the role both interesting and challenging, and distinct from other healthcare environments. Sick and injured patients are commonly found in areas that are difficult to access, including remote and austere locations, or even in precarious situations within their own residences. This can place both the patient and the paramedic at risk of injury, and ongoing vigilance is required to ensure that all involved in patient care are safe and that injury is avoided.

Manual-handling injuries to paramedics are all too commonplace (Roberts et al., 2015). Historically, paramedics and other health professions involved in the physical movement of sick and injured patients have suffered severe injuries than can unfortunately be career-ending. Ambulance services have recognised this risk, and in recent years most Australasian ambulance services have taken a more proactive approach to injury prevention (Paul & Hoy, 2015). Through the use of paramedic education programs focusing on safe manual handling, and the introduction of novel manual-handling assistance devices (see Figure 12.1), a culture of safety is now permeating the profession. Paramedic and patient wellbeing and safety is paramount, and Australasian ambulance services lead the way in ensuring that paramedicine is a healthy place to work.

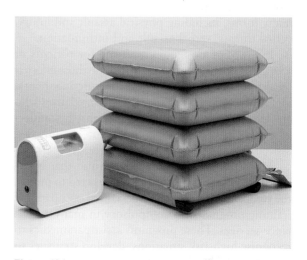

Figure 12.1
The Mangar Elk lifting cushion.

Physical employment standards

Physical employment standards are devised to ensure that an employee's physiological capacities correspond with the specific tasks of the role. The design and implementation of non-arbitrary, scientifically validated physical employment standards can provide benefits to staff, the wider ambulance service and, importantly, patients (Milligan et al., 2016). This is especially relevant in areas of healthcare where patient access, clinical interventions and extraction to definitive care may be time-critical, such as out-of-hospital emergency care.

All Australasian ambulance services require paramedics to satisfy a physical employment standard when commencing their role. Undergraduate paramedicine students may also be required to complete these assessments prior to undertaking clinical placement with ambulance services, most often at their own cost. Physical capacity assessments are mostly task specific (i.e. they relate to the paramedic's ability to perform the core functions of out-of-hospital care). While this is often the case, it is recognised that some services assess physical capacities that may not seem to align with the role. This is identified as an area for improvement and that needs research. Similarly, few ambulance services reassess paramedics after they satisfy the initial requirements, although reassessment is slowly becoming more common. Nonetheless, paramedics must meet the standard of the ambulance service they choose to work with. Common assessments are shown in Table 12.1.

Physical employment standards are developed to minimise the risk to patients, paramedics and the ambulance service as an organisation. They are an important part of becoming a paramedic and demonstrating a commitment to safe out-of-hospital practice, assurance of delivery of patient care and minimising risk of injury.

Table 12.1: Common physical capacity assessments

Assessment	Capacity tested
Submaximal VO$_2$max (beep test/bike/treadmill)	Maximal aerobic capacity
Planking, sit ups	Core abdominal strength
Lifting objects to various heights	Ability to safely carry paramedic equipment
Dynamometry	Grip strength, lifting/holding, leg/lower back strength
Static push/pull/holds	Various joint/muscle group strength

Physical activity

Becoming a paramedic is, to a degree, a lifestyle choice. The previous sections have highlighted the relative risk to paramedics in carrying out their duties, as well as the need to meet an initial physical employment standard. Additionally, it is likely that ongoing assessment of physical capacity will be implemented by most Australasian ambulance services in the future. At a minimum, it is incumbent upon paramedics to maintain a reasonable degree of physical fitness. This is stipulated in most paramedic position descriptions (Ambulance Victoria, 2018).

Paramedic rostering in contemporary Australasian ambulance services offers a reasonable degree of flexibility and free time. Rotating shiftwork rosters often allow for numerous days off in a row, whereby paramedics can theoretically achieve a consistent and predictable approach to maintaining their own wellness. The reasoning for extended days off (compared to the general working population) is to enable recovery from fatiguing shiftwork and exposure to complex and emotionally demanding case types; enabling this recovery is essential. Paramedics are generally afforded more annual leave than the average worker for the same reasons.

Despite these opportunities, maintaining regular physical activity during a career as a paramedic can be difficult (Neil-Sztramko et al., 2016). This is irrespective of the current level of physical activity, be it purely recreational through to elite-level sport participation. This is especially the case when the paramedic is first exposed to regular shiftwork (Nea et al., 2015). Sleep deprivation and cumulative fatigue can see the motivation and energy to undertake physical activity wane, and primarily sedentary behaviour can insidiously become the norm. A reasonable degree of discipline is required to ensure that exercise is regularly undertaken. The benefits of regular physical activity are widely published; however, the applicability of this evidence is of special importance to paramedics.

In light of the higher risk of mental health issues in the field of paramedicine, regular exercise has proven to improve mental health, in spite of significant stressors (Korge & Nunan, 2018). Frequent exercise can increase the levels of mood-elevating hormones and neurotransmitters, while minimising the effect of those that depress mood. Similarly, regular physical activity can mediate the effects of physiological and emotional stress, through acclimatisation of the body to sympathetic stimuli, and enhanced ability to control and moderate an elevated stress response (Rosenbaum et al., 2015).

Importantly, physical fitness has shown a trend to reduce risk of injury in emergency service workers

(Pollack et al., 2017). Intuitively, this makes sense, and a person who is physical actively should in theory be able to manage demanding physical tasks more safely. Although there is limited data showing a statistically significant decrease in injury rate as a result of a formal physical fitness program, it is not unreasonable to translate findings from athletes and other professions, where a clear link has been established (Gabbett, 2016). This is an area of research need, particularly with regard to the specificity of types of fitness activities (e.g. aerobic fitness versus weight training and its role in reducing work-related injury) and how they relate to the manual-handling injury risk.

Many paramedics already undertake regular physical activity prior to joining the profession and have a head start. It is advisable to seek the counsel of experienced paramedics who are also active in an effort to understand how to weave an exercise program into a complex alternating timetable of activity and recovery while undertaking shiftwork. Conversely, if physical activity is not part of your normal routine, consider seeking the advice of a professional exercise physiologist or an ambulance service health and wellness liaison (where applicable) to commence a physical wellness regimen; the benefits are numerous and likely to be beyond those highlighted in this section.

Nutrition

There are many factors that contribute to wellbeing in emergency service workers. An established area of research in the general community is the role of high-quality nutrition in the prevention of disease, and also its contribution to overall wellness. The impact of nutrition on disease processes has progressed significantly in recent times. Specifically, a number of studies have examined the impact of shiftwork on the ability to access high-quality nutrition (Anstey et al., 2016; Bonnell et al., 2017). This is especially relevant to paramedics. Shiftworkers are at a higher risk of suffering from conditions such as obesity, type II diabetes and cardiovascular and inflammatory diseases (Hegg-Deloye et al., 2015). There are a number of reasons postulated for this, including poor sleep patterns, limited physical activity, high injury rates and poor nutrition.

The dynamic nature of paramedicine, and the requirement to be able to respond at any and all times of the day or night, means that rest and meal breaks can be difficult to access. Paramedic crews are constantly mobile, the workload is unpredictable and as such the ability to plan a meal is often

challenging. In one study, paramedics reported a number of barriers to accessing high-quality nutrition. These include mobility of the role, reliance on easily accessible food (e.g. takeaway food), leaving pre-prepared meals at the ambulance station and then being out on jobs all shift, lack of meal breaks and influence of other paramedics (e.g. partner) on meal choices (Anstey et al., 2016).

In isolation, intermittent consumption of low-quality nutrition may seem insignificant; however, increased consumption can be insidious, especially as cumulative fatigue from shiftwork mounts, leading to a lack of motivation to seek high-quality meals. Acknowledging the identified difficulties in planning and accessing good food, it is still important to consider the impact of a poor diet on paramedic wellness. Careful planning and a willingness to be flexible with regard to food types can allow paramedics to eat well; a number of strategies can be employed to ensure paramedics eat well while on duty. Below are some suggestions describing a relatively straightforward approach to ensuring good nutrition is part of your overall wellness plan.

- Plan meals for your block of shifts well in advance.
- Consider planning meals with your partner (where possible).
- Consider allocating time on days off to cook up batches of pre-prepared meals.
- Don't assume that you will be able to cook meals at work.
- If you plan to reheat a meal, have a 'Plan B'.
- Ensure some meals do not require re-heating.
- Choose meals with a balance of macronutrients (fat, carbohydrates and protein).
- Learn how to read nutrition panels on pre-packaged food.
- Carry meals with you in the ambulance, with due consideration to safe storage and infection control.
- Actively avoid reliance on 'fast food', no matter how nutritious the label says it is.
- Prepare non-processed nutritious snacks that are low in sugar.
- Allow yourself some favourite snacks, but be wary of high-sugar content and the metabolic effect.

Adequate and high-quality nutrition can be accessed if you plan carefully. The cumulative effect of shiftwork, fatigue and a constantly mobile workspace means you are at risk of suffering the consequences of poor nutrition. Speak with paramedics that have experienced difficulties in accessing high-quality food while working in paramedicine.

Alcohol and other drugs

In this chapter, we have discussed the variety of stressors—both mental and physiological—to which paramedics may be exposed. There is significant evidence that demonstrates paramedics are at risk of use and/or abuse of alcohol and other drugs (Pilgrim et al., 2017). Within the role of paramedicine, there are many factors that build this risk profile. These include but are not limited to:

- ongoing exposure to stressful events
- disrupted sleep patterns and fatigue
- ad hoc ability to undertake structured physical activity and exercise
- unsociable shift timings
- a tendency to socialise with other paramedics
- ready access to restricted medications (e.g. opioids, stimulants, benzodiazepines).

The combination of one or more of the above may build to a 'perfect storm', and a number of studies demonstrate the tendency for healthcare workers to turn to alcohol and other drugs in order to 'cope' with the demands of their profession (Pilgrim et al., 2017). In the vast majority of circumstances, paramedics and other emergency services workers engage in safe and responsible use of legal substances such as alcohol. However, in some instances dangerous alcohol and/or drug use, with a tendency towards abuse, has been reported among this population (Independent Broad-Based Anti-Corruption Commission, 2017). The health consequences of the use and abuse of legal substances such as alcohol and tobacco and illegal substances including so-called 'recreational drugs' are well documented. Paramedics should be cognisant of the health consequences of frequent use of any high-risk substance, and there are many avenues for support should you have concern for yourself or someone else (see Box 12.3). Open communication with colleagues regarding substance use is a great way to monitor and gauge use of substances

of potential abuse; paramedics are some of the most compassionate and understanding health professionals. Additionally, most ambulance services provide a peer support/counselling service to employees that is free and confidential.

The use and/or abuse of alcohol and other drugs can unquestionably affect a paramedic's ability to provide safe patient care. Paramedicine is among the most trusted of professions in Australasia (New South Wales Ambulance, 2014). Paramedics are not only deeply trusted by the public that they serve, but also by their ambulance colleagues, their employer, medical and nursing staff, and other health professionals. With this trust comes significant responsibility. As such, over recent years ambulance services have aligned their policies with other high-risk professions by implementing a zero-tolerance approach to alcohol and other drugs in the workplace. While it may be culturally acceptable to use alcohol and other drugs in personal time, the use of or being affected by these substances when providing patient care is not. Screening for alcohol and other drugs occurs almost universally during the application process when first commencing work as a paramedic, and random drug testing is now commonplace (Ambulance Victoria, 2017) (see Box 12.4).

As previously mentioned, becoming a paramedic is, to a certain degree, a lifestyle choice. Paramedics come from all walks of life and as such, what is perceived as acceptable will differ between individuals. While acknowledging that substance use can be seen as a normal component of a modern society, patients rightly expect those providing their care to be unaffected by any substance. Thus, it is important that paramedics carefully consider not only the personal health consequences of high-risk substance use, but also what effect this may have on their ability to provide exemplary patient care. Many substances remain present in the body long after

---

BOX 12.3 Drug and alcohol support services in Australia and New Zealand

- Australia:
  › Alcohol and Drug Foundation: 1300 85 85 84
  › Lifeline: 13 11 14
- New Zealand:
  › Alcohol Drug Helpline: 0800 787 797
  › Lifeline: 0800 LIFELINE (0800 5433 5463)

BOX 12.4 Common substances tested for by ambulance services

- Methamphetamine
- Marijuana
- Opioids including morphine, fentanyl and codeine
- Alcohol
- Other recreational drugs such as ketamine and MDMA ('ecstasy')

they have been used, and a positive drug test result may compromise a career.

Change and adaptation to a career in paramedicine can be challenging for many people. The first few years are a steep learning curve academically, operationally and emotionally. Be aware that the profession is one that demands a reasonable commitment, and that parts of the job will infiltrate your personal life. A high level of commitment to personal wellness is vital, as is reflection on the impact the role has on you as a person. Seek assistance openly and frequently. And, as mentioned earlier, there are a number of support services that can assist in adaptation to your new career and life (see Box 12.3).

Summary

While a range of occupational, psychological and social factors may have an impact on paramedics in their workplace, it is possible to take steps to reduce the risk of any adverse effects. Being aware and recognising occupational risk factors (such as lack of access to regular physical activity and high-quality nutrition, exposure to stress, occupational violence and injury) can help paramedics make safe choices and decisions to support their health and wellbeing. The decision-making process and patient care can be influenced by a range of factors confronting paramedics; therefore, optimal wellbeing, in all its forms, is vital to ensure the safety of patients and paramedics alike. Undergraduate students face particular challenges that can affect their wellbeing and it is important that support is accessible during this period of their journey. Self-awareness and monitoring help to recognise stress and other physical and mental health concerns, and lead to improvements in managing your wellness and promoting growth and resilience.

References

Alexander, D. A., & Klein, S. (2001). Ambulance personnel and critical incidents: impact of accident and emergency work on mental health and emotional well-being. *The British Journal of Psychiatry*, *178*(1), 76–81.

Ambulance Victoria. (2017). *Ambulance Victoria's response to the IBAC Operation Tone Report*. [ONLINE] Retrieved from: https://www.ambulance.vic.gov.au/ambulance-victorias-response-to-the-ibac-operation-tone-report/. (Accessed 5 May 2018).

Ambulance Victoria. (2018). *Graduate Paramedic Position Description*. [ONLINE] Retrieved from: https://www.ambulance.vic.gov.au/wp-content/uploads/2019/05/Position-Description-Graduate-Ambulance-Paramedic-Various-December-2018.pdf. (Accessed 5 May 2018).

Anstey, S., Tweedie, J., & Lord, B. (2016). Qualitative study of Queensland paramedics' perceived influences on their food and meal choices during shift work. *Nutrition & Dietetics*, *73*(1), 43–49.

Asbury, E., Rasku, T., Thyer, L., Campbell, C., Holmes, L., Sutton, C., & Tavares, W. (2018). IPAWS: the international paramedic anxiety wellbeing and stress study. *Emergency Medicine Australasia: EMA*, *30*(1), 132.

Bonnell, E. K., Huggins, C. E., Huggins, C. T., McCaffrey, T. A., Palermo, C., & Bonham, M. P. (2017). Influences on dietary choices during day versus night shift in shift workers: a mixed methods study. *Nutrients*, *9*(3), 193.

Clohessy, S., & Ehlers, A. (1999). PTSD symptoms, response to intrusive memories and coping in ambulance service workers. *The British Journal of Clinical Psychology*, *38*(Pt. 3), 251–265.

Clompus, S. R., & Albarran, J. W. (2016). Exploring the nature of resilience in paramedic practice: a psycho-social study. *International Emergency Nursing*, *28*, 1–7.

Covey, S. R. (1992). *Principle-centered leadership*. Simon and Schuster.

Davy, J., & Göbel, M. (2018). The effects of extended nap periods on cognitive, physiological and subjective responses under simulated night shift conditions. *Chronobiology International*, *35*(2), 169–187.

Donnelly, E., & Siebert, D. (2009). Occupational risk factors in the emergency medical services. *Prehospital and Disaster Medicine*, *24*(5), 422–429.

Dowson, D., & Zee, P. (2005). Working hours and reducing fatigue-related risk: good research vs good policy. *JAMA*, *294*(9), 1104–1109.

Gabbett, T. J. (2016). The training–injury prevention paradox: should athletes be training smarter and harder? *British Journal of Sports Medicine*, *50*, 273–280.

Gallagher, S., & McGilloway, S. (2007). Living in critical times: the impact of critical incidents on frontline ambulance personnel—a qualitative perspective. *International Journal of Emergency Mental Health*, *9*(3), 215–223.

Halpern, J., & Maunder, R. (2011). Acute and chronic workplace stress in emergency medical technicians and paramedics. In J. Langan-Fox & C. Cooper (Eds.), *Handbook of Stress in the Occupations*. Cheltenham: Edward Elgar.

Hamilton, L. (2009). Managing emotion, work and stress. In P. O'Meara & C. Grbich (Eds.), *Paramedics in Australia: contemporary challenges of practice*. Sydney: Pearson Education Australia.

Hegg-Deloye, S., Brassard, P., Prairie, J., Larouche, D., Jauvin, N., Poirier, P., Tremblay, A., & Corbeil, P. (2015). Prevalence of risk factors for cardiovascular disease in paramedics. *International Archives of Occupational and Environmental Health*, *88*(7), 973–980.

Hegg-Deloye, S., Brassard, P., Jauvin, N., Prairie, J., Larouche, D., Poirier, P., Tremblay, A., & Corbeil, P. (2014). Current state of knowledge of post-traumatic stress, sleeping problems, obesity and cardiovascular disease in paramedics. *Emergency Medicine Journal, 31*(3), 242–247.

Independent Broad-Based Anti-Corruption Commission. (2017). *Operation Tone: Special report concerning drug use and associated corrupt conduct involving Ambulance Victoria paramedics.* [ONLINE] Retrieved from: http://www.ibac .vic.gov.au/docs/default-source/special-reports/operation -tone-special-report-september-2017.pdf?sfvrsn=2. (Accessed 5 May 2018).

Intensive Care Society, The. (2005). *Standards for critical incident reporting in critical care.* Retrieved from: http://icmwk.com/wp-content/uploads/2014/02/ critical_incident_reporting_2006.pdf.

James, S. M., Honn, K. A., Gaddameedhi, S., & Van Dongen, H. P. (2017). Shift work: disrupted circadian rhythms and sleep—implications for health and well-being. *Current Sleep Medicine Reports, 3*(2), 104–112.

Jansen, N., Van Amelsvoort, L., Kristensen, T., Van den Brandt, P., & Kant, I. (2003). Work schedules and fatigue: a prospective cohort study. *Occupational and Environmental Medicine, 60*(Supp1), i47–i53.

Korge, J., & Nunan, D. (2018). Higher participation in physical activity is associated with less use of inpatient mental health services: a cross-sectional study. *Psychiatry Research, 259*, 550–553.

Lupien, S. J., McEwen, B. S., Gunnar, M. R., & Heim, C. (2009). Effects of stress throughout the lifespan on the brain, behaviour and cognition. *Nature Reviews. Neuroscience, 10*(6), 434.

Maguire, B. J. (2018). Violence against ambulance personnel: a retrospective cohort study of national data from Safe Work Australia. *Public Health Research & Practice, 28*(1), e28011805.

Maguire, B. J., O'Meara, P. F., Brightwell, R. F., O'Neill, B. J., & Fitzgerald, G. J. (2014). Occupational injury risk among Australian paramedics: an analysis of national data. *The Medical Journal of Australia, 200*(8), 477–480.

Martini, F. (2006). *Fundamentals of anatomy and physiology* (7th ed.). San Francisco, CA: Pearson Benjamin Cummings.

Mayhew, C., & Chappell, D. (2009). Ambulance officers: the impact of exposure to occupational violence on mental and physical health. *The Journal of Occupational Health and Safety, Australia and New Zealand, 25*(1), 37–49.

Milligan, G. S., Reilly, T. J., Zumbo, B. D., & Tipton, M. J. (2016). Validity and reliability of physical employment standards. *Applied Physiology, Nutrition, and Metabolism, 41*(6), S83–S91.

Mitchell, J. (1983). When disaster strikes … The critical incident stress debriefing process. *JEMS: A Journal of Emergency Medical Services, 8*(1), 36–39.

Nea, F. M., Kearney, J., Livingstone, M. B. E., Pourshahidi, L. K., & Corish, C. A. (2015). Dietary and lifestyle habits and the associated health risks in shift workers. *Nutrition Research Reviews, 28*(2), 143–166.

Neil-Sztramko, S. E., Gotay, C. C., Demers, P. A., & Campbell, K. L. (2016). Physical activity, physical fitness, and body composition of Canadian shift workers: data from the Canadian health measures survey cycles 1 and 2. *Journal of Occupational and Environmental Medicine, 58*(1), 94–100.

New South Wales Ambulance. (2014). *Paramedics voted most trusted profession.* [ONLINE] Retrieved from: https:// www.parkeschampionpost.com.au/story/2378869/ in-paramedics-we-trust-the-most-trusted-profession/. (Accessed 5 May 2018).

Oades, L. G., Slade, M., & Jarden, A. (2017). Wellbeing and recovery. *Wellbeing, Recovery and Mental Health*, 324.

Paul, G., & Hoy, B. (2015). An exploratory ergonomic study of musculoskeletal disorder prevention in the Queensland Ambulance Service. *Journal of Health, Safety and Environment, 31*(3), 1–13.

Pearlin, L. I. (1989). The sociological study of stress. *Journal of Health and Social Behavior, 30*, 241–256.

Pilgrim, J. L., Dorward, R., & Drummer, O. H. (2017). Drug-caused deaths in Australian medical practitioners and health-care professionals. *Addiction (Abingdon, England), 112*(3), 486–493.

Pollack, K. M., Poplin, G. S., Griffin, S., Peate, W., Nash, V., Nied, E., Gulotta, J., & Burgess, J. L. (2017). Implementing risk management to reduce injuries in the US Fire Service. *Journal of Safety Research, 60*, 21–27.

Reynolds, L., & O'Donnell, M. (2016). The role of pre-hospital care and paramedics: the emerging professionalisation of urgent care. *Understanding the Australian Health Care System*, 271.

Roberts, M. H., Sim, M. R., Black, O., & Smith, P. (2015). Occupational injury risk among ambulance officers and paramedics compared with other healthcare workers in Victoria, Australia: analysis of workers' compensation claims from 2003 to 2012. *Occupational and Environmental Medicine, 72*(7), 489–495.

Rosenbaum, S., Vancampfort, D., Steel, Z., Newby, J., Ward, P. B., & Stubbs, B. (2015). Physical activity in the treatment of post-traumatic stress disorder: a systematic review and meta-analysis. *Psychiatry Research, 230*(2), 130–136.

Ruotsalainen, J. H., Verbeek, J. H., Mariné, A., & Serra, C. (2014). Preventing occupational stress in healthcare workers. *The Cochrane Database of Systematic Reviews,* (12), CD002892.

Sofianopoulos, S., Williams, B., Archer, F., & Thompson, B. (2011). The exploration of physical fatigue, sleep and depression in paramedics: a pilot study. *Journal of Emergency Primary Health Care, 9*(1).

Spelten, E., Thomas, B., O'Meara, P. F., Maguire, B. J., FitzGerald, D., & Begg, S. J. (2017). Organisational interventions for preventing and minimising aggression directed toward healthcare workers by patients and patient advocates. *The Cochrane Database of Systematic Reviews,* (5), CD012662.

SECTION 7:
Legal, Ethical and Professional Considerations

In this section:

Laws, ethics and professional codes of conduct bind paramedics, as with all other health professionals. The law around consent is particularly relevant to paramedic practice. The theory is explored in some detail and contextualised in an example case.

CHAPTER 13

Legal and Ethical Considerations in Clinical Decision-Making

By Brian Stoffell

OVERVIEW

- Clinical reasoning is focused on the development of safe and accurate differential diagnoses on the basis of the patient's history and vital signs, a process that always occurs within legal and ethical boundaries.

- Understanding the legal and ethical standards of conduct created by boards under the national authority will help paramedics to orientate themselves in complex decision-making situations.

Introduction

The paramedic workplace is characterised as rich in stimuli but lacking in clinical information: the clinical problems are multiple and ill-defined, with definitive diagnostic tools in short supply. Throughout this text we describe the decision-making that occurs when clinicians are confronted with patients, and in particular the clinical reasoning challenges faced by paramedics. We also discuss how novice paramedics can gather information and contextualise their knowledge of disease processes.

In Part 2 of this text we cover paramedic practice and detail the steps involved in patient assessment and history gathering, while only briefly considering that some patients might refuse to allow the paramedic to assess them or initiate treatment. That consideration raises the ethical and legal considerations at work when assessing and treating a patient.

The decision-making process starts with the patient but incorporates both the clinical picture and wider factors. This reality is far more complex than a simple protocol-driven treatment plan. How legal and ethical standards need to be integrated with clinical understanding is the focus of this chapter. We concentrate on a case demonstrating two areas of health law impacting on clinical decision-making: the emergency treatment of a non-competent adult; and consent or refusal of treatment by a competent adult.

Ethics and the law

Faced with diagnostic uncertainty, it is reasonable for novice clinicians to seek direction from law or professional conduct codes: good clinical decisions need to be consistent with what is legally and ethically acceptable.

When *ethics* enters the conversation, its ambiguity must be dealt with immediately. The word's roots are in the critical evaluation of human behaviour (in the 4th century BCE, the Greek word *ethikos* meant 'character'). Later, the acceptance that there are customary practices accepted in all societies figuring in our assessment of people's actions broadened the concept of ethics (the Latin term *mores* for customary practices gives us the word 'morality'). In the intervening 25 centuries, a number of different meanings have been attached to the word 'ethics'. It is wise to distinguish between three current meanings to identify what a busy clinician should address in professional life:

1. a philosophical discipline focused on the language of moral evaluation and theoretical models

2. a deep personal sense of attachment to certain values (standards), often connected to conscience

3. codes of professional conduct that call themselves *ethics codes*.

The idea that an urgent clinical decision might await the resolution of some philosophical debate about the nature of justice, or the scope of benevolence, is of course ridiculous. What Plato wrote about justice in his *Republic* (4th century BCE), and what hundreds of philosophers have canvassed about justice since, are still in active debate. This never-ending conversation is characteristic of philosophy: it is fine for the classroom but not for the roadside. So ethics as moral philosophising is not

BOX 13.1 Paramedicine board of australia code of conduct

1.2 Professional values and qualities
While individual practitioners have their own personal beliefs and values, there are certain professional values on which all practitioners are expected to base their practice. These professional values apply to the practitioner's conduct regardless of the setting, including in person and electronically, e.g. social media, e-health etc.

Practitioners have a duty to make the care of patients or clients their first concern and to practise safely and effectively. They must be ethical and trustworthy. Patients or clients trust practitioners because they believe that, in addition to being competent, practitioners will not take advantage of them and will display qualities such as integrity, truthfulness, dependability and compassion. Patients or clients also rely on practitioners to protect their confidentiality.

Practitioners have a responsibility to protect and promote the health of individuals and the community.

Good practice is centred on patients or clients. It involves practitioners understanding that each patient or client is unique and working in partnership with patients or clients, adapting what they do to address the needs and reasonable expectations of each person. This includes cultural awareness: being aware of their own culture and beliefs and respectful of the

beliefs and cultures of others, and recognising that these cultural differences may impact on the practitioner–patient/client relationship and on the delivery of services. Good practice also includes being aware that differences such as gender, sexuality, age, belief systems and other anti-discrimination grounds in relevant legislation may influence care needs, and avoiding discrimination on the basis of these differences.

Effective communication in all forms underpins every aspect of good practice.

Professionalism embodies all the qualities described here and includes self-awareness and self-reflection. Practitioners are expected to reflect regularly on whether they are practising effectively, on what is happening in their relationships with patients or clients and colleagues, and on their own health and wellbeing. They have a duty to keep their skills and knowledge up to date, refine and develop their clinical judgement as they gain experience, and contribute to their profession.

Practitioners have a responsibility to recognise and work within the limits of their competence and scope of practice. Scopes of practice vary according to different roles; for example, practitioners, researchers and managers will all have quite different competence and scopes of practice …

Source: Paramedicine Board of Australia (2018).

our focus. Nor is bioethics, a discipline that continues those same theoretical debates but uses exclusively healthcare examples (Stoffell, 1994).

Our second meaning, ethics as conscientious adherence to values, is absolutely central to personal ethics, especially where those personally held values, principles or standards, genuinely guide behaviour. There are numerous examples of how conscientious adherence to personal standards has led to dire consequences for the person acting, but one example will do here. Conscientious objection to conscription for military service would get you jailed in Australia in the 1960s and 70s, as in many countries.

What about our third meaning, codes? The principles that are given masthead status in discussions about healthcare ethics must be operational and clear, because lives and careers are on the line. Something concrete and prescriptive needs to be in place, as indeed it is. Consider the following declaration of values and qualities in the opening section from the shared Australian Health

Practitioner Regulatory Agency (AHPRA) Code of Professional Conduct, which paramedics in Australia currently work under (see Box 13.1). This AHPRA code provides a framework for the evaluation of paramedic conduct. This ethical framework also operates in cases where tribunals and courts are making assessments of conduct.

It should be appreciated that an ethics code, authorised in legislation and issued by a board, plays the central role in the evaluation of professional conduct. How your conduct is assessed can have a profound impact on your career. It is fair to conclude that in professional life law and ethics (professional ethics) are intimately connected. Nonetheless, a broader domain of ethics does exist, and so not all evaluations of behaviour as 'unethical' can be expected to relate to codes of conduct. Codes **do not** stipulate that what you do in professional life must be guided by love, deep compassion, or exhibit generosity and heartfelt kindness. However, for some people those qualities might be the very core of ethical values, and as such those values will have a role in the way they size-up situations and people.

The terms 'ethical' and 'unethical' are not defined in the National Law, so what should they be taken to mean? If they were understood in a very broad way, encompassing all forms of ethical evaluation from the realm of personal ethics, then those personal evaluations would all be licensed to play a role in professional tribunals and courts: it would be chaos. Thankfully that is not the case. Here is an example of how 'unethical' appears in section 139B of the National Law (NSW) in the definition of 'unsatisfactory professional conduct', which is defined as including:

> *(l) Any other **improper or unethical conduct** relating to the practice or purported practice of the practitioner's profession.*
> Health Practitioner Regulation National Law (NSW) No 86a

In the *Health Practitioner Regulation National Law (South Australia) Act 2010* (Schedule 2, section 5), the definition of 'unprofessional conduct' refers to behaviour that is 'inconsistent with the practitioner being a fit and proper person to hold registration in the profession'. The legal scope given to the vague terms 'improper' and 'unethical', and to the 'fit and proper person' standard, is provided by the members of the NSW Civil and Administrative Tribunal in *Health Care Complaints Commission v Picones* (2018) NSWCATOD 56:

> *The assessment of what constitutes improper or unethical conduct is based upon their ordinary meaning. 'Improper' conduct does not need to be intentional and includes conduct not in conformity with standards of professional conduct: HCCC v Phung (No 1) [2012] 1 NSWDT 3 at [68]; HCCC v Fisher [2016] NSWCATOD 62 at [57]; HCCC v Flekser [2016] NSWCATOD 1 at [119]. Improper and unethical conduct may be dishonest, disreputable to the profession, in breach of explicit professional standards such as codes of conduct, guidelines and competencies, and may also be determined by reference to the views of reasonable members of the profession: Slezak, Dr Peter [2011] NSWMPSC 10 at [83] and [87]. Making a false statement to a professional body or regulatory inquiry may constitute improper and unethical conduct: HCCC v Mitchell [2015] NSWCATOD 15 at [59].*

Guidance for a health practitioner on appropriate professional conduct or practice is found in their nationally approved code, set against a broader background of professional opinion about what is proper conduct. There is a direct parallel here with the role of professional opinion in establishing standards for treatment or standards of care (see, for example, section 41 of the South Australian *Civil Liability Act 1936*). Finally, both ethical conduct and standards of care will be 'determined by … reasonable members of the profession', with one significant proviso: in disputed cases it will be the court who decides what is reasonable.

Legislation provides the basis for boards to create conduct codes, but it also gives the force of law to ethical notions that are core values in liberal democratic societies. The most prominent of these values is self-determination, a value protected in consent law in Australia.

Consent

Consent law creates a legally enforceable claim—a legal right—in a situation where there would otherwise merely be a moral claim to be allowed to make free and informed choices about whether or not to undergo treatment. The core value can be expressed actively as the moral claim *to determine what happens to your body* and is variously referred to as autonomy, self-determination or personal sovereignty. We, the audience for the claim, are being exhorted to respect (give due weight to) a protected area of action. This very ancient claim is captured in legal notions like 'trespass to the person' (where the physical integrity of the body is being protected against incursion). It is also reflected in phrases like 'dominion over one's body' and health practitioners are often reminded that they need approval via consent to touch patients. Autonomy should be understood as control of territory; it is not a concept trying to label some nebulous psychological faculty like the will (autonomy = *auto-nomos*, our realm of control wherein we make

---

REFLECTIVE BOX

1. If a reduced dose of naloxone would wake the patient but retain the euphoric effects of the narcotic, should it be considered? Or should you provide a dose of naloxone that completely reverses the condition?

2. Should any line of enquiry be made to see whether the patient's friend has documents to back up his view that the patient would not want the treatment to be administered?

3. What legislation exists in your jurisdiction to allow the appointment of substitute decision-makers in medical matters?

CASE STUDY

Case 10504, 2250 hrs.

Dispatch details: An unconscious young male at a domestic address. The caller identifies that the patient may have been using heroin.

Initial presentation: On arrival the crew find the male patient unconscious, with a central cyanosis, a respiratory rate of 4, decreased tidal volume but a clear airway. He has a pulse that is palpable at the wrist at a rate of 130. The patient's two housemates state that the three of them injected heroin shortly before the patient fell unconscious. The crew support the patient's respiration by bag-mask ventilation and he becomes less cyanosed. As one crew member draws up the naloxone, one of the patient's friends says: 'I'm pretty sure he wouldn't want to be treated with that stuff. Isn't there anything else you can do?' Despite these concerns, the crew administer 0.4 mg of naloxone IM and 6 minutes later the patient is alert and oriented to place and time. He refuses all offers of further care or transport.

laws for ourselves). Our freedom to act may not be constrained by anything other than physical capacity, fear and desire, but in demanding respect for individual self-determination or autonomy we are demanding a protected space for choices where others are excluded by law. Just how limited that space is in healthcare choices can be seen easily.

In Australia, consent law (in both common law and statute) protects a very limited area of choice: an adult may either **accept** or **reject** proposed treatments. This entails of course that they may later **withdraw** their consent. Within this narrow space there is emphatically no right (enforceable claim) to **demand** treatments that are not offered; at best our freedom of choice is among options that are offered. Recent legal history—in the United Kingdom, United States, Australia and Canada—suggests that the dominant public concern is with cases where **refusal** of treatment is at issue. This narrow space for choice can be augmented by newly minted legal options, like physician-assisted suicide being added to treatment options in Victoria or the legal creation of substitute decision-makers (advance care directive [ACD] legislation), can add agents to the list of those empowered to choose. These proxies, substitute decision-makers or surrogates (once referred to as appointees exercising medical power of attorney) enter when an agent's capacity

is lost, so how does a patient's level of capacity impact on respect for their self-determination?

In the case study, the patient is unconscious when the crew arrives so his decision-making capacity is not in operation. Doing everything possible to save his life will, if successful, protect and preserve his capacities for self-determination (remember that capacities are like abilities: not always in operation). The professional and legally sanctioned imperative is to provide active treatment and avoid harm. The facts in the case make it abundantly clear that emergency treatment must be provided to safeguard the patient by avoiding any further threat to his physical or mental wellbeing. The legal doctrine of emergency is a common law creation that provides healthcare personnel with a justification to intervene without the patient's prior consent. In *Marion's care*, Justice McHugh said:

> *Consent is not necessary … where a surgical procedure or medical treatment must be performed in an emergency and the patient does not have the capacity to consent and no legally authorised representative is available to give consent on his or her behalf.*

NT v JWB (Marion's Care) *(1992) 175 CLR 218, 310.*

Since the initial presentation in the case study was an unconscious patient in need of urgent and necessary treatment, the doctrine of emergency/necessity applies, providing the paramedic with legal authority to touch the patient and administer the life-saving naloxone. This course of action is also ethically sound since it aims to prevent further harm. Once the patient has regained consciousness, his capacity to make decisions regarding further treatment would need to be assessed. So the practitioner acted ethically as well as legally in treating the patient with naloxone because there is good evidence that without it he was at risk of death. Does his friend's suggestion about what the patient may have preferred have any weight? There are plainly situations where authorised substitute decision-makers (working under ACD law) can affect your treatment, but this is not the case here.

Now consider the situation of a patient who was initially conscious and able to consent to treatment, but then subsequently deteriorates. Here the paramedic might consider that the patient's changing condition necessitates the administration of additional treatments not previously anticipated or discussed with the patient. The scope of the original consent does not extend to include these additional treatments. However, again, if it can be shown that the new measures were provided out of necessity (the medical necessity created by the situation), and given to protect the life and health of a patient no longer capable of consent, then the justification is exactly the same (*Hunter and New England Area Health Services v A* (2009) 74 NSWLR 88[31–33] C.F.R.). Bear in mind that conscious, capable patients may issue clear instructions about future treatments that are not to be used. In the *Consent to Medical Treatment and Palliative Care Act 1995* (SA) section 13(1)(c) it is clear that medical treatment cannot be legally administered if the practitioner is aware that the unconscious patient 'refused to consent to the treatment' by a prior refusal.

> ## PRACTICE TIP
>
> If a conscious patient you are treating for, say, chest pain has a cardiac arrest and you are treating them for something that they understood and consented to, you don't have to stop and obtain their consent before defibrillating.

Refusal of treatment

The clinical reasoning process employed in the management of the patient in the case study is relatively straightforward: the patient self-administered an accidental overdose of an opioid narcotic. Non-invasive management of the patient's airway and ventilation removed an immediate threat and evidence-based practice supported the use of intramuscular naloxone.

Once the patient has regained consciousness, as occurs in the second part of the case, what should be done becomes more problematic.

Respecting self-determination means defending the patient's right to *refuse* treatment. Chief Justice Martin of the Western Australian Supreme Court described it as follows:

> *The corollary of [self-determination] is that an individual of full capacity is not obliged to give consent to medical treatment, nor is a medical practitioner or other service provider under any obligation to provide such treatment without consent, even if the failure to treat will result in the loss of the patient's life … the principle is applied without regard to the reasons for the patient's choice, and irrespective of whether the reasons are rational, irrational, unknown or even non-existent …*
>
> Brightwater Care Group (Inc) v Rossiter *(2009) WASC 229 (20 August 2009) at 24–27.*

The key point here is the notion of competence or capacity (these terms are used interchangeably) and paramedics therefore need an understanding of how competence is assessed. Transport is a form of treatment and a patient who is deemed to be competent needs to consent to transport just as they would any other form of treatment. So in the case study, once the patient has woken up and asks you to cease treatment, you are ethically and legally bound to follow that instruction, provided you think he is competent to make the decision. That his decision is not the one you would personally make is irrelevant. The ethical or code-based parameters around informed consent are all about process (see Box 13.2), but they would be pointless unless a simple imperative were not followed: accept and respect decisions made within the legal power of patients or their substitute decision-makers.

Elements of consent from a paramedic perspective

Consent is one of the most difficult concepts to apply in the paramedic setting. There are four elements of consent and each must be satisfied for consent to be deemed lawfully satisfied.

1. The consent is voluntary (un-coerced).
2. The patient has the capacity to make the decision about the treatment.
3. The patient has been provided with sufficient information.
4. The consent covers the treatment that is to be provided.

BOX 13.2 Informed consent practice

Informed consent is a person's voluntary decision about healthcare that is made with knowledge and understanding of the benefits and risks involved.

Good practice involves:

a. providing information to patients in a way they can understand before asking for their consent

b. providing an explanation of the treatment/care recommended, its likely duration, expected benefits and cost, any alternative(s) to the proposed care, their relative risks/benefits, as well as the likely consequences of no care

c. obtaining informed consent or other valid authority before undertaking any examination or investigation, providing treatment/care (this may not be possible in an emergency) or involving patients in teaching or research, including providing information on material risks

d. consent being freely given, without coercion or pressure

e. advising patients, when referring a patient for investigation or treatment/care, that there may be additional costs, which they may wish to clarify before proceeding

f. obtaining (when working with a patient whose capacity to give consent is or may be impaired or limited) the consent of people with legal authority to act on behalf of the patient, and attempting to obtain the consent of the patient as far as practically possible

g. being mindful of additional informed consent requirements when supplying or prescribing products not approved or made in Australia, and

h. documenting consent appropriately, including considering the need for written consent for procedures that may result in serious injury or death.

Source: Paramedicine Board of Australia (2018).

Voluntariness

We have discussed the right of individuals to make healthcare decisions for themselves. This right includes the notion that the patient is not coerced into making decisions. Coercion imposes threats or pressure that negate voluntariness. In situations where a third party may be influencing the patient's decision, the paramedic should consider the nature of the relationship and gauge the patient's vulnerability to undue influence by the third party (e.g. husband, wife or religious adviser). It is particularly important that paramedics do not themselves engage in coercive behaviour; for example, by persuading a patient to do what is convenient for the paramedic but not in the best interests of the patient (*Re T (Adult: Refusal of Medical Treatment)* (1992) 4 All ER 649).

PRACTICE TIP

'If you don't come to hospital with us, I'll call the police and tell them you have illicit drugs here' is an example of coercion and hence is unacceptable.

Sufficient information

It is both an ethical and a legal requirement that where possible paramedics provide their patients with information regarding their condition, the options for treatment, the broad nature and effects of that treatment and the risks associated with the treatment or its absence. This requirement includes covering risks identified by the patient, even though they may be highly unlikely to occur. (*Rogers v Whittaker* (1992) 175 CLR 479, 490). The High Court has said that medical service providers should, where feasible, ensure that the competent patient is 'given full information as to the consequences of any decision to discontinue treatment before [the patient] makes that decision', and reiterated that providers have a legal duty to do so (*Brightwater Care Group (Inc) v Rossiter* (2009) 40 WAR 84 at 30–32). For a statutory statement of the duty to explain see the *Consent to Medical Treatment and Palliative Care Act 1995* (SA) section 15.

PRACTICE TIP

'If you don't come with us, you're certainly going to die' probably isn't a fair and balanced view of the information. You need to explain all the possible risks and how likely they are.

Treatment-specific consent

After the patient has been advised of the nature and effect of the proposed treatment (including the risks and benefits) and consent is given, that consent only applies to the treatment described. The nature of paramedic work is such that further treatment that has not been specifically consented to may be required; for example, their condition deteriorates and they are no longer able to consent to the new treatment. In this case, provided the treatment is administered out of necessity and it is not practicable to obtain consent from a substitute decision-maker, the paramedic may administer the treatment. This treatment is given on the presumption that it is in the patient's best interests. (See *Hart v Herron* (1984) Aust Torts Reports 80-201 on subsequent unauthorised treatments.)

Competence/capacity

The validity of the patient's consent to, or refusal of, treatment is dependent on the patient's capacity; that is, their ability to understand the nature and effect of their decision. The issue in the case study is whether the now conscious patient has the decision-making capacity to refuse transport. Settling this issue involves a test. In law it is presumed as a starting point that adults are competent (*Re C (Adult: Refusal of Medical Treatment)* (1994) 1 All ER 819, 822). The presumption is also embodied in the New Zealand Code of Health and Disability Services Consumers' Rights, Right 7(2). The onus to disprove the presumption is on the healthcare practitioner (*Re MB (Medical Treatment)* (1997) 2 FCR 426).

There are several factors that can erode a person's decision-making capacity, on either a temporary or a permanent basis. For example, a person with an intellectual disability may not be able to understand the nature and effect of proposed treatment or the risks and benefits of consenting or refusing consent. A temporary loss of capacity might be caused by conditions that result in hypoxia. Drug or alcohol intoxication can also impact on a person's decision-making capacity (*Re B (Adult: Refusal of Medical Treatment)* (2002) 2 All ER 449; Re T *(Adult: Refusal of Medical Treatment)* (1992) 4 All ER 649). However, the responsibility to demonstrate that a condition impairs the patient's decision-making capacity remains with the paramedic. Presence of the condition itself is not enough to prove lack of competence: the paramedic must assess the patient's capacity to reach a decision.

In the case study, even though you may doubt that the patient is fully competent after his near respiratory arrest, you cannot just work on that assumption: you have to check and justify.

Assessment of competence

The legal test of competence will contain the following elements:
- the ability to take in, retain and comprehend the treatment information
- the ability to believe that information and weigh up risks and benefits of the treatment before consenting or refusing consent.

For a statutory version of this process see the *Consent to Medical Treatment and Palliative Care Act 1995* (SA) section 4(2) and (3).

Retention and understanding of the treatment information could be assessed by asking the patient to repeat, in their own words, the treatment information that has been given to them by the paramedic.

Assessment also includes whether they believe the information. It is difficult to imagine that a patient might disbelieve a paramedic's explanation of proposed treatment, but there are several mental health conditions where the patient does not believe that they are unwell.

Weighing up the risks and benefits is also part of the assessment. Again, it is possible to ask the patient to explain, in their own words, what they believe are the risks and benefits of the proposed treatment. The test is merely to check that the patient has noted the risks and benefits. There is no requirement for the patient's ultimate choice to match the choice that the paramedic would themselves make. The paramedic may believe that the patient's choice is illogical or irrational, but this is not relevant in determining whether or not the patient has demonstrated that they are capable of weighing up the risks and benefits. For example, you may have told a patient that without a particular treatment they are certain to die. The patient may say, 'Okay, I understand that without this treatment I will die, but I choose not to have the treatment anyway'. This response demonstrates the patient's understanding that treatment refusal will result in their death.

The importance of the decision

A patient's competence also needs to be considered in light of the gravity of the potential consequences of treatment refusal. In other words, a patient's capacity to make decisions may alter with the seriousness of the decision to be made. For example, in the case *Hunter and New England Area Health Services v A*, Justice McDougall said:

It is necessary to bear in mind that there is no sharp dichotomy between capacity on the one hand and want of capacity on the other. There is a scale, running from capacity at one end through reduced capacity to lack of capacity at the other.

In assessing whether a person has capacity to make a decision, the sufficiency of the capacity must take into account the importance of the decision (as Lord Donaldson pointed out in Re T). The capacity required to make a contract to buy a cup of coffee may be present where the capacity to decide to give away one's fortune is not.

(2009) 74 NSWLR 88, [24]

In the case study, the patient needs to be competent to make an informed decision about a very significant issue because there is a substantial risk that harm may come to him when the naloxone wears off if he does not go to hospital for observation.

Clinical and legal considerations in context

In the case study, the legal position starts from an underlying presumption that the now conscious patient is competent to refuse consent for transport. However, that starting point could be immediately undermined by the patient's clinical history: a narcotic overdose and resultant period of unconsciousness. The paramedic therefore needs to determine whether the patient is capable of making a decision to consent or reject the recommended treatment, and this requires not only an assessment of the patient's orientation to time and place but also his level of understanding of the nature and effect of his decision (*Re T (Adult: Refusal of Medical Treatment)* (1992) 4 All ER 649, 641). While assessment of competence is a legal test, it is the paramedic who is required to make the assessment, taking into consideration the gravity of the risk involved.

The lack of precise legal direction in this situation is a common problem for paramedics and there is no simple answer that covers all circumstances. Being aware that a 'scale of capacity' exists, and that a lack of capacity may only be demonstrated *after* the patient has suffered harm, places paramedics in a difficult position. Trying to fit legislation to the circumstance may not clarify the situation either. For example, mental health law in some jurisdictions provides a mechanism allowing paramedics to transport a patient who has refused treatment and transport; however, the patient *must* be suffering from a mental illness as defined in the local mental health act *and* meet strict criteria before the relevant mechanism can be invoked.

In reality, if the paramedic feels that the clinical risks of not transporting the patient are too significant, it falls to the paramedic to convince the patient to agree to transport. The legalities and logistics of involuntary transport are simply too complicated and lengthy to be effective in the field in most acute cases, and the ability to communicate with the patient and engage them in your treatment plan will be a more effective strategy in the situation.

A third party who is willing and competent to supervise the patient is commonly seen as a means of mitigating some of the risks of non-transport, but this should be done only *after* the paramedic has decided that the patient has the requisite decision-making capacity to refuse transport. If the patient is not being transported because of a competent refusal, and the patient consents to informing a third party of the paramedic's diagnosis, a third party can be involved. However, the third party must be effectively informed as to the clinical risks, signs and symptoms to watch for and the proposed action plan in case of the patient's deterioration.

In the case study there are others present, any one of whom could act as a third party. However, they have by their own admission been using heroin, which may diminish their ability to perform a useful function, arguing powerfully against the paramedic relying on them.

The clinical question is this: are you sure on reasonable grounds that the patient is competent to refuse transport, or are you sure that they are not fit to competently refuse? He is either competent or incompetent on these bases:

- incompetent secondary to the effects of hypoxia precipitated by his near respiratory arrest
- incompetent secondary to the effects of hypercarbia precipitated by his near respiratory arrest
- incompetent secondary to the effects of the original drug overdose
- incompetent secondary to another factor (e.g. hypoglycaemia, electrolyte disturbance, infection).

If the patient is deemed to be incompetent, then the duration of effect of the causative agent comes into question. In other words, could he reasonably be expected to regain his capacity to demonstrate competence in the near future? Hypoxia and hypercarbia rapidly correct with the restoration of normal ventilation, and their metabolic consequences rapidly correct too. The original overdose may still impair the patient's ability to make a competent

---

PRACTICE TIP

A repeated and consistent instruction to the paramedics to go away does not necessarily constitute evidence of competence. The patient needs to demonstrate competence associated with the refusal of care. An extreme example is a patient with a significant head injury. It is worth noting that a patient who has lost two points on the Glasgow Coma Scale may still be capable of saying 'yes', 'no' and expletives.

decision: although the naloxone has improved his conscious state it does not necessarily mean that it has improved to a point where he is capable of demonstrating competency. Hypoglycaemia, infection, electrolyte imbalance or other unrelated conditions could also be coexisting. Obtaining a blood glucose level will exclude hypoglycaemia, but the ability to assess electrolyte levels is not readily available in the field.

Legal consequences for the paramedic

The legal consequence surrounding decisions about competence impact on both the individual paramedic and the employing ambulance service. The paramedic has a duty to conduct a thorough clinical assessment that is reasonable in the circumstances and must inform the patient of the assessment findings and recommendations for treatment and transport. If the patient refuses the recommendation, the paramedic informs them of the associated risks and then must determine if the patient's decision is competently reached, remembering the logic: the patient is to be deemed competent if no clear basis can be established to show incompetence. If the patient subsequently suffers harm related to the initial condition, then it is unlikely that the paramedic or their agency would be considered liable for the harm.

In situations like the case study there is powerful reason to provide thoroughly documented evidence that the paramedic acted reasonably, in terms of both the assessments undertaken and the decisions reached on the basis of those assessments. This evidence will support the view that it was not their acceptance of the patient's refusal that led to damage for the patient (*Neal v Ambulance Service of New South Wales* (2008) NSWCA 346, 24). However, if the paramedic assesses a patient as requiring further treatment but does not offer to transport the patient for that treatment, the subsequent adverse outcomes are very likely to expose the paramedic and/or their agency to a negligence action (Forrester & Griffiths, 2015, pp. 106–113).

Case study evaluation

You have made a thorough assessment, including an assessment of the patient's competence. You have documented this assessment and clearly communicated the risk profile to the patient. You, your partner and the bystanders have witnessed the thorough professional briefing.

Having considered the ethics and legal requirements in the case, the crew need to make a decision about how to support a course of action when confronted with a patient who rejects any further treatment. Consider the two actions listed in Table 13.1. They are a framework based solely on addressing the ethical and legal concepts covered above.

The case facts advise only that following treatment with naloxone the patient is alert and aggressively refusing all offers of further care and transport. In dealing with this patient's refusal to be transported, subsequent actions will hinge entirely on the paramedic's evaluation of the patient's competence. Either:

- It has been determined that the patient is competent and therefore able to make decisions regarding further treatment and transport.
  Or
- It has been determined that the patient is not capable of understanding the nature and consequences of his decision about further treatment and transport.

Currently, the paramedics don't have enough information to make a decision regarding further treatment or transport, but they will be able to assess his level of understanding and evaluate his competence with more questioning and interaction. There are many clinical benefits to be gained for this patient in going to hospital. For example, access to withdrawal support can be provided in addition

Table 13.1: Possible paramedic actions when a patient refuses transport to hospital

Action 1: Patient not transported to hospital	
Ethics	Upholds autonomy
Code	Respect for the patient and consent of the patient
Law	Respect the right of the patient to make decisions regarding treatment and transport

Action 2: Patient transported to hospital	
Ethics	Having judged the patient as not competent, the paramedics believe that his autonomy cannot be expressed in his opinion and they revert to the justification of acting in his best interests as they perceive them
Code	Respect for the patient and consent of the patient
Law	Duty of care to provide treatment and transportation in accordance with the standards expected

to a full clinical review. Despite this, the paramedics cannot transport the patient against his will unless it has been determined that he is not able to make a competent decision.

Documentation

One final legal and professional requirement is to document the assessment and communication with the patient. It is essential that the case sheet is comprehensively completed with details about the patient's assessment, including their competence, and your communication with the patient regarding any recommendations for further treatment. In the past a patient's refusal of treatment or transport was something that paramedics may not have considered a significant issue. The presence of adequate documentation demonstrating a detailed and thorough assessment of both the clinical problem and the patient's competence has proved extremely useful when assessing these cases.

Summary

The ethical and legal principles of healthcare rarely impact on the process of clinical decision-making: making good decisions inherently aligns clinical practice with ethical and legal behaviour. There are cases, however, where the decision-making process can be supported by referring to the ethical and legal principles that support paramedic practice. The widely held assumptions that patients understand their condition and agree to the most appropriate clinical care are quickly tested in the out-of-hospital environment where social factors, drug use, mental health and personal freedoms commonly interact with emergency healthcare. A clear understanding of the principles of autonomy, non-maleficence, beneficence and justice will not only allow paramedics to understand why and how good clinical practice is supported by the law, but also act as a guide where the clinical situation is unclear or when the rights of the patient to refuse care are raised.

References

Forrester, K., & Griffiths, D. (2015). *Essentials of health Law for health professionals* (4th ed.). Sydney: Elsevier.

Paramedicine Board of Australia. (2018). *Code of Conduct (interim)*. June. https://www.paramedicineboard.gov.au/Professional-standards/Codes-guidelines-and-policies.aspx.

Stoffell, B. (1994). Ethical praxis. *Health Care Analysis, 2*(4), 306–310.

PART TWO
PARAMEDIC PRACTICE

SECTION 8:
The Paramedic Clinical Approach

In this section:

A sound clinical approach underpins every episode of patient care. A systematic and structured clinical approach as discussed in Chapter 14 sets the paramedic up with all the information required to make an informed clinical decision about the patient's care. The patient-centred interview forms part of the structured clinical approach and is a means to not only gather pertinent information from the patient, but to establish trust and rapport. Chapter 15 offers a step-by-step approach to the patient-centred interview and provides examples and strategies for eliciting information.

CHAPTER 14

The Structured Clinical Approach

By Linda Ross

OVERVIEW

- A structured clinical approach is an effective and comprehensive method for assessing all patients.
- The clinical approach that has been developed for use in hospitals and clinics is optimised for gathering information in low-stimulus environments where the roles of clinicians and patients are well defined. This does not adequately describe the paramedic's clinical decision-making environment.
- To safely and effectively gather information in the high-stimulus environment in which paramedics

work, paramedics must be aware of the strengths and weaknesses of using a structured approach.
- Understanding and utilising the process of the clinical assessment can lower the cognitive load that paramedics have to deal with. It allows them to concentrate on the content, or the information generated by the assessment, and to incorporate that into their decision-making process.

Introduction

This chapter focuses on the **process** of gathering the information that paramedics need in order to make effective clinical decisions.

In the dynamic out-of-hospital environment using a **structured clinical approach** gives you a road map to guide you from the moment you are dispatched, through the patient encounter, to patient treatment and to handover at hospital. The structured clinical approach is heavily focused on the initial phase of the patient encounter but is fluid and can be interrupted, reinstated or repeated at any stage necessary as dictated by the situation. Employing this process for every patient will reliably provide you with the information you need to safely apply the knowledge and clinical skills you have attained during your education and training.

Casting a wide net to capture information is an essential skill for modern paramedics as the rapid expansion of the paramedic scope of practice, diverse populations and burdens of disease has created clinical challenges far beyond what paramedics experienced as little as a decade ago. Increasingly, patients have complex or multiple chronic health problems with overlapping pathologies and symptoms as opposed to a single, sudden episode with a clear cause. Simultaneously, the choice of treatment pathways and interventions available to paramedics have also become much greater and more complex. In addition, the unpredictable and mobile nature of paramedic work also means that diagnostic equipment is limited by what is safe, practical and mobile. In short, paramedics are expected to

make timely, accurate, high-stakes clinical decisions with little support in highly dynamic and often emotive situations. It is this overwhelming complexity that makes a structured clinical approach so valuable.

The structured clinical approach

Although the terminology and steps may vary between ambulance services, education providers and practitioners the major steps in the structured clinical approach can be summarised as follows:

1. primary survey
2. information gathering
3. vital signs survey
4. physical exam/secondary assessments
5. differential diagnosis/main presenting problem.

The patient-centred interview, discussed in the next chapter, provides a framework for your interaction with the patient while gathering information, taking assessments and explaining findings and treatments as part of your clinical approach.

The primary survey

The primary survey (see Fig 14.1) is the perfect example of a tool that can be used to reduce the decision-making load while simultaneously providing essential information. It is used to quickly establish whether a patient is dead or dying or alive. Faced with an unconscious patient, the primary survey removes any tendency for the paramedic to start considering complex causes and directs them to

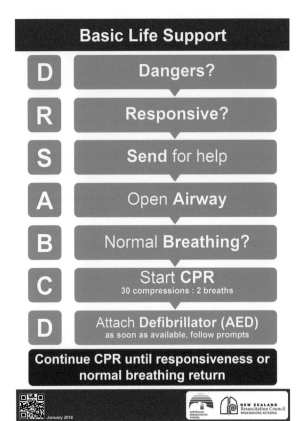

Basic Life Support

D — Dangers?

R — Responsive?

S — Send for help

A — Open Airway

B — Normal Breathing?

C — Start CPR
30 compressions : 2 breaths

D — Attach Defibrillator (AED)
as soon as available, follow prompts

Continue CPR until responsiveness or normal breathing return

January 2016

NEW ZEALAND Resuscitation Council WHAKAHAUORA AOTEAROA

Figure 14.1
ANZCOR Basic Life Support Flowchart.
Source: ANZCOR Basic Life Support Flowchart. January 2016. https://resus.org.au/guidelines/flowcharts-3/

just *one* task: DRSABCD (Australian Resuscitation Council, 2016).

D = dangers to patient, bystanders or rescuer need to be removed or reduced.

R = response; is the patient able to make a purposeful response to voice or touch?

S = send for help/backup or situation report

A = airway; check and clear

B = breathing; if yes continue, if no commence intermittent positive pressure ventilation

C = circulation; if yes continue, if no commence chest compressions

D = defibrillation if indicated

If A, B and C are intact, controlling any obvious external haemorrhage (H) is the paramedic's next priority.

Over the past decade two additional aspects have been added to some versions of the primary survey: disability (D) and exposure (E). To assess disability the responder needs to conduct a rapid neurological assessment, while to assess exposure the responder

has to expose the patient to reveal any injuries. Although these aspects fit neatly into the primary survey in an alphabetical sense, for paramedics both involve complex assessments and procedures (e.g. to be conducted safely, exposing a trauma patient can take several minutes and a small team). Thus, in the primary survey these additional aspects are generally more suitable for first responders who have limited clinical decisions and interventions to initiate. For paramedics, disability and exposure are explored in the vital signs survey and secondary survey, which are conducted once the primary survey has been completed and any actions it specifies have been commenced.

Since more than 90% of ambulance service patients are conscious when paramedics arrive (Queensland Ambulance Service [QAS], 2011), the primary survey quickly exhausts its ability to guide the decision-making process. Thus, to determine how sick the conscious patient may be, paramedics rely on history gathering and patient assessments.

Information gathering

Paramedics use both communication techniques and physical observations to gather information as a basis for their clinical decision-making. Physical observations such as the vital signs survey and secondary survey are discussed below. Patient history gathering and the nuances of the patient-centred interview are discussed in detail in the next chapter. Depending on the patient's condition, paramedic experience level and the number of clinicians on scene, information may be gathered in a stepped approach or concurrently.

The vital signs survey

While the primary survey establishes whether a patient is dead/dying or alive, the vital signs survey (VSS) provides a qualitative measure of *how sick or well* the patient is. It is defined as a series of clinical measurements and observations used to determine a patient's current and trending health status. Vital signs assist paramedics in determining likely causes of a patient's condition and inform suitable treatment pathways. In addition, they act as a valuable baseline for future comparisons and the detection of improvement

> ### PRACTICE TIP
>
> Most vital signs surveys specify a 'normal' range, but some patients fall outside these values even when they are healthy. The very fit, the very slight or the very old may have heart rates and blood pressures that fall outside of the 'normal' range, but don't assume that outside of 'normal' is a healthy variant: explore the patient's background (previously assessed heart rates and blood pressures) to ensure what is discovered does not have a pathological cause.

or deterioration. The human body is capable of maintaining relatively normal activities despite significant injury or illness. It does this by various compensatory mechanisms such as increasing the heart rate, redistributing blood from the skin to the vital organs, or altering the rate or rhythm of ventilation. As a result, a patient may outwardly appear relatively well despite a severe underlying injury or illness. An alteration in a patient's vital signs can provide objective evidence of the body's response to physical and psychological stress or changes in physiological function.

The order and composition of the VSS may vary slightly between ambulance services but is essentially made up of three components: a respiratory status assessment (RSA), a cardiovascular status assessment (CVSA) or perfusion status assessment (PSA), and a neurological status assessment or Glasgow Coma Scale (GCS). In addition to observing and talking to the patient, the VSS requires the paramedic to take physical measurements such as the patient's pulse rate, respiratory rate and blood pressure (see Fig 14.2).

The RSA considers measurements and observations which are indicative of the respiratory state, ranging from normal to severe respiratory distress (see Table 14.1). For example, a patient sitting forward with hands on knees is indicative or someone in severe respiratory distress as is an elevated respiratory rate. While these assessments in isolation do not indicate much, when coupled with the full RSA they are indicative of an accurate level of respiratory distress.

The PSA considers measurements and observations which are indicative of the patient's level of perfusion, ranging from normal to extremely poor and nil (see Table 14.2). A patient with a low blood pressure who is cool, pale and clammy would be considered to have compromised perfusion which, as discussed in Chapter 2, is necessary for vital organ function.

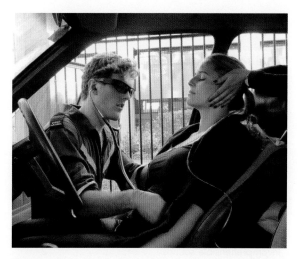

Figure 14.2
Vital sign survey assessment of a road accident patient.

Table 14.1: Respiratory status assessment

	Normal	Mild respiratory distress	Moderate respiratory distress	Severe respiratory distress
Appearance	Calm, quiet	Calm or anxious	Distressed, anxious	Distressed, exhausted
Speech	Normal flowing sentences	Full sentences	Limited to short phrases between breaths	Limited to words only, or unable to speak
Breath sounds	Quiet	Cough, mild wheeze or basal crackles	Cough inspiratory/ expiratory wheeze or mid-zone crackles	No cough, inspiratory/ expiratory wheeze, full field crackles, stridor, no breath sounds
Respiratory rate	12–16 bpm	16–20 bpm	> 20 bpm	> 20 or < 8 bpm
Respiratory rhythm	Regular cycles with expiratory phase slightly longer	Prolonged expiratory phase	Prolonged expiratory phase	Prolonged expiratory phase
Respiratory effort	Normal	Slight	Use of accessory muscles	Use of accessory muscles, braced arms
Heart rate	60–100 bpm	60–100 bpm	100–120 bpm	> 120 bpm, < 60 bpm (late)
Skin	Normal	Normal	Pale, sweaty	Pale, sweaty
Conscious state	Normal	Normal	Usually normal	Altered or unconscious

Source: Adapted from Ambulance Victoria Clinical Practice Guidelines (2019).

Table 14.2: Perfusion status assessment

	Normal	Borderline	Inadequate	Extremely poor	Nil
Heart rate	60–100 bpm	50–100 bpm	< 50 or > 100 bpm	< 50 or > 110 bpm	Absence of carotid pulse regardless of heart rate
Blood pressure	> 100 mmHg	80–100 mmHg	60–80 mmHg	< 60 mmHg	Undetectable
Skin	Warm, pink, dry	Cool, pale, clammy	Cool, pale, clammy	Cool, pale, clammy	Cool, pale, clammy
Conscious state	Alert	Alert	Usually orientated	Usually altered	Altered or unconscious

Source: Adapted from Ambulance Victoria Clinical Practice Guidelines (2019).

Table 14.3: Conscious status assessment

Eye opening	Score
Spontaneous	4
To voice	3
To pain	2
None	1

Verbal response	Score
Orientated	5
Confused	4
Inappropriate words	3
Incomprehensible sounds	2
None	1

Motor response	Score
Obeys command	6
Localises to pain	5
Withdraws (pain)	4
Flexion (pain)	3
Extension (pain)	2
None	1

Source: Adapted from Ambulance Victoria Clinical Practice Guidelines (2019).

The 15-point GCS is almost universally accepted as a useful tool for assessing a patient's conscious state (see Table 14.3). Eye opening, responses to voice and pain are used to determine the level of consciousness of a patient. Some ambulance services utilise a simpler four-point assessment tool known as AVPU, whereby patients are categorised as being alert (A), responding to voice (V) or pain (P), or unresponsive (U).

The physical examination/secondary assessments

This stage will include any secondary assessments of the patient. The assessments conducted will be determined by the nature of the condition. For example, for patients presenting with traumatic injuries this stage includes a head-to-toe physical examination looking for evidence of injuries. Commonly called the *secondary survey*, this can be a challenging process on fully clothed patients who are anxious and in pain. It may be appropriate to do this more thoroughly once in the back of the ambulance, or once initial pain relief has been administered. For patients suffering a medical complaint, this stage may include measurements such as blood glucose level (BGL), temperature and ECG recordings.

It is also important to include questions here to determine if there is any pain, discomfort or unusual sensations or feelings. For example, the patient may feel nauseous, have tingling in their fingers or pain in a specific location. A structured approach in the form of a mnemonic is commonly used to explore these aspects; DOLOR is discussed in more detail in the next chapter.

The differential/provisional diagnosis

While not always possible to definitively diagnose a patient's condition in the out-of-hospital environment devoid of blood work results, x-ray and other diagnostic tools, paramedics are required to form a provisional opinion based on the evidence they have collected. The sum of information gathered from the patient, bystanders and scene, VSS and secondary assessments needs to be evaluated and

> **PRACTICE TIP**
>
> Exposing a trauma patient to the environment to conduct a secondary survey is not always possible or wise, but rather than neglect this step entirely until a 'full' survey can be completed, try to conduct the survey as best you can through the patient's clothes if access is limited. Broken bones and other injuries that are hidden can often be identified by gentle, systematic palpation. The survey can be completed once the patient is more accessible.

interpreted by the paramedic. Using their knowledge, experience and clinical reasoning skills they should in most instances be able to suggest a provisional working diagnosis. They may be required to compare and contrast various conditions which could account for the patient's presentation and determine the most likely cause. This diagnosis will form the basis of their treatment pathway. There will, however, be instances when the cause cannot be identified and the paramedic will need to treat the patient based on their signs and/or symptoms alone.

References

Ambulance Victoria. (2019). *Clinical Practice Guidelines.* https://www.ambulance.vic.gov.au/paramedics/clinical -practice-guidelines/.

Australian Resuscitation Council. (2016). *ANZCOR Guideline 8 cardiopulmonary resuscitation (CPR).* https://resus.org.au/guidelines/.

Queensland Ambulance Service (QAS). (2011). *Department of Safety Annual Report.* Brisbane: Queensland.

The Patient-Centred Interview

By Linda Ross

OVERVIEW

- Like other medical consultations, the paramedic–patient encounter is inherently unbalanced in that the paramedic holds the scientific knowledge required to diagnose the patient, but requires the patient to describe their symptoms and history in order to apply this knowledge. The patient is unlikely to understand the significance or importance of all their symptoms in enabling the paramedic to reach a diagnosis.

- Effective paramedic–patient communication is fundamental to collecting sufficient information to determine an accurate diagnosis and gaining the support of the patient for the preferred treatment.
- The use of a structured patient interview plan can provide a 'map' to ensure important data is gathered while the patient's concerns are considered.

Introduction

Despite advances in medicine and technology, the ability to communicate effectively and gain an accurate history from patients remains an essential skill for any health professional. While media and public impressions of paramedic practice can be limited to the care of critically ill unresponsive patients, the reality is that low- and medium-acuity cases are far more prevalent (Eastwood et al., 2015). Paramedics in Victoria, for example, utilised resuscitation skills on average 1.4 times per year from 2003–2012 (Dyson et al., 2015). So, while practising resuscitation is important, the patient-centred interview, in contract, is a skill required much more frequently. This skill is performed on a daily basis and is an essential component of paramedic practice. Medical practitioners across a number of specialties will testify that there are many conditions where the physical examination or laboratory investigations may not yield anything useful, and it is the patient's story that offers the only route to reach a potential diagnosis (Groopman, 2007). That is not to say that patients always know what is wrong with them or how to articulate their symptoms correctly; their stories can be distorted by past experiences, anxiety, fear, pain, bias and hidden agendas. Paramedics must therefore explore the patient's perceptions and experiences of their illness, taking into account biopsychosocial factors, in addition to making physical assessments. This requires an open-minded, flexible and tolerant approach.

Good clinicians are able to elicit a relevant patient history and use this in conjunction with physical findings to formulate a diagnosis and/or treatment pathway while simultaneously establishing rapport with the patient (Norfolk et al., 2007). This chapter outlines a structured approach to conducting a patient-centred interview.

The structured patient-centred interview

In Part 1 we described some of the underlying challenges of delivering emergency healthcare as a paramedic. We outlined the role of paramedics in modern society and the characteristics of patients requiring paramedic care. We also discussed interpersonal communication and patient-focused care and the importance of these things in paramedic practice. The patient-centred interview incorporates both these elements and has a dual purpose. The primary purpose is to gain relevant information regarding the patient's condition, which in conjunction with physical findings, will inform management of the patient. A second purpose is to develop rapport with the patient, which is critical to the patient–paramedic relationship. Rapport is the development of a therapeutic relationship based on mutual understanding, respect, empathy and trust (O'Toole, 2008). Developing rapport through a well structured and mannered patient-centred interview can improve patient cooperation and eventual outcomes (Hojat et al., 2011).

In the previous chapter we introduced the structured clinical approach, a 'road map of patient assessment' designed to give paramedics a step-by-step approach to collecting the information necessary to make the most appropriate assessment and management plan. While not listed as an explicit step in the structured clinical approach, the patient-centred interview is used as a means to elicit some of the information required to complete a thorough patient assessment and often occurs concurrently with physical assessments such as the vital signs survey. The timing, breadth and depth of the patient-centred interview may be determined by the severity and nature of the patient's condition. Paramedics are then able to piece together findings and use clinical knowledge, reasoning and experience to determine and implement the best management options.

Patient-centred interview versus history taking

In this chapter we use the phrase 'patient-centred interview' rather than 'history taking'. While a patient-centred interview contains elements of history taking, or gathering, it is much more than that. The patient-centred interview involves a two-way encounter in which both parties interact and share information to reach a mutually acceptable understanding of what has happened, what is currently happening and what will happen.

The patient-centred interview setting

In most locations where medicine is practised roles and processes are clear and orderly. Emergency departments, for example, have clearly delineated spaces, procedures, rules and roles. Similarly, general practitioner consultation rooms are private and the layout makes it obvious where the patient is to sit and what role they are to assume. Compare this with the crowded noisy environment in the case study where friends are surrounding a patient in a public place.

The paramedic's workplace is different in every case and is frequently a place of high stimulus and little information. In this often noisy, emotional and unfamiliar environment the paramedic can easily become distracted when assessing the patient (see Fig 15.1). Having some structure around the patient-centred interview portion of the patient assessment can be helpful to guide the paramedic and ensure they gather all relevant details.

Paramedic–patient interview structure

Using the various social models that describe the clinician–patient interview, numerous researchers have developed guidelines and checklists to assist clinicians to conduct effective patient interviews and gain accurate diagnostic information (Cohen-Cole,

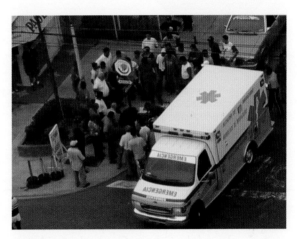

Figure 15.1
The complex paramedic workplace.
Source: Giancarlo Rossi/CC BY-SA (https://creativecommons.org/licenses/by-sa/3.0)

 CASE STUDY

Case 11274, 1147 hrs.

Dispatch details: A 72-year-old female is complaining of chest pain.

Initial presentation: The paramedic crew finds the patient sitting on a chair at a crowded food court in a major shopping centre. She is pale but conscious and surrounded by concerned friends. The patient is telling everyone she is 'fine', but friends tell the crew that the patient suddenly complained of feeling unwell and that she had chest pain.

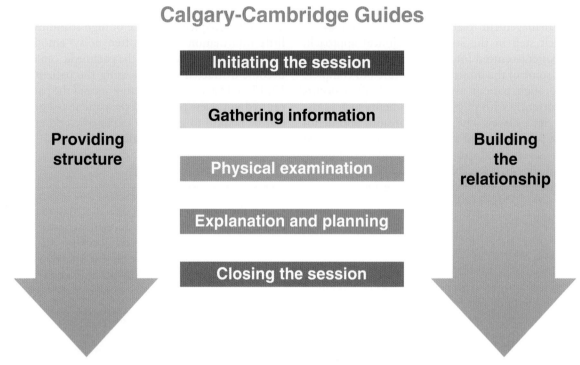

Figure 15.2
Structuring the patient interview provides the clinician with a road map to guide and provide landmarks where specific communication tools need to be used. Performed effectively, it addresses the patient's need to feel their story is understood.
Source: Adapted from Kurtz et al. (2003).

1991; Makoul, 2001; Novack et al., 1992; Riccardi & Kurtz, 1983; Stillman et al., 1976). For the unique nature of the paramedic–patient interview we have adapted the Calgary-Cambridge guide (see Fig 15.2; Kurtz et al., 2003). This guide has been chosen because it does not simply overlay communication skills on top of the traditional model of taking a medical history. Instead, it integrates the communication tasks into the process of gathering a history and recognises that there are phases in the patient interview where the paramedic needs specific, detailed information, and moments when the patient should be encouraged to tell their story. It also recognises that the sometimes intrusive and intimate nature of the physical examination (pulse, blood pressure, chest auscultation etc.) is part of information gathering as well as being intertwined with communication and rapport development.

The framework provides a logical, structured approach to the patient-centred interview that directs the paramedic towards a conclusion but also ensures that important information is not missed (Nolan, 2000). It recognises that specific communication skills need to be used at specific times and for specific goals. Apart from providing landmarks that the

paramedic can return to if interrupted, by dividing the interview into distinct phases, it also delineates points where the paramedic's communication style needs to change if it is to be effective. Finally, the framework decreases the cognitive load for the paramedic by dividing the interview into small acts, each of which is finished before the next is started.

This structured framework divides the patient-centred interview into five basic steps (see Fig 15.2).

1. Initiating the session
2. Gathering information
3. Physical examination
4. Explanation and planning
5. Closing the session

Each of these can be further divided by activities and tasks. Performed correctly, these steps should provide the paramedic with accurate information collected in a form that is easier to contextualise while also addressing the patient's concerns.

Step 1: Initiating the session
The first few moments of the interview shape the patient's view of the clinician's competence (see

BOX 15.1 First impressions count

Real communication occurs when the evaluative tendency is avoided, when we listen with understanding. It means to see the expressed idea and attitude from the other's point of view, to sense how it feels to him, to achieve his frame of reference in regard to the thing he is talking about.

Rogers (1961)

For the paramedics involved, cases commence when the dispatch is received. For patients, however, the events leading up to a call may stretch back weeks or even years. Failing to appreciate why a patient has engaged an ambulance service and what that process will do to their communication style impedes many paramedics from conducting a successful patient interview. Probably the most obvious impact of the patient's state of mind on their ability to communicate effectively is the case of a patient who is experiencing severe pain. In such a case no-one would be surprised that a normally quiet and reserved person could respond with anger or impatience towards those trying to assist them.

If you fail to gain a patient's trust or you make them feel as if you do not understand their situation, they may consider you unprofessional and not good at your job. Remember, the patient does not know how well you followed the guidelines or how accurately you performed their chest auscultation. They only know how much you seemed to listen and care.

Box 15.1). In terms of stimulus versus information, this is the phase where possibly the greatest imbalance exists, and communication in this early stage cannot simply conform to social conventions and politeness. The information and trust gained at this point will have ongoing effects on the accuracy and efficiency of the interview (Silverman et al., 2013).

Preparation

Paramedics usually work in teams so there is an opportunity to brief cases before being confronted with a patient. The journey to a case is an opportunity to read the dispatch details and start preparing a list of likely differential diagnoses. It is imperative at this point, however, to keep an open mind as dispatch details can often differ from the reality of the situation. For the case study the crew might consider the common causes of chest pain and

determine what questions they will need to ask. This process can highlight causes which the paramedic will need to include in their investigation and elimination process.

Observation

Given the stress of driving under 'lights and sirens', it is easy to arrive at a case and continue the sense of urgency. Effective paramedics use structure to reduce stimulus and seek to gain information wherever they can. While collecting equipment from the vehicle, take a moment to observe the environment: is it a well-kept house with an immaculate garden or is it overgrown and poorly tended? This can give you clues as to the patient's normal level of activity and the expectations they will have regarding treatment and outcome. Numerous photos of family members can indicate levels of social support. Take a moment to absorb your surroundings, as they will add context to what you find during the patient interview and examination.

Establishing initial rapport: introduction and role clarification

While patients are often relieved at the arrival of paramedics, this is not always the case. Research suggests that patient responses to medical emergencies are much more complex and, unless these responses are considered, the paramedic risks making assumptions that will restrict their ability to gain an accurate history (Gallagher et al., 2005). Patients often face a series of events (onset of pain) and decisions (take medication, call family, call emergency number) before the paramedics arrive. For many patients, the arrival of two (or more) uniformed medical professionals carrying equipment only confirms their worst fears: that they are, in fact, seriously ill. A calm demeanour and relatively standard greeting can help normalise the situation for the patient. Start by introducing yourself and your partner: *Hello, my name is Sarah and this is my partner, Tom. We are paramedics and here to help you. What is your name?*

Paramedics should also remember that patients who have called for help have reached a point where they have admitted that they or their family can no longer cope with their illness or the situation confronting them (Morgans et al., 2008). This can evoke feelings such as vulnerability, shame, embarrassment, fear, anxiety and hopelessness.

Identifying yourself as a paramedic can be vital when dealing with patients such as children, older people, new immigrants or drug-affected patients who may struggle to differentiate one uniform from another. Not knowing who has arrived or what role they play can be extremely unsettling. The patient

145

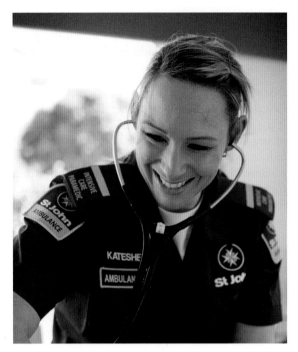

Figure 15.3
Patients can be surprised or even concerned when young paramedics arrive to assist them, in case they are inexperienced. As a result, young paramedics need to portray themselves professionally to instil confidence in the patient.
Source: Image courtesy St John New Zealand.

themselves may not even know you have been called by someone else. Paramedics should not assume that the patient knows who they are or why they are there.

The shift to university education has dramatically altered the demographic of paramedics practising in Australia and New Zealand, and some patients may be surprised when young paramedics arrive to manage their health emergency (see Fig 15.3). For these patients, presenting a calm, professional and assertive introduction may overcome their suspicion that the paramedic is too inexperienced to manage their condition. Referring to the patient respectfully by the name they have provided will also go a long way towards establishing trust. Refrain from the use of generic names such as Darl, Pet, Sweetie, Mate etc.

Effective communication at this point of the interview is dependent on the paramedic's ability to analyse and accept the patient's frame of reference. Everyone brings their past experiences, prejudices and social status to a communication exchange. In the out-of-hospital environment these factors determine how the patient and paramedic will express themselves. This is further complicated by the stress of the situation and other environmental stimulus. Effective paramedics consider their own

and the patient's backgrounds to determine what the patient is trying to express and what methods they will use to communicate effectively in return. Recognising biases and an ability to put them to one side at times is vital to establishing communication and rapport with patients from all backgrounds in a wide variety of situations.

Remember, patients are almost certainly unaware of the paramedic's adherence to clinical guidelines when being treated: they do not know whether the correct drug was administered, in the correct dose, at the correct time. Instead, they will judge the paramedic's clinical ability on the rapport they built. Ask any patient how their stay in hospital was or how they were treated by paramedics and they will invariably tell you about how caring, empathetic and nice they were—not if they were clinically competent or not. It is difficult to overstate the importance at this stage of gaining the support, trust and involvement of the patient in helping you gather information and develop a management plan.

Identifying the reasons for the consultation
It's nice to meet you, Mrs Ramsey. Why have you called an ambulance today?

The key here is to seek the patient's perspective of the events that have led up to this point and why you were called. Many patients have already explained their situation to the emergency call-taker and assume the paramedics are fully aware of it, so paramedics need to phrase this carefully. You may like to always open with the same question or have a variety of opening questions depending on the circumstances. *I understand you're not well; can you tell me about what's happening today? We are here to help you; can you tell us what's wrong today?* A question that displays both understanding and concern, as well as asks for the main presenting problem, will be most effective. Whatever question is chosen, clinicians need to carefully consider the effect of how they start the interview as it will impact the entire encounter (Silverman et al., 2013).

Environmental control
Considerations of where the interview should be conducted are not addressed in the Calgary-Cambridge Guide as most medical interviews are scheduled to occur in private locations. Interviews conducted by paramedics, however, can occur in public spaces (see Fig 15.1). The ability to elicit frank and honest answers from patients and to conduct a physical examination is dependent on how comfortable the patient feels in that environment, and paramedics may need to exclude bystanders or move the patient as necessary. Even when the patient is physically and psychologically comfortable,

paramedics can create a more conducive interview setting by reducing background noise or adjusting lighting. Importantly, assuming a position close to the patient and at the same height reduces the power imbalance inherent in the interview and suggests that the paramedic is not only focused on the patient but is also willing to devote time to their assessment (Silverman et al., 2013).

Step 2: Information gathering

With the tone of the interview set, the next stage addresses two overlapping needs: the patient's need to convey what they feel is important about their illness/situation; and the paramedic's need to identify the underlying problem. Accordingly, the paramedic adaptation of the Calgary-Cambridge Guide divides this phase into two distinct components that require different communication skills. In the initial patient-centric phase the skill of active listening is essential; while controlling the subsequent paramedic-centric phase with directed questions ensures the collection of accurate information specific to the disease/injury process. Importantly these phases may not necessarily proceed in order with the patient-centred interview moving fluidly between phases as dictated by the situation.

Patient-centric phase

As already discussed, patients assess and engage with the paramedic based on their belief that the paramedic 'understands' what is happening to them. For this to occur, the patient must have the opportunity to present their explanation of the illness. Skilful listening helps the paramedic identify the main presenting problem, make accurate determinations and convey empathy and support (Mauksch, 2017). Listening doesn't simply comprise being able to recite what a patient has said, however. For the patient to feel you are listening, they need to feel you are giving them your full attention. Most of the cues patients use to determine whether the paramedic is listening come from the paramedic's body language (Silverman et al., 2013) (Fig 15.4). Important among these is eye contact; taking notes has been shown to reduce the patient's belief that the clinician is paying full attention to all their concerns (Ruusuvuori, 2001). While historically interruptions were considered counterproductive, a timely interjection can serve a useful purpose. Interjections may be used to build rapport, show support or concern, to clarify or garnish more information or to paraphrase what has been conveyed so far before proceeding (Mauksch, 2017). Paramedics must therefore find the right balance of listening and speaking in this phase. By the end of this phase

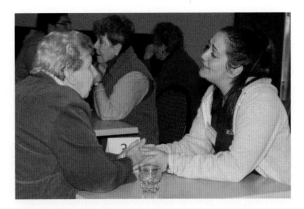

Figure 15.4
Nonverbal rapport.
Nonverbal cues such as body position, eye contact, nodding and facial expressions can convey understanding and compassion vital in the establishment of rapport.

the paramedic should have a sense of the patient's perspective on their illness.

The shift from the patient-centric phase to the paramedic-centric phase of information gathering reflects the shift from an understanding of the illness to determining the underlying disease. Before this commences it is important to provide the patient with a summary of your understanding of the illness. Critically, this demonstrates to the patient that you have absorbed and understood their explanation. At once, this paraphrasing demonstrates your listening and understanding of the patient's perspective. Importantly, this is not the time to challenge any of the patient's ideas—regardless of how inaccurate you perceive them to be.

Paramedic-centric phase

Determining the underlying disease process requires the paramedic to assume more control over the interview but does not mean that the patient becomes completely passive. The aim is to gather 'accurate, complete and mutually agreeable' information (Silverman et al., 2013). Whereas the patient-centric phase required a single open question (*How can we help you today?*), this phase requires careful use of closed and open questioning techniques.

Open questions allow the patient to introduce information on conditions that the clinician may not have considered previously: *Tell me about this pain you've been having.* They have been shown to produce more information more quickly than a series of closed questions (Takemura et al., 2005).

Closed questions are specific and can usually be answered with a single word: *Is the pain sharp or dull? Do you have pain at the moment?* They are invaluable when trying to differentiate between conditions. An important skill in phrasing closed questions is not to suggest to the patient that one answer is better than another. Patients will have their own explanations and expectations of their condition and may tend to align their answers if they feel these fit with their explanation.

Key history

The sequencing and progression of symptoms can be strongly indicative of a particular disease process: shortness of breath from acute pulmonary oedema (APO) tends to manifest in the early hours of the morning after several hours of lying supine, whereas asthma presents acutely at any time but rarely when the patient is asleep or not being exposed to a trigger. Thus, identifying when particular symptoms occurred and their severity can help identify the underlying disease. If the patient has been allowed to describe their illness, much of this information will already have been obtained. The patient's opening statement will often present much of the key history.

Investigating signs and symptoms

The information gained from the patient by questioning them more specifically about their signs and symptoms can be pivotal in providing a more complete picture of the patient's condition. A number of mnemonics have been developed to assist clinicians to investigate a patient's signs and symptoms as part of the patient-centred interview. Such mnemonics are a good way to ensure all the necessary information has been gathered. The most commonly used mnemonic in paramedic practice is **DOLORS**. Other mnemonics are shown in Box 15.2.

BOX 15.2 History-gathering mnemonics

WWQQAA + B
Where
When
Quality
Quantity
Aggravating and relieving factors
Associated manifestations
Beliefs

OPQRST
Onset
Provocation
Quality
Region, relief, radiation, recurrence
Severity
Time

Description of pain/discomfort/problem
Onset
Location
Other signs and symptoms
Relief
Scale/score

Description

The description or nature of the pain or condition provides the paramedic with a good sense of the main presenting problem from the patient's perspective described in their own words. Always start with an open question so you don't lead the patient:

Paramedic: Mrs Ramsey, we understand you are having an issue with your chest? Can you describe what it feels like?

Patient: I have a very heavy feeling in my chest.

Shifting to a closed question can add more specific information:

Paramedic: Would you describe this heavy feeling as either sharp or dull?

Patient: Definitely a dull heavy feeling.

> **PRACTICE TIP**
>
> Try to use the patient's terminology to describe their symptoms as they may use different words or attach different meaning to some words. For example, patients may answer 'no' when asked if they have any pain because they would describe it as an ache or heaviness. Continue to use their descriptors when questioning further or reassessing presence or severity.

Onset

This may have been covered in the opening statement but now is the time to gain more detail. Again, start with an open question:

Paramedic: When did this heaviness begin?

Patient: About an hour ago when I was walking around the shops.

Focus with a closed question:

Paramedic: What were you doing immediately before that?

Patient: Having lunch.

And another:

Paramedic: Did the heaviness come on suddenly or did it build up gradually?

Patient: No, it just hit me suddenly.

Location

By this time some paramedics may be forming a strong hypothesis for the cause of the pain (cardiac, pleuritic or musculoskeletal) and may rush this stage by asking a closed question, such as: *Is the pain just in your chest or does it radiate anywhere else?* To gain accurate information it is better to ask an open question first:

Paramedic: Mrs Ramsey, can you point to where the heaviness is?

Patients will either point to a specific location or illustrate a large area. This is a valuable differential tool that can then be clarified with a closed question:

Paramedic: So, the heaviness is right across your chest and down your left arm?

Patient: Yes.

Other signs and symptoms

How this question is phrased is often an indicator of whether a paramedic is able to assume the patient's perspective. 'Signs and symptoms' are paramedic terms and most patients would not be sure what the paramedic was seeking if they were asked: *Do you have any other signs and symptoms?*

A better way to gain this information is to start with an open question:

Paramedic: When the heaviness started, did you feel anything else that is not normal for you?

Patient: I felt a little dizzy and like I was going to vomit.

If there are specific symptoms that help differentiate between diseases, these can be asked about in closed questions. Only enquire about one symptom at a time, otherwise it can be difficult to identify which symptom the patient is agreeing to:

Paramedic: So, you felt dizzy and like you were going to vomit. Were you sweaty?

Patient: A little, just for a couple of minutes.

Paramedic: Did you feel short of breath?

Relief

You want to find out if anything the patient has done prior to your arrival relieves the pain such as position, rest or medication. Start with an open question again before going for specific closed questions to refine the responses based on what you want to know.

Paramedic: Mrs Ramsey, does anything relieve the heaviness for you?

Patient: No.

Focus with a closed question:

Paramedic: Now that you are sitting and resting, is it less?

Patient: A little.

Scale/score

This step in the mnemonic may not be applicable to all cases as it is specifically seeking a baseline pain score.

Paramedic: How would you rate this heaviness?

Patient: It's really bad.

Focus with a closed question:

Paramedic: Can you give it a score out of 10 for me; 10 being the worst pain imaginable and 0 being no pain at all?

Patient: Eight

While the example questions given above are specific to the case study and chest pain, mnemonics such as DOLORS can be adapted to suit other conditions and are best used as a guide or trigger for questions central to forming a full clinical picture of the patient's condition.

Step 3: Physical examination

Hopefully by this point paramedics would have gained the trust and compliance of the patient. However, before doing any physical examination it is still necessary to explain the procedures and ask for permission; remember informed consent from Chapter 13 on legal and ethical considerations. Paramedics will need to balance their need for information against preserving the patient's comfort and dignity. Assessments should be avoided if unnecessary (e.g. taking a blood glucose level [BGL] on a conscious paediatric patient with a broken arm and no evidence of diabetes) or delayed (e.g. lifting a patient's top to auscultate their chest in the back of the ambulance or another private setting rather than in a public place). Initial physical assessments have been described in the previous chapter. More assessments that are specific to particular conditions will be described in subsequent chapters.

Step 4: Explanation and planning

After completing the assessment but before commencing the treatment plan is the time to present your findings and preliminary diagnosis to the patient and seek to align their expectations with your clinical opinion.

Paramedic: I know you were hoping it is not your heart playing up, Mrs Ramsey, but your description, my assessments and experience all indicate that it is the most likely cause at this stage. We will need to treat you for this now and take you up to the hospital for further tests. Is that okay with you?

It is imperative that the patient is given an explanation of your assessment in terms they can comprehend and that they are included in the decision-making based on your recommendation.

Step 5: Closing the session

Patients presenting with acute pain or injuries are less likely to resist treatment or transport to hospital, but the increasingly chronic nature of paramedic work now requires paramedics to explain to patients that transport to hospital may not always be the most appropriate option for their condition. Such a difference between the patient's perceived outcome (transport to hospital) and the paramedic's preferred management (referral to another treatment pathway) can be a source of conflict for paramedics who lack the insight and communication skills to develop the patient interview to the point of shared understanding. Closing the session is thus increasingly necessary for paramedics whose scope of practice allows them to 'treat and leave' patients as opposed to the traditional role of 'treat and transport'. (Please be aware that individual services may have guidelines and procedures around the transport of patients who have received a pharmaceutical intervention.) An important aspect of closure is to provide the patient with a pathway for the expected outcome of treatment as well as what should be considered an inadequate response to treatment. For example, in the case of a young male treated with an antiemetic for acute gastroenteritis:

Paramedic: This medication will not make you feel normal but it should reduce the nausea and vomiting. The vomiting should subside over the next 12 hours. If it persists any longer, make an appointment to see your GP.

Summary

The patient-centred interview is an essential part of paramedic practice. The use of a well-structured patient-centred interview can facilitate the garnishing of vital information about the illness from the patient's perspective and assist in the establishment of rapport. Rapport building in this early stage of the patient–paramedic encounter cannot be underestimated as it will impact the entire episode of care. Patient-centred does not imply the communication is one way, however, and paramedics need to employ exceptional communication skills to guide and shape the interview for mutual benefit. It is important that the patient-centred interview conclude with a summary of mutually agreed upon information and a discussion about a plan of action.

References

Cohen-Cole, S. A. (1991). *The medical interview: a three function approach*. St Louis, MO: Mosby-Year Books.

Dyson, K., Bray, J., Smith, K., Bernard, S., Straney, L., & Finn, J. (2015). Paramedic exposure to out-of-hospital cardiac arrest is rare and declining in Victoria, Australia. *Resuscitation, 89*, 93–98.

Eastwood, K., Morgans, A., Smith, K., Hodgkinson, A., Becker, G., & Stoelwinder, J. (2015). A novel approach for managing the growing demand for ambulance services by low-acuity patients. *Australian Health Review, 40*, 378–384.

Gallagher, T. J., Gregory, S. W., Bianchi, A. J., Hartung, P. J., & Harkness, S. (2005). Examining medical interview asymmetry using the expectation status approach. *Social Psychology Quarterly, 68*(3), 187–203.

Groopman, J. (2007). *How Doctors Think*. Melbourne: Scribe Publications.

Hojat, M., Louis, D. Z., Markham, F. W., Wender, R., Rabinowitz, C., & Gonnella, J. S. (2011). Physicians' empathy and clinical outcomes for diabetic patients. *Academic Medicine: Journal of the Association of American Medical Colleges, 86*(3), 359–364.

Kurtz, S., Silverman, J., Benson, J., & Draper, J. (2003). Marrying content and process in clinical method teaching: enhancing the Calgary-Cambridge guides. *Academic Medicine: Journal of the Association of American Medical Colleges, 78*(8), 802–809.

Makoul, G. (2001). Essential elements of communication in medical encounters: the Kalamazoo Consensus Statement. *Academic Medicine: Journal of the Association of American Medical Colleges, 76*(4), 390–393.

Mauksch, L. (2017). Questioning a Taboo. Physicians' interruptions during interactions with patients. *JAMA, 317*(10), 1021–1022.

Morgans, A., Archer, F., & Allen, C. (2008). Patient decision making in prehospital health emergencies: determinants and predictors of patient delay. *Journal of Emergency Primary Health Care, 6*(3).

Nolan, T. W. (2000). System changes to improve patient safety. *British Medical Journal, 18*(320), 771–773.

Norfolk, T., Birdi, K., & Walsh, D. (2007). The role of empathy in establishing rapport in the consultation: a new model. *Medical Education, 41*(7), 690–697.

Novack, D. H., Dube, C., & Goldstein, M. G. (1992). Teaching medical interviewing: a basic course on interviewing and the physician-patient relationship. *Archives of Internal Medicine, 152*, 1814–1820.

O'Toole, G. (2008). *Communication: core interpersonal skills for health professionals*. Sydney: Churchill Livingstone.

Riccardi, V. M., & Kurtz, S. M. (1983). *Communication and counselling in healthcare*. Springfield, IL: Charles C. Thomas.

Rogers, C. R. (1961). *On becoming a person: a therapist's view of psychotherapy*. Boston: Houghton Mifflin.

Ruusuvuori, J. (2001). Looking means listening: coordinating displays of engagement in doctor-patient interaction. *Social Science & Medicine, 52*(7), 1093–1108.

Silverman, J., Kurtz, S., & Draper, J. (2013). *Skills for communicating with patients* (3rd ed.). Boca Raton: CRC Press.

Stillman, P. L., Sabars, D. L., & Redfield, D. L. (1976). Use of paraprofessionals to teach interviewing skills. *Pediatrics, 57*, 769–774.

Takemura, Y., Sakurai, Y., Yokoya, S., Otaki, J., Matsuoka, T., Ban, N., Hirata, I., Miki, T., & Tsuda, T. (2005). Open-ended questions: are they really beneficial for gathering medical information from patients? *The Tohoku Journal of Experimental Medicine, 206*, 151–154.

SECTION 9:
The Paramedic Approach to the Patient With a Respiratory Condition

In this section:

Quickly determining the cause of a patient's respiratory distress is one of the most difficult clinical reasoning challenges that paramedics face. Shortness of breath can be caused by a multitude of pathologies and can occur in life-threatening forms at almost any age. The cause may be acute or chronic, or a combination of both. Dispatches to patients who are complaining of respiratory distress are among the most common calls for paramedics, and the ability to quickly determine the cause is necessary not only because the condition can quickly progress to a life-threatening situation, but also because misdiagnosis and treatment can actually worsen the condition.

Performing effective clinical reasoning in this situation is made even more difficult by the anxiety and distress the symptoms cause for the patient. The impact of breathlessness on the patient's ability to talk can also make it extremely difficult to gain an accurate history.

Very broadly, respiratory distress can be categorised by one of three causes:

1. inability to ventilate adequately—unable to move air in and out of the lungs and alveoli (choking, asthma, anaphylaxis, drug overdose, pneumothorax, pleural effusion)

2. inability to externally respirate—unable to move oxygen and carbon dioxide from the alveoli into the blood (acute pulmonary oedema, bronchitis, pneumonia, chronic obstructive pulmonary disease, pulmonary embolism)

3. inability to internally respirate—inability of the blood to deliver sufficient oxygen to the cells (anaemia, carbon monoxide poisoning).

In many cases, however, it is a combination of these that lead to the call for an emergency ambulance.

In order to manage these patients effectively you need to be able to quickly differentiate between the causes of respiratory distress and know which can be corrected in the field. This section reviews common causes of respiratory distress and links the pathophysiology to paramedic management of these common conditions.

CHAPTER 16

Airway Obstruction

By Hugh Grantham

OVERVIEW

- Airway obstruction can be partial or complete.
- Airway obstruction is more common among children and people with eating or swallowing disorders.
- Choking and aspiration are serious hazards for those with severe learning and/or physical disabilities (Thacker et al., 2008).
- Adults with mental illness are more at risk of airway obstruction due to medication side effects, behavioural changes and concurrent neurological disorders (Aldridge & Taylor, 2012).
- Immediate management of an airway obstruction is lifesaving.

- There has been controversy as to the safest approach to relieving complete airway obstruction.
- Consequences of a choking event include local trauma, aspiration and negative pressure pulmonary oedema.
- Patients whose early obstruction has been relieved should be assessed for precipitating factors leading to the airway obstruction and associated iatrogenic injury.

Introduction

Airway obstruction occurs when there is a partial or complete acute blockage of the upper airway, usually above the vocal cords, but may include subglottic causes (Levin & Smith, 2010). It results in varying degrees of inadequate ventilation and respiration, ranging from mild partial airway obstruction with no notable physiological compromise to complete airway obstruction resulting in choking. Certain groups of people have a higher risk of airway obstruction, including children (due to anatomical and cognitive differences), people with dysphagia (swallowing impairment) and anyone in an altered conscious state (Aldridge & Taylor, 2012).

Pathophysiology

Airway obstruction

An airway obstruction can be partial or complete. A partial airway obstruction allows some airflow past the point of obstruction, while a complete obstruction does not allow any airflow. Causes of obstruction include both endogenous and exogenous factors (see Box 16.1).

If a solid object is lodged above the vocal cords in the supraglottic region above the cricopharyngeus muscle which closes the top of the oesophagus, it may cause obstruction by its physical presence acting as a mechanical obstruction and also by precipitating laryngeal spasm associated with the direct contact. Complete obstruction can occur with a mechanical obstruction above the vocal cords, but an incomplete obstruction with stridor is far more likely. Patients with a complete obstruction are silent as there is no air moving past the object and the patient will generally lose consciousness quickly.

A choking episode associated with laryngeal spasm and a coughing fit from inhaled liquids is different from one precipitated by a solid piece of food or a foreign body. In the inhaled liquid situation the inability to breathe is caused by a coughing fit and may be exacerbated by the vocal cords being held closed by spasm.

There are also predisposing factors that heighten an individual's risk of airway obstruction.

Dysphagia

Dysphagia (difficulty swallowing) following a cerebrovascular accident (CVA) in older adults and the tendency of young children to place items in their mouths represent significant cohorts at risk of choking but the possibility of choking in other age groups should not be ignored, with drugs and alcohol both affecting conscious state and reducing an individual's ability to protect their airway.

Swallowing

Although performed unconsciously, swallowing is a complex reflex that involves the coordinated constriction and relaxation of several muscle groups to ensure that food is passed into the oesophagus and the airway remains protected. The process relies on an appropriately masticated bolus of food or a mouthful of liquid being propelled to the back of the mouth where the swallowing reflex is initiated.

BOX 16.1 Causes of airway obstruction

Endogenous factors

- Airway oedema in the setting of:
  › anaphylaxis
  › angiotensin-converting enzyme (ACE) inhibitor reaction
- Mucus plug
- Tongue placement
- Infection (e.g. epiglottitis, croup)

Exogenous factors

- Inhalation of food during eating
- Inhalation of other foreign objects
- Airway burns
- Inhalation of poisonous gases
- Trauma

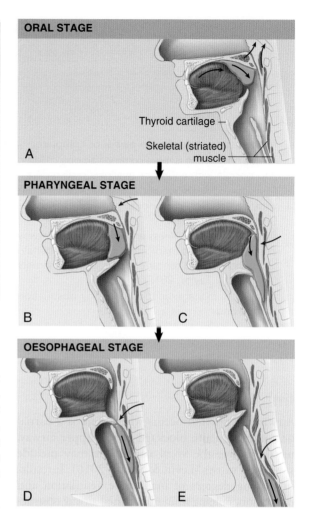

Figure 16.1
Stages of swallowing.
A–C Oropharyngeal stage. **A** During this stage, a bolus of food is voluntarily formed on the tongue and pushed against the palate and into the oropharynx. Notice that the soft palate and uvula prevent food from entering the nasopharynx. **B** After the bolus enters the oropharynx, involuntary reflexes push the bolus down towards the oesophagus. **C** The upward movement of the larynx and downward movement of the bolus close the epiglottis and thus prevent food from entering the lower respiratory tract. **D–E** Oesophageal stage. **D** Involuntary reflexes of skeletal and smooth muscle in the wall of the oesophagus move the bolus through the oesophagus towards the stomach. **E** After the bolus has passed, the epiglottis moves upwards, opening the larynx and trachea to respiration.
Source: Craft, Gordon & Tiziani (2011); Patton & Thibodeau (2010).

As the food is passed into the superior pharynx three pharyngeal constrictor muscles working in sequence propel it through the pharynx and past the larynx. As this is initiated, the larynx is pulled up, allowing the epiglottis to effectively seal off the entrance to the larynx and the cricopharyngeus muscle relaxes opening the top of the oesophagus (see Fig 16.1; Hall, 2012).

Choking most often occurs when this process is not carried out successfully. Solids that have not been chewed properly or a foreign body that is too large and inflexible to pass smoothly through the pharynx may catch in the supraglottic region, obstructing airflow and causing choking. Lacking the viscosity and form of a food bolus, fluids swallowed at a time when inhalation is occurring can enter into the larynx and precipitate a cough reflex or a laryngeal spasm, which can be seen as a choking episode.

The failure to chew food appropriately and swallowing too quickly can be associated with individuals with an intellectual disability (Samuels & Chadwick, 2006), while an impaired level of consciousness due to the effects of drugs or alcohol is thought to predispose individuals to choking and a failure to maintain a clear airway if regurgitation or vomiting occurs. This concern about a failure to maintain a clear airway is the rationale for managing patients with an impaired conscious level in a lateral position.

A failure to correctly initiate the swallowing reflex and maintain a gag reflex is often associated with stroke and other neurological problems such as motor neuron disease and Parkinson's disease (Goh et al., 2016), thus this group of patients is at increased risk of choking (Logemann, 1998). It is for this reason that patients who have had a stroke are assessed for their ability to swallow and demonstrate a gag reflex as part of the early clinical assessment. Another high-risk group is those who are receiving enteral feeding usually via percutaneous endoscopic gastrostomy (PEG) tube who have been noted to have a higher risk of choking if the feeding regimen is not strictly adhered to (Goh et al., 2016).

Airway oedema and inflammation

A shift of fluid into the dermis, the subcutaneous or submucosal tissues around the airway can also result in a narrowing of the airway. Depending on the pathology, the swelling can occur at different points along the airway and the presentation can be varied.

Anaphylaxis

The airway can be compromised during an anaphylaxis episode due to angio-oedema of the tongue or larynx, or both. Refer to Chapter 28 for more about this process.

Infection

There are several infective processes that affect the upper airway and have the potential to result in either a partial or a complete occlusion. These include:

- epiglottitis
- croup (laryngotracheobronchitis)
- peritonsillar abscess
- retropharyngeal abscess.

Epiglottitis is most often caused by a bacterial infection that affects the epiglottis. It can, however, be caused by burns or trauma to the epiglottis. It involves swelling of both the epiglottis and the surrounding tissues. Once considered a paediatric disease, widespread Hib vaccinations have significantly reduced epiglottitis in Western countries (Guldfred et al., 2008) but elderly immigrants from poorer areas should be included in the list of possible patients suffering this infection (Briem et al., 2009). The inflamed epiglottis can cause either a partial or a complete occlusion of the entrance to the trachea. Patients will often present with fever, a hoarse voice, a severely sore throat, pain on swallowing (if possible), dysphagia/aphagia, drooling (due to aphagia) and the need to sit up and lean forwards to allow drainage of their mouth (Price et al., 2005).

Croup is caused by a range of viral or bacterial infections. Most commonly it is caused by viruses, in particular the parainfluenza virus (Malhotra & Krilov, 2001; Peltola et al., 2002). Croup is most often seen in children aged 6 months to 3 years, but it may also be seen into adolescence (Thomas & Friedland, 1998). The male-to-female ratio of occurrence of croup is 3 to 2 (Knutson & Aring, 2004). Croup generally presents in the days following the onset of an upper respiratory tract infection with a low-grade fever. It involves oedema of the larynx, trachea and bronchi. Due to the cartilaginous rings maintaining the structure of the trachea and bronchi, the partial obstruction occurs at the level of the larynx. A distinctive barking cough and inspiratory stridor are the most obvious signs of croup (Gardner, 2008). These are also the most obvious signs to a clinician of a partial airway obstruction resulting from the oedema. Emergency out-of-hospital management involves nebulised adrenaline which will produce an improvement at 30 minutes, while steroids have been shown to make a difference at 6 hours (Bjornson et al., 2013; Russell et al., 2011).

PRACTICE TIP

Patients with suspected epiglottitis should be managed with as little intervention as possible in the out-of-hospital setting. Allow the patient to remain in their preferred position as much as possible.

A peritonsillar abscess (quinsy) is the collection of pus between the tonsils and the muscular wall of the pharynx. It is often a complication of acute tonsillitis and occurs more frequently in adults. Usually the inflammation is on one side only, but it can occur bilaterally, resulting in a significant narrowing of the airway in severe cases. A retropharyngeal abscess occurs in the lymph nodes located posterior to the pharynx. Peritonsillar abscesses and retropharyngeal abscesses are caused by bacteria.

CASE STUDY 1

Case 12564, 1234 hrs.

Dispatch details: A 78-year-old man in a cafe is having difficulty breathing.

Initial presentation: When the paramedics arrive at the cafe they find the patient sitting down. He is conscious, cyanosed and unable to speak. There is also a marked stridor, which ceases with a decrease in ventilatory effort shortly after the paramedics arrive. The patient becomes drowsy with the decrease in ventilation.

Glandular fever or infective mononucleosis may present with severe swelling of the tonsils and surrounding tissues to the point of causing an airway obstruction (Chan & Dawes, 2001). Emergency management in the out-of-hospital field is limited but nebulised adrenaline is worth considering in extreme situations where near obstruction with stridor exists. A rare but important cause of airway obstruction is an infection in the floor of the mouth and pharynx called Ludwig's angina. This requires aggressive and early antibiotic therapy and has been known to cause complete obstruction (Candamourty et al., 2012; Pak et al., 2017).

 ASSESS

Patient history

In this case the history is suggestive of a choking episode that occurred while the patient was eating. The fact that he is relatively elderly raises the possibility that he may have a chewing problem associated with poor dentition. Other risk factors that might also be found in the elderly include an impaired gag reflex, possibly associated with acute/chronic stroke, a progressive neurological disease or confusion associated with dementia. In all adults there is also the possibility that the gag reflex was impaired by drugs or alcohol.

The patient would probably have adopted the universal choking sign, which entails holding both hands around the front of his neck. Initially he had signs of a partial airway obstruction with a marked stridor caused by turbulent airflow around the obstruction. Complete obstruction then occurred, as demonstrated by the absence of air movement and therefore respiratory or vocal noise.

Airway

The patient's oropharynx may appear clear. The blockage may be in the laryngopharynx or even beyond the epiglottis in the subglottic region. Over time, depending on the size of the occlusion, the tissues around the site may become inflamed. Paramedics must keep in mind that if this blockage is not the result of a foreign object, they must consider pathophysiological causes for the airway obstruction.

Breathing

The mechanical act of ventilation is not possible without a portal to the environment to allow for the volume changes. The airway needs to be cleared of the obstruction to allow the chest wall to expand and the diaphragm to descend in order to draw air into the lungs. In this case, the patient's ventilatory effort decreases following a period of increased effort, indicating a complete

HISTORY

Ask!

Ask bystanders:
- What was the patient eating?
- How did the choking episode start?

RESPIRATORY STATUS

Look for!
- In the conscious patient, look for the universal sign of choking: both hands around the throat.
- Look for obvious effort to manually engage the thoracic muscles to expand the chest and the open mouth, again another effort to encourage airflow into the lungs.

obstruction that has resulted in hypoxia and a reduction in the respiratory drive. This occurs concurrently with a decreasing conscious state, also due to hypoxia.

Cardiovascular

This patient will have a sympathetic response to the stress of the situation. A conscious patient will be tachycardic. As an unconscious patient becomes more hypoxic, a bradycardic response may be seen prior to cardiac arrest.

Initial assessment summary

Problem	Choking, most likely on food
Conscious state	Initially alert, now getting drowsy
Position	Sitting in a chair
Heart rate	Tachycardic; exact reading not taken at this stage
Blood pressure	Not taken at this stage
Skin appearance	Flushed face, evidence of cyanosis appearing around the lips
Speech pattern	Unable to speak
Respiratory rate	At first sounded moderately fast (according to the stridor heard), no successful ventilation now
Respiratory rhythm	None
Respiratory effort	Marked ventilatory attempt now failing
Chest auscultation	Auditory stridor in the upper airway heard without auscultation
Pulse oximetry	80%
Temperature	Not taken at this stage
History	Patient eating at a cafe; other history unknown.

D: None.
A: The patient has a complete airway obstruction with a decreasing conscious state.
B: Respiratory effort is being made but there is no ventilation.
C: Heart rate is elevated but accurate assessment of heart rate and blood pressure are superseded by the urgent need to clear the airway.

The patient is in an immediately life-threatening state. In working through the primary survey, upon establishing that the airway is completely compromised all further assessment should be withheld until this problem is solved.

② CONFIRM

The essential part of the clinical reasoning process is to seek to confirm your initial hypothesis by finding clinical signs that should occur with your provisional diagnosis. You should also seek to challenge your diagnosis by exploring findings that do not fit your hypothesis: do not just ignore them because they do not fit.

In this particular case the history and presentation demonstrate progression from partial obstruction to complete obstruction: the classic presentation of hands clutching at the front of the throat, the flushed face from coughing, plus the possibility of cyanosis if it has been going long enough.

What else could it be?
Laryngeal spasm
Laryngeal spasm is possible and might have been precipitated by inhaling liquid (a drink or vomit). If this were laryngeal spasm, it should relax in time and will always relax if the patient becomes significantly hypoxic. Laryngeal spasm associated with aspiration should classically present with a coughing fit, as the fluid goes through the larynx, and then possibly stridor, as the spasm becomes established. In extreme cases complete obstruction could occur but this would be unlikely.

> **DIFFERENTIAL DIAGNOSIS**
>
> **Choking associated with mechanical obstruction**
> Or
> - Laryngeal spasm
> - Acute anaphylaxis

Acute anaphylaxis

Acute obstruction of the airway is often associated with fatal anaphylactic reactions. Assessing the patient for small airway changes (wheezes are often difficult to hear when the patient has a stridor or complete obstruction), concurrent angio-oedema, skin manifestations and gastrointestinal disturbances reveal none of these symptoms, but the diagnosis should not be entirely discarded too early. This patient has presented with stridor, decreasing consciousness, tachycardia and a history of potentially having eaten something. Ascertaining whether he has a history of severe allergies or anaphylaxis is important at this stage.

3 TREAT

Emergency management

Initially, management of a supraglottic partial obstruction with stridor may require minimal intervention if the patient is still well oxygenated, encouraging the patient to cough and clear their own obstruction.

Back blows

If it becomes necessary to intervene because of complete obstruction or signs of deteriorating oxygen delivery, the ANZCOR Guideline 4 (2016) recommends commencing with five back blows. The aim is to provide a shockwave through the chest and hopefully dislodge the obstruction, which can then be coughed up. Small patients can be placed across the paramedic's lap with the patient's head below their chest, to allow gravity to help clear the obstruction if it can be displaced.

Chest thrusts

If simple back blows fail to displace the obstruction, then chest thrusts are recommended and should be performed according to local guidelines and training. Abdominal thrusts are still recommended in some parts of the world but are not supported in Australia because of the risk of associated injuries (ANZCOR Guideline 4, 2016).

Positive pressure ventilation

Positive pressure ventilation with an appropriate bag and mask is worth attempting if back or chest blows have been ineffective. It may force the obstruction into a main bronchus and allow normal ventilation of the other lung, or it may assist in forcing air past the obstruction and allow lung inflation, but generating sufficient pressure and coordinating with the patient's own respiratory effort are often difficult. In most cases either the obstruction will allow sufficient airflow to maintain cerebral perfusion and the patient will remain conscious (albeit distressed) or the obstruction will limit ventilation and produce hypoxia and unconsciousness. In the latter case, it is necessary to inspect the airway prior to using forceful ventilation, as the foreign body may be able to be removed. If no obstruction can be seen on inspection (i.e. it is below the larynx), positive pressure can be used to try to force the obstruction down into one of the two main bronchi of the lungs and at least allow the paramedics to ventilate one lung.

Manual clearance

In the unconscious patient, a foreign body or piece of food in the supraglottic region can often be removed easily with Magill forceps and a laryngoscope. It is sometimes possible to remove material from between the cords with care in this situation. The risk of damaging the cords is balanced by the clinical urgency of establishing an airway. This procedure can be done only in an unconscious patient (who will tolerate laryngoscopy).

If no foreign body can be seen above the cords and an endotracheal tube can successfully be passed through the cords, as a last-ditch manoeuvre advancing the endotracheal tube and pushing the obstructing body into the right main

PRACTICE TIP

In some parts of the world the Heimlich manoeuvre (Heimlich, 1975) is still recommended despite reported cases of iatrogenic injuries associated with this procedure, including spleen damage and a ruptured stomach and liver (Cecchetto et al., 2011; Chillag et al., 2010; Redding, 1979). Because much of the ambulance dispatch processes and advice is generated in countries where the Heimlich manoeuvre is still taught, it is possible that call-takers following this algorithm may advise this procedure. This is no longer considered evidence-based practice.

bronchus is recommended. In this situation the patient will survive on one lung and the obstructing object can be retrieved in hospital later.

Surgical airway

A surgical airway procedure, either a cricothyroidotomy or a formal surgical cricothyroidotomy, may be considered if the obstruction is at the level of the larynx or above and cannot be removed. A large-bore needle placed through the cricothyroid membrane has been advocated as a simple procedure for administering oxygen in patients with a complete obstruction. This requires a high-pressure oxygen source which is connected intermittently to introduce oxygen into the airway. It is a very short-term intervention and is not intended to produce ventilation; therefore, it will not clear carbon dioxide. Many authors, particularly those drawing on military experience, are recommending a definitive surgical cricothyroidotomy over the needle cricothyroidotomy (Collopy et al., 2015; DiGiacomo et al., 2003; Scrase & Woollard, 2006). Practice should be guided by local guidelines and procedures.

For this patient, if attempts at dislodging with back blows and chest thrusts prove ineffective, it is most likely that the obstruction can be removed with Magill forceps and a laryngoscope. Paramedics carry out this procedure frequently, particularly in elderly patients who have attempted to swallow large pieces of poorly chewed food.

4 EVALUATE

Post removal of the foreign body the evaluation returns to the start of the primary survey approach. Unless the hypoxic event has been profound, most patients will recommence breathing spontaneously after the object has been removed. With a profound respiratory acidosis occurring as a result of inadequate ventilation, an increased rate and depth of breathing are to be expected, and with provision of high-flow oxygen the patient's oxygen saturations may return to normal quickly.

A full return of conscious state may be delayed until CO_2 levels drop. Some degree of hypoxic brain injury is to be expected and although intubation may be considered, it is advisable to allow the patient a reasonable timeframe to restore their own conscious state before complicating their treatment with this option. The benefits of out-of-hospital intubation and rapid sequence intubation (RSI) have been studied with mixed results, with authors suggesting that published adverse findings of out-of-hospital intubation may be due to study design (Fouche et al., 2014); nevertheless, a cautious considered approach to out-of-hospital intubation is recommended.

Both lungs should be auscultated in the initial assessment and then again during re-evaluation and follow-up. Negative pressure pulmonary oedema can result in crepitations, but isolated coarse crackles as a result of aspiration of food or fluid into the small airways are probably more common. As the respiratory status returns to normal so should the cardiovascular observations. A failure to return to normal could suggest the insult has precipitated an acute coronary syndrome: not unlikely in an elderly patient. For this reason 12-lead ECG is part of the evaluation process, as is a detailed ischaemic heart disease history.

This patient's neurological status is of great interest as he suffered enough of a hypoxic episode to impair his level of consciousness. Once again, he would be expected to return to a normal conscious state with clear higher functions in the ongoing evaluation: a failure to do so is indicative of more sustained damage or a secondary neurological pathology precipitated by the event. Note that although no mention was made of cervical spine precautions, the sharp back blows generally given as part of the efforts to clear a conscious patient's airway have the potential to cause bony damage to the spine of elderly patients and any resulting damage should be part of the evaluation.

PRACTICE TIP

Tachycardia associated with hypoxia and stress is common in partial airway obstruction but severe hypoxia will cause the heart rate to slow. The development of bradycardia in a partial obstruction indicates deterioration and the failure of the patient to ventilate adequately 'around' the obstruction. In this circumstance the crew should prepare to perform a laryngoscopy once the patient loses consciousness. The presentation of an unconscious bradycardic patient at a dining table who is difficult to ventilate strongly suggests a choking incident.

AIRWAY ASSESSMENT

Look for!
- Is the airway still clear?
- Is there evidence of increasing oedema and swelling?
- Does the patient have a hoarse voice? (In conscious patients the quality of voice is a very sensitive indicator of laryngeal oedema.)

Ongoing management

Once a foreign body has been removed from a patient's airway, they should be able to breathe. The patient will have, however, suffered a severe hypoxic insult and may require positive pressure ventilation via a bag and mask. They will have a significant metabolic acidosis and respiratory acidosis by this stage so their drive to breathe will be particularly strong. Absence of spontaneous ventilation would be concerning and indicates impairment of the respiratory centres, either by excessively high CO_2 levels or, more likely, by diffuse hypoxic damage, which may or may not reverse.

The patient's airway may have been subjected to trauma and may be in the process of becoming oedematous and swollen. Its patency needs to be continually reassessed and early intubation should be considered if there is any doubt. In addition, there is no guarantee that all the material will have been cleared from the patient's airway and they may have a degree of aspiration. This will need following up with chest x-rays and observation at hospital.

Finally, negative pressure pulmonary oedema is a possible complication for these patients. Starling's law of the capillary describes the forces moving fluid out of a capillary, which include negative tissue pressure. Although the negative tissue pressures in pulmonary capillaries under normal respiratory patterns are relatively minor, when a patient is struggling to breathe against an obstruction, significant negative pressures can be generated resulting in pulmonary oedema.

Hospital admission

Even if a patient is able to sit up and talk after the event they should be observed in a safe environment at hospital, looking for signs of progressive airway oedema, pulmonary oedema or aspiration.

Follow-up

As part of the follow-up process, not only should a patient's progress be monitored but a retrospective review of the factors precipitating the choking episode should be considered. Does the patient have a chewing problem? Do they have an impaired gag reflex associated with a neurological condition? Parkinson's disease, motor neuron disease and stroke can all be associated with an impaired gag reflex. Finally, does the patient have any evidence of dementia or cognitive impairment?

 CASE STUDY 2

Case 10223, 1200 hrs.

Dispatch details: A 92-year-old female in a residential care institution has had repeated choking episodes and this morning was seen to go blue. The patient is now pink and breathing.

Initial presentation: The patient is a frail old lady who is being managed in the dementia wing. Accompanying her is a relative who says that she gave the patient tea to drink before she had a severe choking episode and went blue.

 ASSESS

1209 hrs Primary survey: The patient is conscious and talking.

1212 hrs Vital signs survey: Perfusion status: HR 92 bpm, sinus rhythm; BP 130/90 mmHg; skin pink, warm, dry; capillary refill normal; ECG demonstrates sinus tachycardia. Respiratory status: calm, RR 28 bpm, clear air entry, L = R, normal work of breathing, speaking in sentences with a normal-sounding voice, SpO_2 96% on room air. Conscious state: GCS = 14, confused (normal state).

1218 hrs Pertinent hx: Her granddaughter is somewhat embarrassed that the paramedics have been called. She says that this sometimes happens when her grandmother tries to drink tea too quickly and that she is fine and normal now.

Both the granddaughter and the staff of the residential care unit apologise for calling the ambulance crew (they were called when the patient was blue) and are strongly of the opinion that the patient should not be taken to hospital.

At this stage moving the patient to hospital would involve a change of environment for this confused elderly patient and does not appear to be clinically warranted. Furthermore, an emergency ambulance would be unavailable for other cases. It seems reasonable to accept the word of the staff and relatives and classify this as an ambulance-is-not-required case.

2 CONFIRM

In many cases paramedics are presented with a collection of signs and symptoms that do not appear to describe a particular condition. A critical step in determining a treatment plan in this situation is to consider what other conditions could explain the patient's presentation.

What else could it be?
Pulmonary aspiration
The patient appears to be relatively normal now, except for a raised respiratory rate of 28 bpm. Such a rise is quite understandable immediately after the event but it should have settled in the 8 minutes it took for the ambulance to respond. One possible explanation for this raised rate is a significant aspiration which would predispose the patient to an aspiration pneumonia.

Cerebrovascular accident
A new-onset CVA is possible and may be difficult to detect against a background of dementia confusion. The absence of any gross motor localising signs does not rule out a CVA. As part of the assessment this patient warrants a detailed examination of the chest, including auscultation (unfortunately, many elderly patients have basal crepitation as a background anyway) and an evaluation of her gag reflex.

3 TREAT

In this case the paramedics are evaluating a treatment and transport decision. If they assume that the crepitation that can be heard, particularly at the left base, is new and that the patient's raised respiratory rate does not settle with time, it would appear that she has aspirated some tea and so an aspiration pneumonia is a possibility. Further medical attention should be considered, including a chest x-ray and a discussion about antibiotics. Attitudes to prescribing antibiotics at this stage may vary between prophylactic antibiotics and a wait-and-see approach.

However, the wishes of the patient and her family will impact on treatment decisions. While the possible aspiration needs attention and this is obtained in hospital, there may be a clear direction stating that the patient refuses to go to hospital or receive invasive therapy. If this is the case, the paramedics have a responsibility to arrange an alternative timely follow-up in the patient's own environment. This means contacting the patient's treating GP and initiating a joint management plan. Continuing observation of the patient's respiratory rate and pattern will give clinical insight into the severity of the problem. Evaluating the patient's views as documented in the notes will give insight into the patient's wishes and status. Evaluating the practicality of any alternative arrangements including their timeliness and robustness will provide input into the treatment decisions and options.

4 EVALUATE

Evaluating the effect of any clinical management intervention can provide clues to the accuracy of the initial diagnosis. Some conditions respond rapidly to treatment so patients should be expected to improve if the diagnosis and treatment were appropriate. A failure to improve in this situation should trigger the clinician to reconsider the diagnosis.

USING THE MNEMONIC DENT

(Define, Explore, Narrow and Test)
Define:
- What is the patient's main presenting problem?
- Is this a choking episode?
- Does it fit the definition?

Explore your hypothesis and try to narrow it down.
What else could it be?
- Pulmonary aspiration
- Cerebrovascular accident

If this patient has not aspirated, her respiratory rate would be expected to return to baseline once any anxiety has resolved. If she has aspirated, it will take several hours for any infection to develop and her observations are unlikely to change during transport.

 CASE STUDY 3

Case 18432, 1740 hrs.

Dispatch details: An 18-year-old male at a barbecue is choking and has acute abdominal pain.

Initial presentation: The crew arrives to find an 18-year-old male at a barbecue on private property: he is lying down, complaining of abdominal pain. He is pale and sweaty and appears to have a reduced conscious state. His friends seem to be concerned, but they are speaking loudly and showing signs of unsteadiness and coordination problems. There are a significant number of empty beer bottles around them.

 ASSESS

1756 hrs Chief complaint: 'I have pain in my stomach.'

1758 hrs Vital signs survey: Perfusion status: HR 130 bpm regular; P 75/50 mmHg; skin pale, warm, dry; extended capillary refill time. Respiratory status: RR 28 bpm, adequate air entry, no increase in the work of breathing, speaking in sentences, SpO$_2$ 98% on room air. Conscious state: GCS = 15.

1803 hrs Pertinent hx: His friends volunteer that he choked on a chop and suggest that this was because he was drunk. Fortunately, they remembered seeing a movie in which somebody was saved by having their abdomen squeezed hard from behind and so they did this and the obstruction was coughed up. The patient was initially fine but over the next hour started to complain more and more of abdominal pain, hence the call for the ambulance.

The patient appears to have had a choking episode on food, possibly precipitated by swallowing difficulties due to alcohol. His friends seem to have removed the obstruction but called the ambulance when he began to develop increasing abdominal pain. It is possible that he has suffered a ruptured stomach as a consequence of the rescue attempt.

 CONFIRM

In many cases paramedics are presented with a collection of signs and symptoms that do not appear to describe a particular condition. A critical step in determining a treatment plan in this situation is to consider what other conditions could explain the patient's presentation.

What else could it be?
Abdominal wall bruising
A bruised abdominal wall would be consistent with increasing pain but would not be expected to produce the signs of hypovolaemic shock.

Fractured ribs

Fractured ribs could be consistent with pain but on their own should not produce the signs of hypovolaemic shock. The possibility of a pneumothorax should be considered and explored. A tension pneumothorax associated with a fractured rib could give a very similar presentation. Careful examination of the patient's chest is required: signs of reduced movement, hyperresonance and decreased sounds on one side and distension of the jugular veins and deviated trachea would lead one to this diagnosis.

Liver or spleen rupture

A ruptured liver or spleen could well be associated with this presentation. It is worth noting that 18 years is a typical age for glandular fever when the spleen is enlarged and susceptible to mechanical damage. Both of these would account for hypovolaemic shock and pain and would present with the clinical signs found in this patient.

All of the above have been reported as a consequence of rescue attempts in choking people. In the setting of a barbecue in which a large amount of beer has been consumed, the patient's stomach could be full of food, beer and gas and would be particularly prone to rupture if suddenly compressed. Gastric acid in the peritoneum would cause pain and effectively an intraperitoneal burn. Irritation of the diaphragm and irritation of the peritoneum each time the patient breathed would cause the breathing pattern to be shallow. The raised respiratory rate could be explained by a metabolic acidosis secondary to the poor perfusion associated with hypovolaemic shock. The impact of the effects of alcohol might make it difficult to elicit a good history and might mask some of the clinical signs of pain.

The lack of any significant respiratory dysfunction or abnormal breath sounds is strongly suggestive that an airway obstruction no longer exists. This requires the patient's abnormal cardiovascular observations to be viewed with more concern. The combination of tachycardia and borderline low blood pressure following abdominal trauma is concerning and needs to be managed.

③ TREAT

The treatment for hypovolaemia is to replace volume while transporting the patient to a place of definitive care. Where a suspected haemorrhage cannot be controlled, it is increasingly recommended that fluid administration be limited until the bleed can be managed. While doing this it is important to remember that this episode started with choking and to continue to monitor the patient's airway to ensure continued patency and no secondary oedema.

1806 hrs: The paramedics insert an IV cannula and commence an infusion of 10 mL/kg of an isotonic crystalloid (normal saline).

1809 hrs: The paramedics consider and administer analgesia for the abdominal pain.

④ EVALUATE

Evaluating the effect of any clinical management intervention can provide clues to the accuracy of the initial diagnosis. Some conditions respond rapidly to treatment so patients should be expected to improve if the diagnosis and treatment were appropriate. A failure to improve in this situation should trigger the clinician to reconsider the diagnosis.

This patient's vital signs remain unchanged. That his heart rate and blood pressure have not responded to 10 mL/kg of IV fluid or effective pain relief is suggestive of an uncontrolled internal haemorrhage. 'Chasing' a normal set of vital signs in a patient with an uncontrolled haemorrhage is counterproductive: the fluid administered maintains the haemorrhage by maintaining the pressure while concurrently diluting the clotting factors. The crew wisely decide to limit any further fluid administration, update the receiving hospital about the patient's condition and insert a second IV line en route to aid resuscitation if it becomes necessary. The rate of bleed appears to be slow and it could be expected that the patient won't deteriorate significantly before arrival at the hospital in 10–15 minutes.

Summary

The diagnosis of an acute choking episode is fairly straightforward and its management escalates in increasingly vigorous and invasive attempts to remove the obstructing foreign body. The consequences of an inhaled foreign body require careful evaluation as there may be secondary events (myocardial infarction) or developing consequences from the obstruction (aspiration, airway oedema or negative pressure pulmonary oedema).

References

Aldridge, K., & Taylor, N. (2012). Dysphagia is a common and serious problem for adults with mental illness: a systematic review. *Dysphagia*, *27*, 124–137.

ANZCOR Guideline 4. (2016). Retrieved from https://resus.org.au/glossary/choking-guideline-4/

Bjornson, C., Russell, K., Vandermeer, B., Klassen, T. P., & Johnson, D. W. (2013). Nebulized epinephrine for croup in children. *The Cochrane Database of Systematic Reviews*, (10), CD006619, https://www.ncbi.nlm.nih.gov/pubmed/24114291.

Briem, B., Thorvardsson, O., & Petersen, H. (2009). Acute epiglottitis in Iceland 1983–2005. *Auris, Nasus, Larynx*, *36*(1), 46–52.

Candamourty, R., Venkatachalam, S., Babu, M. R. R., & Kumar, G. S. (2012). Ludwig's Angina—An emergency: a case report with literature review. *Journal of Natural Science, Biology, and Medicine*, *3*(2), 206–208. doi: 10.4103/0976-9668.101932.

Cecchetto, G., Viel, G., Cecchetto, A., Kusstatscher, S., & Montisci, M. (2011). Fatal splenic rupture following Heimlich maneuver: case report and literature review. *American Journal of Forensic Medicine and Pathology*, *32*(2), 169–171.

Chan, S. C., & Dawes, P. J. (2001). The management of severe infectious mononucleosis tonsillitis and upper airway obstruction. *Journal of Laryngology & Otology*, *115*(12), 973–977.

Chillag, S., Krieg, J., & Bhargava, R. (2010). The Heimlich maneuver: breaking down the complications. *Southern Medical Journal*, *103*(2), 147–150.

Craft, J., Gordon, C., & Tiziani, A. (2011). *Understanding pathophysiology*. Sydney: Elsevier.

Collopy, K. T., Kivlehan, S. M., & Snyder, S. R. (2015). Surgical cricothyrotomies in prehospital care. Surgical airway placement is indicated when you cannot intubate or ventilate. *EMS World*, *44*(1), 42–49.

DiGiacomo, C., Neshat, K. K., Angus, L. D., Penna, K., Sadoff, R. S., & Shaftan, G. W. (2003). Emergency cricothyrotomy. *Military Medicine*, *168*(7), 541–544.

Fouche, P. F., Simpson, P. M., Bendall, J., Thomas, R. E., Cone, D. C., & Doi, S. A. R. (2014). Airways in out-of-hospital cardiac arrest: systematic review and Meta-analysis. *Prehospital Emergency Care*, *18*(2), 244–256. doi: 10.3109/10903127.2013.831509.

Gardner, J. (2008). Viral croup in children. *Nursing*, *38*(4), 57–58.

Goh, K.-H., Acharyya, S., Ng, S. Y.-E., Boo, J. P.-L., Kooi, A. H.-J., Ng, H.-L., Li, W., Tay, K.-Y., Au, W.-L., Tan, L. C.-S. (2016). Risk and prognostic factors for pneumonia and choking amongst Parkinson's disease patients with dysphagia. *Parkinsonism and Related Disorders*, *29*, 30–34. https://doi.org/10.1016/j.parkreldis.2016.05.034.

Guldfred, L. A., Lyhne, D., & Becker, B. C. (2008). Acute epiglottitis: epidemiology, clinical presentation, management and outcome. *Journal of Laryngology & Otology*, *122*(8), 818–823.

Hall, J. (2012). *Guyton and Hall textbook of medical physiology* (12th ed.). St Louis: Saunders.

Heimlich, H. J. (1975). A life-saving maneuver to prevent food-choking. *JAMA*, *234*(4), 398–401.

Knutson, D., & Aring, A. (2004). Viral croup. *American Family Physician*, *69*(3), 535–540.

Levin, R., & Smith, G. (2010). Choking prevention among young children. *Pediatric Annals*, *39*(11), 721–724.

Logemann, J. (1998). *Evaluation and treatment of swallowing disorders* (2nd ed.). Austin: Pro-Ed.

Malhotra, A., & Krilov, L. R. (2001). Viral croup. *Pediatrics in Review*, *22*(1), 5–12.

Pak, S., Cha, D., Meyer, C., Dee, C., & Fershko, A. (2017). Ludwig's Angina. *Cureus*, *9*(8), e1588.

Patton, K. T., & Thibodeau, G. A. (2010). *Anatomy & Physiology* (7th ed.). St Louis: Mosby.

Peltola, V., Heikkinen, T., & Ruuskanen, O. (2002). Clinical courses of croup caused by influenza and parainfluenza viruses. *Pediatric Infectious Disease Journal, 21*(1), 76–78.

Price, I. M., Preyra, I., Fernandes, C. M., Woolfrey, K., & Worster, A. (2005). Adult epiglottitis: a five-year retrospective chart review in a major urban centre. *Canadian Journal of Emergency Medicine, 7*(6), 387–390.

Redding, J. (1979). The choking controversy: critique of evidence on the Heimlich maneuver. *Critical Care Medicine, 7*(10), 475–479.

Russell, K. F., Liang, Y., O'Gorman, K., Johnson, D. W., & Klassen, T. P. (2011). Glucocorticoids for croup. *The Cochrane Database of Systematic Reviews,* (1), CD001955.

Samuels, R., & Chadwick, D. (2006). Predictors of asphyxiation risk in adults with intellectual disabilities and dysphagia. *Journal of Intellectual Disability Research, 50*(5), 362–370.

Scrase, I., & Woollard, M. (2006). Needle vs surgical cricothyroidotomy: a short cut to effective ventilation. *Anaesthesia, 61*(10), 962–974. doi: 10.1111/j.1365-2044.2006.04755.x.

Thacker, A., Abdelnoor, A., Anderson, C., White, S., & Hollins, S. (2008). Indicators of choking risk in adults with learning disabilities: a questionnaire and interview study. *Disability and Rehabilitation, 30*(15), 1131–1138.

Thomas, L. P., & Friedland, L. R. (1998). The cost-effective use of nebulized racemic epinephrine in the treatment of croup. *The American Journal of Emergency Medicine, 16*(1), 87–89.

CHAPTER 17

Asthma

By John Craven

OVERVIEW

- Characterised by wheezing, breathlessness, chest tightness and coughing, the spectrum of patient presentations for asthma ranges from mild symptoms to respiratory and cardiac arrest.
- There were 441 deaths from asthma in Australia in 2017 (Australian Institute of Health and Welfare [AIHW], 2017).
- In severe asthma, airflow restriction compromises alveolar ventilation and respiration, leading to hypoxia and hypercapnia.
- The increased resistance to airflow can trap gas in the lungs and, with repeated efforts to ventilate,

patients can raise intrathoracic pressures so high that venous return to the heart is restricted. This can result in loss of blood pressure and loss of consciousness.
- Asthma is diagnosed clinically. Diagnosis relies heavily on an accurate history and respiratory assessment.
- Asthma is considered one of the atopic illnesses; there are many similarities between asthma and the allergy/anaphylaxis pathophysiology pathway.

Introduction

Although asthma is a common disease it is difficult to clearly define, and diagnosis is based primarily on symptoms, examination findings and clinical response to treatment. Asthma is now understood to be a complex collection of diseases that share the commonality of being inflammatory disorders of the small airways. Inflammation produces mucus, bronchiole wall oedema and airway smooth muscle hyperactivity which causes airflow restriction to and from alveoli as a result of airway constriction and obstruction.

Pathophysiology

Understanding airway physiology and the changes that occur with inflammation is important to understanding asthma.

The upper airway is subject to large pressure changes and high rates of airflow. The bronchi are structurally reinforced by cartilage and lined with mucus-secreting ciliated columnar epithelial cells, which help trap and remove foreign bodies, contaminants and microorganisms.

The smaller bronchioles are structurally different. They are made up of smooth muscle and elastic tissue, are lined ciliated cuboidal epithelial cells and do not contain cartilage. Cells in the terminal bronchioles secrete surfactant that has an important role in decreasing surface tension in the smallest airways and alveoli, which allows them to retain

considerable elastic response. Between the inner and outer layers of the bronchioles are numerous cells of the immune system such as mast cells, eosinophils and neutrophils (see Fig 17.1). When the immune cells detect a pathogen, they initiate an inflammatory response (see Ch 4). The release of inflammatory mediators (histamine, eosinophilic and neutrophilic chemotactic factors, leukotrienes, prostaglandin and cytokines) from the immune cells causes:

- bronchoconstriction due to contraction of the smooth muscle lining the airway
- mucus plugging due to increased mucus secretion into the lumen of the bronchiole by goblet cells
- oedema of the airway walls which occurs secondary to vascular congestion and increased capillary permeability (Curtis & Ramsden, 2011).

As a result, the airway lumen narrows and airflow resistance increases. These responses are aimed at trapping, destroying and removing pathogens, preventing their progression deeper into the airway, and reflect a normal immune reaction (Murphy & O'Byrne, 2010; see Box 17.1).

In the asthmatic patient, however, the complex interaction between the inflammatory mediators is overly sensitive and produces a response far in excess of normal and often in response to otherwise innocuous stimuli such as pollens or weather changes. Small airway inflammation is not unique to asthma as it occurs in response to chest infections and in other respiratory diseases, but asthma is characterised by

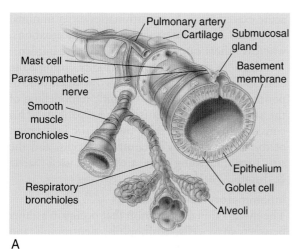

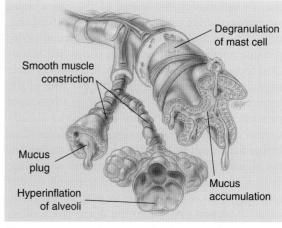

A

B

Figure 17.1
A Normal lung with clear airways. **B** Thick mucus, mucosal oedema and smooth muscle spasm causing obstruction of small airways occurs in asthma, breathing becomes laboured and expiration is difficult due to the airway restrictions.
Source: Des Jardins & Burton (2006).

BOX 17.1 Asthma triggers

There has been considerable research into the reason why this immune-based condition occurs. The body's normal immune response protects against antigens through antibody recognition of the antigen, followed by the release of a cascade of inflammatory mediators that are designed to isolate and destroy the antigen. Allergic reactions are excessive reactions by these antibodies, and diseases such as asthma, anaphylaxis and hay fever share the common pathway of a supposedly protective reaction that has overreacted and become harmful. The tendency to produce the particular type of antibodies associated with allergies has some genetic component but also appears to be related to the amount of exposure to potential allergens, with more appearing better than less.

Many of the triggers that cause asthma are typical antigens associated with allergies: house mites, animal hair and pollen. Drugs that interfere with the inflammatory response (such as aspirin, ibuprofen and ACE inhibitors) can also upset the delicate inflammatory pathway, but interestingly non-antigen–based triggers such as cold air, exercise, stress and smoke can also trigger an inflammatory response in the lungs. Although they may differ in a chemical sense, the clinical manifestations of both the immunological and the non-immunological pathways result in the same presentation.

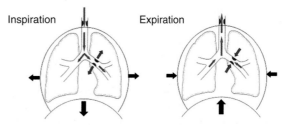

Figure 17.2
Mechanism of dynamic hyperinflation in the setting of severe airflow obstruction. With narrowing of the small airways and forced expiration, there Is premature closure of the small airways, trapping gas In the alveoli. This leads to hyperinflation and Inability of the asthmatic to empty their lungs and Inspire fresh air.

a hyperresponsive inflammatory reaction that can occur in areas of the lung not directly affected by a pathogen or allergenic trigger (Rodriguez-Roisin, 1997).

Gas trapping

Understanding the concept of dynamic hyperinflation or gas trapping is the key to understanding the respiratory dysfunction caused by asthma and many of the symptoms of the disease (see Fig 17.2).

On inspiration the pressure outside the lung is higher than inside. This causes the air to go in. The lower pressure in the pleural cavity keeps the alveoli open. On expiration, contraction of the chest and diaphragm increases the intrathoracic pressure, which raises the alveoli pressure and causes the air to move out. In asthmatics, the lumen of the bronchioles are narrowed due to inflammatory processes (oedema, mucus, bronchoconstriction) and the pleural cavity pressure increases with each breath as asthmatics used forced expiration, rather than elastic, as their respiratory distress worsens. As the pressure of the bronchiole drops during expiration, the increased pressure of the pleural cavity squeezes the already narrow lumen of the terminal bronchioles shut before the alveoli fully empties, trapping gas within the alveoli. Worsening disease correlates with more bronchiole inflammation and more alveoli unable to empty. This is not an issue on inspiration as the negative pleural cavity pressure opens the airways again and allows for further air to flow to the alveoli. This is known as gas trapping and leads to dynamic hyperinflation.

Thus, severe asthmatics suffer respiratory compromise as they are unable to empty their lungs effectively to draw fresh oxygenated air back into the lungs. The symptoms of tight chest and breathlessness relate to this persistent hyperinflation of the lungs, and as gas trapping worsens, the asthmatic must work harder to maintain effective respiration. Wheeze is created when the narrowing of the bronchiole lumen is such that turbulent flow of air occurs rather than laminar. Wheeze is predominantly expiratory due to the narrowing on expiration but may become biphasic with worsening disease; however, it will resolve when air movement fails altogether to produce a silent chest. The musical quality of a wheeze that is absent is stridor, which occurs due to the collection of many individual bronchioles that each contribute a noise to create a polyphonic sound.

As a result of the varying severity of disease, mild-to-moderate asthma can present with a combination of slight increase in the work of breathing with or without a cough, and either with or without wheezes. The progression from mild to severe (and life-threatening) asthma involves an increase of airflow restriction that progressively compromises the ability to exchange oxygen and CO_2, leading to hypoxia, hypercarbia and eventual circulatory failure.

Airway remodelling

The form of asthma seen out-of-hospital and in hospital emergency departments is primarily an acute exacerbation. Some asthmatics suffer minimal symptoms in the intervals between exacerbations, whereas others carry a significant disease burden.

Mortality and significant morbidity during acute exacerbations is strongly associated with chronic or poorly controlled asthma. Chronic remodelling of the smaller airways occurs in these patients. This consists of two major components: the infiltration of the airway wall by inflammatory cells, and the structural thickening of the airway wall itself (Saetta & Turato, 2001).

Inflammatory cell infiltration

The dysfunctional interaction that occurs in asthma between mast cells, eosinophils, neutrophils and lymphocytes is still not completely understood, but histological examinations of chronic asthmatic airways usually reveal excessive populations of eosinophils. The abundance of eosinophils almost certainly contributes to hyperreactive inflammatory response, but more recently a small group of asthmatics have been found to also have excessive populations of neutrophils within their airway walls. This group of asthmatics typically suffers from severe symptoms but it remains unclear if the neutrophils are the cause of symptom severity, are a response to the medications used to treat severe asthma or are unrelated to the disease severity (Saetta & Turato, 2001).

Structural changes

While the exact contribution that the increased populations of eosinophils and neutrophils plays in the chronic development of the disease remains unclear, significant structural changes can also occur. Hypertrophy of smooth muscle, deposits of collagen, proliferation of mucus-secreting cells, vascular congestion and thickening of the basement membrane that attaches the epithelial tissue to the airway are all evident on histological examination. By adding to the bulk of the airway wall, all these factors place pressure on the lumen and reduce the diameter of the airway, but some also add to the degree of constriction (bronchospasm) and obstruction (mucus production) when an acute episode occurs. The thickening of the basement membrane may be of particular importance in asthma, as it is not shared by other chronic airways diseases such as chronic obstructive pulmonary disease (COPD) (Saetta & Turato, 2001).

CASE STUDY 1

Case 10364, 1030 hrs.

Dispatch details: A 5-year-old female with a recent upper respiratory tract infection.

Initial presentation: The patient is sitting upright in her mother's arms on the sofa in the lounge room at home. She is conscious, alert and breathing rapidly with a marked rise and fall of the chest. She appears distressed. Her mother says that she had a runny nose yesterday and was coughing a lot overnight but was settling with her salbutamol inhaler. This morning she hasn't improved despite frequent dosing with her puffer and was having more trouble breathing.

1 ASSESS

Patient history

Patients presenting with significant disturbances of conscious state, breathing or perfusion need rapid intervention. Paramedics must quickly recognise situations when they do not have the luxury of obtaining a full clinical history. As described in Chapter 14, a rapid decision must be made to either follow the emergency model of rapid assessment or the medical interview model.

In a breathless patient, obtaining history can be difficult and questioning needs to be focused on differentiating causes so that management can be quickly and appropriately initiated. Less-distressed patients can be more thoroughly questioned.

Approximately 95% of exacerbations of asthma in children under 6 years are triggered by viral respiratory tract infections, whereas in children over 6 years viral infections account for roughly two-thirds and allergic reactions account for one-third (Dondi et al., 2017) (see Box 17.2).

When the patient's mother in Case Study 1 is questioned further, she says the patient has not been prescribed a preventer but has previously had two admissions to hospital with asthma. Both admissions lasted a couple of days and ICU care was not required.

Peak expiratory flow measurement and spirometry

Peak expiratory flow (how quickly a patient can exhale) can be simply measured with a peak flow meter. It was very popular several decades ago as a cheap and straightforward attempt at objectively assessing and monitoring what is otherwise a clinical condition. Unfortunately, it has not been shown to be as effective or reliable as once presumed. Peak expiratory flow (PEF) is effort dependent and results vary wildly depending on both the patient and the instrument. Thus, prediction of severity of asthma was generally no better than clinical assessment (Sly et al., 1994; Brusasco, 2003). PEF has mostly been replaced in health systems by portable spirometry devices, which in addition to PEF provide expiratory flow times (forced expiratory volume [FEV_1], maximal mid expiratory flow [MMEF]), lung volumes (FVC) and ratios (FEV_1/FVC). The role of either PEF measurement or spirometry in the out-of-hospital setting or the assessment of acute asthma has not been established but can be useful if the diagnosis is uncertain or in monitoring response to treatment (National Asthma Council, 2019).

HISTORY

Ask!

- Have you had any previous episodes of asthma or shortness of breath?
- Have you needed hospital or intensive care management in the past?
- Is this as bad as your asthma ever gets?
- What medications have you used and how often?
- Are the symptoms getting better or worse?
- What do you think may have triggered this episode?

BOX 17.2 Asthma classifications

Intermittent asthma

Untreated asthma is classified as *intermittent* if all of the following apply.

- Daytime asthma symptoms occur less than once per week.
- Night-time asthma symptoms occur less than twice per month.
- Exacerbations are infrequent and brief.
- FEV_1 (forced expiratory volume in 1 second) is at least 80% predicted and varies by less than 20%.

Mild persistent asthma

Untreated asthma is classified as *mild persistent* if one or more of the following applies (and more severe signs and symptoms are not present).

- Daytime asthma symptoms occur more than once per week but not every day.
- Night-time asthma symptoms occur more than twice per month, but not every week.
- Exacerbations occur occasionally and may affect activity or sleep.
- FEV_1 is at least 80% predicted and varies by 20–30%.

Moderate persistent asthma

Untreated asthma is classified as *moderate persistent* if one or more of the following applies (and more severe signs and symptoms are not present).

- Daytime asthma symptoms occur every day, but do not generally restrict physical activity.
- Night-time asthma symptoms occur at least once per week.
- Exacerbations occur occasionally and may affect activity or sleep.
- FEV_1 is 60–80% predicted and varies by more than 30%.

Severe persistent asthma

Untreated asthma is classified as *severe persistent* if one or more of the following applies.

- Daytime asthma symptoms occur every day and restrict physical activity.
- Night-time asthma symptoms occur every day.
- Exacerbations are frequent.
- FEV_1 is 60% predicted or less, and varies by more than 30%.

Source: National Asthma Council (2019).

PRACTICE TIP

Paramedics face a challenge when assessing a severely breathless patient who cannot answer questions if no relative, carer or bystander is present. Limiting your questions as much as possible and asking questions requiring a yes/no response can help. Writing 'yes' and 'no' on a sheet of paper and asking the patient to point to the relevant response is another useful technique. However, do not spend excessive amounts of time doing this: the patient needs treatment! Further history can be obtained when the patient is less breathless.

EtCO$_2$ measurement

End-tidal carbon dioxide ($EtCO_2$) monitoring is the non-invasive measurement of exhaled CO_2. This has become more common in the unwell non-intubated patient (Jabre et al., 2009), although the effectiveness of $EtCO_2$ monitoring in improving asthma outcomes has yet to be validated (Howe et al., 2011).

Self-management

Most asthma sufferers or their carers will have a good understanding of their illness and will have initiated management. Assessing the patient's strategies and success in managing their shortness of breath will provide valuable information. A patient who is still quite unwell after significant self-medication is of concern.

Initial assessment summary

Problem	Acute shortness of breath
Conscious state	Alert
Position	Sitting upright
Heart rate	Radial pulse 134
Blood pressure	97/70 mmHg
Skin appearance	Flushed, warm
Speech pattern	Able to speak in sentences
Respiratory rate	42 bpm
Respiratory rhythm	Prolonged respiratory phase
Chest auscultation	Generalised expiratory wheezes, L = R
Pulse oximetry SpO$_2$	96% on room air

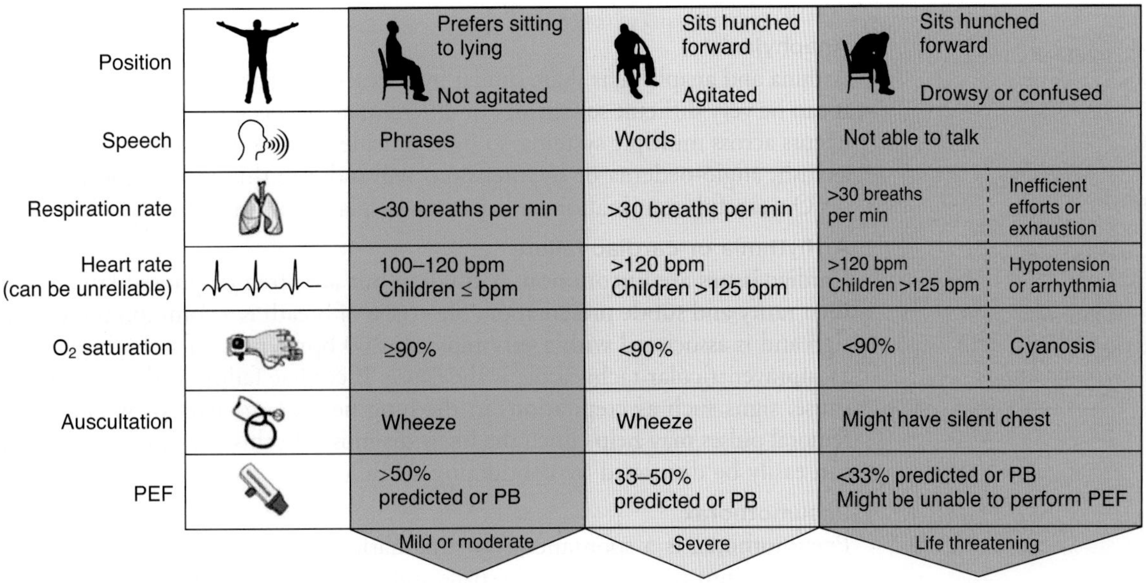

Position		Prefers sitting to lying Not agitated	Sits hunched forward Agitated	Sits hunched forward Drowsy or confused	
Speech		Phrases	Words	Not able to talk	
Respiration rate		<30 breaths per min	>30 breaths per min	>30 breaths per min	Inefficient efforts or exhaustion
Heart rate (can be unreliable)		100–120 bpm Children ≤ bpm	>120 bpm Children >125 bpm	>120 bpm Children >125 bpm	Hypotension or arrhythmia
O₂ saturation		≥90%	<90%	<90%	Cyanosis
Auscultation		Wheeze	Wheeze	Might have silent chest	
PEF		>50% predicted or PB	33–50% predicted or PB	<33% predicted or PB Might be unable to perform PEF	
		Mild or moderate	Severe	Life threatening	

Figure 17.3
Assessment of acute asthma severity.
Adapted from: Papi et al. (2018).

Temperature	36.8°C
Capillary refill (seconds)	2
Pain score	0/10
Motor/sensory function	Normal
History	Asthma Worsening overnight despite salbutamol puffers

D: There is no danger to the ambulance crew or patient.
A: The patient is conscious with no airway obstruction.
B: Respiratory rate is elevated and the work of breathing is increased. There is an expiratory wheeze in both lungs that is equal left to right.
C: Heart rate is elevated; blood pressure is within normal limits.

The patient is presenting with dyspnoea at rest and has a history of asthma. The presence of the wheeze combined with the increased work of breathing are consistent with acute asthma.

Figure 17.3 outlines the assessment of acute asthma severity.

② CONFIRM

The essential part of the clinical reasoning process is to seek to confirm your initial hypothesis by finding clinical signs that should occur with your provisional diagnosis. You should also seek to challenge your diagnosis by exploring findings that do not fit your hypothesis: don't just ignore them because they don't fit.

Asthma is diagnosed on its clinical presentation. There are no definitive tests. As such it is important to consider and exclude other possible causes before commencing treatment. However, the presence of wheezes with respiratory distress, combined with the relative safety of the first-line treatment, will see many paramedics commence treating for asthma while they exclude other causes.

RESPIRATORY STATUS

Look for!
- Increased work of breathing
- Ability to speak full sentences
- Prolonged expiratory phase

CARDIO-VASCULAR STATUS

Look for!
- Tachycardia: early
- Bradycardia: late!
- Cyanosis: late!
- Altered conscious state: late!

What else could it be?

Anaphylaxis

Asthma and anaphylaxis share similar hyperreactive inflammatory responses and it can be very difficult sometimes to differentiate between the two. Anaphylaxis occurs across multiple systems, so signs outside of the respiratory system (such as rash, angio-oedema or hypotension) will indicate this as a diagnosis.

On careful examination, this patient displays no signs of anaphylaxis.

Arrhythmia or cardiac failure

Cardiac issues are uncommon in children but are often diagnosed late due to their rarity and subtle presentation. Shortness of breath is a common presenting sign and is associated with a very rapid (> 200 bpm) pulse if arrhythmia such as supraventricular tachycardia is the cause. If cardiac failure is the underlying cause, signs such as crepitations in the lung fields, large liver or weak/absent femoral pulses may help clinch the likely diagnosis. In this situation, arrhythmia can easily be dismissed by conducting an ECG.

Pneumothorax

Pneumothorax is a spontaneous or traumatic rupture of the lung tissue that allows air into the intrathoracic space and restricts ventilation of a portion of the lung. It is rare in small children and more common in teenagers, particularly when tall and thin. It is more commonly associated in children with chronic lung disease such as cystic fibrosis or with connective tissue disorders such as Marfan's syndrome.

Airway narrowing and bronchoconstriction across both lung fields do not match the pathophysiology of a pneumothorax that, if present, should have been noted during the chest auscultation as an area of poor ventilation. This has been excluded in this patient.

Inhaled foreign body

A foreign body such as a polystyrene bead or peanut may present with no history and symptoms of respiratory distress in small children. It can be clinically differentiated from asthma by localised symptoms such as solitary, monophonic wheeze and isolated decreased air entry, as opposed to the generalised wheeze of asthma.

Pneumonia

Young people with pneumonia often present initially with fever, lethargy and respiratory distress. Wheeze is generally absent and the classic signs of bronchial breath sounds, dull percussion and productive cough often take some time to develop. Coughing in asthma is a relatively common sign but is non-productive, generally described as 'tight', 'dry' or 'wheezing' and tends to commence early in the illness.

Anxiety and panic attacks

Anxiety and panic attacks often have hyperventilation and breathlessness as common symptoms. It can be very difficult to differentiate from asthma, particularly as the breathlessness of asthma can lead to anxiety. The presence of a wheeze, the prolonged expiratory phase and the use of accessory muscles are more specific asthma symptoms, and breathlessness as a presenting symptom of anxiety is exceedingly rare in prepubescent children. In teenagers and adults, spirometry can be a very useful diagnostic tool.

3 TREAT

Assessment of severity

Asthma, like many disease processes, comes in a range of severities. By assessing the severity of the asthma episode, the paramedic is able to tailor the management to the disease. Acute asthma exacerbations are stratified into mild, moderate,

Table 17.1: Rapid primary assessment of acute asthma in adults and children

Mild/moderate	Severe	Life-threatening
Can walk, speak whole sentences in one breath (For young children: can move around, speak in phrases) Oxygen saturation > 94%	Any of these findings: ● use of accessory muscles of neck or intercostal muscles or 'tracheal tug' during inspiration or subcostal recession ('abdominal breathing') ● unable to complete sentences in one breath due to dyspnoea ● obvious respiratory distress ● oxygen saturation 90–94%	Any of these findings: ● reduced consciousness or collapse ● exhaustion ● cyanosis ● oxygen saturation < 90% ● poor respiratory effort, soft/absent breath sounds

Notes:
- If features of more than one severity category are present, record the higher (worse) category as overall severity level.
- The severity category may change when more information is available (e.g. pulse oximetry, spirometry) or over time.
- The presence of pulsus paradoxus (systolic paradox) is not a reliable indicator of the severity of acute asthma.
- Oxygen saturation measured by pulse oximetry. If oxygen therapy has already been started, it is not necessary to cease oxygen to do pulse oximetry.
- Oxygen saturation levels are a guide only and are not definitive; clinical judgment should be applied.
- Definitions of severity classes for acute asthma used in this handbook may differ from those used in published clinical trials and other guidelines that focus on, or are restricted to, the management of acute asthma within emergency departments or acute care facilities.

Source: National Asthma Council (2019).

BOX 17.3 Principles of management

Asthma
- Improve the efficiency of ventilation for maximum gas exchange
- Provide maximum inspired oxygen for patients with impaired ventilation
- Reduce bronchospasm
- Reduce mucosal oedema and mucus production

---

severe and life-threatening (see Table 17.1). For practical purposes, mild and moderate asthma categories are usually combined. Symptoms and signs should be correlated with degree of severity, and with experience patterns in the presentation of different severities of illness can be quickly recognised because there is an association between many of the signs. As a rule, patients are treated as the most serious category that their symptoms fall into, with the proviso that an isolated severe sign should be taken as either a sign of unrecognised severity of illness or the possibility of a different condition altogether.

Emergency management
Treatment is aimed at relieving bronchospasm, settling inflammation and generally improving ventilation and the symptoms of the acute asthma (see Box 17.3 and Table 17.2).

Position
Most dyspnoeic patients will position themselves to improve their ventilation, which is generally in an upright position which aids the mechanics of chest wall and diaphragm movement and allows for augmentation with the accessory respiratory muscles. Disrupting this positioning in a severe asthmatic, particularly trying to lie them flat, may have disastrous consequences and you may have to adapt your assessment to the patient's position rather than trying to move them to your preferred position. As a general rule, and provided it is safe to do so, assess and initiate treatment of respiratory patients in the position you find them.

Table 17.2: Medications

Duration	Role	Pharmacological class	Agent
Short term	*Relievers*	Short-acting beta$_2$ agonist relievers	Salbutamol Terbutaline sulfate
		Inhaled corticosteroid/rapid-onset long-acting beta$_2$ agonist combinations[†]	Budesonide/eformoterol fumarate dihydrate
	Other short-term medicines (symptomatic and acute asthma treatment)	Systemic corticosteroids	Prednisolone or prednisone Methylprednisolone sodium succinate Hydrocortisone
		Anticholinergic bronchodilators (in acute asthma)	Ipratropium bromide
		Magnesium sulfate (in acute asthma)	Magnesium sulfate
Long term	*Preventers*	Inhaled corticosteroids (glucocorticosteroids)	Beclomethasone dipropionate Budesonide Ciclesonide Fluticasone propionate
		Inhaled corticosteroids/long-acting beta$_2$ agonist combinations	Budesonide/eformoterol fumarate dihydrate Fluticasone furoate/vilanterol trifenatate Fluticasone propionate/eformoterol fumarate dihydrate Fluticasone propionate/salmeterol xinafoate
		Leukotriene receptor antagonists	Montelukast
		Cromones (mast cell stabilisers)	Sodium cromoglycate Nedocromil sodium
	Other long-term medicines	See: **asthmahandbook.org.au/resources/medicines-guide**	

*Please note this is an abridged version of the complete table provided in the full online Australian Asthma Handbook.

[†]The budesonide/eformoterol fumarate dihydrate combination is only used as reliever for adolescents and adults on maintenance-and-reliever regimen

Notes: Before prescribing any medicine, check the Therapeutic Goods Administration-approved product information.

Pharmaceutical Benefits Scheme criteria for some asthma medicines differ between age groups and indications.

Source: National Asthma Council (2019).

Bronchodilators
Short-acting beta-adrenergic agonists

The cornerstone of acute treatment of asthma is the use of short-acting beta$_2$ adrenoceptor agonists (SABAs) such as salbutamol (see Table 17.3). The agent binds to the beta$_2$ adrenoceptors that are prolific on bronchiole smooth muscle cells and cause muscle relaxation, leading to bronchodilation. Nebulisation of salbutamol was previously the drug delivery mode of choice, leading to a proliferation of expensive nebuliser machines in homes, but it has been shown that puffer and spacer delivery of salbutamol is just as effective as nebulisation in all severities of acute exacerbations. Puffer and spacer use has the advantage of being cheap, portable and a good reinforcement for patient and carers in the appropriate use of their asthma medication. Nebulisation is still recommended for severe/life-threatening disease due to the advantage of co-administration of oxygen, but in the poorly ventilating patient with life-threatening asthma there remains the question of the amount of salbutamol that is being inhaled versus nebulised into the environment. A nebulised 5 mg dose of salbutamol is considered to be clinically equivalent to 12 puffs of salbutamol, with children under 6 years recommended to have either 6 puffs

Table 17.3: Treatments to consider for mild, moderate, severe and life-threatening asthma

Treatment	Mild	Moderate	Severe	Life-threatening/near fatal
Oxygen	Yes	Yes	Yes	Yes
SABA (puffer or nebulised)	Yes	Yes	Yes	Yes
Ipratropium bromide (puffer or nebulised)	No	No	Yes	No
IV salbutamol	No	No	Yes	Yes
Steroids	No	Yes	Yes	Yes
Magnesium sulfate (MgSO$_4$)	No	No	Yes	Yes
IM or IV adrenaline	No	No	No	Yes
IPPV/intubation	No	No	No	Yes

Source: Adapted from QAS (2011) and Holly & Boots (2009).

or 2.5 mg nebulised aliquots. In recent times, 'rescue puffers' have become a popular treatment schedule in emergency departments, with 12 (or 6) puffs given 20 minutes apart for moderate to severe asthmatics. The dosing and the regimentation of it allows patient therapy to be maximised and side effects to be minimised, and the assessment of the response to treatment becomes more reproducible (Idris et al., 1993).

Side effects of SABA are common, particularly with aggressive dosing, and there is a move away from the reflex delivery of 10 mg nebulised doses. Watch out for tachycardia, tremor and psychomotor agitation. While SABAs are designed to be predominantly beta$_2$, there is some cross-binding to other adrenoceptors, particularly beta$_1$ (hence tachycardia as a common side effect). In addition, as SABA increase oxygen use of all cells in the body, large doses increase total body oxygen requirement which can be counterproductive for the patient and lactic acidosis can result (Tomar et al., 2012) (see Box 17.4).

Salbutamol is very well absorbed through the respiratory tract when inhaled, and clinically significant doses can be delivered quickly and effectively. Administering salbutamol via intravenous route has become less common and is now generally reserved for patients with significant ventilation issues and life-threatening asthma. There is no evidence that IV salbutamol is more effective than inhaled salbutamol (Travers et al., 2014). IV salbutamol also has a high incidence of side effects and takes considerably more time required to draw up and administer in comparison with inhaled salbutamol.

Adrenaline in asthma predates the use of SABA. While adrenaline remains recommended for use in asthma in many out-of-hospital services, it is not used or recommended within hospital services. Adrenaline has far more activity at alpha adrenoceptors than beta adrenoceptors, particularly when compared with SABA, and has a higher rate of side effects at clinically effective dosing levels. Several small studies have shown it to be no more effective than SABA (Walker, 2009). It is best used in situations of respiratory arrest, where inhaled medication cannot be delivered, and in situations where other options are exhausted or unavailable.

Anticholinergics

Bronchioles are innervated by the parasympathetic nervous system. Blocking parasympathetic tone with anticholinergic agents causes the smooth muscles of the bronchiole walls to relax and decreases secretions into the airway lumen. It is recommended that ipratropium bromide be added to SABA for moderate-to-severe asthma patients (National Asthma Council, 2019). The dosing is 4 puffs or 250 mg nebulised for under 6 years old and 8 puffs or 500 mg for

---

BOX 17.4 Using a metered-dose inhaler for acute asthma

Administration of salbutamol by health professional for a patient with acute asthma

1. Use a salbutamol pressurised metered-dose inhaler (100 microgram/actuation) with a spacer that has already been prepared (see notes).
2. Shake inhaler and insert upright into spacer.
3. Place mouthpiece between the person's teeth and ask them to seal lips firmly around mouthpiece.
4. Fire one puff into the spacer.
5. Tell person to take 4 breaths in and out of the spacer.
6. Remove the spacer from mouth. Shake the inhaler after each puff before actuating again. (This can be done without detaching the pressurised metered-dose inhaler from the spacer.)

Notes:

The process is repeated until the total dose is given. Different doses are recommended for patients and carers giving asthma first aid in the community.

New plastic spacers should be washed with detergent to remove electrostatic charge (and labelled), so they are ready for use when needed. In an emergency situation, if a pre-treated spacer is not available, prime the spacer before use by firing at least 10 puffs of salbutamol into the spacer. (This is an arbitrary number of actuations in the absence of evidence that would enable a precise guideline.)

Priming or washing spacers to reduce electrostatic charge before using for the first time is only necessary for standard plastic spacers. Treatment to reduce electrostatic charge is not necessary for polyurethane/antistatic polymer spacers (e.g. Able A2A, AeroChamber Plus, La Petite E-Chamber, La Grande E-Chamber) or disposable cardboard spacers (e.g. DispozABLE, LiteAire).

For small children who cannot form a tight seal with their lips around the spacer mouthpiece, attach a well-fitted mask to the spacer.

Source: National Asthma Council (2019).

---

over 6 years old and adults. In isolation, ipratropium has a moderate effect only; it appears most useful as an augmentation in severe cases of asthma, but is particularly efficacious in older patients with COPD, asthma or chronic bronchitis.

Aminophylline

Aminophylline causes bronchiole smooth muscle relaxation and bronchodilation by blocking intracellular phosphodiesterase (Stanley & Tunnicliffe, 2008). The drawback is that it has a very narrow therapeutic margin with significant side effects in toxicity (agitation, tachycardia and tremor through to seizures and arrhythmias) and was mostly dropped from use in the 1990s. However, it is effective in severe asthma and is still carefully used in extreme situations.

Magnesium

In contrast to aminophylline, the administration of a single dose (1–2 g) of IV or IO magnesium sulfate ($MgSO_4$) over 20–30 minutes is becoming a more widely accepted management strategy for asthma and is increasingly used by paramedics (Kokotajlo et al., 2014). Intravenous $MgSO_4$ is supported in the literature as an adjunct to standard treatment for asthma patients with severe or life-threatening exacerbation of their asthma (Kew et al., 2014). There is little evidence to support the use of nebulised $MgSO_4$ (Knightly et al., 2017). Magnesium is a smooth muscle relaxant with a relatively short therapeutic life (usually up to an hour); however, in a critically unwell asthma patient that may be long enough to buy time for other therapies (SABA, steroids, aminophylline) to be administered and have effect.

Oxygen

Increasing the percentage of inspired oxygen (FiO_2) can improve the hypoxia caused by inadequate ventilation in severe acute asthma. High-flow oxygen via a Hudson or non-rebreather mask should routinely be administered to all asthmatics with moderate-to-severe symptoms; once the patient has stabilised, the oxygen can be then weaned to the lowest required amount.

While a high FiO_2 will assist in managing hypoxia, it will not reduce hypercapnia and a rising pCO_2 is a clear sign of impending respiratory arrest.

Steroids

Corticosteroids are used extensively and effectively in the management of asthma to suppress the inflammatory response. As a rule, steroids generally take approximately 4 hours to have clinical effect in asthma. This can be expedited by 20–30 minutes by using IV steroids (hydrocortisone or dexamethasone); however, IV steroids are generally only indicated when there is impaired conscious state, severe breathlessness or vomiting. Once a clinically effective dose has been administered, there is little advantage in giving further or extra doses in the acute setting. Outcomes are improved when steroids are administered early (Stanley & Tunnicliffe, 2008) and many parents will initiate the first dose of prednisolone at home prior to seeking medical attention. There is currently some debate if prednisolone alters outcomes in children with mild-to-moderate viral-induced wheeze.

(4) EVALUATE

Evaluating the effect of any intervention can provide clues to the accuracy of the initial diagnosis. Some conditions respond rapidly to treatment and patients with these conditions should be expected to improve if the diagnosis and treatment were appropriate. A failure to improve in this situation should trigger the clinician to reconsider the diagnosis.

Bronchodilation with SABAs treats only one component of the triad that causes airflow restriction (bronchospasm, airway swelling, airway obstruction), but this is generally very effective in reducing symptom severity and allowing the patient to breathe more easily. Normally, you would expect to see improvement in a patient within 5–10 minutes. Signs of improvement include:

- reduced work of breathing
- increased air entry with decreased wheeze (or presence of wheeze if the chest was previously silent)
- coughing, which may become more apparent as the patient is able to generate higher expiratory flows
- heart rate, which may remain tachycardic due to the beta$_1$ effects of the SABAs.

Oxygen saturations often temporarily dip immediately following SABA administration, particularly in severe asthma. It is thought to be due to temporary ventilation/perfusion (V/Q) mismatch and is not clinically significant. It is generally accompanied by an improvement in clinical picture and often taken as a sign of effective treatment.

The bronchodilatory effect of SABA is limited as there is no change in the underlying inflammatory process or the chronic airway changes, and the symptoms may return once SABA is metabolised (1–2 hours). Regardless of the degree of improvement, this patient must be transported to hospital.

Ongoing management

Non-invasive ventilatory support

It is paradoxical to apply additional respiratory pressure to a patient already struggling to exhale, but continuous positive airway pressure (CPAP) is widely used to provide ventilatory support in diseases such as acute pulmonary oedema and COPD. Adding positive end expiratory pressure (PEEP) appears to support the collapsing airways during exhalation and reduce gas trapping in the alveoli, allowing a more proficient exhalation and less hyperinflation. This is balanced against the exhaustion that severe asthmatics suffer from their profound respiratory effort. A number of small studies suggest that this management strategy may be effective for asthma but identifying which patients will benefit and whether biphasic positive airway pressure (BiPAP) is a better option (Brandao et al., 2009) are still unclear. A review of these few trials indicates that this strategy has not been found to reduce the risk of death or need for intubation; however, the review did find that it may reduce hospital admissions, length of hospital stay and length of ICU stay (Lim et al., 2012).

Over the last decade, high-flow nasal cannula (HFNC) has increasingly been used for patients with respiratory distress, replacing CPAP. Its use is well established in neonatal respiratory disease and bronchiolitis, benefiting from small children's preference for nasal breathing. HFNC generates some PEEP if the mouth is closed and improves respiratory effort. The use in severe asthma and other respiratory disease has less evidence base but some early studies are promising (Baudin et al., 2017).

Invasive ventilatory support

Patients who are unable to maintain adequate ventilation will eventually lose consciousness and suffer respiratory arrest. Attempting to ventilate patients is difficult as they are generally extremely hyperinflated and require a long passive expiratory phase, which is difficult to do when the patient is hypoxic to begin with. In the past, asthmatics who required mechanical ventilation had poor outcomes but that has improved enormously with modern ventilators and improved techniques. If hand ventilating a severe asthmatic, allow 3–4 seconds of expiration to each second of inspiration.

Antibiotics

The prevalence of chest infections in acute asthma exacerbations is substantial but they are primarily viral and therefore not appropriate for antibiotic treatment (British Thoracic Society, Scottish Intercollegiate Guidelines Network, 2016). Antibiotics are usually restricted to patients displaying symptomology consistent with pneumonia or other bacterial infection.

In-hospital tests

Unless asthma is life-threatening, in hospital tests often do not contribute to clinical management. Tests are mostly indicated if there is concern over alternative diagnoses, such as a chest x-ray to exclude pneumonia or pneumothorax.

Follow-up

It is important that asthma sufferers receive good education. An effective asthma management plan has been shown to improve symptom control and reduce hospital presentations (National Asthma Council, 2019). Allergy testing has some use if there are allergen-related triggers but does not alter disease management for most asthmatics.

 CASE STUDY 2

Case 11442, 2012 hrs.

Dispatch details: A 21-year-old male in severe respiratory distress with a history of asthma.

Initial presentation: On a cold winter's night the ambulance crew locate the patient in the lounge of his fourth-floor student apartment. He is sitting upright on the edge of a kitchen chair. He has both palms on the table in front of him with his arms extended. He is conscious and talking.

 ASSESS

2024 hrs Chief complaint: 'My asthma … has been … playing up … for a couple of weeks. I went … to training tonight … for football … and during … training … I couldn't catch … my breath. My puffers … aren't working'.

2025 hrs Vital signs survey: Perfusion status: HR 128, BP 158/91 mmHg, skin cool and pale.

Respiratory status: anxious, struggling to breathe, respiratory rate 30, SpO_2 90%, air entry, L = R, soft inspiratory and expiratory wheeze all lung fields, use of accessory muscles (tripod position against table edge), speaking in words, prolonged expiratory phase, complains of shortness of breath.

Conscious state: GCS = 15, anxious.

2027 hrs Pertinent hx: The patient's asthma was diagnosed as a child. He frequently uses his puffer and has suffered a number of flare-ups. It is difficult to obtain much information due to his breathlessness. He shows you a preventer puffer (it is out of date) and you notice a packet of cigarettes on the table.

② CONFIRM

What else could it be?

Anxiety

Breathlessness causes anxiety. The patient clearly has signs of obstructive respiratory disease that cannot be explained by anxiety alone. Relaxation alone will often improve asthma, but this patient is exhibiting severe symptoms and needs active treatment.

Anaphylaxis

The absence of upper airway symptoms, erythematous rash, urticaria and any gastrointestinal symptoms suggests the condition is confined to the lungs. His relatively high blood pressure points away from cardiovascular compromise.

Cardiac arrhythmia

While cardiac arrhythmias such as supraventricular tachycardia can be associated with shortness of breath, the respiratory compromise is due to poor cardiac output and perfusion. An ECG recording will exclude this diagnosis. The symptoms in this patient point towards a primary lower respiratory issue.

Chest infection

An exacerbation of this patient's asthma caused by an acute infection is possible and likely. Smoking significantly increases the risk of respiratory compromise with asthma. This does not alter the initial management, which should be initiated promptly and without delay.

③ TREAT

2028 hrs: The patient is commenced on supplemental oxygen at 8 L/minute and given 5 mg of salbutamol with 500 micrograms of ipratropium bromide via a nebuliser mask. The crew are concerned with his condition and insert a cannula in his right hand while this is occurring.

2034 hrs: The patient is still sitting upright but is now staring straight ahead and is no longer responding to verbal requests. He is not speaking and is reaching exhaustion.

Perfusion status: HR 154 bpm, sinus tachycardia, BP 150/90 mmHg, skin warm and pink.

Respiratory status: pale, struggling to breathe, RR 30 bpm, SpO_2 91% on 8 L O_2, air entry poor with minimal wheeze, poor inspiratory effort, use of accessory muscles (tripod position), not speaking, prolonged expiratory phase.

Conscious state: GCS = 13.

2036 hrs: Aware that the patient is deteriorating and not ventilating well, the crew administer 2 g of magnesium sulfate as a slow push. Adrenaline is also drawn up (1 mg). A repeat nebuliser of 5 mg of salbutamol and 500 micrograms of ipratropium is commenced when the previous is finished. He is aided to

> **USING THE MNEMONIC DENT**
>
> Define:
> - What is the patient's main presenting problem?
> - Is this asthma?
> - Does it fit the definition?
>
> Explore your hypothesis and try to narrow it down.
>
> What else could it be?
> - Anxiety
> - Anaphylaxis
> - Cardiac arrhythmia
> - Chest infection

PRACTICE TIP

Check for a pulse! Has the patient lost consciousness because hyperinflation has occluded blood returning to the heart? If this is the case, a period of apnoea may allow gas to escape and attempting to force inspiration will only worsen the condition. If the patient remains pulseless after 1 minute of apnoea, there is little alternative to commencing the cardiac arrest guidelines, but a spontaneous tension pneumothorax should also be considered.

PRACTICE TIP

It takes energy for a patient to maintain their ventilatory effort in severe asthma. Patients will often deteriorate as they become tired. Watch out for the asthmatic who gradually becomes quiet; this may be a sign that you need to intervene.

sit more upright. One of the paramedics opens the airway kit and begins setting up for emergency intubation.

2039 hrs: The patient develops a flushed face: a sure sign the magnesium is having an effect as it also causes vasodilation. His blood pressure dips to 122/71 mmHg but his heart rate remains steady at 132 bpm.

2043 hrs: The patient begins to respond. His breaths become deeper and he looks more alert. The wheezing in his chest becomes louder as more air moves through his lungs.

Perfusion status: strong pulse, HR 134 bpm, sinus tachycardia, BP 119/79 mmHg, skin warm and pink.

Respiratory status: work of breathing improved but remains markedly increased, RR 28 bpm, SpO$_2$ 93%, air entry equal with some improvement in air entry and marked wheeze throughout.

2046 hrs: A third nebuliser of 5 mg salbutamol and 500 micrograms of ipratropium is commenced. The patient is now jittery—a sign of salbutamol toxicity (see Box 17.5)—and the crew need to balance the need for therapy against the developing side effects.

As he has stabilised, a decision is made to move the patient. He is able to ambulate to the elevator with assistance and is then loaded onto a stretcher in an upright position. The crewmembers with the patient spend a moment organising themselves so they have repeat doses of medication and airway support equipment to hand before they pull away, with lights and sirens.

4 EVALUATE

Evaluating the effect of any clinical management intervention can provide clues to the accuracy of the initial diagnosis. Some conditions respond rapidly to treatment. These patients should be expected to improve if the diagnosis and treatment are appropriate. A failure to improve in this situation should trigger the clinician to reconsider the diagnosis.

This patient's deterioration is not an indication of a misdiagnosis but rather that initial therapy was not sufficient, nor had time enough, to reverse his condition. This result is not unexpected in severe disease. The crew had to decide between three options: change management (working on a different diagnosis), wait (allow the therapy to work) or escalate the therapy (correct diagnosis but more therapy required). These are difficult decisions to make, particularly in time-critical illness. Decision-making is aided by systematically assessing the patient to gather appropriate clinical information, formatting the information into a diagnosis and having a clear plan of escalation of therapy.

Future directions

Further work is occurring to delineate the different subtypes of asthma. A diagnosis of 'viral-induced wheeze' is now commonly used for young children that only suffer episodes of asthma when provoked by viral respiratory tract infections. There is ongoing research into whether this group benefits from steroids therapy.

There is a move away from intravenous salbutamol in the hospital system and adrenaline in the out-of-hospital arena in favour of magnesium sulfate and aminophylline for severe asthma, but further work is needed to clearly establish therapeutic superiority.

Summary

Paramedics deal with the whole spectrum of asthma; from parents seeking advice on coughing children to respiratory failure and arrest. Life-threatening asthma is a relatively rare occurrence, but with over 400 deaths occurring annually, it is expected that competent paramedics will be able to recognise and manage severe asthma when it occurs.

References

Australian Institute of Health and Welfare. (2019). *Asthma. Cat. no. ACM 33.* Canberra: AIHW. https://www.aihw.gov.au/reports/chronic-respiratory-conditions/asthma. (Accessed 23 April 2020.)

Baudin, F., Buisson, A., Vanel, B., Massenavette, B., Pouyau, R., & Javouhey, E. (2017). Nasal high flow in management of children with status asthmaticus: a retrospective observational study. *Annals of Intensive Care, 7,* 55.

Brandao, D. C., Lima, V. M., & Filho, V. G. (2009). Reversal of bronchial obstruction with bi-level positive airway pressure and nebulization in patients with acute asthma. *The Journal of Asthma, 46.*

British Thoracic Society, Scottish Intercollegiate Guidelines Network. (2016). *British guideline on the management of asthma: quick reference guide.* BTS.

Brusasco, V. (2003). Usefulness of peak expiratory flow measurements: is it just a matter of instrument accuracy? *Thorax, 58*(5), 375.

Curtis, K., & Ramsden, C. (2011). *Emergency and trauma care for nurses and paramedics.* Sydney: Elsevier.

Des Jardins, T., & Burton, G. G. (2006). *Clinical manifestations and assessment of respiratory disease* (5th ed.). St Louis: Mosby.

Dondi, A., Calamelli, E., Piccinno, V., Ricci, G., Corsini, I., Biagi, C., & Lanari, M. (2017). Acute asthma in the pediatric emergency department: infections are the main triggers of exacerbations. *BioMed Research International, 2017,* https://www.ncbi.nlm.nih.gov/pubmed/29159184. 9687061.

Holly, A. D., & Boots, R. J. (2009). Review article: management of acute severe and near-fatal asthma. *Emergency Medicine Australasia: EMA, 21*(4).

Howe, T. A., Jaalam, K., Ahmad, R., Sheng, C. K., & Rahman, N. H. N. A. (2011). The use of end-tidal capnography to monitor non-intubated patients presenting with acute exacerbations of asthma in the emergency department. *The Journal of Emergency Medicine, 41*(6), 581–589.

Idris, A. H., McDermott, M. F., Raucci, J. C., Morrabel, A., McGorray, S., & Hendeles, L. (1993). Emergency department treatment of severe asthma: metered-dose inhaler plus holding chamber is equivalent in effectiveness to nebulizer. *Chest, 103*(3), 665–672.

Jabre, P., Jacob, L., Auger, H., Jaulin, C., Monribot, M., Aurore, A., Margenet, A., Marty, J., & Combes, X. (2009). Capnography monitoring in nonintubated patients with respiratory distress. *The American Journal of Emergency Medicine, 27*(9), 1056–1059.

Kew, K. M., Kirtchuk, L., & Michell, C. I. (2014). Intravenous magnesium sulfate for treating adults with acute asthma in the emergency department. *The Cochrane Database of Systematic Reviews,* (5), CD010909.

Knightly, R., Milan, S. J., Hughes, R., Knopp-Sihota, J. A., Rowe, B. H., Normansell, R., & Powell, C. (2017). Inhaled magnesium sulfate in the treatment of acute asthma. *The Cochrane Database of Systematic Reviews,* (11), CD003898.

Kokotajlo, S., Degnan, L., Meyers, R., Siu, A., & Robinson, C. (2014). Use of intravenous magnesium sulfate for the treatment of an acute asthma exacerbation in pediatric patients. *The Journal of Pediatric Pharmacology and Therapeutics, 19*(2), 91–97.

Lim, W. J., Mohammed Akram, R., Carson, K. V., et al. (2012). Non-invasive positive pressure ventilation for treatment of respiratory failure due to severe acute exacerbations of asthma. *The Cochrane Database of Systematic Reviews,* (12), CD004360.

Murphy, D. M., & O'Byrne, P. M. (2010). Recent advances in the pathophysiology of asthma. *Chest, 137*(6), 1417–1426.

National Asthma Council. (2019). *Asthma Management Handbook Version 2.0.* March. Retrieved from: www.asthmahandbook.org.au.

Papi, A., Brightling, C., Pedersen, S. E., & Reddel, H. K. (2018). Asthma. *The Lancet,* . doi: 10.1016/S0140-6736 (17)33311-1.

Queensland Ambulance Service (QAS). (2011). *Ambulance service clinical practice manual.* Queensland Government.

Rodriguez-Roisin, R. (1997). Acute severe asthma: pathophysiology and pathobiology of gas exchange abnormalities. *The European Respiratory Journal, 10,* 1359–1371.

Saetta, S., & Turato, G. (2001). Airway pathology in asthma. *The European Respiratory Journal, 18*(4), 18s–23s.

Sly, P. D., Cahill, P., Willet, K., & Burton, P. (1994). Accuracy of mini peak flow meters in indicating changes in lung function in children with asthma. *British Medical Journal, 308*, 572–574.

Stanley, D., & Tunnicliffe, W. (2008). Management of life-threatening asthma in adults. *Continuing Education in Anaesthesia, Critical Care & Pain, 8*(3), 95–99.

Tomar, R. P. S., Cola, L. T., & Vasudevan, R. (2012). Metabolic acidosis due to inhaled salbutamol toxicity: a hazardous side effect complicating management of suspected cases of acute severe asthma. *Medical Journal, Armed Forces India, 68*(3), 242–244.

Travers, A. H., Milan, S. J., Jones, A. P., Camargo, C. A., Jr, & Rowe, B. H. (2014). Addition of intravenous beta(2)-agonists to inhaled beta(2)-agonists for acute asthma. *The Cochrane Database of Systematic Reviews,* (12), CD010179.

Walker, D. (2009). Update on epinephrine (adrenaline) for pediatric emergencies. *Current Opinion in Pediatrics, 21*(3), 313–319.

CHAPTER 18

Acute Pulmonary Oedema

By Hugh Grantham

OVERVIEW

- Pulmonary oedema can be associated with chronic fluid overload or acute cardiac failure.
- The treatment of pulmonary oedema is different for the acute and chronic presentations.
- Acute pulmonary oedema can present with moist crackles in both lungs, hypertension, tachycardia and profound hypoxia but it can also present more subtly as wheezing.

- The principles of treatment are maintenance of patient oxygenation and perfusion while addressing the cause of the acute failure.
- Pulmonary oedema may be associated with myocardial infarction, acute valve rupture and a variety of unusual clinical settings. The majority of acute presentations are associated with acute failure of the left ventricle secondary to hypoxia.

Introduction

Pulmonary oedema is the presence of serous fluid in the interstitial spaces between the alveoli and the pulmonary capillaries and within the alveoli, bronchioles and bronchi. **Acute pulmonary oedema** (APO) is a sudden accumulation of serous transudate fluid (extravascular fluid low in protein count), most commonly caused by left ventricular failure resulting in an acute alteration of the osmotic or tissue pressures affecting capillary fluid balance. Another cause can be an alteration in the permeability of the capillary membrane. **Chronic pulmonary oedema** is a gradual accumulation of oedema fluid associated with chronic fluid overload, and often associated with left ventricular failure.

Pathophysiology

The pathophysiology of pulmonary oedema revolves around the balance of forces controlling fluid flow into and out of the pulmonary capillaries (Hall, 2010; see Fig 18.1). At the arteriole end of the capillaries the blood hydrostatic pressure (35 mmHg) and the interstitial fluid osmotic pressure (1 mmHg) exert an overall force out of the vessel. There is no interstitial fluid hydrostatic pressure exerted at this end of the capillary; however, the proteins within the capillary do exert a blood colloid osmotic (or oncotic) pressure resulting in a pulling force of 26 mmHg into the capillary. So there is 36 mmHg of pressure forcing fluid out of the capillary and 26 mmHg of pressure forcing fluid into the capillary. This means there is an overall pressure of 10 mmHg forcing fluid out of the capillary. At the venous end the blood hydrostatic pressure has dropped to 16 mmHg, but the interstitial fluid osmotic pressure, the interstitial fluid hydrostatic pressure and the blood colloid oncotic pressure have all remained the same. So now there is an outward force of 17 mmHg and an inward force of 26 mmHg. Therefore, there is now an overall inwards pressure of 9 mmHg, resulting in a fluid shift into the capillaries.

The forces responsible for the movement of fluid out of the capillary are:
- hydrostatic (the force exerted on the fluid [and vice versa] by the tissues around it; e.g. the vessel walls during diastole and systole)
  - blood hydrostatic pressure
  - interstitial fluid hydrostatic pressure
- negative tissue pressure (a reflection of negative intrathoracic pressure associated with inspiration)
- tissue oncotic pressure (the osmotic pressure of the surrounding tissues drawing fluid into or out of the capillaries)
  - interstitial fluid osmotic pressure
  - blood colloid osmotic (oncotic) pressure.

In the normal healthy state the force drawing fluid into the capillary is just exceeded by the force driving fluid out of the capillary and the resulting imbalance is cleared by the lymphatic system and evaporation. The lymphatic system is capable of dealing with quite a large imbalance but eventually will be overcome and pulmonary oedema will be established (Hall, 2010; see Fig 18.2).

Recently, the role of the endothelial glycocalyx layer in the control of fluid movement in and out of capillaries has been studied and seems to play an important role in oedema formation that was not previously appreciated in Starling's model (Collins et al., 2013).

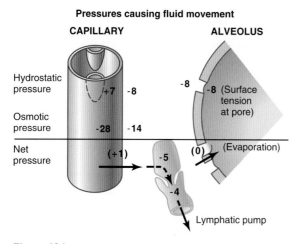

Figure 18.1
Pressures causing fluid movement.
Hydrostatic and osmotic forces in mmHg at the capillary (left) and alveolar membrane (right) of the lungs. Also shown is the tip end of a lymphatic vessel (centre) that pumps fluid from the pulmonary interstitial spaces. If the left ventricle fails to eject all the blood it receives, the volume of blood in the pulmonary circuit will increase and cause a corresponding increase in hydrostatic pressure 'pushing' fluid into the interstitial and alveolar spaces.
Source: Hall (2010).

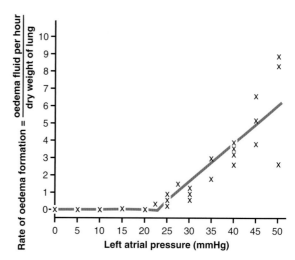

Figure 18.3
Rate of fluid loss into the lung tissues when the left atrial pressure (and pulmonary capillary pressure) is increased.
Experiments in animals have shown that the pulmonary capillary pressure normally must rise to a value at least equal to the colloid osmotic pressure of the plasma inside the capillaries before significant pulmonary oedema will occur and fluid will begin to accumulate in the lungs. This fluid accumulation will increase more rapidly with further increases in capillary pressure.
Source: Hall (2010).

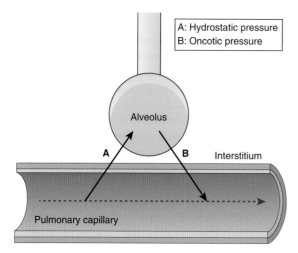

Figure 18.2
Pulmonary fluid dynamics.

Cardiogenic causes of pulmonary oedema

Chronic pulmonary oedema can be a consequence of chronic fluid retention which may be precipitated by reduced urine output. In this situation a patient who is retaining fluid will have a raised preload. In order to manage the raised preload and the resultant increased stretch on the ventricular myocardium, the Frank-Starling mechanism will be in play. This mechanism describes the increased force of contraction secondary to the increased stretch of myocardial muscle. This reactive mechanism will only compensate up to a point and then it will no longer maintain appropriate cardiac output to manage the increased intravascular volume.

Under these circumstances the volume within the left ventricle cannot be completely shifted into the aorta, meaning blood volume within the left atrium, pulmonary arteries and capillaries will increase, translating to an increase in blood hydrostatic pressure. If this blood hydrostatic pressure increased to above 25 mmHg, there would be no opportunity for the fluid that shifted out of the capillary at the arteriole end to return, resulting in interstitial oedema in the pulmonary tissues (see Fig 18.3).

A patient with chronic pulmonary oedema will have a thickened respiratory membrane due to interstitial oedema, which will in turn reduce the efficiency of oxygen exchange. In addition to the thickening of the respiratory membrane pulmonary oedema may progress to oedema within the alveoli and terminal airway structures, which will further compromise respiratory function. Patients with chronic fluid overload have shortness of breath and moist crackles in their lower lung fields.

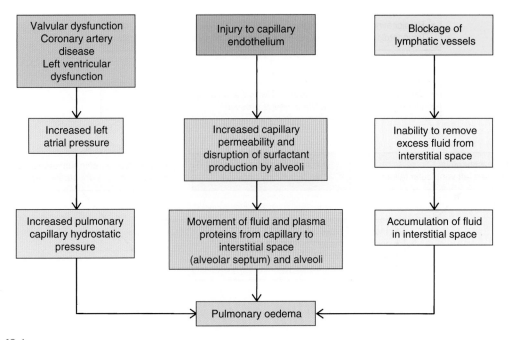

Figure 18.4
Causes of acute pulmonary oedema.
By far the most common cause of acute pulmonary oedema that will present to paramedics is the result of left ventricular failure. Injury to the alveolar surface from inhaled gases or fluids or as a result of a systemic inflammatory response should be considered in young patients without a cardiac history and is technically not oedema but an inflammatory exudate. Unfortunately, out-of-hospital management of acute pulmonary oedema revolves around reducing cardiac workload and there is little that can be done to directly manage exudate or ARDS in this setting. Early recognition and maximising inspired oxygen are the two primary keys to managing ARDS for paramedics.
Source: McCance & Huether (2014).

Acute pulmonary oedema is a rapid-onset pulmonary oedema that is associated with poor left ventricular function (Cleland et al., 2010; see Fig 18.4). A reduction in left ventricular function results in a back pressure on the pulmonary system, which in turn increases the hydrostatic pressure in the pulmonary capillaries beyond 25 mmHg. Once again the process commences with a thickening of the pulmonary membrane due to interstitial oedema and reduction in gas exchange and progresses to pulmonary oedema in the alveoli and respiratory tree.

Although acute pulmonary oedema can be associated with acute problems with heart valves and heart muscle (myocardial infarction, ruptured valves and inefficient cardiac rhythms) the majority of acute pulmonary oedema cases are precipitated by myocardial hypoxia. Myocardial hypoxia causes a stiff left ventricle that will not relax properly and therefore will not fill properly in diastole. The cause of the stiff left ventricle is a lack of adenosine triphosphate (ATP), which is necessary to break the bonds between the myosin and actin filaments in muscle. Without ATP, the muscle is effectively

prevented from relaxing (a similar process to rigor mortis), which prevents the heart from effectively filling.

Patients with a mild degree of chronic pulmonary oedema or another cause of hypoxia are prone to episodes of acute pulmonary oedema. Acute pulmonary oedema classically occurs at night when presumably the respiratory pattern in sleep promotes a further drop in oxygen concentrations. In acute pulmonary oedema the situation is exacerbated by a sympathetic response to the drop in the partial pressure of oxygen. A sympathetic response will result in vasoconstriction, which will effectively squeeze the existing blood volume into a smaller space. The patient is now pale and sweaty, tachycardic and hypertensive with distended neck veins. The distended neck veins translate to a raised preload, which increases the hydrostatic pressure in the left side of the heart and eventually the pulmonary capillaries.

The situation can be further exacerbated as pulmonary oedema fluid dilutes the surfactant that was secreted by the type 2 cells in the alveoli. With a reduction in the amount of surfactant present in

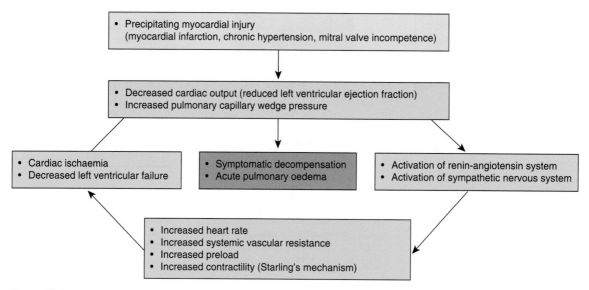

Figure 18.5
Pathophysiology of acute pulmonary oedema.

the alveoli the work of breathing is increased. The loss of surfactant results in a decrease in lung compliance due to the collapse of the alveoli. The work of breathing is increased not only as a response to the hypoxaemia, but also due to the need to overcome the surface tension required to reinflate the alveoli. In extreme pulmonary oedema the frothy cough is 'pink' because of a small amount of red blood cells in the fluid.

A vicious cycle is established with increasing hypoxia causing increased sympathetic drive, which in turn increases the heart rate and vasoconstriction, exacerbating the pulmonary oedema (see Fig 18.5). This cycle is complicated by the increase in difficulty in achieving ventilation due to a relative lack of surfactant causing the patient to work even harder to breathe.

Other causes of pulmonary oedema

Pulmonary oedema can also be associated with significant changes to the intrathoracic pressure (Kapoor, 2011; Bhaskar & Fraser, 2011). This is the explanation for pulmonary oedema occurring as a consequence of partial airway obstruction when the intrathoracic pressure has to be far more negative in order to overcome the obstruction.

This is a rare cause of pulmonary oedema associated with obstruction from occluded endotracheal tubes, inhaled foreign bodies and suffocation. Because the cause of the pulmonary oedema is completely different from the usual hydrostatic pressure aetiology, the treatment needs to differ as well (see Fig 18.4). These patients do not need

treatment aimed at correcting a hydrostatic pressure imbalance and will usually respond to removing the obstruction and correcting any associated hypoxia.

Pulmonary oedema is reported at high altitude and is thought to be precipitated by hypoxia and pulmonary vasospasm at that altitude. In this situation the treatment will be slightly different with an emphasis on restoring the partial pressure of oxygen delivered to the myocardium, by returning to a lower altitude or simulating a return to a lower altitude with a portable hyperbaric unit (Hopkins et al., 2005; Noelkel, 2002). Acetazolamide is a well-established prophylactic treatment (Nieto Estrada et al., 2017) and is taken by many individuals when travelling at high altitude; it counteracts the respiratory alkalosis associated with a raised respiratory rate by promoting the urinary excretion of bicarbonate.

A rare cause of pulmonary oedema is associated with scuba diving (Slader et al., 2001). The exact aetiology is not clear but a

> ### PRACTICE TIP
>
> The oedematous thickening of the respiratory wall lining causes narrowing of the airways. Some elderly patients may present with a wheeze, with no history of asthma or bronchitis. In the setting of hypertension, dependent oedema and cardiac disease, these patients must be managed cautiously: any physical exertion can increase their cardiac demand and venous return. This will increase their hypoxia, and the increased volume of blood returning to the heart will exert higher hydrostatic pressures, increasing the interstitial oedema and causing the interstitial fluid to shift into the alveoli and terminal airways.

combination of hydrostatic pressure externally raising the central venous pressure and a degree of negative intra-pleural pressure associated with breathing at depths has been suggested.

Fluid in the lungs secondary to a chemical burn (chlorine and other chemicals; Pillai et al., 2005) may present similarly to acute pulmonary oedema but is not pulmonary oedema. This is because the fluid is an exudate precipitated by the burn and is not a transudate present because of hydrostatic or pressure changes (Kosmidou et al., 2008). Treatments aimed at changing the hydrostatic pressure in the pulmonary capillary are not going to

be effective in these situations. Treatment should be confined to maintaining adequate tissue oxygenation through providing supplementary oxygen and managing the inflammatory process.

Fluid can also be present in the lungs as a consequence of capillary leakage in acute respiratory distress syndrome (ARDS), which is part of a systemic inflammatory response. This is a secondary complication resulting from an initial injury to the capillary endothelium and possibly involving changes to the glycocalyx. In this setting the systemic inflammatory response increases capillary permeability, causing a loss of fluid from those capillaries (Kosmidou et al., 2008). Once again the treatment will differ from the standard management of acute pulmonary oedema because the issue is not hydrostatic force but the permeability of the capillary.

CASE STUDY 1

Case 10711, 0214 hrs.

Dispatch details: A 78-year-old male is complaining of acute shortness of breath and chest pain.

Initial presentation: The ambulance crew find the patient sitting on the edge of his bed. He looks up at them as they enter the room, appearing anxious and distressed, with an obvious increase in the work of breathing and sweat streaming down his face. His pyjamas appear damp with sweat. He says that he woke up in the middle of the night to go to the toilet and suffered a sudden-onset shortness of breath, which is worsening. He is complaining of mild chest pain and is having difficulty speaking more than a few words.

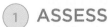

ASSESS

Patient history

This patient developed acute shortness of breath in the early morning hours. The history of sudden onset of acute shortness of breath is compatible with acute pulmonary oedema. The time of onset is very typical and is thought to be associated with changes in ventilation patterns during sleep. The patient has reduced his myocardial oxygenation with a change in respiration during sleep. The reduction in myocardial oxygenation has given him a stiff left ventricle and an inability to pump. This in turn has created back pressure on the pulmonary vascular system and precipitated pulmonary oedema. The situation has been exacerbated by his sympathetic response to poor oxygenation, and he is tachycardic, hypertensive, pale and sweaty. His neck veins will be distended and he has a high central venous pressure giving him a high preload.

Ask!
- What is your previous history?
- What are your routine medications? (Is he already on treatment for chronic heart failure; i.e. digoxin, diuretics and ACE inhibitors?)
- What is your preferred sleeping position in terms of the number of pillows? (orthopnoea)
- Were you well when you went to bed?

Look for!
- Respiratory rate
- Signs of sympathetic engagement (pulse, BP, skin colour, pupil size)
- Evidence of pulmonary oedema, lung sounds
- Evidence of chronic right heart failure, peripheral oedema, ascites

This episode of acute pulmonary oedema is probably associated with an underlying chronic hypoxia, the most likely cause of which is some degree of chronic pulmonary oedema. He may also have signs of chronic right heart failure (peripheral oedema and ascites).

Initial assessment summary

Problem	Acute shortness of breath and chest pain
Conscious state	Alert and orientated; GCS = 15
Position	Sitting upright
Heart rate	146 bpm, regular
Blood pressure	180/100 mmHg
Skin appearance	Pale, diaphoretic
Speech pattern	Speaking 3–4 words at a time
Respiratory rate	36 bpm
Respiratory rhythm	Regular even cycles
Respiratory effort	Mild increase in the use of accessory muscles
Chest auscultation	Bilateral coarse crackles bases to midzones
Pulse oximetry	91% on room air
Temperature	36.9°C
Motor/sensory function	Normal
History	Angina, hypertension, hyperlipidaemia. Became short of breath (SOB) after getting up to go to the toilet; sleeps semi-recumbent on three pillows

D: The major danger to this patient at this point would be any physical exertion.

A: The patient is conscious with no current upper airway obstruction.

B: Respiratory function is currently compromised. He is having difficulty ventilating due to the collapse of the alveoli and the presence of serous transudate fluid in the terminal airways. He also has compromised gas exchange due to the thickening of the respiratory membranes between the capillaries and the alveoli.

C: This patient is hypertensive, tachycardic, pale and diaphoretic. His cardiovascular system is under considerable strain. Myocardial infarction also needs to be considered as a precipitating event.

This patient appears to be presenting with acute pulmonary oedema from cardiogenic causes.

2 CONFIRM

The essential part of the clinical reasoning process is to seek to confirm your initial hypothesis by finding clinical signs that should occur with your provisional diagnosis. You should also seek to challenge your diagnosis by exploring findings that do not fit your hypothesis: do not just ignore them because they do not fit.

Although this patient has a presentation typical of acute pulmonary oedema there are other causes of acute shortness of breath that can present similarly.

What else could it be?

Acute bronchospasm

A nocturnal presentation of bronchospasm could be a possible diagnosis and if there is a background of chronic bronchitis the lungs might sound moist as well as wheezy. This patient does not have a history of either acute or chronic lung disease and the rapid development of moist crackles in both lung zones would favour acute pulmonary oedema over acute bronchospasm. Sympathetic

DIFFERENTIAL DIAGNOSIS

Acute pulmonary oedema
Or
- Acute episode of bronchospasm associated with asthma and COPD
- Acute presentation of pneumonia
- Acute metabolic acidosis
- Pulmonary embolism
- Arrhythmia

engagement and hypoxaemia can both be compatible with an acute episode of bronchospasm.

Pneumonia

An acute pneumonia could present with moist chest sounds and shortness of breath. It would be usual to expect the patient to be febrile, although in an elderly patient this is not always as obvious. It would be usual to expect a productive cough of thick sputum as opposed to bilateral dependent inspiratory crackles, and pneumonia tends to start on one or other side as opposed to being balanced and bilateral.

Acute metabolic acidosis

It is possible that the shortness of breath is a response to metabolic acidosis, which in turn is a response to either general or a local area of poor perfusion. Ischaemic bowel, for instance, can give a very marked metabolic acidosis. Moist chest sounds should not be a feature of shortness of breath associated with metabolic acidosis, nor should profound hypoxia, as the patient is breathing much harder than usual. A sympathetic response is not necessarily part of metabolic acidosis but may be associated with the cause of the metabolic acidosis (poor perfusion). This patient does not give a history of anything that would precipitate a metabolic acidosis and the lung signs are not consistent with a metabolic acidosis.

Pulmonary embolism

A large pulmonary embolism can present with acute shortness of breath associated with acute hypoxia. However, moist chest sounds would not be expected in this case. A sympathetic response is entirely consistent with pulmonary embolism although a large pulmonary embolism tends to affect cardiac output, making hypertension less likely.

Arrhythmia

The patient's tachycardia, hypertension and shortness of breath need to be further investigated and excluded with cardiac monitoring. Supraventricular tachycardia, ventricular tachycardia and myocardial infarction all need to be excluded or managed as potential causes of this patient's acute pulmonary oedema.

The musical tone of a wheeze is most often caused by bronchospasm narrowing the small airways. Any form of airway inflammation can trigger bronchospasm but the most common cause is asthma. In the early stages of acute pulmonary oedema, the movement of fluid from the intravascular space can cause the airway walls to swell and narrow. The fluid shift could also trigger an inflammatory response that causes bronchospasm.

③ TREAT

Emergency management

Treatment is aimed at restoring myocardial oxygenation and reducing hydrostatic pressure on the pulmonary capillaries. Box 18.1 outlines the principles of management for acute pulmonary oedema.

Reassurance

Reassurance has a significant clinical role to play by reducing excessive sympathetic drive and therefore cardiac workload, vascular tone and, in turn, venous return pressure.

Posture

Helping the patient to sit up and providing something to lean on and thus stabilise their shoulders will improve ventilation. Stabilising the shoulders enables the patient to adopt a tripod position and recruit accessory muscles

> ## BOX 18.1 Principles of management
>
> **Acute pulmonary oedema**
> - Give reassurance
> - Help with posture
> - Obtain a history and examination
> - Treat hypoxia with oxygen therapy and CPAP
> - Administer GTN if blood pressure and rhythm adequate
> - Obtain IV access
> - Monitor vital signs, pulse oximetry and ECG rhythm
> - Perform a 12-lead ECG

to help ventilation. Adopting a sitting position stops abdominal contents from pushing on the diaphragm, making it easy to breathe. Sitting with the legs dependent over the side of the bed allows for venous pooling in the legs, thereby lowering the central venous pressure and reducing preload. Although compromises will have to be made, attempts to maintain this posture in transport have definite clinical advantages.

Oxygen

One of the precipitating factors in this patient's acute episode is myocardial hypoxia and adding oxygen will raise the partial pressure of oxygen reaching the myocardium. Because the terminal airways are partially obstructed by fluid and the pulmonary membrane is thickened, gas exchange will be impaired, so a higher partial pressure of oxygen at the alveoli will be needed to achieve adequate oxygenation. In practice, improved oxygen concentrations can be delivered via a simple mask (which should be capable of an inspired oxygen concentration of about 45%), a rebreather mask with a built-in reservoir bag (which in ideal situations may give a concentration up to 80%) or a closed-circuit bag and mask (which in ideal circumstances offers the possibility of a concentration of 100%). Many patients have difficulty tolerating a bag and mask because it is difficult to achieve an adequate minute volume with an oxygen supply of only 15 L per minute. For this reason some ambulance services employ oxygen gauges that go up to 25 L per minute. The practical considerations of assisting ventilation with perfectly timed positive pressure assistance with only two paramedics often mean that a compromise is made and an oxygen mask (either standard or rebreather) is used.

Continuous positive airway pressure

Continuous positive airway pressure (CPAP) has been used as a mainstay of hospital management of acute pulmonary oedema for some time and is now being employed in paramedic management (Ducros et al., 2011). CPAP works by splinting the alveoli open, allowing more effective exhalation and supporting the process of inhalation with positive pressure (Plaisance et al., 2007). The pressure used is low (5 or 10 cm of water) so does not represent a significant increase on the 1 atm (atmosphere) of pressure that the patient is already experiencing. Positive airway pressures are maintained throughout the respiratory cycle. CPAP can be effectively applied in the field and maintained to hospital (Hubble et al., 2008; Kallio et al., 2003; Dieperink et al., 2009). Although the pressure is relatively low it does raise intrathoracic pressure, potentially affecting venous return to the heart. Pulse and blood pressure should therefore be monitored.

CPAP is different from positive end-expiratory pressure (PEEP), in which the patient breathes against an increased resistance in expiration. Although

> ## PRACTICE TIP
>
> CPAP/PEEP does not drive fluid back from the alveoli into the interstitial spaces. It simply maintains the alveoli open, stopping them from collapsing, therefore enabling gas exchange to occur.

PEEP splints airways open in the same way that CPAP does, it increases the work of breathing by providing resistance to expiration and no assistance to inhalation. CPAP will thus be superior to controlled PEEP in assisting this patient. Occasionally-uncontrolled PEEP, created by maintaining pressure on the bag (not allowing the bag to completely inflate) at the same time that the patient breathes out, has been tried but the inability to accurately control what has to be a very small pressure difference makes this practice potentially harmful.

Nitrates

Glyceryl trinitrate (GTN) is a mainstay of treatment for acute pulmonary oedema, although other nitrates are also used. The aim of GTN treatment is to lower vascular tone down to normal, but no further, and return the vascular space to a normal volume. By allowing the vascular space to expand the fluid contained within it is at a normal central venous pressure and the preload returning to the heart is reduced. GTN effectively treats the adverse consequences of the sympathetic stimulation and vasoconstriction that form one of the vicious cycles of acute pulmonary oedema. Blood pressure is used as a guide to the frequency of doses, with most treatment guidelines recommending a minimum systolic blood pressure of 100 mmHg before GTN should be considered. A guideline that focuses solely on blood pressure, of course, does not account for differences in rate and rhythm or the importance of maintaining adequate preload when right heart infarct or ischaemia is suspected. In practice, caution should be used when there is evidence of right heart ischaemia and when ventricular filling is dependent on preload as in ventricular tachycardia, rapid ventricular response to atrial fibrillation and, to a lesser extent, extreme sinus tachycardia.

Salbutamol

Salbutamol may have a role to play if true bronchospasm is present; however, it is likely that much of the wheeze will be due to airway oedema and therefore not responsive to bronchodilators. When considering the use of salbutamol the possibility of reducing oxygen delivery should be balanced against any potential benefits that the salbutamol might offer.

Diuretics

Diuretics have a role to play in the management of chronic fluid overload and thus may sometimes be seen in the setting of acute pulmonary oedema if a background of chronic fluid overload is felt to be part of the precipitating circumstances. Diuretics are not a logical treatment for the acute component of acute pulmonary oedema (Cleland et al., 2010). In the purely acute setting the patient is not fluid overloaded but the vascular space is contracted, causing a temporary rise in central venous pressure. Once the vasoconstriction has been addressed with GTN or another nitrate and the vascular space returned to normal size, the patient will have the same volume (or less) and therefore the same central venous pressure in their vascular space as they had prior to the acute event. Also, addressing hypoxaemia will oxygenate the heart, improving the effectiveness of the pump in shifting the fluid forwards.

Opiates

Opiates reduce anxiety and slow the respiratory rate, reducing respiratory drive and thus providing symptomatic relief, which is particularly valuable in palliative care situations. There is little evidence that opiates provide any additional benefit in terms of haemodynamic effects (Cleland et al., 2010). Their use in acute pulmonary oedema is now extremely rare (Cleland et al., 2010), although in the past they were given to relieve anxiety and were said to provide vasodilation (which was most likely only ever seen in response to the decrease in sympathetic drive due to the anxiolytic effects of the opiates).

A presentation of acute pulmonary oedema to the extent that the patient is coughing up pink frothy sputum is not only frightening for the patient but also challenging for the paramedic. Such patients tend to be anxious and extremely difficult to reassure as they have an overwhelming dyspnoea. The challenge of managing an extremely scared, possibly confused and anxious patient will complicate the treatment, often resulting in a series of compromises in terms of oxygen administration. Time spent reassuring the patient and endeavouring to get them comfortable with CPAP is well invested.

This patient will benefit from reassurance, posture, oxygen (preferably with CPAP) and nitrates en route to hospital.

4 EVALUATE

Evaluating the effect of any clinical management intervention can provide clues to the accuracy of the initial diagnosis. Some conditions respond rapidly to treatment so patients should be expected to improve if the diagnosis and treatment were appropriate. A failure to improve in this situation should trigger the clinician to reconsider the diagnosis.

This patient should be improving and should be able to breathe more easily and therefore have a reduced work and rate of breathing. Observing the rate and respiratory effort will be one of the most useful feedback signs. Respiratory fatigue needs to be differentiated from respiratory improvement: the patient's level of consciousness and interaction will be a useful guide in this area. As the patient's situation improves the sympathetic drive will lessen and his skin colour should improve and diaphoresis should resolve. Other signs to monitor include an improvement in oxygen saturation and a reduction in tachycardia. Moist crackles in the chest tend to clear from the top downwards if the patient is sitting up and will clear rapidly enough to be worth monitoring over the course of his clinical treatment by the paramedics.

Adverse signs to consider include increasing respiratory distress, worsening hypoxia and the development of arrhythmia. This patient's cardiovascular system is under considerable strain and a myocardial infarction would not be unusual.

Hospital admission

On arrival at hospital it is likely that the patient will already have started to improve. The oxygen therapy using CPAP will be continued, nitrates will continue to be administered but possibly via an infusion (which allows greater control) and hopefully the need for further intervention and intubation will be avoided (Marco et al., 2008). Hospital investigation will include a chest x-ray to confirm the clinical findings of left ventricular failure and pulmonary oedema and a baseline for blood count urea, electrolytes and liver function tests. Blood tests for markers of acute coronary syndrome (troponin, cardiac enzymes) and also a blood gas may be taken if the patient is still acutely short of breath. A 12-lead ECG is indicated looking for either underlying acute coronary syndrome causes or ischaemic damage secondary to the cardiovascular system strain that the patient has been enduring. Hospital management will be guided by the patient's response to treatment with oxygen (CPAP) and nitrates. Many patients settle within a few hours of the commencement of this regimen.

Long-term impact

The long-term impact of this episode of acute pulmonary oedema depends on whether any damage was done due to the myocardial workload. If the precipitating cause was borderline chronic failure and this can be treated, it is quite possible that there will be no specific long-term impact of this acute episode. Nevertheless, a patient who develops acute pulmonary oedema does so because they have underlying pathology. Once the acute pulmonary oedema has been managed a detailed clinical review is indicated looking for the precipitating circumstances.

Acute pulmonary oedema across the lifespan

Acute pulmonary oedema is much more likely in elderly people with preexisting comorbidities that contributed to creating myocardial hypoxia or cardiac dysfunction in an acute setting. The exceptions to this trend are those people who develop acute pulmonary oedema due to unusual circumstances (altitude, drowning, negative pressure pulmonary oedema, ARDS) or who have an underlying cardiac condition (valve problem, myocardial dysfunction, arrhythmia).

 CASE STUDY 2

Case 15528, 2354 hrs.

Dispatch details: A 68-year-old female with acute-on-chronic shortness of breath. She has a previous history of lung disease and has become acutely short of breath this evening.

Initial presentation: On arrival the paramedics find an elderly lady sitting on the edge of her bed with acute shortness of breath. She appears anxious and is adopting a tripod position.

1 ASSESS

0007 hrs Vital signs survey: Her airway is clear and she has a respiratory rate of 26. The respiratory pattern has a prolonged exploratory phase. She is tachycardic with a pulse of 110 and her blood pressure is 140/90 mmHg. Although her skin is pale she is not excessively sweaty. Her neck veins appeared dilated and the jugular venous pressure (JVP) is raised. She is alert and anxious. Auscultation of her chest reveals bilateral wheezes.

0009 hrs Pertinent hx: She gives a previous history of COPD, which has been associated with her heavy smoking until the last few years. Among her medications are bronchodilators, which she says help her breathing a bit, but are not dramatically effective.

2 CONFIRM

In many cases paramedics are presented with a collection of signs and symptoms that do not appear to describe a particular condition. A critical step in determining a treatment plan in this situation is to consider what other conditions could explain the patient's presentation.

The patient has an exacerbation of shortness of breath with some evidence of a raised JVP. Her chest sounds are wheezes rather than moist crackles and her clinical history is of chronic lung disease with a degree of bronchospasm that is relieved by bronchodilators. The presentation is not clear as these symptoms could well be ascribed to her respiratory condition but could also be early-onset acute pulmonary oedema. The initial phase of pulmonary oedema can present as a wheeze. This may be due to airway obstruction secondary to oedema or there may actually be bronchospasm precipitated by an inflammatory response, which in turn has been triggered by the oedema.

The raised JVP could be indicative of chronic fluid overload. It could also be indicative of right ventricular failure secondary to pulmonary hypertension secondary to chronic pulmonary hypoxia. A third explanation for the raised JVP could be raised intrathoracic pressure associated with gas trapping and COPD with exacerbation. In this situation the neck veins are not going to be particularly helpful.

If this is early-onset acute pulmonary oedema the clinical trajectory is progression to overt classical pulmonary oedema over a relatively short time period.

What else could it be?

Bronchospasm

Bronchospasm as an acute element on top of a background respiratory condition is possible. The wheezing and prolonged expiratory phase are entirely consistent with bronchospasm, but could also be consistent with the wheezing associated with early pulmonary oedema (see Fig 18.6). The patient's history of chronic lung disease is relevant and might be considered supporting evidence for bronchospasm. However, she indicates that bronchodilators are not particularly effective, from which we could infer that the bronchospasm component of her respiratory disease is relatively small.

Acute infection

An exacerbation of her respiratory disease caused by an acute infection is possible and likely. Inflammation associated with the infection could present as a wheeze due to either primary oedema or triggering bronchospasm. The absence of a productive cough or a temperature means relatively little in the acute phase. If she has been on long-term steroids for her chest condition her ability to mount an inflammatory response will also be blunted.

At this stage it is extremely difficult to be sure whether this is a cardiac or respiratory condition. The diagnosis will become clear as the condition progresses and responds to treatment.

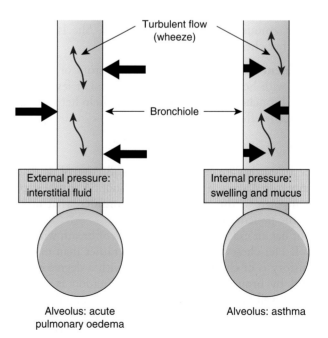

Figure 18.6
Differentiation of turbulent flow in asthma.

③ TREAT

Due to the somewhat ambiguous presentation, treatment is aimed at covering both eventualities while the paramedics observe clinical developments.

0010 hrs: The crew apply oxygen via a nebuliser mask with salbutamol and then gain IV access.

0014 hrs: Perfusion status: HR 125 bpm; BP 150/95 mmHg; skin pale, warm, slightly diaphoretic.

Respiratory status: RR 32, becoming more distressed, crackles heard bilaterally from bases to midzones, no wheeze heard, speaking in phrases.

Conscious state: GCS = 15.

Administering oxygen to avoid hypoxia (target 94–98%) is beneficial to both respiratory and cardiac aetiologies. Salbutamol is effective against bronchospasm but may actually worsen the acute failure by increasing the tachycardia. This patient's wheeze may be a result of fluid in the interstitial spaces narrowing the terminal airways and not bronchospasm. The increased workload on the heart in the form of tachycardia, secondary to salbutamol administration, has resulted in a decreased stroke volume and increased pulmonary congestion. This has led to shift of fluid into the alveoli.

0015 hrs: Salbutamol is ceased and GTN is administered. The crew carry the patient to the stretcher (no physical exertion is asked of the patient) for transport.

0020 hrs: Perfusion status: HR 125 bpm; BP 150/90 mmHg; skin pale, warm, dry.

Respiratory status: RR 28 bpm, crackles bilaterally to midzones, speaking in phrases.

Conscious state: GCS = 15.

0021 hrs: The paramedics give another dose of GTN.

0025 hrs: Perfusion status: HR 110 bpm; BP 140/85 mmHg; skin pale, warm, dry.

Respiratory status: RR 26 bpm, crackles bilaterally to midzones, speaking in phrases.

Conscious state: GCS = 15.

Careful monitoring of the physiological parameters, oximetry and ECG is appropriate, as is gaining an IV access point in case of deterioration.

④ EVALUATE

Evaluating the effect of any clinical management intervention can provide clues to the accuracy of the initial diagnosis. Some conditions respond rapidly to treatment so patients should be expected to improve if the diagnosis and treatment were appropriate. A failure to improve in this situation should trigger the clinician to reconsider the diagnosis. In this case the patient has deteriorated and this is a cue that the diagnosis may be flawed.

CASE STUDY 3

Case 11946, 1220 hrs.

Dispatch details: A 70-year-old male with shortness of breath and a previous history of cardiac problems and failure.

Initial presentation: The patient is sitting in his lounge room. His skin colour is normal.

 ASSESS

1230 hrs Vital signs: His airway is clear and he is able to speak in long sentences. His respiratory rate is 18 and he has a recurring cough. His pulse is 96 and his blood pressure is 150/90 mmHg. He has a normal skin colour and temperature. He has marked swelling of his ankles that extends to just below the knee. He has bilateral moist crackles at his lung bases. Oxygen saturations are 96%. His neck veins are distended and his JVP is raised.

1232 hrs Pertinent hx: The patient says that he has been getting gradually more short of breath for the last 12 hours and that the swelling has been getting worse over the last few days. He gives a history of chronic heart failure and is taking a variety of medications for this including digoxin, frusemide and captopril. He has severe arthritis, which was originally thought to be gout, and has recently begun taking a non-steroidal anti-inflammatory drug for this.

 CONFIRM

In many cases paramedics are presented with a collection of signs and symptoms that do not appear to describe a particular condition. A critical step in determining a treatment plan in this situation is to consider what other conditions could explain the patient's presentation.

What else could it be?
Acute pulmonary oedema
Although the paramedics were called because of the patient's acute shortness of breath, his history is of a more chronic exacerbation of shortness of breath. He has evidence of fluid retention with marked peripheral oedema and a raised JVP, which could be an indication of fluid overload or right heart failure, or both. He would appear to have pulmonary oedema as evidenced by the moist crackles.

Acute pulmonary oedema does not seem likely because of the gradual onset, lack of significant respiratory and cardiovascular embarrassment and lack of sympathetic response. It is possible for acute pulmonary oedema to complicate a background of chronic pulmonary oedema, in which case it would be relatively mild and early in its development, and although distressing him enough to call for an ambulance has not promoted a dramatic sympathetic response.

Acute renal failure
It is possible that renal failure precipitated by the non-steroidal anti-inflammatory drug was the last straw in the sequence of events. If this were the case he may have abnormal electrolytes, particularly a high potassium level (hyperkalaemia).

USING THE MNEMONIC DENT

Define:
- What is the patient's main presenting problem?
- Is this chronic pulmonary oedema?
- Does it fit the definition?

Explore your hypothesis and try to narrow it down.

What else could it be?
- Acute pulmonary oedema
- Acute renal failure
- Bilateral chest infection

High potassium can sometimes be detected through its effects on the T-wave of the ECG (high and peaked), but the significance of this observation is that high potassium can be associated with arrhythmia and therefore he might be at risk of a significant arrhythmia or even arrest. He gives no history of acute chest pain but a 12-lead ECG is still indicated in case he has undergone an acute coronary event. His pulse and blood pressure seem normal, implying adequate cardiac function.

The possibility of an acute deterioration in renal function precipitated by the anti-inflammatory drugs is worth considering but will not have an impact on his out-of-hospital care.

Infection

Infection is unlikely because the patient does not have a temperature and his lung signs are bilateral: infections tend to occur in localised areas so the affected areas will produce specific sounds. It would be highly unusual for the fields of both lungs to be equally affected.

3 TREAT

The patient clearly needs a clinical review either at hospital or with his own GP. His clinical state and shortness of breath are probably enough to warrant hospital investigation where x-rays and rapid access to blood tests are available. His need for emergency out-of-hospital intervention is less pressing.

1234 hrs: The paramedics withhold supplementary oxygen as the patient's oxygen saturations are being maintained at a reasonable level (94–98%). GTN is withheld as the patient's physiological status does not indicate a need for GTN.

The patient should undergo cardiac monitoring. IV access may be indicated if the paramedics suspect the potential for deterioration.

4 EVALUATE

Evaluating the effect of any clinical management intervention can provide clues to the accuracy of the initial diagnosis. Some conditions respond rapidly to treatment so patients should be expected to improve if the diagnosis and treatment were appropriate. A failure to improve in this situation should trigger the clinician to reconsider the diagnosis.

In this case the patient is stable and does not need immediate treatment. However, his condition could worsen with the exertion of being transferred to a stretcher. Increasing dyspnoea on exertion does not help identify a particular disease but the activity can generate previously opaque symptoms such as abnormal breath sounds.

Ongoing management

Ongoing management will be divided between assessing the cause of the patient's deterioration and adjusting the patient's medical therapy to return the fluid balance to normal. Assessment of the patient's renal function via a blood test is a high priority. Repeat 12-lead ECGs and cardiac enzymes are appropriate, as is a chest x-ray to further evaluate the extent of failure. Once again management will be slow and considered rather than rapid and urgent.

CASE STUDY 4

Case 00864, 0415 hrs.

Dispatch details: A 75-year-old female with acute shortness of breath. The call comes from her husband, who thinks she is dying.

Initial presentation: On arrival the crew find the patient lying in bed. She is unable to prop herself up on the pillows and is barely conscious.

① ASSESS

0423 hrs Vital signs: Her airway appears clear and she has a raised respiratory rate of 30 with moist rattling breaths. Her skin is pale and she is so sweaty that the monitor dots will not stick. Her pulse is thready and a radial pulse is not detectable. Her brachial pulse is 130 and seems to be irregular. Her blood pressure is not easy to obtain but turns out to be 70/40 mmHg. Auscultation of her chest confirms that the moist rattles extend to both sides and cover the whole chest. She is coughing some pink frothy sputum. The pulse oximeter is unable to take a reading and the ECG monitored through large pads shows a sinus rhythm with multiple multifocal ectopics. There is evidence of old Q waves and new ST elevation.

0425 hrs Pertinent hx: Her husband gives a history of multiple myocardial infarctions in the past and many admissions to hospital for chest pain and acute failure. She was a little more short of breath than usual on going to bed last night. She woke him in the early hours acutely short of breath and it is his impression that she has got worse since he called the ambulance. Her medication list is extensive and he offers to collect all the tablets for the paramedics.

② CONFIRM

In many cases paramedics are presented with a collection of signs and symptoms that do not appear to describe a particular condition. A critical step in determining a treatment plan in this situation is to consider what other conditions could explain the patient's presentation.

What else could it be?
The patient appears to be time-critical and could be classified as being in pre-arrest. The history and presentation are consistent with acute pulmonary oedema associated with poor myocardial function. Although she has the skin signs of sympathetic engagement, she has a very low blood pressure. Failure to maintain a blood pressure under the influence of maximal sympathetic stimulation is a reflection of the extent of her cardiac dysfunction. Not only does she have evidence of acute failure but the ECG is showing marked ST elevation, which must be presumed to be evidence of fresh ischaemic damage until proven otherwise.

Patients with acute pulmonary oedema maintain a high blood pressure due to the maximum sympathetic stimulation and the Frank-Starling mechanism.

USING THE MNEMONIC DENT

Define:
- What is the patient's main presenting problem?
- Is this acute pulmonary oedema?
- Does it fit the definition?
Explore your hypothesis and try to narrow it down.
What else could it be?
- Septic shock
- Hypovolaemic shock

Failure to maintain a blood pressure under these circumstances is indicative of an imminent arrest. The patient does not have enough cardiac function (due to a failure of the Frank- Starling mechanism) to respond to her sympathetic stimulation due to her underlying cardiac disease and profound myocardial hypoxia.

Septic shock
Septic shock is a possibility and could result in extremely low blood pressure and tachycardia. The chest signs could be explained only by a rapidly progressing pneumonia completely involving both lungs, which would be very unusual, particularly with this short onset time. If this were septic shock, then it is possible that she could be poorly perfused to the extent that she was pale and sweaty as opposed to the usual vasodilated appearance.

Hypovolaemic shock
Hypovolaemia could account for the shock but is not consistent with the lung findings. This patient also has no signs of revealed or concealed blood loss.

③ TREAT

The patient is acutely compromised and is in a near state of arrest. Apart from rapid mobilisation, the priority is to establish myocardial function with some cardiac output. GTN is out of the question for this patient.

0426 hrs: Reversing the profound myocardial hypoxia with positive pressure ventilation support might improve cardiac function, so positive pressure ventilation supporting the patient's own native respiratory rate is a strategy that is worth investing a lot of effort in. It ties up one crew member completely to do it properly. It will be extremely difficult to manage this case without backup. Paramedics must also be wary of increasing intrathoracic pressures above the already low pressures in the venous vessels returning to the heart.

0427 hrs: Having ascertained that this patient is in pre-arrest, it is imperative to get access before implementing other treatment or disturbing the patient.

If improving the ventilation with positive pressure support fails to produce an improvement, inotropes could be considered. Using an inotrope to support cardiac function is a very difficult judgment call as the increased myocardial workload might increase the extent of ventricular failure. Ideally this should be done in an emergency department or intensive care department, and the out-of-hospital aim is to try to get the patient to that setting.

0430 hrs: HR 135 bpm, BP 70/40 mmHg, RR 28 bpm, chest auscultation remains unchanged.

0431 hrs: The paramedics withhold fluid due to the chest auscultation indicating fluid in the lungs. Instead they elect to give low-dose inotropes at regular intervals. They administer 10 micrograms of adrenaline IV and plan to repeat this dose at 2-minute intervals, titrating the dose to effect; alternatively, they might commence an infusion via a syringe driver or pump at 5 micrograms per min.

0432 hrs: HR 125 bpm, BP 80/45 mmHg, RR 28 bpm, chest auscultation unchanged.

0433 hrs: Given the good result after the first dose, the paramedics elect to continue with incremental inotropes. They may consider slightly increasing the dosage. An infusion of inotropes can also be considered.

This patient is very delicate and needs to be carefully transferred and closely monitored en route to hospital.

EVALUATE

Evaluating the effect of any clinical management intervention can provide clues to the accuracy of the initial diagnosis. Some conditions respond rapidly to treatment so patients should be expected to improve if the diagnosis and treatment were appropriate. A failure to improve in this situation should trigger the clinician to reconsider the diagnosis.

In this case the patient has failed to improve with first-line management and remains dangerously poorly perfused. Failing to respond to basic care is not unusual in patients who are this ill with acute pulmonary oedema and acute pulmonary oedema is still the primary diagnosis.

Ongoing management

Evaluation of a patient such as in Case study 4 will be challenging because they will be too sick to demonstrate most of the signs that the paramedics would like to monitor. Their level of consciousness will give an indication of brain perfusion and oxygenation. A pulse oximeter is a useful evaluation tool because if perfusion improves to the point where it starts to read, this would indicate a significant improvement in the patient's status. ECG monitoring through large pads will provide information on rates but hopefully as myocardial oxygenation improves the frequency of ectopics will decrease. The most common cause of multifocal ectopics is myocardial hypoxia. BP assessment will be difficult and probably not useful during resuscitation. The return of a peripheral pulse at the wrist coinciding with the pulse oximeter beginning to monitor would indicate a BP of at least 80 mmHg and therefore an improvement. The feel of the bag when using it to assist ventilation with positive pressure will provide some feedback on lung condition and surfactant disbursement. Initially the lungs might feel extremely stiff but an improvement in compliance would be a positive sign.

Although presenting with acute pulmonary oedema, this is essentially one of the symptoms of the larger issue of cardiogenic shock. Like any resuscitation the key elements are quality of handover, clarity of communication and teamwork.

Future research

The use of CPAP in the field is in its infancy and there is still a role for research into the optimum role and use of CPAP. Management of oxygen delivery and ideal target partial pressures of oxygen in acute pulmonary oedema also require further research. The role of hypoxia in the pathogenesis of acute pulmonary oedema is now well understood but the optimum re-oxygenation strategy avoiding hypoxia may well generate research questions.

Summary

Management of acute pulmonary oedema has undergone considerable change over the last 20 years with the move away from diuretics and morphine to oxygen and nitrates. Acute pulmonary oedema is a very different problem from chronic fluid overload oedema: it presents differently and is managed differently. Acute pulmonary oedema can present with very similar signs to the acute exacerbation of respiratory disease in the initial phase.

The initial response to acute pulmonary oedema is sympathetic engagement, which will produce hypertension and perversely exacerbate the pulmonary oedema. Care must be taken in managing these patients, as any exertions or further stimulation of their sympathetic nervous system can result in a significant worsening of their condition. Severe pulmonary oedema can be a symptom of cardiogenic shock and, although the sympathetic system is still engaged, a hypertensive response is not possible.

References

Bhaskar, B., & Fraser, J. (2011). Negative pressure pulmonary edema revisited: pathophysiology and review of management. *Saudi Journal of Anaesthesia, 5*(3), 308–313.

Cleland, J. G. F., Yassin, A. S., & Khadjooi, K. (2010). Acute heart failure: focusing on acute cardiogenic pulmonary oedema. *Clinical Medicine, 10*(1), 59–64.

Collins, S. R., et al. (2013). Special article: the endothelial glycocalyx: emerging concepts in pulmonary edema and acute lung injury. *Anesthesia and Analgesia, 117*(3), 664–674.

Dieperink, W., et al. (2009). Treatment of presumed acute cardiogenic pulmonary oedema in an ambulance system by nurses using Boussignac continuous positive airway pressure. *Emergency Medicine Journal, 26*(2), 141–144.

Ducros, L., Logeart, D., Vicaut, E., Henry, P., Plaisance, P., Collet, J.-P., Broche, C., Gueye, P., Vergne, M., Goetgheber, D., Pennec, P.-Y., Belpomme, V., Tartière, J.-M., Lagarde, S., Placente, M., Fievet, M.-L., Montalescot, G., Payen, D., CPAP collaborative study group (2011). CPAP for acute cardiogenic pulmonary oedema from out-of-hospital to cardiac intensive care unit: a randomised multicentre study. *Intensive Care Medicine, 37*(9), 1501–1509.

Hall, J. E. (2010). *Guyton & Hall textbook of medical physiology* (12th ed.). Philadelphia: Saunders.

Hopkins, S. R., Garg, J., Bolar, D. S., Balouch, J., & Levin, D. L. (2005). Pulmonary blood flow heterogeneity during hypoxia and high-altitude pulmonary edema. *American Journal of Respiratory and Critical Care Medicine, 171*(1), 83–87.

Hubble, M., Richards, M., & Wilfong, D. (2008). Estimates of cost effectiveness of prehospital continuous positive pressure in the management of acute pulmonary edema. *Prehospital Emergency Care, 12*(3), 277–285.

Kallio, T., Kuisma, M., Alaspää, A., & Rosenberg, P. H. (2003). The use of prehospital continuous positive airway pressure treatment in presumed acute severe pulmonary edema. *Prehospital Emergency Care, 7*(2), 209–213.

Kapoor, M. (2011). Negative pressure pulmonary oedema. *Indian Journal of Anesthesia, 55*(1), 10–11.

Kosmidou, I., Karmpaliotis, D., Kirtane, A. J., Barron, H. V., & Gibson, C. M. (2008). Vascular endothelial growth factors in pulmonary edema: an update. *Journal of Thrombosis and Thrombolysis, 25*(3), 259–264.

Marco, F. D., Tresoldi, S., Maggiolini, S., Bozzano, A., Bellani, G., Pesenti, A., & Fumagalli, R. (2008). Risk factors for treatment failure in patients with severe acute cardiogenic pulmonary oedema. *Anaesthesia and Intensive Care, 36*(3), 351–359.

McCance, K., & Huether, S. (2014). *Pathophysiology: the biologic basis for disease in adults and children* (7th ed.). Philadelphia: Mosby.

Nieto Estrada, V. H., Molano Franco, D., Medina, R. D., Gonzalez Garay, A. G., Martí-Carvajal, A. J., & Arevalo-Rodriguez, I. (2017). Interventions for preventing high-altitude illness: part 1. Commonly-used classes of drugs. *The Cochrane Database of Systematic Reviews*, (6), CD009761.

Noelkel, N. F. (2002). High-altitude pulmonary edema. *The New England Journal of Medicine, 346*(21), 1606–1607.

Pillai, L., Ambike, D., Saifuddin, H., Vishwasrao, S., Pataskar, S., & Kulkarni, S. (2005). Severe lung injury following inhalation of nitric acid fumes. *Indian Journal of Critical Care Medicine: Peer-Reviewed, Official Publication of Indian Society of Critical Care Medicine, 9*(4), 244–247.

Plaisance, P., Pirracchio, R., Berton, C., Vicaut, E., & Payen, D. (2007). A randomized study of out-of-hospital continuous positive airway pressure for acute cardiogenic pulmonary oedema: physiological and clinical effects. *European Heart Journal, 28*(23), 2895–2901.

Slader, J. B., Jr, Hattori, T., Ray, C. S., Bove, A. A., & Cianci, P. (2001). Pulmonary edema associated with scuba diving: case reports and review. *Chest, 120*(5), 1686–1694.

CHAPTER 19

Chronic Obstructive Pulmonary Disease

By Ziad Nehme

OVERVIEW

- Chronic obstructive pulmonary disease (COPD) is a leading cause of morbidity and mortality worldwide, with projections it will become the third leading cause of death worldwide by 2020.
- In Australia and New Zealand, COPD is the sixth- and fifth-highest cause of death, respectively, and affects as many as 14% of people aged 40 years or more.
- Cigarette smoking is the single most important risk factor for the development of COPD. Half of all smokers develop some degree of airflow limitation and persistent respiratory symptoms, and approximately 15–20% develop COPD.
- Individuals with COPD often have a reduced quality of life and require frequent hospitalisations as the disease progresses.
- COPD is a preventable disease but it can take up to 20 years of smoking before it becomes symptomatic. Diagnosis is usually too late to reverse the underlying tissue damage.

- The pulmonary component of COPD is characterised by chronic airflow limitation that is not fully reversible.
- An acute exacerbation of COPD is associated with acute worsening of airflow limitation and dyspnoea. These acute exacerbations are usually caused by respiratory infections and often generate a call for an emergency ambulance.
- COPD has a range of significant extra-pulmonary and systemic effects that vary from person to person and can lead to a variety of co-existing illnesses and conditions.
- Determining the cause of sudden dyspnoea in a patient with COPD is challenging due to their already altered respiratory function and the systemic nature of the disease.
- Bronchodilators and steroids are currently the mainstay of therapy for exacerbations of COPD.

Introduction

Chronic obstructive pulmonary disease (COPD) is a common, preventable and treatable disease that is characterised by persistent respiratory symptoms in response to a combination of structural pulmonary changes, including small airways disease and parenchymal destruction (GOLD, 2018). Internationally, COPD is a leading cause of morbidity and mortality, and is expected to become the third-highest cause of death in the world by 2020 (GOLD, 2018). In Australia and New Zealand, COPD is the sixth- and fifth-highest cause of death, respectively, and affects as many as 14% of people aged 40 years or more (Toelle et al., 2013; Shirtcliffe et al., 2012; Yang et al., 2018). The burden of disease from COPD is also up to five times higher among Indigenous Australians and Māori peoples.

Although medical literature favours the terms 'emphysema' and 'chronic bronchitis' as two distinct and major precipitators, COPD is a highly heterogeneous disorder which is typically characterised by a combination of these pathologies evolving at different rates over time (GOLD, 2018). Emphysema, or destruction of the lung tissues (alveoli), is a pathological term used to describe only one component of the several structural changes present in COPD. Similarly, chronic bronchitis is present in only a minority of people when this definition is used in isolation. This highlights the complex and heterogeneous nature of COPD pathogenesis, which can vary considerably from person to person.

The primary cause of COPD is long-term tobacco smoking, but exposure to occupational pollutants can also contribute to this debilitating disease. The chronic inflammatory response of the lungs to noxious particles or gases can be severe. In addition to lung structural changes, established COPD results in a number of systemic changes which increase the risk of death and disability from a range of co-existing disorders. The slow development of the disease usually means that the effects are well-established and mostly irreversible by the time a diagnosis is made (see Fig 19.1), but the disease can be managed effectively in most patients provided they adhere to their prescribed medications and modify their lifestyle (e.g. cease smoking).

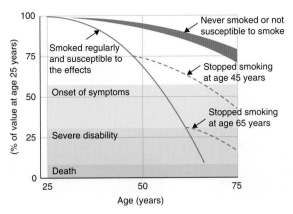

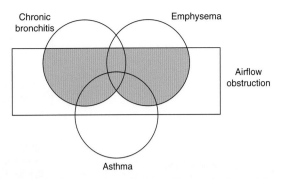

Figure 19.2
COPD is a heterogeneous condition, involving three main phenotypes: asthma, chronic bronchitis and emphysema.

Figure 19.1
The time course of smoking and the changes with smoking cessation at 45 and 65 years of age. Notice that for the smoker who quit at age 45, the serious progression of COPD is much slower than that for the smoker who quit at age 65. In both cases, the disease progression is slower than for those who continue smoking.
Source: Craft, Gordon & Tiziani (2011); Fletcher & Peto (1997).

While adherence to medications and lifestyle modifications can enable people with COPD to remain living in the community, their lung function may be so compromised that common respiratory infections can lead to intractable dyspnoea. While a common and logical link exists between COPD and infections causing an acute exacerbation, the systemic changes associated with the disease mean that infections are not the only cause of acute dyspnoea in COPD patients. Understanding and assessing for the presence of these other diseases is essential if paramedics are to deliver safe and effective treatment in the out-of-hospital setting.

Pathophysiology

COPD involves progressive, largely irreversible damage to the airways with resulting airflow limitation (GOLD, 2018). The principal aetiology responsible for these changes is the inhalation of noxious gases, the most common of these being cigarette smoke. Exposure to these irritants activates a number of inflammatory processes in the lower airways that permanently alter the structure and function of the tissue.

Emphysema and chronic bronchitis are typically described as two of the most common precipitators of COPD. Although they have distinct pathologies themselves, there is a high degree of overlap in most patients. In addition, the underlying inflammatory response in COPD shares much of the same pathophysiology as asthma (see Fig 19.2). Chronic

inflammation of the airways leads to irreversible structural changes and airway damage through a process of ongoing injury and repair (see Fig 19.3). The changes occur throughout the airway structures, including the proximal and distal portions of the airway, the lung parenchyma and the pulmonary vasculature (see Fig 19.4). COPD is a complex and highly heterogeneous condition, meaning that a number of different pathological changes can be occurring simultaneously, but evolving at different rates over time. As such, the condition varies considerably from person to person.

The hallmark physiological abnormalities of COPD include mucus hypersecretion, airflow limitation and gas-trapping, gas exchange abnormalities, pulmonary hypertension and other systemic effects (GOLD, 2018).

Emphysema

Emphysema is a pathological term used to describe the breakdown of alveolar tissue due to a loss of elastin. This occurs without significant scar tissue being formed and the end effect is a loss of gas exchange surface area and lung elasticity. It is the loss of elastic recoil that normally assists with expiration that causes inhaled air to become 'trapped' in alveoli, leading to airflow limitation (McCance & Huether, 2014). The loss of surface area for gas exchange also leads to progressively worsening chronic hypoxaemia and hypercapnia (see Figs 19.5 and 19.6).

The loss of elastin and the breakdown of the alveolar walls occurs due to an imbalance between the inflammatory mediators triggered by smoking (specifically the protease and antiprotease mediators). The breakdown of tissue can be exacerbated if an individual has an inherited deficiency of the enzyme alpha$_1$-antitrypsin: this enzyme inhibits the breakdown of proteins, and homozygous individuals who

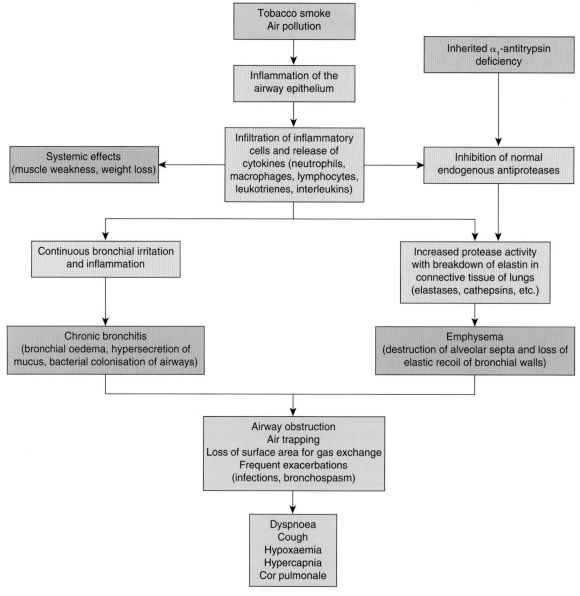

Figure 19.3
Pathogenesis of chronic bronchitis and emphysema (COPD).
Source: McCance & Huether (2014).

have alpha₁-antitrypsin deficiency have a 70–80% likelihood of developing emphysema (McCance & Huether, 2014). Alpha₁-antitrypsin deficiency is the most likely cause of emphysema in individuals who are non-smokers or who develop the disease before the age of 40.

The enlargement of the alveoli increases the residual volume of the lungs and causes hyperinflation of the chest. Even without changes to airway resistance this hyperinflation reduces the effectiveness of both the diaphragm and the accessory muscles during inspiration and leads to an increase in the

work of breathing throughout the ventilatory cycle (O'Donnell & Parker, 2006; Yang et al., 2018).

Although widely used as a clinical term, emphysema is a pathological process used to describe only one of the many structural changes occurring in patients with COPD. In fact, only 10% of patients with COPD have emphysema as the sole physiological finding (Marsh et al., 2008).

Chronic bronchitis

Chronic bronchitis is defined as the presence of productive cough and increased sputum production

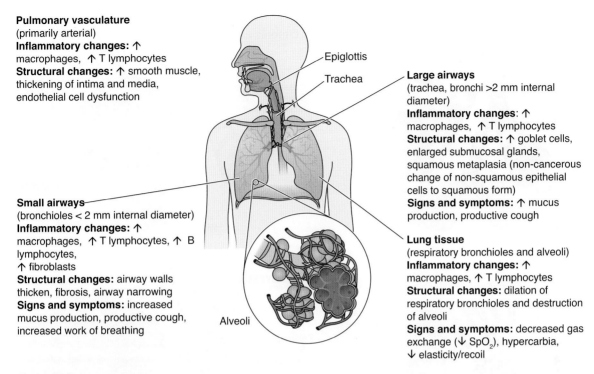

Pulmonary vasculature
(primarily arterial)
Inflammatory changes: ↑
macrophages, ↑ T lymphocytes
Structural changes: ↑ smooth muscle,
thickening of intima and media,
endothelial cell dysfunction

Epiglottis

Trachea

Large airways
(trachea, bronchi >2 mm internal
diameter)
Inflammatory changes: ↑
macrophages, ↑ T lymphocytes
Structural changes: ↑ goblet cells,
enlarged submucosal glands,
squamous metaplasia (non-cancerous
change of non-squamous epithelial
cells to squamous form)
Signs and symptoms: ↑ mucus
production, productive cough

Small airways
(bronchioles < 2 mm internal diameter)
Inflammatory changes: ↑
macrophages, ↑ T lymphocytes, ↑ B
lymphocytes,
↑ fibroblasts
Structural changes: airway walls
thicken, fibrosis, airway narrowing
Signs and symptoms: increased
mucus production, productive cough,
increased work of breathing

Alveoli

Lung tissue
(respiratory bronchioles and alveoli)
Inflammatory changes: ↑
macrophages, ↑ T lymphocytes
Structural changes: dilation of
respiratory bronchioles and destruction
of alveoli
Signs and symptoms: decreased gas
exchange (↓ SpO_2), hypercarbia,
↓ elasticity/recoil

Figure 19.4
Inflammation is the underlying pathology involved in COPD. A specific pattern of inflammation that involves
neutrophils, macrophages and lymphocytes characterises the disease and over time leads to structural
changes in the lung tissue and function. These changes cause the classic signs and symptoms of COPD.
Source: Adapted from Castro & Kraft (2008); GOLD (2018).

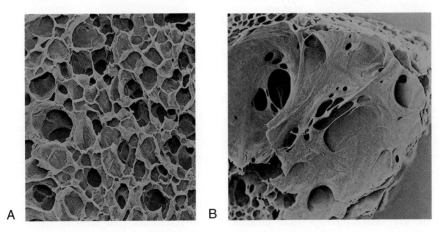

Figure 19.5
The effects of emphysema on the gas exchange units. **A** Normal lung with many small alveoli. **B** Lung tissue
affected by emphysema. Notice that the alveoli have merged into larger air spaces, reducing the surface area
for gas exchange.
Source: Thibodeau (2010).

for at least 3 months of the year for 2 consecutive years (GOLD, 2018). Compared with the tissue breakdown associated with emphysema, the inflammatory mediators in chronic bronchitis result in more typical bronchial reactions: mucosal swelling and increased mucus production (see Fig 19.6). The prolonged inflammatory reactions to the inhaled irritants are different from the acute changes associated with short-term infections. In the case of chronic bronchitis, the airways become

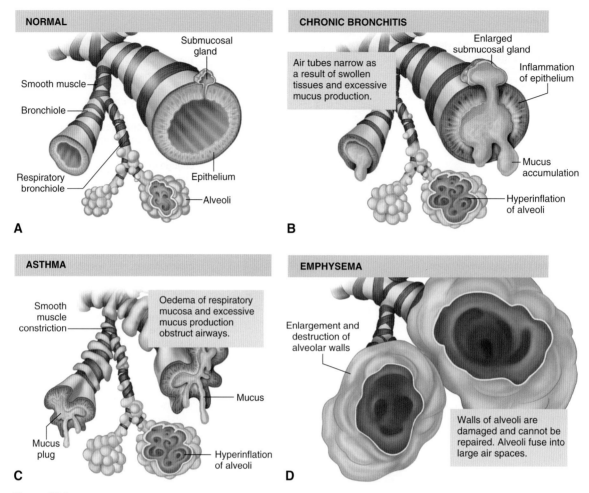

Figure 19.6
Examples of chronic disorders involving pulmonary obstruction.
Source: Patton & Thibodeau (2010).

oedematous and permanently narrowed, the mucus-secreting cells become enlarged and more numerous (producing a more tenacious sputum) and the cilia lining the airway become impaired (McCance & Huether, 2014). Together these changes make further infections not only more likely but also more severe. Bronchospasm and hypertrophy of the bronchial smooth muscle are characteristics that chronic bronchitis shares with chronic asthma, and the two diseases are difficult to differentiate if the patient suffers from both. As the disease becomes more established, the lungs are unable to exchange gas efficiently and hypercapnia and hypoxaemia develop.

Pulmonary hypertension

Late in the course of COPD, worsening alveolar hypoxia and ventilation-perfusion (V/Q) mismatch leads to the activation of hypoxic pulmonary vasoconstriction: a compensatory mechanism designed to redirect blood flow away from poorly ventilated alveoli in order to improve gas exchange (O'Driscoll et al., 2017). Chronic exposure to pulmonary vasoconstriction results in structural changes to the small pulmonary arteries, including intimal hyperplasia and smooth muscle hypertrophy (GOLD, 2018). The inflammatory response in the pulmonary arteries also resembles that seen in the airways, with the destruction of the capillary beds further contributing to the pressure in the pulmonary vasculature. Over time persistent pulmonary hypertension causes right ventricle enlargement, dysfunction and subsequent right heart failure (GOLD, 2018). The terms 'pulmonary heart disease' or '*cor pulmonale*' are commonly attributed to development of right heart failure precipitated by pulmonary hypertension. Ankle oedema is a late feature seen in patients with COPD and cor pulmonale (Yang et al., 2018).

Right ventricle dilation may also impair left ventricle function by shifting the interventricular septum towards the left ventricle, impairing left ventricle filling (O'Donnell & Parker, 2006).

Systemic effects

While often considered a respiratory disease, COPD is also associated with a number of extra-pulmonary pathologies. The mechanism behind these effects is not always clear, but it is most likely to be an extension of the inflammatory processes into the systemic circulation, impacting on skeletal muscle function and endothelial function (Hansel et al., 2009). Cachexia and skeletal muscle wasting are commonly seen in COPD and may be directly related to the circulating inflammatory mediators as well as the significant decline in physical activity brought about by the disease. The risk factors for COPD, such as smoking, ageing and inactivity, also increase the risk of concomitant diseases including ischaemic heart disease, heart failure, osteoporosis and diabetes (GOLD, 2018). Chronic exposure to hypoxaemia in COPD leads to the production of excess red blood cells, a condition called polycythaemia. Combined with long sedentary periods and inactivity, polycythaemia can increase the risk of thrombosis, including deep vein thrombosis, pulmonary embolus, stroke and acute coronary syndromes.

Acute exacerbations of COPD

The natural history of COPD is characterised by progressive deterioration of the condition with episodes of acute deterioration in symptoms referred to as an exacerbation. Acute exacerbations of COPD are commonly triggered by infectious and non-infectious precipitants. They are associated with worsening respiratory symptoms and are a leading cause of unscheduled out-of-hospital and emergency care. Although as many as 30% of acute exacerbations of COPD have no known trigger, the majority are caused by viral or bacterial (or both) respiratory tract infections (Ko et al., 2016). Non-infectious triggers, such as air pollution, meteorological factors, concomitant conditions (e.g. pulmonary embolism,

heart failure) and non-compliance with long-term therapy are also thought to exacerbate COPD (Ko et al., 2016).

Patients with acute exacerbations of COPD will often present with tachypnoea, tachycardia, use of accessory muscles, tracheal tugging and cyanosis. However, their clinical presentation can vary considerably, and is dependent on a number of factors such as the patient's age, co-existing illness, baseline severity of airflow limitation, and the underlying trigger. There is no confirmatory diagnostic test for exacerbations of COPD, so assessment of the patient should focus on evaluating the severity of the episode, providing symptomatic relief and managing the underlying precipitant were possible (e.g. infection). The assessment should involve determining the normal status of the disease in the patient and the precipitants of this exacerbation.

Definitions

The Global Initiative for Chronic Obstructive Lung Disease (GOLD) defines COPD as a progressive, preventable and treatable disease which is characterised predominantly by airflow limitation which is not fully reversible (GOLD, 2018). In clinical practice, the diagnosis of COPD is based on the presence of three criteria: 1. the presence of symptoms such as exertional breathlessness, cough and sputum production; 2. a history of smoking, or exposure to other noxious agents, and; 3. after using a bronchodilator, the proportion of vital capacity that can be expired in the first second of forced expiration is less than 70% (referred to as the FEV_1/FVC ratio, which is estimated using spirometry).

An exacerbation of COPD is defined as an event in the natural course of the disease that is characterised by a change in the patient's baseline dyspnoea, cough and/or sputum that is beyond normal day to day variations, is acute in onset, and may warrant a change in regular medication.

(GOLD, 2018)

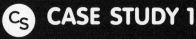

CASE STUDY 1

Case 10587, 0835 hrs.

Dispatch details: A 68-year-old male who has difficulty breathing.

Initial presentation: The ambulance crew find the patient sitting upright at his kitchen table. His skin is pale and he is complaining of shortness of breath. He is on oxygen via nasal prongs. He has a 10-year history of COPD and has had a productive cough for 4 days.

 ASSESS

Patient history

This case suggests an exacerbation of COPD. Exacerbations of COPD are highly variable in their presentation, which reflects the heterogeneity of the underlying pathology. As it is virtually impossible to determine the baseline severity of COPD in the out-of-hospital setting, particularly during acute exacerbations, the Modified Medical Research Council Dyspnoea Scale can be used to provide paramedics with a snapshot of the effect of COPD and breathlessness on daily activities (Celli et al., 2004; see Table 19.1). The assessment provides an important insight into the baseline severity of COPD, which is valuable for contextualising the severity of exacerbations. Importantly, a higher Modified Medical Research Council Dyspnoea Scale grade correlates with an increased risk of mortality (Celli et al., 2004).

In an acute exacerbation it is also important to identify symptoms such as fever, increased cough and/or sputum production, the nature of the sputum (colour, purulence), chest pain suggestive of pulmonary embolism (PE) or pneumothorax, coexisting illnesses and compliance with the use of existing pharmacological therapies. Winter months see an increase in viral infections and can further increase exacerbation frequencies (Yang et al., 2018). It is often difficult to distinguish the cause of the respiratory distress in the patient with COPD, particularly in the out-of-hospital setting with limited access to

Table 19.1: Modified Medical Research Council Dyspnoea Scale

Grade	Description
0	I only get breathless with strenuous exercise
1	I get short of breath when hurrying on level ground or walking up a slight hill
2	On level ground, I walk more slowly than people of the same age because of breathlessness, or I have to stop for breath when walking at my own pace on the level
3	I stop for breath after walking about 100 metres or after a few minutes on level ground
4	I am too breathless to leave the house or I am breathless when dressing or undressing

Source: Celli et al. (2004); Yang et al. (2018).

investigative procedures such as chest x-ray and blood analysis. Assessment of the patient must be thorough and use all available means at the paramedic's disposal.

Airway

It is important to ensure that the upper airway is clear. It is also prudent to ensure that the cause of the respiratory distress is not due to a foreign body, food or excessive secretions that may be difficult to clear.

Breathing

If there is sufficient air movement, bronchospasm and airway narrowing will usually present with severe wheezing and a prolonged expiratory phase or, if air movement is insufficient, there may be no wheeze heard (Shujaat et al., 2007). Sputum changes in volume, thickness and colour should be assessed. Purulent sputum reflects an increase in inflammatory mediators and may indicate the presence of bacteria (GOLD, 2018). In this case study, the patient has bilateral wheezes on auscultation.

Patients adopt a rapid shallow breathing pattern, where expiratory flow is further limited and the expiratory time during spontaneous respirations is insufficient to allow the end-expiratory and residual volume to return to baseline, resulting in lung hyperinflation. This hyperinflation, where there is an acute and variable increase in the end-expiratory lung volume with a reduction in inspiratory capacity, is called dynamic hyperinflation (O'Donnell & Parker, 2006). The degree of dynamic hyperinflation is due to the severity of airflow limitation, the tidal volume and the expiratory time.

Dynamic hyperinflation impacts on respiratory mechanics and gas exchange. Normal tidal volumes shift towards total lung capacity, and there is a corresponding reduction in inspiratory capacity and inspiratory reserve volume. This has the effect of limiting tidal volume expansion despite the increasing inspiratory effort seen in patients with COPD (O'Donnell & Parker, 2006). The respiratory muscles compensate adequately while breathing at rest; however, during exercise or exacerbation, patients with dynamic hyperinflation can quickly overwhelm respiratory muscles leading to fatigue and weakness. As a result of expiratory flow limitation, intrapulmonary pressures remain positive at the end of the expiration cycle, a process called intrinsic or 'auto' peak end-expiratory pressure. At the commencement of the next cycle of ventilation, inspiratory muscles need to work harder to create the negative intrathoracic pressures required to initiate inspiration (O'Donnell & Parker, 2006).

The neural drive to breathe increases during exacerbations, but the ability of the respiratory muscles to respond when they are already under increased load, weaker and functionally impaired due to dynamic hyperinflation may not increase in the same proportion as the neural response (O'Donnell & Parker, 2006). The end result is increased loading and functional weakness of the muscles of respiration. The accessory muscles of breathing are maximally recruited and in severe respiratory failure the diaphragm weakness may present as paradoxical breathing (O'Donnell & Parker, 2006).

In this case study, the patient is presenting with a prolonged expiratory phase and a mild increase in the use of his accessory muscles, indicating that expiratory flow limitation and dynamic hyperinflation are underway.

Cardiovascular

Tachycardia, as seen in this patient, is common in severe unstable COPD and is associated with the increased work of breathing and hypoxaemia (Yang et al., 2018). Haemodynamic instability is a sign of a severe exacerbation (GOLD, 2018), which is often the result of dynamic hyperinflation reducing right ventricular preload and venous return (O'Donnell & Parker, 2006).

HISTORY

Ask!

- How long have you had lung disease?
- What medications are you taking and how long have you been taking them? (This can be an important indication as to the onset and severity of COPD.)
- Are you or were you a smoker? How long have you been smoking? How much do you smoke?
- Do you have home oxygen? If so, what flow rate? What is the duration of use each time you require it?
- How frequently have you been admitted to hospital for exacerbations of COPD? When was the last time? Have you ever been admitted to ICU?
- What other treatments have you received on previous ED presentations (e.g. non-invasive ventilation)?
- When did you start to experience the symptoms leading to this episode?
- Has there been any change or limitation to your daily activities?
- Do you have a cough? Is the cough worse than usual? If so, is it dry or productive?
- Have you produced sputum? If so, what are the changes in the character (colour, volume, thickness)?

HISTORY

Look for!

Signs of severe exacerbations, which might include:

- use of accessory respiratory muscles
- paradoxical chest wall movement
- worsening or central cyanosis
- development of peripheral oedema
- haemodynamic instability
- signs of right heart failure
- drowsiness/altered conscious state.

Signs of right heart failure, peripheral oedema (ankle swelling) and elevated jugular venous pressure (JVP) may be evident. Signs may also be evident in the ECG, with P pulmonale, right axis deviation, dominant R waves in V1–V2, right bundle branch block and ST depression and flattened T waves in V1–V3. However, differentiating acute from chronic ECG changes may be difficult in this setting. The development of right heart failure in COPD has a poorer prognosis (GOLD, 2018). In this case study, the patient has mild tachycardia but no other signs of haemodynamic instability are present.

Skin

Cyanosis, particularly central cyanosis, is a sign of a severe exacerbation and may indicate impending respiratory failure (GOLD, 2018). Fever may be present; however, fewer than 50% of patients with an acute exacerbation have fever (Shujaat et al., 2007). High fever may be associated with pneumonia (Shujaat et al., 2007). This patient has a mild fever but is not showing any signs of cyanosis.

Conscious state

Drowsiness, confusion and altered conscious state are signs of a severe exacerbation (GOLD, 2018). Patients with impending respiratory failure due to an exacerbation of COPD will have hypoxaemia with varying degrees of carbon dioxide retention and acidosis (O'Driscoll et al., 2017). In the out-of-hospital setting, without access to blood gas analysis, altered conscious state may be the only sign of impending respiratory failure. This patient does not have an altered conscious state.

Initial assessment summary

Problem	Shortness of breath
Conscious state	GCS = 15
Position	Sitting
Heart rate	108 bpm
Blood pressure	115/70 mmHg
Skin appearance	Pale, warm, dry
Speech pattern	Phrases
Respiratory rate	34 bpm
Respiratory rhythm	Prolonged expiratory phase
Respiratory effort	Mild increase in accessory muscle use
Chest auscultation	Bilateral wheeze
Pulse oximetry	88%
Temperature	37.8°C
Motor/sensory function	Normal
History	Recent chest infection

D: There are no obvious dangers.
A: The patient is conscious with no current airway obstruction.
B: Respiratory function is currently increased but the tidal volume remains adequate. Needs frequent reassessment.
C: Heart rate is elevated but there is sufficient blood pressure.

The patient is displaying the respiratory and cardiovascular symptoms of an infective exacerbation of COPD.

2 CONFIRM

The essential part of the clinical reasoning process is to seek to confirm your initial hypothesis by finding clinical signs that should occur with your provisional diagnosis. You should also seek to challenge your diagnosis by exploring findings that do not fit your hypothesis: don't just ignore them because they don't fit.

The causes of dyspnoea are numerous and the symptom of dyspnoea is common to a number of disease processes. It is often difficult to differentiate an exacerbation of COPD from other causes of dyspnoea due to the limitations of out-of-hospital assessment tools.

What else could it be?

Asthma

COPD can coexist with asthma, and while the underlying mechanism of the chronic inflammation differs, the acute presentation of respiratory symptoms (e.g. wheeze, cough and dyspnoea) and fixed airflow limitation can be common between them. Although it can be difficult to differentiate between them, a key often lies in the patient's medical history. COPD is seen more commonly in the older population, presents as chronic airflow limitation that does not completely resolve and is often accompanied by chronic sputum production. Asthma occurs in response to a precipitant (allergen, weather, exercise), generally responds well to beta$_2$ agonists and inhaled steroids (Global Initiative for Asthma, 2018) and is not usually associated with sputum production. Although asthma often begins in childhood, late-onset asthma (> 40 years old) is not uncommon: it may occur in up to 10% of lifetime non-smokers and is often associated with gastro-oesophageal reflux disease (GOLD, 2018). Although the aetiologies are different, first-line management of acute exacerbations of both diseases in the out-of-hospital setting is similar.

Congestive heart failure

It can be difficult to distinguish heart failure, particularly left-sided failure, from an acute exacerbation of COPD. This difficulty is compounded as approximately one-third of heart failure patients have concurrent COPD (Hawkins et al., 2011). Both conditions are common to smokers, with the prevalence of COPD greater in patients with heart failure than the general population. The systemic inflammation associated with COPD may contribute to atherosclerosis, leading to adverse cardiac events (GOLD, 2018).

Delineating between an acute exacerbation of COPD and acute heart failure requires the paramedic to be diligent and thorough in the history and physical examination. Indications that heart failure is the underlying cause of dyspnoea could include: a past history of heart failure; the presence of crackles on auscultation; the presence of paroxysmal nocturnal dyspnoea and the absence of dyspnoea on exertion; a third heart sound (S3) gallop; and atrial fibrillation on the electrocardiogram (Wang et al., 2005).

Pneumonia

The signs of dyspnoea, cough and sputum production are also common to patients with pneumonia. Differentiating between the two may be possible only with x-ray imaging. Pneumonia patients have been found to have higher fevers and a more acute onset of illness (Shujaat et al., 2007). However, the differentiation between the two conditions is not clinically meaningful in the out-of-hospital setting, and treatment is usually focused on the symptomatic relief of symptoms.

Pleural effusion

Pleural effusion may exacerbate dyspnoea in COPD. It may also be secondary to other exacerbating pathologies such as pneumonia. Auscultation may reveal decreased or absent breath sounds which is usually limited to one side (Shujaat et al., 2007).

Pneumothorax

Lung diseases with chronic airflow limitation, such as COPD and asthma, are associated with the majority of secondary spontaneous pneumothorax cases

---

DIFFERENTIAL DIAGNOSIS

Exacerbation of COPD
Or
- Asthma
- Congestive heart failure
- Pneumonia
- Pleural effusion
- Pneumothorax
- Pulmonary embolism
- Acute coronary syndrome or arrhythmia

(Bintcliffe & Maskell, 2014). In fact, COPD is responsible for almost 60% of all cases of secondary spontaneous pneumothoraces, and the risk increases with worsening airflow limitation. Pneumothorax should be suspected if there is a reduction in lung expansion and a decrease in air entry to one side (Bintcliffe & Maskell, 2014).

Pulmonary embolism

Approximately one in six patients with a preliminary diagnosis of acute COPD will be found to have a pulmonary embolism (Aleva et al., 2017). In the out-of-hospital setting, pulmonary embolism can be difficult to distinguish from an exacerbation of COPD. Clinical factors associated with an increased risk of pulmonary embolism in patients with COPD are pleuritic chest pain, hypotension, syncope and the absence of signs of respiratory tract infection (Aleva et al., 2017).

Acute coronary syndrome or arrhythmia

The nature of any cardiac pain should be explored. The ECG may assist in identifying any ischaemia or arrhythmia.

This patient has obvious worsening dyspnoea beyond his normal daily variations. He has had a recent cold, a precipitant of an exacerbation and an indication of a potentially more severe episode. His elevated temperature is also suggestive of an underlying infection. His dyspnoea is still present despite treatment with his usual medications and oxygen.

Chest auscultation has revealed a wheeze, which may not respond as effectively to bronchodilators in COPD as in asthma. His oxygen saturations (SpO_2) at 88% are on the low end of the target range for patients on home oxygen: the target range is SpO_2 between 88 and 92% (Yang et al., 2018). He has no cardiac history, but given that he is on home oxygen therapy, he may have underlying pulmonary hypertension and right heart failure (Yang et al., 2018). The ECG may also assist in identifying signs of heart failure.

How severe is the exacerbation?

Clinically the patient is tachypnoeic, tachycardic and pale with SpO_2 of 88% on 3 L/min, which would indicate moderate respiratory distress. However, he is most likely to have severe COPD, being on home oxygen therapy, where exacerbations may be life-threatening (GOLD, 2018). This may potentially lead to worsening respiratory failure, with subsequent respiratory acidosis, hypoxaemia and hypercapnia, where prognosis is poorer (Yang et al., 2018). There are no signs of crackles consistent with heart failure on chest auscultation. He has not described any chest pain. The severity of the exacerbation must also take account of the work of breathing, speech, accessory respiratory muscle use, retractive breathing and signs of an extremely severe exacerbation with imminent respiratory failure, fatigue and paradoxical respirations.

(3) TREAT

Emergency management

Management of an acute exacerbation is directed at relieving dyspnoea and associated symptoms. Exacerbations with an increased volume and/or change in the colour of sputum and/or fever may benefit from antibiotics (Yang et al., 2017). In the out-of-hospital setting, optimal management involves correcting hypoxia, treating airflow limitation (bronchospasm, inflammation) and optimising ventilation.

Position

The patient with an acute exacerbation of COPD will most likely adopt an upright sitting or tripod position (elbows or hands resting on knees or other surface), which helps to optimise respiratory mechanics (Kim et al., 2012). This assists with the use of accessory muscles and the work of breathing. The patient should be encouraged into this position if not already in it. It is unlikely that hypotension will be present unless there is another factor complicating the presentation. If this is the case, a recumbent position may be possible but it will most likely depend on the patient's respiratory function.

It is important to note that when moving or transferring a patient with an acute exacerbation of COPD, this alters the sitting position they have adopted to maximise their ventilation. The patient may experience a worsening of their condition during or after they have moved; if necessary, allow them to assume a more physiologically favourable position when feasible and safe to do so. This can include allowing them to sit with their feet off the stretcher once they are in the ambulance.

Oxygen therapy

The deleterious effects of high-concentration oxygen therapy in acute exacerbations of COPD have been widely documented. Acute COPD patients who arrive at hospital with a high PaO_2 (> 75 mmHg) are more likely to develop hypercapnia and acidosis, and have an increased dependence on in-hospital care, including non-invasive ventilation (NIV) and ICU admission (Plant et al., 2000; Wijesinghe et al., 2011). An out-of-hospital randomised controlled trial conducted in Australia showed that maintaining peripheral SpO_2 within the range of 88–92% reduces mortality and acidosis in patients with acute exacerbations of COPD (Austin et al., 2010). Unfortunately, a number of studies point to the uncontrolled use of oxygen therapy by paramedics and other emergency practitioners, because of either misdiagnosis or a misunderstanding of the risks associated with hyperoxia in COPD patients (O'Driscoll et al., 2017).

Between 20 and 50% of patients with acute exacerbations of COPD are at risk of carbon dioxide retention if they are given excessive amounts of oxygen (O'Driscoll et al., 2017). Although it is paramount to administer supplemental oxygen to COPD patients with clinical evidence of hypoxia and hypoxaemia, its overzealous use can also lead to hypercapnia. The mechanisms involved in oxygen-induced hypercapnia are complex and have not been completely elucidated. Literature as far back as the 1940s suggested that patients with COPD were dependent on low blood oxygen to stimulate breathing (known as the 'hypoxic drive'), and removal of the stimulus with supplemental oxygen would lead to hypoventilation and the subsequent retention of carbon dioxide (Abdo & Heunks, 2012). Despite being widely taught to medical professions, a reduction in ventilation drive after oxygen administration contributes to only a transient increase in blood carbon dioxide levels (Abdo & Heunks, 2012; O'Driscoll et al., 2017).

There are a number of other mechanisms which can help explain oxygen-induced hypercapnia. First, oxygen therapy inhibits hypoxic pulmonary vasoconstriction, a compensatory mechanism designed to redirect blood flow away from poorly ventilated alveoli. Inhibition of pulmonary vasoconstriction leads to an increase in dead space and decreases the amount of carbon dioxide that can participate in gas exchange. Second, because deoxygenated haemoglobin has a higher capacity for carbon dioxide carriage, administration of excessive amounts of oxygen can lead to a reduction in the amount of carbon dioxide offloading in the lungs (i.e. the 'Haldane effect'). Finally, supplemental oxygen 'washes out' the nitrogen-rich gas that is present in the lungs during room air breathing. Remember that nitrogen is poorly soluble and helps to inhibit the collapse of the alveoli during gas exchange. In the absence of nitrogen, pure oxygen (which is highly soluble) can be completely absorbed into the blood stream leading to alveolar collapse, a process called absorption atelectasis. Absorption atelectasis can occur with a fraction of inspired oxygen as low as 30% and promotes worsening V/Q mismatch (Abdo & Heunks, 2012; O'Driscoll et al., 2017).

The Thoracic Society of Australia and New Zealand recommends that acute exacerbations of COPD be treated with oxygen at either 1–2 L/min via nasal cannulae or 2–4 L/min via Venturi mask, titrated to a SpO_2 target of 88–92% (Beasley et al., 2015). A Venturi mask is an oxygen delivery device commonly used in hospitals which entrains room air and a constant flow of oxygen through a specially engineered chamber in the device. Unlike other oxygen delivery masks, Venturi masks provide a constant flow of oxygen to the patient and minimise variations in the fraction of inspired oxygen due to variations in respiratory rates or tidal volumes (O'Driscoll et al., 2017). Although a standard oxygen face mask can also be used to deliver oxygen therapy (at a rate between 5 and 15 L/min), there is a possible risk of carbon dioxide rebreathing in patients with moderate to high respiratory rates. For instance, a person breathing at a rate of 30 breaths per minute and with a tidal volume of 500 mL exhales 15 L of carbon dioxide rich gas every minute into the mask. This should be considered when titrating oxygen flow rates using face masks.

The administration of bronchodilators in the out-of-hospital setting may require the use of an oxygen-driven nebuliser. In these situations, when the nebuliser has delivered the medications treatment should revert to nasal cannula unless higher flow rates are required to achieve the target SpO_2 (88–92%). Importantly, nasal cannulae can deliver a wide fraction of inspired oxygen at flow rates between 1 and 6 L/min and are usually preferred by patients over facemasks (O'Driscoll et al., 2017). Concerns about nasal dryness (or other complications) with higher flow rates are usually not justified with short-term use.

Emergency practitioners will sometimes express reluctance with targeting a lower than normal SpO_2 (88–92%) if the diagnosis of COPD is uncertain. Interestingly, several studies conducted during flight have found that the average SpO_2 at cruising altitude drops to 93% for healthy volunteers and as low as 87% for patients with COPD (Humphreys et al., 2005; Akero et al., 2005). These reductions in SpO_2 are well tolerated and do not cause breathlessness or other symptoms. Some international guidelines indicate that an SpO_2 threshold of 85% is the safe lower limit of hypoxaemia before the development of symptoms (O'Driscoll et al., 2017).

Bronchodilator therapy

An acute exacerbation of COPD involves increased airflow limitation and airway resistance, of which bronchospasm is a significant component. A single or combined use of short-acting and long-acting bronchodilators is recommended as the initial drug therapy in acute exacerbations of COPD (GOLD, 2018). Although the immediate effect of bronchodilators is small, they usually provide an improvement in clinical symptoms in patients with severe obstruction (Yang et al., 2018). Current guidelines recommend initial treatment with a short-acting beta$_2$ agonist, such as salbutamol (Ventolin), followed by a muscarinic receptor antagonist if the initial response is slow (GOLD, 2018). Beta$_2$ agonists have been shown to reduce dynamic hyperinflation at rest and during exercise, and improve exercise performance. They can be administered as needed or on a regular basis.

Anticholinergics act by blocking the effect of acetylcholine on muscarinic receptors, inhibiting cholinergic reflex bronchoconstriction and reducing vagal cholinergic tone (GOLD, 2018). Ipratropium is a non-selective short-acting anticholinergic that acts on the muscarinic receptors M_1, M_2 and M_3. M_3 receptors mediate the bronchoconstriction and mucus-secretion actions of acetylcholine on airways (Hansel et al., 2009). Although the blockade of M_3 receptors is the main effect of antimuscarinic drugs, the non-selective nature of ipratropium also blocks the inhibitory neuronal receptor M_2, which can lead to vagally induced bronchoconstriction (GOLD, 2018). In comparison, long-acting muscarinic receptor antagonists such as tiotropium have prolonged binding to M_3 receptors with faster dissociation from M_2 receptors, therefore optimising the duration of the bronchodilator effect (GOLD, 2018).

Bronchodilators can be administered via pressurised metered dose inhaler (pMDI) and spacer or nebulisation. The recommended dose of salbutamol and ipratropium via pMDI is 400–800 micrograms and 80 micrograms, respectively. The recommended dose for nebulisation is 2.5–5 mg salbutamol and 500 micrograms ipratropium (Yang et al., 2018). The dose interval is titrated to the response and can range from hourly to six-hourly. There is no conclusive evidence to support the superiority of nebulised administration of bronchodilators over pMDI delivery (van Geffen et al., 2016).

The crew elect to commence the patient on salbutamol 5 mg and ipratropium 500 micrograms via nebuliser mask at 6 L/min of supplemental oxygen.

Corticosteroids

In acute exacerbations of COPD, systemic glucocorticoids shorten recovery time, improve lung function and reduce the length of hospital stay (Walters et al., 2014). Glucocorticoids reduce the number of inflammatory cells in the airways: eosinophils, T-lymphocytes, mast cells and dendritic cells. The major action of glucocorticoids is to switch off the multiple activated inflammatory genes that encode cytokines, chemokines, adhesion molecules, inflammatory enzymes and receptors (Barnes, 2009).

Glucocorticoids can be given either orally or intravenously, although both routes provide similar levels of effectiveness (Walters et al., 2014). In addition, inhaled glucocorticoids are an alternative to oral or intravenous glucocorticoids in patients with moderate-to-severe disease and frequent exacerbations (GOLD, 2018). Hyperglycaemia is the most common adverse effect of steroid therapy and may be more common in patients with preexisting diabetes mellitus (Wedzicha, 2009).

IV steroid therapy should be initiated after the first-line therapy of oxygen (if required) and bronchodilators. The recommended regimen of glucocorticoids is a five-day course of 30–50 mg of oral prednisolone. In the acute setting, the first dose may be provided by paramedics or emergency department staff, although there is no evidence to support the optimal timing of its administration.

Non-invasive ventilation

International guidelines recommend a trial of NIV for patients with impending respiratory failure or persistent hypoxaemia that is refractory to oxygen therapy (Yang et al., 2018; GOLD, 2018). NIV, in the form of either continuous positive airway pressure (CPAP) or bilevel positive airway pressure (BiPAP), has demonstrated improvement in respiratory physiology with success rates between 80 and 85% (GOLD, 2018). Patients with hypercapnic respiratory failure receiving NIV therapy experience a 46% reduction in the risk of death and a 65% reduction in the risk of endotracheal intubation (Osadnik et al., 2017). NIV has also been associated with reduced length of hospital stay, a lower incidence of complications and an improvement in pH and PaO_2 (Osadnik et al., 2017). Unfortunately, the data supporting the use of NIV in the out-of-hospital setting is limited. However, there is a series of small clinical trials conducted in the out-of-hospital setting which show that NIV was associated with a reduction in mortality and intubation rates for patients with acute respiratory failure (Goodacre et al., 2014). At this time, there is limited availability of BiPAP technology in the out-of-hospital setting. In comparison, portable CPAP devices are now widely available in the out-of-hospital setting and may be a suitable alternative to BiPAP ventilation.

Indications for the initiation of NIV in patients with acute exacerbations of COPD include: 1. severe dyspnoea that responds inadequately to initial emergency therapy; 2. confusion, lethargy or evidence of hypoventilation; 3. persistent or worsening hypoxaemia despite supplemental oxygen, worsening hypercapnia ($PaCO_2 > 70$ mmHg), or severe or worsening respiratory acidosis (pH < 7.3); and 4. assisted mechanical ventilation is required (Yang et al., 2018).

Invasive ventilation

There are a number of situations where NIV is contraindicated or unlikely to benefit patients with acute exacerbations of COPD. This includes patients who are unable to protect their airway, have severe hypoxaemia that is refractory to initial treatment ($PaO_2 < 60$ mmHg), bronchiectasis with copious secretions, severe pneumonia and haemodynamic instability (Yang et al., 2018). The limited monitoring in the out-of-hospital setting reduces the applicability of a number of these measures, so the paramedic is reliant on the clinical manifestations of severe respiratory failure (and local guidelines) in determining the need for intubation. Intubation may be required in the patient with a clinical appearance of fatigue, confusion, lethargy or evidence of hypoventilation, impending respiratory collapse or deterioration in conscious state (GOLD, 2018). Patients who are unable to tolerate NIV or present with persistent vomiting (airway risk) may also require rescue mechanical ventilation.

Intubation of a patient with severe exacerbation of COPD is not without potential complications, such as the inability to appropriately pre-oxygenate (and remove nitrogen). There is also a risk of developing ventilator-acquired infections which can increase the risk of death. Almost 40% of acute exacerbations requiring intubation and mechanical ventilation will not survive to hospital discharge (Wildman et al., 2009). Paramedics and emergency staff need to assess the value of invasive ventilation in the context of a number of factors, including the patient's wishes, the likely reversibility of the precipitating event and the availability of intensive care facilities (GOLD, 2018).

Resuscitation

Patients with COPD who lose cardiac output should be managed using standard resuscitation guidelines. The Australian and New Zealand Committee on Resuscitation (ANZCOR) recommend additional treatments in patients with evidence of gas-trapping (bronchospasm). If dynamic hyperinflation of the lungs is suspected, compression of the chest wall and/or a period of apnoea (e.g. withholding ventilations) may relieve gas-trapping (ANZCOR, 2011). If ventilation continues to be difficult, intubation should be prioritised.

(4) EVALUATE

Evaluating the effect of any clinical management intervention can provide clues to the accuracy of the initial diagnosis. Some conditions respond rapidly to treatment so patients should be expected to improve if the diagnosis and treatment were appropriate. A failure to improve in this situation should trigger the clinician to reconsider the diagnosis.

Is the patient:
- Improving after initial treatment (bronchodilators ± O_2)?
- Deteriorating after initial treatment?
  › Look for and eliminate possible cause of deterioration.
  › Consider other causes of respiratory distress: acute pulmonary oedema, pulmonary embolism, pneumonia, pneumothorax (tension) and cardiac arrhythmia. Findings such as cardiac arrhythmias may be secondary to

beta$_2$ agonists or hypoxia. Be diligent in monitoring the patient who has cardiac disease.

› Check for hypotension. Determine the cause and manage according to local guidelines.

› Does the patient have profound airflow limitation and bronchospasm? Consider IV bronchodilators (salbutamol). There is no evidence to support their use in exacerbation of COPD and they should be reserved for patients who are in immediate life-threat.

› If NIV is available and patient is still conscious and breathing, consider this.

● Now unconscious?

› Start primary survey.

› Monitor for respiratory arrest, decreasing conscious state, exhaustion and fatigue. Provide assisted ventilation. Provide a ventilation rate of 5–8 L/min with a long expiratory pause to allow for expiration and prevent worsening hyperinflation.

› Consider intubation.

● Now pulseless?

› Check monitor.

› Not ventricular tachycardia or ventricular fibrillation?

› If assisted positive pressure ventilation (APPV) initiated and patient loses output, allow 1 minute of apnoea.

› If a carotid pulse is present but no BP, adrenaline and fluid should be administered according to local guidelines (adrenaline 50 micrograms IV, NaCl 20 mL/kg).

› Commence CPR.

Hospital admission

When patients with acute exacerbations of COPD attend the emergency department, medical staff need to determine the need for admission. International guidelines recommend that patients with the following indications are considered for hospitalisation, including: 1. the presence of severe symptoms such as sudden worsening of resting dyspnoea, high respiratory rate, decreased oxygen saturation, confusion or drowsiness; 2. the presence of acute respiratory failure; 3. the onset of new physical signs such as cyanosis or peripheral oedema; 4. failure to respond to initial treatment; 5. the presence of serious comorbidities such as heart failure or new arrhythmias; and 6. insufficient home support (GOLD, 2018). Patients in acute respiratory failure that is refractory to NIV or where NIV is contraindicated may be admitted to the ICU. This decision will take into account quality of life and likely outcomes for patients who have end-stage COPD.

During admission and post-discharge, a course of antibiotics may be prescribed for patients with clinical signs of infection, particularly purulent sputum, increased sputum amount or change in sputum colour (GOLD, 2018; Yang et al., 2018). Patients with a higher severity exacerbation are likely to experience a greater benefit from antibiotics than those with a milder form (Vollenweider et al., 2012). Additional hospital treatments include: fluid therapy, as patients can be dehydrated—or conversely diuretic therapy where cardiac impairment is evident; nutritional supplements for patients with a low body mass index; prophylaxis for DVT; and sputum clearance therapy (GOLD, 2018).

There is limited clinical data available to determine the optimal hospital duration (GOLD, 2018). In general patients will be admitted for 1 or 2 days. They may be discharged from the ED, but this depends on conditions at home and support being in place. The patient will be discharged when they have been clinically stable for 12–24 hours and the patient, doctor and family or carers are confident they can manage competently at home and have a full understanding of the correct use of their medications. Criteria for clinical stability include inhaled beta$_2$ therapy is required no more frequently than every 4 hours and arterial blood gases (ABGs) have been stable for 12–24 hours. If the patient was previously ambulant, they should be able to walk across a room; and they should be able to sleep without frequently being awoken by dyspnoea. Discharge should include appropriate follow-up arrangements for outpatient or home visits, review of prescription medication, spirometry, smoking cessation therapy and a personalised action plan as required (GOLD, 2018). Pulmonary rehabilitation is also being increasingly used to reduce readmission rates and improve quality of life outcomes (Puhan et al., 2016).

Investigations

In hospital, investigations are further aimed at evaluating the severity of the exacerbation and identifying alternative diagnoses and the causative nature of this episode. Spirometric measurement may be undertaken to assess the severity of the exacerbation. An $FEV_1 < 1.0$ L, or < 40% predicted, indicates a severe exacerbation (Yang et al., 2018). ABG also provides important information about the severity of the exacerbations, and indications for NIV. A PaO_2 < 60 mmHg indicates respiratory failure, while a $PaCO_2$ > 45 mmHg indicates ventilatory failure. A decreased pH indicates that the compensatory mechanisms are depleted and mechanical ventilation may be needed (Yang et al., 2018). In addition, a full blood examination is routine and may identify polycythaemia or anaemia. An increased white blood cell count may indicate an infection but should be considered in the presence of long-term steroid use. Electrolytes are evaluated as patients with exacerbations may present with hypokalaemia and hyponatraemia (GOLD, 2018). Finally, chest x-rays and electrocardiography help to identify alternative diagnoses and complications, such as pulmonary oedema, pneumothorax, pneumonia and arrhythmias (Yang et al., 2018). Chest x-rays may also assist in evaluating the effectiveness of treatment.

Follow-up

COPD and its associated comorbidities are treatable, but not curable. The disease is progressive, particu-larly if the exposure to noxious gases (predominantly cigarette smoking) continues. Treatment is therefore aimed at smoking cessation if required, controlling the symptoms, reducing the frequency of exacerbations and improving the patient's quality of life. Management of COPD is based on the severity of the disease: as the severity increases treatment modalities are increased and tend to become cumulative (see Fig 19.7).

Long-term oxygen therapy is a principal non-pharmacological therapy for very severe (stage 4) COPD where chronic hypoxaemia is present (GOLD, 2018). Long-term oxygen therapy (> 18 hours/day) has been shown to prolong survival, possibly by halting the progression of pulmonary hypertension. It may also be beneficial for haemodynamics, haematological characteristics, exercise capacity, lung mechanics and mental state (GOLD, 2018). The criteria for initiating oxygen therapy in chronic hypoxaemia are PaO_2 < 55 mmHg, or $PaO_2 \leq 59$ mmHg in the presence of pulmonary hypertension, right heart failure or polycythaemia (GOLD, 2018; McKenzie et al., 2011). There is no benefit in routine oxygen therapy for patients with mild to moderate hypoxaemia at rest or on exertion (Long-Term Oxygen Treatment Trial Research et al., 2016).

Currently there are no recommended pharmacotherapies for pulmonary hypertension associated with COPD (GOLD, 2018). Diuretics may be used to reduce right ventricular filling pressure and oedema, but close monitoring of the patient's volume status is required to avoid volume depletion. Vasodilators have not demonstrated a sustained effect on pulmonary hypertension in COPD and may worsen oxygenation and cause systemic hypotension. However, in severe persistent pulmonary hypertension refractory to oxygen therapy a trial of a vasodilator may be indicated (Yang et al., 2018). When reviewing the patient's medication look for these types of medications and identify why the patient is receiving them. In particular, consider other possible indications where these drugs are prescribed (e.g. hypertension, heart failure).

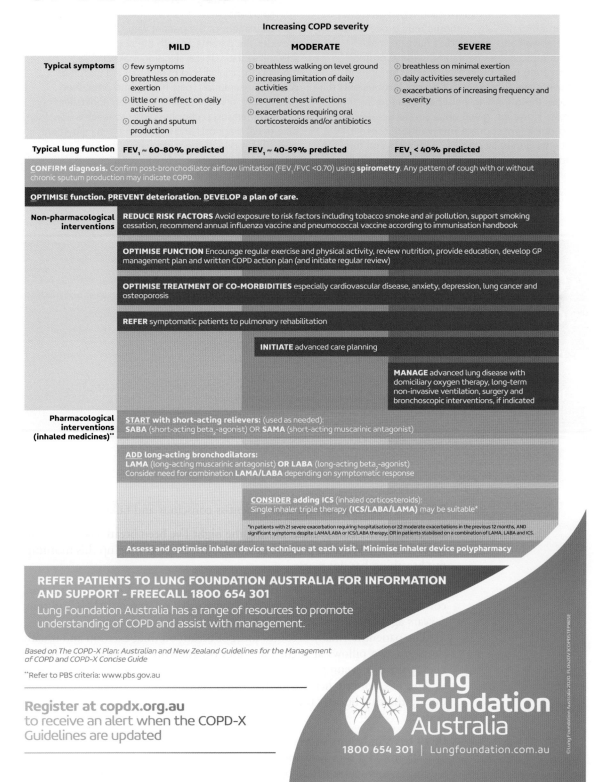

Figure 19.7
Stepwise management of stable COPD.
Source: Lung Foundation Australia (June 2020).

COPD ON THE ROAD

Patients presenting with breathing difficulties are one of the most frequent case types attended by paramedics. Initially, patients may present as very unwell and paramedics have to make some rapid assessments and initiate prompt interventions to prevent further deterioration. Patients are also likely to be very anxious and this places the attending paramedics under further stress. However, given an accurate assessment and quick, appropriate intervention, these patients generally stabilise within several minutes and can be maintained en route to hospital. Continuous reassessment will determine their response to management and guide ongoing management.

Assessment of the patient with COPD provides the paramedic with the opportunity to fully utilise their clinical decision-making skills, juggling the clinical information gained from the patient presentation, past history and prescribed medications and combining it with an understanding of the underlying pathophysiology to reach a differential diagnosis and implement a management plan. This is one of the cases where the full repertoire of the paramedic's knowledge and skills is required to ensure the best patient outcome.

CASE STUDY 2

Case 11449, 0825 hrs.

Dispatch details: A 61-year-old female with severe respiratory distress.

Initial presentation: On arrival the crew are led inside a private house by the patient's husband and find the patient sitting on the side of the bed.

ASSESS

0835 hrs Primary survey: The patient is conscious and talking.

0836 hrs Chief complaint: 'During the night I've been breathless. I get some relief from my Ventolin puffer, but not totally. Since getting up this morning, my breathing has got worse.'

0837 hrs Pertinent hx: The patient has a past history of COPD, hypertension, coronary artery disease (with an acute myocardial infarction [AMI] and stent 5 years ago) and intermittent angina responsive to GTN spray.

The patient normally becomes short of breath on mild exertion and usually sleeps on two pillows at night. She does occasionally get angina, but has no chest pain this evening.

She has noticed her ankles have been getting more swollen than usual during the day, but her breathing has been no worse than normal before this episode.

0840 hrs Vital signs survey: Perfusion status: HR 118, sinus tachycardia, BP 160/95 mmHg, skin pale and clammy, temperature 36.5°C.

Respiratory status: RR 28 bpm, decreased air entry, L = R, scattered expiratory wheeze across all fields, fine inspiratory crackles to mid-zone, increased work of breathing, speaking single words, SpO_2 85% on room air.

Conscious state: GCS = 15.

Paramedic:	What is different about this episode of shortness of breath?
Patient:	I've been short of breath during the night before, but usually it's relieved by my Ventolin.
Paramedic:	Have you had a cough, or been coughing up sputum?
Patient:	I have had a cough, a bit worse than normal, but I haven't been coughing up any sputum. It's been a fairly dry cough for about a week now.
Patient:	What are your normal medications?'

The patient shows the paramedics a shoebox filled with the following medications: Ventolin MDI, Spiriva MDI, Coversyl, Plavix, Panadol, Nitrolingual Spray.

(2) CONFIRM

In many cases paramedics are presented with a collection of signs and symptoms that do not appear to describe a particular condition. A critical step in determining a treatment plan in this situation is to consider what other conditions could explain the patient's presentation.

There is definitely some component of COPD contributing to the patient's current episode of respiratory distress. There is an expiratory wheeze audible on auscultation and the patient has received some relief from her Ventolin.

What else could it be?

The patient reports a more recent history of shortness of breath during the night, with a dry cough and worsening ankle oedema during the day. She already requires several pillows to sleep and has preexisting ischaemic heart disease, with a previous AMI and hypertension. In addition, fine end inspiratory crackles on auscultation suggest there is a component of heart failure contributing to her condition. The wheeze may also be associated with her heart failure.

The patient has been prescribed a short-acting beta$_2$ agonist (Ventolin) and a longer-acting beta$_2$ agonist (Serevent), but no glucocorticoids or home oxygen. This would suggest that she has moderate-stage COPD. The prescription of Coversyl suggests her hypertension requires medical management and may be associated with chronic heart failure, and the Plavix reflects a secondary prevention measure for her previous AMI.

Heart failure

As discussed above, there is probably an element of heart failure contributing to the patient's current episode. There are indications of both left heart failure (fine inspiratory crackles) and right heart failure (peripheral oedema/swollen ankles).

Pneumonia

While chest infections are a common cause of COPD exacerbations, it is less likely to be the problem in this patient. She does not have a productive cough or a fever, and there are no coarse crackles on auscultation.

Acute coronary syndrome/arrhythmia

There may be an element of cardiac ischaemia contributing to the patient's heart failure. While the patient has not mentioned cardiac chest pain, she should be queried about any recent history of ischaemic chest pain. A 12-lead ECG will help rule out ischaemia or an arrhythmia and may identify other pathologies such as P pulmonale or pulmonary embolism.

USING THE MNEMONIC DENT

Define:
- What is the patient's main presenting problem?

Explore:
- Is this COPD?
- What else could it be?
  - › Heart failure
  - › Pneumonia
  - › Acute coronary syndrome/arrhythmia
  - › Pneumothorax
  - › Pleural effusion
  - › Pulmonary embolism

Narrow:
- What else might be going on?
- What information regarding the possible severity of the patient's COPD, and other conditions, can be gained from seeing her medications?

REFLECTIVE BOX

1. COPD is a heterogeneous condition, involving three main phenotypes. What are they?
2. Emphysema is a pathological term referring to what structural change occurring in patients with COPD?
3. What clinical features indicate the presence of an acute exacerbation of COPD?
4. What is the target oxygen saturation in patients presenting with an acute exacerbation of COPD?
5. Hypoxic pulmonary vasoconstriction is a compensatory mechanism that occurs in patients with COPD. What purpose does it have?
6. Detail three potentially detrimental effects of excessive oxygen administration in patients with COPD.
7. Emphysema is present in the majority of patients with COPD. True or false?
8. The predominant physiological feature of COPD is dynamic hyperinflation. True or false?
9. The diagnosis of COPD is confirmed using spirometry. True or false?
10. Steroid therapy is the first-line treatment of COPD in the out-of-hospital setting. True or false?

Pneumothorax
The patient has equal air entry, and there has been no history of chest pain. It is unlikely this is contributing to the patient's current exacerbation.

Pleural effusion
Chest auscultation may reveal absent or diminished breath sounds over a particular area of the chest. The patient would generally complain of chest pain on breathing. None of these signs and symptoms are evident in this patient.

Pulmonary embolism
There is no evidence of thromboembolic disease in this patient and she is not bed-bound. It would be relevant to enquire if she has had any calf pain to further eliminate this as a likely differential diagnosis. If the patient maintains a low systolic blood pressure, and a persistently low SpO_2 despite adequate oxygen therapy, pulmonary embolism should be given greater consideration.

TREAT

Although beta$_2$ agonists may increase myocardial oxygen consumption, it is unlikely that short-term treatment in the acute setting would translate into poorer patient outcomes. A review investigating the effects of nebulised beta$_2$ agonists in heart failure patients reported that the intervention appeared to be safe, and may improve pulmonary function and resorption of pulmonary oedema (Maak et al., 2011). In addition, the use of short-acting bronchodilators is common in the hospital setting for patients admitted with heart failure (Dharmarajan et al., 2013). It would also be sensible to treat the heart failure in conjunction with the COPD as it is likely that both pathologies are contributing to the patient's current presentation.

0842 hrs: The patient is administered oxygen therapy at 8 L/min and commenced on nebulised salbutamol 5 mg/2.5 mL and ipratropium bromide 500 micrograms/2 mL.

0845 hrs: The symptoms start to subside slightly, but the patient is still experiencing moderate respiratory distress.
Perfusion status: HR 128 bpm, sinus tachycardia, BP 165/98 mmHg, skin pale and clammy.
Respiratory status: RR 24 bpm, decreased air entry, L = R, expiratory wheeze resolved, but more audible fine inspiratory crackles to mid-zone, increased work of breathing, speaking short phrases, SpO_2 89% on oxygen 8 L/min.
Conscious state: GCS = 15.

0846 hrs: Given the patient's persisting shortness of breath, and the more audible fine inspiratory crackles, the paramedics elect to manage possible signs of heart failure with GTN 600 micrograms administered sublingually. They also opt to increase the oxygen flow rate to 10 L/min, targeting an SpO_2 at the upper end of the acceptable range in the COPD patient (90–92%).

0855 hrs: Before loading the patient onto the stretcher, a reassessment shows the following.
Perfusion status: HR 120, sinus tachycardia, BP 140/80, skin pale and dry.
Respiratory status: RR 22 bpm, slightly decreased air entry, L = R, fine inspiratory crackles to bases, normal work of breathing, speaking in sentences, SpO_2 91% on oxygen 10 L/min.
Conscious state: GCS = 15.

0905 hrs: Once the patient is in the ambulance, a reassessment shows the following.

Perfusion status: HR 130 bpm, sinus tachycardia, BP 140/80 mmHg, skin pale and dry.

Respiratory status: RR 28 bpm, slightly decreased air entry, L = R, fine inspiratory crackles to bases, increased work of breathing, speaking in short phrases, SpO_2 88% on oxygen 10 L/min.

Conscious state: GCS = 15.

How should this patient's deterioration be managed?

There may be a number of factors contributing to the patient's deterioration. First, she is now in a less favourable posture, with her feet elevated and diaphragm partially splinted. There may not be much that can be done to remedy this, and she may need some time to compensate for this change. However, if possible the patient should be placed in the best possible position on the stretcher, sitting upright, with her legs placed more dependent. Second, if the external environment is cold, transferring the patient into the cold may precipitate worsening of the dyspnoea, associated with increased airflow limitation. Third, there may be an element of anxiety for some patients as they face the prospect of leaving their home and confronting possible hospital admission. COPD patients may have frequent exacerbations requiring hospital attendance and may exhibit stress and anxiety when faced with this possibility.

If the patient's dyspnoea persists and there is no improvement in her vital signs, further intervention may be required. Depending on the presenting signs and symptoms, this may mean reviewing oxygen therapy (be wary of the potential for oxygen-induced hypercapnia), beta$_2$ agonist if expiratory wheeze returns and GTN if heart failure worsens. At some stage during transport, oral or IV steroids can be administered as per local guidelines. If the patient continues to deteriorate or shows evidence of respiratory muscle fatigue following these interventions, out-of-hospital NIV should be considered.

0923 hrs at hospital: Perfusion status: HR 104 bpm, sinus tachycardia, BP 145/80 mmHg, skin warm and pink.

Respiratory status: RR 22 bpm, slightly decreased air entry, L = R, normal work of breathing, fine inspiratory crackles to bases, speaking in sentences, SpO_2 92% on oxygen 10 L/min.

Conscious state: GCS = 15.

4 EVALUATE

Evaluating the effect of any clinical management intervention can provide clues to the accuracy of the initial diagnosis. Some conditions respond rapidly to treatment so patients should be expected to improve if the diagnosis and treatment were appropriate. A failure to improve in this situation should trigger the clinician to reconsider the diagnosis.

Future research and trends

While there has been significant progress in understanding the natural history and pathophysiology of COPD, there remains considerable knowledge gaps in its assessment and treatment. In 2015, a COPD expert task force established a research agenda describing the critical knowledge gaps in COPD (Celli et al., 2015). The research recommends almost 100 critical research questions which are needed to help establish a strong foundation for the diagnosis and management of COPD. In summary, the agenda recommends:

1. studies examining optimal patient-centred outcomes (in the absence of patient-centred outcomes, there is a need to develop reliable surrogate outcomes)
2. studies examining the role of computed tomography scanning in COPD patients
3. studies examining the use of risk assessment screening tools to help guide diagnosis and treatment of COPD
4. studies examining the relationship between COPD phenotypes and long-term outcomes
5. studies evaluating the relationship between COPD and comorbidities
6. studies examining the impact of smoking cessation on the progression of COPD
7. studies targeting the effects of pharmacological interventions on specific subgroups of COPD
8. studies examining the effectiveness of pulmonary rehabilitation programs
9. studies examining the effectiveness of long-term oxygen therapy and long-term non-invasive mechanical ventilation for COPD patients
10. studies describing the impact of palliative care and end-of-life discussions on outcomes in COPD.

Unfortunately, there is also very little research describing the effectiveness of pharmacological interventions during acute exacerbations of COPD. In particular, the out-of-hospital management of acute COPD remains largely supportive, and despite one clinical trial assessing the impact of oxygen therapy on patients with acute COPD (Austin et al., 2010), there are very few randomised controlled trials conducted in the out-of-hospital setting that help guide optimal management of acute exacerbations of COPD.

Summary

COPD is an irreversible disease that has increasing prevalence throughout the community. Exacerbations of COPD are the primary cause for hospitalisation of people with COPD.

It can be difficult to obtain a full history from a patient presenting with severe respiratory distress due to their inability to speak. In addition, there are a number of differential diagnoses that are not always easy to eliminate. However, there can be diagnostic clues in the patient's clinical signs and current medications. Paramedics must therefore use their knowledge and assessment skills to arrive at the best diagnosis and implement appropriate out-of-hospital interventions.

References

Abdo, W. F., & Heunks, L. M. (2012). Oxygen-induced hypercapnia in COPD: myths and facts. *Critical Care: The Official Journal of the Critical Care Forum, 16,* 323.

Akero, A., Christensen, C. C., Edvardsen, A., & Skjonsberg, O. H. (2005). Hypoxaemia in chronic obstructive pulmonary disease patients during a commercial flight. *The European Respiratory Journal, 25,* 725–730.

Aleva, F. E., Voets, L., Simons, S. O., De Mast, Q., Van Der Ven, A., & Heijdra, Y. F. (2017). Prevalence and localization of pulmonary embolism in unexplained acute exacerbations of COPD: a systematic review and meta-analysis. *Chest, 151,* 544–554.

Austin, M. A., Wills, K. E., Blizzard, L., Walters, E. H., & Wood-Baker, R. (2010). Effect of high flow oxygen on mortality in chronic obstructive pulmonary disease patients in prehospital setting: randomised controlled trial. *British Medical Journal, 341*(c5462).

Australian and New Zealand Committee on Resuscitation (ANZCOR). (2011). *Guideline 11.10: Resuscitation in special circumstance.* Retrieved from: http://www.resus.org.au.

Australian Lung Foundation. (2017). *Stepwise management of stable COPD.* Retrieved from: http://lungfoundation.com.au/health-professionals/guidelines/copd/stepwise-management-of-stable-copd/.

Barnes, P. J. (2009). Corticosteroids. In P. J. Barnes, N. C. Thomson, J. M. Drazen & S. I. Rennard (Eds.), *Asthma and COPD* (2nd ed.). San Diego, CA: Elsevier.

Beasley, R., Chien, J., Douglas, J., Eastlake, L., Farah, C., King, G., Moore, R., Pilcher, J., Richards, M., Smith, S., & Walters, H. (2015). Thoracic Society of Australia and New Zealand oxygen guidelines for acute oxygen use in adults: 'Swimming between the flags'. *Respirology (Carlton, Vic.), 20,* 1182–1191.

Bintcliffe, O., & Maskell, N. (2014). Spontaneous pneumothorax. *British Medical Journal, 8*(348), g2928. doi:10.1136/bmj.g2928.

Castro, M., & Kraft, M. (2008). *Clinical asthma*. St Louis: Mosby.

Celli, B. R., Cote, C. G., Marin, J. M., Casanova, C., Montes De Oca, M., Mendez, R. A., Pinto Plata, V., & Cabral, H. J. (2004). The body mass index, airflow obstruction, dyspnea, and exercise capacity index in chronic obstructive pulmonary disease. *The New England Journal of Medicine, 350*, 1005–1012.

Celli, B. R., Decramer, M., Wedzicha, J. A., Wilson, K. C., Agusti, A., Criner, G. J., Macnee, W., Make, B. J., Rennard, S. I., Stockley, R. A., Vogelmeier, C., Anzueto, A., Au, D. H., Barnes, P. J., Burgel, P. R., Calverley, P. M., Casanova, C., Clini, E. M., Cooper, C. B., Coxson, H. O., Dusser, D. J., Fabbri, L. M., Fahy, B., Ferguson, G. T., Fisher, A., Fletcher, M. J., Hayot, M., Hurst, J. R., Jones, P. W., Mahler, D. A., Maltais, F., Mannino, D. M., Martinez, F. J., Miravitlles, M., Meek, P. M., Papi, A., Rabe, K. F., Roche, N., Sciurba, F. C., Sethi, S., Siafakas, N., Sin, D. D., Soriano, J. B., Stoller, J. K., Tashkin, D. P., Troosters, T., Verleden, G. M., Verschakelen, J., Vestbo, J., Walsh, J. W., Washko, G. R., Wise, R. A., Wouters, E. F., Zuwallack, R. L., & Research, A. E. T. F. F. C. (2015). An official American Thoracic Society/ European Respiratory Society statement: research questions in COPD. *The European Respiratory Journal, 45*, 879–905.

Craft, J., Gordon, C., & Tiziani, A. (2011). *Understanding Pathophysiology*. Sydney: Elsevier.

Dharmarajan, K., Strait, K. M., Lagu, T., Lindenauer, P. K., Tinetti, M. E., Lynn, J., Li, S. X., & Krumholz, H. M. (2013). Acute decompensated heart failure is routinely treated as a cardiopulmonary syndrome. *PLoS ONE, 8*, e78222.

Fletcher, C., & Peto, R. (1977). The natural history of chronic airflow obstruction. *British Medical Journal, 1*, 1645–1648.

Global Initiative for Asthma. (2018). *Global strategy for asthma management and prevention*. Retrieved from: www.qinasthma.org.

GOLD. (2018). *Global strategy for the diagnosis, management, and prevention of chronic obstructive pulmonary disease*. Global Initiative for Chronic Obstructive Lung Disease (GOLD). Retrieved from: www.goldcopd.org.

Goodacre, S., Stevens, J. W., Pandor, A., Poku, E., Ren, S., Cantrell, A., Bounes, V., Mas, A., Payen, D., Petrie, D., Roessler, M. S., Weitz, G., Ducros, L., & Plaisance, P. (2014). Prehospital noninvasive ventilation for acute respiratory failure: systematic review, network meta-analysis, and individual patient data meta-analysis. *Academic Emergency Medicine: Official Journal of the Society for Academic Emergency Medicine, 21*, 960–970.

Hansel, T. T., Tan, A. J., Barnes, P. J., & Kon, O. M. (2009). Anticholinergic bronchodilators. In P. J. Barnes,

N. C. Thomson, J. M. Drazen & S. I. Rennard (Eds.), *Asthma and COPD* (2nd ed.). San Diego, CA: Elsevier.

Hawkins, N., Petrie, M., MacDonald, M., Jhund, S., Fabbri, L., Wikstrand, J., & McMurray, J. (2011). Heart failure and chronic obstructive pulmonary disease. *Journal of the American College of Cardiology, 57*(21), 2127–2138.

Humphreys, S., Deyermond, R., Bali, I., Stevenson, M., & Fee, J. P. (2005). The effect of high-altitude commercial air travel on oxygen saturation. *Anaesthesia, 60*, 458–460.

Kim, K. S., Byun, M. K., Lee, W. H., Cynn, H. S., Kwon, O. Y., & Yi, C. H. (2012). Effects of breathing maneuver and sitting posture on muscle activity in inspiratory accessory muscles in patients with chronic obstructive pulmonary disease. *Multidisciplinary Respiratory Medicine, 7*, 9.

Ko, F. W., Chan, K. P., Hui, D. S., Goddard, J. R., Shaw, J. G., Reid, D. W., & Yang, I. A. (2016). Acute exacerbation of COPD. *Respirology (Carlton, Vic.), 21*, 1152–1165.

Long-Term Oxygen Treatment Trial Research Group, Albert, R. K., Au, D. H., Blackford, A. L., Casaburi, R., Cooper, J. A., Jr, Criner, G. J., Diaz, P., Fuhlbrigge, A. L., Gay, S. E., Kanner, R. E., Macintyre, N., Martinez, F. J., Panos, R. J., Piantadosi, S., Sciurba, F., Shade, D., Stibolt, T., Stoller, J. K., Wise, R., Yusen, R. D., Tonascia, J., Sternberg, A. L., & Bailey, W. (2016). A randomized trial of long-term oxygen for COPD with moderate desaturation. *The New England Journal of Medicine, 375*, 1617–1627.

Maak, C. A., Tabas, J. A., & McClintock, D. E. (2011). Should acute treatment with inhaled beta agonists be withheld from patients with dyspnea who may have heart failure? *The Journal of Emergency Medicine, 40*, 135–145.

Marsh, S. E., Travers, J., Weatherall, M., Williams, M. V., Aldington, S., Shirtcliffe, P. M., Hansell, A. L., Nowitz, M. R., McNaughton, A. A., Soriano, J. B., & Beasley, R. W. (2008). Proportional classifications of COPD phenotypes. *Thorax, 63*, 761–767.

McCance, K., & Huether, S. (2014). *Pathophysiology: the biologic basis for disease in adults and children* (7th ed.). St Louis: Mosby.

McKenzie, D., Abramson, D., Crockett, A., Glasgow, N., Jenkins, S., McDonald, C., Wood-Baker, R., & Frith, P., on behalf of The Australian Lung Foundation. (2011). *The COPD-X Plan: Australian and New Zealand Guidelines for the management of Chronic Obstructive Pulmonary Disease*. Version 2.26.

O'Donnell, D. E., & Parker, C. M. (2006). Pathophysiology of COPD exacerbations. *Thorax, 61*, 354–361.

O'Driscoll, B. R., Howard, L. S., Earis, J., & Mak, V. (2017). BTS guideline for oxygen use in adults in healthcare and emergency settings. *Thorax, 72*, ii1–ii90.

Osadnik, C. R., Tee, V. S., Carson-Chahhoud, K. V., Picot, J., Wedzicha, J. A., & Smith, B. J. (2017). Non-invasive ventilation for the management of acute hypercapnic respiratory failure due to exacerbation of chronic obstructive pulmonary disease. *The Cochrane Database of Systematic Reviews*, (7), CD004104.

Patton, K. T., & Thibodeau, G. A. (2010). *Anatomy & physiology* (7th ed.). St Louis: Mosby.

Plant, P. K., Owen, J. L., & Elliott, M. W. (2000). One-year period prevalence study of respiratory acidosis in acute exacerbations of COPD: implications for the provision of non-invasive ventilation and oxygen administration. *Thorax, 55*, 550–554.

Puhan, M. A., Gimeno-Santos, E., Cates, C. J., & Troosters, T. (2016). Pulmonary rehabilitation following exacerbations of chronic obstructive pulmonary disease. *The Cochrane Database of Systematic Reviews*, (12), CD005305.

Shirtcliffe, P., Marsh, S., Travers, J., Weatherall, M., & Beasley, R. (2012). Childhood asthma and GOLD-defined chronic obstructive pulmonary disease. *Internal Medicine Journal, 42*, 83–88.

Shujaat, A., Minkin, R., & Eden, E. (2007). Pulmonary hypertension and chronic cor pulmonale in COPD. *International Journal of Chronic Obstructive Pulmonary Disease, 2*(3), 273–282.

Thibodeau, G. A. (2010). *The human body in health and disease* (5th ed.). St Louis: Mosby.

Toelle, B. G., Xuan, W., Bird, T. E., Abramson, M. J., Atkinson, D. N., Burton, D. L., James, A. L., Jenkins, C. R., Johns, D. P., Maguire, G. P., Musk, A. W., Walters, E. H., Wood-Baker, R., Hunter, M. L., Graham, B. J., Southwell, P. J., Vollmer, W. M., Buist, A. S., & Marks, G. B. (2013). Respiratory symptoms and illness in older Australians: the Burden of Obstructive Lung Disease (BOLD) study. *The Medical Journal of Australia, 198*, 144–148.

van Geffen, W. H., Douma, W. R., Slebos, D. J., & Kerstjens, H. A. (2016). Bronchodilators delivered by nebuliser versus pMDI with spacer or DPI for exacerbations of COPD. *The Cochrane Database of Systematic Reviews*, (8), CD011826.

Vollenweider, D. J., Jarrett, H., Steurer-Stey, C. A., Garcia-Aymerich, J., & Puhan, M. A. (2012). Antibiotics for exacerbations of chronic obstructive pulmonary disease. *The Cochrane Database of Systematic Reviews*, (12), CD010257.

Walters, J. A., Tan, D. J., White, C. J., Gibson, P. G., Wood-Baker, R., & Walters, E. H. (2014). Systemic corticosteroids for acute exacerbations of chronic obstructive pulmonary disease. *The Cochrane Database of Systematic Reviews*, (9), CD001288.

Wang, C. S., Fitzgerald, J. M., Schulzer, M., Mak, E., & Ayas, N. T. (2005). Does this dyspneic patient in the emergency department have congestive heart failure? *JAMA, 294*(15), 1944–1956.

Wedzicha, J. A. (2009). Acute exacerbations of COPD. In P. Barnes, N. Thomson, J. Drazen & S. Rennard (Eds.), *Asthma and COPD* (2nd ed.). San Diego, CA: Elsevier.

Wijesinghe, M., Perrin, K., Healy, B., Hart, K., Clay, J., Weatherall, M., & Beasley, R. (2011). Pre-hospital oxygen therapy in acute exacerbations of chronic obstructive pulmonary disease. *Internal Medicine Journal, 41*(8), 618–622. https://doi.org/10.1111/j.1445-5994.2010.02207.x.

Wildman, M. J., Sanderson, C. F., Groves, J., Reeves, B. C., Ayres, J. G., Harrison, D., Young, D., & Rowan, K. (2009). Survival and quality of life for patients with COPD or asthma admitted to intensive care in a UK multicentre cohort: the COPD and Asthma Outcome Study (CAOS). *Thorax, 64*, 128–132.

Yang, I. A., Brown, J. L., George, J., Jenkins, S., McDonald, C. F., McDonald, V., Smith, B., Zwar, N., & Dabscheck, E. (2018). *The COPD-X Plan: Australian and New Zealand Guidelines for the management of Chronic Obstructive Pulmonary Disease: 2017 update. Med J Aust, 207*(10), 436–442. doi: 10.5694/mja17.00686.

CHAPTER 20

Pneumothorax

By Toby St Clair

OVERVIEW

- By impeding effective ventilation, the presence of air between the lungs and the chest wall can be a cause of respiratory compromise.
- Although commonly associated with trauma, a pneumothorax can occur spontaneously or as a result of disease.
- A pneumothorax can be categorised as spontaneous or traumatic, and further subcategorised to simple, open or tension.

- Pneumothorax is often difficult to identify based solely on auscultation.
- A simple pneumothorax may not need active intervention beyond analgesia, assessment and transport.
- Tension pneumothorax can cause cardiovascular collapse due to decreased venous return and requires accurate assessment and timely management.

Introduction

Pneumothorax is defined as air in the pleural space between the visceral and parietal pleura. The consequences of air entering the pleural space can range from minor to seriously life-threatening, with the severity and clinical consequence depending on the patient's age and health, the underlying aetiology and, importantly, the size and type of the pneumothorax (Porth & Martin, 2014).

Pathophysiology

The movement of air in and out of the lungs of the healthy individual depends on the contraction and relaxation of the major and accessory muscles of inspiration. Contraction of the external intercostal muscles raises the anterior ribs, while contraction of the diaphragm flattens in a downward motion, together increasing the overall volume of the thoracic cavity. This change in volume creates an area of low pressure within the lungs, causing atmospheric air to be inspired and equalise the pressure differential. Relaxation of the inspiratory muscles allows the elasticity of the chest wall and diaphragm to reduce the volume of the chest, forcing air back out into the atmosphere (McCance & Huether, 2010).

The lungs are bound to the chest wall and diaphragm, not by connective tissue but rather a pleural membrane. The visceral (inner) pleura and the parietal (outer) pleura are one continuous membrane forming sealed envelopes surrounding each lung. The visceral pleura, attached to the lungs' surface, doubles back at the hilar region and forms the parietal pleura, which is attached to the chest wall surface (Beachey, 2018).

Between the two pleural layers there is a potential space referred to as the pleural space. The pleural space contains a thin layer of serous pleural fluid that lubricate the membranes and allows near-frictionless movement as the pleural layers slide over one another during ventilation. The intrapleural pressure is sub-atmospheric as a result of the chest wall and lungs recoiling in opposite directions and thus forming a vacuum within the potential space (Beachey, 2018). However, as the space is only a 'potential' space this concept can be confusing. A more accurate way to describe the negative pressure is that the elasticity of lung tissue wants to draw the lungs smaller than they are, even at rest. Simultaneously, the structures of the chest wall want to expand the chest wall larger than it is at rest. As a result, there is a constant tension between the chest wall and the lungs, with each trying to pull away from the other. Any separation is prevented as there is no air or fluid to fill the potential space.

If the seal between the chest wall and the lungs is somehow broken, however, the tension between the two will be released and the lungs will be able to collapse away from the chest wall (see Fig 20.1).

The accumulation of air in the pleural space is referred to as a pneumothorax. Air can enter the pleural cavity through one of three mechanisms:

1. communication between the bronchial/

> ## PRACTICE TIP
>
> The mediastinum and all the structures within it pose a threat to the airtight integrity of the pleural space. Oesophageal ruptures from vomiting or high-pressure mechanical ventilation can provide a pathway for air to enter the pleura while both the chest wall and the lungs are intact (Dehours et al., 2013).

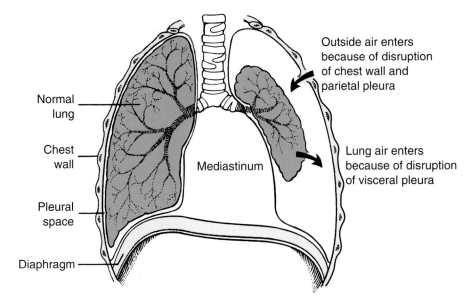

Figure 20.1
Air entering the pleural space due to damage to either the chest wall (open) or the lung wall (closed) enables the natural elasticity of the lung to collapse the lung away from the chest wall. This leads to decreased ventilation and subsequent gas exchange in the affected lung.
Source: Craft, Gordon & Tiziani (2011).

alveolar space and the pleural space (a breach of the lung wall)

2. direct or indirect communication between the atmosphere and the pleural space (a breach of the chest wall)

3. the presence of gas-producing organisms in the pleural space.

Pneumothorax is a relatively common condition that can occur in people of any age and the results can vary from asymptomatic to mild chest discomfort and breathlessness or ultimately life-threatening cardiorespiratory collapse (see Box 20.1). The extent of the impact depends on the nature and size of the pneumothorax and therefore on the degree of ventilation/perfusion (V/Q) mismatch (McCance & Huether, 2010). There is a broadly used classification system (see Box 20.2) but it only identifies the cause and does not address the severity.

A *primary spontaneous pneumothorax (PSP)* typically occurs in the absence of any apparent underlying disease, although the likelihood of PSP increases in people who smoke. It can also be associated with a connective tissue disease such a Marfan's syndrome, but the disease may not be diagnosed prior to the occurrence of PSP. The exact cause of PSP is often unknown but may be associated with the rupture of a subpleural bleb or bulla (Porth & Martin, 2014). These thin areas of lung tissue allow the tissue to stretch and form small balloon- or bubble-like abnormalities that pouch

> ## BOX 20.1 Common signs and symptoms associated with pneumothorax
>
> - Dyspnoea, tachypnoea
> - Tachycardia
> - Hyperresonance on the affected side
> - Hyperinflation of the chest wall on the affected side
> - Chest pain
> - Subcutaneous emphysema
> - Open wound with sucking sound on inspiration (open pneumothorax)
> - Oxygen desaturation

out in the pleural space. In many cases the increased pressure of a cough or a sneeze can produce PSP in the weakened lung tissue. The amount of air that moves into the pleural space as a result is generally small and doesn't progress after the initial injury. However, this doesn't preclude that PSP has the potential to move air into the pleural space with each subsequent inspiration and cause a *tension pneumothorax* to develop, with catastrophic results (see below). Although PSP may be associated with pain and shortness of breath, the symptoms are variable and generally improve quickly. Patients can be asymptomatic following as little as 24–48 hours (Brown et al., 2016).

BOX 20.2 Classification of pneumothorax

Spontaneous
- Primary: no apparent underlying disease
- Secondary: clinically apparent underlying disease

Traumatic
- Iatrogenic: secondary to a medical procedure
- Accidental: secondary to blunt or penetrating trauma

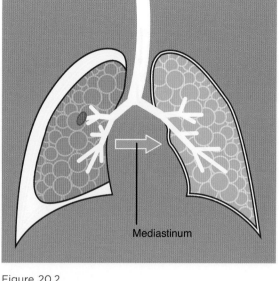

Figure 20.2
Closed pneumothorax.
A breach in the lung wall allows air to escape into the pleural space and the lung to collapse away from the chest wall. Lung disease and blunt trauma (especially when it causes a fractured rib that tears the lung wall) are common causes. The amount of air in the pleural space remains constant so the condition is referred to as a 'simple' rather than a 'tension' pneumothorax; the amount of air trapped between the lung and the chest wall increases with each inspiration and eventually creates sufficient intrathoracic pressure to prevent venous return to the heart and cause circulatory collapse.
Source: Quick et al. (2014).

A *secondary spontaneous pneumothorax (SSP)* occurs in association with clinically apparent pulmonary disease. As a consequence SSP most often presents later in life, commonly in the 60–65 age group, unlike PSP which typically occurs between the ages of 10 and 30 years (Onuki et al., 2017). Chronic obstructive pulmonary disease (COPD) is the most common preexisting lung condition associated with SSP, but other associated conditions include cystic fibrosis, asthma, neoplasms and infection. That there is significant underlying lung disease among these patients means a relatively minor SSP can often present as a life-threatening condition.

A *traumatic pneumothorax* may be caused by penetrating or non-penetrating trauma, resulting in an open or closed pneumothorax (McCance & Huether, 2010). An open traumatic pneumothorax occurs when a penetrating wound allows air to enter the pleural space directly through an opening in the chest wall. Air will preferentially enter the pleural space through a wound, as opposed to via the upper airway and trachea, when the wound diameter approaches two-thirds of the patient's tracheal diameter (Greaves et al., 2006). In this circumstance the chest wall will expand normally; however, air will preferentially move into the pleural

CATEMENIAL PNEUMO-THORAX

Catamenial pneumothorax is a type of spontaneous pneumothorax that typically occurs in women aged 30–40 with a history of endometriosis. The cause is largely unknown but is thought to be linked to pleural and diaphragmatic endometriosis. Patients with catamenial pneumothorax develop chest pain and dyspnoea within 24–72 hours of the onset of the menstrual flow. It is usually recurrent and correlated with menses (Porth & Martin, 2014).

space to equalise the lower thoracic pressure resulting in impaired lung expansion and ventilation.

A closed traumatic pneumothorax is most often caused by a fractured rib that is driven inwards lacerating the pleura. It may also occur without fracture when the blunt impact is delivered at full inspiration with the glottis closed, leading to a massive increase in intra-alveoli pressure and subsequent rupture of the alveoli. A penetrating injury may also cause a closed pneumothorax if there is no free communication with the atmosphere (Walls et al., 2018; see Fig 20.2).

An *iatrogenic traumatic pneumothorax* can occur secondary to certain medical procedures. (The term 'iatrogenic' meaning 'resulting from the actions of a clinician'.) The most common medical procedures leading to this type of pneumothorax are thoracentesis, pleural biopsy, transthoracic needle biopsy, transbronchial lung biopsy, subclavian vein catheterisation and positive pressure ventilation (McCance & Huether, 2010). An *iatrogenic traumatic pneumothorax* is often not clearly outwardly

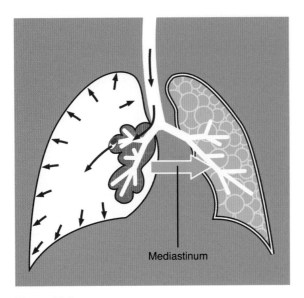

Mediastinum

Figure 20.3

Tension pneumothorax.

Compared with a simple pneumothorax where the volume of air in the pleural space is stable, in a tension pneumothorax the damaged lung or chest wall can create a 'one-way valve' where air is sucked into the pleural space by the negative pressure created with each inspiratory effort. This air is unable to escape on expiration. The escalating volume eventually collapses the affected lung almost completely and exerts pressure on the mediastinum. The inferior vena cava can become completely compressed and allow no return of blood to the heart. This situation of increasing respiratory distress with decreasing blood pressure and conscious state in the setting of chest trauma requires urgent decompression of the affected side.

Source: Quick et al. (2014).

visible and may be complicated by bleeding into the pleural space along with lung contusion. As such, a high index of suspicion, regular assessment and observations are required for any patient involved with a mechanism of injury capable of causing pneumothorax.

Although rare, pneumothorax of any aetiology has the potential to progress to a *tension pneumothorax* (see Fig 20.3). A pneumothorax becomes a tension pneumothorax when the intrapleural pressure exceeds the atmospheric pressure throughout expiration and possibly during inspiration (Greaves et al., 2006). This is due to the continued accumulation of air within the thoracic cavity, which is unable to escape. In spontaneously breathing patients tension pneumothorax occurs in the presence of a one-way valve mechanism (e.g. tissue flap or lung tissue acting as a pressure valve in association with a penetrating chest wound, lower airway narrowing in

asthma or application of an occlusive dressing to a wound associated with an open pneumothorax). The progression of tension pneumothorax risk is increased greatly in the setting of positive pressure ventilation. In either case air enters the pleural space during inspiration but does not exit during exhalation, leading to an increasing accumulation of pressure within the pleural cavity (Greaves et al., 2006). As this accumulation of air increases, intrathoracic pressure increases and starts to compress the vessels returning blood to the heart; ultimately the pressure on the affected side may be so great that it displaces the mediastinum further impairing cardiac function. This reduction in venous return to the heart results in reduced cardiac output and hypotension. As the tension pneumothorax extends, the unaffected lung is compressed, resulting in a rapid and catastrophic deterioration of the patient's respiratory function. A tension pneumothorax is a life-threatening condition requiring immediate decompression of the affected side using a cannula, a pneumocath or blunt thoracostomy. The decision which technique to use and where to insert the needle varies depending on local guidelines, often either the second intercostal space (ICS) mid-clavicular line or fifth ICS anterior or mid-axillary line.

Box 20.3 outlines the signs of a tension pneumothorax. Most of these signs could be the result of trauma to any region or could simply be the result of bleeding or pain, while others are late signs. Traditionally tracheal deviation and jugular venous distension were taught as key signs for tension pneumothorax; however, they have been shown to be poorly sensitive in the diagnosis of tension pneumothorax. Jugular vein distension is further

BOX 20.4 Pulsus paradoxus

Pulsus paradoxus is a condition in which the systolic blood pressure drops by more than 10 mmHg during inspiration. It is clinically identified when taking a radial pulse. The heart rate may appear irregular as beats will not be palpated during inspiration. On auscultation, however, beats associated with the missed radial beats can be heard. This is due to the decrease in blood pressure and the lack of transmission of the wave of pressure during the lower systolic blood pressure. Pulsus paradoxus is associated with tension pneumothorax, pericarditis, cardiac tamponade and obstructive lung disease.

unlikely to be present in the hypovolaemic trauma patient. Importantly, in some cases central hypoxia from pulmonary collapse is the primary pathology, and cardiac output and blood pressure are maintained until respiratory arrest (Inocencio et al., 2017). Maintaining a high index of suspicion of tension pneumothorax in patients who have suffered chest trauma is the key to making an effective clinical decision. If other causes have been treated such as severe pain and poor perfusion and the symptoms remain, a strong suspicion of tension pneumothorax should be adopted.

Diagnosis of pneumothorax can be complicated in the out-of-hospital setting by factors such as excessive noise, anxious bystanders, poor lighting levels, environmental conditions and patient position (Cantwell et al., 2009). Combined with the patient who has concurrent distracting traumatic injuries, diagnosis based on vital signs must be made following judicious analgesia and steps to support perfusion made.

 CASE STUDY 1

Case 05152, 1815 hrs.

Dispatch details: A 19-year-old football player in severe respiratory distress.

Initial presentation: On arrival the crew are directed to a fit-looking 19-year-old male sitting upright in the changing rooms. He is conscious and obviously tachypnoeic.

 ASSESS

Patient history

The patient says that he was completing a series of hill sprints during pre-season training with his team. On the fourth hill he felt a click in the left side of his chest but no pain. At the top of the hill he felt short of breath but instead of recovering he actually 'got slightly worse': 'I thought I was having a heart attack or something'. He was helped back to the changing rooms and his respiratory distress has not eased.

He says that he didn't feel any pain at the time but now can feel a mild sharp pain in the mid-axillary line of his left chest about level with his nipple when he inspires. Both the patient and the team coach insist that he has not been involved in any physical contact or tackling drills: 'It's pre-season training: we're just doing running'. He states that he has never experienced anything

HISTORY

Ask!

- Where was the impact?
- Are your symptoms progressing?

like this previously and has no medical history; he also has no allergies and takes no medications.

Airway
The patient's airway appears clear.

Breathing
The patient is sitting upright. He appears anxious but is cooperative and is breathing in even cycles at 34 bpm. On auscultation there are no obvious wheezes or crackles but there may be slightly reduced breath sounds on the left upper field. Chest excursion is good and appears equal. The patient's work of breathing appears slightly elevated but the tidal volume appears normal, if not above normal.

Cardiovascular
This patient is tachycardic but not hypotensive. There are multiple factors that could cause this physiological response, including pain, anxiety, hypovolaemia, hypoxia and sympathetic nervous system activation. With no obvious mechanism of injury, hypovolaemia can be considered a low probability, as respiratory distress is rarely the primary presenting problem in this condition.

Central nervous system
This patient is conscious and alert. Profound hypercapnia and hypoxia will lead to depression of conscious state but for the moment at least he has no alterations of conscious state.

Initial assessment summary

Problem	Acute shortness of breath
Conscious state	Alert and oriented; GCS = 15
Position	Sitting upright against wall
Heart rate	120 bpm, regular
Blood pressure	120/85 mmHg
Skin appearance	Pale, warm
Speech pattern	Short sentences
Respiratory rate	34 bpm
Respiratory rhythm	Adequate tidal volume
Respiratory effort	Mild increase in the use of accessory muscles
Chest auscultation	Nil wheeze, nil crackles, ? decreased breath sounds on upper left side
Pulse oximetry	93% on room air
Temperature	36.9°C
Motor/sensory function	Normal
History	Nil
Pain	Minimal
Physical examination	Unremarkable

D: There are no dangers.
A: The patient is conscious with no current airway obstruction.
B: The patient is ventilating effectively with an apparently clear chest but remains short of breath. There are slightly decreased breath sounds in the upper left lobe.
C: Heart rate is significantly elevated but blood pressure is normal.

The patient is displaying respiratory distress despite effective ventilation and perfusion. There is no history of trauma.

② CONFIRM

The essential part of the clinical reasoning process is to seek to confirm your initial hypothesis by finding clinical signs that should occur with your provisional diagnosis. You should also seek to challenge your diagnosis by exploring findings that do *not* fit your hypothesis: don't just ignore them because they don't fit.

The patient who presents with established shortness of breath but who is able to ventilate normally and has neither wheezes nor crackles presents a diagnostic challenge for the paramedic. Pathologies such as asthma and acute pulmonary oedema present with abnormal breath sounds that guide treatment, but in their absence the possible list of alternatives must be expanded to ensure a cause is not missed.

What else could it be?

Asthma
Adult-onset asthma is not uncommon but usually presents with mild chronic symptoms (such as a nocturnal cough) before a severe episode. Shortness of breath in asthma, however, occurs from bronchospasm causing increased airway resistance, and in this patient the above-average tidal volume, even respiratory cycle and lack of wheezes all indicate normal airway patency (see Ch 17).

Anaphylaxis
Shortness of breath in anaphylaxis follows the same inflammatory pathway as asthma (see Ch 17) and would require an increased work of breathing, a prolonged expiratory phase and wheezes to be definitive. It is worth checking the other systems for potential signs but this patient has no skin rash, erythema, angio-oedema or change of voice.

Anaemia
A loss of red blood cells due to a minor recurring hidden bleed (e.g. gastro-intestinal bleeding) or disease can be sufficient to cause respiratory distress at rest. The process develops over time, however, and is unlikely to present as acute and then not respond to rest. Anaemia is not supported when the patient's conjunctiva and gums are examined and they appear pink, not pale.

Acute pulmonary oedema/acute myocardial infarction
Failure of the mitral valve, the sudden onset of an arrhythmia or decreased left ventricular function from an infarction can all cause acute pulmonary oedema (APO). However, the ECG reveals only sinus rhythm with no ST changes, and the likelihood of infarction in a person of this age is highly unlikely. The pain is also well localised, described as 'sharp' and changes with ventilation. Although acute myocardial infarction (AMI) may present with 'pleuritic' pain (see Ch 21), without the supporting signs for fluid accumulation in the lungs (crackles) this diagnosis is not supported.

Pleural effusion
An abnormal accumulation of fluid between the lungs and the chest wall can allow an area of alveoli to collapse and no longer be ventilated. This fluid accumulation generally takes time to develop, however, and is unlikely to present as suddenly as in this instance. Effusions are most often caused by infection and the patient has no recent history of respiratory infection.

Haemothorax
Bleeding into the pleural space has the same effect as a pleural effusion in creating a V/Q mismatch in the area of the lung compressed by the fluid and can develop quickly. In the absence of trauma, however, it is an unlikely diagnosis. Blood and pleural fluid drain with gravity so they tend to compromise ventilation in the lower lung lobe and affect breath sounds and percussion

---

DIFFERENTIAL DIAGNOSIS

Shortness of breath despite normal ventilation
Or
- Asthma
- Anaphylaxis
- Acute pulmonary oedema/acute myocardial infarction
- Anaemia
- Pleural effusion
- Haemothorax
- Primary spontaneous pneumothorax
- Tension pneumothorax
- Anxiety

PRACTICE TIP

Most cases of PSP are confirmed by upright posteroanterior chest x-ray, while CT scans along with ultrasonography have proved effective in detecting small pneumothorax.

(dull) in this area. In this case, the compromised breath sounds are in the upper fields.

Primary spontaneous pneumothorax

Spontaneous damage to the lung wall is up to seven times more common in males than in females and most commonly occurs in taller individuals aged between 10 and 20 years (Luh, 2010). The pathology is not well understood and while blebs or infections increase the risk they are not always associated, and any situation that increases intrathoracic pressure (e.g. deep breathing, coughing) can be considered an adequate cause. Localised pain is common but it can resolve well before the pneumothorax is healed (Luh, 2010). The size of the pneumothorax will determine the extent to which it compromises lung function, and the collapsed area may stay in the site of tissue damage or migrate (commonly to the upper regions of the chest cavity). Hyperresonance of the affected area is common but is not a skill commonly practised by paramedics. This diagnosis is supported by nearly all the clinical findings in this case.

Tension pneumothorax

While a simple pneumothorax rarely requires out-of-hospital intervention, it can evolve into a life-threatening tension pneumothorax. A progression of symptoms (increasing respiratory distress with decreasing perfusion and ultimately a decrease in conscious state) indicates a tension pneumothorax, but in this case the patient appears stable.

Anxiety

As described in Chapter 52, the diagnosis of behavioural disturbances should be made when all physical causes of the condition have been eliminated. In this case there is a supporting physical diagnosis. Without any physical cause, the patient's respiratory rate and volume would result in hypocapnia and this would produce tetany and paraesthesia in the hands. Both of these are absent in this case. This patient's SpO_2 is also bordering on abnormally low, supporting the conclusion that a pathological abnormality is present. The patient may indeed be anxious, but this is not the primary cause of his respiratory distress.

While is it impossible to definitively exclude several of the causes in the field, the sudden onset of symptoms combined with a normal work of breathing and no obvious lung pathology are suggestive of a simple closed pneumothorax. There is no cardiovascular compromise but that doesn't preclude a tension pneumothorax developing later.

TREAT

Emergency management

The principles of management of a simple pneumothorax are outlined in Box 20.5.

Safety

There are no issues of safety.

Position

As with all cases of respiratory distress, the patient should be helped to find a position of comfort and then managed around that presentation as the situation allows. Ventilatory efficiency is best when the thorax is vertical, so most patients will prefer this position and will probably resist being placed supine.

Oxygen

Air in the pleural space will allow the area of lung around it to collapse and create an area where the alveoli are perfused but no longer ventilated. If sufficiently large, this V/Q mismatch will reduce the oxygen in arterial blood and lead to a sensation of air hunger or shortness of breath. In the out-of-hospital setting

> ## BOX 20.5 Principles of management
>
> **Simple pneumothorax**
>
> Safety: Remove any dangers.
>
> Position: Allow the patient to find the most efficient position.
>
> Oxygen: Increase the fraction of inspired oxygen to combat the V/Q mismatch.
>
> Pain relief: Allow pain-free ventilation.
>
> Transport: For definitive care and diagnosis.
>
> Monitor: For signs of a tension pneumothorax (see Ch 20 for management).

where reduction of the pneumothorax is not always practical, the best method to manage the V/Q mismatch is to increase the fraction of inspired oxygen with high-flow oxygen via a rebreather mask. The subsequent increase in partial oxygen pressure in the alveoli may be sufficient to rectify the hypoxaemia.

Pain relief

Pain from a spontaneous pneumothorax can vary considerably in intensity and in the more severe case it may impede the patient ventilating adequately. Pain relief should be titrated according to the patient's condition and local guidelines.

Transport

This patient should be transported to the most appropriate facility indicated by the local network. The receiving hospital should be advised of the patient's condition and impending arrival. This will enable the hospital to assemble the appropriate team to manage him expediently on arrival. In rural and remote locations this will enable activation of the relevant retrieval system.

4 EVALUATE

Evaluating the effect of any clinical management intervention can provide clues to the accuracy of the initial diagnosis. Some conditions respond rapidly to treatment so patients should be expected to improve if the diagnosis and treatment were appropriate. A failure to improve in this situation should trigger the clinician to reconsider the diagnosis.

Continuous reassessment of the patient with a pneumothorax is essential in order to identify trends in the patient's condition, which may indicate deterioration and in particular the development of a tension pneumothorax. The diagnosis of a tension pneumothorax is clinical and if suspected must be immediately decompressed by the paramedic. Any patient who has a pneumothorax and develops respiratory and cardiovascular collapse is clinically diagnosed as having a tension pneumothorax.

Ongoing management

Evolution from a simple to a tension pneumothorax is difficult to predict. The crew should recruit back-up if they are not able to perform a chest decompression should the patient deteriorate. Up to 2% of patients with a spontaneous pneumothorax will also experience a haemothorax and the accumulation of blood in the pleural space could contribute to a deterioration (Luh, 2010). Where a haemothorax does occur the bleeding is usually associated with scar tissue from a previous pneumothorax (Luh, 2010).

With no reliable method of predicting in the out-of-hospital setting whether a simple pneumothorax will progress to a tension pneumothorax, any significant deterioration should be treated as if it is a tension pneumothorax.

Hospital admission

Patients with a small pneumothorax will be admitted and assessed by x-ray, ultrasonography and or CT scan and often the pneumothorax will be left to reduce over time. In this case, however, the patient requires a chest drain or lateral intercostal catheter to allow the lung to expand. An intercostal catheter connected to either an underwater seal drain or a Heimlich valve will allow air to leave the chest without re-entering.

Long-term impact

Recovery from pneumothorax is dependent on the aetiology and severity of the insult. Whether the pneumothorax was an isolated incident or associated with comorbidities or concurrent injuries is a significant factor. Ongoing sequelae can include recurrence of the pneumothorax and reduced lung compliance due to scar tissue. Even following optimal treatment to fully expand lungs, 20–60% of PSP patients suffer relapse (Tan et al., 2017).

 CASE STUDY 2

Case 10211, 0720 hrs.

Dispatch details: A 32-year-old female with sudden shortness of breath. The patient's best friend is waiting with her.

Initial presentation: On arrival the patient's friend meets the crew outside the patient's house and leads them to the patient. She is sitting upright on the edge of a bed. She is conscious, and slightly anxious.

 ASSESS

0734 hrs Chief complaint: She complains of right-side chest pain that she describes as 'sharp' and catching each time she breathes in. The pain is well localised.

0734 hrs Vital signs survey: GCS = 15, RR = 22, mild dyspnoea increasing slightly on speaking or exertion. Tidal volume is restricted due to increasing pain on inspiration. Breath sounds are slightly decreased on the right side. SpO_2 = 94% on room air. HR = 95 regular and strong. BP = 125/70 mmHg. The rhythm strip shows sinus rhythm. The patient says she has right-sided chest pain, sharp in quality. Her pain score is 3 out of 10, increasing to 7 out of 10 on inspiration. She has no physical injuries.

0738 hrs Pertinent hx: The patient states that she was undertaking her regular morning yoga class when she suddenly felt localised right-sided chest pain. This was accompanied by mild trouble taking a breath. She has a history of asthma, which is well-controlled with medications, and takes the contraceptive pill. She has no other personal or family history of serious illness, and no known allergies. She rang her friend, who convinced her that she should go to hospital in case it was her asthma 'playing up', prompting the ambulance call.

② CONFIRM

In many cases paramedics are presented with a collection of signs and symptoms that do not appear to describe a particular condition. A critical step in determining a treatment plan in this situation is to consider what other conditions could explain the patient's presentation.

Unlike Case study 1, where the primary complaint was shortness of breath, the presentation here is pain caused by breathing. The patient notices she is more short of breath when she tries to speak longer sentences. Her SpO_2 is also lower than it should be for her age and history.

What else could it be?

Asthma

As in Case study 1 the normal work of breathing and lack of wheezes make this diagnosis unsupported.

Acute coronary syndrome

Acute coronary syndrome is always worth considering as a differential diagnosis, but this patient's age, combined with the location and nature of the pain, would indicate this to be an unlikely diagnosis. Acute coronary syndrome would not explain the changes in breath sounds that have been observed.

Pulmonary embolism

Pulmonary embolism (PE; see Ch 21) can present with both pain and shortness of breath, and use of the oral contraceptive pill increases the risk of forming clots that could lodge in the lungs. The pain from PE (if present at all) tends to be dull and poorly localised and would explain the unequal breath sounds.

Thoracic aortic dissection

While a sharp pain is typical of a thoracic aortic dissection, the location is not consistent, nor is the changing intensity of pain with ventilation. It is also unsupported by the unequal chest sounds. Thoracic dissection can sometimes occlude one of the major arteries supplying the upper limbs, producing a different blood pressure in each arm. Although not always present, a significant difference in brachial blood pressure strongly suggests a dissection thoracic aneurysm. In this case bilateral blood pressure is equal.

Pleurisy

Infection of the pleura can cause friction between the lungs and the chest wall. This can cause a sharp, well-localised pain similar to that which this patient is experiencing, but it would be expected to follow a history of infection. Pleurisy also creates a distinct 'rub' when you auscultate over the site of pain as the patient breathes. The lack of rub and signs of infection effectively rule this diagnosis out.

Musculoskeletal trauma

This is probably the most logical and common diagnosis for this type of pain, even allowing for the low-intensity exercise. Described in more detail in Chapter 36, musculoskeletal pain can usually be elicited on palpation but in this case that is not possible. While the pain could cause the patient to reduce her tidal volume, the pain alone doesn't explain the unequal breath sounds.

DIFFERENTIAL DIAGNOSIS

Spontaneous pneumothorax
Or
- Asthma
- Acute coronary syndrome
- Pulmonary embolism
- Thoracic aortic dissection
- Pleurisy
- Musculoskeletal trauma

TREAT

0740 hrs: The patient remains sitting upright.

Although not primarily indicated in this setting ($SpO_2 > 93\%$ on room air), because of the provisional diagnosis of a pneumothorax it is prudent to give the patient oxygen prior to her exerting herself to move to the stretcher for transport.

0742 hrs: A decrease in pain will most likely increase the patient's tidal volume and improve the arterial oxygen content. The paramedics may choose from a variety of pain management strategies including intravenous, intramuscular, intranasal and inhaled agents according to local guidelines.

0745 hrs: The patient needs to be transferred to hospital for further investigation of the cause of her chest pain and shortness of breath.

④ EVALUATE

Evaluating the effect of any clinical management intervention can provide clues to the accuracy of the initial diagnosis. Some conditions respond rapidly to treatment so patients should be expected to improve if the diagnosis and treatment were appropriate. A failure to improve in this situation should trigger the clinician to reconsider the diagnosis.

During transport to hospital continuous monitoring of the patient through regular and repeated assessments will identify trends regarding her response to treatment and whether or not the treatment regimen needs to be modified. It is important to assess the effect of analgesia and reassurance on the patient's respiratory effort and effectiveness. Although unlikely, it is possible that the pneumothorax may increase in size, causing increasing respiratory distress. Progression of a spontaneous pneumothorax to a tension pneumothorax is very rare but should still be considered.

Summary

A pneumothorax is generally considered to be a result of trauma to the chest, but it can occur spontaneously and in this instance is more common in patients with existing lung disease. A pneumothorax causes respiratory distress by allowing a section of lung to collapse and become non-ventilated while remaining perfused. The extent of hypoxaemia is dependent on the size of the pneumothorax.

Spontaneous pneumothorax presents a clinical challenge because shortness of breath is usually associated with abnormal breath sounds but in this case the auscultation will reveal only possibly decreased breath sounds over the affected area and this may be difficult to detect. While some groups such as tall males, females with a history of endometriosis and people with connective tissues disorders are at higher risk of developing a pneumothorax, pneumothorax should always be considered in a differential diagnosis of the patient in respiratory distress who presents with normal tidal volumes and breath sounds (Box 20.6).

BOX 20.6 Out-of-hospital Point Of Care Ultrasound (POCUS)

Chest ultrasonography has a great potential for increasing the sensitivity of the initial diagnostic assessment concerning pneumothorax and haemothorax in trauma patients (Staub et al., 2018). The absence of lung slide (visual friction between the *in-contact* visceral and parietal pleura) on chest ultrasonography has been shown to be superior or equivalent to supine anteroposterior chest radiographs (x-ray) and CT in detection of pneumothoraces (Bloch et al., 2011). Paramedic-performed out-of-hospital ultrasound is a novel skill that has gained popularity in some services in recent years. In this setting POCUS can provide additional information that can assist with management and guide transport to the most appropriate facility (Meadley et al., 2017).

References

Beachey, W. (2018). *Respiratory care anatomy and physiology—foundations for clinical practice* (4th ed.). St Louis: Mosby.

Bloch, A., Bloch, S., Secreti, L., & Prasad, N. (2011). A porcine training model for ultrasound diagnosis of pneumothoraces. *The Journal of Emergency Medicine, 41*(2), 176–181.

Brown, S. G. A., Ball, E. L., Perrin, K., Read, C. A., Asha, S. E., Beasley, R., Egerton-Warburton, D., Jones, P. G., Keijzers, G., Kinnear, F. B., Kwan, B. C. H., Lee, Y. C. G., Smith, J. A., Summers, Q. A., Simpson, G., & the PSP Study Group. (2016). Study protocol for a randomized controlled trial of invasive versus conservative management of primary spontaneous pneumothorax. *BMJ Open, 6*, e011826. doi: 10.1136/bmjopen-2016-011826.

Cantwell, K., Burgess, S., Patrick, I., Jones, C., Cameron, P., Fitzgerald, M., & Niggemeyer, L. (2009). Pre-hospital tension pneumothorax: has it improved? *Injury, 40*, S15.

Craft, J., Gordon, C., & Tiziani, A. (2011). *Understanding pathophysiology*. Sydney: Elsevier.

Dehours, E., Valle, B., Bounes, V., & Lauque, D. (2013). A pneumomediastinum with diffuse subcutaneous emphysema. *Visual Diagnosis in Emergency Medicine, 44*(1), e81–e82.

Greaves, I., Porter, K., Hodgetts, T., & Woollard, M. (2006). *Emergency care: a textbook for paramedics*. London: Elsevier.

Inocencio, M., Childs, J., Chilstrom, M. L., & Berona, K. (2017). Ultrasound findings in tension pneumothorax: a case report. *Journal of Emergency Medicine, 52*(6), e217.

Luh, S. (2010). Diagnosis and treatment of primary spontaneous pneumothorax. *Journal of Zhejiang University SCIENCE B (Biomedicine & Biotechnology), 11*(10), 735–744.

McCance, K., & Huether, S. (2010). *Pathophysiology: the biologic basis for disease in adults and children* (6th ed.). St Louis: Mosby.

Meadley, B., Olaussen, A., Delorenzo, A., Roder, N., Martin, C., St Clair, T., & Williams, B. (2017). Educational standards for training paramedics in ultrasound: a scoping review. *BMC Emergency Medicine, 17*, 18.

Onuki, T., Ueda, S., Yamaoka, M., Sekiya, Y., Yamada, H., Kawakami, N., Araki, Y., Wakai, Y., Saito, K., Inagaki, M., & Matsumiya, N. (2017). Primary and secondary spontaneous pneumothorax: prevalence, clinical features, and in-hospital mortality. *Canadian Respiratory Journal: Journal of the Canadian Thoracic Society, 2017*, 6014967.

Porth, C., & Martin, G. (2014). *Pathophysiology: concepts of altered health states* (9th ed.). Philadelphia: Lippincott Williams & Wilkins.

Quick, C. R. G., Reed, J. B., Harper, S. J. F., Saeb-Parsy, K., & Deakin, P. J. (2014). *Essential surgery: problems, diagnosis and management*. Edinburgh: Churchill Livingstone.

Staub, L., Biscaro, R., Kaszubowski, E., & Maurici, R. (2018). Chest ultrasonography for the emergency diagnosis of traumatic pneumothorax and haemothorax: a systematic review and meta-analysis. *Injury, 49*(3), 457.

Tan, J., Yang, Y., Zhong, J., Zuo, C., Tang, H., Zhao, H., Zeng, G., Zhang, J., Guo, J., & Yang, N. (2017). Association between BMI and recurrence of primary spontaneous pneumothorax. *World Journal of Surgery, 41*, 1274–1280.

Walls, R., Hockberger, R., & Gausche-Hill, M. (2018). *Rosen's emergency medicine – concepts and clinical practice* (9th ed.). Philadelphia.: Elsevier. Chapter 38 Thoracic Trauma (Raja, S.).

CHAPTER 21

Pulmonary Embolism

By Jarrod Wakeling

OVERVIEW

- Pulmonary embolism (PE) is not a disease entity by itself, but is a complication of venous thrombo-embolism (VTE), most commonly a deep vein thrombosis (DVT).
- Emboli formed as a consequence of VTE result from the influence of factors in Virchow's triad; vessel wall injury, venous stasis or a hypercoagulable state.

- Hypoxaemia occurs frequently, but is not seen in all PE patients.
- Computed tomography pulmonary angiography (CTPA) is the gold standard diagnostic test for PE.
- Treatment of a PE typically involves oxygen therapy, analgesia, anticoagulant medications and, in some circumstances, a fibrinolytic or surgical embolectomy.

Introduction

The sudden occlusion of the blood supply to a portion of the lungs can produce a range of non-specific symptoms that extend from minor to life-threatening, and as such the provisional diagnosis of a pulmonary embolism (PE) can be challenging in the out-of-hospital environment. Even though paramedic management of a PE is largely supportive, patients with this condition can quickly deteriorate, with a 70% mortality rate within the first hour of patients presenting with PE and severe cardiovascular compromise (Lehnert et al., 2017). Overall, the fatality rate for untreated PE is as high as 25% (McRae, 2010).

The symptoms that a PE can produce are wide-ranging, non-specific and can mimic a number of other disease processes. A comprehensive understanding of the risk factors and presenting symptoms, complemented by a high index of suspicion, is necessary if paramedics are to recognise a patient presenting with a PE.

Pathophysiology

Pulmonary arteries can become blocked by a number of mechanisms. Amniotic fluid expelled into the venous system during birth and fat displaced by long bone fractures are possible causes, but by far the most common cause is a venous thrombo-embolism (VTE). A VTE commonly forms in the lower extremities before breaking loose, travelling through the right side of the heart and becoming lodged in the pulmonary arteries. As such, PE is not a disease entity by itself, but is a complication of a deep vein thrombosis (DVT). VTE has an annual incidence of approximately 1.0 per 1000, with peak incidence seen in males > 80 years at 1.0 per 100 (Bersten & Soni, 2019). Forty per cent of patients with a DVT will develop a PE and 90% of PEs develop from a DVT (Bersten & Soni, 2019). Children (< 18 years) presenting with a PE is increasing with a peak incidence in the community being 4.9 per 100,000 (Konstantinides et al., 2020). This is due to improved complex illness survival and the increasing use of oestrogen-containing oral contraceptives (Kline, 2020).

Although emboli may be formed from blood constituents, tumour, fat or air, those formed as a consequence of VTE usually result from the influence of factors in Virchow's triad (Ouellette et al., 2012; see Fig 21.1). Virchow's triad describes the three main contributors to the formation of a DVT: 1. hypercoagulability—any disorder that promotes blood clotting; 2. stasis—any condition that slows or causes a period of stagnation of blood flow through the veins; and 3. endothelial injury—injuries to the endothelial cells that line the vessels trigger a clotting cascade. Once a thrombus forms, it is at risk of dislodging and travelling through the right side of the heart and lodging in the pulmonary vasculature.

Most pulmonary emboli are caused by thrombi originating in the deep veins of the lower limbs, but other sources of emboli are the veins of the pelvis and upper limbs, and even the heart. The effect of the embolus depends on the size and location of the region it occludes. A PE creates an area of ventilation/perfusion (V/Q) mismatch where the alveoli are ventilated but not perfused (see Fig 21.2 and Box 21.1 with Figs 21.3 and 21.4). A

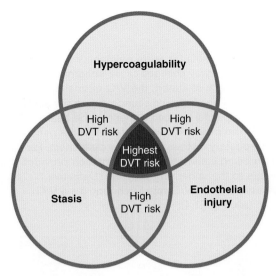

Figure 21.1
Virchow's triad describes the three main contributors to the formation of a DVT: 1. hypercoagulability; 2. stasis; and 3. endothelial injury.

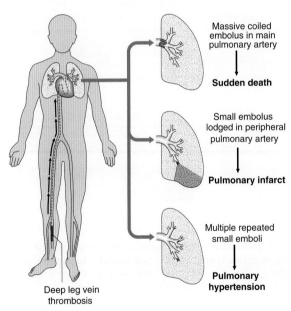

Figure 21.2
Blocking the arteries carrying deoxygenated blood to the lungs creates an area of lung that remains ventilated but not perfused. If the mismatch is sufficiently large it may lead to hypoxaemia. The loss of perfusion can also lead to systemic hypotension as it reduces blood flow to the left side of the heart. Locally, the poorly perfused lung tissue may become ischaemic and die.
Source: Cross (2013).

large PE, often associated with an occlusion involving > 30–50% of the pulmonary artery bed, is likely to create two concerning symptoms that are directly associated with an increased morbidity and mortality; those being hypoxaemia and hypotension

(Konstantinides et al., 2020). Hypoxaemia results due to a significant portion of lung tissue not participating in oxygen delivery in the affected pulmonary capillary bed leading to deoxygenated blood mixing with newly oxygenated blood ready for systemic perfusion. Hypotension is likely to occur as result of the obstruction PE adversely affecting cardiac preload and/or right ventricular failure.

Additional symptoms that can also be seen relate to the direct lung injury itself. The lungs receive oxygenated blood from the bronchial arteries and lung tissue is also dependent on deoxygenated blood from the pulmonary arteries for survival. During a PE the lung tissue in the area in which blood flow is occluded will be injured and may become infarcted. This process of anaerobic metabolism pathway accounts for the pain associated with some presentations of PE. Unlike large emboli, which occlude a significant area of lung tissue and cause sudden respiratory and circulatory compromise, smaller emboli can migrate more deeply into the lung whereby symptoms can evolve over hours or even days. The resultant inflammatory response to injured tissue can irritate the pleura (causing pain) and produce a fever, pleural effusions, friction rub and malaise. The breakdown of lung tissue in this area may also contribute to haemoptysis.

Differentiating the severity of a PE can be challenging in the out-of-hospital setting due to varying symptoms and this can signify confusion relating to both treatment and transport pathways. Below is a simple, yet conclusive account of PE severity that is frequently used in hospitals to aid in diagnostic and treatment modalities.

- *Massive PE:* haemodynamic instability characterised by hypotension. Patients present with acute respiratory and cardiovascular symptoms (see Fig 21.5). These patient presentations have a 25–30% mortality rate despite treatment (Bersten & Soni, 2019). This further increases to 65% mortality if CPR is required at any stage (Bersten & Soni, 2019).
- *Sub-massive PE:* haemodynamically stable with evidence of right ventricular dysfunction. Patients often present with acute respiratory symptoms and haemodynamic stability; however, this can quickly progress to haemodynamic instability. These patients have a higher incidence of right ventricular thrombosis and mortality when compared to PE patients with normal right ventricular function (Bersten & Soni, 2019).
- *Mild PE:* haemodynamically stable with no right ventricular dysfunction. Patients can have varying non-specific symptoms that may present suddenly

BOX 21.1 Ventilation/perfusion mismatch

Red blood cells are exposed to the thin alveolar-capillary membrane for at least 0.75 of a second but it takes only a third of this time for the partial pressure of oxygen to equalise and the blood to become fully oxygenated. For this process to occur the alveoli require both ventilation (V) with external air and perfusion (Q) of deoxygenated blood. A number of respiratory diseases cause their symptoms by altering this 'match' of ventilation and perfusion (V/Q). Asthma and other diseases that obstruct the airways lead to an area that is perfused but not ventilated. PE has the opposite effect: creating a zone where the alveoli are ventilated normally but do not receive any blood (see Fig 21.3).

Unlike asthma (or acute pulmonary oedema) where the airway changes cause abnormal sounds that can be auscultated, the V/Q mismatch in a PE creates no abnormal sounds during the acute phase (a pleural rub can sometimes be heard later). The paramedic will be faced with a patient in respiratory distress but with a clear chest. Far from being confusing, this presentation provides a clue to the underlying problem. Definitive assessment of a V/Q mismatch requires a V/Q scan (see Fig 21.4).

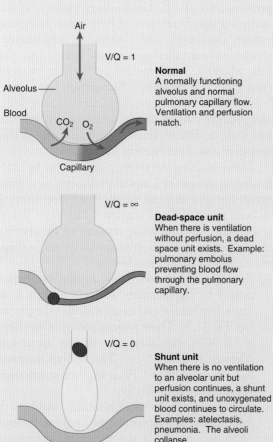

Normal
A normally functioning alveolus and normal pulmonary capillary flow. Ventilation and perfusion match.

$V/Q = 1$

Dead-space unit
When there is ventilation without perfusion, a dead space unit exists. Example: pulmonary embolus preventing blood flow through the pulmonary capillary.

$V/Q = \infty$

Shunt unit
When there is no ventilation to an alveolar unit but perfusion continues, a shunt unit exists, and unoxygenated blood continues to circulate. Examples: atelectasis, pneumonia. The alveoli collapse.

$V/Q = 0$

Figure 21.3
V/Q mismatch. The first alveoli pictured above represents normal ventilation and perfusion matching. The second alveoli is typical of PE: ventilated but not perfused The third alveoli is typical of asthma: perfused but not ventilated.
Source: Carroll (2007).

Single Breath	Equilib
POST	LPO
ANT	RAO

Figure 21.4
V/Q mismatch seen by measuring the uptake of radioactive isotopes injected into the bloodstream. Ventilation is assessed as the patient inhales a radiolabelled compound, which becomes distributed throughout the lung. In this case, the distribution appears uniform except for a portion of the lower left lobe in which there is a lack of ventilation (red arrow). Perfusion is assessed after the patient has been injected with a radiolabelled compound that is distributed throughout the pulmonary vasculature. In the bottom two panels, various views indicate multiple areas in which perfusion is diminished (red arrow); these areas are different from the area of decreased ventilation. There is thus a V/Q mismatch that gives a high probability for PE. Because in most cases the patient's lungs are ventilated but not perfused, giving an affected patient oxygen therapy increases the PaO_2 minimally.
Source: Klatt (2015).

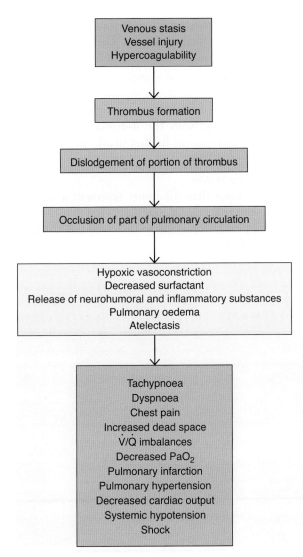

Figure 21.5
Pathogenesis of massive PE caused by a thrombus (pulmonary thromboembolism).
Source: McCance & Huether (2010).

BOX 21.2 Risk factors for venous thrombosis

Recent surgery
Joint replacement, cancer surgery, fracture, major gastrointestinal surgery, gynaecological surgery, inpatient day surgery

Acute illness
Congestive cardiac failure, acute respiratory failure, inflammatory conditions such as inflammatory bowel disease and rheumatological disease

Malignancy
Increased risk in chemotherapy, hormone therapy and surgery

Hormonal risk factors
Oral contraceptive pill, hormone replacement therapy

Miscellaneous
Increased age (> 60 years), increased body mass index, prolonged travel, heparin-induced thrombocytopenia, antiphospholipid antibody syndrome

Inherited risk factors
High risk: antithrombin, protein C + S deficiency
Moderate risk: factor V Leiden and prothrombin gene mutations
Source: McRae (2010).

or gradually over hours to days. These patients have low mortality and recurrence rates with appropriate diagnosis and treatment (Bersten & Soni, 2019).

A number of pathological processes occur as a result of direct obstruction including an increase in pulmonary vascular resistance, localised vasoconstriction secondary to hypoxia and the release of pro-inflammatory mediators which also increase resistance of blood flow through the lungs. Common comorbidities such as coronary artery disease or cardiopulmonary disease are associated with a higher incidence of respiratory failure, cardiac dysfunction, morbidity and mortality when compared to patients without these conditions.

Some emboli get lodged at the bifurcation of the pulmonary trunk into the left and right pulmonary arteries. These emboli are termed 'saddle emboli' as they sit across the bifurcation (Lee et al., 2005). Because they occlude the main entry path of blood into the lungs they have the potential to block blood flow to most of the lungs. In severe cases these emboli will occlude so much blood supply that no cardiac output from the left side of the heart is possible and the patient will present as a pulseless electrical activity (PEA) cardiac arrest.

Risk factors

While a pulmonary embolism can occur in any patient, there is a group of known risk factors that should raise the diagnostic suspicion of a PE when any of the symptoms are displayed (see Box 21.2).

Recent surgery

Day surgery increases the risk of VTE by a factor of 10, while the risk following inpatient surgery increases by a factor of 70 (McCance & Huether, 2010). Importantly, the risk is maximal 3 weeks post-surgery and remains elevated for up to 12 weeks, so most patients presenting with symptoms at this time will have been discharged from hospital and are likely to be encountered by paramedics.

Acute illness

The inflammatory and clotting responses are intrinsically linked so acute illnesses can raise the risk of hypercoagulability. Combined with dehydration and immobility, the risk of PE in this group is significantly raised and when a fever is present it can be difficult to differentiate the symptoms from acute sepsis.

Malignancy

Cancer patients represent between 15 and 20% of all VTE presentations with chemotherapy, surgery and hormone therapy all contributing to the risk (McCance & Huether, 2010). This is most likely to have been compounded by immobility.

Pregnancy and oral contraceptive pill (OCP)

The incidence of PE is 10 times higher during and after pregnancy, with the 4–6-week postpartum phase representing the highest incidence (McCance & Huether, 2010).

Extended travel

Flights longer than 12 hours represent a fivefold increase in risk of VTE, but flights less than 4 hours don't appear to represent an increased risk (Kuipers et al., 2007).

 CASE STUDY 1

Case 11008, 1023 hrs.

Dispatch details: A 32-year-old female with breathing problems, severe respiratory distress and chest pain.

Initial presentation: On arrival the patient is sitting on the couch and looking 'unwell'. She is alert, pale and anxious, short of breath and clutching the right side of her chest.

 ASSESS

HISTORY

Ask!
- When did the symptoms start?
- Are there any risk factors present?
- Do you have any pain (location and nature)?

Patient history

The patient is an obese 32-year-old female who is typically well with no reported past medical history, allergies and is only prescribed the oral contraceptive pill. She reports the acute onset of dyspnoea while watching TV and this has progressively worsened over the last few hours. Associated symptoms include right-sided pleuritic chest pain and a non-productive cough. The patient reports that she smokes approximate 15 cigarettes a day and has done so for the past 15 years, and that she has been increasingly inactive and depressed as a result of losing her job a few weeks ago. She has not experienced recent extended air travel or surgery.

Airway

Airway concern and intervention is rarely required and is only likely to be associated with a *massive PE* whereby profound hypoxaemia and/or hypotension is seen.

Breathing

Paramedic assessment of breathing has traditionally focused on identifying the presence of diseases for which paramedics intervene directly (i.e. upper airway obstruction, asthma, acute pulmonary oedema, pneumothoraces and chronic obstructive pulmonary disease). A significant component of this assessment is the chest auscultation and the presence of adventitious breath sounds; these include wheezes, stridor, crackles and diminished and/or absent breath sounds. There is a range of conditions in which the patient will present with respiratory distress without clear adventitious sounds making the differential diagnosis more challenging. The grouping of pneumothorax, PE and pleural effusion is especially difficult to determine as the work of breathing and tidal volume may be normal.

This patient is short of breath with no adventitious chest sounds and presents with a SpO_2 of 94% on room air. This is suggestive of mild hypoxaemia, especially in a young patient with nil preexisting lung disease. SpO_2 of 92.5% or below has been shown to be sensitive to detecting low-risk patients with a PE (Nordenholz et al., 2011). Interestingly, hypercapnia is rarely associated with PE (or pneumothorax and effusions) as the increased respiratory rate allows the highly soluble CO_2 to escape. In fact, early in the presentation of all these conditions the level of CO_2 dissolved in the blood may be lower than normal (Bersten & Soni, 2019).

Cardiovascular

Cardiovascular impairment is typically seen only in *massive PEs*; however contributing factors such as age, preexisting cardiovascular disease and complicating disease processes such as sepsis can all impair perfusion and cardiac function.

Massive PE will cause blood flow obstruction to the right side of the heart, promote pulmonary vasoconstriction secondary to hypoxaemia and cause an adaptive neural hormonal response to the decrease in cardiac output. All these factors will lead to an increasing pulmonary vascular resistance and right heart strain. The non-conditioned and thin right ventricular wall adaptation to a *massive PE* insult is limited and pulmonary artery pressures exceeding 40 mmHg are likely to lead to right ventricular failure.

Pleuritic and ischaemic cardiac chest pain can often be seen in unison, especially in PEs that have cardiac compromise. Excessive myocardial needs and decreased myocardial perfusion due to low cardiac output states are the main contributors to ischaemic cardiac chest pain.

The patient's ECG demonstrates sinus tachycardia; although this is a non-specific finding, it is associated with acute PE. There are a number of specific ECG findings in addition to sinus tachycardia associated with acute PE. These findings are consistent with right heart strain and include:

- S wave in lead I, Q wave in lead III and T-wave inversion in lead III
- T-wave inversion in leads V1–V4
- incomplete RBBB (Kline, 2020).

These right heart strain signs are generally associated with *massive PEs* and although their presence can aid in PE diagnosis, their absence does not exclude a PE (Kline, 2020).

Conscious state

In acute PE conscious state is likely to be impaired only due to profound hypoxaemia and/or hypotension. This patient's vital signs, in particular SpO_2 and perfusion, are inconsistent with causing an altered level of consciousness.

Physical examination

Examination of the patient's chest wall does not demonstrate any tenderness or abnormality over the site of pain consistent with traumatic cause. The patient's lower legs are equal in size and appearance and there is no pain

RESPIRATORY STATUS

Look for!
- General appearance; skin, speech and level of distress
- Chest sounds, respiratory rate, depth and work of breathing
- Oxygen saturation and responsiveness to supplementary oxygen if required
- Signs of cardiovascular compromise

indicative of a DVT. This is a common contributor to a PE and should be a routine consideration as part of thorough patient assessment involving acute dyspnoea. She describes the pain as dull but severe (8/10), changing on inspiration and localised to an area directly under her breast on the right side and confined to a palm-sized area.

Initial assessment summary

Problem	Moderate respiratory distress and pleuritic chest pain
Conscious state	Alert and oriented; GCS = 15
Position	Sitting upright on the couch holding the right side of her chest
Heart rate	118 bpm, regular; good pulses, equal bilaterally
Blood pressure	105/70 mmHg
Skin appearance	Pale, cool and dry
Speech pattern	Speaking in short sentences
Respiratory rate	26 bpm
Respiratory rhythm	Regular even cycles
Respiratory effort	Use of accessory muscles with a mild increase in WOB
Chest auscultation	Clear breath sounds, good bilateral air entry apices to bases, normal inspiratory/expiratory cycles; has a dry cough
Pulse oximetry	94% on room air
Temperature	37.2°C
Motor/sensory function	Normal
History	No medical history

D: Nil
R: Yes
A: Patent
Cx: Nil traumatic cause
B: Yes—with adequate ventilation
C: Yes
Hx: Nil visible external haemorrhage
D: Conscious
E: Patient is inside in a warm environment.

The patient is conscious; however, she is short of breath, displays pallor and looks unwell. She is complaining of dyspnoea and pleuritic chest pain. She is tachycardic, presenting in moderate respiratory distress with clear lung fields and a lower than expected SpO_2 for a young healthy patient without any preexisting lung diseases.

DIFFERENTIAL DIAGNOSIS

Pulmonary embolism
Or
- Asthma /anaphylaxis
- Acute pulmonary oedema
- Pneumothorax/pleural effusion
- Sepsis/pneumonia/ pleurisy
- Acute coronary syndrome/acute myocardial infarction
- Anxiety

2 **CONFIRM**

The essential part of the clinical reasoning process is to seek to confirm your initial hypothesis by finding clinical signs that should occur with your provisional diagnosis. You should also seek to challenge your diagnosis by exploring findings that do *not* fit your hypothesis: don't just ignore them because they don't fit.

There is no definitive test for PE in the field and the diagnosis is rather a combination of history, symptoms, clinical signs and simple investigations contextualised by risk factors. Many elements of the presentation of an acute PE are shared with other common diseases, so before leaping to any conclusions it is essential to consider other possible causes for this patient's acute dyspnoea.

What else could it be?

Asthma/anaphylaxis

Asthma can be easily excluded in this patient's presentation; the lack of an audible wheeze or diminished tidal volume combined with normal inspiratory/ expiratory cycles make an asthma diagnosis unlikely. Anaphylaxis requires a potential trigger with two of the Respiratory, Abdominal, Skin and/or Hypotension (RASH) criteria to aid the anaphylaxis diagnosis. A comprehensive patient assessment mitigates anaphylaxis as a likely differential diagnosis. This patient does not have preexisting history of either condition which adds to the evidence of each disease process being an unlikely cause of the patient's presentation.

Pulmonary oedema

The onset of acute respiratory distress can be seen in both cardiogenic and non-cardiogenic causes of pulmonary oedema. It would be a reasonable assumption that oedema leading to moderate respiratory distress and mild hypoxaemia would generate audible crackles on chest auscultation. Given the patient's age, nil known cardiac, liver or renal impairment, or recent history of near drowning, aspiration or progressive chest infection, the differential diagnosis of pulmonary oedema is again less likely.

Pneumothorax/pleural effusion

A conclusive diagnosis of a spontaneous pneumothorax, in particular a simple pneumothorax, without suspicion of other disease processes can be somewhat difficult for out-of-hospital clinicians. This patient presentation has many similarities consistent with a spontaneous pneumothorax: dyspnoea, pleuritic chest pain and mild hypoxaemia. A comprehensive patient assessment reveals that the risk factors, medication and past medical history is more consistent with a pulmonary embolus. Also, the chest sounds expected in a patient with moderate respiratory distress and mild hypoxaemia in a simple pneumothorax would be diminished with impaired tidal volumes. A chest x-ray should easily diagnose a simple pneumothorax.

A pleural effusion in a young and fit 32-year-old female with nil past medical history is not a common occurrence. It would be expected that there would be a clear delineation between chest sounds, whereby a pleural effusion causing moderate respiratory distress and mild hypoxaemia would have diminished breath sounds and likely 'muffled' sounds over the effusion. Again, a chest x-ray should easily diagnose a pleural effusion.

Sepsis/pneumonia/pleurisy

Although sepsis can occur without a fever, this is generally a late sign and sepsis and pneumonia are almost always preceded by a period of malaise and flu-like symptoms. The sudden onset, combined with a lack of prodromal symptoms and fever, lower the probability that sepsis/pneumonia/pleurisy is the cause. Careful auscultation would also reveal an area of consolidation if pneumonia was present.

Acute coronary syndromes (ACS)

Out-of-hospital clinicians can utilise their experience, knowledge and a comprehensive patient assessment including evaluating the patient's past medical history, risk factors, prodromal symptoms, current presenting symptoms and serial 12-lead ECGs to make an informed decision about the likelihood of an ACS presentation. Unfortunately, definitive exclusion can only be conclusively performed in hospital with cardiac investigations, including cardiac enzymes and repeat 12-lead ECGs. A comprehensive assessment of this patient presentation would inform the out-of-hospital clinician that ACS is unlikely; the patient's age, risk factors, atypical right-sided pleuritic chest pain, mild hypoxaemia and moderate respiratory distress in the presence of a clear chest

Table 21.1 Frequency of signs and symptoms in PE

Symptoms	Frequency in PE
Dyspnoea (rest or exertional)	60%
Pleuritic chest pain	60%
Cough	10%
Fever	15%
Calf or thigh pain	44%
Calf or thigh swelling	41%
Signs	Frequency in PE
Tachypnoea	60%
Tachycardia	40%
Crackles on auscultation (rales)	18%
Atelectasis	30%
Jugular venous distension	10%

Source: Lee et al. (2005).

would clearly suggest a PE as the primary differential diagnosis. In terms of treating this patient as per an ACS pathway or to 'pay-off' is fraught with risks that don't necessarily outweigh the benefits. Aspirin, an anti-emetic and analgesia is reasonable and poses a number of benefits for the patient with minimal risk. Conversely, nitrates have the real potential to adversely affect perfusion and worsen the patient's presenting condition. This patient is unlikely to have a blockage related to atherosclerotic plaque.

Anxiety

Behavioural diagnoses should be considered only when all physical causes for the presentation can be eliminated. For this patient that is clearly not the case but there is still no definitive link to PE and the inconsistency of symptoms (see Table 21.1) is disconcerting for most clinicians.

Wells score

The variable nature of PE symptoms and the overlap with other conditions has led to the development of several clinical prediction rules for PE. The Wells score is a commonly used clinical predictive tool for PE. Points are given for the presence or absence of risk factors and symptoms (see Table 21.2). The Wells score is a diagnostic algorithm for PE that assists emergency department (ED) clinicians to determine which diagnostic tests to perform, but it is also effective in the out-of-hospital setting.

Using the Wells criteria, this patient has a score of 6 even though her symptoms are non-specific ([alternative diagnosis less likely than PE = 3] + [heart rate > 100 bpm = 1.5] + [immobilisation = 1.5] = 6). In addition, she has several positive risk factors:

- smoking
- oral contraceptive pill
- obesity
- inactivity (recent).

The patient's clinical presentation is consistent with a PE. An informed out-of-hospital decision can be made based on a comprehensive patient assessment and care evaluation of the patient's risk factors, clinical presentation and Wells score.

Table 21.2 The simplified Wells score for pulmonary embolism

Variable	Points
Clinical signs and symptoms of deep vein thrombosis (minimum of leg swelling and pain on palpation of the deep veins)	3.0
Alternative diagnosis less likely than pulmonary embolism	3.0
Heart rate > 100 bpm	1.5
Immobilisation (> 3 days) or surgery within the previous 4 weeks	1.5
Previous pulmonary embolism or deep vein thrombosis	1.5
Haemoptysis	1.0
Malignancy (receiving treatment, treated in last 6 months or palliative)	1.0
Clinical probability of PE unlikely: score ≤ 4 points	
Clinical probability of PE likely: score > 4	

Source: McRae (2010).

 TREAT

Emergency management

Paramedic care for the patient presenting with a PE involves:

1. identifying the likely PE diagnosis with a comprehensive patient assessment

2. care and treatment to aid hypoxaemia, pain and/or perfusion support

3. prompt transport to an appropriate facility capable of managing a PE (likely ICU capable).

Position

Complementing V/Q is the main aim of positioning a patient presenting with a PE or any cardio-respiratory illness. This patient presents as haemodynamically stable; therefore, a sitting position is appropriate.

Oxygen

This patient presents as 'unwell', with moderate respiratory distress and mild hypoxaemia. This consideration and understanding the disease process of a PE suggests adjunct oxygen therapy and increasing the fraction of inspired oxygen (FiO_2) will benefit this patient. The increased alveolar partial pressure of oxygen *may* offset the hypoxaemia and improve the level of respiratory distress. A common approach would include delivering 10–15 L/min of oxygen through a non-rebreather mask with the view to titrate the FiO_2 delivery as the patient's condition improves.

Analgesia

Analgesia has a number of beneficial effects.

- It is humane to provide analgesia to a patient presenting in acute severe pain.
- It can mitigate the adverse effects created by severe pain, in particular the overactive sympathetic response.
- It may improve ventilation, especially when deep inspiration exacerbates the pain and decreases tidal volume.
- It may have some helpful anxiolytic properties.

A common approach would be the administration of intravenous fentanyl 25–50 micrograms as required.

Haemodynamic support

Maintaining adequate perfusion is pertinent to mitigate further complications and patient deterioration. It is important to appreciate that a PE with cardiovascular compromise is a form of both obstructive and cardiogenic shock. Therefore, normal saline and an inotrope (often adrenaline) are titrated together to increase intravascular volume and support preload as well as improve cardiac contractility. The patient at this stage has adequate perfusion and does not need immediate intervention; however, having both the normal saline and an inotrope (ideally by infusion) ready is recommended.

 EVALUATE

Evaluating patient trends and the effect of clinical intervention is a universally adopted approach that is imperative to confirm or refute a differential diagnosis, identify the effectiveness of intervention and gain insight into the clinical course of the patient's condition. It will allow the clinician either to justify their initial clinical impression or to adapt; to continue with the management plan or to change and allow a more informed decision regarding patient transport and escalation of patient care if required.

The goals of patient care with this case study is to improve hypoxaemia, level of respiratory distress and pain, and identify any changes or signs of deterioration.

Ongoing management

The primary aim of PE treatment in hospital is to first diagnose, identifying the size, location and severity. Once this is known, the patient can then receive a targeted treatment plan consistent with best care to ideally dissolve the clot and promote reperfusion to the affected area. The ongoing patient care will also aim to minimise the likelihood of PE reoccurrence.

For the patient outlined in this case study, a PE presentation without cardiovascular compromise or *mild PE* anticoagulant therapy is the likely treatment plan. Subcutaneous low-molecular-weight heparin (LMWH) or IV unfractionated heparin is most commonly used, and therapy often continues for up to 3 months after symptom resolution. A targeted INR of > 2.0 is a common approach with anticoagulant therapy in PE patients (Bersten & Soni, 2019).

Patients who present with *a massive PE or submassive PE* require both prompt and immediate resolution of the clot to mitigate further cardiovascular compromise, morbidity and mortality. There are a few considerations for the way a hospital team will treat patients and this will depend on a number of patient factors and clinical symptoms. These patients will also receive anticoagulant therapy and fibrinolysis and/or surgical embolectomy. Inferior vena cava filters are indicated for patients who are contraindicated to anticoagulant therapy, who experience recurrent PE despite adequate anticoagulation and those undergoing open embolectomy (Bersten & Soni, 2019).

Intra-aortic balloon counterpulsation and extracorporeal membrane oxygenation (ECMO) are also a consideration for critically unwell, dying patients with a *massive PE* (Bersten & Soni, 2019).

Investigations

Blood tests (PE specific)

If the presentation is consistent with PE but the probability assessment (e.g. Wells score) suggests PE is unlikely, a D-dimer test is usually performed. D-dimer is a fibrin degradation product—a small fragment of protein present in the blood after a blood clot has been degraded by fibrinolysis. A negative result rules out PE, but because the test is not specific to PE a positive result is not definitive of PE. A positive D-dimer can also be seen as a result of trauma, surgery, malignancy, acute myocardial infarction, pneumonia and heart failure (Bersten & Soni, 2019).

Clinicians who have a high suspicion of a PE (despite a Wells score of < 4) in the presence of a positive D-dimer test will initiate further diagnostics and investigation.

Routine and thorough blood tests will be performed in all patients with suspicion of a PE to aid in identifying contributing factors and disease process diagnosis (e.g. cardiac enzymes, inflammatory markers, clotting profile).

Imaging

A chest x-ray is useful in reaching an alternative diagnosis: pneumothorax, pneumonia, pulmonary oedema, fractures and pleural effusions. It is not reliable in PE diagnosis, and a radiologist is often required to identify the signs consistent with a PE. These signs include focal oligaemia, a peripheral wedge-shaped density above the diaphragm or an enlarged right descending pulmonary artery (Bersten & Soni, 2019).

Computed tomography pulmonary angiography (CTPA) is considered the 'gold standard' for PE diagnosis (Estrada-Y-Martin & Oldham, 2011; Bersten & Soni, 2019) and uses CT to obtain an image of the pulmonary arteries and map the extent and location of any emboli. CTPA has 90% sensitivity and is useful in detecting an alternative diagnosis; for example, pneumonia in up to 22% of cases (Kline, 2020). Unfortunately, not all patients can undergo CTPA (e.g. pregnancy, renal impairment or anaphylaxis to contrast) and therefore other diagnostics will be considered (Bersten & Soni, 2019).

A V/Q scan (see Fig 21.4) is a valid adjunct when CTPA is either inconclusive or contraindicated. It has a sensitivity of 96% and is considered a viable diagnostic tool for PE (Kline, 2020; McCance & Huether, 2010).

Lung ultrasound and MRI are also adjunct diagnostic considerations (less common) of PE and have 85% and 75% sensitivity respectively (Kline, 2020).

Ultrasound of the lower limbs is routinely performed if there are symptoms of a DVT or confirmed PE diagnosis as 90% of PEs originated from DVTs (Bersten & Soni, 2019).

Other tests

The echocardiograph, along with other cardiac and pulmonary function tests, is also used to aid in identifying PE severity. These investigations are important in influencing the recommended treatment pathway for the PE patient (Bersten & Soni, 2019; Kline, 2020).

The 12-lead ECG can provide valuable information to a clinician in the setting of a PE. It is important to appreciate that the 12-lead ECG is a poor predictor of a PE and a normal ECG does not rule out a PE; a normal ECG is seen in one-third of PE patients (Bersten & Soni, 2019). The ECG can indicate the additional cardiac workload and stress that is caused by a PE. Tachycardia, evidence of atrial enlargement and right-sided heart strain can be suggestive of the cardiovascular strain and severity of a PE (Bersten & Soni, 2019).

A 12-lead ECG with a diagnostic STEACS or pericarditis can also assist in an alternative diagnosis.

Hospital admission

Duration of stay in hospital for a patient presenting with a PE is highly variable. Numerous considerations including age, comorbidities, severity of the PE, responsiveness to treatment and whether the PE is associated with another disease process can all influence the duration of the hospital stay.

The patient depicted in the case study is likely to receive intravenous anticoagulant therapy, a hospital admission and, depending on the responsiveness to treatment, will receive ongoing assessment and management as an outpatient with her general practitioner (GP).

Follow-up

PE-specific follow-up generally involves assessment and determination of the effectiveness of anticoagulation. An uncomplicated PE may be anticoagulated for 3–6 months.

The contributing cause of the PE can be a result of varying disease processes. The identification of the PE could be the trigger to investigate and diagnose other conditions, such as coagulopathies, malignancies and immune diseases. As a result the patient may receive specialist referral and ongoing care and treatment unrelated to the PE.

CASE STUDY 2

Case 11009, 0835 hrs.

Dispatch details: A 24-year-old pregnant female complaining of shortness of breath and chest pain.

Initial presentation: On arrival the crew are greeted by the patient's distressed mother and directed to the location of the patient.

 ASSESS

0855 hrs Primary survey: The patient looks 'unwell'—short of breath and with pallor.
D: Nil dangers
R: Yes
A: Patent
Cx: Nil traumatic cause
B: Yes—with adequate ventilation
C: Yes
Hx: Nil visible external haemorrhage
D: Conscious
E: Warm environment in the house.

0855 hrs Chief complaint: 'I woke up really short of breath and with chest pain (20 minutes ago). I'm worried about my baby because I'm 35 weeks pregnant.'

0857 hrs Vital signs survey: Perfusion status: HR 130 bpm; BP 80/50 mmHg
Skin: Cool, pale, clammy
Conscious state: conscious
Capillary refill: 2 seconds centrally and 4 seconds peripherally
   Respiratory status: Patient is anxious and distressed, speaking in phrases, has a RR of 36, clear air entry on chest auscultation L = R and no adventitious sounds, increased work of breathing with accessory muscle use, inspiratory and expiratory cycles are normal.
   Glasgow Coma Scale score: GCS of 15.

0903 hrs Secondary assessments:
SpO_2: 85% on room air
Temperature: 37.0°C
BGL: 6.1
Pupils: PEARL
   12-lead ECG: reveals a sinus tachycardia with a Q wave in lead I, S wave and T-wave inversion in lead III and T-wave inversion in V1–V4.

0903 hrs Previous history: Nil
Medication: Folic acid since deciding to have a baby
Allergies: Nil
Risk factors: Nil

Pregnancy: G1P0, 35 + 2 gestation with all appropriate antenatal care and nil diagnosed complications. Baby is cephalic and normal vaginal delivery is anticipated and booked in at the hospital.

Secondary survey: Thorough medical and head-to-toe secondary survey identifies the following.
Chest pain: 8/10; description = sharp that is exacerbated by deep inspiration; onset = 0830 hrs; location = right-sided chest; other signs and symptoms = dyspnoea, light headed and dry cough; relief = nil
Bilateral lower leg oedema = normal for the patient during the pregnancy
Obvious right calf swelling = red, tender to touch and identified 2 days ago.

② CONFIRM

A thorough patient assessment gives a paramedic all the information to be able to make an informed decision about the patient's presenting condition. As part of this process it is important to consider and challenge the various and relevant differential diagnosis to the patient's presenting condition.

What else could it be?
Many PE symptoms are often non-specific and can easily correlate to other disease processes. This case study clearly identifies a number of concerning abnormal signs and symptoms; in particular respiratory distress, hypoxaemia, chest pain and inadequate perfusion. It is important to evaluate the potential disease processes and identify a likely differential diagnosis.

Pneumonia
The patient presentation is not consistent with a typical pneumonia presentation. The symptom onset is acute, with sudden hypoxaemia and moderate respiratory distress, clear chest sounds, a non-productive cough, afebrile and no recent coryzal symptoms.

Pneumothorax
PE and pneumothorax symptoms can have many similarities; in particular sudden onset of pleuritic chest pain, dyspnoea, hypoxaemia and inadequate perfusion. It can also be difficult to conclusively differentiate between the two disease processes. The thorough patient assessment in this case study certainly supports a PE diagnosis rather than a pneumothorax. It would be expected that a spontaneous pneumothorax transitioning towards a tension pneumothorax would have a clear delineation between PE breath sounds; diminished or absent breath sounds and unequal chest wall expansion is expected. Additionally, a pregnant female with signs consistent with DVT and presenting with such symptoms supports a PE diagnosis.

Pericarditis
Inflammation of the pericardial sac around the heart can cause some of the above symptoms, including pain, tachycardia and tachypnoea. Many of the symptoms, however, are inconsistent with pericarditis. These include sudden onset of profound hypoxaemia, inadequate perfusion and without the presence of coryzal symptoms or fever. Pericarditis can also have unique ECG symptoms characterised by PR depression and ST elevation in the inferior leads and PR elevation and ST depression in lead aVR which is again inconsistent with this case study.

Acute coronary syndromes
Many of the non-specific symptoms seen in this case study can be seen in an acute coronary syndrome presentation. These include atypical chest pain, dyspnoea and inadequate perfusion secondary to cardiogenic shock (pump failure).

This case study also signifies many aspects inconsistent with an ACS presentation. First, the patient's age, sex, lack of risk factors and comorbidities class

> **USING THE MNEMONIC DENT**
> Define:
> - What is the patient's main presenting problem?
>
> Explore:
> - What else could it be?
>   - Pneumonia/bronchitis
>   - Pneumothorax
>   - Pericarditis
>   - Acute coronary syndromes
>
> Narrow:
> - Is this pulmonary embolism?
> - Does it fit the definition?

this patient as 'low risk' for coronary vessel occlusion related to an atherosclerotic plaque. The chest pain and ECG changes are also more consistent with a pleuritic or PE-causing event. Profound hypoxaemia seen in an ACS presentation is typically associated with acute left ventricular failure and cardiogenic acute pulmonary oedema, and given that the patient has a clear chest and nil fine crackles it is again inconsistent with this patient's presentation.

An interesting consideration for this patient's presentation would be the notion of 'paying off' and treating as per ACS. It would be highly recommended to consult with perinatal specialist and/or emergency consultant given that this patient is pregnant and is likely to require an emergency caesarean section due to fetal distress and for ongoing care of the patient. They can also provide guidance on the use of an anti-emetic, analgesia and perfusion support.

③ TREAT

There are number of patient symptoms that require prompt treatment, including the following.

- **Position:** Semi-recumbent position with a 15–30° left lateral tilt is the happy medium to maximise V/Q in a patient with hypoxaemia and inadequate perfusion. This positioning will ideally aid both the patient and the fetus.
- **Hypoxaemia:** High-flow oxygen therapy via a non-rebreather mask at 10–15 L/min is a common approach and should be maintained throughout patient care to support the critical illness and unborn fetus. By increasing the alveolar partial pressure of oxygen this may assist and ideally overcome (to some degree) the presenting hypoxaemia. Intubation in the out-of-hospital setting should be reserved as an absolute last resort with the priority of getting the patient to definitive care to treat the underlying cause of the hypoxaemic respiratory failure.
- **Inadequate perfusion:** The patient's cause of inadequate perfusion is likely to be due to the obstruction, decreased preload and/or right ventricular failure. This is a form of cardiogenic shock and a common treatment approach in the out-of-hospital setting would involve 250 mL normal saline boluses and an adrenaline (inotrope/vasopressor) infusion. This approach should be titrated aiming for systolic blood pressure of 100 mmHg. The fact this patient is pregnant adds to the importance of maintaining adequate perfusion; however, guidance from a perinatal and/or ED specialist is highly recommended given vasopressors can adversely affect fetal circulation.
- **Pain:** This patient requires analgesia for a number of differing reasons including:
  - › that it is humane to the patient to treat acute severe pain
  - › physiological benefits relating to the patient's presentation
  - › minimising the level of stress, anxiety and the additional use of unnecessary oxygen and energy requirements.

  The analgesic of choice should again be discussed with the receiving hospital as opioids can pose issues to the fetus if there is to be an emergency caesarean section performed.
- **Transport:** Prompt transport to an appropriate hospital with notification is of the utmost importance in this patient's presentation.

④ EVALUATE

All critically unwell patients require:
- timely reassessment
- a challenge of the initial differential diagnosis

- regular evaluation of the interventions provided. This ensures that:
- the correct treatment path is followed or appropriately adapted to
- the interventions provided are working or it is identified that they are not working.

Research

A review in 2008 (Jiménez & Yusen) described a number of prognostic prediction rules for PE and showed that rules such as the Pulmonary Embolism Severity Index and the more conservative Home Management Exclusion Criteria could identify patients with acute symptomatic PE who were at low risk of fatal or nonfatal adverse outcomes. It suggested that clinicians should incorporate such predictive models into treatment algorithms for patients with acute symptomatic PE diagnosed in the ED. The utility of these tools is yet to be validated in the out-of-hospital setting. A later study (Zondag et al., 2012) compared the performance of two clinical decision rules—the Hestia criteria and the simplified Pulmonary Embolism Severity Index (sPESI)—to select patients with acute PE for outpatient treatment. It concluded that although both rules classified different patients as eligible for outpatient treatment, with similar low risks for 30-day mortality, they could both select patients at low and high risk.

Summary

Pulmonary embolism is a potentially fatal disease that often presents in the community. It is often characterised by a set of non-specific symptoms, which makes diagnosis difficult, especially in the out-of-hospital setting. The unintuitive combination of respiratory distress, lack of adventitious lung sounds and hypoxaemia is a strong clue that PE may be present. The inclusion of a thorough patient assessment, adopting probability assessment scores (e.g. Wells score) and a high index of suspicion can guide the diagnostic process. Out-of-hospital care is vital as paramedics are often the first medical contact for the PE patients. Paramedic care primarily involves a differential diagnosis of a PE, severity of the PE (e.g. cardiac compromise), maintaining oxygenation, analgesia, perfusion support and prompt transport to an appropriate receiving hospital with notification. The receiving hospital will then have the ability to formally diagnose a PE, identify the severity and initiate a treatment plan to ideally dissolve the clot and restore perfusion to the affected area.

References

Bersten, A., & Soni, N. (2019). *Oh's intensive care manual* (6th ed.). Elsevier.

Carroll, R. G. (2007). *Elsevier's integrated physiology*. St Louis: Mosby.

Cross, S. S. (2013). *Underwood's pathology: a clinical approach* (6th ed.). Edinburgh: Churchill Livingstone.

Estrada-Y-Martin, R., & Oldham, S. (2011). CTPA as the gold standard for the diagnosis of pulmonary embolism. *International Journal of Computer Assisted Radiology and Surgery, 6*(4), 557–563.

Jiménez, D., & Yusen, R. D. (2008). Prognostic models for selecting patients with acute pulmonary embolism for initial outpatient therapy. *Current Opinion in Pulmonary Medicine, 14*(5), 414–421.

Klatt, E. C. (2015). *Robbins and Cotran atlas of pathology* (3rd ed.). Philadelphia: Saunders.

Kline, J. A. (2020). Venous thromboembolism including pulmonary embolism. In J. E. Tintinalli, O. Ma, D. M. Yealy, G. D. Meckler, J. Stapczynski, D. M. Cline & S. H. Thomas (Eds.), *Tintinalli's emergency medicine: a comprehensive study guide*, ninth ed. New York, NY: McGraw-Hill.

Konstantinides, S. V., Meyer, G., Becattini, C., Bueno, H., Geersing, G. J., Harjola, V. P., & Kucher, N. (2020). 2019 ESC Guidelines for the diagnosis and management of acute pulmonary embolism developed in collaboration with the European Respiratory Society (ERS) The Task Force for the diagnosis and management of acute pulmonary embolism of the European Society of Cardiology (ESC). *European Heart Journal, 41*(4), 543–603.

Kuipers, S., Cannegieter, S. C., Middeldorp, S., Robyn, L., Büller, H. R., & Rosendaal, F. R. (2007). The absolute risk of venous thrombosis after air travel: a cohort study of 8755 employees of international organisations. *PLoS Medicine, 4*, e290.

Lee, C., Hankey, G., Ho, W., & Eikelboom, J. (2005). Venous thromboembolism: diagnosis and management of pulmonary embolism. *Medical Journal of Australia, 182*(11), 569–574.

Lehnert, P., Møller, C. H., Mortensen, J., Kjaergaard, J., Olsen, P. S., & Carlsen, J. (2017). Surgical embolectomy compared to thrombolysis in acute pulmonary embolism: morbidity and mortality. *European Journal of Cardio-Thoracic Surgery*, *51*(2), 354–361.

McCance, K., & Huether, S. (2010). *Pathophysiology: the biologic basis for disease in adults and children* (6th ed.). St Louis: Mosby.

McRae, S. (2010). Pulmonary embolism. *Australian Family Physician*, *39*(7), 462–466.

Nordenholz, K., Ryan, J., Atwood, B., & Heard, K. (2011). Pulmonary embolism risk stratification: pulse oximetry and pulmonary embolism severity index. *Journal of Emergency Medicine*, *40*(1), 95–102.

Ouellette, D., Setnik, G., Beeson, M. S., Garg, K., Amorosa, J., Kamangar, N., Sutherland, S., Harrington, A., Tino, G., Talavera, F., O'Connor, R., Lin, E., Mosenifar, Z., & Stern, E. (2012). Pulmonary embolism. *eMedicine*. Retrieved from http://emedicine.medscape.com/article/300901-overview. (Accessed 12 November 2012).

Zondag, W., den Exter, P. L., Crobach, M. J., Dolsma, A., Donker, M. L., Eijsvogel, M., Faber, L. M., Hofstee, H. M., Kaasjager, K. A., Kruip, M. J., Labots, G., Melissant, C. F., Sikkens, M. S., & Huisman, M. V., on behalf of The Hestia Study Investigators. (2012). Comparison of two methods for selection of out of hospital treatment in patients with acute pulmonary embolism. *Journal of Thrombosis and Haemostasis*, *109*(1).

SECTION 10
The Paramedic Approach to the Patient With a Cardiac Condition

In this section:

Disease of the organs contained by the chest wall can produce a confusing spectrum of pain and symptoms. The chest wall itself can also be affected by injury and disease and, overlaying the organs within, it can add to the complexity of diagnosing chest pain in the field. The most serious cause of chest pain is generally considered to be a blockage to a coronary blood vessel (acute coronary syndrome). The subsequent damage to the myocardium (the muscle of the heart) can lead to arrhythmias and ultimately cardiac arrest.

Differentiating the wide variations of cardiac chest pain from other sources of chest pain with equipment limited by portability is a challenging but essential paramedic skill. Over the past decade the ability of paramedics to directly intervene in managing myocardial ischaemia has progressed from providing cautious pain relief to direct intervention in dissolving clots in the affected vessels or bypassing emergency departments to direct patients to cardiac theatres where the clots are removed mechanically. The ability to determine which patients receive these expensive and potentially dangerous interventions reflects the growing complexity of paramedic practice and its integration into broader medical practice. The ability of paramedics to manage the arrhythmias and cardiac arrests that can evolve from cardiac disease has also become more complex and effective.

While the electrocardiogram (ECG) plays an important role in identifying which patients can be administered drugs to dissolve coronary occlusions or directed to cardiac catheterisation, the ECG is least accurate early in the development of cardiac chest pain and therefore of less help to paramedics than other medical professionals. Determining the nature of chest pain in the emergency setting relies on a strong knowledge of anatomy, disease pathology and risk factors and the ability to gain a succinct history to identify which patients require management of acute coronary syndrome.

The chapters in this section take readers through the progression of acute coronary syndrome, from the onset of pain to the subsequent development of potentially life-threatening arrhythmias and into the cohort of patients who ultimately go into cardiac arrest. Chapter 24 steps readers through the clinical reasoning process to determine whether chest pain is related to the heart. Chapter 25 provides the links between myocardial ischaemia and disturbances of heart rhythm and why some rhythms are more dangerous than others. Finally, Chapter 26 reveals the causes (not just ischaemic) of cardiac arrest and how recent changes to management are improving patient outcomes.

CHAPTER 22

Chest Pain

By Hugh Grantham

OVERVIEW

- Chest pain is a common presentation in ambulance practice but a final diagnosis of ischaemia occurs in fewer than 10% of cases.
- The underlying pathology of a proportion of chest pain presentations is an acutely obstructed coronary artery that can lead to cardiac arrest.
- Cases presenting as chest pain include many non-ischaemic causes of chest pain.
- Distinguishing an obstructed coronary artery from other causes of chest pain in the out-of-hospital environment is difficult.

- Features distinguishing myocardial infarction on an ECG are not always present.
- The principles of management of acute coronary syndrome seek to resolve the imbalance between oxygen supply and oxygen demand in myocardial tissue.
- Early identification and early access to reperfusion strategies are essential to positive outcomes.
- The consequences of myocardial ischaemia include angina, arrhythmia, altered muscle function and infarction.

Introduction

Coronary artery disease (CAD) is the leading cause of death in Western societies (AIHW, 2011) and must be considered a possible cause of any adult presentation of chest pain. But while cardiac ischaemia can lead to cardiac arrest in a matter of minutes, chest pain caused by ischaemia actually makes up less than 10% of the final diagnoses of all patients who initially present with chest pain (Bhuiya et al., 2010).

For the layperson, diagnosis of cardiac ischaemia appears to be highly supported by technology and, in the hospital setting, this assumption is reasonably valid. In the community setting, however, the technology is far less definitive than the general population appreciates, and the weight of diagnosis falls on the patient's description of their own symptoms and the clinical presentation perceived by the paramedic. Distinguishing ischaemic chest pain from all other causes of chest pain requires a thorough understanding of the pathology of cardiac ischaemia but also the clinical reasoning process used to initiate safe and effective treatment.

Although access to life-saving clinical interventions for cardiac ischaemia is growing, definitive interventions such as coronary arterial stenting and bypass remain limited and expensive. Despite the lack of definitive diagnostic tools available to them, paramedics play a vital role in providing early access to these treatments through their in-field diagnosis and selection of appropriate treatment pathways (Ducas et al., 2012).

This chapter briefly describes the process by which ischaemic chest pain presents and what factors should be considered essential in making a safe diagnosis.

Pathophysiology

The chest cavity contains organs that differ remarkably in their structure and function. Packed tightly together, these organs are subject to a wide array of potential diseases that can develop in isolation or as a syndrome across the entire body. Worryingly for the paramedic, innervation of sensory nerves to most of the organs of the chest cavity is poor and the pain produced by a disease can refer away from the site or present as belonging to another organ. In the emergency setting, the condition of greatest concern is the sudden occlusion of a coronary artery, as it can quickly lead to the development of fatal cardiac arrhythmias. But it can be difficult to differentiate ischaemic pain from pain caused by diseases of the lungs, the great vessels of the chest, the chest wall itself or even the organs of the upper abdomen.

Myocardial cells require just 1.3 mL of oxygen per 100 mL of blood but are normally supplied with six times this amount (Hall, 2012). Anatomically, therefore, the heart has more than sufficient blood supply to meet its metabolic demands, but the processes of ageing and disease can narrow the arteries supplying blood to the myocardium and lead to an imbalance between myocardial oxygen supply and myocardial oxygen demand (see Fig 22.1

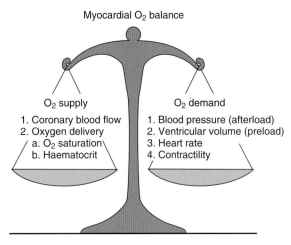

Figure 22.1
Myocardial ischaemia occurs when the tissue demand for oxygen exceeds supply. The principle behind the management of ischaemia is to reduce demand (lower blood pressure, reduce activity) while increasing oxygen supply (inspired oxygen, lysis of thrombus).
Source: Fleisher (2012).

Table 22.1 Factors determining myocardial oxygen supply and demand

Determinants of myocardial oxygen supply	Determinants of myocardial oxygen demand
Blood pressure (higher blood pressure increases coronary perfusion pressure)	Blood pressure (higher blood pressure increases afterload)
Length of diastole	Heart rate
Intraluminal coronary artery size	Contractility
Haemoglobin value	Amount of myocardial tissue (increase in hypertrophy)
Dissolved oxygen content of blood	Sympathetic tone

and Table 22.1). Less commonly (and usually combined with CAD) diseases can also lead to an increased myocardial metabolic demand. In either circumstance, the result is ischaemia of the myocardial cells. If the ischaemia is severe and prolonged, the myocardial cells can begin to dysfunction (causing arrhythmias; see Ch 23) or they can die and/or limit the effectiveness of the heart as a pump.

Arteriosclerosis and stable atherosclerosis produce a fixed obstruction that limits supply. An increase in demand may then produce ischaemia. A dynamic coronary obstructive component also exists with clot formation (over unstable atherosclerotic plaques) and/or vasospasm suddenly reducing supply.

Arteriosclerosis refers to the gradual stiffening of the walls of the arteries with age (see Box 22.1). This can occur due to the loss of elastic tissue or the growth of smooth muscle in the vessel walls. Although arteriosclerosis occurs naturally with age it can be accelerated by hypertension, diabetes and other diseases. Atherosclerosis is a particular form of arteriosclerosis where fatty lesions develop between the intima and media of the vessel walls (see Figs 22.2 and 22.3). These lesions can grow large enough to occlude blood flow, or they can rupture and cause the sudden development of a clot that occludes the blood vessel. Atheroma occurs when erosion, rupture or fissuring of an atherosclerotic plaque disrupts the endothelium and exposes platelets to the underlying connective tissue (Sanders, 2007). A localised blood clot can form and the reduction in blood flow may be sufficient to cause myocardial ischaemia, particularly when myocardial oxygen demand increases (Kumar & Cannon, 2009).

As an indication of how oversupplied with blood the heart is, the vessels can become up to 70% occluded before symptoms of ischaemia may present (Hall, 2012). For decades, arteriosclerosis and atherosclerosis were considered somewhat separate diseases with distinct profiles and treatment pathways. The past decade has seen a growing recognition that the pathophysiologies of arteriosclerosis and atherosclerosis overlap significantly and that the traditional terms may not accurately describe the underlying causes or specific risks. As a thrombus overlying a plaque can form and lyse many times before causing an infarct, the term acute coronary syndrome (ACS) has been introduced. For paramedics it should also reinforce the dynamic nature of ischaemic chest pain and the potential for symptoms to evolve and make a diagnosis more or less clear.

In the past the development of arteriosclerosis was considered to be slow and linear with the disease progressing asymptomatically until the occlusion prevented sufficient blood flow to maintain myocardial perfusion at higher workloads. When the workload was removed the balance between oxygen supply and oxygen demand was re-sorted and symptoms would resolve. This 'fixed stenosis' created the typical picture of angina where reducing workload (by rest or medications) relieved symptoms effectively and there was no death of myocardial tissue. If a patient with known angina presented with pain of a different intensity, nature or form of relief it was usually referred to as unstable angina, with the inference that it was primarily arteriosclerotic in nature. Conversely, the sudden rupturing

BOX 22.1 Definitions

- *Angina:* Reversible myocardial hypoxia occurring with exertion and improving with rest is termed stable angina (McCance & Huether, 2013). Patients often live with stable angina for years treating it symptomatically with glyceryl trinitrate (GTN) when required. It should be considered a fixed and irreversible occlusion of the lumen that doesn't present with symptoms at rest.
- *Unstable angina (UA):* In patients with a history of angina, a pattern of increasing frequency of pain or pain occurring at rest is described as unstable angina (McCance & Huether, 2013). It should not be considered as simply the extension of the fixed stenosis of angina as it could be the result of a ruptured atherosclerotic plaque with a superimposed thrombus creating a dynamic stenosis (Daga et al., 2011). Until the return of negative biomarkers is provided, in-field assessment and management of unstable angina should be equivalent to an NSTEMI (see below).
- *Acute myocardial infarction (AMI):* AMI occurs when there is myocardial cell death secondary to obstruction of blood flow. Myocardial infarction may occur in the absence of ST elevation. This is known as a non-ST elevation myocardial infarction (NSTEMI). NSTEMI may have no ECG changes or may present with ST depression or T wave changes (Aroney et al., 2006). A myocardial infarction associated with classic ECG changes of ST elevation is described as an ST elevation myocardial infarction or STEMI (see Fig 22.3). Although NSTEMIs may involve the death of less tissue compared with STEMIs, the 6-month mortality of both is comparable (Daga et al., 2011).
- *Acute coronary syndrome (ACS):* This term describes the spectrum of ischaemic disease from unstable angina through to STEMI and was developed to encourage clinicians to recognise that the conditions share a common pathology (a disrupted atherosclerotic plaque with superimposed thrombus), the progression is unpredictable and the principles of management are common (Aroney et al., 2006).

of an atherosclerotic plaque and the formation of a thrombus over the rupture causes a non-fixed stenosis and was considered the common cause of nearly complete vessel occlusion. This classically causes the sudden presentation of symptoms that do not resolve with rest or medications that lower myocardial oxygen demand.

The most common mechanism for complete occlusion of the coronary artery is rupturing of the surface of the plaque. This allows a new focus for platelet aggregation, thus precipitating blood clotting at the site. Much of the acute management is aimed at retarding the progression of this clot. Another potential mechanism of occlusion is an unstable plaque that mechanically obstructs the blood vessel when the proximal end becomes free and the other is anchored, creating a flap that obstructs flow (Hall, 2012).

Coronary artery spasm can also restrict the flow to the extent that it creates an acute coronary ischaemia or acute coronary syndrome. Notable causes of coronary artery spasm include the use of sympathomimetic stimulant drugs. For example, cocaine has been shown to cause coronary artery spasm in young people (Menyar, 2006). In addition, severe coronary artery spasm has been recognised in females under extreme emotional stress, presenting as myocardial ischaemia (Golabchi & Sarrafzadegan, 2011).

Nitric oxide released from the endothelium of coronary arteries in response to stress (pulsatile distension with the pulse) is thought to produce vasodilation in the downstream vessels by activating the intracellular production of cyclic guanine monophosphate (CGMP), which controls the smooth-muscle tone by reducing the level of free intracellular calcium. Vessels that have become rigid due to extensive atherosclerosis will have not only a reduction in flow but also a reduction in distension and thus creation of nitric oxide. An upstream atherosclerotic lesion may therefore also cause downstream vasoconstriction, further reducing myocardial oxygen supply. This mechanism explains the ability of GTN to reverse coronary artery spasm by providing an alternative source of nitric oxide to distal coronary arteries that still have the ability to constrict and dilate (Bryant et al., 2011).

Restriction of coronary artery flow due to either obstruction associated with atherosclerosis or spasm results in a decrease in myocardial perfusion, creating myocardial hypoxia.

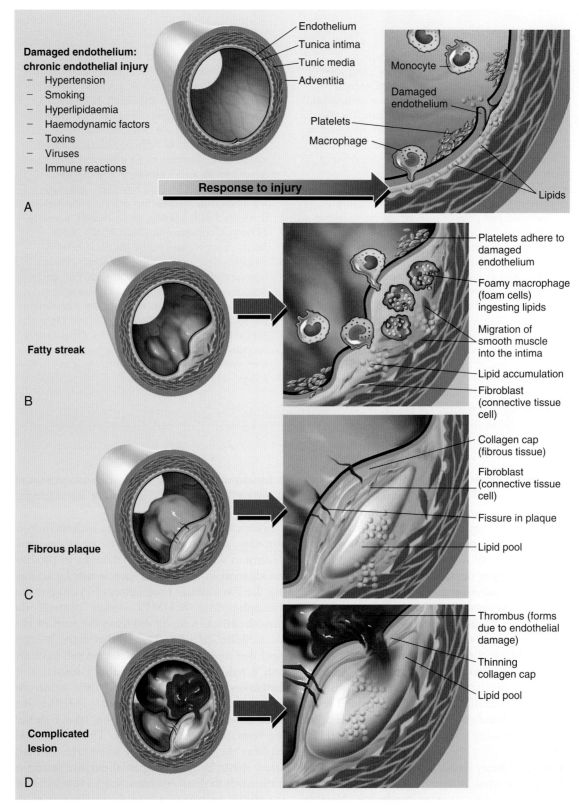

Figure 22.2
Atherosclerosis causing a narrowing of the coronary arteries is present in the majority of cases of ischaemic heart disease. Atherosclerosis is an accumulation of cholesterol and triglycerides within the vessel wall that leads to stiffening of the vessel wall and occlusion of the lumen (McCance & Huether, 2013). **A** Damaged endothelium. **B** Diagram of fatty streak and lipid core formation. **C** Diagram of fibrous plaque. Raised plaques are visible: some are yellow; others are white. **D** Diagram of complicated lesion; thrombus is red; collagen is blue. Plaque is complicated by red thrombus deposition.
Source: Craft et al. (2011).

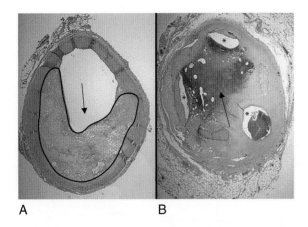

Figure 22.3
Coronary artery atherosclerosis.
A Coronary artery with 60–70% occlusion (black outline and arrow demonstrate narrowing of lumen) due to atherosclerosis. This degree of occlusion may lead to angina. **B** Severe coronary artery disease and evidence of past thrombus (black arrow), with only three small lumens (*) providing blood flow to the myocardium.
Source: Craft et al. (2011).

Myocardial perfusion and myocardial workload

Normal perfusion of the myocardium occurs in diastole. Blood is delivered to the myocardium via the right and left coronary arteries, which originate from the aorta just above the aortic valve. During systole, the entry points into the coronary arteries are partially occluded by the open aortic valve leaflets. During diastole, the backward movement of blood towards the heart down the pressure gradient results in an increased supply of blood to the coronary arteries. The pressure in the coronary arteries is a reflection of the pressure in the aorta. The terminal branches of the coronary arteries and the myocardial capillary bed are subject to external pressure as the myocardium contracts. The perfusion pressure within the myocardial capillary bed allows perfusion of the myocardium only when the external pressure drops in diastole. As the heart is perfused in diastole, the diastolic pressure is effectively the perfusion pressure of the coronary circulation. Reduction in diastolic pressure and increase in heart rate, which reduces the relative diastolic period, reduce the myocardial blood flow (McCance & Huether, 2013).

Myocardial ischaemia can alter the flow of depolarisation/repolarisation across the myocardium and this can be detected by an ECG in as many as 68% of cases (O'Connor et al., 2010) but also as few as 13%, depending on the type of ECG and the location of the occlusion. Death and rupture of myocardial cells due to lack of blood supply result in myocardial cell contents moving into the blood where they can be detected. Together, these two effects provide the diagnostic criteria for cardiac ischaemia: an abnormal ECG and a rise in cardiac enzymes.

There is currently no ability to test for a rise in cardiac enzymes in the field. However, the enzymes can take hours to reach detectable levels in the blood after the onset of pain and their diagnostic utility to the paramedic is likely to always be limited. Similarly, the sensitivity of early ECGs is as low as 13%. The net effect of these two facts is that paramedics will never be able to rely solely on diagnostic tests to determine which patients are suffering a myocardial infarction and so will need to combine an accurate history with the clinical presentation.

Determining the nature of chest pain is further complicated by the lack of any dedicated pain receptors in the heart. Pain is normally sensed by nociceptors responding to noxious stimuli and stimulating the transmission of an impulse to the brain that identifies the response as pain. In the case of myocardial ischaemia, the build-up of waste products is thought to be the stimulus, but the lack of dedicated pathways can lead to pain being interpreted as originating anywhere from the heart to the neck and arms. The reason for this distribution of pain is that both the heart and the arms originate in the neck during embryonic life; as a result they share the same spinal cord segments and the brain can misinterpret the stimuli (Hall, 2012).

The lungs suffer a similar lack of direct sensory innervation but parts of the chest wall (especially the parietal pleura) are heavily supplied with nociceptors. Muscles, bones and joints are also well innervated, and palpation or movement is generally able to replicate the pain. It is for these reasons that the location, nature and response to movement of chest pain can be key factors during in-field assessment.

The pathophysiology of ACS reinforces both the uncertainty and the seriousness involved in the assessment of chest pain (see Fig 22.4). Simultaneously, the relatively low frequency that chest pain is ischaemic in nature (< 10%) and the cost and limitations of providing comprehensive cardiac care to every patient require that some degree of triage has to occur in both the out-of-hospital and the ED settings. While diagnosis of chest pain will always fall on the conservative and safe side of certainty, paramedics should be aware of the clinical reasoning errors and predispositions to diagnosis that allow ischaemic chest pain to be missed and non-ischaemic pain to be treated inappropriately.

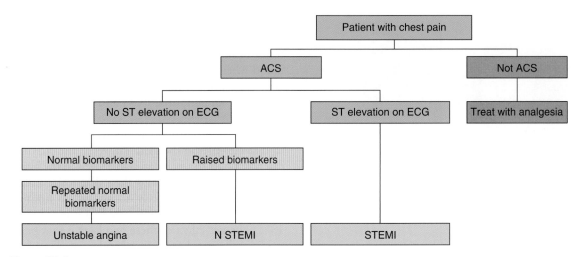

Figure 22.4
Approach to the diagnosis of patients with ACS.
Patients with ACS make up only a small portion of all patients who present with chest pain. Once the pain has been identified as ischaemic in nature, the presence of ST elevation identifies an infarct is present. Where ST elevation is absent, clinicians must wait for the return of cardiac biomarkers to distinguish between unstable angina and NSTEMI. In the out-of-hospital setting unstable angina and NSTEMI cannot be separated.
Source: Adapted from Daga et al. (2011).

Cs CASE STUDY 1

Case 12334, 0934 hrs.

Dispatch details: A 55-year-old businessman complaining of sudden-onset central chest pain radiating down his left arm.

Initial presentation: The ambulance crew finds the patient sitting down. His skin is pale and clammy, and he is conscious but anxious. He appears to be distressed and is pressing a clenched fist against his chest.

1 ASSESS

Patient history

A patient presenting with this history and examination findings appears to have classical myocardial ischaemia, but the diagnosis of ACS is not so simple. The risk factors for developing ischaemic chest pain are well established (gender, age, familial history, hypertension, diabetes) but counterintuitively they do not help with distinguishing the cause of chest pain once it develops (Han et al., 2007; O'Connor et al., 2010; Green & Hill, 2012). Risk factors are far more important in managing patients prior to them developing ischaemia and then once it has been diagnosed and managed acutely (to minimise the likelihood of reoccurrence). In the patient history do not overemphasise risk factors or underemphasise undiagnosed chronic symptoms.

Perhaps equally counterintuitive is the presence of prodromal symptoms. The formation of a thrombus over an atherosclerotic plaque (an atheroma) has typically been described as being both sudden and unexpected. While this suits the classic view of a plaque remaining stable until rupture, it is now clear that plaques and atheromas tend towards instability prior to rupture (Kumar & Cannon, 2009). One study identified that 45% of patients who suffered their first AMI had prodromal symptoms in the year prior (Løvlien et al., 2009). This is often difficult to identify as the patients themselves only retrospectively recognise the symptoms as ischaemic, but a chronic or repeated series of self-resolving symptoms does not reduce the likelihood of the cause being ischaemic and a prelude to an AMI. Interestingly, the same study found that prodromal symptoms predicted the symptoms that occurred during the acute stage of the AMI.

Airway
Unless the ischaemia causes tachycardic or bradycardic rhythms that do not produce sufficient cerebral perfusion to maintain consciousness, ischaemic chest pain is not a cause of airway compromise.

Breathing
Tachycardic or bradycardic rhythms that fail to produce an adequate blood pressure will generate symptoms of poor perfusion (altered consciousness, dizziness, nausea) before any respiratory symptoms. Shortness of breath with chest pain can be caused by anxiety but it can provide numerous diagnostic clues. Acute pulmonary oedema (see Ch 18) with chest pain indicates a failing left ventricle and increases the likelihood of an ischaemic cause (Kumar & Cannon, 2009). Severe dyspnoea with clear lung fields and pleuritic pain suggests a lung problem rather than a cardiac problem (pneumothorax, pulmonary embolism or pleural effusion; see Chs 20 and 21).

Cardiovascular
Depending on the extent and location of an atheroma, the normal rhythms of the heart can be disturbed and cause either tachycardic or bradycardic rhythms. Bradycardia should never be ignored as the response to poor perfusion or anxiety should be an increase in heart rate. Bradycardia indicates structural damage to either the propagation or the conduction of normal rhythm and, outside of drug effect, ischaemia is the most likely cause. While pain of any sort can generate a sympathetic response and subsequent tachycardia, it would be extremely unwise not to include low blood pressure and high or low heart rate as suggestive of ischaemic chest pain.

Electrocardiogram
The technical and objective nature of the ECG promises a degree of certainty that is lacking elsewhere in the assessment of ischaemic chest pain. Unfortunately even ECG findings need to be considered in context with the clinical presentation and the limitations of the device (see Fig 22.5). ST segment elevation of > 1 mm in the limb leads and 2 mm in the praecordial leads (see Fig 22.6 and Box 22.2) is considered diagnostic for myocardial infarction, but a lack of ST elevation or depression, particularly in the acute stages, must not be considered negative for cardiac ischaemia: two-thirds of all cases of AMI do not have any early ST elevation (Kumar & Cannon, 2009). Similarly, the presence of ST elevation in one or more leads is the result of AMI in only 15–31% of cases where ST elevation is detected (Brady, 2006). Common non-ischaemic causes of ST elevation include left ventricular hypertrophy (LVH), benign early repolarisation, pericarditis, left bundle branch block (LBBB) and ventricular paced rhythms. The presence of Q waves and alterations to T waves are also inconsistent.

The upgrading to 12-lead ECGs (from 3-lead) conducted by many ambulance services over recent years has improved the diagnostic utility of the ECG but

HISTORY
Ask!
- Description: 'What is the pain like?'
- Onset: 'When did it start?'
- Location: 'Where is the pain?'
- Other signs and symptoms: 'Are there any other associated signs and symptoms?'
- Radiation: 'Does the pain radiate? If so, to where?'

PRACTICE TIP
Dyspnoea is not a typical sequela of ischaemic chest pain if the lung fields are clear. Always suspect lung pathology in severe dyspnoea.

PRACTICE TIP
Tachycardia can be the result of anxiety and pain but any alterations to heart rate and perfusion should never be ignored in the setting of chest pain.

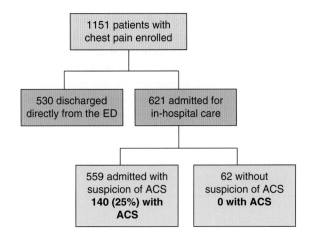

Figure 22.5
The challenge facing all primary clinicians is balancing the potential seriousness of chest pain with the uncertain nature of ACS symptoms. This chart illustrates that in one study nearly half of all patients with chest pain were discharged straight from ED, while of those admitted with suspected ACS, only 25% were eventually determined to have ACS.
Source: Kamali et al. (2014).

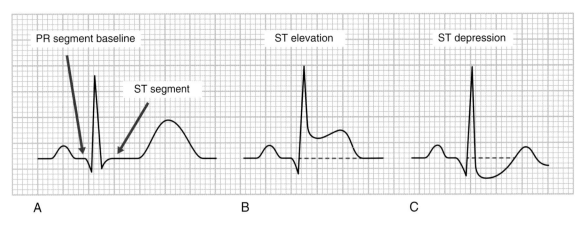

Figure 22.6
ST segment deviations.
A Use of the PR segment as a baseline. **B** The ST segment is elevated with respect to the PR segment baseline. **C** The ST segment is depressed with respect to the PR segment baseline.

BOX 22.2 ST changes

Interpreted correctly, a 12-lead ECG describes the net flow of electricity around the heart. Occlusions of coronary vessels leading to ischaemia subsequently change the electrical flow. Diagnostically, the most significant of these changes are to the ST segment (see Fig 22.6).

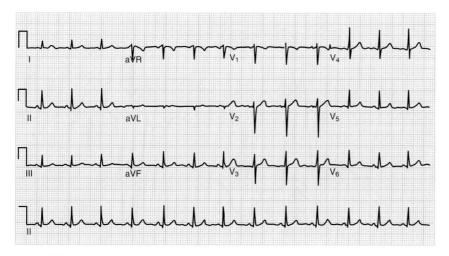

Figure 22.7
Normal electrocardiogram.
The heart rate is approximately 78 beats per minute, with minor irregularity. Sinus arrhythmia is present. The axis is approximately +60 degrees. The PR, QRS and QT intervals are approximately 140, 90 and 360 msec, respectively. P wave morphology, duration and axis are normal. The transition is between leads V3 and V4. No abnormal Q waves are present. ST segments are isoelectric and T waves are concordant with QRS complexes.
Source: Goldman & Ausiello (2008).

the posterior, lateral and apical walls of the left ventricle remain poorly examined or unexamined even on a 12-lead ECG (Kumar & Cannon, 2009). For experienced clinicians the apparent lack of utility of ECGs in detecting AMI is not overly concerning as it is the patient's clinical presentation that provides most of the diagnostic clues (Kamali et al., 2014). In a patient with the clinical signs of cardiac ischaemia the lack of ST elevation is not surprising (only one-third of AMI = STEMI) (see Fig 22.7), and for a patient with a non-ischaemic clinical picture but an incidental finding of ST elevation it is likely to be from other causes. However, in the patient with both an ischaemic clinical presentation and ST elevation the utility of the ECG is truly revealed, with a number of recent of studies proving the transmission of STEMI ECGs to receiving hospitals can reduce the time to revascularisation of the vessel (Diercks et al., 2009).

While limited accessibility to revascularisation centres has historically limited the procedure to patients with ST elevation, there are indications that NSTEMI patients also benefit from the procedure (2012 Writing Committee Members et al., 2012). The next step in improving AMI outcomes is likely to be a result of NSTEMI patients receiving more invasive therapies.

The presence of arrhythmias and conduction blocks is an equally important aspect of ECG investigation. In addition to being indicative of ischaemia, these findings can also direct treatment or withhold the use of certain medications.

ST elevation in two or more anatomically contiguous leads has been shown to be sensitive to acute vessel obstruction (STEMI) and is used to predict the need for urgent revascularisation therapy (percutaneous intervention or thrombolysis). The current 12-lead diagnostic criteria for STEMI used by most ambulance services are:

- 1 mm elevation in two or more contiguous limb leads
- 2 mm elevation in two or more contiguous chest leads
- new-onset left bundle branch block (LBBB) when compared with the previous ECG (O'Gara et al., 2013).

PRACTICE TIP

Anatomically appropriate ST elevation with chest pain can be used to rule ischaemia in, but a lack of ST elevation should never be used to rule ischaemia out.

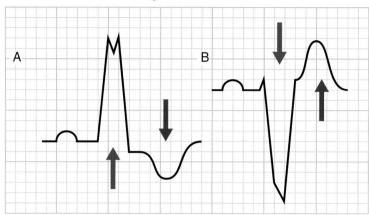

Discordant
ST segments and T waves

Normal for LBBB and paced rhythm

Figure 22.8
Left bundle branch block.
The disruption to the electrical pathway caused by LBBB makes it difficult to discern ischaemic-related ST segment changes. Typically the QRS complex (blue arrow) will be wider than usual and the ST segment (red arrow) will move away from the baseline. As such, many current STEMI criteria list a 'new' LBBB as the equivalent to ST elevation.
Source: With permission, Tom Bouthillet, ems12lead.com.

Sgarbossa (2000) conducted ECG analysis of LBBB cases with myocardial infarction (MI) and identified specific criteria that significantly increase the chances of identifying MI in the presence of LBBB (see Fig 22.8). The criteria are based on analysis of three ECG criteria: ST elevation ≥ 1 mm in leads with a positive QRS; ST depression ≥ 1 mm in V1 to V3 with a negative QRS; and discordant ST/S or ST/R ratio of ≤ –0.25. The third criterion has recently been established as a more accurate way of determining the presence of infarction in the presence of LBBB and replaces the old criterion of discordant ST elevation of ≥ 5 mm. It is likely this criterion will increasingly be used to determine urgent treatment pathways where ischaemic pain occurs with LBBB.

Causes of ST segment change other than ischaemia
There are a number of other conditions that can produce ST elevation but do not represent acute ischaemia, such as: a normal variant high take-off, drug-induced changes, electrolyte changes, pericarditis and ventricular aneurysm. Readers are advised to familiarise themselves with a detailed text on ECG interpretation, which is beyond the scope of this book.
ST segment changed due to early repolarisation
Early repolarisation with benign elevation of the ST segments is sometimes seen in young fit individuals with no other symptoms. The patient in Case study 1 does not fit this demographic and has symptoms.
ST segment changed due to bundle branch block
Interpretation of ST segments in the presence of a bundle branch block (particularly left) can be flawed because the two ventricles are repolarising at different times as opposed to at the same time and balancing the electrical potential (giving a straight line). Unless this patient has a markedly wide QRS complex, this can be excluded by looking at the ECG.

ST segment changes due to pericarditis

As a rule pericarditis tends to produce more widespread changes rather than focal changes and is associated with pain. This patient does not fit this clinical picture.

ST segment changes due to electrolyte imbalance or drugs

Although abnormal ST segments can be associated with abnormal electrolytes and the impact of drugs, these changes tend to be more global and not focal as in this patient's case. The paramedics have no reason to suspect that this patient would have abnormal electrolytes or is taking drugs that could impact on his ECG.

Posterior infarcts: where depression can be elevation

On a standard 12-lead ECG no leads directly view the posterior aspect of the heart. Infarction of tissue in this area will often appear as an ST depression in the anterior chest leads where they are looking through the heart to view the damaged myocardium from the inside. Placement of posterior leads is more accurate but ST depression in leads V1–V4 with a R:S ratio > 1 in V1 or V2 is often considered diagnostic of a posterior STEMI.

Pain

The location and nature of the pain, combined with other symptoms, will most often form the basis of the diagnosis (Kamali et al., 2014) and the use of a mnemonic to structure the patient interview can assist in gaining all the required information (see Ch 15). Caution is advised, however, as a number of factors can be inappropriately weighted in the assessment and there are many causes of chest pain other than ischaemia (see Table 22.2).

Description

'Heavy', 'crushing', 'dull' and 'pressure' are typical terms used to describe ischaemic pain, while a 'sharp' or 'stabbing' pain that changes with ventilation is classically categorised as pleuritic or related to the chest wall. While any of the classic descriptors must be considered as positive predictors of ACS, atypical descriptions should be regarded as the rule rather than the exception. Up to 22% of AMI patients describe their pain as sharp, stabbing or pleuritic in nature, while up to half do not complain of chest pain at all (Green & Hill, 2012). Patients with diabetes and females are more prone to atypical presentations and must always be treated with a higher index of suspicion for ACS (Dorsch et al., 2001; Lefler & Bondy, 2004).

A clenched fist held over the chest is known as Levine's sign and was historically thought to be a strong indicator of ischaemic chest pain, but is in fact demonstrated in only 11% of cases and is not sensitive in more than 35% of cases. In fact, the palm sign (a flat palm over the chest) is more prevalent (35%) and shows equivalent sensitivity (Marcus et al., 2007).

Physiologically, chest wall tenderness should be strongly suggestive of a musculoskeletal injury and not ischaemic pain, but it has been reported in up to 15% of patients who were subsequently diagnosed with AMI. This not only reinforces the difficulty of ruling out ACS using any single item, but should also remind clinicians that in their anxiety patients may report what they think the pain should be rather than what it actually is. Language, gender and cultural differences can also confuse the accuracy of the communication. Severity (usually on a scale of 0–10) can be a useful tool in measuring the effectiveness of analgesia, but a study of more than 2000 patients complaining of chest pain on arrival of the paramedics found severity is not useful in differentiating ischaemic pain from non-ischaemic pain (Galinski et al., 2015).

Onset

Pain that manifests suddenly is typically associated with plaque rupture and subsequent thrombus formation and as such is considered to be associated

Table 22.2 Potential causes of chest pain

Type	Cause
Non-ischaemic cardiovascular	Aortic dissection*
	Myocarditis
	Pericarditis
	Hypertrophic cardiomyopathy
Musculoskeletal/chest wall	Costochondritis
	Rib fracture
	Herpes zoster
	Neuropathic pain
	Neoplasms
Pulmonary	Pneumonia/pleurisy
	Pulmonary embolism
	Pneumothorax
Gastrointestinal	Cholecystitis/biliary colic
	Peptic ulcers (perforating and non-perforating)
	Duodenal ulcers
	Oesophageal spasm/rupture
	Pancreatitis
	Gastro-oesophageal reflux disease
Behavioural	Depression
	Anxiety
	Psychiatric

*Can also cause myocardial ischaemia if it blocks main coronary arteries.
Source: Adapted from Kumar & Cannon (2009).

with ACS. In many cases, however, the plaque may become unstable over a period of days to weeks and the pain may rise and fall several times before patients call for an ambulance. Again, the sudden onset of pain and other symptoms should be considered consistent with ACS, but other presentations should not be used as the sole basis to rule out ACS.

Pain that increases with physical exertion such as walking is a positive predictor of ACS (Green & Hill, 2012) but conducting in-field stress tests is strongly discouraged. Similarly, a disrupted plaque can create a sufficient occlusion to cause pain at rest. Recent studies have revealed that there is no circaseptal (weekly) variation in the onset of ACS but there is a circadian variation: while the number of chest pain presentations to the ED was lowest between midnight and 9 am, this period had the highest proportion of chest pain patients who were diagnosed with ACS (Ekelund et al., 2012).

Location
Retrosternal pain is the 'classic' presentation but the area of pain and the ability to accurately localise the pain are important predictors of ACS. Larger areas of pain are more predictive of ACS, while the ability to point to the pain with a finger has a high specificity for non-ischaemic pain (Marcus et al., 2007).

Other signs and symptoms
There are a number of other symptoms that can be predictors of ACS and paramedics should enquire specifically about each while remaining cognisant of their sensitively (true positive rate) and specificity (true negative rate).

Likelihood ratios (LR) greater than 10 are considered to strongly indicate the presence of a disease, while LR < 0.1 would be considered suitable to rule out a disease. The highest LR is 'radiation to both shoulders' (4.07), with 'exertional pain' (2.07) and 'nausea and vomiting' (2.0) being near equivalent ahead of 'pain that changes with movement' (0.3) (Goodacre et al., 2002; Kamali et al., 2014). On this basis, nausea, vomiting and diaphoresis cannot be considered as predictive of AMI or ACS, and in isolation no single symptom makes either diagnosis highly likely or unlikely (Goodacre et al., 2002; Kamali et al., 2014). Shortness of breath and dizziness are also more common in non-ACS than ACS (Pelter et al., 2012).

Radiation
Radiation to both arms has the strongest LR of predicting ACS or AMI. The typical radiation pattern is to the medial aspect of the left arm and may include the neck. Referred pain to these regions reflects the common embryological origins of the structures but referred pain can be found in the epigastric region, the back, the jaw or even the ear (Sanders, 2007).

Initial assessment summary

Problem	Sudden onset of central chest pain radiating down the left arm
Conscious state	GCS = 15
Position	Sitting
Heart rate	110 sinus tachycardia
Blood pressure	130/90 mmHg
Skin appearance	Pale and clammy
Speech pattern	Sentences
Respiratory rate	22 bpm
Respiratory rhythm	Even cycles
Respiratory effort	Normal
Chest auscultation	Clear air entry bilaterally
Pulse oximetry	97% on room air
Temperature	36.9°C
Motor/sensory function	Normal
History	The patient was watching TV when the pain struck
ECG	Sinus tachycardia, nil ST elevation/depression, normal T waves, no Q waves, no bundle branch blocks

D: There are no dangers.
A: The patient is conscious with no current airway obstruction.
B: Respiratory function is currently normal but needs frequent reassessment. The respiratory rate is elevated but ventilation is normal.
C: Heart rate is elevated and there is a sufficient blood pressure.

The patient is conscious and ventilating normally but with a slightly increased rate. His heart rate is elevated and he is complaining of pain that is typical of cardiac ischaemia.

2 CONFIRM

The essential part of the clinical reasoning process is to seek to confirm your initial hypothesis by finding clinical signs that should occur with your provisional diagnosis. You should also seek to challenge your diagnosis by exploring findings that do *not* fit your hypothesis: don't just ignore them because they do not fit.

The ability to definitively confirm or deny ischaemic chest pain in the out-of-hospital setting is extremely limited, and although this patient presents with classic symptoms, differential diagnoses should be explored.

What else could it be?

Angina

The pain from angina is the result of a fixed stenosis from arteriosclerosis and as such tends to develop slowly as myocardial workload is increased through activity and subsides as demand is reduced. The progressive nature of the disease means it rarely presents as severe, first-time pain. An exception to this is a form of angina caused by coronary artery spasm known as Prinzmetal's angina (Keller & Lemberg, 2004). This relatively rare variant of a temporary stenosis can occur suddenly but is usually responsive to drugs that relax vascular smooth muscle, such as nitrates or calcium channel blockers. In the field, Prinzmetal's angina is indistinguishable from ACS. Similarly, angina requires repeated presentations and either a stress test or an angiogram to diagnose. First-time presentations of sudden-onset chest pain that is ischaemic in nature at rest should never be described as angina. Angina can cause changes to both the ST segment and T waves while pain is present, but these will usually resolve as the pain subsides.

Thoracic aortic dissection

A dissecting aneurysm of the aorta, creating a false passage within the wall of the aorta, is associated with severe chest pain that is classically described as tearing or ripping in nature and radiating from the sternum to between the shoulder blades posteriorly (Green & Hill, 2012) (see Table 22.3). The risk factors are similar to those for CAD but the pain is usually most intense as it commences (as the layers of the aorta separate). Depending on the location and

---

DIFFERENTIAL DIAGNOSIS

Acute coronary syndrome
Or
- Angina
- Thoracic aortic dissection
- Pulmonary embolism
- Spontaneous pneumothorax
- Pneumonia/pleurisy
- Oesophageal disorders/ gastritis
- Cholecystitis/perforated peptic ulcer/pancreatitis
- Costochondritis/ musculoskeletal pain
- Shingles
- Panic disorder (anxiety attack)
- Acute pericarditis

Table 22.3 Classic pain presentations according to disease

Disorder	Pain (location)	Pain (character)	Pain (radiation)	Associated symptoms
Angina pectoris	Retrosternal or epigastric	Crushing, tightness, squeezing, pressure	Right or left shoulder, right or left arm/hand, jaw	Dyspnoea, diaphoresis, nausea
Massive pulmonary embolism	Whole chest	Heaviness, tightness	None	Dyspnoea, unstable vital signs, feeling of impending doom
Segmental pulmonary embolism	Focal chest	Pleuritic	None	Tachycardia, tachypnoea
Aortic dissection	Midline, substernal	Ripping, tearing	Intrascapular area of back	Secondary arterial branch occlusion
Pneumothorax	One side of chest	Sudden, sharp, lancinating, pleuritic	Shoulder, back	Dyspnoea
Oesophageal rupture	Substernal	Sudden, sharp, after forceful vomiting	Back	Dyspnoea, diaphoresis, may see signs of sepsis
Pericarditis	Substernal	Sharp, constant or pleuritic	Back, neck, shoulder	Fever, pericardial friction rub
Pneumonia	Focal chest	Sharp, pleuritic	None	Fever, may see signs of sepsis
Perforated peptic ulcer	Epigastric	Severe, sharp	Back, up into chest	Acute distress, diaphoresis

Note: Atypical presentations are common with all listed life-threatening disorders.

Source: Kumar & Cannon (2009).

extent of the aneurysm, vessels branching off the aorta can become occluded. Ischaemia to one or both limbs can occur, but the aneurysm can also occlude one or both of the main coronary arteries and cause an AMI. The description and location of this patient's pain are not typical of a dissecting aneurysm and the condition is relatively rare. A dissecting thoracic aneurysm requires chest radiography to rule out, but in this case ACS should be considered as more likely.

Pulmonary embolism

Pulmonary embolism (PE) can present with a wide variety of symptoms including chest pain. The pain tends to be poorly localised initially and becomes more pleuritic in nature as the pleural surfaces become inflamed, but this is not a reliable progression. If the embolism is located laterally, the pain will tend to occur in that location. Although there are classic signs of PE on an ECG, they are not common. PE is a difficult diagnosis to exclude in the field but ACS is more common and, in the absence of hypoxia and hypotension, ACS is the more serious diagnosis in this patient that cannot be excluded.

Spontaneous pneumothorax

Patients presenting with a spontaneous pneumothorax often complain of the sudden occurrence of sharp pain (usually after an event such as coughing or minor chest trauma) that is exacerbated by ventilation. The pain can be well localised but does not cause chest wall tenderness unless related to trauma. Dyspnoea may occur if the pneumothorax is large and this may be detected as decreased breath sounds on the affected side. Pneumothorax is also difficult to exclude conclusively in the field but the history, nature of pain and lack of dyspnoea all suggest that the more common and more serious diagnosis of ACS should stand for this patient.

Pneumonia/pleurisy

Pleuritic chest pain associated with an inflamed pleural surface tends to produce pain that is exacerbated by deep breaths and coughing. Pleuritic pain is usually a consequence of an underlying infection, but PE and other pathologies can present with pleuritic pain. This patient does not have a history of pleuritic pain and even if there was a component of pleuritic pain to his history, it does not rule out ACS.

Oesophageal disorders/gastritis

Gastro-oesophageal disorders make up almost half of all causes of chest pain that are ultimately found to not be cardiac in nature (Karnath, Holden & Hussain, 2004). Spasm of the oesophagus usually presents with a sharp, central pain immediately after attempting to swallow a bolus of food or medication. Oesophageal spasm is easily confused with ischaemic pain as it responds to nitrates (Karnath et al., 2004; Green & Hill, 2012).

Gastritis typically presents as well-localised, burning epigastric pain that is usually worse after meals and is aggravated by lying supine. It is not associated with radiation to the arms. While the classic presentation of gastritis is distinct from ischaemic pain, it is not always perfectly 'typical' in nature and clinicians should be suspicious of recently diagnosed heartburn that occurs suddenly later in life and is not responsive to proton-pump inhibitors. For this patient there is no strong evidence to suggest that gastritis is a better diagnosis than ACS.

Cholecystitis/perforated peptic ulcer/pancreatitis

Disorders of the gastrointestinal tract can rarely be completely excluded in the field due to the variable nature and progress of pain in the early stages, but there are some conditions that are commonly confused with ischaemic pain.

Cholecystitis can present centrally and be mistaken for ACS. Murphy's sign is a reliable sign of cholecystitis, while a wave-like pain pattern is suggestive of biliary colic. The pain from a perforated peptic ulcer tends to be exacerbated after meals and shares a 'boring' quality with pancreatitis. While all these conditions may eventually evolve into states of poor perfusion or sepsis, in the early stages they can be difficult to differentiate from ACS. Until they manifest clearly, ACS should remain the working diagnosis.

Costochondritis/musculoskeletal pain

Costochondritis describes inflammation of the cartilaginous joint between the ribs and the sternum. The pain typically has a dull background with a sharp 'catch' on ventilation or movement. Visual inspection is usually unremarkable and it can be difficult to elicit the pain by palpation, but it is otherwise distinct and not usually associated with any changes to vital signs or ECG.

Pain from muscle or rib damage is usually sharp, well localised and unilateral. Visual inspection should always be conducted and a lack of recent trauma should not exclude the diagnosis, as pathological conditions can weaken connective tissue. Musculoskeletal pain that is isolated to the left shoulder can sometimes generate anxiety in patients who become concerned it may be a sign of AMI. Referred ischaemic pain will not be exacerbated by palpation or movement of the shoulder joint and in this patient's case the pain does not change on examination, so ACS remains the diagnosis.

Shingles

The herpes zoster virus typically creates a burning sensation along the dermatome of the infected nerve root. The pain often develops before any skin lesions become visible, but the nature of the pain is not typical for ACS.

Panic disorder

Palpitations, dyspnoea, chest tightness and nausea are all symptoms that overlap ACS and panic disorder. Panic disorder must be considered a diagnosis of exclusion that is only reached when all other causes have been excluded. Even in the overly anxious patient with a history of panic disorder, ignoring the classic signs of ACS is dangerous as they are more likely than other patients to have ACS.

Acute pericarditis

Inflammation of the pericardium can occur spontaneously and produces a sharp and persistent retrosternal pain that may radiate in a pattern similar to ACS (Green & Hill, 2012). Changes in the pain with movement and pericardial friction rub are diagnostically significant and the ECG is likely to show PR depression and widespread ST segment elevation and T wave inversion (see Box 22.3). Sinus tachycardia is common and pain severity is variable. Together, the anatomically inconsistent ST changes, PR segment depression and friction rub are diagnostically sensitive and specific, but none are present in this patient's case.

Pleuritic chest pain is the most common symptom in acute pericarditis. A prodrome of fever, myalgia and malaise is also common, especially in younger patients. On physical examination, a pericardial friction rub is pathognomonic.

BOX 22.3 ECG criteria for pericarditis

- ST segment elevation that is concave upwards, occurring in all leads except aVR
- T waves concordant with ST segment deviation
- PR segment depression, sparing V1 and aVR
- PR segment elevation and ST depression in aVR

An increase in cardiac troponin is also frequently observed in acute pericarditis, reflecting biochemical evidence of inflammatory myocardial cell damage.

The patient is complaining of pain that is typical of cardiac ischaemia. A number of alternative conditions could generate a similar pain pattern, but none fit the presentation and clinical signs better than ischaemic pain. With no previously diagnosed angina, the provisional diagnosis must be ACS. The lack of ischaemic changes on the ECG does not rule this out.

③ TREAT

Principles of ACS management

From the most basic actions to the most complex, the principles of management of ACS are based on reducing the imbalance between myocardial oxygen demand and supply (see Table 22.4). Initial strategies focus on reducing demand by reducing anxiety, activity and pain. Supply strategies primarily aim to reduce the luminal occlusion by retarding and then reversing the clotting process by using thrombolytic agents or percutaneous coronary artery angioplasty to remove the clot and/or dilate fixed atherosclerotic occlusions (Mehta et al., 2001). Early recognition of patients requiring urgent revascularisation is associated with improved patient outcomes and this responsibility falls largely in the hands of the first clinician to assess the patient. The principles of management for a suspected MI are outlined in Box 22.4.

Emergency management

Position and reassurance

Reducing systemic oxygen demand will allow for a reduced heart rate and subsequently reduce myocardial oxygen demand. Lowering an elevated heart rate will also increase the period of diastole (when the heart muscle receives its blood flow) and may also contribute to increasing myocardial oxygen supply. Placing patients in a seated or recumbent position will minimise their systemic oxygen demand. Providing adequate reassurance can also reduce sympathetic drive and lower heart rates driven up by anxiety.

Table 22.4 Principles of management of cardiac ischaemia

Demand reduction			Supply increase		
Aim	Action	Agent	Aim	Action	Agent
Reduce systemic demand for oxygen	Scene management	Seated or recumbent positioning	Normalise oxygen delivery	Increase FiO$_2$ if hypoxia is present	Inhaled oxygen
Normalisation of elevated heart rate	Reduce sympathetic drive	Analgesia, reassurance	Limit further development of thrombus	Antiplatelet therapy; antithrombin therapy	Aspirin, clopidogrel, low-molecular-weight heparin, enoxaparin
Reduce left ventricle pre- and afterload	Vasodilation	Nitrates	Removal of clot	Breakdown of clot by lysis	Thrombolytics
Normalisation of heart rhythms	Restore sinus rhythm	Antiarrhythmics, synchronised cardioversion		Removal of clot	Percutaneous coronary intervention (PCTI) with/without stent, coronary artery bypass graft surgery (CABGS)
			Revascularisation	Reduce fixed stenosis	

BOX 22.4 Principles of management

Suspected myocardial infarction
- Reassurance
- Avoid hypoxia
- Obtain history and examination
- Early 12-lead ECG
- GTN if blood pressure and rhythm adequate
- Aspirin if not allergic and not already on it
- Early reperfusion via thrombolytics or angioplasty
- Expectant management of reperfusion arrhythmias

Antiplatelet therapy

Aspirin inhibits platelet aggregation, with studies showing that aspirin given within the first 4 hours reduces the mortality from MI (ISIS-2, 1988). Subsequent recommendations have directed that it should be given as soon as possible provided the patient has no contraindications (allergy; ISIS-2, 1988). A single loading dose of 300 mg should be administered once any sensitivities to the drug have been excluded (NICE, 2010). Routine administration of a second type of antiplatelet medication, a $P2Y_{12}$ inhibitor such as clopidogrel or ticagrelor, is now widely recommended (NICE, 2010; Dörler et al., 2011). $P2Y_{12}$ inhibitors have a more potent effect on platelet aggregation, selectively inhibiting the binding of adenosine diphosphate (ADP) to the platelets and preventing the activation of the GPIIb/IIIa complex, which is responsible for platelet aggregation. A minimum 300 mg dose is recommended in conjunction with aspirin in ACS, particularly when percutaneous angioplasty is contemplated (Sabatine et al., 2005; Van de Werf et al., 2006; NICE, 2010; Dörler et al., 2011). A third group of drugs known as IIb/IIIa glycoprotein inhibitors are administered intravenously in some centres during the acute phase. These drugs are routinely administered during percutaneous coronary intervention to reduce clotting, but they are not usually given until PCTI is confirmed as their prolonged effect can delay surgery for up to a week. It is unlikely that they will transition into an out-of-hospital protocol.

Antithrombin therapy

Attacking a separate stage of the clotting cascade, antithrombin medications are not common agents in the out-of-hospital setting but are being increasingly administered in hospitals. Unfractionated heparin has been largely replaced by newer low-molecular-weight heparins such as enoxaparin and fondaparinux or direct thrombin inhibitors such as bivalirudin (Dumaine et al., 2007).

Nitrates

Glyceryl trinitrate (GTN) is a vascular smooth-muscle relaxant that causes vasodilation, reducing myocardial oxygen demand and thereby reducing preload and afterload. GTN is one of the few drugs where the intended effect (rather than a side effect) is to lower blood pressure. As such, caution should always be used when administering GTN to patients displaying signs of very poor perfusion (very high or low heart rate, low blood pressure).

Most ambulance services use a blood pressure of 100 mmHg or 110 mmHg systolic as a cut-off value for administration of GTN, although clinical judgment comes into play as patients who are normally hypertensive may well be poorly perfused with a blood pressure above the cut-off value. Similarly, very fast or slow rhythms indicate that the patient may have little ability to compensate if the GTN causes blood pressure to fall significantly. The use of GTN in

---

PRACTICE TIP

Patients with evidence of right ventricular ischaemia are much more susceptible to the effects of a reduction in preload and a corresponding reduction in right ventricular stretch (Bryant et al., 2011).

patients with a right-sided infarct may produce a marked drop in cardiac output as these patients are dependent on right ventricular filling which is in turn dependent on preload. GTN lowers preload by causing vasodilation. Some services have a caution with regards to the use of GTN in this circumstance while others have a rule not to use it in this circumstance.

A small group of patients have an exaggerated response to GTN and many experienced clinicians withhold the 'first' GTN administration until the patient is semi-recumbent. An exaggerated effect also occurs when GTN is given when erectile dysfunction medication is active (usually taken as administered in the last 24 hrs). The result is a precipitous fall in blood pressure.

Pain relief

Depending on the extent and nature of the occlusion, GTN may not be able to fully restore blood flow and relieve the pain or discomfort. Careful use of opioids such as morphine or fentanyl can assist in reducing pain further; however, they can have a synergistic effect with GTN on blood pressure so should be used in small titrated doses intravenously and only when nitrates are not offering any further reduction in pain. An IV dose of 2–2.5 mg of morphine or 20–25 micrograms of fentanyl for an adult is a reasonable starting point, and doses can always be added to once safety has been confirmed.

Oxygen

Increasing the fraction of inspired oxygen (FiO_2) by use of a mask connected to an oxygen supply is a logical strategy when trying to correct an imbalance in myocardial oxygen supply and demand and has been a standard treatment for chest pain for decades (Burgess, 2010). Recent research indicating that oxygen administration may be associated with higher rates of mortality from AMI has triggered a number of new trials (Stub et al., 2012) and recommendations that oxygen should be withheld unless profound hypoxia ($SpO_2 < 94\%$) is present (Cabello et al., 2010). The physiological effect of oxygen on damaged tissue is still unclear but there is growing evidence to suggest that high levels of oxygen can trigger cell death when reperfusion of the injured tissue finally occurs (Zweier, 2006).

Monitoring

The provision of 12-lead ECGs in many ambulances has improved the ability of paramedics to detect a wide range of STEMIs but any patient diagnosed with ACS should be monitored until handover at hospital regardless of their initial ECG finding or the sophistication of the ECG. The development of arrhythmias in ACS is a poor sign and requires early identification and management. Even 3-lead ECGs provide the ability to detect arrhythmias. A distinct advantage of 12-lead monitors is that many hospitals will admit patients with a STEMI found on a 12-lead directly to the cardiac team for PCTI. This system has now been implemented in a number of centres and has significantly reduced the time from arrival at hospital to revascularisation (Ducas et al., 2012).

A reflection of how the history and clinical presentation dominate the assessment of chest pain is that many experienced paramedics start the process of transport very early and confirm the diagnosis with a 12-lead ECG once in the ambulance. The benefits of a short scene time and a direct admission should be weighed against the optimum history and examination, but this is one case where a short scene time is very appropriate.

4 EVALUATE

Evaluating the effect of any clinical management intervention can provide clues to the accuracy of the initial diagnosis. Some conditions respond rapidly to treatment so patients should be expected to improve if the diagnosis and treatment were appropriate. A failure to improve in this situation should trigger the clinician to reconsider the diagnosis. The effects of antiplatelet agents in the short period between administration and handover are unlikely to directly improve the patient's condition. Any improvement in pain or discomfort is likely to come from the effects of nitrates or analgesics. Provided they are titrated against the patient's perfusion, it should be possible to use nitrates and opioids to reduce pain for most patients to near zero.

Even short periods of ischaemia can cause abnormal automaticity to develop in myocardial cells and the subsequent generation of arrhythmias such as ventricular tachycardia or ventricular fibrillation. These can be expected in patients showing signs of poor perfusion, but they can also occur quickly in patients who appear otherwise stable. Experienced paramedics often prepare medications and equipment to manage this situation once they have made the diagnosis of ACS.

Is the patient:
- Adequately perfused?
  › Level of consciousness
  › Skin colour/sweating
  › Pulse rate and quality
  › Blood pressure
  › ECG changes and rhythm
- Improving or deteriorating?
  › Responding to treatment
  › Developing life-threatening arrhythmias

Ensure that the receiving hospital/catheter laboratory is notified if the patient has ST elevation.

Investigations

ECG

Repeat ECGs to detect evolution of an infarct are routine, as is continuous monitoring to detect arrhythmias.

Biomarkers

Even when the ECG provides evidence of infarction, blood tests seeking the biochemical markers of myocardial cell death will be ordered soon after arrival at hospital. In the case of NSTEMI these will determine the subsequent management, but in all infarcts they provide an indication of the age of the infarct and whether it is stable, progressing or resolving. There are several biomarkers of infarct but cardiac troponin I is both sensitive and specific (Collinson et al., 2012; see Box 22.5). Because it can take up to 6 hours after the onset of pain for detectable levels to develop, a single normal troponin level cannot be used to rule out infarct without a second negative sample being taken several hours later (between 3 and 8 hours depending on local policy). Newer, more sensitive assays may allow earlier detection in the future and exclude false positives from sepsis, renal failure, right heart strain, heart failure and myocarditis (Roongsritong et al., 2004).

Other blood tests

Ruling out anaemia is important, as is determining a clotting profile. Disturbances of electrolytes (especially magnesium and potassium) can increase the risk of arrhythmias.

Chest x-ray

Chest x-rays are routinely performed primarily to exclude pathologies such as aortic dissection, fractures and neoplasms, but they may also detect early signs of congestive heart failure.

Echocardiogram

Infarcted myocardium does not contract normally and the echocardiogram can be used to detect abnormal wall movement.

Angiography

The injection of radio-opaque dyes to detect lesions is indicated in high-risk patients or those with elevated biomarkers. The process may identify patients with vessels that are calcified or otherwise unsuitable for stenting and may require bypass surgery.

CT angiography

Computed tomography angiography (CTA) is a less invasive method of examining the coronary vessels and could provide a more cost-efficient model of

BOX 22.5 Conditions associated with elevated troponin levels in the absence of ischaemic heart disease

- Cardiac contusion
- Cardio-invasive procedures (surgery, ablation, pacing, stenting)
- Acute or chronic congestive heart failure
- Aortic dissection
- Aortic valve disease
- Hypertrophic cardiomyopathy
- Arrhythmias (tachy- or brady-)
- Apical ballooning syndrome
- Rhabdomyolysis with cardiac injury
- Severe pulmonary hypertension, including pulmonary embolism

- Acute neurological disease (e.g. stroke, subarachnoid haemorrhage)
- Myocardial infiltrative diseases (amyloid, sarcoid, haemochromatosis, scleroderma)
- Inflammatory cardiac diseases (myocarditis, endocarditis, pericarditis)
- Drug toxicity
- Respiratory failure
- Sepsis
- Burns
- Extreme exertion (e.g. endurance athletes)

Source: Green & Hill (2012).

assessing low to medium risk patients (Samad et al., 2012).

Ongoing management

Once basic management has been initiated the subsequent plan requires confirmation of infarction. In the case of STEMI the 12-lead ECG is sufficient to trigger reperfusion therapies of either thrombolytics or angioplasty (with or without stent) (see Fig 22.9). For the patient with NSTEMI the return of raised cardiac enzymes will be required to confirm the need for reperfusion (see Fig 22.10).

Indications for percutaneous intervention (PCI) include:

- patient presenting within 12 hours of symptom onset, and anticipated time from first medical contact to balloon inflation is 2 hours or less (including time taken for transport)
- contraindications to fibrinolytic therapy
- patient presenting within 12–24 hours of symptom onset with ongoing symptoms/signs of ischaemia or haemodynamic instability.

Reperfusion therapies

The current recommendation is for patients presenting with ST elevation less than 12 hours from the onset of pain to be treated with reperfusion therapy, by either PCI or thrombolysis. Thrombolysis is currently not recommended for NSTEMI due to poor outcomes compared with PCI (Daga et al., 2011; Papadakis & McPhee, 2012) and patients should be directed to PCI (NICE, 2010).

Thrombolysis

In urban centres where access to angioplasty is available, the administration of thrombolytic medications such as tissue plasminogen activator (tPA), streptokinase, alteplase or reteplase is generally

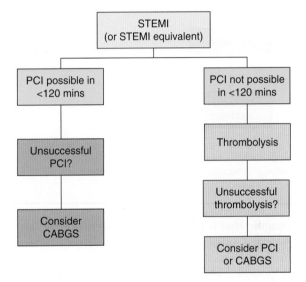

Figure 22.9
Approach to the management of STEMI.
Source: Adapted from Daga et al. (2011).

withheld, but in rural and remote areas this therapy provides the best opportunity to reduce the occlusion and preserve myocardial tissue in STEMI. Paramedics in some rural ambulance services are trained to administer this group of medications, primarily after diagnosing STEMI on a 12-lead ECG. In urban areas most ambulance services have moved towards rapid access to angioplasty and omit thrombolytics as patients who receive this treatment prior to angioplasty experience worse outcomes than those who receive only angioplasty (McDonald et al., 2008).

Angioplasty

Angioplasty involves the dilation of a stenosis using a balloon placed across the lesion under radiological

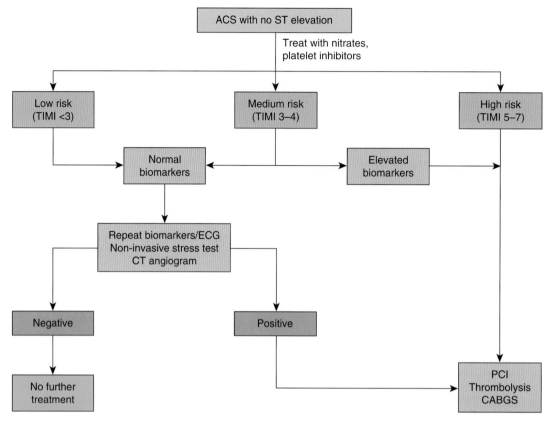

Figure 22.10
Approach to management of NSTEMI.
Source: Adapted from Daga et al. (2011).

imaging that is then inflated to stretch the lesion. Access is usually achieved via the femoral artery in the groin. Angioplasty should occur as soon as possible. Once flow is obtained the artery is stented, which entails leaving a spring-like splint behind to prevent the stenosis re-occluding (see Fig 22.11). Some stents gradually release a drug to inhibit platelet aggregation. Many metropolitan systems have rapid access to angioplasty, making it the preferred primary response (ARC, 2016); however, in the absence of rapid-access angioplasty, thrombolysis is commonly used as the primary response.

The period immediately following reperfusion from either angioplasty or successful thrombolysis is often associated with arrhythmias. Patients should be monitored at this time and a defibrillator must be at hand in case they develop ventricular fibrillation or ventricular tachycardia.

PCI is now recommended for NSTEMI patients who score as high risk on scales such as the TIMI risk score (see Box 22.6) or the Global Registry of Acute Cardiac Events (GRACE). This move towards early intervention in NSTEMIs is likely to impact paramedics over the next decade, with early hospital notification and deciding on clinical pathways without the support of ECG evidence becoming more common.

Beta-blockers
Early administration of beta-blockers (within 24 hours of onset of pain) improves patient outcomes for both STEMI and NSTEMI (Miller et al., 2007). Calcium channel blockers are an alternative if there is a sensitivity/allergy to beta-blockers.

Hospital admission

Patients presenting with ischaemic pain but no ST changes will undergo a number of investigations while staff await the results of the cardiac enzyme test and will often be admitted on the basis of the nature of pain, even when all the tests are returned as negative. Exclusion of MI involves a holistic process, which comprises the history, examination, serial ECGs, serial cardiac enzymes and further testing (e.g. exercise stress tests). This process can take some hours and in many cases is done in a chest pain assessment unit.

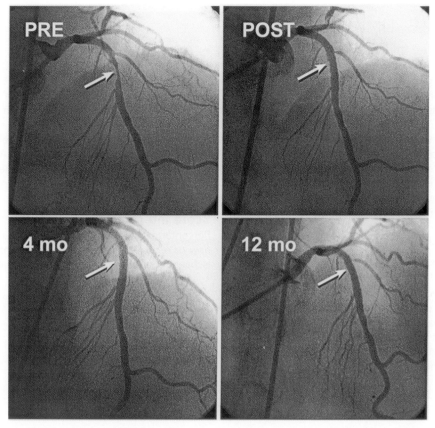

Figure 22.11
Angiographic images before and after placement of a sirolimus-eluting stent. The left anterior descending artery contains a tight stenosis (arrow, upper left panel). After stent implantation (upper right panel), the stenosis is abolished (arrow). Follow-up at 4 and 12 months (bottom panels) reveals a completely open lumen, with no evidence of restenosis (arrows).
Source: Goldman & Ausiello (2008).

Follow-up

Discharge planning and rehabilitation are now recognised as significant factors in reducing the rates of re-occlusion and progression of CAD (NICE, 2010). The era where large portions of myocardium were lost due to infarct has largely passed and patients without substantial occlusions who have been treated early can return to normal lifestyles. Without regular assessment and modification of risk factors, however, the likelihood of re-infarction is high. Multiple small infarcts also threaten long-term left ventricular failure and are a significant health burden for the individual and for the health system caring for them.

ACS across the lifespan

Although ACS is classically associated with older patients with relevant comorbidities, it is still possible for patients as young as 18 to experience the syndrome. Some cases of MI in younger patients are due to either congenital abnormality or interactions with other factors such as drugs, while other cases have the same aetiology as older patients.

The impact of early out-of-hospital care for ACS is particularly relevant to the outcome of MI, allowing better and earlier recovery if the coronary artery obstruction is identified and addressed quickly. Paramedics can have a very significant impact on patients' quality and duration of life following an acute coronary episode. With improving approaches to management of coronary syndrome patients will live longer with more functioning myocardium, reducing the burden of chronic heart failure.

A patient in this younger age demographic with an acute cardiac event may well put off calling an ambulance due to a combination of embarrassment and denial. Some patients may be reluctant to share information about their use of erectile dysfunction drugs unless questioned directly and in a supportive manner that explains the reason for the questioning.

BOX 22.6 TIMI risk score

TIMI stands for 'Thrombolysis In Myocardial Infarction' and is the name of an academic research organisation that was founded in 1984 and has conducted numerous practice-changing clinical trials in patients with cardiovascular disease or risk factors for cardiovascular disease. In patients with unstable angina/NSTEMI, the TIMI risk score is a simple prognostication calculation that categorises the patient's risk of death and ischaemic events and provides a basis for therapeutic decision-making. The need to obtain biomarker results precludes its usefulness for paramedics but it is used to guide decision-making in the ED.

TIMI score calculation
Score 1 point for each of the following:
- Age ≥ 65
- Aspirin use in last 7 days (patient experiences chest pain despite aspirin use in past 7 days)
- At least 2 angina episodes within the last 24 hours
- ST changes of at least 0.5 mm on admission ECG

- Elevated serum cardiac biomarkers
- Known coronary artery disease (CAD) (coronary stenosis ≥ 50%)
- At least 3 risk factors for CAD, such as: hypertension > 140/90 mmHg or on antihypertensives, current cigarette smoker, hypercholesterolaemia, diabetes mellitus, family history of premature CAD (CAD in male first-degree relative or father younger than 55, or female first-degree relative or mother younger than 65).

Score interpretation
Percentage risk at 14 days of all-cause mortality, new or recurrent MI, or severe recurrent ischaemia requiring urgent revascularisation:
- Score 0–1 = 4.7% risk
- Score 2 = 8.3% risk
- Score 3 = 13.2% risk
- Score 4 = 19.9% risk
- Score 5 = 26.2% risk
- Score 6–7 = at least 40.9% risk

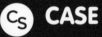

CASE STUDY 2

Case 10940, 1505 hrs.

Dispatch details: A 62-year-old woman with back pain.

Initial presentation: The crew are led inside a private house and find the pale and sweaty patient sitting on a chair in the kitchen. A friend of the patient is in attendance.

 ASSESS

1515 hrs Primary survey: The patient is conscious and talking.

Chief complaint: 'I've had back pain for an hour and it hasn't gone away with paracetamol.'

1517 hrs Vital signs survey: Perfusion status: HR 108 bpm; sinus rhythm; BP 130/90 mmHg; skin cool, pale and sweaty.
    Respiratory status: RR 18 bpm; good normal air entry bilaterally; speaking in full sentences; denies shortness of breath; oxygen saturations 98% on room air.
    Conscious state: GCS = 15.

1521 hrs Pertinent hx: The patient gives a history of upper back pain that has been coming and going for about a week. She hasn't had it before. An hour ago, however, while having a coffee with her friend the pain suddenly returned, worse than ever. The pain has not changed since and has not responded to treatment with paracetamol or one of her friend's indigestion tablets. There is no radiation of the pain and she is unable to accurately pinpoint its location. She describes the pain as a dull ache.

1524 hrs Past medical hx: She is a smoker and has a family history of ischaemic heart disease on her father's side. She takes no medications and 'never goes to the doctor'.

1525 hrs Physical exam: Taking a deep breath does not alter the pain, nor does movement of her arms or neck. Inspection of the area reveals no rash, bruising or swelling. She appears discomforted by the pain but not overly anxious. She rates the pain as 6/10. Her 12-lead ECG shows sinus rhythm with inverted T waves in leads I and V4–V6. BGL = 7.2 mmol.

Females are more likely to develop atypical presentations of ischaemic pain and postmenopausal women do not have the protection against developing CAD that occurs with gender prior to menopause. A positive finding of ST elevation on the ECG would confirm the underlying cause but in this case the ECG is not so specific. While this pain is definitely not 'classic' for ischaemia, an inability to confidently attribute it to another cause means it has to be treated as such.

② CONFIRM

In many cases paramedics are presented with a collection of signs and symptoms that do not appear to describe a particular condition. A critical step in determining a treatment plan in this situation is to consider what other conditions could explain the patient's presentation.

What else could it be?
Musculoskeletal trauma
Osteoporosis is common among women in late middle age and fractures can occur from seemingly normal forces such as lifting and bending. Point tenderness is associated with almost all fractures and careful palpation of the spine should reveal any localised pain. The lack of response to ventilation or movement is not suggestive of musculoskeletal pain but a closer examination should be conducted. In this case, there is no localised tenderness.

Dissecting aneurysm
Sudden-onset chest pain radiating through to the back is typical of a dissecting thoracic aneurysm, although the pain is usually described as 'tearing' or 'ripping' and is worse at onset. The repeated nature of the pain does not rule an aneurysm in or out. Unequal brachial blood pressures can indicate a thoracic aneurysm, but that is not present in this case. Definitive diagnosis of a dissecting aneurysm requires a CT scan.

Nonspecific ECG changes and nonspecific chest pain
Sudden-onset, central, 'crushing' chest pain that radiates to one or both arms does occur, but more often paramedics are confronted with chest pain presentations (as in this case) that lack a conclusive cause. ECGs are similarly wide-ranging, and between the clear extreme of ST elevation and a normal ECG lies a host of changes that could be attributed to ischaemia or could just be normal variations.

Changes to T wave shape and direction are among the early signs of ischaemia, with peaked and widened T waves usually preceding the development of ST

> ### DIFFERENTIAL DIAGNOSIS
> **ACS**
> Or
> - Musculoskeletal trauma
> - Dissecting aneurysm
> - Nonspecific ECG changes and nonspecific chest pain

elevation. T wave inversion is generally described as a sign of a fully resolved infarct, however, and widespread T wave inversion is also common in paediatrics, cardiomyopathy, pericarditis, left ventricular hypertrophy and bundle branch blocks.

The key in this case is that the T wave inversion is occurring in only the lateral leads (I, V4, V5 and V6). Unlike widespread T wave inversion that is caused by structural changes (such as hypertrophy), this anatomical grouping suggests an (at least partial) occlusion to the vessel supplying this region of the heart. The narrow and symmetrical inverted T waves produced by myocardial ischaemia can also be distinguished from the deep and wide T waves of structural cause (Hayden et al., 2002).

While neither the atypical chest pain nor the atypical ECG changes are definitive, the combined presentation adds weight to the diagnosis of ACS. Underpinning the diagnosis is the overt sympathetic response and change to the patient's vital signs. While anxiety can cause these changes, the combination of altered vital signs (especially the changes to the skin), pain that could be ischaemic in nature and an abnormal ECG that is consistent with cardiac ischaemia make a strong case for ACS.

③ TREAT

1528 hrs: This patient has not been administered nitrates previously and is showing signs of poor perfusion. The crew wisely choose to place her on their stretcher prior to administering a conservative dose of GTN. If the GTN dose causes a significant drop in blood pressure, having the patient on the stretcher allows the crew to lay the patient flat.

Aspirin and other anticoagulants are contraindicated in suspected cases of dissecting aneurysm, and while an aneurysm cannot be ruled out the symptoms are not definitive and the benefits of anticoagulation therapy in ACS outweigh the risks of worsening the aneurysm in this case. The patient is not hypoxic so receives no supplemental oxygen.

④ EVALUATE

Evaluating the effect of any clinical management intervention can provide clues to the accuracy of the initial diagnosis. Some conditions respond rapidly to treatment so patients should be expected to improve if the diagnosis and treatment were appropriate. A failure to improve in this situation should trigger the clinician to reconsider the diagnosis.

The patient's symptoms start to subside and within 2 minutes she is calmer and says the pain has partially resolved. She rates her pain 3/10.

Pain relief from nitrates should not be considered diagnostic of ACS: one study of more than 400 patients initially managed for ACS found that patients ultimately diagnosed as not having ACS were more likely to report pain relief from nitrates compared with those ultimately found to have active ACS (41% compared with 39%; Henrikson et al., 2003).

1530 hrs: Perfusion status: HR 92 bpm; sinus rhythm; BP 120/80 mmHg; skin cool, pale, dry.

Respiratory status: RR 18 bpm; good normal air entry bilaterally; speaking in full sentences; patient denies shortness of breath; oxygen saturations 98% on room air.

Conscious state: GCS = 15.

Although this patient's blood pressure has fallen significantly following her initial dose of nitrates, her perfusion has actually improved (heart rate lower, no longer sweaty). A repeated, conservative dose of nitrates is warranted and subsequent IV analgesia if required to achieve patient comfort.

The paramedics should consider notifying the receiving hospital of the patient's abnormal ECG finding to reduce triage delays.

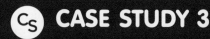

CASE STUDY 3

Case 13914, 2340 hrs.

Dispatch details: A 19-year-old male at a nightclub venue is complaining of chest pain and shortness of breath.

Initial presentation: The crew find the patient sitting on the footpath outside the nightclub. He is distressed and sweaty.

1 ASSESS

2356 hrs Primary survey: The patient is conscious and talking.

Chief complaint: 'I had chest pain for a little while but now I feel like I can't breathe.'

2358 hrs Vital signs survey: Perfusion status: HR 190 bpm, narrow complex tachycardia, BP 120/90 mmHg, skin cool and pale.

Respiratory status: RR 30 bpm; good air entry bilaterally; speaking in full sentences; patient denies shortness of breath but says his chest feels tight; oxygen saturations 100% on room air; normal work of breathing.

Conscious state: GCS = 15.

0004 hrs Pertinent hx: The patient states that he developed chest pain inside the venue, went outside for fresh air but felt worse. The patient and his friends are adamant that he has taken nothing unusual or illegal. The patient holds a flat palm over his chest to indicate where he feels the discomfort. He describes the pain as a 'tightness' and says it extends up to his neck. The pain has not changed since it appeared suddenly and does not change with ventilation, palpation or movement.

0005 hrs Past medical hx: The patient has never had chest pain previously and has no significant medical history.

0007 hrs Physical examination: No obvious rashes, swelling or signs of trauma. Both pupils are dilated and sluggish. There are no obvious IV marks. On ECG, narrow complex junctional tachycardia (see Ch 23) with ST elevation of 2 mm is noted in leads V2 and V3.

Although this is not the typical picture of ACS caused by the sudden occlusion of a coronary artery, the description of the pain is very typical of ACS. In this case the patient's very high heart rate is likely to be the cause of the imbalance between myocardial oxygen supply and demand, but it raises the question of treating with both nitrates and aspirin.

<table>
<tr><td>

DIFFERENTIAL DIAGNOSIS

ACS
Or
- Chest pain that is not associated with ACS

</td></tr>
</table>

② CONFIRM

In many cases paramedics are presented with a collection of signs and symptoms that do not appear to describe a particular condition. A critical step in determining a treatment plan in this situation is to consider what other conditions could explain the patient's presentation.

Such is the oversupply of blood to the myocardium that it takes a significant occlusion to a vessel to upset the balance between supply and demand. There are circumstances where a combination of a rise in demand and a mild reduction in supply are capable of producing myocardial ischaemia and subsequent chest pain. In this case the patient has developed a re-entry tachycardia that is causing a fixed, elevated heart rate (see Ch 23). At this rate the diastolic filling time is severely reduced while the myocardial demand is raised. This arrhythmia is neither uncommon nor especially dangerous in young people, and could be due to a minor structural abnormality within the heart. It could also have been triggered by use of stimulants such as caffeine, pseudoephedrine (cold and flu tablets), methamphetamine or cocaine. Denial of drug use is common when patients are confronted in public places but the ingestion could be accidental, and it is the clinical signs rather than an admission of guilt that should guide the clinician. While the speed of the arrhythmia has generated a supply–demand imbalance, methamphetamines and cocaine have both been shown to cause vasospasm of coronary arteries capable of producing a myocardial infarct (Jiao et al., 2009; Chen, 2007; Hung et al., 2003; Menyar, 2006; Waksman et al., 2001).

③ TREAT

The description of the pain and the presentation fits concisely into the definition of ACS but there are a number of complicating factors that need to be considered prior to treatment.

Nitrates are routinely recommended for ACS in an effort to lower both pre- and afterload and to reduce myocardial workload. The 'safety net' for administering this drug, which lowers blood pressure, is that the patient can generate a higher heart rate if the GTN causes their blood pressure to fall too far. This patient's heart rate is disengaged from normal sympathetic and parasympathetic feedback: it is fixed by an internal re-entry circuit and will not change if blood pressure rises or falls. Administering nitrates to this patient risks a catastrophic fall in blood pressure with no ability to compensate.

The appropriate solution is to revert the arrhythmia (see Ch 23), allow the heart rate to return to normal and then reassess if the ischaemia has resolved. In most ambulance services this reversion of rate is restricted to paramedics trained in intensive care, but it should be the first line of treatment rather than triggering the ACS guidelines (ARC, 2011). In areas where there is no ability to revert the arrhythmia in the field, urgent transport to hospital and judicious pain relief are the only options.

1540 hrs: The paramedics revert the arrhythmia according to local guidelines (see Ch 23).

④ EVALUATE

Evaluating the effect of any clinical management intervention can provide clues to the accuracy of the initial diagnosis. Some conditions respond rapidly to treatment so patients should be expected to improve if the diagnosis and treatment were appropriate. A failure to improve in this situation should trigger the clinician to reconsider the diagnosis.

1542 hrs: Perfusion status: HR 110 bpm, sinus tachycardia, BP 120/90 mmHg, skin normal.

Respiratory status: RR 30 bpm, good air entry bilaterally, speaking in full sentences. The patient states he is no longer short of breath or has chest tightness. Oxygen saturations 100% on room air, normal work of breathing.

Conscious state: GCS = 15.

In most cases ischaemia due to grossly elevated heart rate will resolve once the arrhythmia has been reverted, but it is worth considering that in addition to producing vasospasm both cocaine and methamphetamine can cause a prothrombotic state and accelerated atherosclerosis (Jiao et al., 2009). A disrupted coronary plaque cannot be ruled out in any patient, regardless of age, and the benefits of aspirin are such that the combination of ischaemic pain and ECG changes should trigger administration provided there are no contraindications if symptoms persist once the arrhythmia has been reverted.

Future research

Future research into the diagnosis and management of ACS includes research into the potentially harmful consequences of hyperoxaemia as opposed to targeted oxygen delivery (Nolan, 2011).

Further systems-based research studying the effects of reduced time delay until re-establishment of perfusion is needed to fine-tune the response to ACS. In the past decade there have been a number of projects where hospitals have been notified about incoming STEMI patients to reduce 'door-to-balloon time'. Although most of these studies have reduced this time by up to one-third there has been no corresponding improvement in patient mortality (Menees et al., 2013). The focus is now likely to shift to educating the public in order to reduce 'pain to balloon time'.

High-sensitivity biomarkers that are revealed within 30 minutes of infarct may allow the diagnosis of NSTEMI in the field. Heart-type fatty acid binding protein (hFABP) assays appear sensitive within 30 minutes and may provide a quick and portable test (McCann et al., 2008). The role that endothelial dysfunction and inflammatory mediators play in the development of unstable atherosclerotic plaques is also likely to be the target of new therapies and interventions. There is growing evidence that isolated ST elevation in aVR in patients who otherwise have no ST elevation (NSTEMI) is predictive of poor outcomes and this may become an indicator for early PCI in these patients (Barrabes et al., 2003).

Summary

The management of ACS has undergone significant development, with early treatment options being available in the field. With the increasing treatment options comes an increasing level of clinical risk of iatrogenic effects. The assessment of clinical risk involves integration of the history and examination with a thorough working knowledge of interpreting 12-lead ECGs. Abnormal and unusual presentations of myocardial ischaemia necessitate keeping an open mind to the possibility of myocardial ischaemia. Conversely, there are a number of conditions that may mimic myocardial ischaemia, which necessitates careful evaluation before commencing on an invasive treatment pathway.

References

2012 Writing Committee Members, Jneid, H., Anderson, J. L., Wright, R. S., Adams, C. D., Bridges, C. R., Casey, D. E., Jr, Ettinger, S. M., Fesmire, F. M., Ganiats, T. G., Lincoff, A. M., Peterson, E. D., Philippides, G. J., Theroux, P., Wenger, N. K., Zidar, J. P., Anderson, J. L., & American College of Cardiology Foundation; American Heart Association Task Force on Practice Guidelines. (2012). 2012 ACCF/AHA focused update of the guideline for the management of patients with unstable angina/non–ST-elevation myocardial infarction (updating the 2007 guideline and replacing the 2011 focused update): a report of the American College of Cardiology Foundation/American Heart Association Task Force on practice guidelines. *Circulation, 126.*

Aroney, C., Aylward, P., Kelly, A., Chew, D., & Clune, E. (2006). Acute coronary care syndrome guidelines working group. Guidelines for the management of acute coronary syndromes. *The Medical Journal of Australia, 8*(8), S1–S30.

Australian Institute of Health and Welfare (AIHW). (2011). *Cardiovascular disease: Australian facts, 2011. Cat. no. CVD 53.* Canberra: AIHW.

Australian Resuscitation Council (ARC). (2016). *Guidelines: Acute Coronary Syndrome.* ARC.

Barrabes, J. A., Figueras, J., Moure, C., Cortadellas, J., & Soler-Soler, J. (2003). Prognostic value of lead aVR in patients with a first-time non-ST elevation acute myocardial infarction. *Circulation, 108,* 814–819.

Bhuiya, F. A., Pitts, S. R., & McCaig, L. F. (2010). Division of health care statistics. Emergency department visits for chest pain and abdominal pain: United States, 1999–2008. *NCHS Data Brief, 43,* 1–8.

Brady, W. J. (2006). ST segment and T wave abnormalities not caused by acute coronary syndromes. *Emergency Medicine Clinics of North America, 24*(1).

Bryant, B., Knights, K., & Salerno, E. (2011). *Pharmacology for health professionals.* Sydney: Elsevier.

Burgess, S. (2010). Oxygen therapy for acute myocardial infarction. *Australasian Journal of Paramedicine, 8*(2).

Cabello, J. B., Burls, A., Emparanza, J. I., Bayliss, S., & Quinn, T. (2010). Oxygen therapy for acute myocardial infarction. *The Cochrane Database of Systematic Reviews,* (12), CD007160.

Chen, J. P. (2007). Methamphetamine-associated acute myocardial infarction and cardiogenic shock with normal coronary arteries: refractory global coronary microvascular spasm. *Journal of Invasive Cardiology, 19,* E89–E92.

Collinson, P., Goodacre, S., Gaze, D., Gray, A., & RATPAC Research Team. (2012). Very early diagnosis of chest pain by point-of-care testing comparison of the diagnostic efficiency of a panel of cardiac biomarkers compared with troponin measurement alone in the RATPAC Trial. *Heart (British Cardiac Society), 98*(4).

Craft, J., Gordon, C., & Tiziani, A. (2011). *Understanding pathophysiology.* Sydney: Elsevier.

Daga, L. C., Kaul, U., & Mansoor, A. (2011). Approach to STEMI and NSTEMI. *JAPI, 59,* 19–25.

Diercks, D. B., Kontos, M. C., Chen, A. Y., Wiviott, S. D., Pollack, C. V., Jr, Wiviott, S. D., Rumsfeld, J. S., Magid, D. J., Gibler, W. B., Cannon, C. P., Peterson, E. D., & Roe, M. T. (2009). Utilization and impact of pre-hospital electrocardiograms for patients with acute ST-segment elevation myocardial infarction: data from the NCDR (National Cardiovascular Data Registry) ACTION (Acute Coronary Treatment and Intervention Outcomes Network) Registry. *Journal of the American College of Cardiology, 53*(2), 161–166.

Dörler, J., Edlinger, M., Alber, H. F., Altenberger, J., Benzer, W., Grimm, G., Huber, K., Pachinger, O., Schuchlenz, H., Siostrzonek, P., Zenker, G., Weidinger, F., & Austrian Acute PCI Investigators. (2011). Clopidogrel pre-treatment is associated with reduced in-hospital mortality in primary percutaneous coronary intervention for acute ST-elevation myocardial infarction. *European Heart Journal, 32*(23), 2954–2961.

Dorsch, M. F., Lawrance, R. A., Sapsford, R. J., Durham, N., Oldham, J., Greenwood, D. C., Jackson, B. M., Morrell, C., Robinson, M. B., Hall, A. S., & for the EMMACE Study Group. (2001). Poor prognosis of patients with symptomatic myocardial infarction but without chest pain. *Heart (British Cardiac Society), 86*(5), 494–498.

Ducas, R. A., Wassef, A. W., Jassal, D. S., Weldon, E., Schmidt, C., Grierson, R., & Tam, J. W. (2012). To transmit or not to transmit: how good are emergency medical personnel in detecting STEMI in patients with chest pain? *Canadian Journal of Cardiology, 28*(4), 432–437.

Dumaine, R., Borentain, M., Bertel, O., Bode, C., Gallo, R., White, H. D., Collet, J. P., Steinhubl, S. R., & Montalescot, G. (2007). Intravenous low-molecular-weight heparins compared with unfractionated heparin in percutaneous coronary intervention: quantitative review of randomized trials. *Archives of Internal Medicine, 167*(22), 2423–2430.

Ekelund, U., Akbarzadeh, M., Khoshnood, A., Björk, J., & Ohlsson, M. (2012). Likelihood of acute coronary syndrome in emergency department chest pain patients varies with time of presentation. *BMC Research Notes, 8*(5).

Fleisher, L. A. (2012). *Anesthesia and uncommon diseases* (6th ed., pp. 28–74). Philadelphia: Saunders.

Galinski, M., Saget, D., Ruscev, M., Gonzalez, G., Ameur, L., Lapostolle, F., & Adnet, F. (2015). Chest pain in an out-of-hospital emergency setting: no relationship between pain severity and diagnosis of acute myocardial infarction. *Pain Practice, 15*(4), 343–347.

Golabchi, A., & Sarrafzadegan, N. (2011). Takotsubo cardiomyopathy or broken heart syndrome: a review article. *Journal of Research in Medical Sciences, 16*(3), 340–345.

Goldman, L., & Ausiello, D. A. (2008). *Cecil Medicine* (23rd ed.). Philadelphia: Saunders Elsevier.

Goodacre, S., Locker, T., Morris, F., & Campbell, S. (2002). How useful are clinical factors in the diagnosis of acute, undifferentiated chest pain? *Academic Emergency Medicine: Official Journal of the Society for Academic Emergency Medicine, 9*(3).

Green, G. B., & Hill, P. (2012). Chest pain: cardiac or not. In J. Tintinalli (Ed.), *Tintinalli's emergency medicine: a comprehensive study guide* (7th ed.). Sydney: McGraw-Hill.

Hall, J. (2012). *Guyton and Ball textbook of medical physiology* (12th ed.). St Louis: Saunders.

Han, J. H., Lindsell, C. J., Storrow, A. S., Luber, S., Hoekstra, J. W., Hollander, J. E., Peacock, W. F., Pollack, C. V., Gibler, W. B., & EMCREG i*trACS Investigators. (2007). The role of cardiac risk factor burden in diagnosing acute coronary syndromes in the emergency department setting. *Annals of Emergency Medicine, 49*(2).

Hayden, B. E., Brady, W. J., Perron, A. D., Somers, M. P., & Mattu, A. (2002). Electrocardiographic T-wave inversion: differential diagnosis in the chest pain patient. *The American Journal of Emergency Medicine, 20*(3), 252–262.

Henrikson, C. A., Howell, E. E., Bush, D. E., Miles, J. S., Meininger, G. R., Friedlander, T., Bushnell, A. C., & Chandra-Strobos, N. (2003). Chest pain relief by nitroglycerine does not predict active coronary artery disease. *Annals of Internal Medicine, 139,* 979–986.

Hung, M. J., Kuo, L. T., & Cherng, W. J. (2003). Amphetamine-related acute myocardial infarction due to coronary artery spasm. *International Journal of Clinical Practice, 57,* 62–64.

ISIS-2 (Second International Study of Infarct Survival) Collaborative Group. (1988). Randomized trial of intravenous streptokinase, oral aspirin, both, or neither among 17,187 cases of suspected acute myocardial infarction: ISIS-2. *Journal of the American College of Cardiology, 12*(6 Suppl.A).

Jiao, X., Velez, S., Ringstad, J., Eyma, V., Miller, D., & Bleiberg, M. (2009). Myocardial infarction associated with Adderall XR and alcohol use in a young man. *Journal of the American Board of Family Medicine, 22*(2), 197–201.

Kamali, J., Soderholm, M., & Ekelund, U. (2014). What decides the suspicion of acute coronary syndrome in acute chest pain patients? *BMC Emergency Medicine, 14,* 9.

Karnath, B., Holden, M., & Hussain, N. (2004). Chest pain: differentiating cardiac from non-cardiac causes. *Hospital Physician,* April.

Keller, K. B., & Lemberg, L. (2004). Prinzmetal's angina. *American Journal of Critical Care, 13*(4), 350–354.

Kumar, A., & Cannon, C. P. (2009). Acute coronary syndromes: diagnosis and management, part I. *Mayo Clinic Proceedings, 84*(10), 917–938.

Lefler, L. L., & Bondy, K. N. (2004). Women's delay in seeking treatment with myocardial infarction: a meta-synthesis. *Journal of Cardiovascular Nursing, 19*(4), 251–268.

Løvlien, M., Johansson, I., Hole, T., & Schei, B. (2009). Early warning signs of an acute myocardial infarction and their influence on symptoms during the acute phase, with comparisons by gender. *Gender Medicine, 6*(3), 444–453.

Marcus, G. M., Cohen, J., Varosy, P. D., Vessey, J., Rose, E., Massie, B. M., Chatterjee, K., & Waters, D. (2007). The utility of gestures in patients with chest discomfort. *American Journal of Medicine, 120*(1), 83–89.

McCance, K. L., & Huether, S. E. (2013). *Pathophysiology: the biologic basis for disease in adults and children* (7th ed.). St Louis: Mosby.

McCann, C. J., Glover, B. M., Menown, I. B. A., Moore, M. J., McEneny, J., Owens, C. G., Smith, B., Sharpe, P. C., Young, I. S., & Adgey, J. A. (2008). Novel biomarkers in early diagnosis of acute myocardial infarction compared with cardiac troponin T. *European Heart Journal, 29*(23).

McDonald, M. A., Fu, Y., Zeymer, U., Wagner, G., Goodman, S. G., Ross, A., Granger, C. B., Van de Werf, F., Armstrong, P. W., & ASSENT-4 PCI Investigators. (2008). Adverse outcomes in fibrinolytic-based facilitated percutaneous coronary intervention: insights from the ASSENT-4 PCI electrocardiographic substudy. *European Heart Journal, 29*(7), 871–879.

Mehta, S. R., Salim, Y., Peters, R. J. G., Bertrand, M. E., Lewis, B. S., Natarajan, M. K., Malmberg, K., Rupprecht, H,-J., Zhao, F., Chrolavicius, S., Copland, I., Fox, K. A. A., & for the Clopidogrel in Unstable angina to prevent Recurrent Events trial (CURE) Investigators. (2001). Effects of pretreatment with clopidogrel and aspirin followed by long-term therapy in patients undergoing percutaneous coronary intervention: the PCI-CURE study. *The Lancet, 358*(9281), 527–533.

Menees, D., Menees, D. S., Peterson, E. D., Wang, Y., Curtis, J. P., Messenger, J. C., Rumsfeld, J. S., & Gurm, H. S. (2013). Door-to-balloon time and mortality among patients undergoing primary PCI. *The New England Journal of Medicine, 369.*

Menyar, A. (2006). Drug-induced myocardial infarction secondary to coronary artery spasm in teenagers and young adults. *Journal of Postgraduate Medicine, 52*(1), 51–56.

Miller, C. D., Roe, M. T., Mulgund, J., Hoekstra, J. W., Santos, R., & Pollack, C. V. (2007). Impact of acute beta-blocker therapy for patients with non–ST-segment elevation myocardial infarction. *American Journal of Medicine, 120*(8).

NICE. (2010). *National clinical guideline centre (UK). Unstable angina and NSTEMI: the early management of unstable angina and non-ST-Segment-Elevation myocardial infarction. NICE clinical guidelines No. 94.* London: Royal College of Physicians. Revised 2013.

Nolan, J. P. (2011). Advances in post-resuscitation care. *Clinical Medicine, 11*(6), 605–608.

O'Gara, P. T., Kushner, F. G., Ascheim, D. D., Casey, D. E., Jr, Chung, M. K., de Lemos, J. A., Ettinger, S. M., Fang, J. C., Fesmire, F. M., Franklin, B. A., Granger, C. B., Krumholz, H. M., Linderbaum, J. A., Morrow, D. A., Newby, I. K., Ornato, J. P., Ou, N., Radford, M. J., Tamis-Holland, J. E., Tommaso, C. I., Tracy, C. M., Woo, Y. J., & Zhao, D. X. (2013). 2013 ACCF/AHA guideline for the management of ST-Elevation myocardial infarction. *Journal of the American College of Cardiology, 61*(4), e78–e140.

O'Connor, R. E., Bossaert, L., Arntz, H. R., Brooks, S. C., Diercks, D., Feitosa-Filho, G., Nolan, J. P., Vanden Hoek, P. I., Walters, D. I., Wong, A., Welsford, M., Woolfrey, K., & Acute Coronary Syndrome Chapter Collaborators. (2010). Part 9: acute coronary syndromes 2010 international consensus on cardiopulmonary resuscitation and emergency cardiovascular care science with treatment recommendations. *Circulation, 122*(16, Suppl. 2), S422–S465.

Papadakis, M. A., & McPhee, S. J. (Eds.), (2012). *Medical diagnosis and treatment* (51st ed.). New York: McGraw-Hill.

Pelter, M. M., Riegel, B., McKinley, S., Moser, D. K., Doering, L. V., Meischke, H., Davidson, P., Baker, H., Yang, W., & Dracup, K. (2012). Are there symptom differences in patients with coronary artery disease presenting to the ED ultimately diagnosed with or without ACS? *The American Journal of Emergency Medicine, 30*(9), 1822–1828.

Roongsritong, C., Warraich, I., & Bradley, C. (2004). Common causes of troponin elevations in the absence of acute myocardial infarction: incidence and clinical significance. *Chest, 125*(5), 1877–1884.

Sabatine, M. S., Cannon, C. P., Gibson, C. M., Jose, L. L.-S., López-Sendón, J. L., Montalescot, G., Theroux, P., Lewis, B. S., Murphy, S. A., McCabe, C. H., Braunwald, E., & Clopidogrel as Adjunctive Reperfusion Therapy (CLARITY)-Thrombolysis in Myocardial Infarction (TIMI) 28 Investigators. (2005). Effect of clopidogrel pretreatment before percutaneous coronary intervention in patients with ST-elevation myocardial infarction treated with fibrinolytics: the PCI-CLARITY Study. *JAMA, 294*(10), 1224–1232.

Samad, Z., Hakeem, A., & Mahmood, S. S. (2012). A meta-analysis and systematic review of computed tomography angiography as a diagnostic triage tool for patients with chest pain presenting to the emergency department. *Journal of Nuclear Cardiology, 19.*

Sanders, M. J. (2007). *Mosby's paramedic textbook* (rev 3rd ed.). St Louis: Mosby.

Sgarbossa, E. B. (2000). Value of the ECG in suspected acute myocardial infarction with left bundle branch block. *Journal of Electrocardiology, 33*, 87–92.

Stub, D., Smith, K., Bernard, S., Bray, J. E., Stephenson, M., Cameron, P., Meredith, I., & Kaye, D. M. (2012). A randomized controlled trial of oxygen therapy in acute myocardial infarction: air versus oxygen in myocardial infarction study (AVOID study). *American Heart Journal, 163*, 339–345.

Van de Werf, F., Ross, A., Armstrong, P., & Granger, C. (2006). Primary versus tenecteplase-facilitated percutaneous coronary intervention in patients with ST-segment elevation acute myocardial infarction (ASSENT-4 PCI): randomised trial. *The Lancet, 367*(9510), 569–578.

Waksman, J., Taylor, R. N., Bodor, G. S., Daly, F. F. S., Jolliff, H. A., & Dart, R. C. (2001). Acute myocardial infarction associated with amphetamine use. *Mayo Clinic Proceedings, 76*(3), 323–326.

Zweier, J. L. (2006). The role of oxidants and free radicals in reperfusion injury. *Cardiovascular Research, 70*(2), 181–190.

CHAPTER 23

Arrhythmias

By Brett Williams

OVERVIEW

- Arrhythmias may present with signs and/or symptoms ranging from none through to respiratory distress, cardiovascular compromise and sudden cardiac death.
- If at any time a patient presents with no signs of life, commence resuscitation as per the advanced life support guidelines.

- The ECG must be interpreted in conjunction with the patient's history and physical examination findings.
- The key consideration is the presence or absence of compromised perfusion.
- Any wide-complex tachyarrhythmias should be considered to be ventricular tachycardia.

Introduction

Cardiac arrhythmias are among the most complex cases facing any clinician. While the field of paramedicine appears largely well defined and structured, the range of possible arrhythmias, how they are identified and how they should be managed are potentially very subjective and challenge even experienced cardiologists. Arrhythmias that share the same name can present with vastly different ECG traces and produce clinical presentations that range from asymptomatic to cardiac arrest. Variations in cardiac structure, atherogenesis, disease progression, medications and past history can all impede clinical decision-making and ECG trace interpretations.

For paramedics and other clinicians limited by diagnostic equipment and time, clear clinical pathways are described for many arrhythmias. Together, the definition of a particular arrhythmia and the subsequent clinical practice guideline often leave little room for clinical reasoning. It is therefore not necessary for this chapter to list the values that describe the various arrhythmias and their usual course of management. Instead, the chapter will examine the relatively common group of patients who present in the out-of-hospital setting and who do not fit the classic definition, presentation and management pathway. It is for these patients in particular that paramedics require their clinical reasoning skills.

The term **arrhythmia** has been used for centuries to describe an abnormal rhythm and in 1978, following the rapid expansion of medical communication across borders, the World Health Organization and the International Society of Cardiology convened a taskforce to define terms related to cardiac rhythms (WHO ISC Task Force, 1978). The term 'arrhythmia' was given the broadest possible definition: any rhythm other than a sinus rhythm. Importantly, it was also suggested that the term should be used to describe the entire array of non-sinus rhythms, rather than an individual rhythm.

The terms 'arrhythmia' and 'dysrhythmia' are often used interchangeably within the out-of-hospital environment. This stems from discussion in the literature around the technical definition of the two terms (Royster, 1990). For the purposes of this chapter the term 'arrhythmia' will be used when describing the collective group of non-sinus rhythms.

Pathophysiology

Within the muscular structure of the heart there is a collection of cells that do not contract or play any direct mechanical role in the movement of blood. Rather, they are integral to cardiovascular function and it is these cells that generate and conduct the electrical impulses that stimulate the mechanical work of the heart. Cardiac myocytes (or contractile cells) are the most common cells of the heart and contract to generate the compressive force that moves blood out of each of the heart's chambers. Autorhythmic cells propagate and conduct the impulses that trigger the mechanical action. They can be further divided into pacemaker cells (e.g. sinoatrial [SA] or atrioventricular [AV] node) that propagate the impulses, and specialised conduction cells that conduct the impulses to the myocardial cells.

Over the past 50 years cardiovascular science has gained a greater understanding of how the contractile and pacemaker cells of the heart work and interact (Park & Fishman, 2011). Technological innovations have revealed how ion channels control the function of both groups of cells and this knowledge has given rise to medications that allow clinicians to manage an increasing number of arrhythmias.

Impulse formation and conduction

Human cells generate some degree of electrochemical gradient between the contents within their cell walls and the environment outside the cell. This voltage difference across the cell membrane is known as the *membrane potential* and is maintained by the action of ion pumps, channels, transporters and exchangers (Park & Fishman, 2011). In addition to maintaining a resting membrane potential, muscle and nerve cells can, to varying degrees, generate an electrochemical wave known as an *action potential* to signal or activate other cells (Park & Fishman, 2011).

For myocardial cells the receipt of an action potential primarily triggers the cell to contract, but the membranes of myocardial cells are also connected to allow the action potential to flow to other myocardial cells and thus spread the electrical wave (and mechanical contraction) throughout the myocardium (see Fig 23.1). As such, the heart effectively works as a single unit. This concept, called cardiac syncytium, occurs due to the presence of gap junctions, allowing the action potential to be propagated (transferred) from one cell to another through the movement of a small number of positively charged ions (property of conductivity).

While myocardial cells are able to pass action potentials onto other myocardial cells, they are not able to generate action potentials spontaneously; that is, they do not normally possess 'automaticity'. Automaticity is a property of the cardiac pacemaker cells. Being modified myocardial cells, these cells do not have the ability to contract but are able to move spontaneously from their resting membrane potential (RMP) to their threshold potential where the ion channels will open and trigger depolarisation (see Fig 23.2). The depolarisation of the pacemaker cells triggers the depolarisation of the surrounding myocardial cells and another wave of excitation–contraction will sweep across the heart. Action potentials allow rapid signal propagation across the cell membrane. In the heart, each type of cardiac cell (e.g. nodal, atrial, ventricular, Purkinje) has a characteristic action potential that is determined by the panel of ion channels expressed (see Fig 23.3).

During a normal cardiac cycle, the pacemaker potential is generated within the sinoatrial node and conducted along the internodal conduction tracts to the atrioventricular junction, consisting of the atrioventricular node and the bundle of His (see Fig 23.4). After being held for a short period of time, the impulse travels through the bundle branches to the Purkinje network and finally to the ventricular myocardium.

Cardiac myocytes rely on the autorhythmic cells to generate action potentials. Understanding the five phases of the action potential is very important in the pathophysiology and management of arrhythmias. Figure 23.5 illustrates the five phases a myocyte transitions through during a depolarisation/repolarisation cycle. Sodium (Na^+), calcium (Ca^{++}) and potassium (K^+) are the three key ions involved in the process. Each ion requires a specific voltage-gated channel

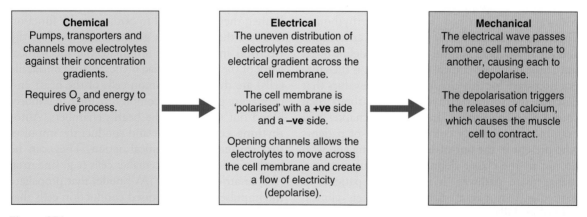

Chemical
Pumps, transporters and channels move electrolytes against their concentration gradients.

Requires O_2 and energy to drive process.

Electrical
The uneven distribution of electrolytes creates an electrical gradient across the cell membrane.

The cell membrane is 'polarised' with a **+ve** side and a **−ve** side.

Opening channels allows the electrolytes to move across the cell membrane and create a flow of electricity (depolarise).

Mechanical
The electrical wave passes from one cell membrane to another, causing each to depolarise.

The depolarisation triggers the releases of calcium, which causes the muscle cell to contract.

Figure 23.1
The mechanical action of the heart is intrinsically linked to the ability of the cells to shift electrolytes against their concentration gradient across the cell membrane. Creating this chemical imbalance requires energy but creates an electrical difference across the cell membrane, with the inside of the cell more negatively charged than the outside (the cell is described as polarised). If the cell is triggered to open specific ion channels embedded in the membrane, the electrolytes will flow according to their chemical and electrical gradients and the cell will depolarise. The electricity generated will trigger the next cell to depolarise and trigger the movement of calcium into the cell to trigger contraction. Most antiarrhythmic medications act to alter the behaviour of one or more ion channels and thus make the cell less or more excitable, or less or more contractile.

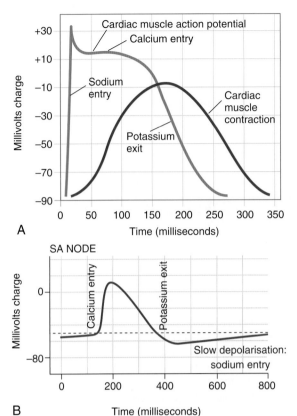

A

B

Figure 23.2
A Myocardial cells wait at their RMP for an external stimulus to open sodium channels and allow the positive electrolytes to flow in and depolarise the cell. This triggers the release of calcium, which causes the cell to contract and generate pressure to expel blood from the chambers of the heart.
B By contrast, pacemaker cells do not contract but without stimulus move from RMP towards spontaneous depolarisation. This depolarisation triggers waiting myocardial cell to depolarise.
Source: Craft et al. (2011); Patton & Thibodeau (2010); Boron & Boulpaep (2009).

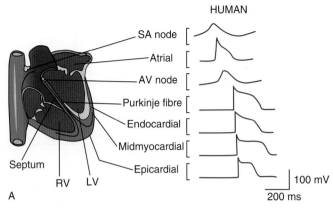

A

Figure 23.3
Schematic of action potential waveforms and propagation at various points in the human heart.
Source: Saksena & Camm (2011).

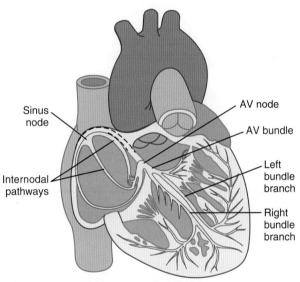

Figure 23.4
The cardiac conduction system.
Source: Hall (2012).

to open, allowing movement of the relevant ion. In other words, the channel will not open until a specific voltage is reached. Importantly, once the cell has reached phase 1 it cannot create another action potential until approximately halfway through phase 3: this is referred to as the *absolute refractory period*. The action and pacemaker RMP and threshold potentials are also affected by the autonomic nervous system, hormones, drugs, electrolyte concentrations, ischaemia and hypoxia.

Arrhythmia mechanisms

The primary bradyarrhythmia mechanisms include dysfunction or failure of the SA node to spontaneously propagate an action potential. Blocks within the AV node may also stop an action potential

reaching the ventricles. Excessive parasympathetic activity, disease or a lack of blood supply to either the SA or the AV nodes can reduce their function (see Fig 23.6), as too will drugs that block the inward flow of sodium and calcium.

The primary tachyarrhythmia mechanisms are excessive sympathetic activity or drugs that enhance the inward flow of sodium and calcium. Arrhythmias can also be generated when myocardial cells (usually through injury from ischaemia) develop automaticity and spontaneously trigger an action potential (see Table 23.1). If this occurs at a rate faster than the SA node, this activity will become the pacemaker that sets the rate of the heart. Re-entry

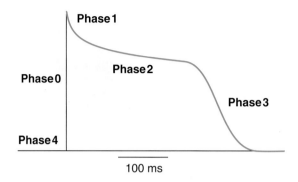

100 ms

Phase	Pacemaker potential	Action potential
0	• Slow influx of Ca⁺⁺ • Voltage at start of phase 0 approx. −50 mV	• Influx of Na⁺ • Voltage at start of phase 0 approx. −90 mV
1	• Not present	• Fast Na⁺ channels close • Efflux of K⁺ • Voltage at start of phase 1 approx. +20–30 mV
2	• Not present	• Ca⁺⁺ slowly enters the cell • Ca⁺⁺ released from sarcoplasmic reticulum • Efflux of K⁺ continues • Voltage at start of phase 2 approx. 0 mV
3	• Ca⁺⁺ channels close • Efflux of K⁺	• Ca⁺⁺ channels close • Continued efflux of K⁺ • Voltage at start of phase 3 approx. 0 mV
4	• Influx of Ca⁺⁺ and Na⁺ • Slow efflux of K⁺ • Does not maintain a steady voltage, continues to increase until threshold potential is reached • The slope of phase 4 determines the depolarisation rate	• Na⁺ and K⁺ pumps activated • Ca⁺⁺ returned to sarcoplasmic reticulum • Generally maintains voltage of −90 mV

Figure 23.5
Ion movement during pacemaker and action potentials.
Source: (Top image) Saksena & Camm (2011).

circuits within a small area of cells can also create tachyarrhythmias.

Under normal conditions, an impulse travels throughout the entire cardiac conduction system and, due to the absolute refractory period, dies out. In arrhythmias caused by a re-entry mechanism, this does not occur: rather, as the impulse passes through the conduction system, it is delayed and/or blocked at one point, but conducted normally throughout the remainder of the system. This mechanism allows cells within the relative refractory period to again be depolarised and may occur on a macro or micro level. At a macro level, an accessory or anatomical pathway will typically be implicated, such as the bundle of Kent in Wolff-Parkinson-White syndrome. Usually a fibrous insulating barrier is present between the atria and the ventricles. In some patients, this fibrous barrier is not complete and so the impulse can pass between the ventricles and the atria via the alternative anatomical pathway. At a

micro level, a functional circuit can be formed within the atria or the ventricles and is typically caused by ischaemia. These conditions slow the conduction of the impulse through the cell; if slowed enough it will re-excite cells that are in the relative refractory period.

The enhanced automaticity mechanism occurs in autorhythmic cells due to an increase in the slope of phase 4 of the pacemaker potential through the influx of potassium. Increasing the slope causes the autorhythmic cell to reach its threshold potential sooner and is often caused by adrenergic stimulation. Abnormal automaticity occurs in cardiac myocytes that do not normally possess this property and is often caused by hypoxia, ischaemia or hypercarbia. Due to the less negative resting potential and influx of sodium and calcium, the threshold potential is reached.

Arrhythmias that arise due to triggered activity occur when a cardiac myocyte membrane potential is triggered more than once from a single impulse.

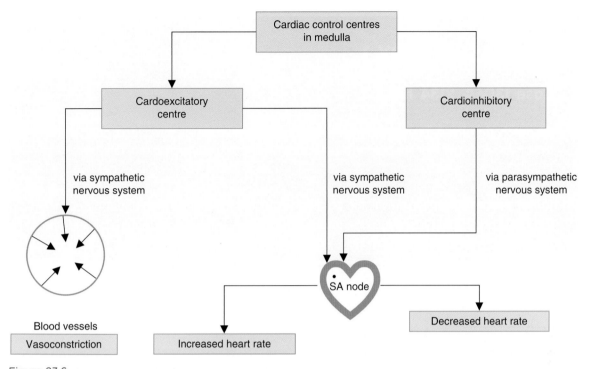

Figure 23.6
Autonomic innervation of the cardiovascular system.
The sympathetic nervous system increases both heart rate and vasoconstriction, while the parasympathetic nervous system decreases heart rate.
Source: Craft et al. (2011).

Table 23.1 Sources of arrhythmias

Infection	Sepsis causes release of adrenaline and noradrenaline leading to increased sinus rates Infection can trigger paroxysmal atrial fibrillation in susceptible patients
Disease	Thyrotoxicosis: tachycardia Valvular heart disease (atrial fibrillation/flutter, supraventricular tachycardia) Pericarditis: tachycardia Left ventricular failure: tachycardia Fibrosis/calcification of heart tissue
Ischaemia/infarction	Sinus tachycardia/bradycardia AV blocks (bradycardia) Ventricular tachycardia
Electrolyte imbalance	Hyperkalaemia: bradycardia (sinus and AV blocks) Hypokalaemia: tachycardia Hypomagnesaemia: bradycardia Hypocalcaemia: bradycardia
Drugs	Beta-blockers, calcium channel blockers: bradycardia Tricyclics (tricyclic antidepressants): sinus tachycardia, ventricular tachycardia Amphetamines/cocaine/caffeine: sinus tachycardia, supraventricular tachycardia

Source: Adapted from Ninio (2000).

It is termed *after-repolarisation* and is further subdivided into early and delayed after-repolarisation. Early after-repolarisation occurs during phase 2 or 3 of the action potential and a classic example is torsades de pointes. Delayed after-repolarisation occurs after the completion of depolarisation and results in some ventricular tachycardias and digitalis-induced arrhythmias.

CASE STUDY 1

Case 13064, 2134 hrs.

Dispatch details: A 55-year-old male has collapsed while walking in a local park. Bystanders indicate that the patient is pale, diaphoretic and complaining of difficulty breathing.

Initial presentation: On arrival, the paramedics locate the patient lying under a tree in the local park. He acknowledges the paramedics' arrival, but appears to be confused and presents with difficulty breathing. He is extremely pale and diaphoretic.

HISTORY

Ask!

- When did the complaint start?
- Has this happened before?
- Do you have any significant previous medical history?
- Do you smoke/drink/take drugs? What is your job? Where do you live and with whom?
- Does your family have any significant illnesses (diabetes, for instance)?
- Do you have any other symptoms in other body systems?

BREATHING

Look for!

- Respiratory rate, rhythm and effort

① ASSESS

Patient history

Confusion is a common side effect of poor cerebral perfusion and it can make obtaining (or trusting) a history difficult. It is important to take note of other sources of information available, such as evidence of surgery, medications that the patient may be carrying, information from bystanders and/or persons who know the patient, medical alert necklace/bracelet/card and evidence of a pacemaker or implantable cardioverter-defibrillator (ICD).

In addition to the standard goals of history taking and physical examination, the initial key question to resolve is whether the patient has compromised perfusion. Key signs and/or symptoms consistent with compromised perfusion include altered level of consciousness, shortness of breath or respiratory distress and the presence of poor perfusion/shock or chest pain. These signs and symptoms principally result from poor cardiac output and, if left untreated, may result in cardiac arrest.

After completing a patient history, the paramedics obtain the following information.

- The patient was walking in the park when he was seen to hold his chest and collapse onto the grass. Prior to this, bystanders state that he appeared to be walking at a brisk pace and did not show any signs of distress.
- At no point was the patient unconscious.
- The patient cannot answer any questions due to his confusion.
- He has no obvious surgical scars.
- He has no medications with him.
- Bystanders state that his condition appears to be deteriorating and after providing basic first aid, there was no improvement.

Airway

Patients with an altered level of consciousness are at risk of airway obstruction and must receive ongoing assessment and active management. This patient is demonstrating a clear airway by his ability to talk normally.

Breathing

The presence of respiratory distress, inadequate respiratory effort and pulmonary oedema require immediate intervention. This patient appears to have a raised respiratory rate that could be due to a metabolic (lactic) acidosis secondary to reduced perfusion. Respiratory compromise secondary to left ventricular failure is a possibility, but is unlikely to have developed this quickly.

Cardiovascular

The cardiovascular assessment should seek to resolve the question of compromised perfusion (haemodynamic instability). Evidence of an altered level of consciousness, hypotension (BP < 90 mmHg systolic), shock (hypotension, pale/cool/clammy skin and diaphoresis) and/or heart failure (shock and/or pulmonary oedema) are suggestive of compromised perfusion and require immediate intervention. This patient is clearly presenting with compromised perfusion and so requires immediate intervention.

An elevated heart rate is a normal physiological compensatory response when the blood pressure and/or perfusion falls. Clinicians need to investigate whether the elevated heart rate is the primary problem or a compensatory response. It is suggested that in an adult without impaired cardiac function, a heart rate of less than 150 bpm is unlikely to cause compromised perfusion. Therefore, careful consideration should be given to other diagnostic differentials.

Electrocardiograph

The ECG is key to the diagnosis of an arrhythmia; however, it is important to note that the presence or absence of an arrhythmia must be interpreted in the context of the patient, their history and clinical presentation (see Fig 23.7). Should the patient present as having compromised perfusion, exact interpretation of the ECG should not delay the onset of initial management.

Categorising any arrhythmia as fast, slow, wide or narrow can provide a shortlist of possibilities. For ease of management, tachyarrhythmias are divided first into regular or irregular arrhythmias, then second into narrow QRS complex (≤ 0.12 sec) or wide QRS complex (> 0.12 sec) (see Table 23.2). This simplified and stepped approach allows the clinician to quickly identify the tachyarrhythmia and instigate a management strategy, particularly when a patient is haemodynamically compromised.

RISK FACTORS

- Previous cardiac history
- Ejection fraction < 35%
- Patient > 35 years old
- Family history
- Syncope
- Compromised perfusion

PRACTICE TIP

Signs of compromised perfusion include:
- altered level of consciousness
- respiratory distress
- shock
- hypotension
- chest pain
- acute heart failure

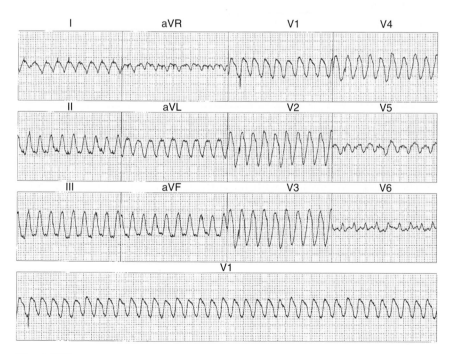

Figure 23.7
A 12-lead ECG of sustained ventricular tachycardia in an older man with coronary artery disease.
Source: Saksena & Camm (2011).

Table 23.2 Basic arrhythmia assessment

	Fast		Slow	
	Regular	Irregular	Regular	Irregular
Narrow QRS complex (≤ 0.12 sec)	Sinus tachycardia Supraventricular tachycardia Atrial flutter	Atrial fibrillation	Sinus bradycardia Sinoatrial/ atrioventricular blocks	Atrial fibrillation
Wide QRS complex (> 0.12 sec)	All of above with bundle branch block Ventricular tachycardia	All of above with bundle branch block	All of above with bundle branch block Idioventricular	Atrial fibrillation with bundle branch block

Neurological

Patients with an arrhythmia who present with an altered level of consciousness require immediate management. The altered level of consciousness results from compromised cardiac output and increased myocardial demand. Although this patient appears to have some compromise to his cerebral perfusion, he is not so badly affected that he is unconscious.

Initial assessment summary

Problem	Collapsed while walking in the park
Conscious state	GCS = 13 (E4, V4, M5)
Position	Lying under a tree
Heart rate	170 weak, regular
Blood pressure	85/50 mmHg
Skin appearance	Extremely pale and sweaty
Speech pattern	Phrases
Respiratory rate	36 bpm
Respiratory rhythm	Even cycles
Respiratory effort	Elevated
Chest auscultation	Equal air entry bilaterally, no adventitious sounds
Pulse oximetry	92% on room air
Temperature	36.7°C
Motor/sensory function	Normal
History	Walking briskly in the park, seen to clutch his chest and collapse
ECG	Wide-complex regular tachycardia, which appears to be ventricular tachycardia (QRS 0.16 sec)

D: The patient has been made safe by bystanders.

A: The patient is conscious with no current airway obstruction, but needs frequent reassessment.

B: The respiratory rate is elevated but ventilation appears normal.

C: Heart rate is elevated and there is insufficient blood pressure to maintain adequate cerebral perfusion. The ECG indicates an arrhythmia that could be a possible cause.

Considering the wider picture, this patient has a clinical appearance and history that is compatible with ventricular tachycardia, which is providing enough perfusion for him to remain conscious but not enough to maintain orientation.

DIFFERENTIAL DIAGNOSIS

Ventricular tachycardia

Or

- Supraventricular tachycardia (SVT) with bundle branch block (BBB)

2 CONFIRM

The essential part of the clinical reasoning process is to seek to confirm your initial clinical hypothesis by finding clinical signs that should occur with your provisional diagnosis. You should also seek to challenge your diagnosis by exploring findings that do *not* fit your hypothesis: don't just ignore them because they don't fit.

This patient is presenting with an arrhythmia that is greater than 100 bpm, regular and has a QRS complex of greater than 0.12 sec. Using Table 23.2, this would indicate that the patient could be presenting with one of two arrhythmias: ventricular tachycardia or supraventricular tachycardia with a bundle branch block (BBB).

What else could it be?

SVT with BBB

Distinguishing between ventricular tachycardia and supraventricular tachycardia with aberrancy (often BBB) can be difficult and clinicians are strongly advised to manage the patient as if the arrhythmia were ventricular tachycardia, particularly if there is any uncertainty. Importantly, there is a significantly lower risk for the patient to manage supraventricular tachycardia with aberrancy as if it were ventricular tachycardia than to manage ventricular tachycardia as if it were supraventricular tachycardia with aberrancy. Primary cardiac causes of ventricular tachycardia include ischaemia, acute myocardial infarction and structural defects. Potential reversible causes may include electrolyte disturbances or medications/drugs.

Evidence of one or more of the following findings is associated with an increased likelihood of the arrhythmia being a ventricular tachycardia:

- QRS complex width > 0.14 sec
- RS interval > 0.1 sec (high specificity for ventricular tachycardia)
- negative concordance in praecordial leads (strongly favours ventricular tachycardia as this is evidence of a highly unusual axis of depolarisation)
- positive aVR likely to be due to significant axis deviation
- patient > 35 years of age
- patient has a previous cardiac or ventricular tachycardia history
- evidence of P waves occurring independently of the QRS complexes seen as minor irregularities in the overriding ECG
- evidence of fusion beats where an atrial contraction initiates a ventricular contraction, which is then incorporated into the VT beat.

This patient has a QRS complex width of > 0.14 sec and is older than 35 years of age. This strongly supports the ECG interpretation of ventricular tachycardia.

3 TREAT

Emergency management

The management of all tachyarrhythmias is aimed at controlling the rate and/or rhythm. This allows for a reduction in the oxygen demand of the cardiac tissue and improved cardiac output. The increase in cardiac output leads to an increase in blood pressure and finally end-organ perfusion. This will be evidenced by improved mental status, a reduction in respiratory distress, increasing blood pressure and reduction of pale, diaphoretic skin.

While developing a management plan, it is important to recognise the potential risks associated with each intervention. All interventions associated with the management of arrhythmias have the potential to adversely impact the patient.

Principles of management for wide-complex tachycardias (with pulse) are outlined in Box 23.1.

Safety

Management of patients presenting with arrhythmias may require the use of medications, defibrillation, synchronised cardioversion or pacing. At all times

---

PRACTICE TIP

Consider long QT as a cause of ventricular tachycardia/ventricular fibrillation. Selected causes of long QT include:

- congenital (long QT syndrome)
- electrolyte abnormalities (hypokalaemia, hypomagnesaemia, hypocalcaemia)
- medications (tricyclic antidepressants, antipsychotics, phenothiazines)
- organophosphates.

> ## BOX 23.1 Principles of management
>
> **Wide-complex tachycardias (with pulse)**
> - Provide supportive care.
> - Identify and manage underlying cause.
> - If compromised perfusion, undertake synchronised cardioversion.
> - If cardioversion unsuccessful, consider amiodarone.
> - Transport patient to an appropriate facility.

consideration should be given to the safety aspects of these skills and procedures, particularly in a moving vehicle.

Position

This patient is presenting with compromised perfusion and respiratory distress. He should be postured supine and receive supplemental oxygenation, and intravenous access should be gained. Posture and intravenous fluid can be used to increase central venous pressure and thus venous return to the heart. The improved filling pressure will increase ventricular stretch and force of contraction, producing increased cardiac output unless the heart is already overstretched and the patient already in failure. Optimising the patient's preload will help reduce the possible haemodynamic risks that can be associated with sedation before cardioversion.

Synchronised cardioversion

Synchronised cardioversion, like a direct current countershock (defibrillation), involves passing an electrical current through the heart, forcing cardiac myocytes and autorhythmic cells to depolarise at one time. Cardioversion will then potentially allow one of the autorhythmic cells to resume primary pacemaker control of the heart.

Unlike the unsynchronised delivery of a direct current countershock, the current delivered during cardioversion is synchronised with the R wave. This eliminates the risk of the current being delivered during the relative refractory period of the action potential and therefore the risk of ventricular fibrillation is also reduced.

Initial biphasic energy settings for cardioversion will differ, depending on the arrhythmia present. This patient is presenting with monomorphic ventricular tachycardia, so an initial setting of 100 joules is appropriate. Should the initial attempt be unsuccessful, energy levels should be increased incrementally and attempted up to a maximum of three times before considering pharmacological intervention.

If synchronised cardioversion is contemplated, sedation to the point of creating amnesia would be good patient care. Sedation of this patient presents a number of challenges if the patient is already haemodynamically compromised. While considering the use of sedating medication, the following questions must be considered.

- Does the patient have a predicted difficult airway for management?
- What is the most appropriate pharmacological intervention, considering the compromised nature of the patient's perfusion?
- What are the potential risks?
- If sedation is required, is waveform capnography available?
- What is the plan to manage the patient's airway, should it become compromised?
- Is the out-of-hospital team briefed and have individual roles been delineated?
- Is all of the equipment prepared?

BOX 23.2 The Vaughan-Williams classification of antiarrhythmic drugs

The Vaughan-Williams classification of antiarrhythmic medications was initially described as four distinct groupings (classes I–IV), based on their effect on the action potential. Later, due to the inability of the system to classify all antiarrhythmic medications, a fifth class was added.

- Class I agents block fast sodium channels, decreasing the depolarisation rate of phase 0 of the action potential and increasing the refractory period. Class I agents are further subdivided into Ia (prolong the action potential), Ib (no change to the duration of the action potential) and Ic (slight prolonging of the action potential).
- Class II agents include beta-adrenoceptor antagonists. These agents decrease the ability

of the sympathetic nervous system and therefore slow impulse conduction, prolong the duration of the action potential and reduce automaticity.

- Class III agents, including amiodarone, prolong the action potential (plateau phase) by blocking the efflux of potassium during repolarisation.
- Class IV agents slow the voltage-gated calcium channels, decreasing the plateau phase and reducing contractility.
- Class V is a mixture of antiarrhythmic medications and includes digoxin and adenosine.

Note: Amiodarone, although placed in class III, has actions that spread across classes I, II, III and IV.

Pharmacological intervention

Patients who present with a wide-complex tachycardia and compromised perfusion should, if cardioversion is unsuccessful, be administered amiodarone 300 mg intravenously over 10–20 minutes (a compromise between the urgency of the situation and the recommended rate of infusion in a controlled situation), followed by a second cardioversion attempt. Amiodarone is a class III Vaughan-Williams antiarrhythmic agent (see Box 23.2).

4 EVALUATE

Any patient presenting with an arrhythmia requires continuous assessment, cardiac monitoring and the acquisition of a 12-lead ECG. Should the patient present with no signs of compromised perfusion (haemodynamically stable), they should be transported to an appropriate facility for further assessment and management.

This patient requires sedation prior to cardioversion. The administration of sedation is likely to impact the patient's central nervous, respiratory and cardiovascular systems. Optimising the central venous pressure and thus preload will mitigate some of the negative haemodynamic effects of sedation, but the patient will require close ongoing monitoring if the rhythm is not reverted by the interventions discussed above.

Ongoing management

On arrival at the emergency department, if the patient is presenting with compromised perfusion, the initial priority will be to control the arrhythmia with synchronised cardioversion. Consideration will also be given to pharmacological intervention and management of reversible causes. If the patient is stable, additional assessment may be conducted,

allowing for an exploration of potential causes of the arrhythmia. This may include:

- 12-lead ECG to confirm the diagnosis of ventricular tachycardia
- laboratory tests such as troponin, urea, creatinine, electrolytes and thyroid function; if the patient was prescribed medications such as digoxin, additional blood testing would be completed to exclude toxicity

- chest x-ray to investigate structural defects
- consultation with a cardiologist.

If the aetiology of a regular, monomorphic, wide-complex tachycardia cannot be established and the patient is stable, consideration may be given to the use of adenosine as a treatment and/or diagnostic tool. For stable ventricular tachycardia the preferred management strategy is administration of antiarrhythmic medications (Vaughan-Williams class I [lignocaine] or class III [amiodarone]) or elective cardioversion.

Hospital admission

Following acute management in the ED, the patient will be transferred for further evaluation. A 12-lead ECG completed at rest will assist in the diagnosis of congenital abnormalities, electrolyte disturbances or structural disease. Cardiac stress testing and ambulatory monitoring are often used for patients with ventricular arrhythmias and assist with diagnosis of myocardial ischaemia, structural disease/changes and diagnosis of arrhythmias. Where patients are believed to have structural heart disease, it is recommended they undergo an echocardiograph. Electrophysiological testing may also be recommended in patients with coronary heart disease.

The primary goal of long-term management of arrhythmias is to reduce morbidity and mortality. Management may consist of a reduction in cardiac re-modelling following myocardial infarction, ongoing management of electrolyte disturbance risks, antiplatelet and anticoagulant therapy, consideration of an implantable cardioverter-defibrillator in patients with low ejection fractions, radiofrequency catheter ablation or revascularisation of coronary arteries.

Arrhythmias across the lifespan
Neonates

The normal heart rate for a neonate is 100–160 bpm. A rate less than 100 bpm requires intervention and a rate greater than 160 bpm should be investigated further. Arrhythmias are seen in approximately 1–5% of neonates and the most common symptomatic arrhythmia is supraventricular tachycardia (Dubbin, 2000). When managing arrhythmias in neonates, clinicians should use a similar approach to that used for all paediatric patients.

Bradycardia in neonates is predominantly caused by hypoxia and requires appropriate airway and respiratory support. The bradycardia should resolve quickly following the instigation of effective airway and respiratory support. If effective management of the airway and ventilation does not resolve the bradycardia and further resuscitation is not required,

consideration should be given to an assessment of the ECG and potential differential diagnoses (congenital, sepsis, acidosis, trauma, hypovolaemia etc.). If unstable, consideration should be given to specific arrhythmia bradycardia management (atropine, pacing etc.). Transportation and notification to a tertiary facility specialising in neonatal services is key.

Tachyarrhythmias may have an extremely rapid ventricular rate (240–300 bpm), increasing the difficulty of ECG interpretation and diagnosis. Specialist medical support is required and clinicians should carefully consider the risks prior to initiating any interventions. As with other tachyarrhythmias, two classifications should be used: narrow complex and broad complex. Narrow complex is significantly more common than wide complex, and both should be managed as per the paediatric treatment guidelines. As with bradycardia, transport to a facility with a specialist neonatal service is important. Out-of-hospital clinicians generally have limited experience and knowledge relating to the management of neonates with arrhythmias. Due to this, consideration should be given to consultation with a specialist facility prior to the initiation of management outside of standard neonatal resuscitation.

During pregnancy

Throughout pregnancy there are a number of compensatory alterations to the maternal anatomy and physiology. Specifically, the cardiac alterations include increased heart rate, increased cardiac output, alterations in the size and position of the heart, changes in systemic vascular resistance and alterations in blood pressure.

Importantly, the criteria by which arrhythmias are diagnosed and the majority of management strategies are identical for pregnant and non-pregnant females. When assessing and managing a pregnant patient, follow the standard approach and management strategies, noting the following:
- There is an increased risk of arrhythmia in patients with underlying cardiac disease.
- Differential diagnoses should be considered, both related and unrelated to the pregnancy.
- All medications used in the management of arrhythmias cross the placenta.
- Patients who present as haemodynamically unstable require management. Remember that compromised maternal perfusion will result in fetal compromise.
- Consideration should be given to the fetus when managing arrhythmias in this subgroup of patients, but the mother's health should remain the primary consideration. Transportation to a facility that has the appropriate specialist services should be considered.

- Appropriate positioning of the mother should be considered to reduce the risk of supine hypotension syndrome, resulting from compression of the descending aorta by the fetus.

Athletes

Athletes have an overall lower risk of adverse health events, but may present with arrhythmias and/or sudden cardiac death. The vast majority of young athletes (< 35 years of age) who die suddenly are male and are found to have a structural cardiac pathology, including cardiomyopathy, congenital coronary artery anomalies, myocarditis, Marfan's syndrome or valvular heart disease. Notwithstanding this, 2–5% present at autopsy with no structural cardiac defect (Link & Estes, 2010). While the majority of young athletes who die suddenly do not present with symptoms, those who do complain of chest pain, palpitations, respiratory distress, dizziness and weakness. In older athletes (> 35 years of age) who die suddenly the majority are again male and engaged in strenuous activity. Approximately half complain of symptoms preceding the collapse and all present with structural cardiac defects.

The most common arrhythmia found in athletes is sinus bradycardia and this is strongly correlated with fitness. Despite this, other causes may be present and careful examination is recommended.

When confronted with an athlete presenting with an arrhythmia or symptoms suggestive of an arrhythmia, the standard approach to assessment and management should be undertaken.

Wolff-Parkinson-White

Wolff-Parkinson-White conduction occurs when an accessory conduction pathway is present between the atria and the ventricles. The additional pathways allow the electrical impulse to bypass the AV node and potentially cause a tachyarrhythmia. Wolff-Parkinson-White conduction presents with a shortened PR interval and delta wave. When the pathway is associated with a supraventricular tachycardia, it is known as Wolff-Parkinson-White syndrome. In athletes, there is no increased occurrence, but potentially increased risk due to high sympathetic drive.

Long QT syndrome

Long QT syndrome can be either acquired (i.e. medications, AMI, electrolyte disturbances) or genetic and despite its origin it can result in polymorphic ventricular tachycardia (torsades de pointes; see Box 23.3). Management consists of direct current countershock and magnesium (in addition to standard advanced life support measures).

BOX 23.3 Polymorphic ventricular tachycardia and torsades de pointes

Polymorphic ventricular tachycardia is easily distinguished from monomorphic ventricular tachycardia by assessing the morphology of the QRS complex. Monomorphic ventricular tachycardia presents with essentially similar-shaped QRS complexes, whereas in polymorphic ventricular tachycardia the complexes are irregular. Torsades de pointes (twisting of the points) is a polymorphic ventricular tachycardia and presents with a varying axis. Examination of the ECG will reveal a QRS complex that appears to be twisting around the isoelectric line. Torsades typically has a prolonged QT interval seen on the non-tachycardia baseline ECG and usually resolves spontaneously; however, patients are also at risk of ventricular fibrillation.

Management of these arrhythmias consists of defibrillation as per ventricular fibrillation. Other management strategies are determined by the presence or absence of a prolonged QT interval. The QT interval is the time from the start of ventricular depolarisation to the end of repolarisation; increasing this interval is associated with an increased relative refractory period. Because the QT interval is affected by heart rate, a formula is used to correct for the rate when assessing for prolonged QT. The corrected QT interval (QTc) is calculated using Bazett's formula: corrected QT = QT/square root of the R-R interval. The corrected values should be ≤ 0.44 sec in adult males and ≤ 0.46 sec in adult females.

Management to prevent the recurrence of torsades consists of eliminating medications that prolong the QT interval, managing electrolyte disturbances or other underlying cause (if identifiable) and intravenous magnesium.

Polymorphic ventricular tachycardia with a normal QTc (not always possible to examine in the out-of-hospital setting as an ECG is required where the patient has a sinus rhythm) is predominantly caused by ischaemia and should be managed as per monomorphic ventricular tachycardia. Due to the mechanism, magnesium is unlikely to be effective. Intravenous amiodarone and beta-blockers should be considered.

Prevention includes the use of beta-blockers and, in a small subset of patients, an implantable cardioverter-defibrillator. Long QT syndrome is associated with cardiac arrest in young people and should be sought out in other family members once a case has been suspected. Other family members can be managed prophylactically to prevent further arrests.

Commotio cordis

Commotio cordis is defined as sudden cardiac death in an individual with no structural cardiac disease following a blow to the chest. Factors that increase the risk of commotio cordis include male gender; small, hard and round objects striking the chest; a direct strike to the left side of the chest; and increased velocity of the strike. The object striking the chest causes a focal ventricular depolarisation during the upstroke of the T wave (relative refractory period), resulting in ventricular fibrillation. The majority of cases occur in individuals younger than 16 years of age and rarely occur in patients older than 21. It is probable that this is due to the increased compliance of the chest wall in younger patients, allowing the force to be more readily transferred through to the myocardium. Management is as per the standard advanced cardiac life support treatment guidelines.

 CASE STUDY 2

Case 12487, 1850 hrs.

Dispatch details: A 25-year-old male complaining of chest pain and palpitations.

Initial presentation: The paramedics arrive outside a local gym and are taken inside by the patient's friend. The patient is seated in the reception area.

---

1 ASSESS

1900 hrs Primary survey: The patient is conscious and alert.

Chief complaint: 'I have pain in my chest and my heart feels like it's racing. The same thing happened a few days ago.'

1903 hrs Vital signs survey: Perfusion status: HR 185 bpm, BP 110/70 mmHg, skin warm and pink, ECG (see Fig 23.8).
   Respiratory status: RR 16 normal effort, good air entry, L = R, SpO$_2$ 98% on room air.
   Conscious state: GCS = 15, dizzy.

1907 hrs Pertinent hx: The patient's heart started racing during a workout. He describes it as 'pounding'. He then had the onset of chest pain that he rates 1/10. A similar thing happened a week ago but he doesn't recall what his doctor said it was. He was given medication that made him feel like he was going to die and he stresses that he doesn't want it again. It did stop the pounding though. He has not followed up with his GP. He has no previous medical or family history, is generally fit and healthy and is currently not taking any medications.

2 CONFIRM

In many cases paramedics are presented with a collection of signs and symptoms that do not appear to describe a particular condition. A critical step in determining a treatment plan in this situation is to consider what other conditions could explain the patient's presentation.

DIFFERENTIAL DIAGNOSIS

SVT
Or
- Stimulants
- Electrolyte or acid–base abnormalities
- Psychological stress
- Compensatory sinus tachycardia
- Hyperthyroidism

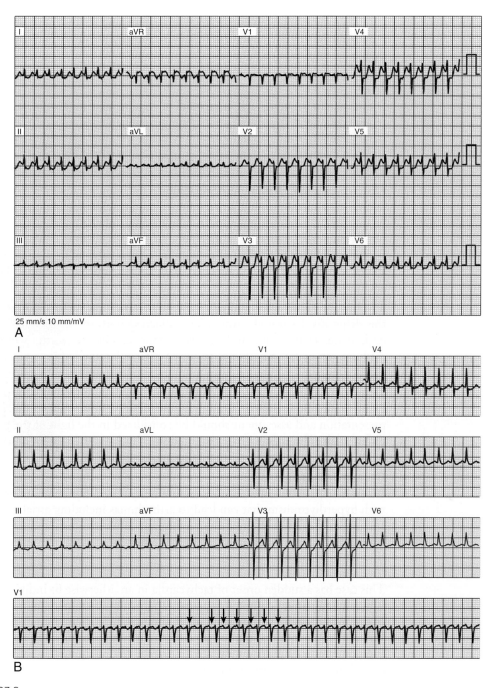

25 mm/s 10 mm/mV

A

B

Figure 23.8
A Narrow-complex supraventricular tachycardia at a rate of 240 bpm with no retrograde or antegrade P wave visible in the R-R cycle. The tachycardia was subsequently confirmed to be type 1 atrioventricular nodal re-entrant tachycardia on electrophysiological study. **B** Narrow-complex supraventricular tachycardia at a rate of 206 bpm with the retrograde P wave clearly visible in the mid-R-R cycle, especially in lead V1. The tachycardia was subsequently confirmed to be atrioventricular re-entrant tachycardia with a retrograde posteroseptal accessory pathway on electrophysiological study.
Source: Saksena & Camm (2011).

This patient is presenting with symptoms of, and an ECG consistent with, a paroxysmal atrial tachycardia otherwise known as an SVT. This could be due to a congenital extra conduction pathway.

What else could it be?

Stimulants
Stimulant drugs, such as amphetamines or cocaine, may lead to the presentation of arrhythmias and patients should be questioned in a respectful manner to investigate this possibility. Supporting evidence may include drug paraphernalia, changes in pupil size or intravenous injection marks. The actual arrhythmia may be a paroxysmal atrial tachycardia or simply a sinus tachycardia.

Electrolyte or acid–base abnormalities
Within the out-of-hospital setting electrolyte or acid–base abnormalities may be difficult to confirm, but careful consideration of the patient's medications, history and presentation may offer some insight. Electrolyte abnormalities may be responsible for instability of the cardiac cell membrane leading to increased automaticity and arrhythmias associated with both extra depolarisation and re-entry.

Psychological stress
The history of the event and the patient's presentation will assist in excluding this diagnosis. Increased automaticity affecting both the firing rate of the SA node (sinus tachycardia) and cell membrane stability across the whole myocardium can occur in response to raised catecholamine levels.

Compensatory sinus tachycardia
This may occur in the presence of trauma, hypoxia, infection or sepsis. The ECG should be reviewed, attempting to identify P waves, and the patient's presentation and assessment should be considered in the light of the potential differentials. The approximate maximal sinus tachycardia rate for an adult can be calculated by subtracting the patient's age from 220.

Hyperthyroidism
A rare but possible cause of tachycardia is increased automaticity associated with hyperthyroidism that can lead to arrhythmias including atrial fibrillation and supraventricular tachycardia. A history of weight loss, tachycardia and hyperreflexia might suggest hyperthyroidism, which could be confirmed with thyroid function tests in hospital.

This case has a sudden onset of tachycardia in an otherwise fit individual. This is highly suggestive of supraventricular tachycardia. If the patient has a history of previous episodes with sudden onset and spontaneous resolution this would support the diagnosis of supraventricular tachycardia. In addition, he described the side effects of adenosine when stating he felt as though he was going to die following drug administration (see Box 23.4).

③ TREAT

1910 hrs: The paramedics have the patient perform the Valsalva manoeuvre (see Box 23.5) but it is not successful in reverting the arrhythmia.

1912 hrs: The paramedics gain IV access and administer adenosine.

When administering adenosine, the patient must be reassured that they are safe and that the feeling they are experiencing will pass. Midazolam may be considered prior to administration where local guidelines permit. If adenosine administration fails to revert the rhythm, or if the patient is rapidly deteriorating, synchronised cardioversion can be considered.

1915 hrs: After performing the Valsalva manoeuvre the patient's ECG reverts to a sinus rhythm. He indicates that his chest discomfort is resolving.

BOX 23.4 Adenosine

Adenosine is a class V antiarrhythmic agent with a half-life of approximately 10 seconds. It works by hyperpolarising the pacemaker potential within the AV node, slowing the transit of impulses through the nodal tissues (negative dromotropic effect). Following administration, patients may complain of an 'impending doom' and present with symptoms such as chest pain, respiratory distress, nausea or dizziness. Some patients require a small (0.5–1.5 mg) dose of midazolam before administration of adenosine. Due to its very short half-life, adenosine should be administered via a rapid intravenous push and flushed with at least 20 mL of saline:

- First dose: 6 mg adenosine with saline flush (55–60% of patients will revert with a 6 mg dose).
- Second dose: If arrhythmia does not revert after 1–2 minutes, 12 mg with saline flush will increase the reversion rate to 90%.
- Third dose: If arrhythmia does not revert after 1–2 minutes, 12 mg with saline flush will increase the reversion rate to 96%.

BOX 23.5 The Valsalva manoeuvre

The Valsalva manoeuvre is considered a first-line management strategy for regular, narrow-complex tachyarrhythmias. Successful reversion of a supraventricular tachycardia through the use of the Valsalva manoeuvre is approximately 15–25% (Mottram & Svenson, 2011). To perform the Valsalva manoeuvre, place the patient head down with their feet elevated for several minutes, then instruct them to blow into a 10-mL syringe (enough pressure to slowly move the plunger) for 15 seconds. This increases intrathoracic pressure, which reduces venous return to the heart and therefore reduces cardiac output. A sympathetic stimulation then occurs in response to the reduced cardiac output. When the Valsalva chest pressure is released, the increased venous return suddenly and dramatically increases cardiac output. It is the parasympathetic response to the rapidly increasing cardiac output in a situation where the sympathetic tone is increased that produces the vagal response. The vagal response causes a reduction in conduction velocity through the AV node. The possible outcomes from the Valsalva manoeuvre include successful reversion or a transient slowing of the rate, revealing a sinus rhythm or a flutter wave.

If the Valsalva manoeuvre is unsuccessful, it should be repeated. A carotid sinus massage may also be considered; however, it is painful if performed properly and it is not recommended in elderly patients (or in an unknown patient over the age of 50) because of the possibility of displacing an atheroma causing an embolic stroke.

Perfusion status: HR 70 bpm; BP 125/85 mmHg; skin dry, warm and pink; ECG sinus rhythm.

Respiratory status: RR 12 bpm, normal effort, good air entry, L = R, SpO_2 97%.

Conscious state: GCS = 15.

4 EVALUATE

Evaluating the effect of any clinical management intervention can provide clues to the accuracy of the initial diagnosis. Some conditions respond rapidly to treatment so patients should be expected to improve if the diagnosis and treatment were appropriate. A failure to improve in this situation should trigger the clinician to reconsider the diagnosis. This patient requires transport for a medical review. En route to hospital he should receive continuous cardiac monitoring, completion of a 12-lead ECG and regular vital signs assessment.

CASE STUDY 3

Case 18064, 2124 hrs.

Dispatch details: A 75-year-old male has had a syncopal episode. He is at home and his wife advises that he is not alert and is pale and diaphoretic.

Initial presentation: The crew are led inside a private house and find the patient sitting on the lounge.

 ASSESS

2137 hrs Primary survey: The patient does not respond to their voices, but he does groan following a painful stimulus.

Chief complaint: The patient's wife states that he had been complaining of feeling unwell for about 30 minutes and got up to go to bed. He then fainted.

2138 hrs Vital signs survey: Perfusion status: HR 32 bpm; sinus bradycardia; BP 80/50 mmHg; skin cool, pale, diaphoretic.

Respiratory status: RR 28 bpm, good air entry, L = R, no adventitious sounds, SpO$_2$ non-sensing.

Conscious state: GCS = 8 (E2, V2, M4).

Blood glucose level: 5.7 mmol/L.

2142 hrs Pertinent hx: The patient has a significant history of cardiac problems, based on his prescribed medications for hypertension, hyperlipidaemia, high cholesterol and diabetes mellitus type 2.

ECG interpretation should follow the same structure as with any arrhythmia (see Table 23.3). Notwithstanding this, the ECG should be examined for P waves and if present, the P wave QRS complex ratio/relationship should be examined.

CONFIRM

In many cases paramedics are presented with a collection of signs and symptoms that do not appear to describe a particular condition. A critical step in determining a treatment plan in this situation is to consider what other conditions could explain the patient's presentation.

DIFFERENTIAL DIAGNOSIS

Sinus bradycardia

Or

- SA node hypoxia
- Sinus bradycardia secondary to parasympathetic stimulation
- Drug toxicity
- Hypothermia

Table 23.3 ECG interpretation for bradycardia

P wave: QRS complex ratio/relationship			
1:1 Sinus bradycardia First-degree AV block	Intermittent block Second-degree AV block type I Second-degree AV block type II	Dropped P wave Sinus arrest and SA exit block	Dissociated Third-degree AV block
No P wave present			

- Junctional escape rhythm
- Ventricular escape rhythm

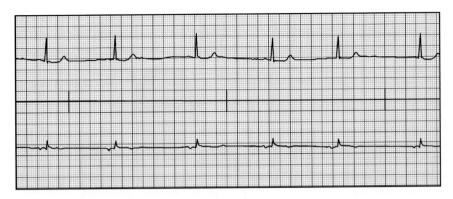

Figure 23.9
Sinus bradycardia.
Source: Saksena & Camm (2011).

What else could it be?

SA node hypoxia

This patient is an elderly diabetic with a significant cardiac history and is on medication for hyperlipidaemia. It would not be surprising if he had ischaemic heart disease, particularly involving the right coronary artery, which is responsible for supplying the SA node. When an opportunity presents itself to perform an ECG (see Fig 23.9), evidence of acute ischaemia in the right coronary artery may confirm this.

Sinus bradycardia secondary to parasympathetic stimulation

A profound sinus bradycardia can be associated with excessive parasympathetic stimulation. Parasympathetic stimulation may be secondary to visceral innervation from urinary retention or bowel obstruction.

Drug toxicity

There are a number of drugs that could be responsible for bradycardia if they are present in too great a concentration. These include beta-blockers, calcium channel blockers and digoxin. The drug concentration may be increased due to patient error or impaired drug clearance, often associated with renal failure. A detailed drug history may identify a possible drug. Renal function tests and levels of some drugs can be obtained at hospital.

Hypothermia

Elderly patients presenting with a decreased conscious state and bradycardia may actually be hypothermic. Clinical examination looking for hypothermia will exclude this, but note that many of the easily applied thermometers (i.e. tympanic membrane thermometer) may have a significant error, particularly at low temperatures.

3 TREAT

The patient should be positioned supine to aid venous return to the heart. All patients should receive continuous cardiac monitoring and intravenous access should be gained. A fluid challenge to increase the central venous pressure (CVP) and preload may improve the patient's perfusion and thus the perfusion of the SA node if positioning has been insufficient to restore adequate perfusion. However, fluid is unlikely to revert the bradycardia and, in this case, it makes no change to the patient's vital signs.

2153 hrs: The crew administer 600 micrograms of atropine IV. Atropine administration to block parasympathetic innovation to the SA node may allow for the sympathetic drive to increase the heart rate. In this case atropine is not

BOX 23.6 Transcutaneous pacing

Patients presenting with significant physiological derangement who are not responding to atropine or who have second-degree type II or third-degree AV block should have transcutaneous pacing pads placed anterior posterior and pacing initiated if they are significantly compromised (see Fig 23.10). In the out-of-hospital setting fixed pacing mode will be used, as the pacing is not affected by movement artefact shutting off the demand pacing function. Once in a stable environment it is safer to employ demand pacing, which will cease when the patient's own rate increases.

Initiating transcutaneous pacing requires a number of considerations and ongoing assessments. The pacer rate should be set initially at 60–70 bpm and then adjusted to produce effective output, balancing rate and oxygen demand versus maintenance of pressure. Electrical capture is evidenced by a pacing spike, followed by a broad QRS complex. The energy setting should be increased quickly until electrical capture is consistently achieved. Mechanical capture is evidenced by palpation of a pulse associated with every QRS complex. Ongoing monitoring is required to ensure that electrical capture and mechanical capture are maintained. Passing electrical currents through a patient's chest may cause discomfort. This is typically managed with small aliquots of a narcotic analgesic and midazolam.

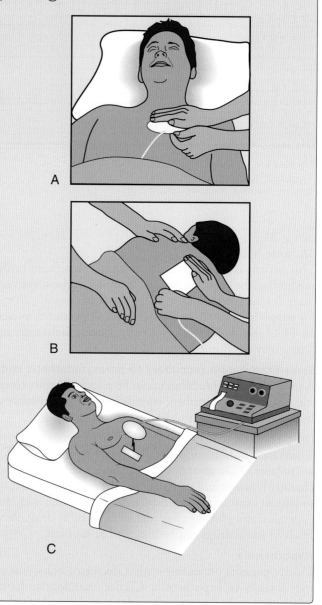

Figure 23.10
Transcutaneous pacemaker.
Pacing electrodes are placed on the patient's anterior **A** and posterior **B** chest walls and attached to an external pacing unit **C**.
Source: Brown & Edwards (2012).

effective (see Box 23.6). Adrenaline can be administered according to local guidelines if atropine is not effective. Adrenaline is a catecholamine and stimulates alpha, beta₁ and beta₂ receptors, resulting in peripheral vasoconstriction and increased inotropic and chronotropic effects.

4 EVALUATE

Evaluating the effect of any clinical management intervention can provide clues to the accuracy of the initial diagnosis. Some conditions respond rapidly to treatment so patients should be expected to improve if the diagnosis and treatment were appropriate. A failure to improve in this situation should trigger the clinician to reconsider the diagnosis.

This patient responds to the adrenaline infusion after several small increases in dose. At this point his heart rate has increased to 58 bpm and his blood pressure is 100/70 mmHg. Although technically still bradycardic, this response reflects a significant improvement and could be considered sufficient. Any further increases in inotrope infusions should be titrated against the onset of side effects such as ectopic beats.

Summary

Arrhythmias are a leading cause of death in Australia and a common presentation within the out-of-hospital environment. Irrespective of the type of arrhythmia, the central question to be answered is around the issue of compromised perfusion. End-organ dysfunction, resulting from compromised perfusion, commonly presents with syncope, altered level of consciousness, respiratory distress, hypotension, shock, chest pain and heart failure. A 12-lead ECG is an important diagnostic tool for patients with an arrhythmia, but the clinician must weigh up the need for immediate management with the additional information provided by the ECG.

When confronted with a patient with an arrhythmia, you should: complete a rapid but thorough assessment; consider and manage reversible causes; provide initial care including appropriate posturing, airway and ventilator support, oxygenation and intravenous access; consider and, if appropriate initiate, specific arrhythmia management; and provide ongoing assessment and transport to an appropriate facility.

References

Boron, W. F., & Boulpaep, E. L. (2009). *Medical physiology* (2nd ed.). Philadelphia: Saunders.

Brown, D., & Edwards, H. (2012). *Lewis's medical-surgical nursing* (2nd ed.). Sydney: Elsevier.

Craft, J., Gordon, C., & Tiziani, A. (2011). *Understanding pathophysiology*. Sydney: Elsevier.

Dubbin, A. M. (2000). Arrhythmias in the newborn. *NeoReviews, 1*(8), e146–e151.

Hall, J. (2012). *Guyton and Ball textbook of medical physiology* (12th ed.). St Louis: Saunders.

Link, M. S., & Estes, N. A. (2010). Athletes and arrhythmias. *Journal of Cardiovascular Electrophysiology, 21*(10), 1184–1189.

Mottram, A. R., & Svenson, J. E. (2011). Rhythm disturbances. *Emergency Medicine Clinics of North America, 29*, 729–746.

Ninio, D. F. (2000). Contemporary management of atrial fibrillation. *Australian Prescriber, 23*, 100–102.

Park, D. S., & Fishman, G. (2011). Basic electrophysiological procedures for the clinician. In I. Saksena & J. Camm (Eds.), *Electrophysiological disorders of the heart* (2nd ed.). Philadelphia: Saunders.

Patton, K. T., & Thibodeau, G. A. (2010). *Anatomy & physiology* (7th ed.). St Louis: Mosby.

Royster, R. L. (1990). Arrhythmia or dysrhythmia. *Anesthesia and Analgesia, 70*(1), 125.

Saksena, S., & Camm, J. A. (2011). *Electrophysiological disorders of the heart* (2nd ed.). Philadelphia: Saunders.

WHO ISC Task Force. (1978). Definition of terms related to cardiac rhythm. *American Heart Journal, 95*(6), 796–806.

CHAPTER 24

Cardiac Arrest

By Hugh Grantham

OVERVIEW

- Out-of-hospital cardiac arrest (OHCA) is common and has poor outcomes (Bernard, 2014).
- Myocardial infarction and coronary heart disease are major risk factors for OHCA and significantly increase mortality risk.
- Changes to cardiac arrest guidelines in the past decade have emphasised the importance of uninterrupted chest compression and have led to improved rates of return of spontaneous circulation (ROSC).
- Survival rates are linked to the underlying cause of cardiac arrest, comorbidities, arrest 'downtime', bystander cardiopulmonary resuscitation (CPR), time to first defibrillation and the type of presenting cardiac arrest arrhythmia (Nolan, 2011).
- Cardiac arrest arrhythmias are divided into shockable rhythms and non-shockable rhythms. Shockable rhythms include ventricular fibrillation (VF) and pulseless ventricular tachycardia (VT); and the non-shockable rhythms are asystole and pulseless electrical activity (PEA).
- The important factors in cardiac arrest management are non-interrupted CPR, effective chest compressions, adequate ventilation and non-delayed defibrillation of shockable rhythms.
- There is no current evidence to suggest that the use of cardiac arrest drugs or advanced airway devices improves patient survival rates post cardiac arrest.
- Paediatric cardiac arrest usually occurs as a result of hypoxia and/or hypovolaemia. The most common cardiac arrest arrhythmia is asystole.
- Shockable arrhythmias are uncommon and usually result from underlying cardiac disease, poisoning or hypothermia.
- Post-resuscitation care following ROSC is targeted at preserving normal cerebral, cardiac and haemodynamic function and is a rapidly developing field.

Introduction

In Australia, in excess of 30,000 people die each year from cardiac arrest, with many victims having no previous symptoms (ABS, 2010). The leading underlying cause of death is ischaemic heart disease, which includes the spectrum of diseases found in acute coronary syndrome.

Out-of-hospital cardiac arrests (OHCAs) encapsulate most of the unique challenges that face paramedics: they occur in the public domain, unexpectedly and often in front of the patient's friends and relatives. Equipment is limited by portability and the responding team members may never have even met each other beforehand. It is for these reasons that adhering to the evidence-based algorithms developed for cardiac arrest (see Fig 11.4) is so important (Australian Resuscitation Council [ARC], 2011). The structure, sequencing and standardisation that the algorithms provide have been demonstrated to improve patient outcomes and they allow people who are unfamiliar with each other to quickly form into a team that works cooperatively.

The vast majority of cardiac arrests occur as a result of coronary artery disease (CAD; Modi & Krahn, 2011) and the standard Basic Life Support (BLS) and Advanced Life Support (ALS) algorithms support this pathology. In effect, they reduce the clinical reasoning required so that paramedics and other clinicians can deliver effective care without becoming overwhelmed by assessment and decision-making. There are, however, a few forms of cardiac arrest that differ in aetiology, requiring some clinical reasoning to identify and manage.

The editors of this text fully endorse the BLS and ALS guidelines and stress they must be applied in all circumstances as every cardiac arrest requires a clear systematic approach. This chapter seeks to add to the understanding of cardiac arrest cases by exploring less typical causes and looking at first how they align with the standard algorithms and second how a deeper understanding can improve patient outcomes.

Chain of survival

Successful outcomes following a cardiac arrest are influenced by a number of key interventions. These interventions are conceptualised in the *chain of survival* (Adgey & Johnston, 1998). Each link in the chain aims to improve survival outcomes in patients suffering from cardiac arrest through a number of connected actions. As with any chain, it is only as strong as its weakest link. The links

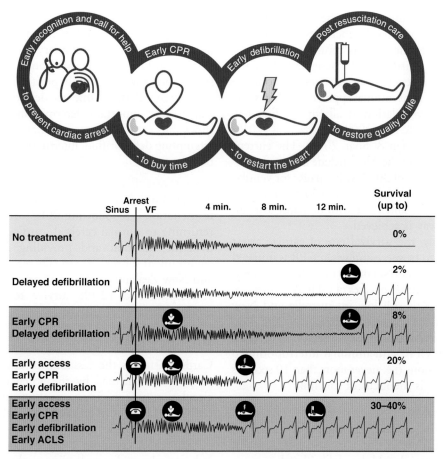

Figure 24.1
The chain of survival illustrates the role and effectiveness of intervention in the patient who has suffered a VF arrest. CPR effectively prolongs the period in which defibrillation is effective and minimises systemic ischaemia.
Source: (Top image): Laerdal. (Bottom image) Adapted from Laerdal (2011).

are: early recognition and call for help; early commencement of CPR; early defibrillation of shockable cardiac arrest arrhythmias; and, where return of spontaneous circulation (ROSC) has occurred, appropriate post-resuscitation care (see Fig 24.1).

Early recognition and call for help

The first link in the chain acknowledges the importance of recognising a patient in cardiac arrest and initiating an early call for help which includes a defibrillator, assistance and the ambulance service.

Early commencement of CPR

The primary goal of CPR is directed at maintaining some supply of oxygenated blood to keep the brain, myocardium and vital organs alive (Mistovitch & Karren, 2010). A lack of effective CPR has been shown to predict negative outcomes in patients regardless of other interventions (Souchtchenko et al., 2013). For every minute that passes between collapse and attempted defibrillation in the early

phase of arrest, mortality increases by 10–12% if CPR is not conducted (Mistovitch & Karren, 2010).

The aim of CPR is to produce blood flow through the body via compression of the chest. Retrograde flow is inhibited due to compression of the veins in the chest (Jung et al., 2006; Rajab et al., 2011). Even when CPR is applied flawlessly, the effectiveness of this action produces blood flow approximate to only 20–30% of the normal cardiac output (Artini et al., 2011). The ability to generate aortic pressure and thus flow requires constant compressions, with flow falling to zero almost instantly compressions are ceased and requiring 10–12 compressions to recommence (Kern et al., 2002).

As such, minimising any interruptions to chest compression has been extensively investigated over the past decade (Souchtchenko et al., 2013) and the emphasis on ventilation during CPR has been reduced for both lay and expert providers.

In addition to interrupting chest compressions, positive-pressure ventilation increases intrathoracic pressures, decreasing venous return and limiting cardiac output during CPR (Berg, 2001). Some groups have even reported success rates that compare favourably with conventional approaches when CPR consists of no ventilation at all for the first few minutes (Bobrow & Ewy, 2009; Bobrow et al., 2010; Kellum, 2007; Nolan & Soar, 2008). The current recommendations of the ARC include a compression-to-ventilation ratio of 30:2 with a pause for ventilation prior to placement of a supraglottic airway or endotracheal tube and 15:1 with no pause after an advanced airway is achieved.

Importantly, the survival rate of cardiac arrest is more likely to be successful when CPR is initiated early by bystanders (Nolan, 2011). Unfortunately, the average proportion of cases of OHCA that receive bystander CPR is still low in Australia and New Zealand; 41% are witnessed by bystanders and 76% of these receive bystander CPR (Beck et al., 2018). High-quality CPR with minimal interruptions to chest compressions (i.e. never more than 10 seconds 'off the chest') is the focus of this link.

Early defibrillation

Numerous studies have advocated the benefit of early defibrillation in order to save lives. Ideally, OHCA patients should be defibrillated as soon as possible and within 5 minutes of their cardiac arrest (Artini et al., 2011). This is achieved in many areas by bystanders using public automatic external defibrillators (AEDs), as in most cases the arrival of an ambulance may take more than 5 minutes.

The first monitored cardiac arrhythmia is a shockable rhythm, ventricular fibrillation (VF) or pulseless ventricular tachycardia (VT) in 27.9% of all cardiac arrests in Australia and New Zealand (Beck et al., 2018). VF and VT occur not only in acute myocardial infarction and primary electrical disturbances, but also secondary to antiarrhythmic drugs, prolonged QT syndromes, re-excitation syndromes and systemic hypoxaemia (Mistovitch & Karren, 2010). Time to defibrillation is the single most important determinant of survival in shockable cardiac arrests. As stated above, when attempting defibrillation, interruptions in CPR must be minimised.

Post-resuscitation care

The final link is aimed at providing effective post-resuscitation care following ROSC. It is targeted at returning to normal cerebral, cardiac and haemodynamic function and providing an optimum environment for recovery to take place. In Australia and New Zealand 27.7% of all arrests have ROSC at hospital and 12.1% survive to discharge at 30 days (Beck et al., 2018).

Pathophysiology

Cardiac arrest is the cessation of effective cardiac output as confirmed by the absence of signs of circulation (unconsciousness, abnormal breathing) (ARC, 2011). Common causes of cardiac arrest are outlined in Table 24.1.

The most common cause of cardiac arrest is ischaemic heart disease leading to the development of VT or VF as the result of a sudden coronary artery occlusion (Modi & Krahn, 2011). Ischaemic myocardial tissue demonstrates an increased automaticity allowing ectopic depolarisation to occur, seen as ventricular ectopics or as VF/VT. Although VT may generate a cardiac output, it is an ineffective rhythm that places a high oxygen demand on the heart while not generating a high perfusion pressure to the coronary vessels. This supply/demand imbalance increases the area of ischaemia and more

Table 24.1 Common causes of cardiac arrest

	Arrhythmias	Metabolic/toxic	Structural internal	Structural external
Typical causes	Coronary thrombosis Cardiomyopathies Scarred myocardial tissue (old infarct)	Hypoxia Beta-blockers Calcium channel blockers Hyperkalaemia Hypokalaemia Hypomagnesaemia Tricyclic antidepressants Digoxin	Mitral valve prolapse Ventricular aneurysm	Hypovolaemia Airway obstruction Tension pneumothorax Severe asthma Pericardial tamponade Pulmonary embolism
Typical ECG	Ventricular tachycardia or ventricular fibrillation	Bradycardia/asystole Ventricular tachycardia/ ventricular fibrillation	Pulseless electrical activity	Pulseless electrical activity

Source: Adapted from Handley (2010).

BOX 24.1 Mechanism of fibrillation

Ventricular fibrillation is characterised by a multitude of aberrant pacemakers propagating action potentials across the ventricles. Like pebbles thrown into a pond each pacemaker generates a wavefront of depolarisation that spreads and encounters other waves. From initially just a single central point (see heart A in Fig 24.2) the first wave emanating from an aberrant myocardial cell causes a depolarisation wave to spread in all directions, leaving all the muscle beneath the electrode in a refractory state. After about 0.25 seconds, part of this muscle begins to come out of the refractory state. Some portions come out of refractoriness before other portions. This state of events is depicted in Figure 24.2A by many lighter patches, which represent excitable cardiac muscle, and dark patches, which represent still refractory muscle. Now another stimulus from the aberrant cell can cause impulses to travel only in certain directions through the heart but not in all directions. Thus, in Figure 24.2A, certain impulses travel for short distances, until they reach refractory areas of the heart, and then are blocked. But other impulses pass between the refractory areas and continue to travel in the excitable areas. When a depolarisation wave reaches a refractory area in the heart, it travels to both sides around the refractory area. Thus, a single impulse becomes two impulses. Then, when each of these reaches another refractory area, it too divides to form two more impulses. In this way, many new wave fronts are continually being formed in the heart by progressive chain reactions until, finally, there are many small depolarisation waves travelling in many directions at the same time. More and more impulses are formed; these cause more and more patches of

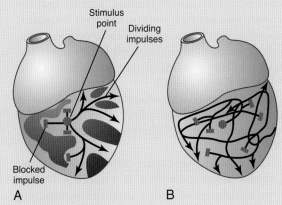

Figure 24.2
Mechanism of fibrillation.
A Initiation of fibrillation in a heart when patches of refractory musculature are present. **B** Continued propagation of fibrillatory impulses in the fibrillating ventricle.
Source: Hall (2012).

refractory muscle, and the refractory patches cause more and more division of the impulses. Therefore, any time a single area of cardiac muscle comes out of refractoriness, an impulse is close at hand to re-enter the area.

Figure 24.2B demonstrates the final state of fibrillation: many impulses travelling in all directions, some dividing and increasing the number of impulses, others blocked by refractory areas. The lack of coordinated electrical flow leads to no effective muscular contraction and no cardiac output. With no effective supply to perfuse the myocardial cells the movement of electrolytes against their concentration gradient becomes limited and the voltage of each depolarisation weakens and asystole eventually develops.

aberrant pacemakers will develop. With multiple pacemakers now generating action potentials, the depolarisation wave radiating outwards from each can encounter tissue in either relatively refractory or absolute refractory periods and re-entry circuits can develop. Electrically inert tissue from previous infarcts can also contribute to the development of re-entry circuits. The deterioration of VT into the chaotic electrical activity of VF should be considered the rule rather than the exception and is described in Box 24.1.

In the cases of VF and VT, myocardial metabolism continues, exhausting oxygen and adenosine triphosphate (ATP) supplies. Acidosis results from

PRACTICE TIP

CPR will maintain circulation, allowing for delivery of oxygen and nutrients to cells and removal of waste, but it does not offer an opportunity for arrhythmia reversion: the paramedic's top priority. Defibrillation is a means by which the heart is given the opportunity to resume a rhythm conducive with cardiac output, which in turn will provide a circulation better than even the best CPR can produce. Therefore, if a defibrillator is readily available, it must be used at the earliest possible time.

increased anaerobic metabolism and the accumulation of CO_2 in the tissues. Cardiovascular collapse causes release of catecholamines, adrenal corticosteroids, antidiuretic hormone and other hormonal responses, which can all lead to hyperglycaemia, electrolyte imbalances, increased lactate levels and thus a tendency towards further arrhythmias (Mistovitch & Karren, 2010).

It is postulated that there are three phases of cardiac arrest: electrical phase, circulatory phase and metabolic phase (Craft et al., 2010; Vilke, 2004):

- The *electrical phase* begins immediately following cardiac arrest and ends after 4 minutes. During the initial stage of cardiac arrest the myocardium still has a good supply of oxygen and glucose, so aerobic metabolism and energy production for cell function are maintained. Throughout this phase the heart is in a good state to respond to early effective CPR and defibrillation. It is during this phase that survival rates can be significant with prompt, effective cardiac arrest management (Bur et al., 2001).

- The *circulatory phase* begins after 4 minutes of cardiac arrest and lasts approximately 10 minutes. Oxygen has been exhausted and the myocardial cells shift from aerobic to anaerobic metabolism. With the reduction in ATP production, cell function diminishes as large amounts of lactic acid accumulate. It is during this phase that the heart may not respond to early defibrillation. It has been suggested that a period of good-quality CPR preceding attempts to defibrillate would produce superior outcomes for patients in this phase, but subsequent studies have refuted this approach and CPR before defibrillation in this group is no longer recommended (Baker et al., 2008; Jacobs et al., 2005; Meier et al., 2010).

- The *metabolic phase* begins approximately 10 minutes following cardiac arrest. The myocardium is now starved of oxygen and glucose, there

is an accumulation of hydrogen ions and the tissues become ischaemic and begin to die. The sodium–potassium pump begins to fail, thus allowing sodium to enter the cells and potassium to leak out of the cells, resulting in profound metabolic acidosis and hyperkalaemia. During this phase, resuscitation is difficult and unlikely to respond to resuscitation attempts as the cells become unable to produce sufficient action potentials to initiate a viable rhythm.

The spontaneous propagation of VT and the deterioration into VF are typical of an isolated area of ischaemia that develops due to an occluded coronary artery. This is by far the most common cause of cardiac arrest, but not the only cause. A profound increase in intrathoracic pressure (severe asthma, tension pneumothorax) can occlude any blood returning to the right atrium. With no input the heart cannot generate any output. In these cases the initial ECG may appear relatively normal, with sinus tachycardia the most common rhythm, but the patient presents in cardiac arrest. Eventually the heart itself will become hypoxic and bradycardia will typically develop. If there is an isolated area of poor myocardial perfusion VT may develop, but many of these cases will simply become more bradycardic with time and eventually fall into asystole. Profound hypovolaemia will cause a similar pattern. Similarly, conditions that cause profound hypoxia (airway occlusion, hanging, anaphylaxis) or a lack of ventilation (severe asthma, spinal injury) will progress from a narrow-complex tachycardia to a wide-complex bradycardia and eventually asystole.

These groups of cardiac arrest where it appears that the initial rhythm should generate a pulse are described as pulseless electrical activity (PEA). Unlike VT/VF arrest where the primary aim is to maintain cerebral perfusion (with CPR) while reverting the arrhythmia with defibrillation and medications, PEA requires the underlying cause to be reversed.

CASE STUDY 1

Case 22343, 0740 hrs.

Dispatch details: A 50-year-old male motorcyclist has collided with a bus. He is now in cardiac arrest.

Initial presentation: On arrival the paramedics find the patient lying supine on the road next to his motorcycle. His helmet has been removed and there are no immediately obvious injuries. Effective chest compressions are being performed by a bystander, who identifies herself as a nurse.

 ASSESS

Patient history

For patients in cardiac arrest with a shockable rhythm, the time to first defibrillation is a predictor of positive outcomes (ARC, 2011). Similarly, minimising downtime to effective CPR has been demonstrated to be associated with ROSC. There is nothing in either of these actions that requires a detailed medical or social history. Later, once the crew are performing their roles effectively, a history may assist in determining underlying cause or treatment.

Airway

This patient is unconscious and is therefore unable to protect his airway. Patients who have arrested through a process of VT to VF may have maintained some cerebral perfusion after they had insufficient blood pressure to remain conscious and upright. Gag reflexes can therefore remain intact for a minute or two after arrest and trismus is not uncommon, but both should no longer be in evidence within a minute of complete cardiac arrest. Jaw thrust and support should be adequate at this stage to inspect and maintain an airway. The inspection should not be so detailed (i.e. laryngoscopy) as to delay initiation of CPR. For this reason, during the initial approach to a patient, only the oropharynx should be visually inspected.

Breathing

This check should also occur quickly. If rise and fall of the chest cannot be easily detected, then it should be assumed that the patient is not breathing, abnormal breathing (agonal gasping) is also taken as a sign of arrest. It is not necessary to check for a pulse (which can be hard to detect) at this stage although many health professionals will still attempt it without causing any more delay at the same time as checking the breathing. Unconsciousness and the absence of normal breathing is the trigger to start chest compressions. The crew instruct the nurse to continue with CPR.

Cardiovascular

The crew establish a baseline time on their monitor and attach the defibrillation pads while CPR continues. They organise who will take over compressions and who will control the monitor during the pulse/rhythm check as soon as the defibrillator is ready. The monitor displays a sinus tachycardia of 165 bpm but there is no pulse.

Initial assessment summary

Problem	PEA cardiac arrest
Conscious state	GCS = 3
Position	Supine
Heart rate (monitor)	160 bpm, sinus tachycardia
Heart rate (pulse)	0
Blood pressure	0
Skin appearance	Cyanosed, dry, cool
Speech pattern	N/A
Respiratory rate	0
Respiratory rhythm	N/A
Respiratory effort	No effort
Chest auscultation	Not yet performed
Pulse oximetry	Not yet performed
Temperature	Not yet performed
Motor/sensory function	N/A
History	The patient was seen riding his motorcycle erratically before slowly colliding with a bus.
Visual inspection	No obvious long bone fractures, head injuries or bleeding.

D: The crew and patient are protected from traffic; there are no spills or other hazards.

R: The patient is unconscious.

S: The crew have requested another crew to assist.

A: The patient is unconscious with no current airway obstruction.

B: Respiratory function is currently absent.

C: There is no cardiac output.

H: There are no external haemorrhages.

The patient was seen riding unsteadily but slowly before colliding with the side of a near-stationary bus. The bike is not severely damaged. The ECG reveals a normally perfusing rhythm but the patient is pulseless and unconscious. The mechanism and pattern of injury as assessed so far do not appear consistent with the presentation. The crew disarm the defibrillator, check for a carotid pulse (not felt) and recommence CPR without delivering a shock and begin the next stage of the PEA resuscitation guideline.

② CONFIRM

The essential part of the clinical reasoning process is to seek to confirm your initial hypothesis by finding clinical signs that should occur with your provisional diagnosis. You should also seek to challenge your diagnosis by exploring findings that do *not* fit your hypothesis: don't just ignore them because they don't fit.

What else could it be?

Exsanguination

Although there is no obvious haemorrhage and the mechanism of injury appears low, it is possible that the patient has ruptured a major vessel or organ (thoracic or abdominal) and is bleeding internally possibly before the event. Fractures of long bones can cause internal bleeding within limbs but it would be unusual for this to produce a PEA arrest so quickly. While CPR and intermittent positive-pressure ventilation (IPPV) are maintained, a member of the crew performs a more-detailed secondary survey but finds no obvious injuries. IV fluids as per the electromechanical dissociation (EMD) guideline will assist in correcting any haemorrhage that is not able to be detected, but alone they will

DIFFERENTIAL DIAGNOSIS

Cardiac arrest of ischaemic cause

Or

- Cardiac arrest from:
  › Exsanguination
  › Pericardial tamponade
  › Spinal injury
  › Drug effects
  › Upper airway obstruction
  › Asthma/anaphylaxis
  › Tension pneumothorax

not lead to a resumption of cardiac output in a patient who has exsanguinated and where the site of bleeding is not controlled.

Pericardial tamponade

Blows to the chest can cause bleeding into the fibrous pericardial sac that surrounds the heart and this can ultimately restrict the heart from expanding to fill with blood. With nothing in the ventricles it is unable to produce any cardiac output but will maintain normal electrical activity for a period. Muffling of the heart sounds occurs as a tamponade develops but once blood is no longer travelling through the heart and causing the valves to open and close there are no sounds to detect. Very few paramedics are trained in pericardiocentesis (needle aspiration of a tamponade) and the procedure is potentially dangerous. If a pericardial tamponade develops in the field, it is generally irreversible and the fluid and inotropes embedded in the EMD guideline are the only tools that may preserve some blood flow. Unable to diagnose and unable to treat a tamponade if it is present, the paramedics continue with the EMD guideline.

Spinal injury

Injuries to the upper cervical area can paralyse the diaphragm and lead to a hypoxic cardiac arrest. However, these types of injuries also disrupt sympathetic innervation of the heart, and bradycardia and low blood pressure are the typical result. It doesn't fit the clinical picture for this patient but neck stabilisation needs to be maintained.

Drug effects

Drugs that slow the heart and cause the development of blocks can ultimately lead to a PEA arrest. This patient's tachycardia is inconsistent with a toxic level of these drugs.

Upper airway obstruction

Patients should be able to be effectively ventilated using normal volumes and pressures. After ensuring the patient is properly positioned and basic airway adjuncts (oropharyngeal or nasopharyngeal airway) have been introduced, higher-than-normal pressures should trigger a more detailed inspection of the airway.

Asthma/anaphylaxis

Hyperinflation of the chest increases intrathoracic pressure, decreasing venous return, and can produce a PEA arrest. Bronchospasm is central to asthma and is associated with high levels of mortality when it occurs from anaphylaxis. (Stings from flying insects are not uncommon for riders and drivers.) This patient shows no signs of a rash and his lips and face do not look overly swollen. A close assessment of the airway reveals higher-than-normal airway pressures and a decreased tidal volume. An inspection of his belongings reveals no medications to suggest either condition.

Tension pneumothorax

Blunt chest trauma (including CPR) is capable of producing a tension pneumothorax (see Ch 35) that will create sufficient intrathoracic pressure to restrict venous return and create a PEA arrest. Like pericardial tamponade, it is possible to detect a pneumothorax by distension of the jugular veins and changes to auscultated sounds, but once fully developed these discrimination signs become absent. However, an obviously distended chest on one side that is not moving a deviated trachea away from that side and hyperresonance on percussion associated with difficulty ventilating the patient indicate a tension pneumothorax.

③ TREAT

Emergency management

Initiate CPR

PEA arrests present a unique set of challenges as crews work through the various reversible causes. While this reasoning process is performed, the PEA guideline must be maintained as it is possible that none of the easily reversible causes is present. Chest compressions at a rate of 100–120 compressions per minute with a 30:2 compression-to-ventilation ratio are required.

Some guidelines suggest withholding any resuscitation for cardiac arrests that occur as a result of trauma and that such attempts are almost always futile (Hopson et al., 2003). In fact, research data suggests otherwise, with one study of nearly 170 patients suffering traumatic arrest revealing that 6.6% survived to make a complete neurological recovery (Leis, 2013), while another study found nearly 7% survived with 2% making a complete neurological recovery—a figure comparable with non-traumatic forms of arrest (Gräsner et al., 2011; see Fig 24.3). Of all the patients found to be in cardiac arrest following trauma, the majority in the studies were found to be in asystole (67–75%) on first assessment followed by PEA (13–26%) and VF (2–6%) (Leis, 2013; Deasy et al., 2012). Patients suffering hypovolaemia were the least likely to survive, while VF and PEA as the initial rhythms produced better outcomes than asystole (Lockey et al., 2006). Patients for whom an ALS crew arrived before a BLS were more likely to survive (Leis, 2013).

During each 2-minute period of CPR it is essential that the crew plan ahead and manage resources to ensure effective cardiac arrest management. A number of elements need to be considered during this period: the paramedics swapping to alternate the CPR duties, gaining IV access and administering

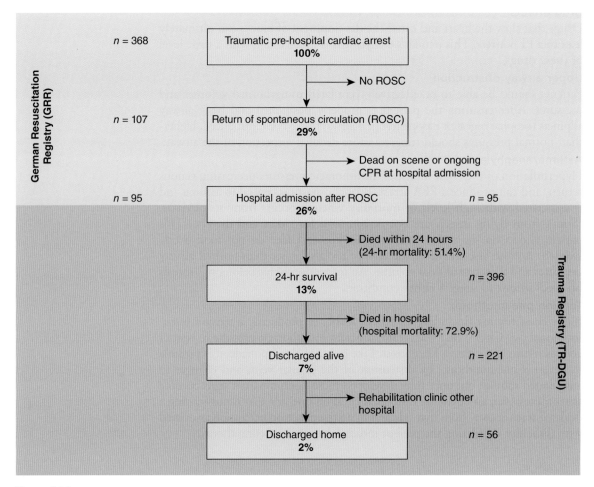

Figure 24.3
Summary of outcomes from the German Resuscitation Registry following traumatic cardiac arrest. The survivor rates are comparable with those of other forms of cardiac arrest.
Source: Gräsner et al. (2011).

Table 24.2 Reversible causes of cardiac arrest (few are feasible in OHCA)

Reversible cause	Treatment options
Hypoxia	Ensure adequate oxygenation with patent airway, adequate ventilation and supplemental oxygen and consider airway adjuncts including advanced airway devices (laryngeal mask airway, endotracheal tube intubation)
Hypovolaemia	Haemorrhage control, IV or IO fluid bolus
Hyperkalaemia, hypokalaemia, hypoglycaemia, hypocalcaemia, pH imbalance and other electrolyte disturbances	Detected by biochemical tests, indicated by patient history or ECG changes. Consider good ventilation to address metabolic/respiratory acidosis/alkalosis. Fluid bolus. Consider sodium bicarbonate for known hyperkalaemia
Hyperthermia/hypothermia	Active cooling or warming
Tamponade (cardiac)	Needle pericardiocentesis or resuscitative thoracotomy
Tension pneumothorax	Decompression
Toxins	Antidotes, dialysis
Thromboembolism	Thrombolytic drugs, percutaneous coronary intervention (PCI)

appropriate cardiac drugs, as well as continuing effective airway management. In most cases, cardiac arrest is managed initially by a two-person team, and in these instances one person should provide high-quality CPR while the other prepares the defibrillator, applies the pads and charges (ARC, 2011).

The third link in the chain of survival emphasises early and immediate defibrillation of shockable arrhythmias. The aim of defibrillation is to cause global depolarisation of the myocardium with the hope that a pacemaker, preferably the SA node, will resume coordination of the myocardium. Consequently, following defibrillation, there will be a period of asystole before electrical coordination takes place, and the myocardium will have a short period of recovery before mechanical capture occurs. This is why it is important to immediately recommence chest compression following defibrillation unless there are obvious signs of life or active patient movement.

Resolve reversible causes

Although this patient has no obvious chest trauma, it is possible that he has suffered a tension pneumothorax as he is difficult to ventilate (see Table 24.2). The decision to attempt decompression without clear signs of tension is a difficult one and practices vary greatly. The benefit of treating a possible pneumothorax must be weighed against the risk of causing one in a patient who did not have one in the first place.

With no breath sounds to assist in determining presence of a pneumothorax or which side to decompress first, the crew choose to decompress the right side. This reduces the chance of damaging the heart or major vessels if a right-sided pneumothorax has pushed the heart to the left. The result of the decompression is negative, so the crew decompress the left side, but it too is negative.

Fluid

Hypovolaemia and raised intrathoracic pressures both reduce venous return and, subsequently, cardiac output. Isotonic fluid (crystalloid or colloid) can act as a volume expander and increase venous return. It should be administered according to local guidelines.

Adrenaline

The effectiveness of adrenaline in any form of cardiac arrest remains unclear, with some studies suggesting that it has little impact on ROSC, while others report improved rates of ROSC but poorer long-term outcomes (Hagihara et al., 2012). The benefits of adrenaline in EMD arrests such as this case are most likely its effect on vessel tone and improving venous return. Adrenaline

PRACTICE TIP

If a previously well (well-oxygenated) patient has a witnessed and monitored arrest, and the initial arrhythmia is VF/VT, then up to three successive stacked shocks can be given if the first shock can occur within 20 seconds. However, this is an extremely rare situation and in most pre-cardiac arrest situations the patient would not have a well-oxygenated heart.

has both alpha- and beta-adrenergic effects. In arrest it is the alpha effects that are desirable as they cause systemic vasoconstriction, which increases coronary and cerebral perfusion pressures. Once adrenaline is given, it is repeated every second arrest cycle or approximately every 4 minutes (reflecting its half-life of 3–5 minutes): 1 mg is given via the IV or intraosseous (IO) route.

Ventilation

Overventilation of cardiac arrest patients in both rate and volume adversely affects the quality of CPR (Adgey & Johnston, 1998) and is common across all levels of clinical expertise (O'Neill & Deakin, 2007). In particular, excessive tidal volumes increase intrathoracic pressure and reduce venous return.

Endotracheal intubation during cardiac arrest remains a controversial topic, as some studies reveal the process of intubation can cause interruptions of CPR for more than 3 minutes, with a mean interruption of 46.5 seconds (Wang et al., 2009). The ARC recommends an interruption of only 5 seconds. Conversely, the ability to protect the airway of non-fasted patients, to deliver effective IPPV to the non-ventilating patient, to limit gastric insufflation and to allow effective management post-ROSC are all undeniable benefits of intubation. Intubation or a supraglottic airway also allows accurate measuring of end-tidal CO$_2$ (EtCO$_2$) values, which are shown to both measure the effectiveness of CPR and predict negative outcomes (EtCO$_2$ < 10 mmHg) (Eckstein et al., 2011).

The disturbing interruptions to CPR are not common to all ambulance services and most likely reflect levels of training and resourcing. A stratified approach using basic airway supports such as oropharyngeal airways should be used initially when resources are limited and ventilations can be adequately delivered. A supraglottic airway can be placed without any interruptions to resuscitation and offers an effective airway but not the airway protection of a cuffed endotracheal tube. Intubation should be delayed until there are adequate resources to maintain resuscitation attempts or the airway is too difficult to manage without intubation or until a return of circulation has been achieved. In this case the patient remains difficult to ventilate and the paramedic in charge of the airway performs a laryngoscopy to ensure there is no obstruction.

After approximately 8 minutes the patient becomes easier to ventilate and a weak pulse returns. Auscultation of the lungs reveals inspiratory and expiratory wheezes and a prolonged expiratory phase. It appears that hypoxia from an acute, severe asthma was the cause of both the accident and the subsequent PEA arrest. Despite not knowing the cause initially, the adrenaline doses in the arrest guideline have treated the underlying cause.

4 EVALUATE

Approaching the ROSC phase with an algorithmic approach similar to the arrest phase has been demonstrated to improve patient outcomes (Sunde et al., 2007). It also provides clinicians with both a pathway and a series of physiological targets to work towards, as opposed to a reactive approach waiting for the patient to deteriorate and then taking corrective action (see Fig 24.4).

Is the patient:

- Haemodynamically stable?
- Adequately oxygenated?
- Appropriately sedated?
- Temperature controlled? (Therapeutic hypothermia if indicated)

In this patient the possibility of developing a pneumothorax from the needle placement remains high, particularly in a patient who is either ventilated or requiring significant negative pressures to ventilate themselves. Ongoing vigilance as to the possibility of this iatrogenic complication is needed.

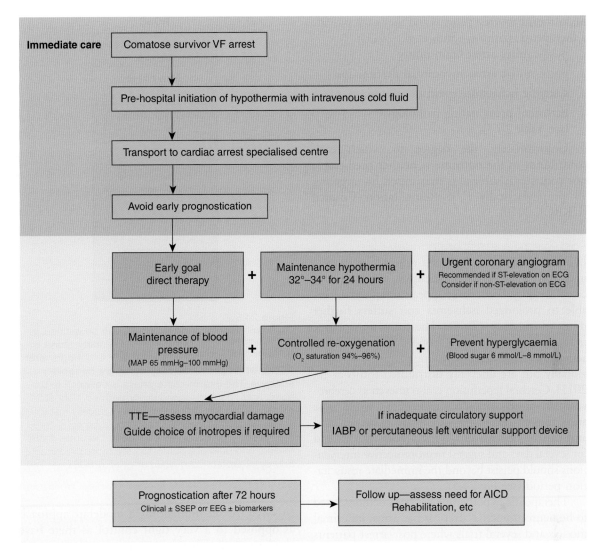

Figure 24.4
An example of an algorithmic approach to ROSC management.
MAP = mean arterial blood pressure; TTE = transthoracic echocardiogram; IABP = intraaortic balloon pump;
SSEP = somatosensory evoked potential; EEG = electroencephalography; AICD = automated internal
cardioverter-defibrillator.
Source: Stub et al. (2011).

Ongoing management

Although ROSC is the initial target of any cardiac arrest and essentially describes the patient as being 'resuscitated', the mortality rate from this point on remains extremely high and the failure of most post-arrest patients to achieve complete neurological recovery reflects the unique pathological process that occurs when perfusion is restored (Stub et al., 2011). Post–cardiac arrest syndrome describes the systemic response that occurs in the hours to days after ROSC and provides a series of targeted therapies

that can improve the likelihood of patient survival. Organs and tissues can suffer significant injury during cardiac arrest due to whole-body ischaemia, but additional damage occurs immediately after reperfusion and will persist for hours or days if not managed effectively (Stub et al., 2011). In recent years several therapies have moved into the out-of-hospital environment and, given their time-dependency, it is likely that more will become available to the paramedic in the future. There are four key components that contribute to mortality in post–cardiac arrest patients and they each provide a therapeutic pathway (Stub et al., 2011):

1. post–cardiac arrest brain injury
2. post–cardiac arrest myocardial dysfunction
3. systemic ischaemia/reperfusion response
4. persistent precipitating pathology
(see Table 24.3).

Unfortunately, the degree to which each contributes to the outcome is neither predictable nor consistent: survival is maximised by targeting all prophylactically (UK Resuscitation Council [UKRC], 2010).

Post–cardiac arrest brain injury

If patients fail to rouse within minutes of ROSC, it is likely that they have incurred some form of cerebral injury. Brain tissue appears uniquely vulnerable to prolonged ischaemia and suffers further injury during reperfusion. The formation of free radicals, shifts in calcium concentration and the activation of cell-death signalling pathways all occur globally but are unevenly distributed (Stub et al., 2011). Cerebral reperfusion is also uneven as cerebrovascular autoregulation is impaired, and while some areas remain ischaemic, others are hyperperfused and can be oedematous. This process can extend for several days and suggest neuroprotective interventions should persist beyond the immediate resuscitation period (see Fig 24.5).

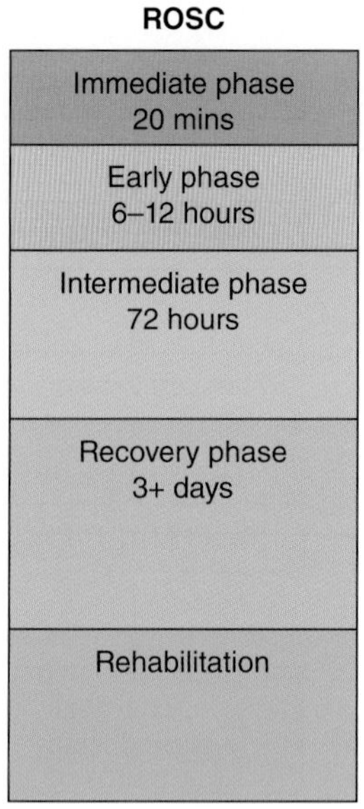

Therapeutic hypothermia has been demonstrated to be neuroprotective after cardiac arrest in animal models and several trials where post-arrest patients were cooled after arrival at hospital have shown positive outcomes (Hypothermia after Cardiac Arrest Study Group [HCASG], 2002; Bernard et al., 2002; Cheung et al., 2006). The best methods for cooling, target temperatures and length of therapeutic hypothermia are not yet clear (Nolan et al., 2012), and trials where cooling was induced by paramedics using ice-cold fluids did not show any clinical benefits (Bernard et al., 2012). The current advice is to aim for a temperature between 32 and 36°C based on a paper that showed equivalent benefit at those two temperatures (Nielsen et al., 2013). Other neuroprotective strategies such as magnesium and calcium channel blockers and prophylactic use of antiseizure medications have also returned non-beneficial findings (Stub et al., 2011; Neumar et al., 2008).

Hyperglycaemia is common during ROSC and is predictive of poor patient outcomes (Nurmi et al., 2012). Normalisation of blood glucose levels should occur as soon as possible, with the Australian and New Zealand Committee on Resuscitation

ROSC

Figure 24.5
The immediate post-arrest phase can be defined as the first 20 minutes after ROSC. The early phase is the period between 20 minutes and 6–12 hours after ROSC, when early interventions might be most effective. The intermediate phase is between 6–12 hours and 72 hours, when injury pathways are still active and aggressive treatment is typically instituted. Finally, a period beyond 3 days could be considered the recovery phase, when prognosis becomes more reliable and ultimate outcomes are more predictable. *Source: Adapted from Neumar et al. (2008).*

(ANZCOR) recommending a moderate approach as opposed to a very tight control as there have also been studies that demonstrated worse outcomes from a very tight control (4–6 mmol).

Current research indicates that excessive arterial oxygen levels during and after cardiac arrest may contribute to post-arrest syndrome, possibly by increasing oxidative stress on vulnerable cells (Neumar, 2011; Henlin et al., 2014). The results remain unclear but early normalisation of arterial oxygen levels is likely to become a focus after ROSC. Definitive clinical trials are needed to determine the ultimate impact of hyperoxaemia on outcome (Neumar, 2011). Currently, due to very little scientific information, ANZCOR recommends a target of 94–98% while further studies are conducted (ANZCOR, 2016).

Post-cardiac arrest myocardial dysfunction

In the minutes following ROSC, myocardial dysfunction and arrhythmias are common as poorly perfused tissue is confronted by high levels of catecholamines, acids and oxidative stresses. Both blood pressure and heart rate should be expected

Table 24.3 Post–cardiac arrest syndrome: pathophysiology, clinical manifestations and potential treatments

Syndrome	Pathophysiology	Clinical manifestations	Potential treatment
Post–cardiac arrest brain injury	● Impaired cerebrovascular autoregulation	● Coma	● Therapeutic hypothermia
		● Seizures	● Early haemodynamic optimisation
	● Cerebral oedema (limited)	● Myoclonus	
	● Post-ischaemic neurodegeneration	● Cognitive dysfunction	● Airway protection and mechanical ventilation
		● Persistent vegetative state	
		● Secondary parkinsonism	● Seizure control
		● Cortical stroke	● Controlled re-oxygenation (SaO$_2$ 94–96%)
		● Spinal stroke	
		● Brain death	● Supportive care
Post–cardiac arrest myocardial dysfunction	● Global hypokinesis (myocardial stunning)	● Reduced cardiac output	● Early revascularisation of AMI
		● Hypotension	
	● ACS	● Arrhythmias	● Early haemodynamic optimisation
		● Cardiovascular collapse	
			● Intravenous fluid
			● Inotropes
			● IABP
			● LVAD
			● ECMO
Systemic ischaemia/ reperfusion response	Systemic inflammatory response syndrome	● Ongoing tissue hypoxia/ ischaemia	● Early haemodynamic optimisation
		● Hypotension	
	● Impaired vasoregulation	● Cardiovascular collapse	● Intravenous fluid
	● Increased coagulation	● Pyrexia (fever)	● Vasopressors
	● Adrenal suppression	● Hyperglycaemia	● High-volume haemofiltration
	● Impaired tissue oxygen delivery and utilisation	● Multi-organ failure	● Temperature control
		● Infection	● Glucose control
	● Impaired resistance to infection		● Antibiotics for documented infection
Persistent precipitating pathology	● Cardiovascular disease (AMI/ACS, cardiomyopathy)	● Specific to cause but complicated by concomitant PCAS	● Disease-specific interventions guided by patient condition and concomitant PCAS
	● Pulmonary disease (COPD, asthma)		
	● CNS disease (CVA)		
	● Thromboembolic disease (PE)		
	● Toxicological (overdose, poisoning)		
	● Infection (sepsis, pneumonia)		
	● Hypovolaemia (haemorrhage, dehydration)		

AMI = acute myocardial infarction; ACS = acute coronary syndrome; IABP = intraaortic balloon pump; LVAD = left ventricular assist device; EMCO = extracorporeal membrane oxygenation; COPD = chronic obstructive pulmonary disease; CNS = central nervous system; CVA = cerebrovascular accident; PE = pulmonary embolism; PCAS = post–cardiac arrest syndrome.

Source: Stub et al. (2011).

to fall as inotropes injected during the arrest are consumed, and early support of blood pressure can maximise myocardial perfusion and prevent arrhythmias. Fluids can be used to expand blood volume and increase blood pressure provided there is no evidence of acute pulmonary oedema.

The use of primary percutaneous coronary intervention (PCI) has been demonstrated to be effective in STEMI (ST elevation myocardial infarction) management in patients who have not suffered cardiac arrest, and the past decade has seen several trials demonstrate a similar benefit for OHCA patients with ST elevation on either their pre- or their post-arrest ECG (Gorjup et al., 2007; Lettieri et al., 2009; Hovdenes et al., 2007). Preferential transport of ROSC patients to centres with PCI facilities is recommended and several centres will perform the procedure even when ST elevation is not present but a coronary cause is considered likely (Stub et al., 2011). The use of thrombolytics following ROSC where ST elevation is apparent but PCI is not available is recommended.

Continued myocardial dysfunction can be supported in hospital by intraaortic balloon pump, extracorporeal membrane oxygenation (ECMO) and left ventricular assist devices (LVAD).

Systemic ischaemia/reperfusion response

Inadequate oxygen delivery to tissues during the arrest phase is unlikely to be fully corrected by CPR and during the early ROSC phase there is widespread release of inflammatory mediators that promote both vasodilation and coagulation. Targeting blood pressures at or above normal levels has been shown to reduce multi-organ failure and infection and shares similarities with the management of severe sepsis (Neumar et al., 2008). A combination of IV fluids and inotropes is recommended, but there is also evidence to support the administration of steroids (Peberdy et al., 2010).

Persistent precipitating pathology

While PCI has the potential to minimise the underlying cause of the majority of cardiac arrests, cardiac arrests from other causes (e.g. asthma, anaphylaxis, tension pneumothorax, pulmonary embolism) need to have concurrent management where possible. In this patient's case, the administration of adrenaline to support blood pressure post-ROSC is likely to be therapeutic, but dosages and other medications should be titrated to ensure bronchospasm is relieved and adequate ventilation is provided.

Long-term outcomes

While the ability to achieve complete neurological recovery for patients who are revived from OHCA remains far less than optimal, the increasing numbers of patients who are achieving ROSC due to better arrest management are providing the opportunity to develop better therapies. Despite these efforts, some patients will not recover any higher neurological function following resuscitation and there is evidence that these patients may make suitable organ donors (Peberdy et al., 2010).

 CASE STUDY 2

Case 51544, 2040 hrs.

Dispatch details: A 25-year-old male has been found in cardiac arrest in his bedroom.

Initial presentation: An ALS crew and intensive care paramedic arrive together and are directed to the patient, who is lying supine on the floor with his distressed father performing ineffective CPR.

1 ASSESS

2054 hrs Primary survey: The patient is unconscious and not breathing. One of the crew members takes over compressions while the other prepares the defibrillator pads. The paramedic inspects the upper airway, which appears clear, and ventilates the patient with two breaths after 30 compressions. Air entry is good. There are no obvious injuries or external haemorrhage.

2055 hrs: Analysis of the rhythm reveals coarse VF. The crew defibrillate the patient and return to CPR with a new operator. (See the adult ALS guidelines in Fig 11.4.)

2 CONFIRM

In many cases paramedics are presented with a collection of signs and symptoms that do not appear to describe a particular condition. A critical step in determining a treatment plan in this situation is to consider what other conditions could explain the patient's presentation. In this particular case the fact that the patient is in arrest is not in dispute, but the potential causes need to be considered as they may be reversible.

What else could be the cause?

As with all cases of cardiac arrest, standard cardiac management strategies should continue (i.e. minimise interruptions in chest compressions, administer early defibrillation of shockable arrhythmias, administer appropriate anti-arrhythmic medications and consider reversible causes of cardiac arrest).

While disrupted atherosclerotic plaques contribute to the majority of VT/VF cardiac arrests, this is unlikely in such a young patient, so the crew look for a reversible cause. Non-cardiac, reversible causes of VF arrest include the following.

- *Tamponade:* this is unlikely without trauma and is not reversible in the field.
- *Tension pneumothorax:* good air entry on ventilation with equal chest rise and breath sounds.
- *Hypovolaemia/exsanguination:* no obvious trauma, no swelling of abdomen or limbs.
- *Asthma/anaphylaxis:* good air entry on ventilation with equal chest rise and breath sounds, no rash or angio-oedema.
- *Airway obstruction:* good air entry on ventilation with equal chest rise and breath sounds.

Pathophysiology

Sudden cardiac arrest without overt heart disease

Cardiac arrest from coronary artery disease is by far the most common cause of sudden cardiac arrest, but there is an increasing understanding that cardiac arrest can occur without overt artery disease (see Table 24.4). The conditions responsible for spontaneously generating non-perfusing rhythms alter the depolarisation or repolarisation of myocardial cells, usually due to inherited, drug or metabolic ion channel dysfunction (Modi & Krahn, 2011). Of these 'channelopathies' or 'primary electric diseases', long QT syndrome is the most well known.

Long QT syndrome describes the ECG presentation of a typically asymptomatic condition that is usually caused by inherited abnormalities of the sodium and potassium channels. Syncope in young adults is a common prodromal sign but unless an ECG is performed the three types of the condition can remain undiagnosed until it triggers a non-perfusing rhythm (see Fig 24.6). The typical arrhythmia produced by long QT syndrome is torsades de pointes: an oscillatory polymorphic VT that is notoriously difficult to correct once

Table 24.4 Causes of sudden cardiac arrest

Cardiac arrest with overt structural heart disease	Coronary disease	Ischaemic heart disease Anomalous coronary circulation Coronary spasm
	Cardiomyopathies	Ischaemic cardiomyopathy Hypertrophic cardiomyopathy Dilated cardiomyopathy Infiltrative (e.g. sarcoid, amyloid) Arrhythmogenic right ventricular cardiomyopathy Takotsubo cardiomyopathy Left ventricular non-compaction cardiomyopathy Myocarditis Corrected congenital cardiomyopathy
	Other	Wolff-Parkinson-White syndrome Commotio cordis
Cardiac arrest without overt heart disease	Primary electric	Long QT syndrome Short QT syndrome Brugada syndrome Early repolarisation syndromes Catecholaminergic polymorphic ventricular tachycardia Idiopathic ventricular fibrillation
	Metabolic imbalance	Hyperkalaemia/hypokalaemia Hypocalcaemia Hypomagnesaemia Acidosis Drug overdose
	Concealed structural	Arrhythmogenic right ventricular cardiomyopathy Myocarditis Coronary spasm Sarcoidosis
	Non-cardiac	Acute intracranial haemorrhage Massive pulmonary embolus Epilepsy

Source: Stub et al. (2011).

BOX 24.2 SUDEPS: sudden unexpected death in epileptics

Epilepsy sufferers are up to nine times more likely to die unexpectedly than the general population (Thom, 2007). While some of these deaths are probably due to traumatic events that occur as a result of unexpected seizures, there is growing evidence that cerebrogenic cardiac arrhythmias also contribute to a number of the deaths. The brain cells in some forms of epilepsy have a similar form of channelopathy as described in long QT syndrome and the pathophysiology may exist in both the heart and the brain in some individuals. For patients who collapse unwitnessed or are found in asystole, it is difficult to determine whether they suffered a sudden cardiac arrest or developed a cardiac arrest following central respiratory depression or positional airway obstruction during the post-ictal period.

established. The condition may be more likely to trigger an arrhythmia at times of emotional or physical stress, and may have contributed to drownings, vehicle accidents and the death of epileptic patients (see Box 24.2). Brugada syndrome is another genetic channelopathy that affects sodium channels and is unlikely to be detected unless an ECG is taken—and even then it can be missed. There are a number of other forms of primary electrical disease but

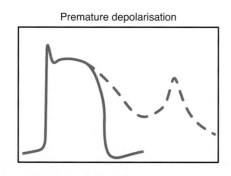

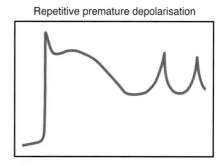

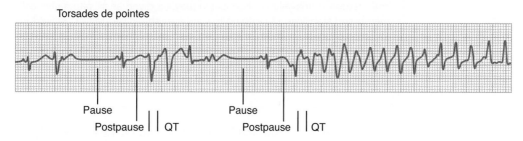

Figure 24.6
Typical propagation of an arrhythmia in long QT syndrome.
When the ventricular muscle fibre action potential is prolonged as a result of delayed repolarisation, a premature depolarisation (*dashed line in top left figure*) may occur before complete repolarisation. Repetitive premature depolarisations (*right top figure*) may lead to multiple depolarisations under certain conditions. In torsades de pointes (*bottom figure*), premature ventricular beats lead to pauses, postpause prolongation of the Q-T interval and arrhythmias.
Source: Hall (2012).

they share the characteristic of sudden, symptomless collapse into a recalcitrant non-perfusing arrhythmia.

Outcomes from this form of cardiac arrest are typically very poor as the rhythms do not revert in the field, and CPR during transport is far less effective in maintaining cellular perfusion (Stub et al., 2014). CPR during transport is also dangerous to the crew performing chest compressions and the refractory nature of the arrest can persist in hospital. In many cases the diagnosis is made post-mortem and only by testing surviving family members to identify expression of the responsible genes.

(3) TREAT

2059 hrs: The crew discover the patient has no medical history, and was seen well and talking only a few minutes before he was found collapsed on the floor. There is no evidence of drug overdose or attempts at self-harm. The patient has been at work all day and has not left the house since arriving home.

2104 hrs: The crew continue to work through the ALS guidelines, ensuring constant CPR. The patient remains in VF with each rhythm check and is defibrillated according to the guidelines each time. The crew administer 300 mg of amiodarone (see Box 24.3). The initial end-tidal CO_2 value was 28 mmHg and remains at that value. The crew are able to palpate a femoral pulse with CPR, which suggests that hypovolaemia is not a factor (note: this pulse wave could equally well be transmuted via the veins as by the arteries).

2115 hrs: It is 20 minutes since the crew arrived and the patient's condition has not changed. The family are increasingly distraught and other family members have arrived on the scene.

BOX 24.3 Amiodarone

Amiodarone causes potassium channel blockade, partial inhibition of sodium channel-mediated depolarisation, a lengthening of the myocardial action potential and a degree of beta blockade. This allows some degree of cell stabilisation and lowers the defibrillation threshold with only a minor effect on myocardial contractility (Birt & Wilson, 1999). Amiodarone has a prolonged half-life measured in weeks. When amiodarone is given in acute situations the plasma level will gradually reduce as the amiodarone redistributes into the fat stores of the body (it has a large volume of distribution). Redistribution to fat stores cannot occur if there is limited perfusion of those fat stores. Where amiodarone is unavailable, lignocaine may be given as an alternative cell membrane stabiliser. Lignocaine has antiarrhythmic properties derived from sodium channel blockade, resulting in membrane stabilisation, but it is not as successful in helping to achieve reversion with defibrillation in arrest as amiodarone (Adgey & Johnston, 1998).

BOX 24.4 Indications for transport with CPR if safe

- Patients who are hypothermic should be considered for transport as their metabolic rate could have lowered sufficiently to allow for preservation of the tissues.
- Women who are heavily pregnant should be transferred to hospital while CPR is continued so that the fetus can be assessed.
- Patients who require interventions only available at hospital and who are potentially viable should be considered for transport.

BOX 24.5 Mechanical CPR devices

The development of mechanical devices capable of providing effective CPR during transport may change the future management of these patients. With the ability to maintain cellular perfusion during transport, there are a number of studies currently using devices to allow time to connect patients suffering refractory cardiac arrests (of both ischaemic and non-ischaemic causes) to extracorporeal membrane oxygenation (ECMO) devices. Once connected, the CPR device can be removed and normal levels of cellular perfusion maintained while the arrhythmia is aggressively managed. Outcomes for this rescue strategy are positive, although the study numbers remain small (Alsoufi et al., 2007; CHEER, 2014).

4 EVALUATE

With the ALS guideline exhausted and the questionable safety and quality of manually performing CPR during transport (see Box 24.4), the crew need to manage the family's expectations while continuing resuscitation and preparing the family for ultimate cessation of resuscitation. The only alternative may be to use a mechanical CPR device that can safely maintain effective CPR during transport (see Box 24.5). Despite disappointing results in terms of overall survival when used in all cardiac arrests (Wik et al., 2014; Rubertsson et al., 2014), this specific circumstance may justify the use of such a device if available.

Future research

Evidence-based medical research from around the world continues to develop and identify cardiac arrest management treatment strategies. Resuscitation councils, including the ARC, are contributing vital data to the International Liaison Committee on Resuscitation (ILCOR) with the aim of facilitating education and knowledge of the critically ill and cardiac arrest patients. As such, cardiac arrest management options will change and develop over time in order to support best practice for all healthcare professionals.

System governance impacts

The establishment of a cardiac arrest epistry across Australia and New Zealand is producing objective data on which to base improvements. The Global Resuscitation Alliance supported by all the ambulance services and the ARC is a program that aims to deliver improved outcomes by focusing on system impacts on the steps in the chain of survival.

Mechanical CPR

Probable areas of change that will be considered include the role of mechanical CPR devices, and ECMO perfusion while undertaking angioplasty, real-time feedback of CPR performance and the ratio of ventilations in the resuscitation cycle, with the current trend towards fewer ventilation efforts and fewer interruptions to compressions.

Metabolic management

Therapeutic hypothermia may prove not to be beneficial in the out-of-hospital setting but normalisation of blood glucose and oxygen levels may be more heavily emphasised.

Cardiac arrest centres

Dedicated trauma centres have proved effective in improving survival from major trauma by focusing equipment and expertise and providing a multidisciplinary team to deal with complex, multi-organ injuries (Nolan et al., 2012). There is already some evidence that ICUs that receive higher numbers of post-arrest patients provide better care (Carr et al., 2009), and the extension of this practice to develop specialist post-arrest centres is likely to continue in the future if paramedics can prove they are able to stabilise post-arrest patients sufficiently to bypass the nearest hospital to access a specialist centre.

Summary

OHCA is common and in Australia is usually associated with ischaemic heart disease but it can be caused by other pathologies. Surviving cardiac arrest can be improved by adhering to the chain of survival and structured post-cardiac arrest care. Cardiac arrest strategies are founded on the adult or paediatric ALS algorithms that use a standardised approach to cardiac arrest management. This has the advantage of enabling treatment to be delivered quickly and effectively without the need for lengthy discussions or debate.

The most important factor in cardiac arrest management is minimising interruptions to CPR, as minimising systemic ischaemia improves not only the changes or ROSC but also the degree of post-arrest syndrome. CPR must be done effectively to achieve the ultimate goal of maintaining brain perfusion and so must be adequate in rate, depth and consistency. Antiarrhythmic drugs such as adrenaline and amiodarone form the basis of the pharmacological management of cardiac arrests.

Consideration of the reversible causes of cardiac arrest should always be at the forefront of the paramedic's mind during patient management—with each cause considered and treated where indicated. Finally, in order to manage all aspects of cardiac arrest, the paramedic must display technical skills to undertake the practical aspects of the arrest as well as non-technical skills to help in crucial aspects such as planning, scene awareness, leadership and communication.

References

Adgey, A., & Johnston, P. (1998). Approaches to modern management of cardiac arrest. *Heart (British Cardiac Society)*, 80(4), 397–401.

Alsoufi, B., Al-Radi, O. O., Nazer, R. I., Gruenwald, C., Foreman, C., Williams, W. G., Coles, J. G., Caldarone, C. A., Bohn, D. G., & Van Arsdell, G. S. (2007). Survival outcomes after rescue extracorporeal cardiopulmonary resuscitation in pediatric patients with refractory cardiac arrest. *Journal of Thoracic and Cardiovascular Surgery*, 134(4), 952–959.

Artini, F., Nath, J., & Bartholomew, E. (2011). *Fundamentals of anatomy and physiology* (9th ed.). San Francisco: Pearson.

Australian Bureau of Statistics (ABS). (2010). *Causes of Death, Australia, 2008*. Canberra: ABS.

Australian Resuscitation Council (ARC). (2011). *Advanced life support: Australian edition* (6th ed.). Perth: Uniprint.

Australian and New Zealand Committee on Resuscitation (ANZCOR). (2016). *ANZCOR Guideline 11.7 – Post-resuscitation Therapy in Adult Advanced Life Support*. ANZCOR.

Baker, P., Conway, J., Cotton, C., Ashby, D., Smyth, J., Woodman, R., & Grantham, H. (2008). Defibrillation or cardiopulmonary resuscitation first for patients with out-of-hospital cardiac arrests found by paramedics to be in ventricular fibrillation? A randomised control trial. *Resuscitation*, *79*(3), 424–431.

Beck, B., Bray, J., Cameron, P., Smith, K., Walker, T., Grantham, H., Hein, C., Thorrowgood, M., Smith, A., Inoue, M., Smith, T., Dicker, B., Swain, A., Bosley, E., Pemberton, K., McKay, M., Johnston-Leek, M., Perkins, G. D., Nichol, G., & Finn, J., on behalf of the Aus-ROC Steering Committee. (2018). Regional variation in the characteristics, incidence and outcomes of out-of-hospital cardiac arrest in Australia and New Zealand: results from the Aus-ROC Epistry. *Resuscitation*, *126*, 49–57.

Berg, R. A. (2001). Adverse hemodynamic effects of interrupting chest compressions for rescue breathing during cardiopulmonary resuscitation for ventricular fibrillation cardiac arrest. *Circulation*, *104*, 2465–2470.

Bernard, S. (2014). Inducing hypothermia after out of hospital cardiac arrest. *British Medical Journal*, *348*.

Bernard, S., Gray, T., Buist, M., Jones, B., Silvester, W., Gutteridge, G., & Smith, K. (2002). Treatment of comatose survivors of out-of-hospital cardiac arrest with induced hypothermia. *The New England Journal of Medicine*, *346*(8), 557–563.

Bernard, S., Smith, K., Cameron, P., Masci, K., Taylor, D. M., Cooper, D. J., Kelley, A. M., & Silvester, W., Rapid Infusion of Cold Hartmanns (RICH) Investigators. (2012). Induction of therapeutic hypothermia by paramedics after resuscitation from out-of-hospital ventricular fibrillation cardiac arrest: a randomized controlled trial. *Circulation*, *122*, 737–742.

Birt, D., & Wilson, I. (1999). Resuscitation from cardiac arrest. *Update in Anesthesia*, *10*.

Bobrow, B., & Ewy, G. (2009). Ventilation during resuscitation efforts for out-of-hospital primary cardiac arrest. *Current Opinion in Critical Care*, *15*(3), 228–233.

Bobrow, B., Spaite, D., Berg, R., Stolz, U., Sanders, A., Kern, K., & Ewy, G. (2010). Chest compression-only CPR by lay rescuers and survival from out-of-hospital cardiac arrest. *JAMA: The Journal of the American Medical Association*, *304*(13), 1447.

Bur, A., Kittler, H., Sterz, F., Holzer, M., Eisenburger, P., Oschatz, E., & Laggner, A. (2001). Effects of bystander first aid, defibrillation and advanced life support on neurologic outcome and hospital costs in patients after ventricular fibrillation cardiac arrest. *Intensive Care Medicine*, *27*(9), 1474–1480.

Carr, B. G., Kahn, J. M., Merchant, R. M., Kramer, A. A., & Neumar, R. W. (2009). Inter-hospital variability in post-cardiac arrest mortality. *Resuscitation*, *80*, 30–34.

CHEER. (2014). *Refractory out-of-hospital cardiac arrest treated with mechanical CPR, Hypothermia, ECMO and Early Reperfusion (CHEER) trial*. Retrieved from www. ambulance.vic.gov.au/Research/Clinical-trials.html. (Accessed 26 May 2014).

Cheung, K., Green, R., & Magee, K. (2006). Systematic review of randomized controlled trials of therapeutic hypothermia as a neuroprotectant in post cardiac arrest patients. *Journal of the Canadian Association of Emergency Physicians*, *8*(5), 329–337.

Craft, J., Gordon, C., & Tiziani, A. (2010). *Understanding pathophysiology*. Sydney: Elsevier.

Deasy, C., Bernard, S., Bray, J., Smith, K., Harriss, L., Morrison, C., & Cameron, P. (2012). Traumatic out-of-hospital cardiac arrests in Melbourne, Australia. *Resuscitation*, *83*(4), 465–470.

Eckstein, M., Hatch, L., Malleck, J., McClung, C., & Henderson, S. O. (2011). End-tidal CO_2 as a predictor of survival in out-of-hospital cardiac arrest. *Prehospital and Disaster Medicine*, *26*(3), 148–150.

Gorjup, V., Radsel, P., et al. (2007). Acute ST-elevation myocardial infarction after successful cardiopulmonary resuscitation. *Resuscitation*, *72*, 379–385.

Gräsner, J., Wnent, J., Seewald, S., Meybohm, P., Fischer, M., Paffrath, T., Wafaisade, A., Bein, B., & Lefering, R., German Resuscitation Registry Working Group, Trauma Registry of the German Society for Trauma Surgery (DGU). (2011). Cardiopulmonary resuscitation traumatic cardiac arrest: there are survivors. An analysis of two national emergency registries. *Critical Care: The Official Journal of the Critical Care Forum*, *15*(6), R276.

Hagihara, A., Hasegawa, M., Abe, T., Nagata, T., Wakata, Y., & Miyazaki, S. (2012). Prehospital epinephrine use and survival among patients with out-of-hospital cardiac arrest. *JAMA: The Journal of the American Medical Association*, *307*(11), 1161–1168.

Hall, J. (2012). *Guyton and Hall textbook of medical physiology* (12th ed.). St Louis: Saunders.

Handley, A. (2010). *Resuscitation council (UK) guidelines 2010*. UK: Resuscitation Council.

Henlin, T., Michalek, P., Tyll, T., Hinds, J. D., & Dobias, M. (2014). Oxygenation, ventilation, and airway management in out-of-hospital cardiac arrest: a review. *BioMed Research International*, doi:10.1155/2014/376871.

Hopson, L. R., Hirsh, E., Delgado, J., Domeier, R. M., McSwain, N. E., & Krohmer, J. (2003). Guidelines for withholding or termination of resuscitation in prehospital traumatic cardiopulmonary arrest: a joint position paper from the National Association of EMS Physicians Standards and Clinical Practice Committee and the American College of Surgeons Committee on Trauma. *Prehospital Emergency Care*, *7*, 141–146.

Hovdenes, J., Laake, J. H., Aaberge, L., Haugaa, H., & Bugge, J. F. (2007). Therapeutic hypothermia after out-of-hospital cardiac arrest: experiences with patients treated with percutaneous coronary intervention and cardiogenic shock. *Acta Anaesthesiologica Scandinavica*, *51*, 137–142.

Hypothermia after Cardiac Arrest Study Group (HCASG). (2002). Mild therapeutic hypothermia to improve the neurologic outcome after cardiac arrest. *The New England Journal of Medicine*, 346, 549–556.

Jacobs, I., Finn, J., Oxer, H., & Jelinek, G. (2005). CPR before defibrillation in out-of-hospital cardiac arrest: a randomized trial. *Emergency Medicine Australasia: EMA*, 17(1), 39–45.

Jung, E., Babbs, C., Lenhart, S., & Protopopescu, V. (2006). Optimal strategy for cardiopulmonary resuscitation with continuous chest compression. *Academic Emergency Medicine: Official Journal of the Society for Academic Emergency Medicine*, 13(7), 715–721.

Kellum, M. (2007). Compression-only cardiopulmonary resuscitation for bystanders and first responders. *Current Opinion in Critical Care*, 13(3), 268–272.

Kern, K., Hilwig, R., Berg, R., Sanders, A., & Ewy, G. (2002). Importance of continuous chest compressions during cardiopulmonary resuscitation: improved outcome during a simulated single lay-rescuer scenario. *Circulation*, 105(5), 645–649.

Laerdal. (2011). *The chain of survival*. Laerdal Medical.

Leis, C. (2013). Traumatic cardiac arrest: should advanced life support be initiated? *The Journal of Trauma and Acute Care Surgery*, 74(2).

Lettieri, C., Savonitto, S., De Servi, S., Guagliumi, G., Belli, G., Repetto, A., Piccaluga, E., Politi, A., Ettori, F., Castiglioni, B., Fabbiocchi, F., De Cesare, N., Sangiorgi, G., Musumeci, G., Onofri, M., D'Urbano, M., Pirelli, S., Zanini, R., & Klugmann, S., on behalf of the Lombard IMA Study Group. (2009). Emergency percutaneous coronary intervention in patients with ST-elevation myocardial infarction complicated by out-of-hospital cardiac arrest: early and medium-term outcome. *American Heart Journal*, 157, 569–575.

Lockey, D., Crewdson, K., & Davies, G. (2006). Traumatic cardiac arrest: who are the survivors? *Annals of Emergency Medicine*, 48, 240–244.

Meier, P., Baker, P., Jost, D., Jacobs, I., Henzi, B., Knapp, G., & Sasson, C. (2010). Chest compressions before defibrillation for out-of-hospital cardiac arrest: a meta-analysis of randomized controlled clinical trials. *BMC Medicine*, 8(1), 52.

Mistovitch, J., & Karren, K. (2010). *Prehospital emergency care* (9th ed.). New Jersey: Pearson.

Modi, S., & Krahn, A. D. (2011). Sudden cardiac arrest without overt heart disease. *Circulation*, 123, 2994–3008.

Neumar, R. W. (2011). Optimal oxygenation during and after cardiopulmonary resuscitation. *Current Opinion in Critical Care*, 17(3).

Neumar, R. W., Robert, W., Nolan, P. J., Adrie, C., Aibiki, M., Berg, R. A., Böttiger, B. W., Callaway, C., Clark, R. S. B., Romergryko, G. G., Jauch, E. C., Kern, K. B., Laurent, I., Longstreth, W. T., Jr, Merchant, R. M., Morley, F., Morrison, L. J., Nadkarni, V., Peberdy, M. A.,

Rivers, E. P., Rodriguez-Nunez, A., Sellke, F. W., Spaulding, C., Sunde, K., & Vanden Hoek, T. (2008). ILCOR consensus statement. Post–cardiac arrest syndrome. *Circulation*, 118, 2452–2483.

Nielsen, N., Wetterslev, J., Cronberg, T., Erlinge, D., Gasche, Y., Hassager, C., Horn, J., Hovdenes, J., Kjaergaard, J., Kuiper, M., Pellis, T., Stammet, P., Wanscher, M., Wise, M. P., Aneman, A., Al-Subaie, N., Boesgaard, S., Bro-Jeppesen, J., Brunetti, I., Bugge, J. F., Hingston, C. D., Juffermans, N. P., Koopmans, M., Kober, L., Langorgen, J., Lilja, G., Moller, J. E., Rundgren, M., Rylander, C., Smid, O., Werer, C., Winkel, P., & Friberg, H., Investigators TTMT. (2013). Targeted temperature management at 33 degrees C versus 36 degrees C after cardiac arrest. *The New England Journal of Medicine*, 369, 2197–2206.

Nolan, J. (2011). Optimizing outcome after cardiac arrest. *Current Opinion in Critical Care*, 17(5), 520–526.

Nolan, J., & Soar, J. (2008). Airway techniques and ventilation strategies. *Current Opinion in Critical Care*, 14(3), 279–286.

Nolan, J., Lyon, R. M., Sasson, C., Rossetti, A. O., Lansky, A. J., Fox, K. A. A., & Meier, P. (2012). Advances in the hospital management of patients following an out of hospital cardiac arrest. *Heart (British Cardiac Society)*, 98, 1201–1206.

Nurmi, J., Boyd, J., Anttalainen, N., Westerbacka, J., & Kuisma, M. (2012). Early increase in blood glucose in patients resuscitated from out-of-hospital ventricular fibrillation predicts poor outcome. *Diabetes Care*, 35(3), 510–512.

O'Neill, J. F., & Deakin, C. D. (2007). Do we hyperventilate cardiac arrest patients? *Resuscitation*, 73, 82–85.

Peberdy, M. A., Callaway, C. W., Neumar, R. W., Romergryko, G., Zimmerman, J. L., Donnino, M., Gabrielli, A., Silvers, S. M., Zaritsky, A. L., Merchant, R., Vanden Hock, T. L., & Kronick, S. L. (2010). 2010 American heart association guidelines for cardiopulmonary resuscitation and emergency cardiovascular care science. Part 9: post–cardiac arrest care. *Circulation*, 122(18 Suppl. 3), S768–S786.

Rajab, T., Pozner, C., Conrad, C., Cohn, L., & Schmitto, J. (2011). Technique for chest compressions in adult CPR. *World Journal of Emergency Surgery*, 6(1), 41.

Rubertsson, S., Lindgren, E., Smekal, D., Östlund, O., Silfverstolpe, J., Lichtveld, R. A., Boomars, R., Ahlstedt, B., Skoog, G., Kastberg, R., Halliwell, D., Box, M., Herlitz, J., & Karlsten, R. (2014). Mechanical chest compressions and simultaneous defibrillation vs conventional cardiopulmonary resuscitation in out-of-hospital cardiac arrest: the LINC randomized trial. *JAMA: The Journal of the American Medical Association*, 311(1), 53–61.

Souchtchenko, S. S., Benner, J. P., Allen, J. L., & Brady, W. J. (2013). A review of chest compression interruptions during out-of-hospital cardiac arrest and strategies for the future. *Journal of Emergency Medicine, 45*(3), 458–466.

Stub, D., Bernard, S., Duffy, S. J., & Kaye, D. M. (2011). Post cardiac arrest syndrome: a review of therapeutic strategies. *Circulation, 123,* 1428–1435.

Stub, D., Nehme, Z., Bernard, S., Lijovic, M., Kaye, D. M., & Smith, K. (2014). Exploring which patients without return of spontaneous circulation following ventricular fibrillation out-of-hospital cardiac arrest should be transported to hospital? *Resuscitation, 85*(3), 326–331.

Sunde, K., Pytte, M., Jacobsen, D., Mangschau, A., Jensen, L. P., Smedsrud, C., Draegni, T., & Steen, P. A. (2007). Implementation of a standardised treatment protocol for post-resuscitation care after out-of-hospital cardiac arrest. *Resuscitation, 73*(1), 29–39.

Thom, M. (2007). The autopsy in sudden unexpected adult death: epilepsy. *Current Diagnostic Pathology, 13,* 389–400.

UK Resuscitation Council (UKRC). (2010). *Resuscitation Guidelines 2010 (Chapter 7 Adult).* UKRC.

Vilke, G. (2004). The three-phase model of cardiac arrest as applied to ventricular fibrillation in a large, urban emergency medical services system. *Academic Emergency Medicine: Official Journal of the Society for Academic Emergency Medicine, 11*(5), 604.

Wang, H. E., Simeone, S. J., Waever, M. D., & Callaway, C. W. (2009). Interruptions in cardiopulmonary resuscitation from paramedic endotracheal intubation. *Annals of Emergency Medicine, 54*(5), 645–652.e1.

Wik, L., Olsen, J.-A., Persse, D., Sterz, F., Lozano, M., Jr., Brouwer, M. A., Westfall, M., Souders, C. M., Malzer, R., van Grunsven, P. M., Travis, D. T., Whitehead, A., Herken, U. R., & Lerner, E. (2014). Manual vs. integrated automatic load-distributing band CPR with equal survival after out of hospital cardiac arrest. The randomized CIRC trial. *Resuscitation, 85*(6), 741–748.

SECTION 11:
The Paramedic Approach to the Patient With a Medical Condition

In this section:

The first-aid principles of supporting **airway, breathing and circulation** continue to be the pillars of emergency medical care regardless of the level of training or skillset of the responder. For the paramedic, airway compromise is intrinsically linked to the patient's conscious state and any patient unable to protect their own airway—regardless of how benign the cause—is at threat of airway occlusion and death from hypoxia.

Paramedics may carry a number of airway support tools such as oropharyngeal airways, laryngeal masks and endotracheal tubes. While these may seem harmless, each device carries significant risks. Far more effective than trying to mechanically maintain a patient's airway is to raise the patient's conscious state so that they can protect it themselves.

Dispatches to patients in an altered conscious state make up a significant proportion of paramedic cases. In order to manage these patients effectively you will need to quickly differentiate between the causes of unconsciousness and know which can be corrected in the field. This section reviews common causes of alterations in conscious state, steps you through the clinical reasoning process to provide a differential diagnosis and links the pathophysiology to the paramedic management of these common conditions.

The human body's immune system is designed to protect against a range of pathogens. Increasingly, however, the immune systems of people in the first world are becoming hyperreactive and generating a response that, rather than providing protection, can actually lead to illness and death. The sudden death of an otherwise healthy individual tends to reverberate through a community and the media. Combined with medical science's inability to predict what food, insect stings or other substances might cause a reaction (and how severe it will be), this can understandably lead the public to react when the first signs of an allergic reaction become apparent.

Mild allergic reactions and life-threatening anaphylaxis are at opposite ends of the clinical continuum and one of the challenges facing paramedics is determining where on this spectrum a particular patient lies. The ability to clinically reason between the extremes is the difference between the burden of unnecessary treatments and transporting patients to hospital, and saving lives with a simple and effective treatment regimen. In order to manage patients effectively you need to be able to quickly differentiate distressing but otherwise harmless localised reactions from life-threatening anaphylaxis. You also need to be able to distinguish anaphylaxis as a cause of airway occlusion, respiratory distress and inadequate perfusion.

This section describes the pathophysiology of anaphylaxis, steps through the clinical reasoning process to provide a differential diagnosis and links the pathophysiology to the paramedic management of life-threatening conditions.

Repeated studies have found that how patients express their pain and how clinicians respond to their complaints of pain are extremely variable and the overall experience is poorly perceived by both parties. To provide effective pain relief clinicians need a deep understanding of the pathology of pain and how it can be accurately assessed, as well as an understanding of the effectiveness of both pharmacological and non-pharmacological methods of pain relief.

This section describes the basic physiology of pain and how it is typically expressed in the out-of-hospital setting and uses the case studies to outline the role of paramedics in providing adequate pain relief—a practice that studies have demonstrated paramedics often struggle to achieve. The section then explores two very common presentations of pain that pose a challenge to clinical reasoning: lower back pain and renal colic.

More than 80% of Australians will experience lower back pain at some time in their life but only a tiny fraction will call for an ambulance. The spine battles the contradictory tasks of providing support, mobility and protection. As a result, the forces experienced by the joints during relatively normal activities such as bending over to brush the teeth can actually be extremely high and sudden damage to the lower spinal segment joints can place pressure on large nerve roots or the spinal cord itself. Without an understanding of the anatomy and mechanics of the spine, the innocuous nature of these injuries can lead clinicians to underestimate their seriousness and undertreat the associated pain and stress.

Back pain can also be an indication of other serious (non-spinal) conditions. The ability to identify chronic exacerbations of back pain or minor muscular (but still painful) injuries is essential in directing patients to appropriate treatment streams. A specific form of back pain that needs to be excluded from musculoskeletal causes and that requires aggressive pain management is renal colic. With paramedics increasingly being required to treat patients and direct them to agencies other than the emergency department, understanding which back complaints have the likelihood of complications is essential.

There are a group of patients who represent specific challenges in terms of assessment and, to a lesser extent, management. Among this group are those who present with abdominal symptoms for which there is no obvious diagnosis, including patients presenting with an acute abdomen or concealed gastrointestinal (GI) haemorrhage. Sepsis is also extremely variable in its presentation, from the classic and obvious presentations to the quite subtle and occult. Unfortunately, the patient who presents with atypical symptoms may still develop the most severe forms of sepsis. The common thread that ties these presentations together is that they contain examples of situations where paramedics might be inclined to underestimate the severity of the case. These topics do not comprise all of the higher risk situations, but they are typical of them. The patients to bear in mind are those with less obvious signs who present looking well but have the potential to deteriorate rapidly. Older patients in particular may not display the changes of vital signs that reflect the severity of their illness.

CHAPTER 25

Hypoglycaemia and Hyperglycaemia

By Jason Bendall

OVERVIEW

- Diabetes is an important clinical problem and paramedics will frequently provide care for individuals with complications arising from diabetes. The most emergent complications of diabetes are clinically important glycaemic crises including hypoglycaemia and hyperglycaemia.

Introduction

Diabetes mellitus (diabetes) is an important chronic medical condition which paramedics will encounter frequently. Diabetes has an estimated prevalence in the adult population of 8.5% and is the 8th leading cause of death (World Health Organization, 2016). Glycaemic emergencies may be associated with either hypoglycaemia or hyperglycaemia.

There are two major types of diabetes, namely type 1 (most commonly due to a failure to produce insulin due to autoimmune destruction of beta cells of the pancreas) and type 2 (due to insulin resistance and reduced insulin production). Type 1 diabetes typically presents with hyperglycaemia associated with excessive thirst (polydipsia), excessive urination (polyuria), excessive hunger (polyphagia), visual disturbances and weight loss. In Australia the majority of type 1 diabetes cases is diagnosed in younger people with the peak age of diagnosis between 10 and 19 years (Australian Institute of Health and Welfare, 2018). Type 1 diabetes accounts for approximately 10% of all diabetes. The initial presentation is diabetic ketoacidosis in about one-third of cases (American Diabetes Association, 2019). Type 1 diabetes requires treatment with insulin to survive.

Type 2 diabetes accounts for the majority of people with diabetes (85%) and is estimated to affect 5% of the Australian population. The majority of diagnoses occur after 45 years of age; however, the prevalence is increasing in younger ages including in children. Type 2 diabetes is often undiagnosed as elevated blood glucose levels develop slowly and may not be severe enough for the person to notice usual symptoms (American Diabetes Association, 2019). The mainstay of treatment for type 2 diabetes is oral hypoglycaemic drugs; however, treatment of type 2 diabetes with insulins is increasingly common.

The goal of diabetes management is to prevent the end-organ damage from hyperglycaemia.

Hypoglycaemia

Pathophysiology

The human brain relies on glucose as its primary energy source and is the highest consumer of glucose of all organs. Tight control of glucose homeostasis is essential for normal neuronal function and production of neurotransmitters. Neurons are particularly susceptible to hypoglycaemia. While hypoglycaemia has many causes, in diabetes it is most commonly associated with insulin therapy and oral hypoglycaemic agents which promote endogenous insulin secretion (i.e. sulphonylureas such as glibenclamide, gliclazide, glimepiride and glipizide) (Australian Medicines Handbook, 2019). Many individuals with diabetes are unaware that they are having a hypoglycaemic episode. If untreated, persistent hypoglycaemia results in brain damage and death. Fortunately, these complications are rare. The severity of hypoglycaemic episodes can be classified as mild (episodes which can be self-treated) or severe (unable to be self-treated). Coma is associated with only 25% of severe episodes (Frier, 2014). While the immediate effects of hypoglycaemia are well known, less considered are the long-term effects including reduced quality of life; impact on relationships, employment and driving; and fear of further episodes (Frier, 2014).

While hypoglycaemia is most commonly associated with diabetes, hypoglycaemia can also occur in individuals without diabetes (e.g. excessive exercise,

PRACTICE TIP

1. Paramedics may identify patients with diabetes even if undiagnosed: diagnostic criteria include a fasting blood glucose of ≥ 7.0 mmol/L (126 mg/dL) OR a random plasma glucose ≥ 11.1 mmol/L (200 mg/dL) with classic symptoms (e.g. polyuria, polydipsia, unexplained weight loss). If identified, referral for further investigation is warranted.
2. The two most common glycaemic emergencies (hypoglycaemia and hyperglycaemia) can be reliably identified by the measurement of blood glucose.

starvation, liver failure, sepsis, drugs, tumours); however, comparatively, hypoglycaemia is rare in individuals without diabetes. Making a diagnosis of hypoglycaemia is now simple with glucometry widely available in out-of-hospital, primary care and first aid settings (and in many homes). Causes of hypoglycaemia in adults are shown in Box 25.1 (Davis et al., 2016).

Definition

Hypoglycaemia is a glycaemic emergency and is defined as a blood glucose level (BGL) < 4.0 mmol/L or at a level which causes signs/symptoms. More severe episodes are typically associated with blood glucose levels < 3 mmol/L. Clinically important hypoglycaemia manifests commonly with:

- intense activation of the sympathetic nervous system causing pallor, sweating, tremor, tachycardia, hypertension and anxiety
- neurological effects including confusion, altered conscious state, changes in behaviour, changes in speech, changes in vision, hemiplegia, coma and seizures

BOX 25.1 Causes of hypoglycaemia in adults

- Drugs
  - › Especially insulin, sulfonylureas, alcohol
- Critical illness
  - › Renal, hepatic and heart disease; sepsis; malnutrition
- Endocrine deficiency
  - › Adrenal > pituitary > thyroid
- Overproduction of insulin or insulin-like material
  - › Insulin-producing islet tumour, non-β-cell tumours
- Other
  - › Pregnancy, strenuous exercise, autoimmune syndromes, reactive hypoglycaemia, inborn errors of metabolism, and inherited enzyme defects
- Iatrogenic
  - › Dialysis, total parenteral nutrition

Source: Davis et al. (2016), Table 47-1.

other features including hunger, headache and malaise.

Management
Restoring blood glucose level to normal

The goal of emergency management of hypoglycaemia is to increase the blood glucose concentration as rapidly as possible. Most commonly this can be accomplished via the administration of a rapidly acting carbohydrate in a form which is safe for the patient. Paramedics must undertake a risk assessment as to whether the patient is able to swallow safely otherwise parenteral treatment should be prioritised (if credentialled and available) to reduce the risk of aspiration. Buccal and sublingual administration of glucose gels have been described (Borra et al., 2018; Hegarty et al., 2017) and may be considered for uncooperative patients or where parenteral therapies are unavailable or impractical.

The use of 10% dextrose solutions (in favour of 50% dextrose) increased in popularity following an out-of-hospital randomised controlled trial in 2005 (Moore & Woollard, 2005). The administration of 10% glucose was associated with lower post-treatment glucose levels and reduced total glucose load. In a more recent study, Kiefer and colleagues (2014) also demonstrated resolution of hypoglycaemia in 8 minutes following administration of 10 g of 10% dextrose (100 mL) with 18% of patients requiring a second dose. Of 162 patients included only one required a third dose. Lower concentration solutions are associated with greater safety in the event of extravasation or inadvertent arterial injection as they are less hypertonic (compared with 50% solutions).

An alternative to intravenous glucose is the administration of glucagon. Glucagon is an endogenous pancreatic hormone secreted from the pancreas (alpha cells) and raises blood glucose by mobilising stored liver glycogen (glycogenolysis) and promoting hepatic generation of glucose (gluconeogenesis) from substrates. Glucagon is available as GlucaGen® HypoKit® containing a vial with 1 mg glucagon and a prefilled syringe (with needle) containing 1 mL sterile water. Common adverse effects include nausea, vomiting and, rarely, allergic reactions. Glucagon is an appropriate therapy if not credentialled to administer intravenous glucose or if there is a delay establishing intravenous access. Glucagon may be ineffective if liver glycogen stores are depleted. Glucagon is contraindicated in patients with rare tumours including:

- phaeochromocytoma (a rare tumour of the adrenal gland)

Table 25.1: Pharmacotherapy for clinically significant hypoglycaemia

Agent	Route	Initial dose	Preparations	Additional considerations
Glucose	Oral	Adult: 15 g Paediatric: < 2 years = 5 g 2–5 years = 10 g ≥ 6 years = 15 g Repeat every 15 minutes	Tablets (variable) Gel (dextrose 40%)*	Ideally in cooperative individuals who are able to swallow safely Buccal/sublingual administration of gel may be considered if parenteral therapy is unavailable or not practical < 2 years ~ 5 g; 2–5 years 10 g
	IV	Adult: 15 g Paediatric: 0.25 g/kg	10% dextrose (10 g/100 mL) 50% dextrose (50 g/100 mL)	10% dextrose is most commonly used as results in lower peak BGL and lower total dose when compared with 50% dextrose Doses of 10 g have been demonstrated to be effective for most patients
Glucagon	IM/ SC	Adult: 1 mg Paediatric: 0.025 mg/kg	1 mg vial requires reconstitution	Reserve for when IV access is not authorised or cannot be obtained or is not practical In children < 25 kg 0.5 mg is a pragmatic and practical dose

IV = intravenous; IM = intramuscular; SC = subcutaneous; BGL = blood glucose level

*Dextrose 40% gel contains 400 mg (0.4 g) glucose per mL

BOX 25.2 Examples of snacks with longer-acting carbohydrate

- 1 slice of bread/toast OR
- 1 glass of milk OR
- 1 piece of fruit OR
- 2 biscuits
- 2–3 pieces of dried apricots, figs or other dried fruit OR
- 1 tub of natural low-fat yoghurt OR
- Normal meal (if due)—must contain carbohydrate

- glucagonoma (a pancreatic tumour that causes increased levels of glucagon)
- insulinoma (a tumour that causes increased levels of insulin).

Pharmacological treatment options for immediate management for hypoglycaemia are described in Table 25.1.

Aftercare

Following successful immediate management of the hypoglycaemic episode, the administration of a longer-acting carbohydrate snack is generally required to prevent recurrence (see Box 25.2). Paramedics should endeavour to identify the most likely cause of the hypoglycaemic episode by taking a thorough history of likely precipitants (e.g. excess insulin, missed/delayed meal, insufficient carbohydrate, unplanned or excess exercise). Paramedics should be aware that if the hypoglycaemia was associated with long-acting insulin (e.g. isophane insulin, insulin detemir, insulin glargine) or sulphonylureas (e.g. glibenclamide, gliclazide, glimepiride and glipizide) there may be an ongoing risk of further hypoglycaemic events for 24–36 hours (Joint British Diabetes Societies [JBDS], 2018).

If glucagon has been administered, a larger snack is recommended (e.g. 2 times recommendations in table above). For individuals using continuous subcutaneous insulin infusions (CSII pumps) (see Figure 25.1) a long-acting carbohydrate is not usually needed following immediate management and recovery, but it is necessary to assess for the cause of the episode. The CSII does not need to be stopped by treating paramedics.

Hyperglycaemia

Hyperglycaemia occurs as a result of impaired glucose homeostasis. The most common cause of hyperglycaemia is diabetes, whether diagnosed or not. An additional cause for paramedics to be aware of is stress-induced hyperglycaemia, a normal, transient and adaptive response in times of stress resulting from increased circulating catecholamines, glucocorticoids (steroids) and glucagon to aid survival. This accounts for the frequent observation of hyperglycaemia in patients with acute medical and trauma presentations in the absence of coexisting diabetes (e.g. cardiac arrest, acute coronary syndromes, traumatic injuries).

Definition

Normal blood glucose levels are between 4 and 7.8 mmol/L; therefore, hyperglycaemia is technically any blood glucose level > 7.8 mmol/L. Pragmatically, blood glucose levels between 4 and 10 are essentially normal. Blood glucose levels are often transiently elevated after meals but should be below 10 within 2 hours of eating. Hyperglycaemia usually occurs slowly, and many instances are asymptomatic. A diagnosis of diabetes can be established when a blood glucose level is ≥ 11.1 with classic symptoms of diabetes.

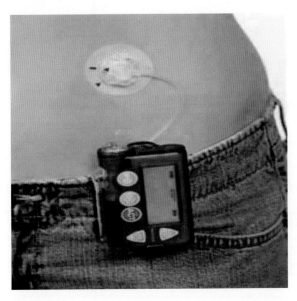

Figure 25.1
Continuous subcutaneous insulin infusion pump.
Source: Kerr & Partridge (2011).

Clinically important hyperglycaemia is more likely to be associated with blood glucose concentrations > 14 mmol/L (but complications can occur below this threshold).

Pathophysiology

There are two main hyperglycaemia emergencies of which paramedics should be aware. The first is diabetic ketoacidosis and the second is hyperglycaemic hyperosmolar states. An overview of the pathophysiology and clinical sequelae of both conditions is shown in Figure 25.2 and Figure 25.3 respectively.

Diabetic ketoacidosis

Diabetic ketoacidosis (DKA) is a serious diabetic complication which occurs most commonly in those with type 1 diabetes but occurs occasionally in those with type 2 diabetes. DKA results from an absolute insulin deficiency (i.e. type 1 diabetes) or relative (e.g. type 2 diabetes) insulin deficiency in the presence of the increased release in counterregulatory hormones (glucagon, catecholamines, cortisol and growth hormone) that causes a worsening of insulin resistance and further impairment of insulin secretion (Pasquel & Umpierrez, 2016). The lack of insulin precludes the uptake of glucose into cells thereby resulting in the need for the body to utilise other sources of energy (e.g. fat). This results in

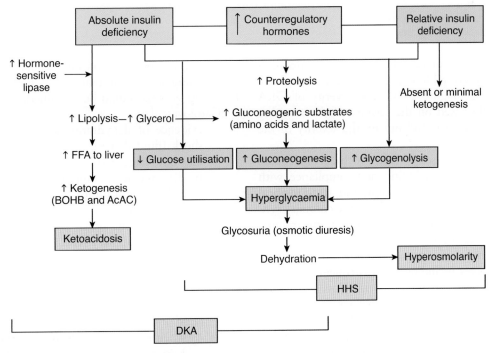

Figure 25.2
Pathogenesis of diabetic ketoacidosis (DKA) and hyperglycaemic hyperosmolar states (HHS).
Source: Davis et al. (2016).

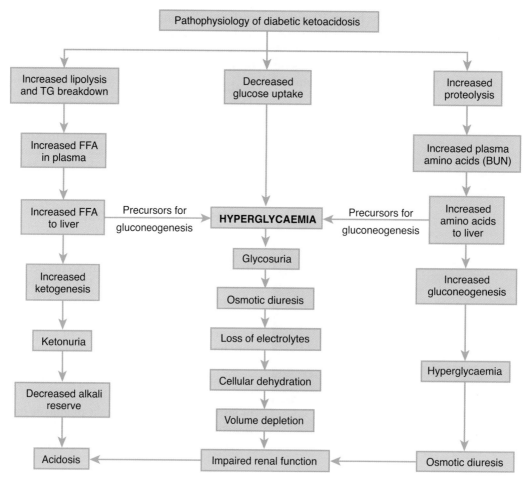

Figure 25.3
Syndrome of diabetic ketoacidosis. BUN = Blood urea nitrogen; FFA = free fatty acids; TG = total glucose concentration.
Source: Maloney & Glauser (2017), Fig 118.1.

the production of ketone bodies which are acids thereby lowering blood pH and causing metabolic acidosis (see Figure 25.3). The severity of DKA is typically based on the severity of the resulting metabolic acidosis and not on the severity of the hyperglycaemia.

Common causes of DKA include inadequate insulin therapy (including non-compliance with insulin therapy) and infections and acute medical or surgical illnesses (e.g. sepsis, acute coronary syndrome, stroke, gastrointestinal conditions, trauma, psychological stress).

The most common symptoms are associated with diabetes including thirst, frequent urination, blurred vision, fatigue and weight loss (recall that about one-third of cases of DKA represent the first presentation of diabetes). Additionally, gastrointestinal symptoms and signs (including nausea, vomiting and abdominal pain) are frequently present and are somewhat correlated with more severe metabolic acidosis.

Findings on examination vary depending on the severity and the precipitant cause; however, the following systems should be examined.

- Cardiovascular:
  › evidence of dehydration or hypovolaemic shock (fluid deficits can be significant and may be as large as 100 mL/kg of bodyweight)
    o dry mucous membranes
    o reduced skin turgor
    o tachycardia
    o hypotension
    o reduced capillary refill.
- Respiratory:
  › increased respiratory rate in an attempt to compensate for metabolic acidosis by reducing blood carbon dioxide levels (usually starts rapid and shallow)
    o when metabolic acidosis becomes severe Kussmaul respiration may ensue (i.e. rapid and deep breathing)
  › fruity-smelling breath (from acetone elimination).

- Neurological:
  › altered conscious state (multifactorial)
    o confusion
    o drowsiness to coma with increasing severity
    o seizures.
- Other systems as suggested by precipitant cause looking for:
  › evidence of sepsis/infection (e.g. respiratory, urinary, central nervous system, gastrointestinal, skin)
  › acute coronary syndromes
  › cerebrovascular accidents (stroke)
  › gastrointestinal haemorrhage
  › pancreatitis.

While history and examination suggest the diagnosis, establishing the definitive diagnosis in the out-of-hospital setting is not generally possible as the diagnosis requires blood gas measurement (to detect metabolic acidosis) and the ability to detect ketones. However, it is possible to measure point-of-care blood ketones using modern blood glucose measurement systems (see Practice point). Hyperglycaemia with symptoms/signs of DKA and detection of ketones make a diagnosis of DKA very likely.

Management

There are four goals to the management of DKA. These are to:

1. restore circulatory blood volume (i.e. treat shock/dehydration)
2. gradually correct hyperglycaemia (i.e. give insulin)
3. detect and correct electrolyte imbalances (mostly sodium and potassium)
4. identify and treat precipitating events/causes.

Paramedics are well placed to recognise/suspect DKA and commence the restoration of the circulating blood volume and replace fluid deficits. Initiating fluids is the cornerstone of initial management: fluids first, insulin second. Disposition for suspected cases of DKA need investigation and management in hospital under the care of specialist physicians (ideally an endocrinologist) with more severe cases requiring management in intensive care units.

Adults

Commence resuscitation with crystalloids (e.g. normal saline or compound sodium lactate [Hartmann's] solution) at 1000 mL/hr over the first hour. If shock is present, an additional bolus may be warranted during the first hour of care. Further fluid management is generally at a rate of 500 mL/hr for hours 2–3 of care (Queensland Health, 2019) (see Table 25.2).

Paediatrics (< 16 years)

The principles and goals of management are the same as in adults. However, children (especially younger children) are at greater risk of complications including cerebral oedema from excessive rehydration so accurate estimates of fluid deficits are required to better guide fluid replacement. It is recommended to replace deficits over 48 hours (more slowly than other clinical conditions).

- Child is shocked (estimated 8% fluid deficit or greater)
  › Child with hyperglycaemia and has tachycardia for age, poor perfusion (e.g. mottled/cool limbs), slow capillary refill, weak peripheral pulses or reduced conscious state)
    o Administer 10 mL/kg crystalloid as a bolus then reassess and repeat if signs of shock persist (to a maximum of 30 mL/kg)
- Child is not shocked (estimated 5–7% fluid deficit)
  › Child with hyperglycaemia who is not in shock but is clinically dehydrated or clinically

---

PRACTICE POINT

Out-of-hospital detection of ketones (see Figure 25.4)

Urine

A urine ketone stick test provides a semiquantitative measure of the ketone body acetoacetate. Provides an average of ketones since last void. Does not detect does the predominant ketone body beta-hydroxybutyrate.

Blood

Many blood glucose monitoring systems can now accurately measure ketones in the blood. They quantitatively measure the predominant ketone beta-hydroxybutyrate. Levels below 0.6 mmol/L are unlikely to be clinically important whereas levels above 1.5 mmol/L are considered clinically important. For individuals with diabetes blood ketone measurement is recommended when blood glucose levels are elevated, when unwell or sick, or when symptoms of DKA are present (e.g. nausea, vomiting, abdominal pain).

Breath

Acetone is a ketone body which is excreted via the lungs. It is described as having a fruity- or pear-like odour and may be detected on the patient's breath.

Table 25.2: Out-of-hospital fluid management for diabetic ketoacidosis in adults

Hour	Rate	Considerations
First hour	1000 mL/hr	Additional bolus can be administered if shock is present
Second hour	500 mL/hr	
Third hour	500 mL/hr	
Fourth hour	250 mL/hr	
Fifth and subsequent hour	125 mL/hr	

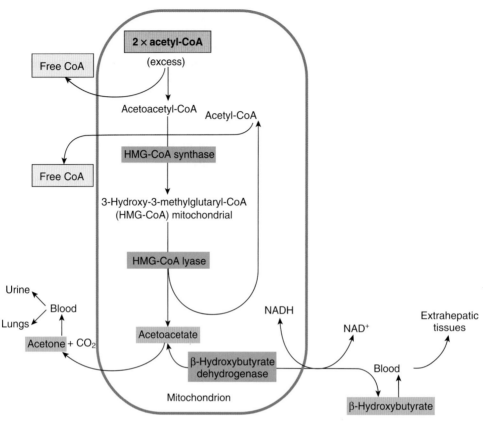

Figure 25.4
Mitochondrial ketogenic pathway. Ketone bodies are in *purple*; enzymes are in *red*. HMG-CoA,
hydroxymethylglutaryl-CoA.
Source: Papachristodoulou et al. (2018).

acidotic (e.g. rapid respiratory rate for age) or vomiting it is recommended that maintenance fluids be administered plus fluid deficit be corrected evenly over 48 hours.

› While many approaches exist for calculating the recommended maintenance, without practice, this can be difficult. A pragmatic fluid regime for non-shocked children is 3-5 mL/kg/hr (see below).
   o 10 kg (assuming 5% deficit): 5 ml/kg/hr (50 mL/hr)
   o 20 kg (assuming 5% deficit): 4 mL/kg/hr (i.e. 80 mL/hr)
   o 50 kg (assuming 5% deficit): 3 ml/kg/hr (i.e. 150 mL/hr)

› Fluids in children should ideally be administered via a fluid pump or via burette or via syringe with 3-way tap). An interactive calculator can be found here http://kidshealthwa.com/guidelines/diabetic-ketoacidosis-fluid-calculator/ to better guide fluid management (Kids Health Western Australia, 2013).

Euglycaemic DKA

In recent years there have been reports of severe diabetic ketoacidosis with normal (or only mildly elevated) blood glucose concentrations (termed euglycaemic DKA) associated with patients taking sodium-glucose co-transporter-2 (SGL2) inhibitors (Australian Diabetes Society, 2018). SGL2 inhibitors include Forxiga (contains dapagliflozin), Xigduo XR (contains dapagliflozin and metformin, controlled-release preparation), Jardiance (contains empagliflozin) and Jardiamet (contains

REFLECTIVE BOX

What if you cannot obtain IV access?
Intravenous access in children is difficult. Reasons for inability include patient reasons (e.g. uncooperative, poor veins, too sick, dehydration) or practitioner reasons (inexperience, confidence, training). What can/should you do? Is intraosseous (IO) access a viable option? How sick would the child need to be before you would use IO in the out-of-hospital setting? How far would you need to be from hospital before using an IO?

empagliflozin and metformin) (Australian Medicines Handbook, 2019) which reduce glucose reabsorption in the kidney. Euglycaemic DKA has been associated with dehydration, fasting, surgery and infections and have mostly presented in the perioperative period.

It is prudent for paramedics to consider DKA in patients taking SGL2 inhibitors who:

- develop abdominal pain, nausea, vomiting, fatigue or clinical acidosis (e.g. increased respiratory rate)
- have capillary ketone (i.e. blood beta-hydroxybutyrate) levels > 0.6 mmol/L in the perioperative period or > 1.5 mmol/L at any other time.

In time capillary ketone testing will become increasingly routine to detect significant levels of blood ketones and identify those at risk of DKA.

Hyperglycaemic hyperosmolar states

Hyperglycaemic hyperosmolar states (HHS) is an important glycaemic emergency typically occurring in older individuals (> 60 years) and those with type 2 diabetes. HHS can occur in the absence of diabetes. Mortality of HHS is higher than DKA reflecting the underlying causes of HHS. Unlike DKA, ketosis is minimal or absent presumably due to sufficient insulin to prevent clinically important ketosis and consequent acidosis. Glycogenolysis, gluconeogenesis and reduced peripheral uptake of glucose result in a significant hyperglycaemic state. Severe hyperglycaemia results in a significant osmotic diuresis with hypovolaemia and consequently impaired renal function.

The clinical manifestations are a state of extreme dehydration, hyperosmolality (from hyperglycaemia, hypernatraemia and renal failure), significant dehydration and generally an altered mental state.

While there are different diagnostic criteria for HHS (usually BGL > 30 mmol/L and osmolality > 320 mOsmol/L without significant acidosis or ketonaemia) establishing a diagnosis of HHS is not practical or possible in most out-of-hospital settings. A pragmatic approach is identifying and referring individuals with hyperglycaemia (> 15 mmol/L) with moderate/severe dehydration without ketosis for fluid resuscitation and emergency department assessment and subsequent management (The Royal Australian College of General Practitioners, 2018). Measuring capillary ketones can help differentiate those at risk of HHS from DKA.

Management of HHS is very similar to DKA with replacing fluid deficits the immediate priority followed by the administration of insulin, correcting electrolyte abnormalities and identifying and treating the cause.

 CASE STUDY

Case 11032, 0115 hrs.

Dispatch details: A 19-year-old male, unconscious; patient is a type 1 diabetic.

Initial presentation: On arrival, the paramedics find a young male slumped over his desk. He is extremely diaphoretic (his clothes are soaked in perspiration), responds only to pain and has loud snoring respirations.

 ## ASSESS

History

The patient's mother states that her son has been studying hard for exams and hasn't been getting much sleep. She awoke at 1 am and saw his bedroom light on. She went to check on him, saw his dinner only half eaten and found him slumped over his desk. The patient has an 8-year history of type 1 diabetes and is now on an insulin (CSII) pump.

While a diagnosis of hypoglycaemia in the unconscious diabetic patient is based on their BGL reading, obtaining an accurate history can assist in adding vital context to aid in determining the need for further assessment and in guiding disposition. Hypoglycaemia causing loss of consciousness can lead to airway obstruction, hypoxia, aspiration and, if untreated, brain injury. Prolonged unconsciousness can also cause compartment syndrome if there is a long lie.

The factors leading to the event can also be predictive of the patient's response to treatment. Accidentally missing one meal suggests the patient will respond well, but if this is one in a series of recent hypoglycaemic events and the patient has been taking normal meals and medication, it suggests progression of the disease and the need for further investigation. Intentional hypoglycaemia is often referred to as factitious (or factitial) and is used in medical parlance to imply covert human activity. In fact, an overdose may be accidental but if it is related to an attempt at self-harm, the dose used may far exceed the normal ranges and the patient may not respond to the standard treatment regimen.

Airway

Hypoglycaemia does not directly lead to airway compromise through swelling or other means, but any decrease in consciousness can lead to airway occlusion, and pathological causes such as hypoglycaemia that restrict the patient's ability to wake can be sufficient to cause hypoxia. The overt link between this patient's history of diabetes and current unconsciousness can lead to premature diagnostic closure and clinicians may miss other causes and fail to follow basic principles of management while they treat the underlying cause.

While definitive management of this patient's airway is returning him to full consciousness, regardless of which hypoglycaemic treatment is chosen, this will take several minutes. In the meantime, the patient should be positioned laterally. While it most likely has a diabetic cause, upper airway should be checked for patency. The airway can usually be maintained with simple manoeuvres but adjuncts may be required.

Breathing

Unlike hyperglycaemia where the generation of a metabolic acidosis stimulates the respiratory centre, hypoglycaemia does not directly lead to specific respiratory changes. Vomiting and aspiration due to a decreased conscious state are a concern, but profound alterations of respiratory rate (e.g. Cheyne-Stokes pattern) indicate underlying brain injury. If hypoxaemia is identified, oxygen should be administered and a cause of hypoxaemia sought.

Circulation

Hypoglycaemia stimulates the sympathetic nervous system causing the release of catecholamines (e.g. adrenaline and noradrenaline) causing tachycardia, peripheral vasoconstriction (pale skin) and sweating (often profuse). While tachycardia is to be expected, bradycardia is an ominous sign and is suggestive of profound hypoxia, probably due to positional airway occlusion. Any absence of tachycardia and pale clammy skin should suggest another cause of altered consciousness than hypoglycaemia.

Environment

The profound diaphoresis that usually accompanies hypoglycaemia can cause a significant temperature loss. Consider hypothermia as a complicating factor in patients who have not been seen for a long period.

Initial assessment summary

Problem	Unconscious
Conscious state	GCS = 7 (E1, M4, V2)
Position	Slumped over his desk
Heart rate	124 bpm
Blood pressure	130/80 mmHg

Skin appearance	Pale, diaphoretic
Speech pattern	No speech
Respiratory rate	18 bpm
Respiratory rhythm	Even cycles
Respiratory effort	Snoring respirations
Chest auscultation	Clear chest bilaterally
Pulse oximetry	95% on room air
Temperature	36.7°C
BGL	1.9 mmol/L
Pupils	Equal and reacting
History	Studying a lot with little sleep; the patient has not eaten his full meal

D: The area has been checked for sharps and the patient's dinner plate and cutlery have been removed.

A: There is evidence of partial airway obstruction. This is relieved by head tilt and lateral posturing; the airway needs ongoing and frequent reassessment until consciousness is restored.

B: There is no current respiratory embarrassment but needs ongoing and frequent reassessment.

C: Heart rate is elevated; blood pressure is high normal and there is poor skin perfusion.

D: Unconscious (GCS = 7), no localising signs, remains at risk of seizures and aspiration.

E: Nil injuries detected.

The patient has the classic signs and symptoms of hypoglycaemia: increased autonomic nervous system (ANS) response including pallor, diaphoresis and tachycardia; he remains normotensive and has dilated pupils.

2 CONFIRM

The essential part of the clinical reasoning process is to seek to confirm your initial hypothesis by finding clinical signs that should occur with your provisional diagnosis. You should also seek to challenge your diagnosis by exploring any findings that do not fit your hypothesis: don't just ignore them because they don't fit. The clinical reasoning process begins as you assess the patient and continues while you consider and attempt to rule out any potential differential diagnoses if the treatment for hypoglycaemia is not working, the patient is presenting as hypoglycaemic yet the BGL is normal or the patient is not a diabetic. In most cases standard hypoglycaemia is relatively easy to establish using a simple BGL, treatment of the patient and evidence of recovery post-treatment. However, there are a few possible differential diagnoses that should be considered.

What else could it be?

Consider other causes of unconsciousness and abnormal behaviour:

- alcohol intoxication
- drug overdose (including agents with sympathomimetic effects)
- infection/sepsis
- stroke
- epilepsy
- adrenal crisis
- depression/psychosis.

This case study reveals a typical case of hypoglycaemia; a patient with known type 1 diabetes on insulin who has not eaten enough at his last meal (both significant risk factors in hypoglycaemia). This, associated with neurological dysfunction (responding only to pain and a BGL measured as 1.9 mmol/L), leaves only one remaining task: to definitely diagnose hypoglycaemia according to Whipple's triad; that is, the patient responds appropriately to treatment for low BGL, then hypoglycaemia is the result. Fortunately, the results from treatments used to correct hypoglycaemia are usually rapid.

③ TREAT
Emergency management
Safety

Wearing personal protective equipment (PPE) is essential, since patients who have a decreased level of consciousness require airway management, and sharps are used for BGL measurement, cannulation and IV treatment. Any patient with a decreased level of consciousness may potentially be combative, complicating treatment. Note the following principles of emergency management.

- Be aware of the risks of using sharps in a patient with a decreased level of consciousness.
- To raise the BGL, use oral glucose/food in the conscious and cooperative patient (i.e. able to swallow safely), and IV glucose/dextrose in patients with an altered mental state. If unable to gain intravenous access, use subcutaneous/intramuscular glucagon.
- Overtreatment with glucose/dextrose will not speed recovery and may actually result in hyperglycaemia.
- Manage other symptoms as necessary.

Should this patient be transported to hospital?

Emergency management of hypoglycaemia is often as simple as performing a BGL test on the patient and initiating treatment: the earlier the treatment commences, the better the patient's probable outcome.

Hypoglycaemia is one of the few cases where some patients can safely be left at home after paramedic treatment. This can be considered for individuals with known diabetes where the cause of hypoglycaemia is evident (e.g. inadequate food intake, above-normal levels of activity). However, those who suffer a hypoglycaemic event and who have not been diagnosed with diabetes should always be referred for further assessment.

Important considerations post-treatment regarding whether a patient should be transported to hospital include the following.

- Does the patient have a history of diabetes? Remember the other potential causes of hypoglycaemia.
- Is the patient responding to treatment?
- Is the patient able to tolerate food/liquids enough to maintain BGL?
- Is there food available?
- Does the patient have a glucometer?
- Does the patient have an insulin pump that is working?
- Does the patient have a concurrent acute illness/injury that may mean glycaemic control is a problem?
- Does the patient live alone?
- Is the patient malnourished and/or alcoholic?
- Is the patient a newly diagnosed diabetic or has the insulin regimen been altered recently? The patient may require stabilisation in hospital.
- Can the patient's carer demonstrate competency/capacity?
- Has the patient experienced repeated episodes of hypoglycaemia with reduced awareness? Will they recognise further episodes?

In this case study the patient is a known diabetic who lives with his carer (his mother) who is likely to have a good understanding of the illness. If his hypoglycaemia is corrected, no underlying pathologies can be identified, he recovers, is fully aware and can demonstrate competency and capacity, then he can be safely left at home post-treatment. You may wish to ascertain details about his insulin pump to ensure there are no issues regarding knowledge of its use.

4 EVALUATE

Evaluating the effect of any clinical management intervention can provide clues to the accuracy of the initial diagnosis. Some conditions respond rapidly to treatment so patients should be expected to improve if the diagnosis and treatment were appropriate. A failure to improve in this situation should trigger the clinician to reconsider the diagnosis.

Reversing hypoglycaemia with oral agents or glucagon may produce no change in the patient for as much as the first 10 minutes after administration. However, once the patient starts to respond, recovery tends to be rapid and is usually fully resolved within a couple of minutes. IV therapy is generally quicker from the time of administration. If a patient fails to respond to treatment within 15 minutes, this should prompt a full reassessment including a new BGL reading. If the BGL remains low, repeat the therapy according to local guidelines. If the reading returns to normal but the patient remains in an altered conscious state, there is likely to be a secondary cause such as hypoxia, hypercapnia, hypothermia, cerebral ischaemia or overdose, and transport for further assessment/management is warranted.

After the patient has recovered, it is feasible to explore some of the factors that may have contributed to the event.

- Does the patient have a BGL record book or glucometer for you to check past records?
- When did the patient last see his GP/endocrinologist for his diabetes management?
- When was the patient's last hypoglycaemic episode and how severe was it?
- Has the patient been unwell lately with a possible infection? Infections pose an increased risk of poor glycaemic control.

Summary

The brain is reliant on a consistent supply of glucose for normal function. The majority of glycaemic emergencies are associated with diabetes mellitus.

Hypoglycaemia and hyperglycaemia can be reliably diagnosed with point-of-care blood glucose measurement systems. Point-of-care blood ketone measurement can assist in the triage and risk stratifications of hyperglycaemic presentations.

The majority of hypoglycaemic presentations are associated with treatment of diabetes with insulin and sulphonylureas. The immediate management priority for hypoglycaemia is to restore blood glucose concentration to normal. The likely cause of hypoglycaemia should be identified: unexplained hypoglycaemia requires referral for further investigation, diagnosis and management (might be an uncommon cause). Stress can induce hyperglycaemia.

Diabetic ketoacidosis might be the first presentation of diabetes for one-third of cases: the absence of diabetes does not exclude diabetic ketoacidosis. Diabetic ketoacidosis and hyperglycaemic hyperosmolar states are associated with significant morbidity and mortality. Both conditions present with significant fluid deficits and require rehydration as a management priority.

Hyperglycaemia associated with moderate to severe dehydration requires referral for further investigation, diagnosis and management. These patients are at risk of serious complications. Coexisting illnesses/medical conditions are a common precipitant for hyperglycaemic emergencies, so be systematic and thorough to identify the most likely and less common causes.

Paramedics are well placed to identify patients with undiagnosed diabetes and should refer at-risk patients for further investigation, diagnosis and management to prevent the long-term harms associated with diabetes.

References

American Diabetes Association. (2019). 2. Classification and diagnosis of diabetes: standards of medical care in Diabetes—2019. *Diabetes Care, 42*(Suppl. 1), S13–S28.

Australian Diabetes Society. (2018). *Severe Euglycaemic Ketoacidosis with SGLT2 Inhibitor Use in the Perioperative Period*. Online. Retrieved from: https://diabetessociety.com.au/documents/2018_ALERT-ADS_SGLT2i_PerioperativeKetoacidosis_v3__final2018_02_14.pdf.

Australian Institute of Health and Welfare. (2018). *Diabetes Snapshot*. Online. Retrieved from: https://www.aihw.gov.au/reports/diabetes/diabetes-snapshot/contents/how-many-australians-have-diabetes/type-1-diabetes.

Australian Medicines Handbook 2019 (online) (2019). Australian Medicines Handbook Pty Ltd, Adelaide. Retrieved from: https://amhonline.amh.net.au/.

Borra, V., Carlson, J. N., De Buck, E., Djärv, T., Singletary, E. M., Zideman, D., Bendall, J., Berry, D. C., Cassan, P., Chang, W. T., Charlton, N. P., Hood, N. A., Meyran, D., Woodin, J. A., & Swain, J. *Glucose administration routes for first aid in case of symptomatic hypoglycemia. Consensus on Science and Treatment Recommendations [Internet] Brussels*, Belgium: International Liaison Committee on Resuscitation (ILCOR) First Aid Task Force, 2018 Aug 27. Retrieved from https://costr.ilcor.org/document/methods-of-glucose-administration-in-first-aid-for-hypoglycemia.

Davis, S. N., Lamos, E. M., & Younk, L. M. (2016). Hypoglycemia and hypoglycemic syndromes. In J. L. Jameson, L. J. De Groot, D. M. De Kretser, L. Giudice, A. Grossman, S. Melmed, J. T. Potts & G. C. Weir (Eds.), *Endocrinology: adult and pediatric* (7th ed.). Elsevier.

Frier, B. M. (2014). Hypoglycaemia in diabetes mellitus: epidemiology and clinical implications. *Nature Reviews. Endocrinology, 10*, 711–722.

Hegarty, J. E., Harding, J. E., Crowther, C. A., Brown, J., & Alsweiler, J. (2017). Oral dextrose gel to prevent hypoglycaemia in at-risk neonates. *The Cochrane Database of Systematic Reviews*, (7), CD012152.

Joint British Diabetes Societies (JBDS) for Inpatient Care Group. (2018). *Hospital management of hypoglycaemia in adults with diabetes* (3rd ed.). Retrieved from https://abcd.care/sites/abcd.care/files/resources/20180508_JBDS_HypoGuideline_Revised_v2.pdf. Online.

Kerr, D., & Partridge, H. (2011). Deus ex machina: the use of technology in type 1 diabetes. *Primary Care Diabetes, 5*(3), 159–165.

Kids Health Western Australia. (2013). *Diabetic Ketoacidosis—Fluid Calculator*. Online. Retrieved from: http://kidshealthwa.com/guidelines/diabetic-ketoacidosis-fluid-calculator/.

Kiefer, M. V., Gene Hern, H., Alter, H. J., & Barger, J. B. (2014). Dextrose 10% in the treatment of out-of-hospital hypoglycemia. *Prehospital and Disaster Medicine, 29*(2), 190–194.

Maloney, G. E., & Glauser, J. M. (2017). *Rosen's emergency medicine: concepts and clinical practice* (9th ed., pp. 1533–1547). Chapter 118.

Moore, C., & Woollard, M. (2005). Dextrose 10% or 50% in the treatment of hypoglycaemia out of hospital? A randomised controlled trial. *Emergency Medicine Journal, 22*(7), 512–515.

Papachristodoulou, D., Snape, A., Elliott, W., & Elliott, D. (2018). *Biochemistry and molecular biology* (6th ed.). London: Oxford University Press.

Pasquel, F. J., & Umpierrez, G. E. (2016). Hyperglycemic crises: diabetic ketoacidosis and hyperglycemic hyperosmolar state. In J. L. Jameson, L. J. De Groot, D. M. De Kretser, L. Giudice, A. Grossman, S. Melmed, J. T. Potts & G. C. Weir (Eds.), *Endocrinology: adult and pediatric* (7th ed.). Elsevier.

Queensland Health. (2019). *Management of diabetic ketoacidosis in adults (age 16 years and over)*. Online. Retrieved from: https://www.health.qld.gov.au/__data/assets/pdf_file/0028/438391/diabetic-ketoacidosis.pdf.

The Royal Australian College of General Practitioners. (2018). *Emergency management of hyperglycaemia in primary care*. Online. Retrieved from: https://diabetessociety.com.au/documents/Emergencymanagementofhyperglycaemiainprimarycare.pdf.

World Health Organization. (2016). *Global Report on Diabetes*. Online. Retrieved from: http://apps.who.int/iris/bitstream/handle/10665/204871/9789241565257_eng.pdf;jsessionid=6A969076FC8BC0008CF09A23291FE5C6?sequence=1.

CHAPTER 26

Stroke

By Helen Webb

OVERVIEW

- Stroke is a leading cause of death and disability in Australia (Stroke Foundation, 2017).
- In Australia, the incidence of stroke is one stroke every 9 minutes. More than 80% of strokes can be prevented.
- The financial cost of stroke in Australia is estimated to be $5 billion per year (Stroke Foundation, 2017).
- Stroke is a common life-threatening condition encountered by paramedics.
- Early identification of acute stroke is essential because acute therapies for stroke have a narrower time window of effectiveness than therapies for myocardial infarction.
- Early recognition of stroke in the community, rapid and accurate assessment of stroke by paramedics,

appropriate out-of-hospital management and prompt transport to an appropriate medical facility result in improved patient outcomes.
- There are a number of stroke mimics that paramedics must be aware of to ensure a diagnosis of stroke is not missed.
- The use of a validated out-of-hospital stroke screening tool has been shown to increase the sensitivity for accurate diagnosis of stroke patients by paramedics.
- Transport of the acute stroke patient to a hospital with a dedicated stroke team and the provision of thrombolytic therapy in appropriate cases reduce stroke mortality and morbidity.

Introduction

Stroke is a leading cause of disability and the third leading cause of death in Australia. Stroke affects both males and females, with little difference between death rates between the sexes. Most deaths due to stroke occur in the older population, with the median age being 86.6 years. However, stroke is one of the top 10 causes of death in persons aged over 45 years and approximately 30% of stroke survivors are of working age (less than 65 years of age). Moreover, around 80% of strokes are preventable. The financial cost is estimated at 5 billion dollars each year (Stroke Foundation, 2017; AIHW, 2018).

Over the past decade a number of significant breakthroughs have occurred in the treatment of stroke and, like the development of acute myocardial infarction (AMI) guidelines previously, early recognition and direction of patients to appropriate centres is the cornerstone of a successful outcome. In this new era of stroke treatment, paramedics play an essential role in the detection and transport of patients. The ability to diagnose a stroke in the out-of-hospital setting is confounded by the number of stroke mimics, but is an essential skill given the limited resources available to manage acute strokes and the devastating cost when the disease is allowed to progress untreated.

Pathophysiology

Stroke occurs when blood supply to a portion of the brain is interrupted. This interruption is caused by either a blockage or a rupture of the arteries that supply the brain (see Fig 26.1).

- Ischaemic strokes occur when vessels are blocked and they account for 80% of strokes. The blockage can be either thrombotic or embolic.
- Haemorrhagic strokes account for the remaining 20% of strokes. Spontaneous intracerebral haemorrhage accounts for 25% of haemorrhagic strokes (see Fig 26.2) while subarachnoid haemorrhage accounts for a further 8% (Boccardi et al., 2017) (see Fig 26.3, Box 26.1 and Table 26.1).

If the area affected is very small, a stroke can occur without any obvious symptoms, but in most cases the lack of blood causes the sudden onset of neurological symptoms. If blood supply is quickly restored the symptoms may resolve and the event is often described as a transient ischaemic attack (TIA; see Box 26.2), but if the symptoms persist beyond 24 hours the diagnosis of a stroke can be made. Approximately 15% of strokes are preceded by a TIA. Magnetic resonance imaging (MRI) on people with TIA lasting in excess of 1 hour have demonstrated that 50% of TIA sufferers have visible areas of infarction. While these persons are not

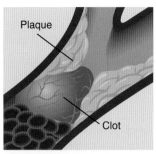

Thrombotic stroke. Cerebral thrombosis is a narrowing of the artery by fatty deposits called *plaque*. Plaque can cause a clot to form, which blocks the passage of blood through the artery.

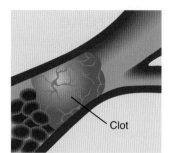

Embolic stroke. An embolus is a blood clot or other debris circulating in the blood. When it reaches an artery in the brain that is too narrow to pass through, it lodges there and blocks the flow of blood.

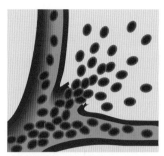

Haemorrhagic stroke. A burst blood vessel may allow blood to seep into and damage brain tissues until clotting shuts off the leak.

Figure 26.1
Major forms of stroke.
Source: Brown & Edwards (2012).

BOX 26.1 Symptoms associated with stroke location

- *Left hemisphere stroke* produces sensory, motor or sensorimotor deficits of the right face and/or arm and/or leg and/or dysphasia; loss of right visual field.
- *Right hemisphere stroke* produces sensory, motor or sensorimotor deficits of the left face and/or arm and/or leg and/or neglect to left side; loss of left visual field.
- *Brainstem stroke* produces vertigo; ataxia; ± nausea, ± vomiting, ± diplopia.
- *Subarachnoid haemorrhage* produces sudden onset 'worst ever' headache; altered level of consciousness and sometimes focal signs.

Table 26.1 Classic stroke presentations

Type	Gender/age	Warning	Time of onset	Common causes	Course/prognosis
Ischaemic (80%)					
Thrombotic	Men more than women, oldest median age	TIA (30–50% of cases). Past history of STROKE/IHD	During or after sleep	Atherosclerosis, smoking, hyperlipidaemia, hypertension	Stepwise progression, signs and symptoms develop slowly, usually some improvement, recurrence in 20–25% of survivors
Embolic	Men more than women	TIA (uncommon) Past history of STROKE	Lack of relationship to activity, sudden onset	Atrial fibrillation, heart valve disease, coagulation disorders	Single event, signs and symptoms develop quickly, usually some improvement, recurrence common without aggressive treatment of underlying disease
Haemorrhagic (20%)					
Intracerebral (12%)	Slightly higher in women	Headache (25% of cases)	Activity (often)	Hypertension	Progression over 24 hours; poor prognosis, fatality more likely with presence of coma
Subarachnoid (8%)	Slightly higher in women, youngest median age	Headache (common)	Activity (often), sudden onset; most commonly associated with head trauma	Hypertension, vascular malformation (berry aneurysms)	Single sudden event usually, fatality more likely with presence of coma

STROKE = cerebrovascular accident; IHD = ischaemic heart disease; TIA = transient ischaemic attack.
Source: Brown & Edwards (2012).

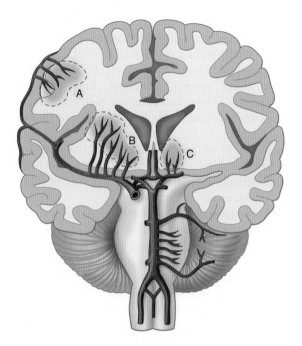

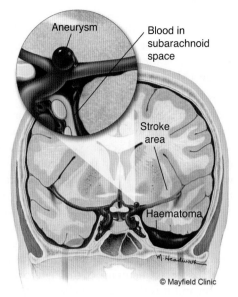

© Mayfield Clinic

Figure 26.2
Typical sites and sources of intracerebral haemorrhage.
Intracerebral haemorrhages most commonly involve the cerebral lobes and originate from penetrating cortical branches of the anterior, middle or posterior cerebral arteries (**A**, **B**, **C**). Infarcts in the pons originate from the basilar artery, while the cerebellar arteries are the source of cerebellar bleeds. Compared with ischaemic stroke they occur more commonly during activity and can be the result of vascular malformations, tumours or the administration of thrombolytic drugs. Hypertension is the most common underlying cause and the symptoms will depend on the location and extent of the haemorrhage. While some haemorrhagic strokes have classically defined symptoms (e.g. subarachnoid haemorrhage) there is no reliable method of differentiating ischaemic stroke from haemorrhagic stroke in the out-of-hospital environment.
Source: Goldman & Ausiello (2007).

Figure 26.3
The subarachnoid space lies between the external surface of the brain and the interior lining of the skull. It is normally filled with a small volume of cerebrospinal fluid (CSF), which creates a small amount of pressure. When arteries that lie in the subarachnoid space rupture, the higher pressure inside the artery forces blood into the space. If the rupture is large, the volume of blood that flows into the space will compress nearby brain tissue and lead to localised ischaemia. The portion of the brain normally supplied by the artery may also become ischaemic. Smaller bleeds may not produce such overt symptoms and the only signs may be from the irritation of the brain meninges by the blood in the space. The sudden rupturing of 'berry aneurysms' that exist at bifurcations of arteries is a common cause of subarachnoid haemorrhage. These thin-walled aneurysms are the result of high blood pressure and some subarachnoid haemorrhages will occur during times of strenuous exercise.
Source: With permission from Mayfield Clinic.

BOX 26.2 Transient ischaemic attack

A TIA is the sudden onset of neurological symptoms that completely resolve within 24 hours and for which a vascular cause is most likely. However, new evidence is challenging this definition, the traditional management plan for TIA and even the use of the term 'TIA'.

TIAs were once treated as relatively benign warning signs. However, research has now revealed that although the majority of TIAs resolve within 1 hour, a significant number cause tissue infarction (Borg & Pancioli, 2002). Patients who have had a TIA are at a much higher risk of a subsequent stroke than previously thought and

many patients will suffer a stroke within the following days: 2.5–5% at 2 days; 5–10% at 30 days; and 10–20% at 90 days (ESO, 2008).

As a result, organisations such as the National Stroke Foundation are recommending that patients who experience a TIA receive the same assessments and investigations as patients who present with active stroke symptoms (NICS, 2009). It is therefore essential that paramedics assess and manage patients whose symptoms have resolved prior to their arrival as they would any other stroke patient.

technically stroke patients, they have an area of cerebral infarction without ongoing neurological deficit. TIA should be considered a sign of impending stroke and be used as an opportunity for stroke prevention (Markus et al., 2017).

Ischaemic stroke

The location and extent of cerebral ischaemia and the clinical presentation are dependent on the location and size of the blocked vessel. Vessel occlusion in ischaemic stroke results in a central core of severe ischaemia surrounded by a less ischaemic region, commonly referred to as the ischaemic penumbra. Unless reperfusion occurs rapidly, usually within 30 minutes, neuronal tissue within the ischaemic core experiences irreversible neuronal damage and necrosis. In the ischaemic penumbra perfusion of neuronal tissue is maintained through collateral circulation and it is this area of ischaemia that may be salvaged if perfusion can be re-established.

The most common causes of ischaemic stroke are atherosclerotic disease of the large and medium-sized extra- and intracranial vessels; cardioembolism; and intracranial small vessel disease. Atherosclerotic lesions of the large and medium-sized extra- and intracranial vessels tend to occur at areas of vessel bifurcations or curves, with the most common locations being the proximal internal carotid arteries, the aortic arch and the vertebral and basilar arteries. Common sites for vessel occlusion within the cerebral circulation are the middle cerebral artery and the posterior cerebral artery (Hall, 2016). Atherosclerotic plaques can become unstable and rupture, resulting in thrombus formation. If the thrombus is large enough, complete obstruction of the vessel lumen can occur, but in many cases part of a thrombus from a proximal plaque rupture breaks away and embolises in a more distal vessel. Thrombotic/embolic stroke associated with atherosclerosis is responsible for 60% of ischaemic strokes.

Cardioembolic stroke is the result of a thrombus originating in the heart and travelling to the cerebral circulation and occluding a vessel causing disruption to blood supply to a part of the brain. Cardioembolic stroke has tripled in frequency in the past few decades in high-income countries. Moreover, cardiac embolism is associated with more severe stroke than other ischaemic stroke subtypes. Risk factors for cardioembolic stroke include atrial fibrillation, systolic cardiac failure, recent myocardial infarction, patent foramen ovale, aortic arch atheroma and infective endocarditis (Kamel & Healey, 2017).

Haemorrhagic stroke

There are two types of haemorrhagic stroke: intra-parenchymal cerebral haemorrhage (also referred to as intracerebral haemorrhage) and subarachnoid haemorrhage. Intra-parenchymal cerebral haemorrhage results from a rupture of a vessel within the intracerebral tissue, predominantly the cerebral lobes, basal ganglia, thalamus, brainstem and cerebellum. These locations are defined as lobar, deep and infratentorial. Deep intra-parenchymal haemorrhage is the most common and accounts for 45% of all intra-parenchymal haemorrhage. Lobar locations account for 30–40%, cerebellar haemorrhage 10% and brainstem 5% respectively (Boccardi et al., 2017).

Intra-parenchymal haemorrhage can have primary and secondary aetiology. The most common primary causes are hypertensive angiopathy and cerebral amyloid angiopathy. Fifty per cent of all intra-parenchymal haemorrhage is caused by hypertension resulting in hypertensive angiopathy. The mechanism causing this type of stroke is predominantly the rupturing of small perforating arteries; for example, the lenticulostriate artery, thalamus perforating arteries and arteries that originate from the basilar artery. Hypertensive angiopathy is the most common cause of intra-parenchymal haemorrhage in persons between 40 and 50 years of age. Recent studies have found systolic blood pressure to be more predictive of risk of stroke than diastolic blood pressure. The threshold for treatment of hypertension is considered greater than 140/90 mmHg. In age groups less than 60 years, 60–69 years and greater than 70 years, a decrease of systolic blood pressure by 10 mmHg was associated with a 54%, 36% and 25% lower risk of stroke respectively (Boccardi et al., 2017; Aiyagari & Gorelick, 2016).

Cerebral amyloid angiopathy (CAA) is a degenerative disorder that arises from β-amyloid protein deposition in the tunica media and adventitia of small to mid-sized cerebral arteries. The cortical and leptomeningeal arteries are often involved. β-amyloid alters the structure of the vessels causing thickening of the basal membrane, stenosis of the vessel lumen and destruction of the internal elastic lamina. The vessel becomes weak and therefore the risk of vessel rupture and haemorrhage increases. CAA accounts for 5–20% of causes of intra-parenchymal haemorrhage and predominantly associated with advancing age (Lin et al., 2018; Boccardi et al., 2017).

Subarachnoid haemorrhage (SAH) accounts for approximately 5% of all strokes. Unlike CAA, SAH predominantly affects the young. Acute SAH (aSAH) occurs when a vessel within the subarachnoid space spontaneously dissects. The majority of aSAH arises through the spontaneous dissection of an aneurysm, while a smaller number are idiopathic: 85% and

BOX 26.3 Risk factors for stroke

- Age: the risk of stroke increases significantly with age—50% of strokes or recurrent strokes occur in those > 74 years.
- Gender: men are at increased risk of stroke, although more women have a stroke due to longer life expectancy in females.
- Family history.
- Ethnicity: Aboriginal and Torres Strait Islander peoples have a higher prevalence of risk factors for stroke.
- Hypertension.
- Smoking: smokers have twice the risk of stroke than non-smokers.
- Atrial fibrillation: high risk of stroke due to thromboembolism.
- Ischaemic heart disease: doubles risk.
- Diabetes: increases risk of ischaemic stroke.
- Excessive alcohol consumption: six or more standard drinks per day increases the risk of stroke.
- Poor diet.
- Lack of exercise.
- Living in regional Australia: regional Australians are 19% more likely to suffer stroke than those living in metropolitan areas (Stroke Foundation, 2017).

10% respectively. The remaining 5% are generally associated with arteriovenous malformations and other vessel diseases. Non-modifiable risk factors related with aSAH include family history, polycystic kidney, Ehlers-Danlos syndrome and female gender. Modifiable risk factors associated with SAH include cigarette smoking, hypertension and high alcohol intake (see Box 26.3). Mortality and morbidity associated with aSAH is considerable. Mortality is as high as 45%, with 12–15% dying before they reach hospital. More than 33% of survivors remain disabled following aSAH. Impaired memory, executive functioning and attention have a deleterious effect on quality of life (Boccardi et al., 2017).

Cellular injury and death in stroke

Decreased cerebral blood flow resulting from ischaemia causes hypoxia of the neuronal cells. Cellular injury and death results from similar biochemical mechanisms in both ischaemic and haemorrhagic strokes. Common biochemical mechanisms include adenosine triphosphate (ATP) depletion, mitochondrial damage, the production of free radicals and cell membrane damage.

Hypoxic cells switch from aerobic to anaerobic metabolism, resulting in decreased adenosine triphosphate stores (ATP), intracellular acidosis and neurotransmitter release. In response to the decrease in ATP, ionic pumps in the cell membranes that regulate intra- and extracellular ion movements fail, resulting in an influx of sodium and calcium ions into the cells. Increased intracellular calcium leads to damage and subsequent death of neuronal cells through multiple mechanisms including the activation of intracellular enzymes, the production of oxygen-free radicals and irreversible damage to the cell mitochondria. Sodium influx results in swelling of neuronal cells, cerebral oedema and raised intracranial pressure. Reperfusion of ischaemic tissue, either spontaneous or following reperfusion therapy, can result in further neuronal cell injury and death (McCance & Huether, 2018).

Clinical manifestations

The sudden disruption of blood supply to various parts of the brain can cause alterations in perception, sensation, movement, personality and expression. These alterations are directly related to the area of the brain affected by the ischaemia (see Fig 26.4). The presence of blood in the tissues, particularly in the subarachnoid space, can also cause symptoms such as pain and photophobia. The location and type of symptoms can provide an indication of which vessel may be involved (see Table 26.2).

Motor deficits

Weakness of the limbs is the most obvious effect of stroke. Because the motor neurons cross sides at the level of the medulla, infarcted tissue on one side of the brain will manifest in an effect on the limb on the opposite side. Initially the affected limb will suffer from a loss of muscle tone (this usually develops into spasticity over days or weeks) and shoulders will tend to drop and rotate inwardly, while hips will rotate externally when the patient is supine. Because the facial muscles are innervated above the medulla, the loss of muscle tone on the face will be on the same side as the lesion. Limb pain is uncommon in acute stroke but there may be alterations of sensation such as paraesthesia. It is also possible for the patient to 'neglect' the affected limb (see the section on spatial awareness below) and allow it to be accidentally injured during transfers and procedures.

Communication

Depending on the area affected, patients can suffer aphasia. Aphasia and dysphasia refer to the inability to understand both spoken and written language. It can take several weeks to determine the extent

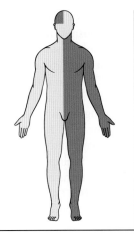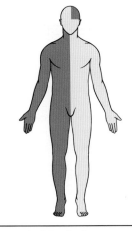

Right-brain damage (stroke on right side of the brain)	**Left-brain damage** (stroke on left side of the brain)
• Paralysed left side: hemiplegia	• Paralysed right side: hemiplegia
• Left-sided neglect	• Impaired speech/language aphasias
• Spatial–perceptual deficits	• Impaired right/left discrimination
• Tends to deny or minimise problems	• Slow performance, cautious
• Rapid performance, short attention span	• Aware of deficits: depression, anxiety
• Impulsive, safety problems	• Impaired comprehension related to language, mathematics
• Impaired judgement	
• Impaired time concepts	

Figure 26.4
Manifestations of right-brain and left-brain stroke.
Source: Brown & Edwards (2012).

of a patient's dysphasia and during the acute phase it can be very difficult to know whether instructions and advice are actually understood. One aspect of an expressive dysphasia is replying 'no' when the patient actually means 'yes', and vice versa. Stroke can also cause dysarthria, a motor speech disorder. Some stroke patients are able to understand language but are unable to make themselves understood due to dysarthria.

Affect, intellect and personality

Changes to personality and emotional expression are common manifestations of stroke and can occur during the acute stage. A 'flat' affect and lack of concern during the acute phase are not uncommon and should be considered as signs of neurological changes—not that the patient is actually unconcerned and therefore not needing treatment. Although not typical during the hyperacute and acute phases, the extent and location of the stroke can affect judgment and reasoning. Patients with a left-sided stroke may take longer to make decisions, while those with a right-sided stroke may appear to act before considering the consequences. This can affect the way patients follow instructions; for example, while being transferred onto and off a stretcher.

Spatial awareness

Stroke can lead to a number of problems with spatial awareness. Depending on the extent and location of the stroke, patients may 'neglect' their affected side and fail to protect it from injury. This can occur due to the brain's inability to process any information from the affected side or to homonymous hemianopsia—blindness in the same half of both visual fields (see Fig 26.5). Patients may also suffer from an inability to recognise objects by name (agnosia). All these factors are important considerations when taking a history or giving a patient instructions on how to move on and off a stretcher.

Stroke mimics

Stroke mimics are neurological or psychiatric conditions that display similar symptomology to that of stroke including seizure, dementia, migraine or headache, vertigo, conversion disorder, electrolyte imbalance, brain tumour or other cerebral disease (Forster et al., 2012). Some of the clinical manifestations of stroke can also be caused by prescription

Table 26.2 Clinical manifestations: specific cerebral artery involvement

Cerebral artery involved	Clinical manifestations
Middle cerebral artery	Contralateral weakness (hemiparesis) or plysis (hemiplegia) Contralateral hemianaesthesia; loss of proprioception, fine touch, localisation Dominant hemisphere: aphasia Non-dominant hemisphere: neglect of opposite side, anosognosia Homonymous hemianopsia
Anterior cerebral artery	Occlusion of stem* Occlusion distal to anterior communicating artery Contralateral sensory and motor deficits of foot and leg, greatest distally Contralateral weakness of proximal upper extremity Urinary incontinence (possibly unrecognised by patient) Sensory loss (discrimination, proprioception) Contralateral grasp and sucking reflexes may be present Apraxia Personality change: flat affect, loss of spontaneity, loss of interest in surroundings, distractibility, slowness in responding Possible cognitive impairment
Posterior cerebral artery and vertebrobasilar arteries†	Alert to comatose Unilateral or bilateral sensory loss Contralateral or bilateral weakness Dysarthria Dysphagia Hoarseness Ataxia Horner's syndrome: miosis, ptosis, decreased sweating Vertigo Unilateral hearing loss Nausea, vomiting Visual disturbances (blindness, homonymous hemianopsia, nystagmus, diplopia)

*There is usually no problem if the stem is occluded near the anterior communicating artery because perfusion from the opposite side is maintained.

†The site of occlusion, the origin of the basilar arteries and the arrangement of the circle of Willis are involved in the type of deficit seen. This can occur from a thrombus or embolus.

Source: Brown & Edwards (2012).

medications, illicit drugs, alcohol, hypotension or hypoglycaemia. Stroke mimics are quite common. One Norwegian study found of the 1881 admissions to a stroke unit, 45% (*n* = 847) were diagnosed as stroke, 16.7% (*n* = 315) as TIA and 38.2% (*n* = 719) as stroke mimics (Faiz et al., 2018). In the out-of-hospital setting, any differential diagnosis of the above should include stroke to ensure that stroke is not missed.

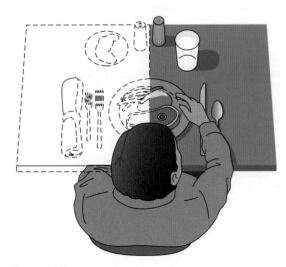

Figure 26.5
Spatial and perceptual deficits in stroke.
Neglect or homonymous hemianopsia can leave a patient unaware or everything on a particular side. This figure shows that food on the left side is not seen and thus is ignored.
Source: Brown & Edwards (2012).

CASE STUDY 1

Case 20105, 2014 hrs.

Dispatch details: A 75-year-old male, confused and with slurred speech.

Initial presentation: The patient's son directs the paramedics into the restaurant where the patient is sitting in a chair. He is sitting upright although supported by a family member. He is conscious but not speaking.

1 ASSESS

Patient history

The acute onset of neurological symptoms is probably the single most important factor in the out-of-hospital diagnosis of stroke. Ischaemic and haemorrhagic strokes are typically acute, sudden events with immediate onset of neurological clinical symptoms and signs. Paramedics should attempt to ascertain as precisely as possible the time of onset of symptoms, as this information is critical in determining a patient's eligibility for reperfusion therapy in the setting of ischaemic stroke. However, often it is impossible to determine the exact time of symptom onset, such as when a patient wakes up with neurological symptoms. In such cases the time of onset is determined as the time at which the patient was last seen without neurological symptoms.

Patients should be questioned regarding the presence of other symptoms (see Table 26.3) and their temporal relationship to those that precipitated the emergency call. Symptoms of ischaemic stroke are dependent on the location and degree of ischaemia. Patients, family members and bystanders should be questioned regarding the observance of any seizure activity and whether the patient had a period of unconsciousness.

Table 26.3 The most common symptoms and signs of stroke and their reliability

Symptom or sign	Prevalence (%)
Acute onset	96
Hemiparesis	87
Facial palsy	79
Sensory loss	62
Dysarthria	48
Disorientation	43
Aphasia	41
Horizontal gaze palsy	37
Visuospatial neglect	14
Visual field loss	7
Headache	3
Seizure	2

Source: Forster et al. (2012).

Seizures in an elderly patient with no history of seizures should always be treated with a suspicion of stroke. Todd's paresis is a transient hemiplegia that can occur in the post-ictal phase following a seizure, but stroke should always be considered as a more likely cause in patients who do not have a history of seizures.

Obtaining a comprehensive and accurate past medical history, including current medication, is essential as this information can determine a patient's eligibility for thrombolytic therapy. The past medical history is also important in assessing for alternative diagnoses, as well as identifying risk factors that the patient may have for stroke. It is common for a person suffering a stroke to display symptoms days to weeks prior to the event. Ascertaining a history of atrial fibrillation, headache, neurological deficits (e.g. limb weakness, difficulty grasping objects) and risk factors for stroke is crucial. Paramedics should inquire about signs and symptoms of TIA. While TIA signs and symptoms often resolve, they can be a precursor to a stroke (Australian Bureau of Statistics, 2017).

Airway
Stroke patients with an altered level of consciousness are at risk of airway obstruction due to mechanical obstruction from the tongue and aspiration of secretions and gastric contents. Conscious patients who present with dysphagia or paralysis of the facial and pharyngeal muscles are unable to effectively manage their secretions and are at risk of airway obstruction and aspiration. Acutely, airway obstruction from either mechanical obstruction or secretions can result in hypoxia. Aspiration of airway secretions and gastric contents can result in delayed complications such as pulmonary infections and is a common secondary complication of stroke.

Breathing
Breathing is generally not affected by stroke directly; however, stroke affecting the respiratory centre in the brainstem or increased intracranial pressure from an intracerebral haemorrhage or cerebral oedema can affect respiration. The most common effect on respiration will be due to airway obstruction, which can result in hypoxia and hypercarbia, both of which worsen cerebral ischaemia.

Neurological
Besides the history, the most important clinical information will be obtained from performing a comprehensive neurological assessment. A detailed assessment can be particularly essential in rural areas where access to treatment may be limited and establishing a baseline neurological assessment can identify a worsening condition. There are a number of screening tools designed to assess acute stroke (see Box 26.4 and Table 26.5), but the components always include assessment of:
- level of consciousness
- visual defects, eye movements and pupil size, response and symmetry
- speech
- facial symmetry
- sensation
- motor strength
- coordination.

Reduced level of consciousness is an uncommon finding in acute ischaemic or intracerebral stroke, but a period of loss of consciousness or a sustained altered conscious state is common in subarachnoid haemorrhage. Deterioration in the level of consciousness may occur over time in all forms of stroke due to the increasing size of the intracerebral haematoma or cerebral oedema.

Changes in pupil size and reactivity are usually late signs of raised intracerebral pressure. A better assessment for stroke is to assess gaze and visual fields. Ask the patient to follow your laterally tracking finger to assess gaze and check the

HISTORY

Ask!
Ask about:
- nature of onset (acute, subacute, chronic, insidious)
- time of symptom onset
- course (static, progressive, relapsing, remitting)
- previous episodes of neurological symptoms
- any seizure activity
- headache
- nausea
- dizziness
- auras.

HISTORY

Assess!
- Conscious state
- Visual fields
- Speech
- Facial symmetry
- Unilateral sensory deficits
- Unilateral motor deficits
- Coordination

BOX 26.4 Out-of-hospital stroke screening tools

A number of validated out-of-hospital stroke screening tools have been developed to assist paramedics in identifying stroke patients, particularly those who may be eligible for reperfusion therapy: these include the Melbourne Ambulance Stroke Screen (MASS), the Pre-hospital Acute Stroke Triage (PAST), the Cincinnati Pre-hospital Stroke Scale (CPSS), Los Angeles Motor Scale for assessment of stroke severity with high likelihood of large vessel occlusion (LAMS, see Table 26.4) and the Los Angeles Pre-hospital Stroke Screen (LAPSS). Other stroke screening tools, such as the Recognition of Stroke in the Emergency Room (ROSIER), initially developed for use in the ED, are also used by some out-of-hospital services. In addition, tools such as FAST have been used to educate the public to recognise stroke symptoms (Stroke Foundation, 2017).

Out-of-hospital stroke screening tools typically use a number of history items designed to identify potential stroke mimics and those unlikely to be candidates for reperfusion therapy, as well as physical assessment items commonly associated with stroke. For the majority of screening tools the criteria for identifying stroke are that all of the history items must be answered 'yes' and the patient has at least one physical assessment item. Most of the tools used in out-of-hospital practice have good sensitivity for identifying stroke and can be undertaken as the initial assessment of patients presenting with neurological symptoms. If the result is positive, paramedics can begin the process of expediting patient transfer as a priority. Unfortunately, however, some tools do not have good sensitivity for stroke identification. It is important to understand that although a patient may have a negative result using an out-of-hospital tool, this does not exclude the diagnosis of stroke; see Table 26.5.

Table 26.4 Las Angeles Motor Scale (LAMS) and the face, arm, speech, time scale for identification of stroke symptoms

LAMS stroke scale	Score
Facial droop: one side of the face does not move as well as the other	0 = absent 1 = present
Arm drift	0 = absent 1 = drifts down 2 = falls rapidly
Grip strength	0 = normal 1 = weak grip 2 = no grip
FAST: Face Arm Speech Time Scale	Description
Facial droop	One side of the face does not move as well as the other
Arm drift	One arm does not move or drifts downwards when held extended
Speech	The patient slurs words, uses the wrong word or cannot speak at all
Time	Get help immediately—immediate transportation to a stroke unit or appropriate facility

Source: Fassbender et al. (2013).

visual fields by wiggling your fingers on both sides of the patient's head simultaneously to assess for inattention or hemianopia.

The acronym FAST is commonly used in the assessment of stroke: face, arms, speech and time.

Facial symmetry is assessed by asking the patient to smile or show their teeth and observing for equal movement of both sides of the face. In normal facial symmetry both sides move equally: an abnormal response occurs if one side does not move. Asking the patient to raise their eyebrows and frown can be useful if Bell's palsy is suspected (see Box 26.5).

Table 26.5 National Institutes of Health Stroke Scale (NIHSS)

NIHSS item	Score
1a. Level of consciousness	0 = alert; keenly responsive 1 = not alert, but arousable by minor stimulation to obey, answer or respond 2 = not alert, requires repeated stimulation to attend, or is obtunded and requires strong or painful stimulation to make movements 3 = responds only with reflex motor or autonomic effects or totally unresponsive, flaccid or flexed
1b. Level of consciousness questions (month and age)	0 = answers both questions correctly 1 = answers one question correctly 2 = answers neither question correctly
1c. Level of consciousness commands (opens and closes eyes; grips and releases non-paretic hand)	0 = performs both tasks correctly 1 = performs one task correctly 2 = performs neither task correctly
2. Best gaze (horizontal movements)	0 = normal 1 = partial gaze palsy 2 = forced deviation or total gaze paresis
3. Visual fields (upper and lower quadrants)	0 = no visual loss 1 = partial hemianopsia 2 = complete hemianopsia 3 = bilateral hemianopsia (blind, including cortical blindness)
4. Facial palsy	0 = normal symmetrical movement 1 = minor paralysis (flattened nasolabial fold, asymmetry on smiling) 2 = partial paralysis (total or near total paralysis of lower face) 3 = complete paralysis of one or both sides (absence of facial movement in the upper and lower face)
5. and 6. Motor arm and leg (drift is scored if the arm falls before 10 seconds or the leg before 5 seconds)	5a and b = left and right arm (respectively) 6a and b = left and right leg (respectively) 0 = no drift, limb holds 90° (or 45°) for full 10 seconds 1 = drift, limb holds 90° (or 45°), but drifts down before full 10 seconds; does not hit bed or other supports 2 = some effort against gravity, limb cannot get to or maintain 90° (or 45°), drifts down to bed, but has some effort against gravity 3 = no effort against gravity; limb falls 4 = no movement UN = amputation
7. Limb ataxia	0 = absent 1 = present in 1 limb 2 = present in 2 limbs
8. Sensory	0 = normal 1 = mild to moderate sensory loss (patient feels pinprick is less sharp on the affected side) 2 = severe to total sensory loss (patient is not aware of being touched on the face, arm or leg)
9. Best language	0 = no aphasia; normal 1 = mild to moderate aphasia (some obvious loss of fluency without significant limitation of ideas) 2 = severe aphasia (all communication is through fragmentary expression; great need for inference) 3 = mute; global aphasia (no usable speech)
10. Dysarthria	0 = normal 1 = mild to moderate (patient slurs at least some words) 2 = severe (patient's speech is so slurred as to be unintelligible in the absence of or out of proportion to any dysphasia or is mute)
11. Extinction	0 = no abnormality 1 = visual, tactile, auditory, spatial or personal inattention or extinction to bilateral simultaneous stimulation in one of these sensory modalities 2 = profound hemi-inattention or hemi-inattention to more than one modality; does not recognise own hand or orients to only one side of space

Source: https://www.mdcalc.com/nih-stroke-scale-score-nihss

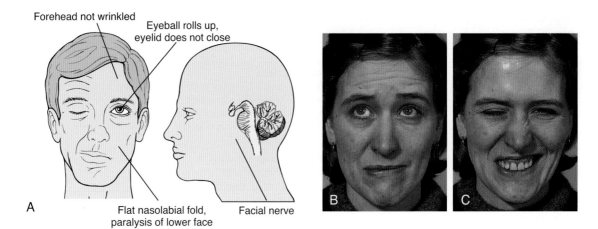

Figure 26.6
Facial characteristics of Bell's palsy.
A and **B** At rest the face may look almost normal but the patient is not able to wrinkle their forehead on the affected side and the right corner of the mouth droops. **C** When the patient is asked to close their eyes and show their teeth, the differences between the affected and unaffected sides become more obvious.
Source: Forbes & Jackson (2003).

BOX 26.5 Bell's palsy

The sudden onset of one-sided facial drop caused by Bell's palsy is understandably often confused with stroke. The condition is not related to cerebral ischaemia but is a disorder of the facial nerve (CN VII) that leads to a temporary paralysis of the muscles on one side of the face (see Fig 26.6). Bell's palsy normally has a gradual onset, unlike a stroke. The cause is unknown and 85% of patients will recover all function within 6 months. Bell's palsy can develop within hours and cause significant facial droop with an inability to close the eyelid (an upward movement of the eyeball when closure is attempted is common). Unlike the facial droop caused by stroke, which is an upper motor neuron lesion, the patient with Bell's palsy will not be able to raise the eyebrow or wrinkle the forehead on the affected side (a lower motor neuron lesion). Bell's palsy should be considered when a patient presents with significant facial droop but no other signs of stroke.

To assess hand grip strength place several of your fingers in the patient's hand and ask them to squeeze your fingers. A normal response is recorded if both hands grip equally or not at all. An abnormal response is recorded if there is unilateral weakness or no grip. Arm drift is assessed by having the patient close their eyes and asking them to extend both arms out in front of them to 90° with the palms facing upwards for 10 seconds. If supine, have the patient hold their arms at a 45° angle for 10 seconds. A normal response is recorded if both arms move or don't move at all. An abnormal response is recorded if one arm does not move or one arm drifts downwards compared to the other. Leg drift is assessed by asking the patient to lift the legs to 30° and hold for 10 seconds. A normal response is recorded if both legs move or don't move at all. An abnormal response is recorded if one leg does not move or one leg drifts downwards compared to the other leg.

Assess leg strength and balance by having the patient stand and walk, if able. Ataxia is indicative of a cerebellar involvement. If the patient is unable to stand, assess for truncal ataxia with the patient in the sitting position.

Assess sensation by touching both sides of the patient's body on the legs, arms and face and check for symmetry.

To assess speech ask the patient to repeat a sentence; for example, 'You can't teach an old dog new tricks'. Dysphasia is present if they use incorrect words, have difficulty articulating words or are unable to speak. Dysarthria is present if the words are poorly formed. Using incorrect words and dysphasia are more sensitive for stroke than slurring alone, as slurring is nonspecific for stroke.

Time is critical in stroke management. It is important to establish the time of onset of the symptoms and to limit time to definitive treatment. Scene time should be minimised and notification to the receiving facility provided with estimated time of arrival provided (Stroke Foundation, 2017).

Cardiovascular

Hypotension is rare following acute stroke and its presence should alert the paramedic to consider other causes of hypotension. Hypertension is an independent risk factor for stroke, and acute stroke patients frequently present with an elevated blood pressure, but hypertension in isolation is not specific for stroke diagnosis. Extreme hypertension is usually a sign of profoundly raised intracranial pressure and is usually associated with a low Glasgow Coma Scale (GCS) score. Conversely, profound hypotension can cause stroke-like symptoms in patients with advanced atherosclerosis in cerebral arteries. In the absence of normal blood pressure, these plaques can restrict normal blood flow. Assessment of cardiac rhythm may indicate the cause of stroke. Cardioembolism as a result of atrial fibrillation is a common cause of ischaemic stroke, accounting for approximately 20% of cases of ischaemic stroke in most populations. The risk of developing atrial fibrillation is age related as shown in Figure 26.7 (Markus et al., 2017).

> ## CARDIOVASCU-LAR STATUS
> **Look for!**
> - Arrhythmia
> - Acute myocardial infarction
> - Prosthetic valves
> - Cardiomyopathy
> - Septal defects
> - Rheumatic valve disease

Initial assessment summary

Problem	Loss of sensation in his right side: query stroke
Conscious state	GCS = 15
Position	Sitting in a lounge chair
Heart rate	84 bpm
Blood pressure	155/95 mmHg
Skin appearance	Pink and dry
Speech pattern	Slurred speech
Respiratory rate	20 bpm
Respiratory rhythm	Even cycles
Respiratory effort	Normal
Chest auscultation	Clear bilaterally
Pulse oximetry	98% on room air
Temperature	37.1°C
Motor/sensory function	The patient has no sensation to touch in the right arm and leg, is unable to lift his right arm or leg, has an absent hand grip on the right and has a right-sided facial droop

D: The patient is sitting in a chair, but his right side needs to be protected.
A: The patient is conscious with no current airway obstruction.
B: Respiratory function is currently normal.
C: Heart rate is normal.

The patient's presentation is consistent with a stroke.

② CONFIRM

The essential part of the clinical reasoning process is to seek to confirm your initial hypothesis by finding clinical signs that should concur with your

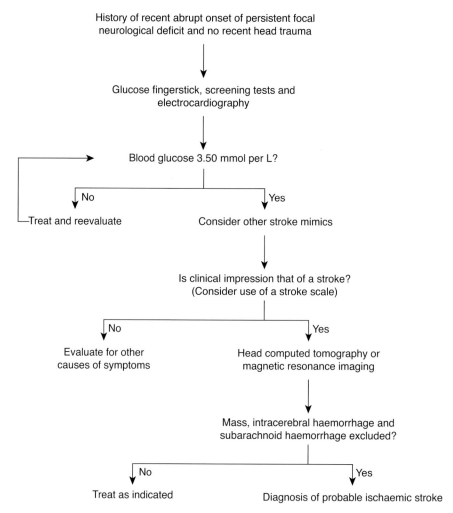

History of recent abrupt onset of persistent focal neurological deficit and no recent head trauma

Glucose fingerstick, screening tests and electrocardiography

Blood glucose 3.50 mmol per L?

No — Treat and reevaluate

Yes — Consider other stroke mimics

Is clinical impression that of a stroke? (Consider use of a stroke scale)

No — Evaluate for other causes of symptoms

Yes — Head computed tomography or magnetic resonance imaging

Mass, intracerebral haemorrhage and subarachnoid haemorrhage excluded?

No — Treat as indicated

Yes — Diagnosis of probable ischaemic stroke

Figure 26.7
Algorithm for the diagnosis of acute stroke.
Source: Yew & Cheng (2009).

DIFFERENTIAL DIAGNOSIS

Stroke
Or
- Seizure
- Hypoglycaemia
- Other metabolic/toxic disturbances
- Syncope/hypotension
- Infection
- Intoxication/overdose

provisional diagnosis. You should also seek to challenge your diagnosis by exploring findings that do *not* fit your hypothesis: don't just ignore them because they don't fit.

Stroke is a clinical diagnosis and is made on the basis of the history and physical assessment. Differentiating between haemorrhagic and ischaemic stroke cannot be made reliably on clinical signs alone and requires neuroimaging—using computerised tomographic (CT) scanning or MRI—to make the diagnosis. Figure 26.7 outlines a typical diagnostic algorithm. The diagnosis of acute stroke should be made with an awareness of stroke mimics and the exclusion of as many as possible.

Stroke mimics: What else could it be?

Stroke mimics are conditions that present with neurological or psychiatric signs and symptoms that can be mistaken for acute stroke. However, stroke mimics are disorders that differ from stroke in clinical presentation. Stroke mimics often present with aphasia and convulsions, which are presentations less aligned with stroke. Stroke mimics less often present with typical stroke presentations which include dysarthria, facial palsy, hemiparesis and horizontal gaze palsy (Forster et al., 2012).

Seizure

Like strokes, seizures have a rapid onset of neurological symptoms and following a seizure the patient may have persistent neurological symptoms similar to a stroke, including Todd's paresis. Approximately 5% of ischaemic stroke patients will experience acute symptomatic seizure, with 50% occurring within the first 24 hours following stroke onset. Haemorrhagic stroke can also be associated with seizure presentation (Alme et al., 2016). Patients presenting with seizure should be transported for further investigation in order to identify or exclude the occurrence of acute stroke.

In the opening case study there is no history of seizure activity having occurred and no past history of a seizure disorder. The patient does not have incontinence, which can be indicative of both seizures and a loss of consciousness.

Hypoglycaemia and other metabolic/toxic disturbances

Brain cells do not have the ability to store large amounts of glucose and a fall in blood glucose level (BGL) can result in the sudden onset of focal neurological signs including decreased level of consciousness, slurred speech, aphasia, blindness and gait disturbances. Severe hypoglycaemia can be associated with hypoglycaemic hemiparesis. This condition is characterised by unilateral motor weakness with concurrent mild or moderate alteration of consciousness. Persons presenting with hypoglycaemia with focal neurological signs should be transported to hospital for further investigation as often there is an underlying cerebral pathology associated with this presentation (Ohshita et al., 2015). Hypoglycaemia can be readily identified by paramedics using glucometry and the condition can be treated effectively with intravenous (IV) glucose or intramuscular glucagon (see Ch 25). A BGL should be taken for any patient suspected of having a stroke in order to exclude hypoglycaemia. Altered level of consciousness is uncommon in acute stroke unless it involves the brainstem, a very large intracerebral haemorrhage or a subarachnoid haemorrhage. An altered level of consciousness should alert the paramedic to look for metabolic/toxic causes including hypoglycaemia and alcohol or drug intoxication.

Syncope/hypotension

Syncope is described as a self-limiting transient loss of consciousness and postural tone due to global cerebral hypoperfusion. In older adults, it is often due to chronic medical conditions, comorbidities and polypharmacy. Syncope can be categorised as neurally mediated syncope, vasovagal syncope, orthostatic hypotension and cardiac syncope (Goyal & Maurer, 2016; Yasa et al., 2018). Motor weakness following syncope is usually generalised rather than unilateral. Syncope and hypotension generally respond to positioning supine and IV fluid replacement.

Infection

Systemic infection and sepsis can present with stroke-like symptoms including weakness, incoordination and abnormal speech, or can worsen already-existing deficits in patients with previous stroke or other neurological conditions such as dementia and Parkinson's disease. In these cases, the neurological symptoms usually have a more gradual onset and there are other signs present indicating infection, such as fever, hyper/hypothermia, tachypnoea, tachycardia, cough and dysuria. Sepsis accounts for 6–20% of stroke mimics. Coma, weakness and speech changes are due to neuro-inflammatory response and blood brain dysfunction. Fever may not be present in older patients (Long & Koyfman, 2017).

Intoxication/overdose

Alcohol and sedatives can cause drowsiness, ataxia and slurred speech but rarely hemiparesis. Even with ingestion of the above, the presence of hemiparesis should direct the diagnosis towards stroke.

Other stroke mimics

Other disorders that may give rise to stroke-like presentations include vertigo, other cerebrovascular conditions, neoplasms, headache and migraine auras, other neurological conditions, urinary system disorders and psychiatric disorders (Faiz et al., 2018; Dawson et al., 2016).

TREAT

Emergency management

Transport

Stroke patients should be managed as a time-critical emergency. Scene time should be minimised and non-essential interventions should not delay transportation. Acute ischaemic stroke patients have demonstrated improved outcomes following early reperfusion therapies (Stroke Foundation, 2017). Treatment should commence within 3–4.5 hours from the onset of an acute ischaemic stroke. The earlier treatment regimens are commenced, the greater the benefit demonstrated. Reperfusion treatment administered in less than 3 hours following the onset of acute ischaemic stroke has been associated with significantly reduced morbidity and mortality at 3–6 months. Optimal outcomes have been noted prior to the 1.5-hour mark. Benefits decrease as time progresses. Reperfusion therapy administered between 4.5 and 6 hours is associated with insignificant benefit (Fassbender et al., 2013; Emberson et al., 2014; Wardlaw et al., 2014).

Stroke patients should, where possible, be transported directly to a facility capable of administering reperfusion therapies, has neurosurgical capability and has a dedicated stroke care unit. The receiving facility should be notified of the patient's pending arrival and an estimated time of arrival provided. Improved outcomes have been demonstrated with pre-notification because of decreased time to administration of reperfusion therapies (Stroke Foundation, 2017). The benefit of upper body elevation during transportation is unclear. Limited evidence has suggested the higher the angle of upper body elevation, the lower the cerebral blood flow velocity in acute ischaemic stroke. Current evidence favours the supine position with 0° of upper body elevation (Hunter et al., 2011; Wojner-Alexandrov et al., 2005).

Airway

The airway in stroke patients can become compromised due to mechanical obstruction or the build-up of secretions, particularly in those with dysphagia. Acutely, obstruction can lead to hypoxia and secretions can result in aspiration, leading to secondary complications such as pneumonia. The airway of the stroke patient requires meticulous management in the out-of-hospital setting. In the patient with a decreased level of consciousness airway adjuncts ranging from oropharyngeal and nasopharyngeal airways to endotracheal intubation may be required to secure a patent airway and provide airway protection (see Box 26.6). Frequent suctioning may be required, even in a conscious patient, to clear airway secretions.

Ventilation

The majority of ischaemic stroke patients have normal breathing, the rare exception being those who have a brainstem stroke affecting the respiratory centres and those with significantly raised intracranial pressure leading to brainstem herniation. In these circumstances suitable patients may benefit from endotracheal intubation and controlled ventilation.

Oxygen therapy

Ischaemic stroke patients who present with hypoxaemia as demonstrated by an arterial oxygen saturation below 94% should receive supplemental oxygen therapy to maintain the SpO_2 above 94% and routine use of oxygen in patients with mild to moderate stroke who are not hypoxaemic may worsen the outcome. Studies have demonstrated no reduction in death or disability at 3 months

BOX 26.6 Advanced airway management in stroke patients

Patients who have suffered a stroke often present with both a decreased conscious state and aspiration. In these circumstances it is worth considering the need (or otherwise) to manage the patient's airway and ventilation with an endotracheal tube. While endotracheal intubation provides control of ventilation and FiO_2 there are a number of risks and drawbacks that should be considered. For example, stroke patients may score low on the GCS due to dysphasia but may otherwise have a good conscious state. They will require significant sedation to enable intubation and this may impact on blood pressure and cerebral perfusion. Intubation also limits the ability to conduct a physical neurological assessment when the patient arrives at hospital. Other issues that should be considered with every intubation include:

• the consequences of a failed intubation
• the consequences of an unrecognised oesophageal intubation.

While these variables can appear confusing and vague, the solution is relatively simple. Where the oxygen saturation cannot be kept above 90–92% using oxygen and non-invasive airway support, the potential harm of widespread cerebral hypoxia outweighs the risks associated with advanced airway management. In case study 4 the patient responds well to oxygen therapy and while he is likely to be intubated at hospital, it can be done in the safest and most supported environment. If the patient had not responded well, intubation should have been considered.

with the routine administration of oxygen in non-hypoxaemic acute stroke patients. Therefore, oxygen administration for non-hypoxaemic acute stroke patients is not recommended (Roffe et al., 2017; Stroke Foundation, 2017).

Control of blood pressure

Acute stroke, either ischaemic or haemorrhagic, rarely results in hypotension, and the presence of hypotension should prompt the paramedic to consider other diagnoses. Hypertension is common following acute stroke and there is controversy regarding when and by how much hypertension should be treated. Lowering the blood pressure during acute stroke can result in decreased cerebral perfusion pressure with subsequent worsening of cerebral ischaemia. Unless there are secondary complications of severe hypertension, such as acute pulmonary oedema or ischaemic chest pain, paramedics should not attempt to reduce the blood pressure. If other complications are present, medications to lower the blood pressure should be used cautiously to prevent precipitous drops in systemic arterial pressure. In addition, paramedics performing advanced airway procedures such as rapid sequence induction (RSI) with intubation should be mindful of the hypotensive effects of the drugs being used and whenever possible prevent precipitous decreases in blood pressure during and following the procedure.

If hypotension or hypovolaemia is observed in the presence of stroke, it should be corrected to support systemic perfusion. However, the blood pressure level to be maintained is uncertain. Further study is required to investigate the volume and duration of parenteral fluid resuscitation in hypovolaemia and concurrent stroke (American Heart Association American Stroke Association, 2018).

Intravenous access

Patients presenting with acute stroke have a life-threatening condition and it is appropriate to establish IV access in any seriously ill patient. While the majority of stroke patients will not require any specific intervention out of hospital, there is the potential for stroke patients to deteriorate acutely and require further intervention. Although obtaining IV access is appropriate in the stroke patient, transport should not be delayed to accomplish it.

Electrocardiograph

A 12-lead ECG is recommended to screen for atrial fibrillation and other potentially lethal dysrhythmias (American Heart Association American Stroke Association, 2018).

Blood glucose levels (BGL)

Hypoglycaemia should be corrected in patients with acute ischaemic stroke (American Heart Association American Stroke Association, 2018).

Prevention of injury and pressure necrosis

Stroke patients are at significant risk of developing pressure necrosis and subsequent ulceration is a common secondary complication of stroke. Likewise, they are at risk of injury if they have a paralysed limb and paramedics should be vigilant in protecting affected limbs from iatrogenic injury during treatment and transfer. If transport is prolonged the patient's position should be changed at least every 30 minutes wherever practical to reduce the risk of pressure necrosis. If it is not possible to change the patient's position, the paramedic should consider providing extra protection to vulnerable areas such as the occiput, sacrum, heels and elbows.

(4) EVALUATE

Evaluating the effect of any clinical management intervention can provide clues to the accuracy of the initial diagnosis. Some conditions respond rapidly to treatment so patients should be expected to improve if the diagnosis and treatment were appropriate. A failure to improve in this situation should trigger the clinician to reconsider the diagnosis.

It is not possible to reliably distinguish between ischaemic and haemorrhagic stroke without the use of neuroradiology. Throughout the out-of-hospital phase of care paramedics need to frequently reassess patients for signs of deterioration. While most ischaemic stroke patients are unlikely to deteriorate, patients with haemorrhagic stroke often have an increase in intracerebral bleeding within the first few hours of stroke and subsequent deterioration in level of consciousness due to increased intracranial pressure. This has particular importance for paramedics working in areas with longer transport times to hospitals or where hospitals are bypassed in favour of regionalised stroke care in major stroke centres.

Patients whose level of consciousness deteriorates may benefit from out-of-hospital endotracheal intubation, controlled ventilation and, in some cases, osmotic diuretics to manage the raised intracranial pressure. In such cases paramedics should consider requesting support from intensive care providers early if the patient is demonstrating signs of clinical deterioration and the journey to the hospital is going to be prolonged.

TAKE CARE!

- Secondary injury can occur easily to paralysed limbs.
- Pressure necrosis and secondary ulceration are common complications of stroke: protect vulnerable areas.

Ongoing management

When a patient arrives at the emergency department (ED) the priority is to perform a rapid clinical assessment and obtain a CT scan to exclude a haemorrhagic stroke. While this is being performed a detailed assessment will be conducted to exclude other diagnoses that may be mimicking stroke and to obtain a stroke severity grading, as well as to obtain information regarding the patient's eligibility for reperfusion therapy.

Thrombolysis with recombinant tissue plasminogen activator (rtPA) drugs initiated within 4.5 hours of symptom onset has been demonstrated to reduce disability from stroke, although the best outcomes will be achieved if thrombolysis can be administered within 3 hours. Trials are currently being conducted that extend the timeframe to 9 hours in selected patients. While systemic thrombolysis with rtPA is the most common form of reperfusion therapy, some institutions are able to perform neuro-interventions including intraarterial rtPA, mechanical clot retrieval and vascular stenting in selected patients. Commonly used rtPA drugs include alteplase and tenecteplase. Patients ineligible for reperfusion therapy who are diagnosed with ischaemic stroke will generally be commenced on anti-platelet therapy such as aspirin ± dipyridamole or clopidogrel. Patients with atrial fibrillation will usually be commenced on anticoagulation therapy with warfarin or dabigatran.

Intracranial aneurysm is a common cause of haemorrhagic stroke. The treatment of intracranial aneurysm has increasingly moved towards intracranial endovascular use of balloon and stent, referred to as the balloon remodelling technique (BRT). Previously wide-necked intracranial aneurysms were considered untreatable; however, improvements in flow diversion techniques and the development of the BRT and stent-assisted coiling technique (SACT) have achieved good outcomes in stroke prevention (Piotin & Blanc cited in Al-Ali, 2015).

Intracranial vasospasm is a phenomenon often seen following subarachnoid haemorrhage and is a significant source of morbidity and mortality in persons suffering aneurysmal subarachnoid haemorrhage. Vasospasm is thought to account for as much as 50% of the deaths in patients who survive the initial aneurysm rupture and subsequent treatment. The main treatment regimens for vasospasm in subarachnoid haemorrhage patients is intraarterial vasodilators and balloon angioplasty (Baurer & Rasmussen cited in Al-Ali, 2015).

Investigations

The most important initial in-hospital investigation in a suspected stroke patient is a CT scan to exclude a haemorrhagic stroke. Other investigations are conducted to exclude stroke mimics and to attempt to identify the underlying cause of the stroke. Common investigations include echocardiography to assess for intracardiac thrombus and other heart conditions, carotid ultrasonography to assess for carotid stenosis, and baseline troponin levels; however, this should not delay initiation of IV alteplase or other reperfusion

> **BOX 26.7 Secondary complications of stroke**
> - Recurrent stroke
> - Seizures
> - Infections (e.g. urinary tract infection, pneumonia)
> - Pressure necrosis/ulceration
> - Falls
> - Deep vein thrombosis/pulmonary embolism
> - Pain
> - Depression

therapies (American Heart Association American Stroke Association, 2018).

Hospital admission

Thorough assessment and testing to identify the cause of the stroke and associated risk factors is an important component of the medical management of the stroke patient. Depending on the issues identified, interventional procedures such as carotid endarterectomy may be recommended. Management of other identified risk factors such as hypertension, diabetes, hypercholesterolaemia and smoking cessation will also be addressed.

Prevention of secondary complications of stroke (see Box 26.7) is an important part of hospital management as these often cause or contribute to death and further disability following stroke. A multidisciplinary approach employed early in the management and rehabilitation of stroke patients can prevent secondary complications and improve stroke outcomes.

Stroke patients often require a prolonged rehabilitation phase, depending on the degree and type of disability caused. Patients may require the services of physiotherapists, occupational therapists, speech therapists, psychologists, orthotists and podiatrists to manage the long-term complications of stroke. Many stroke patients are discharged from acute care medical facilities to specialist rehabilitation facilities for extended periods of rehabilitation.

Stroke across the lifespan

While there has been a significant decrease in the incidence of stroke over the past 20 years due to improved recognition and management of risk factors such as hypertension, diabetes and reduced smoking rates, stroke remains the third leading cause of death and is the highest cause of disability in developed countries (American Heart Association American Stroke Association, 2018). Stroke occurs in people of all ages but is most prevalent in the elderly. The incidence of stroke in the paediatric and young adult population is uncommon and so is frequently misdiagnosed, resulting in delayed diagnosis and treatment. Haemorrhagic stroke, particularly subarachnoid haemorrhage, is more common in younger adults between the ages of 40 and 60 years with a peak incidence during the fifth decade of life (Bauer & Rasmussen cited in Al-Ali, 2015).

Paediatric stroke

Paediatric stroke is an uncommon condition: the reported incidence rate is around 2 to 3 cases per 100,000 children during the first 5 years of life and 8 to 13 per 100,000 from 5 to 14 years. The aetiology of stroke is the same as for adults, being either ischaemic or haemorrhagic. However, the common causes and risk factors for stroke in children are significantly different from those in the adult. Risk factors for paediatric stroke include:

- congenital heart disease
- valvular heart disease
- coagulopathies (e.g. haemophilia, protein C or protein S deficiency)
- arteriopathy
- prothrombotic condition
- arterial aneurysm
- haematological disease
- infection
- severe dehydration (Jeong et al., 2015).

Like in adults the clinical presentation is dependent on the location of the ischaemia or haemorrhage (see Table 26.6). Diagnosis of paediatric stroke is frequently missed due to the rareness and complex differential diagnosis. Common clinical features associated with paediatric stroke include hemiparesis or focal CNS deficits, change in mental status, headache, seizure, speech disorder, vomiting,

Table 26.6 Clinical presentation of paediatric stroke

Presenting symptom	Ischaemic stroke	Haemorrhagic stroke
Hemiparesis	94%	21%
Altered mental status	28%	88%
Headache	22%	59%
Seizure	16%	29%
Fever/Prodrome	35–40%	35–40%

Source: Jeong et al. (2015).

nausea, visual impairment, neck pain and fever (Jeong et al., 2015). The differential diagnoses to be considered in the paediatric population include seizures, metabolic disturbances including hypoglycaemia, toxicological causes, infection and trauma. Where stroke is identified by paramedics as being possible, expeditious extrication and transport to an appropriate facility, including a specialist paediatric hospital if available, should be initiated with appropriate supportive management continued en route. Management of paediatric stroke is similar to that of the adult patient, with attention placed on supportive management of the airway, ventilation and perfusion.

Paediatric stroke is an uncommonly encountered condition in both the out-of-hospital and the in-hospital setting and therefore is frequently overlooked, resulting in delayed diagnosis and treatment. Paramedics should consider stroke as a differential diagnosis in children presenting with neurological symptoms, especially in those with risk factors for stroke.

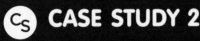

CASE STUDY 2

Case 12439, 1947 hrs.

Dispatch details: A 54-year-old female has collapsed, not alert.

Initial presentation: Paramedics are met at the front door by a concerned husband who directs them to his wife: she is lying on a couch holding her head in her hands and appears to be in severe pain.

① ASSESS

2000 hrs Primary survey: The patient is conscious and tachypnoeic and the radial pulses are easily palpable.

2000 hrs Chief complaint: 'I feel like my head is going to explode.'

2001 hrs Vital signs survey: Perfusion status: HR 106 regular, BP 165/105 mmHg; skin pale, warm, sweating; ECG: sinus tachycardia.

Respiratory status: Airway clear, RR 26 normal effort, good air entry bilaterally, SpO_2 100% on room air.

Conscious state: GCS = 14 (E3, V5, M6), pupils 4 mm and reactive.

Secondary survey: sensation to touch bilaterally, no motor drift of arms or legs, hand grips weak bilaterally but equal.

2005 hrs Pertinent hx: The patient was doing some craft work and while lifting a box of material got a sudden headache that felt like her head was going to explode. The next thing she remembers is waking up on the floor with this incredible headache and feeling nauseated.

On further questioning the patient reports that she had no symptoms prior to the headache commencing. She reports that she feels weak all over, is nauseous and rates the headache a 10/10. She has a past medical history of hypertension for which she takes an angiotensin-converting enzyme (ACE) inhibitor and she is a smoker. She specifically denies any previous similar headaches or migraine history. She denies any recent alcohol use or use of recreational drugs.

The paramedics ask the husband what he witnessed and he states that he heard his wife scream out in pain and that as he was making his way towards the room he heard a bang. When he entered the room he found his wife unresponsive on the floor. He reports that she was unresponsive for 2–3 minutes then awoke and complained of the severe headache and nausea and vomited twice. He says that he didn't witness any seizure activity.

This patient may be experiencing a stroke, particularly a subarachnoid haemorrhage, but do her symptoms fit the definition of a stroke? The patient experienced the sudden onset of a severe headache, followed by a period of unconsciousness, both of which are neurological symptoms that fit the definition of a stroke.

Focal or unilateral sensory and/or motor deficits are common clinical signs of stroke, but stroke can occur without these symptoms, and dysphasia occurs when the stroke affects the patient's dominant cerebral hemisphere, usually the left cerebral hemisphere. The clinical manifestations of stroke are dependent on the area of the brain affected. Using the common out-of-hospital stroke screening tools the patient does not meet the stroke criteria as she does not exhibit any of the items outlined in the motor items assessment. While out-of-hospital stroke screening tools have good sensitivity for stroke diagnosis, they lack specificity.

Stroke is a consideration in this patient so we want to try rule out other conditions that may present with similar symptoms. At this point it would be appropriate to obtain her temperature and BGL: the results are tympanic temperature 36.6°C and BGL 10.3 mmol/L.

② CONFIRM

In many cases paramedics are presented with a collection of signs and symptoms that do not appear to describe a particular condition. A critical step in determining a treatment plan in this situation is to consider what other conditions could explain the patient's presentation.

What else could it be?

Migraine or other headache

Headache is a common medical condition and while sudden onset of a severe headache is the most common presenting symptom in subarachnoid haemorrhage, only about one-quarter of patients with such a presentation are diagnosed with a subarachnoid haemorrhage. Specific inquiry should be made as to whether the patient has experienced an 'unusual' headache in the preceding hours or days, as up to 50% of patients with subarachnoid haemorrhage experience a 'warning leak' in the hours or days before a major haemorrhage. Common non-stroke causes of severe headache include migraine, benign thunderclap headache, cluster headache, intracranial infection and intracranial masses (e.g. tumour). Migraine headache is typically preceded by aura and tends to build gradually, and while paraesthesia or numbness is a common symptom associated with migraine, weakness—particularly focal weakness—is unusual.

Meningitis

Meningitis can present with a severe headache, but the headache is generally of gradual onset. Meningitis is frequently accompanied by other clinical signs such as fever, lethargy, posterior neck pain and nuchal rigidity. While posterior neck pain is common following subarachnoid haemorrhage it typically doesn't manifest until several hours later. The patient in this case reports that she had been well immediately prior to the onset of the headache, making meningitis an unlikely cause.

Seizure

Seizure could explain the patient's loss of consciousness and headache is common following a seizure. To complicate things, seizure is relatively common in subarachnoid haemorrhage, affecting approximately 10–15% of patients. However, in this case the patient's headache preceded the period of unconsciousness and her husband, who arrived almost immediately after she lost consciousness, denied having witnessed any seizure activity.

Syncope

Syncope could explain the brief loss of consciousness in this patient and may have been an autonomic response to severe pain, although the reported period of unconsciousness is somewhat longer than would normally occur with a simple syncopal episode. Loss of consciousness (brief, prolonged or permanent) is common at the onset of subarachnoid haemorrhage, occurring in approximately 50% of cases.

Subarachnoid haemorrhage is a specific subtype of stroke and frequently presents without localising signs that are commonly seen in ischaemic stroke and intracerebral haemorrhage. In approximately 25% of cases, however, subarachnoid haemorrhage does present with focal neurological signs, including hemiparesis, sensory impairment and visual defects.

The patient presents with a history and physical presentation highly suggestive of subarachnoid haemorrhage. While this diagnosis cannot be confirmed in the out-of-hospital environment, it is appropriate to treat the patient as having a subarachnoid haemorrhage until a definitive diagnosis can be established following neuroimaging in hospital.

(3) TREAT

Pain management

The patient presents with 10/10 pain so pain management is an appropriate out-of-hospital intervention. Besides being a humane intervention, providing effective analgesia may result in other therapeutic benefits for this patient.

She is hypertensive and demonstrating other signs of sympathetic activity that may occur in response to pain, including tachycardia, pallor and sweating. The type of analgesia chosen depends on what is available and recommended in the service procedures; however, it is appropriate to choose a medication and route of administration that will have a rapid onset of effect and that can be easily titrated to effect. There are numerous analgesics available to paramedics including oral paracetamol, inhalational agents and narcotic analgesics.

In this case, oral analgesics would not be appropriate as the patient is nauseous and giving anything orally may cause vomiting. A trial of inhalational analgesia such as methoxyflurane is appropriate: it is easy to initiate and has a rapid onset of action if used correctly. Inhalational analgesia is an appropriate initial choice while IV access is being obtained and parenteral analgesics are being prepared. IV narcotic analgesics are also appropriate in this case due to the severity of the pain and the absence of a history of headache being a chronic health problem for the patient. IV morphine at 2.5–5.0 mg repeated up to 2.5 mg at 5-minute intervals or fentanyl 25–50 microgram repeated at 25 microgram at 5-minute intervals titrated to effect is indicated.

Antiemetic

The patient in this case is experiencing ongoing nausea and has been vomiting prior to the ambulance arriving. Nausea and vomiting occur in around 75% of patients presenting with a subarachnoid haemorrhage. It is appropriate to administer an antiemetic in an attempt to relieve the uncomfortable feeling of nausea and to try to prevent further vomiting. Vomiting causes acute rises in blood pressure and intracranial pressure.

IV metoclopramide 10–20 mg, ondansetron 4 mg orally, ondansetron 8 mg IV, promethazine 12.5 mg IV and prochlorperazine 12.5 mg intramuscularly are common antiemetic options available to paramedics and should be used according to service procedures. Caution should be used when administering intramuscular injections to stroke patients as later thrombolysis administered in hospital may result in haematoma at the injection site.

2011 hrs: An IV cannula is placed and the patient receives an antiemetic (e.g. 10-mg IV bolus of metoclopramide or 4 mg of ondansetron) and pain relief (e.g. IV bolus of fentanyl or an IV dose of morphine) while the stretcher is prepared for her extrication and transport.

Transport

The decision as to which hospital to transport to will depend on the location the paramedics are operating in and local protocols. Ideally there should be pre-established systems that will provide clear direction regarding the most appropriate transport destination depending on the resource availability in any particular location.

In this case the provisional diagnosis of subarachnoid haemorrhage may well be accurate, but since there is no way of confirming this in the out-of-hospital setting, transport to the closest hospital with an acute stroke service is the most reasonable option. The patient can undergo neuroimaging at this hospital and if necessary can later transfer to a neurosurgical centre. While invasive interventions such as endovascular coiling and surgical clipping are often required in managing subarachnoid haemorrhages, these interventions usually don't need to be performed immediately.

2018 hrs: The patient is loaded supine with 30° head elevation and transport is initiated to the closest acute stroke unit. The hospital is notified of the patient's presenting complaint, physical exam findings and current vital signs and an estimated time of arrival is given.

> ## TREAT NAUSEA!
> Vomiting causes acute increases in blood pressure and intracranial pressure.

EVALUATE

Evaluating the effect of any clinical management intervention can provide clues to the accuracy of the initial diagnosis. Some conditions respond rapidly to treatment so patients should be expected to improve if the diagnosis and treatment were appropriate. A failure to improve in this situation should trigger the clinician to reconsider the diagnosis.

If blood continues to accumulate rapidly in the subarachnoid space it can lead to increased pain, and if the volume is large it can increase intracranial pressure and impede cerebral perfusion. Any deterioration should trigger a reassessment of hypoxia, hypotension, hypercapnia and hypoglycaemia but it could also be an extension of the haemorrhage. If the reversible causes are not apparent, any deterioration is likely to continue and airway support may be required as the patient's conscious state decreases.

CASE STUDY 3

Case 21209, 1910 hrs.

Dispatch details: A 78-year-old female with dizziness and vomiting at a local restaurant. The patient has a history of hypertension.

Initial presentation: Paramedics are directed to a 78-year-old female lying on the floor of the restaurant with several family members around her.

 ASSESS

1923 hrs Primary survey: The patient is conscious, her airway is clear and she is breathing normally. Her radial pulse is strong.

1923 hrs Chief complaint: 'I was eating dinner when the room suddenly started spinning and I felt sick and started vomiting.'

1925 hrs Vital signs survey: Perfusion status: HR 68 regular, BP 200/110 mmHg, skin pale, warm, no sweating.

Respiratory status: airway clear, RR 20 normal, good air entry L = R, SpO$_2$ 97% on room air.

Conscious state: GCS = 15, pupils 3 mm and reactive.

Secondary survey: equal strength in arms and legs bilaterally, equal sensation to touch in arms and legs bilaterally, no facial droop, speech is normal. BGL is 6.1 mmol/L.

1928 hrs Pertinent hx: Patient has a history of hypertension for which she takes perindopril, but is otherwise healthy. She denies any allergies and lives independently at home with her husband.

The patient was having a birthday dinner with some of her extended family and had just started eating when the room suddenly started spinning and she felt nauseous. She tried to get up to go to the toilet but wasn't able to get her balance and fell back into the chair. Family members assisted her to lie down on the floor and shortly afterwards she began vomiting.

Technically we can't really be certain that this patient is having a stroke as there are many other conditions that could be causing her symptoms.

CLASSICAL BRAINSTEM STROKE PRESENTATION

- Vertigo
- Diplopia
- Nausea
- Vomiting
- Ataxia

However, the history and clinical presentation are suggestive of a stroke and the paramedics should treat for acute stroke until either a definitive diagnosis is made or another more likely diagnosis is arrived at following further assessment. The patient doesn't fit the out-of-hospital screening criteria for stroke as she doesn't present with any of the motor items that typically form part of the screening tools.

The presentation of acute stroke is dependent on a number of factors, including the type of stroke (i.e. ischaemic or haemorrhagic), the stroke location and size. Focal motor signs and dysphasia occur commonly in hemispheric stroke due to ischaemia or an intracerebral haemorrhage, but focal motor signs are less commonly present in brainstem strokes or with subarachnoid haemorrhage.

2 CONFIRM

In many cases paramedics are presented with a collection of signs and symptoms that do not appear to describe a particular condition. A critical step in determining a treatment plan in this situation is to consider what other conditions could explain the patient's presentation.

What else could it be?

Middle ear infection

Middle ear infection can produce symptoms of vertigo, nausea and vomiting, but the symptoms are characteristically gradual in onset and associated with unilateral pain and systemic signs of infection such as fever, malaise and increased heart rate. To be thorough the paramedics record this patient's tympanic temperature: it is 37°C.

Labyrinthitis

Labyrinthitis commonly presents with vertigo, nausea and vomiting, but the symptoms are characteristically gradual in onset. The other distinguishing feature is that the vertigo usually occurs with movement and when the patient remains still the vertigo symptoms resolve, only to return when the patient moves again. In this case the patient's vertigo is continually present and is not dependent on movement or head position.

Syncope

Syncope occurs suddenly and is usually associated with hypotension and skin changes such as pallor and sweating. The symptoms generally resolve rapidly once the patient is placed supine. This patient has been lying supine for a significant period of time so we would expect the symptoms to have resolved; she is also hypertensive.

Anaphylaxis

Anaphylaxis should always be considered when a patient experiences sudden-onset symptoms and may have been exposed to allergens such as food. Nausea and vomiting are symptoms of anaphylaxis and the vertigo could be caused by hypotension from vasodilation. This patient has no history of allergies, she is hypertensive and there are no other signs consistent with anaphylaxis such as urticaria, pruritus, flushing, tachycardia, oedema or respiratory symptoms.

Metabolic/toxicological exposure

Metabolic disturbances, especially hypoglycaemia, and toxicological exposure, including alcohol, are important differential diagnoses. This patient has no history of diabetes and the paramedics recorded a BGL of 6.1 mmol/L during the initial assessment, so this excludes hypoglycaemia as a cause.

3 TREAT

Nausea and vomiting are unpleasant for the patient and potentially pose a risk of airway obstruction, and aspiration and vomiting cause increases in blood

> ### DIFFERENTIAL DIAGNOSIS
>
> **Stroke**
> Or
> - Middle ear infection
> - Labyrinthitis
> - Syncope
> - Anaphylaxis
> - Metabolic/toxicological exposure

pressure and intracranial pressure. Administering an appropriate antiemetic is unlikely to do harm and it may reduce or ameliorate the symptoms of nausea and vomiting. Which medication to administer will be dependent on what the individual service carries, but it would be prudent to administer the antiemetic medication that has the least sedative properties, otherwise it may interfere with accurate assessment of the patient's conscious state. The most commonly carried antiemetics in Australian and New Zealand ambulance services are metoclopramide, prochlorperazine and ondansetron. IV administration is the preferred route of administration due to its rapid onset. In the setting of stroke, where there is the possibility of systemic thrombolysis being experienced, avoid using the intramuscular route as it may result in haematoma formation.

Should the patient be transported?

While there are a number of relatively 'benign' potential diagnoses that could be causing this patient's symptoms, the paramedics have to assume that the patient is having a brainstem stroke until proven otherwise. The most important aspect of treatment for this patient is transport to an appropriate facility, preferably a hospital with an acute stroke unit and the ability to provide reperfusion therapy. There is evidence that patients treated in specialised stroke units have better long-term outcomes, independent of whether they receive reperfusion therapy procedures or not. The patient is conscious with a patent airway, good ventilation and oxygenation and she is adequately perfused. She requires general supportive care, ongoing observation and reassessment, and expeditious transport.

 EVALUATE

Evaluating the effect of any clinical management intervention can provide clues to the accuracy of the initial diagnosis. Some conditions respond rapidly to treatment so patients should be expected to improve if the diagnosis and treatment were appropriate. A failure to improve in this situation should trigger the clinician to reconsider the diagnosis.

Until the benefits of thrombolysis for stroke are fully established, paramedic treatment for stroke is unlikely to impact on the patient's condition during transport. Any deterioration should trigger a reassessment of hypoxia, hypotension, hypercapnia and hypoglycaemia but it could also be an extension of the stroke.

 CASE STUDY 4

Case 17536, 1623 hrs.

Dispatch details: A 78-year-old male found collapsed by his wife. He is unable to move or speak normally.

Initial presentation: Paramedics are directed to a 78-year-old male lying supine on the lounge room floor.

① **ASSESS**

1636 hrs Primary survey: The patient is conscious but has incomprehensible speech. The airway sounds obstructed and gurgling noises are audible, his breathing rate is increased with slightly increased effort and his radial pulse is easily palpable.

1637 hrs Treatment: At this point in the assessment the paramedics have identified a problem in the primary survey: an obstructed airway. The patient is placed into the right lateral position and his oropharynx is very gently suctioned using a Yankauer suction catheter.

1638 hrs Reassess: The airway is clear and the patient's respiratory effort is improved.

1639 hrs Chief complaint: It is difficult to understand the patient's speech so the paramedics obtain a history from the patient's wife. She states that she went out shopping at about 3 pm and when she came home she found her husband collapsed on the floor unable to speak or move properly. She called an ambulance immediately. She reports that he was completely normal when she left to go shopping.

1639 hrs Vital signs survey: Perfusion status: HR 112 bpm, irregular, atrial fibrillation, BP 165/90 mmHg, skin flushed and warm.

Respiratory status: RR 24 bpm, good air entry, coarse mid-field crackles on right, SpO_2 91% on room air.

Conscious state: GCS = 11 (E3, V2, M6), eyes deviated to left, pupils 3 mm and non-reactive.

Secondary survey: incomprehensible speech, unable to lift left or right leg or arm, weak grip with right hand, tympanic temperature 37.1°C, BGL 7.2 mmol/L.

1642 hrs Treatment: During the vital signs survey and patient assessment the paramedics observe that the patient's oxygen saturation is low, indicating hypoxaemia. They place a rebreather mask and commence oxygen therapy at 8 L/minute.

The paramedics also identify that the patient is time-critical and they require assistance to extricate him from the house. In addition, they recognise that the patient has a significantly decreased level of consciousness and is hypoxic, probably due to aspiration. Based on these findings they request assistance from a second crew and intensive care paramedic support.

1643 hrs Pertinent hx: The paramedics are unable to obtain any history directly from the patient and are therefore unable to identify the exact time of onset of symptoms. They therefore assume that the symptoms commenced when he was last seen without neurological symptoms—which is 3 pm, when his wife last saw him.

The wife says that her husband has a history of hypertension, type 2 diabetes mellitus and atrial fibrillation. His medications include perindopril, frusemide, coumadin, metoprolol, atovastatin, gliclazide and metformin.

The patient presents with a number of neurological symptoms including a decreased level of consciousness, fixed eye deviation, dysphasia and bilateral limb paresis. The paramedics cannot ascertain whether the symptoms came on suddenly or occurred gradually over the past 90 minutes.

The patient also presents with a number of risk factors for stroke including age, hypertension, diabetes and atrial fibrillation and he is on an anticoagulant medication. Advancing age, hypertension and diabetes are risk factors for all types of stroke. Atrial fibrillation is a risk factor for ischaemic stroke secondary to cardioembolism, and anticoagulation treatment increases the risk of haemorrhagic stroke.

The patient fits the criteria for stroke using out-of-hospital screening tools as he records a 'yes' to all the history items and has at least one motor item: dysphasia. However, while he also presents with paresis it is bilateral: screening tools generally require any motor deficits to be unilateral. Sensory and motor deficits in acute stroke are usually focal or unilateral but in some cases where there is ischaemia affecting both hemispheres bilateral deficits can be present. Bilateral neurological deficits may also occur following large intracerebral haemorrhages, cerebral oedema and raised intracranial pressure.

Bilateral or generalised neurological symptoms are more consistent with other conditions so it is important to consider alternative diagnoses.

2 CONFIRM

In many cases paramedics are presented with a collection of signs and symptoms that do not appear to describe a particular condition. A critical step in determining a treatment plan in this situation is to consider what other conditions could explain the patient's presentation.

What else could it be?

Seizure

Seizure is a possibility as there were no witnesses to the initial events. Other signs that would indicate a seizure include incontinence, friction burns or abrasions from rubbing against the floor, and bleeding from the tongue, lips or mucosa. While assessment hasn't demonstrated any of these signs, and there is no previous history of seizures, it remains a possibility that the patient has had a seizure.

Trauma

It is important to look for evidence of head trauma as the patient may have had a fall and have a traumatic intracranial haemorrhage. This includes checking carefully for evidence of haematomas, bruising, depressions and wounds around the head and neck to exclude trauma.

Metabolic/toxicological exposure

Hypo- and hyperglycaemia have been excluded as the patient's BGL is normal. The paramedics ask the patient's wife about any history of alcohol use and check the patient's breath for odour that might indicate recent alcohol consumption. They obtain a good medical history, including medications that may indicate a metabolic problem such as renal failure, hepatic failure or electrolyte disturbances. They check the ECG for signs indicating electrolyte disturbances such as hypo- or hyperkalaemia.

The patient's wife said that the patient is taking frusemide, a diuretic medication that causes potassium loss. Patients prescribed frusemide are frequently prescribed a potassium supplement to compensate for the potassium loss, but this hasn't been mentioned. The paramedics ask whether they have all of the patient's medications and also whether there are any medications the patient should be taking but isn't.

Infection/sepsis

Systemic illness secondary to infection (e.g. pneumonia, urinary tract infection, cerebral infection such as meningitis) can present with clinical symptoms similar to acute stroke. However, since the patient was reportedly well 90 minutes earlier it is unlikely he would have deteriorated this quickly from an infection.

Other intracranial lesion

Intracranial lesions such as tumours and cysts can cause cerebral oedema and raised intracranial pressure producing neurological symptoms similar to stroke.

After considering the differential diagnoses the paramedics conclude that the most likely diagnosis is an acute stroke and they continue their out-of-hospital management.

DIFFERENTIAL DIAGNOSIS

Stroke
Or
- Seizure
- Trauma
- Metabolic/toxicological exposure
- Infection/sepsis
- Other intracranial lesion

③ TREAT

1646 hrs: The paramedics prepare for extrication by having a spine board and the stretcher ready for when the back-up crew arrives. They place, secure and check an 18-g IV cannula for patency.

1650 hrs: The upper airway remains clear with the patient in the lateral position and secretions are able to drain. Oxygen saturations have risen to 99%.

1653 hrs: The back-up crew arrives and the patient is extricated and placed in the ambulance.

④ EVALUATE

Evaluating the effect of any clinical management intervention can provide clues to the accuracy of the initial diagnosis. Some conditions respond rapidly to treatment so patients should be expected to improve if the diagnosis and treatment were appropriate. A failure to improve in this situation should trigger the clinician to reconsider the diagnosis.

Until the benefits of thrombolysis for stroke are fully established, paramedic treatment for stroke is unlikely to impact on the patient's condition during transport. Any deterioration should trigger a reassessment of hypoxia, hypotension, hypercapnia and hypoglycaemia but it could also be an extension of the stroke.

Future research

Research into all aspects of stroke, including epidemiology, prevention, assessment, management and rehabilitation, is prominent in all developed countries. Over the past decade extensive research has been conducted on thrombolytic therapy for the management of ischaemic stroke and this has been the driver for improving systems of care, including the importance of out-of-hospital recognition of stroke by paramedics and transport to regionalised stroke centres where available.

Research is ongoing into other reperfusion therapies including intraarterial thrombolysis, mechanical clot removal and vessel stenting, especially for patients with ischaemic stroke who may be ineligible for systemic thrombolysis, or in stroke subtypes in which thrombolysis has been shown to have minimal effect. Much of the neurological injury that occurs following ischaemic and haemorrhagic stroke is from secondary mechanisms that may be ameliorated by the use of neuroprotective therapies including pharmacological treatment and mechanical therapies such as induction of mild hypothermia. These treatments continue to be actively researched.

Research in the out-of-hospital setting is focused on improving out-of-hospital stroke screening tools to improve the sensitivity and specificity for stroke diagnosis. There is ongoing research into the use of sophisticated out-of-hospital stroke response units, including transportable CT scans to reduce the time to stroke diagnosis, and the initiation of reperfusion therapies. Use of portable ultrasound for both diagnosis and treatment in the out-of-hospital setting may hold promise for selected stroke patients and research is continuing in this area. One of the areas of research that may potentially have the biggest impact is in developing strategies to help the public to recognise stroke earlier and to get medical help earlier.

As stroke is such a common, debilitating condition any improvements that result from the research being conducted could potentially have a significant impact on reducing the mortality and morbidity of this frequently devastating disease.

Summary

Stroke is a leading cause of mortality and the leading cause of disability in developed countries. Stroke is a common medical emergency encountered by paramedics in the out-of-hospital setting. Rapid, accurate assessment and transport to an appropriate medical facility, preferably a dedicated stroke unit where available, can improve mortality and morbidity outcomes for patients, independent of thrombolytic therapy. In the subset of patients eligible for reperfusion therapy, transport to a stroke centre capable of initiating reperfusion can improve outcomes in selected patients.

The use of a stroke screening tool by paramedics in the out-of-hospital setting has been shown to improve stroke diagnosis, so paramedics should incorporate a validated out-of-hospital stroke screening tool into their assessment. While current out-of-hospital stroke screening tools have good sensitivity for stroke diagnosis, specificity is not as good and paramedics should be careful of discounting stroke based on screening tools alone. The differential diagnosis of stroke is long and in suspicious cases paramedics should always err on the side of a stroke diagnosis until either an alternative diagnosis is identified or a definitive diagnosis can be made in hospital following further testing.

References

Aiyagari, V., & Gorelick, P. (Eds.), (2016). *Hypertension and stroke pathophysiology and management* (2nd ed.). Switzerland: Springer International Publishing. doi:10.1007/978-3-319-29152-9.

Al-Ali, F., (Ed.), (2015). *Balloon stent for ischemic and hemorrhagic stroke: a new trend for stroke prevention and management, Frontiers Media,* doi:10.3389/978-2-88919-694-4.

Alme, K. N., Engelsen, B. A., Naik, M., & Naess, H. (2016). Identifying patients at risk of acute stroke symptomatic seizure after ischemic stroke. *Acta Neurologica Scandinavica, 136*, 265–271. doi:10.1111/ane.12721.

American Heart Association American Stroke Association. (2018). 2018 Guidelines for the early management of patients with acute ischaemic stroke. *Stroke; a Journal of Cerebral Circulation,* doi:10.1161/STR.0000000000000158. April 2018.

Australian Bureau of Statistics. (2017). *Causes of death in Australia 2015: Stroke, Australian Bureau of Statistics [Online].* Retrieved from http://www.abs.gov.au/ausstats/abs@.nsf/lookup/by%20subject/3303.0~2015~Main...3303.0-causeofdeath,australia,2015.

Australian Institute of Health and Welfare (AIHW). (2018). *Australia's health 2018. Australia's health series no. 16. AUS 221.* Canberra: AIHW. Retrieved from https://www.aihw.gov.au/getmedia/56bb591f-6c56-4397-b928-8de6872e2cdd/aihw-aus-221-chapter-3-7.pdf.aspx.

Boccardi, E., Cenzato, M., Curto, F., Longoni, M., Motto, C., Oppo, C., Perini, V., & Vidale, S. (2017). *Hemorrhagic stroke.* Switzerland: Springer International Publishing. doi:10.1007/978-3-319-32130-1.

Borg, K. T., & Pancioli, A. M. (2002). Transient ischemic attacks: an emergency medicine approach. *Emergency Medicine Clinics, 20*(3), 597–608.

Brown, D., & Edwards, H. (2012). *Lewis's medical-surgical nursing* (2nd ed.). Sydney: Elsevier.

Dawson, A., Cloud, G. C., Pereira, A. C., & Moynihan, B. J. (2016). Stroke mimic diagnoses presenting to a hyperacute stroke unit. *Clinical Medicine, 16*(5), 423–426.

Emberson, J., Lees, K. R., Lyden, P., Blackwell, L., Albers, G., & Bluhmki, E. (2014). Effect of treatment delay, age, and stroke severity on the effects of intravenous thrombolysis with alteplase for acute ischaemic stroke: a meta-analysis of individual patient data from randomised trials. *Lancet, 384*(9958), 1929–1935.

European Stroke Organization (ESO). (2008). *Executive Committee, ESO Writing Committee. Guidelines for Management of Ischaemic Stroke and Transient Ischaemic Attack 2008.* Heidelberg: ESO.

Faiz, K. W., Labberton, A. S., Thommessen, B., Ronning, O. M., Dahl, F. A., & Barra, M. (2018). The burden of stroke mimics: present and future projections. *Journal of Stroke and Cerebrovascular Diseases, 27*(5), 1288–1295.

Fassbender, K., Balucani, C., Walter, S., Levine, S. R., Haass, A., & Grotta, J. (2013). Streamlining of prehospital stroke management: the golden hour. *The Lancet, 12*, 585–596.

Forbes, C. D., & Jackson, W. F. (2003). *Colour atlas and text of clinical medicine* (3rd ed.). London: Mosby.

Forster, A., Griebe, M., Wolf, M. E., Szabo, K., Hennerici, M. G., & Kern, R. (2012). How to identify stroke mimics in patients eligible for intravenous thrombolysis? *Neurol, 259*, 1347–1353. doi:10.1007/s00415-011-6354-9.

Goldman, L., & Ausiello, D. (2007). *Cecil medicine* (23rd ed.). Philadelphia: Saunders Elsevier.

Goyal, P., & Maurer, M. S. (2016). Syncope in older adults. *Journal of Geriatric Cardiology, 13*, 380–386.

Hall, J. E. (2016). *Guyton and Hall: textbook of medical physiology* (13th ed.). Philadelphia: Elsevier.

Hunter, A. J., Snodgrass, S. J., Quain, D., Parsons, M. W., & Levi, C. R. (2011). Head of bed optimization of elevation study: association of higher angle with reduced cerebral blood flow velocity in acute ischemic stroke. *Physical Therapy, 91*(10), 1503–1512.

Jeong, G., Lim, B. C., & Chae, J. (2015). Pediatric stroke. *Journal of Korean Neurosurgical Society, 57*(6), 396–400.

Kamel, H., & Healey, J. S. (2017). Cardioembolic stroke. *Circulation Research, 120*, 514–526. doi:10.1161/circresaha.116.308407.

Lee, S. H. (Ed.), (2017). *Stroke revisited: diagnosis and treatment of ischemic stroke.* Singapore: Springer. doi:10.1007/978-981-10-1424-6.

Lin, C., Arishima, H., Kikuta, K., Naiki, H., Kitai, R., & Kodera, T. (2018). Pathological examination of cerebral amyloid angiopathy in patients who underwent removal of lobar hemorrhages. *The Journal of Neurology, 265*, 567–577.

Long, B., & Koyfman, A. (2017). Clinical mimics: an emergency medicine-focused review of stroke mimics. *The Journal of Emergency Medicine, 52*(2), 176–183.

Markus, H., Cloud, G., & Pareira, A. (2017). *Stroke medicine* (2nd ed.). Oxford University Press. doi:10.1093/med/9780198737889.001.0001.

McCance, K. L., & Huether, S. E. (2018). *Pathophysiology: the biologic basis for disease in adults and children* (8th ed.). St Louis: Elsevier.

National Institute of Clinical Studies (NICS). (2009). *Emergency department stroke and transient ischaemic attack care bundle: information and implementation package.* Melbourne: National Health and Medical Research Council.

Ohshita, T., Imamura, E., Nomura, E., Wakabayashi, S., Kajikawa, H., & Matsumoto, M. (2015). Hypoglycemia with focal neurological signs of stroke mimic: clinical and neuroradiological characteristics. *Journal of the Neurological Sciences, 353,* 98–101.

Roffe, C., Nebatte, T., Sim, J., Bishop, J., Ibes, N., Ferninard, P., & Gray, R. (2017). Effect of routine low-dose oxygen supplementation on death and disability in adults with acute stroke: the stroke oxygen study randomized clinical trial. *JAMA: The Journal of the American Medical Association, 318*(12), 1125–1135.

Stroke Foundation. (2017). *Australian clinical guidelines for stroke management.* Chapter 1 of 8: Pre-hospital care. Retrieved from https://www.magicapp.org/app#/guideline/2142.

Wardlaw, J. M., Murray, V., Berge, E., & Del Zoppo, G. J. (2014). Thrombolysis for acute ischemic stroke, update August 2014. *Stroke; a Journal of Cerebral Circulation, 45,* 222–225. doi:10.1161/strokeaha.114.007024.

Wojner-Alexandrov, A. W., Garami, Z. Y., Chernyshev, O. V., & Alexandrov, A. V. (2005). Heads down: flat positioning improves blood flow velocity in acute ischemic stroke. *Neurology, 64*(8), 1354–1357.

Yasa, E., Ricci, F., Magnusson, M., Sutton, R., Gullina, S., De Caterina, R., Melander, O., & Fedorowski, A. (2018). Cardiovascular risk after hospitalization for unexplained syncope and orthostatic hypotension. *Open Access, 104,* 487–493. doi:10.1136/heartjnl-2017-311857.

Yew, K. S., & Cheng, E. (2009). Acute stroke diagnosis. *American Family Physician, 80*(1).

CHAPTER 27

Overdose

By Joe-Anthony Rotella and Shaun Greene

OVERVIEW

- Many pharmaceutical and recreational drugs have the potential to cause toxicity in overdose. With most overdoses, symptoms occur early but in others, effects can be delayed.
- Ingestion remains the most common route of overdose.
- Risk assessment should encompass drug or substance identity, quantity of exposure, time of exposure and intention (self-harm, accidental, recreational). In situations where a quantity cannot be established, a 'worst case scenario' should be calculated based on empty packets found or medications thought to be missing by the patient's family or friends.
- Adults and adolescents are more likely to overdose with intent to self-harm whereas paediatric patients are more likely to present following accidental exposure.

- Certain drugs have specific antidotes that should be considered as part of treatment where clinically indicated.
- The majority of poisoned patients recover with the provision of good supportive care. Attention to airway, breathing, oxygenation, circulation, blood glucose and conscious state are essential to management of the overdose patient.
- The primary roles for the paramedic when treating the overdosed patient are recognition, attention to airway, breathing and circulation, delivery of time-critical treatment and supportive care.
- Further advice with regards to management should be obtained via the local Poisons Information Centre (Australia, 13 11 26; New Zealand, 0800 POISON [0800 764 766]).

Introduction

The scholar, Paracelsus, is famously credited with the saying 'the dose makes the poison', referring to the concept that it is the amount of exposure to any substance that determines if it is poisonous; there will be a safe level of exposure for humans even with the extremely toxic substances, although that exposure may be very low. Overdose may be accidental (such as in young children exploring their environment), recreational or deliberate in order to self-harm or commit suicide. Up to 5% (Australia) and 1.2% (New Zealand) of hospitalisations are due to deliberate self-harm, placing it in the top five causes of hospital admissions for both men and women (Graudins & Gunja, 2009). While there is a range of important substances implicated in overdose, it is beyond the scope of this book to cover every substance. Instead, in this chapter, we will focus on five substances that are especially important for paramedics to be aware of: alcohol (namely ethanol and the toxic alcohols), methamphetamine (and related amphetamines), opioids, tricyclic antidepressants and quetiapine (an antipsychotic).

Many substances produce a clinical pattern of symptoms and signs known as a *toxidrome*, following exposure to a toxic dose. Typically members of the same class of substance, such as opioids, produce the same or a very similar toxidrome. One example is the opioid toxidrome, which includes miosis (constricted pupils), central nervous system (CNS) depression ranging from drowsiness to stupor to coma, and hypoventilation. It can be useful to view overdose and poisoning through the lens of the toxidrome as it groups patient presentations into syndromes caused by various toxins/agents. This is especially important when—as is typical in the out-of-hospital setting—it can be difficult to identify exactly what substance (or substances) have been taken and how much.

A significant number of overdosed patients who present in the out-of-hospital setting have been exposed to more than one drug—all or some of which may be at a toxic amount. Even for those few drugs where we have a true antidote, the existence of more than one drug in the patient's system can create situations where the patient fails to respond to treatment. Perhaps more so in the overdosed patient than in any other patients, paramedics need to deal with a degree of uncertainty' in their clinical decision-making. As such, this chapter underlines the importance of excellent supportive care (ABC) in managing these patients.

Table 27.1 Acute pharmacological effects of ethanol

CNS	Circulatory	Gastrointestinal
• Euphoria to progressive depression including coma • Impaired transmission of nerve impulses • Inhibited calcium entry into nerve cells, possibly enhancing the inhibitory neurotransmitter GABA • Other targets are NMDA, glycine, serotonin, nicotinic and some potassium channels • Affects the pituitary gland, inhibiting ADH leading to increased urination	Vasomotor neurons are depressed in the medulla causing vasodilation resulting in: • Hypotension • Rapid heat loss with potential for hypothermia • Tachycardia to compensate for hypotension	Excess stimulation of gastric acids and saliva Vomiting

GABA = gamma-aminobutyric acid, NMDA = N-methyl-D-aspartate, ADH = antidiuretic hormone
Source: Marx, Hockberger & Walls (2014).

Pathophysiology

Alcohol (ethanol)

Ethanol is a type of alcohol and is the most commonly used legal recreational substance in Australia. Compared to all other substances, it accounts for the most drug-related presentations to hospital and can prove both a clinical and an occupational challenge for attending paramedics. Ethanol is a CNS depressant, but prior to this can often produce a sense of euphoria with reduced inhibition that can result in poor judgment with adverse actions and consequences. As a result, the ethanol-intoxicated patient may also be a trauma patient.

Ethanol, like all alcohols, is lipid-soluble and is rapidly absorbed following ingestion. The effects of ethanol are summarised in Table 27.1. Several factors can affect the absorption of alcohol (see Box 27.1) and the same dose of alcohol can produce variable effects among individuals. Approximately 90% of alcohol is metabolised by the liver; the remainder is excreted by the lungs and kidneys and in sweat. It is for this reason that the breathalyser was introduced, but the amount measured on the breath is small. Blood alcohol concentration (BAC) in 2 L of breath is equivalent to that in 1 mL of blood. The liver has a relatively fixed rate of metabolism (it takes approximately 1 hour to metabolise 1 standard drink), so rapid ingestion of multiple drinks will result in a high BAC (Bryant & Knights, 2011). In the absence of a clear history, the smell of a patient's breath can provide a clue; however, alcohol intoxication can only be confirmed by measurement of ethanol via breath analysis or a BAC.

Ethanol use can vary from 'social drinking' to alcohol addiction, and familiarity with the distinction between these terms is important as part of patient assessment (see Box 27.2). The most common emergency presentation relating to ethanol relates to acute ethanol intoxication, which produces an alteration in conscious state ranging from euphoria to coma. The term 'acute alcohol (ethanol) poisoning' refers to consumption of ethanol over a relatively short period of time resulting in significant CNS depression that can also cause respiratory compromise. Ethanol affects the conscious state by altering or mimicking the concentrations of inhibitory neurotransmitters in the CNS. Ethanol binds to a receptor site on the chloride channel in brain cells. Once bound, it opens the chloride channel and the inward flow of negative ions makes the cell more negative and less likely to be stimulated (see Fig 27.1). This resembles the effect that the inhibitory neurotransmitter gamma-aminobutyric acid (GABA) has on the CNS. Interestingly, in addition to receptor sites bound by ethanol and GABA, the chloride channel has a distinct receptor site for benzodiazepines, which explains the utility of benzodiazepines for treating alcohol withdrawal (Murray et al., 2015).

While ethanol can cause CNS depression, it is not known to cause significant cardiovascular instability. An open mind should be kept in the case of a patient presenting with arrhythmias or hypotension as other substances or trauma may be the cause.

Toxic alcohols

Toxic alcohols are other types of alcohol that can produce significant poisoning in humans. While much less common than ethanol and other substances taken in overdose requiring treatment in hospital, it is useful for paramedics to be aware of these substances and the potential harms related to exposure.

Isopropanol (also known as isopropyl alcohol)

Isopropanol is a clear liquid with a strong aroma and bitter taste. It is often found in products such as nail polish remover, hand sanitisers, disinfectants, perfumes and rubbing alcohol with concentrations

BOX 27.1 Factors affecting ethanol absorption

Dose
- The higher the concentration of imbibed ethanol, the more rapid the rise in BAC

Type of ingestion
- Peak blood alcohol concentrations are higher if ethanol is ingested as a single dose rather than several smaller doses, due to a higher concentration gradient

Co-ingestion with food
- Ethanol is absorbed most rapidly from the duodenum and jejunum. Meals that are high in fat, carbohydrate or protein slow gastric emptying so can reduce the rate of absorption
- Conversely, having an empty stomach results in rapid passage from the stomach to the duodenum resulting in less first pass metabolism and increased absorption hence the adage of 'don't drink on an empty stomach'

First pass metabolism in the stomach and liver
- Ethanol can be oxidised by alcohol dehydrogenase (ADH) in the stomach prior to absorption and in the liver after absorption, thereby reducing potential blood ethanol concentration
- Drugs such as ranitidine and aspirin inhibit stomach ADH activity thereby reducing first pass metabolism

Alcoholism
- Heavy and/or regular alcohol intake increases alcohol metabolism via induction of liver enzymes so elimination is increased. This possible benefit is lost is advanced liver disease due to loss of liver mass and function resulting in decreased ethanol metabolism

Drugs
- Medications that inhibit ADH such as anti-fungals can decrease ethanol's elimination rate

Source: Cederbaum (2012).

BOX 27.2 Terms associated with alcohol use and abuse

- *Social drinking:* drinking but not to excess with no problems or symptoms evident.
- *Heavy drinking:* regular excessive drinking with no obvious problems or symptoms.
- *Problem drinking:* drinking with evidence of difficulties in personal, family or working relationships but no symptoms of addiction that lead to physical/mental impairment.
- *Alcohol addiction:* drinking with severe impairment of health and intelligence, including loss of control of life, blackouts and stroke (de Crespigny et al., 2011).
- *Binge drinking:* a term that is now discouraged as it means different things to different people; instead, the NHMRC guidelines for drinking alcohol refer to the *single occasion*—drinking more than 4 standard units of ethanol on a single occasion is considered potentially harmful.

varying from 50–70%. When ingested, intoxication presents similarly to ethanol with CNS depression (ranging from mild sedation to coma). Hypotension is rare and usually responds to intravenous fluid (Murray et al., 2015). As little as 1 mL/kg is required to cause symptoms and 3–4 mL/kg can cause significant toxicity including coma. Duration of symptoms can be prolonged in comparison to ethanol and can be further exacerbated when co-ingested with other CNS depressants such as opioids and benzodiazepines. Isopropanol is metabolised to acetone and is excreted partially via the lungs, so a fruity odour may be detected in the patient's breath. Patients are expected to do well with good supportive care alone. A focus on airway is important given the anticipated toxicity, with the most severe cases requiring intubation for airway protection.

Methanol

Similar to ethanol, methanol is colourless and has a typical 'alcohol' smell. It is not widely available in Australia and New Zealand but can be found in model aeroplane fuel and laboratory solvents. It is also a natural byproduct in the distillation of ethanol and while commercial distilleries are tightly regulated, amateur home distillers may inadvertently be exposed to methanol through unsafe practice. Methylated spirits (also known as 'metho') sold in Australia and New Zealand does not contain methanol—it contains ethanol with a bittering agent to render it unpalatable and prevent distillation to obtain pure ethanol.

Formic acid and formaldehyde, the metabolites of methanol, as opposed to methanol itself, are the primary cause of clinical toxicity. Consequently, toxicity following ingestion of methanol is delayed until metabolism occurs. Significant methanol poisoning can present as CNS depression including coma, nausea and vomiting, seizures, visual disturbance

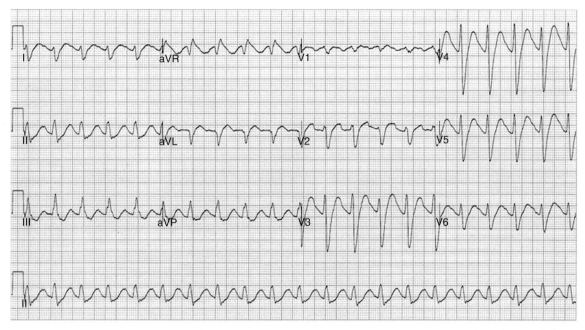

Figure 27.1
ECG changes associated with severe sodium channel blockade.
Source: Burns (2019). Life In the fast lane, https://lifeinthefastlane.com/ecg-library/basics/tca-overdose/

(or even blindness in the most serious cases), shock and metabolic acidosis (Roberts et al., 2015). As methanol toxicity results from its metabolism, agents that block this process can be effective antidotes. Fomepizole, a specific alcohol dehydrogenase inhibitor, is not widely available in Australia so either oral or intravenous ethanol is utilised to prevent methanol being metabolised (alcohol dehydrogenase preferentially metabolises ethanol) (Murray et al., 2015). Haemodialysis is also an essential part of management for patients with severe poisoning. Any delay in diagnosis and treatment is associated with blindness, permanent CNS damage, renal impairment and death.

Ethylene glycol

Ethylene glycol is also colourless but has no odour and has a sweet taste. It is commonly found in antifreeze and brake fluid. Due to its taste, it may be consumed as a substitute for alcohol in patients with problematic drinking or accidentally ingested by children exploring their environment. It may also be used with the intent to self-harm or attempt suicide. Similar to methanol, ethylene glycol is not itself toxic but its metabolites are (glycolic acid and oxalic acid). The effects of ethylene glycol toxicity include CNS depression, nausea and vomiting, seizures, shock and renal failure (Megarbane et al., 2005). Similar to methanol, toxicity can be circumvented using ethanol or fomepizole. Haemodialysis is also an essential part of management for patients with severe poisoning following ethylene glycol ingestion.

Methamphetamine

Methamphetamine is a potent illicit stimulant that is available as a powder or in crystalline form (colloquially referred to as 'ice'). This drug has had significant impacts in healthcare but also in the sociopolitical arena. The death rate from methamphetamine use doubled in Australia from 2009 to 2015, with toxicity related to recreational use being the most common cause of death; however, suicides have also been recorded (Darke et al., 2017). Due to the effects of methamphetamine, healthcare providers also need to be aware of their own safety. Extreme agitation and violence following methamphetamine use necessitate police involvement in some cases.

Methamphetamine, like other amphetamines, is a potent sympathomimetic drug, which enhances catecholamine release, inhibits catecholamine breakdown and blocks reuptake thereby significantly increasing the amount of excitatory neurotransmitters available (Murray et al., 2015). Methamphetamine is well absorbed, whether ingested or insufflated, and clinical effects (see Table 27.2) can persist for 24 hours or longer. Management of methamphetamine intoxication can be life-threatening and attention to management of hyperthermia and agitation are crucial in the out-of-hospital setting. Management of hyperthermia through passive cooling can prevent adverse long-term neurological outcomes. Reducing agitation through administration of parenteral benzodiazepines ameliorates the potential for complications and

Table 27.2 Acute pharmacological effects of methamphetamine

CNS	Cardiovascular	Peripheral sympathomimetic	Complications of toxicity
• Euphoria • Anxiety, dysphoria, agitation and aggression • Paranoid psychosis with visual and tactile hallucinations • Hyperthermia • Rigidity and myoclonic movements • Seizures	• Tachycardia and hypertension • Dysrhythmias • Acute coronary syndrome • Acute cardiomyopathy • Acute pulmonary oedema • Haemoptysis	• Mydriasis • Sweating • Tremor	• Rhabdomyolysis, dehydration and renal failure • Hyponatraemia and cerebral oedema • Aortic and carotid artery dissection • Subarachnoid and intracranial haemorrhage • Ischaemic colitis

Source: Murray et al. (2015).

improves safety for the patient and provider alike. Seizures should be treated with benzodiazepines and supportive airway care. An ECG should be performed to look for evidence of cardiac ischaemia. Early de-escalation of agitation and aggressive management of hyperthermia are likely to lead to improved patient outcomes.

Opioids

Opioids are one of the world's oldest known drugs. Extract from the opium poppy (opium) has been used therapeutically for centuries. Opioids are commonly divided into two groups: those that are legal (prescription) and those that are regarded as illicit (e.g. heroin). While deaths from opioid overdose have previously been related to heroin, there is an increasing number of deaths secondary to prescription opioids such as oxycodone (Pilgrim et al., 2015). For every fatal overdose there are many more non-fatal overdoses, which can cause severe morbidity and added expense for the healthcare system (Doyon, 2011). There is also a high prevalence of mental health problems among opioid-dependent people. Approximately one-third have a lifetime history of attempted suicide, a quarter report major depression and 9 out of 10 report posttraumatic stress disorder (Doyon, 2011).

Use of prescription opioids is steadily rising in Australia. They can be given in liquid form, tablets (standard and slow release) and patches (e.g. fentanyl) in varying strengths. There are risks of dependence, overdose and misuse with these drugs (by crushing and injecting them). The most common method of using heroin is by injecting; however, it can be smoked or the vapour directly inhaled. Intravenous drug users (IVDUs) are at an increased risk of viral infections including hepatitis B and C and HIV. It is estimated that 40% of acute hepatitis B cases are a result of unsafe use of injecting drugs (Doyon, 2011).

> ## BOX 27.3 Opium, opiate, opioid, narcotic: what's the difference?
>
> - *Opium* refers specifically to the dried extract from the seed pod of the opium poppy and includes the pharmacology of morphine and codeine.
> - *Opiate* refers to the derivatives of opium.
> - *Opioid* refers to any substance that can bind to opioid receptors and elicit a response. This also includes the body's endogenous opioids.
> - *Narcotic* means 'sleep-inducing'—this term has been adapted over the years to include illegal versions of many drugs, in particular heroin.
>
> Regardless of the name, the effect on people remains the same.

Irrespective of the type of opioid, the clinical effects following acute exposure on the person remain the same (see Boxes 27.3 and 27.4). Opioids are agonists at opioid receptors distributed throughout the body. There are three types of opioid receptors (mu, kappa and delta), each of which provides some modulation to the pain pathways in the body. The body also has endogenous opioids: endorphins, encephalins, dynorphins and endomorphins 1 and 2. These are the body's 'built-in' form of pain relief (Anderson et al., 2013).

Although opioids are rapidly absorbed after oral administration, not all are orally active because of first-pass metabolism by the liver (morphine is an example). The duration of effect depends on the individual drug; for example, heroin intoxication lasts less than 6 hours whereas clinical effects of

BOX 27.4 Pathophysiology and presentation of opioid overdose

The pharmacological effects of opioids can be both central and peripheral owing to the wide distribution of receptors throughout the body. Central effects include:

- Analgesia (pain relief)
- CNS depression (sedation)
- Respiratory depression
- Cough suppression
- Miosis (pupil constriction)
- Nausea and vomiting (dopamine receptors)
- Hypotension and bradycardia (large doses), ECG changes (QT prolongation and risk of torsades de pointes) with methadone
- Tolerance and dependence (tolerance develops after a few doses; dependence results in withdrawal syndrome after 1–2 days of no use).

Peripheral effects include:

- Decreased gut motility (constipation— opioids are used as an ingredient in anti-diarrhoeal medications)
- Spasm of sphincter muscles (delayed gastric emptying, urinary retention, biliary colic)
- Histamine release (bronchoconstriction, itching) (Osborn et al., 2009; Lee et al., 2011).

BOX 27.5 Symptoms of acute opioid withdrawal syndrome

- Agitation
- Nausea
- Vomiting
- Diarrhoea
- Lacrimation
- Rhinorrhoea
- Diaphoresis
- Pain ++
- Tachycardia
- Hypertension

Patients suffering from withdrawal can be given opioids to treat this, but this can be challenging if a large amount of naloxone is given. Titrated doses of naloxone (if indicated) are far more appropriate as a graduated approach is less likely to precipitate acute withdrawal.

---

opioids such as oxycodone and methadone can last over 24 hours, particularly following overdose. Opioid overdose is fatal when respiratory and CNS depression leads to respiratory arrest; therefore, attention to airway and breathing is a mainstay of treatment. Opioid-naïve patients and those who co-ingest other CNS depressants (including alcohol) are at an increased risk of mortality. Naloxone, an opioid receptor antagonist, can be lifesaving in patients with severe opioid toxicity. However, it is important to remember that provision of an airway and ventilation remain the priorities in management. Patients die from lack of a patent airway and oxygenation, rather than from lack of naloxone. In patients with opioid dependence, excessive naloxone can produce acute withdrawal with agitation, tachycardia and hypertension (see Box 27.5) (Murray et al., 2015). Therefore if naloxone is administered, it should be done so in a rational, titrated manner. As one could imagine, excessive or inappropriate use of naloxone can turn a relatively calm situation into a chaotic one, with the safety of both patient and provider in question. **Naloxone should only**

be administered if there is evidence of hypoventilation (respiratory rate less than 8) or hypoxia (oxygen saturation less than 90% measured on room air; an inspiratory FiO$_2$ of 21%).

Quetiapine

Quetiapine (trade name Seroquel) is a second-generation (or atypical) antipsychotic. It is the leading cause of coma by poisoning requiring admission to intensive care in Australia (Murray et al., 2015). While intended for the treatment of psychotic illness, it is used for other psychiatric problems and recreationally as a 'downer' to counteract the effects of stimulant (or 'upper') effects.

Like other antipsychotics, quetiapine affects multiple receptors and therefore can cause a number of effects in overdose. Quetiapine is an antagonist at mesolimbic dopamine (D$_2$), serotonin (particularly 5-HT$_{2A}$), histaminic (H$_1$), muscarinic (M$_1$) and peripheral alpha (α_1) receptors (Murray et al., 2015). The clinical features therefore include CNS depression including coma (that can be prolonged), sinus tachycardia and hypotension, seizures (rarely) and anticholinergic toxicity. The anticholinergic toxidrome (summarised in Table 27.3) is often delayed and can occur on emergence from sedation.

Management of quetiapine toxicity should focus on good supportive care. Airway management including intubation may be necessary. Hypotension often responds to fluids; however, if an inotrope is required adrenaline should not be administered as the combination of alpha-receptor antagonism from

Table 27.3 Anticholinergic toxidrome

Signs and symptoms
Mad as a hatter (delirium, agitation)
Blind as a bat (mydriasis—dilated pupils, blurred vision)
Hot as a hare (hyperthermia)
Dry as a bone (dry mucous membranes, skin)
Red as a beet (flushed skin)
Sinus tachycardia

Source: Braitberg & Kerr (2009).

quetiapine and beta$_2$-adrenoreceptor agonism from adrenaline can lead to worsened hypotension (Hawkins & Unwin, 2008). Noradrenaline is the inotrope of choice.

Tricyclic antidepressants

Tricyclic antidepressants (TCAs) are a group of drugs prescribed for a variety of disorders including depression, anxiety and neuropathic pain. TCAs act by preventing the reuptake of serotonin and noradrenaline (neurotransmitters in the CNS) in the synaptic cleft of neurons, resulting in increased concentrations of these neurotransmitters. Similar to quetiapine, they also act as antagonists on a variety of CNS-receptors including serotonin, adrenaline, histamine and acetylcholine, often resulting in undesirable side effects (Murray et al., 2015). The clinical effects of TCAs in overdose predominantly feature:

- sodium channel blockade (QRS widening, ventricular arrhythmias) (Body et al., 2011)
- anticholinergic activity (sinus tachycardia, hyperthermia, flushing, dry mucous membranes, delirium, mydriasis as discussed in Table 27.3)
- Alpha-adrenergic blockade (hypotension via peripheral vasodilation).

Patients may appear well initially but can deteriorate rapidly with little warning and develop life-threatening complications. Severe toxicity generally occurs within the first 1–2 hours post-ingestion, with initial signs generally occurring within the first 60 minutes. The commonest early signs of toxicity are CNS depression and sinus tachycardia. The most significant toxic effects of TCAs stem from sodium channel blockade. Degree of clinical toxicity can be predicted by the amount ingested; for instance, an ingestion of > 10 mg/kg can produce significant and potentially life-threatening toxicity (Murray et al., 2015). In a child, this could be as little as one tablet (unfortunately known in clinical toxicology as a 'one pill kill'). Furthermore, the ECG can provide useful clinical evidence regarding the risk of cardiovascular and CNS toxicity, which often cause mortality in TCA overdose.

- QRS > 100 ms is prognostic of seizures.
- QRS > 160 ms is prognostic of ventricular tachycardia (VT) (Parkinson et al., 2011).

Sodium bicarbonate is a lifesaving antidote in overdoses from drugs that cause sodium channel blockade such as TCAs. Sodium bicarbonate provides sodium ions to compete with TCA binding of sodium channels and the bicarbonate affects serum pH to prevent distribution of the TCA from the plasma to organs such as the brain and heart. Sufficient treatment with sodium bicarbonate is confirmed by attainment of a serum pH of 7.50–7.55.

A pitfall in practice is the administration of sodium bicarbonate to patients who have taken overdoses of drugs that do not cause sodium channel blockade (QRS prolongation on ECG). In particular sodium bicarbonate must not be given in cases of toxicity caused by drugs that cause prolongation of the QT interval. This can lead to hypokalaemia, further prolongation of the QT interval and potentially fatal ventricular arrhythmias. Excessive sodium bicarbonate can also lead to hypernatraemia and seizures. Excessive serum alkalisation can cause myocardial dysfunction and shock. As with other areas in toxicology, the antidote must fit the clinical picture. **If QRS prolongation (QRS > 120 ms) in association with evidence of significant clinical toxicity (CNS depression, hypotension, seizures or arrhythmias) IS NOT present, sodium bicarbonate is not indicated.**

CASE STUDY 1

Case 12492, 2225 hrs.

Dispatch details: A 21-year-old male who is unconscious; query intoxicated.

Initial presentation: The ambulance crew find the patient at his 21st birthday party with approximately 100 other people in attendance. There are about 20 guests gathered around the patient, who is lying on the grass. He has been placed in the recovery position by his friends following advice from the emergency call-taker. He responds only by withdrawing to pain. He is making snoring sounds and his breathing is slightly shallow (there is a strong odour of alcohol). He is also pale and diaphoretic and is dry retching. He is covered in vomit and has been incontinent of urine.

ASSESS

Patient history

Estimating the amount of ethanol that the patient has consumed and over what time period can assist in determining whether ethanol is consistent with the patient's condition, but it is rare to get a detailed and accurate answer. The phone numbers of the Poison Information Centre are a vital addition to any paramedic toolkit (see Box 27.6).

Gaining a past medical history may reveal prescription medications or conditions that mean an adverse outcome is more likely when excessive ethanol is imbibed (epilepsy, diabetes). Events immediately preceding the patient's collapse are also worth examining: for example, did the patient suffer any head trauma prior to falling or as a result of falling that could explain their altered conscious state?

This case study reveals a typical presentation of severe ethanol intoxication. The patient is at a party and ethanol is freely available. He presents with signs and symptoms that are classic of severe intoxication, including severe CNS depression, and has no significant past medical history of recent trauma.

Airway

Ethanol presents a dual-pronged challenge to airway patency. As a CNS depressant, ethanol suppresses the protective reflexes of the airway including coughing, swallowing and the gag reflex. Vomiting can occur and when this is combined

---

BOX 27.6 Poison information centres

Poison Information Centres operate 24 hours a day in Australia and New Zealand. Paramedics use them regularly, particularly when a patient has ingested a medication, chemical or plant that is unknown to them. The numbers are:
- Australia: 13 11 26
- New Zealand: 0800 764 766 (0800 POISON)

with a loss of airway reflexes, the risk of aspiration is significant. Predicting the likelihood of vomiting is difficult as it depends on both the volume of ethanol (and other fluids/food) consumed and the period of time over which it has been consumed.

This patient's snoring sounds suggest a significant degree of CNS depression and he should be placed in the lateral position as soon as possible. This should resolve the snoring but a small amount of manual jaw lift/support may be needed. A visual inspection of the upper airway should be sufficient to identify any major obstructions. Persistent airway noises and increased work of breathing are indicative of airway obstruction and need to be managed if present. Otherwise, the insertion of oropharyngeal airways into the mouth of an intoxicated patient should be avoided at this stage, as it is likely to precipitate vomiting.

Breathing

This patient's ethanol level is potentially quite high and it is therefore possible that depression of the medulla and the respiratory centre is occurring. His respiration rate is currently 10 and provided the tidal volume is sufficient, this should be adequate (and can be checked against his SpO_2). Absorption of ethanol is probably still occurring, however, and both the rate and the depth of his breathing could deteriorate.

Circulation

Ethanol is both a mild vasodilator and a diuretic, meaning that it can lead to poor perfusion and inappropriately high urine output, producing mild shock and dehydration. It has fewer cardiovascular effects than benzodiazepines, so profound hypotension should raise suspicions of other drugs. Ethanol's vasodilatory effects direct blood to the skin, so heat loss can develop quickly in cold environments.

Gastrointestinal/urinary systems

Ethanol can trigger the chemoreceptor trigger zone (CTZ) and the vomiting centre. Urinary incontinence is also common due to CNS depression as well as loss of inhibition.

Physical examination

Physical examination and assessment should be undertaken with an open mind. The tendency to reach premature diagnostic decisions is one of the main causes of diagnostic error: *this patient has been drinking ethanol in excess; drinking ethanol in excess leads to unconsciousness—therefore, this patient is intoxicated.* Intoxication increases risk-taking behaviour and the likelihood of falls. Close examination of the patient's face and skull for wounds could reveal injuries from an earlier fall that was possibly unwitnessed.

Initial assessment summary

Problem	Unconscious, possibly intoxicated
Conscious state	GCS = 7 (E1, V2, M4)
Position	Lying on his side on the grass
Heart rate	98 bpm, weak
Blood pressure	105/78 mmHg
Skin appearance	Pale, cool
Speech pattern	Incomprehensible sounds
Respiratory rate	10 bpm
Respiratory rhythm	Even cycles
Respiratory effort	Normal but decreased tidal volume

Chest auscultation	Clear chest
Pulse oximetry	97% on room air
Temperature	36.3°C
History	The patient is covered in vomit and has been incontinent of urine. His friends state that he started drinking at 6.30 pm and has consumed a 750-mL bottle of bourbon and at least 8 or 9 stubbies of beer. They say he is at university full-time and works part-time at a fast-food outlet; he regularly gets drunk at parties but they have never seen him this bad. They assure you that it would be unusual for him to take anything else. There is no evidence of traumatic injury.
BSL	4.7 mmol/L

D: There are no immediate dangers to the patient or crew.

A: The patient is unconscious and his airway is clear.

B: Respiratory rate is slightly depressed but SpO_2 is normal.

C: Heart rate and blood pressure are approaching normal limits.

The patient smells of ethanol, has been seen drinking at the party and has a social history of binge drinking. A physical examination reveals no obvious injuries.

② CONFIRM

The essential part of the clinical reasoning process is to seek to confirm your initial hypothesis by finding clinical signs that should occur with your provisional diagnosis. You should also seek to challenge your diagnosis by exploring findings that do not fit your hypothesis: don't just ignore them because they don't fit.

What else could it be?

Hypoglycaemia

Hypoglycaemic patients can present in a similar way to patients with acute ethanol intoxication. A simple BSL check will allow the paramedic to either detect and correct or rule out hypoglycaemia. A BSL should always be recorded for patients with an altered conscious state.

Hypothermia

Hypothermic patients can present in a similar way to patients with acute ethanol intoxication. A simple check of the patient's temperature will allow the paramedic to either detect and correct or rule out hypothermia. This patient's temperature is slightly low but it is not clinically significant.

Hypoxia

Hypoxia is another condition that can be readily detected and corrected with oxygen, basic airway management and assisted ventilation. Correction of airway compromise, breathing assistance and oxygen should quickly rule out hypoxia as the cause of a decreased GCS. With oxygen saturations of 97% while breathing room air, it is highly unlikely that this patient is hypoxic.

Hypotension

Insufficient cerebral perfusion will cause alterations of consciousness. This patient's blood pressure is slightly low but not enough to explain his condition.

Effects of other drugs or toxins

Ethanol is commonly consumed along with other medications and/or drugs that may interact with it in negative ways. These include:

- antihistamines, antidepressants, opioids, anti-anxiety medications and antipsychotics (these all increase the CNS depressant effects of ethanol)
- oral hypoglycaemics (these may place the patient at risk of hypoglycaemia)

DIFFERENTIAL DIAGNOSIS

Acute alcohol (ethanol) poisoning

Or
- Hypoglycaemia
- Head injury
- Seizure
- Effects of other drugs or toxins
- Effects of other toxic alcohols

- anticonvulsants and anticoagulants (in chronic ethanol abuse where there is impaired liver metabolism these may cause elevated serum concentrations)
- non-steroidal anti-inflammatory drugs (NSAIDs; these may increase gastric irritability)
- nitrates (these may increase the risk of hypotension and syncope due to excess vasodilation)
- anticholinergics and antispasmodics (these may slow gastrointestinal function, which in turn slows absorption of ethanol).

Other toxidromes can be considered as part of the differential diagnoses. One drug in particular that can present in a similar way is an opioid overdose, but this patient's pupils are normal and his respiratory depression is not severe. Combined with the lack of any recent IV injection marks found on physical examination, this is not highly suggestive of an opioid overdose. It is important to note that in mixed drug overdoses which include an opioid, pupils may not be pinpoint, even though opioid-induced reparatory depression is present. Absence of miosis does not rule out exposure to an opioid.

Effects of other toxic alcohols (methanol, ethylene glycol)

Methanol leads to the same ethanol-type odour, tachycardia and hypotension exhibited by this patient but it is not readily available in Australia and New Zealand. It is therefore unlikely that this patient was consuming methanol. Ethanol is the antidote for methanol poisoning (given in hospital only) and a positive outcome is more likely if given early. If methanol poisoning is suspected, early hospital management may have a significant impact upon outcome. Ethylene glycol is an odourless liquid and therefore would be less likely to cause a strong ethanol-type odour on the patient's breath. The hallmark signs of ethylene glycol poisoning are CNS depression, metabolic acidosis and renal failure. The main source of ethylene glycol in Australia and New Zealand is radiator antifreeze/coolant. Although it is unlikely that the patient has ingested ethylene glycol, it cannot be ruled out confidently in the field without a clear history of what was actually ingested.

Head injury

Questioning bystanders regarding the patient's activities prior to the paramedics' arrival is essential. There must also be consideration of a possible mechanism of head injury, so a survey of the scene and where the patient is found is important. The next important step is the secondary survey: a full head-to-toe examination is necessary to ascertain if there is any evidence of trauma or any injuries. No injuries are found in this patient.

TREAT

Emergency management

The principles of management for the unconscious patient are outlined in Box 27.7.

Safety

Negative consequences of ethanol consumption include antisocial and aggressive behaviour, violence, assault and crime. Paramedics should always consider their safety when approaching a scene where one or several people may be intoxicated. It may be necessary to contact the police and have them attend the scene to assist in crowd control. In many cases it is the police that call the ambulance. Wearing personal protective equipment (PPE) including gloves and eyewear is essential due to the high possibility of bodily fluids being present and the fact that antisocial behaviour can include spitting.

Fix the fixable!

Drugs and trauma are obvious causes of an altered conscious state but there are other (largely) reversible causes that should always be addressed prior to

> **PRACTICE TIP**
>
> It is important to approach all patients equally and not to judge or negatively stereotype people just because they have a problem with ethanol or any other drug. It is a medical condition like any other. All patients should be treated with dignity and respect regardless of their choices or lifestyle. If paramedics approach patients in an open, honest and non-judgmental way, patients are more likely to respond by being open and honest in return.

BOX 27.7 Advanced airway management in patients who are intoxicated

Patients who have taken an agent that causes CNS depression may present with or develop a decreased conscious state, which increases the risk of pulmonary aspiration. In these circumstances it is worth considering the need (or otherwise) to manage the patient's airway and ventilation with an endotracheal tube. While endotracheal intubation provides control of ventilation and FiO_2, there are a number of risks and drawbacks that should be considered. For example, the sedative drugs used to enable intubation can exacerbate the respiratory and cardiovascular impacts of the drugs already in the patient's system. These will need to be managed if the intubation is successful, but if it is unsuccessful, the crew will be faced with a worse situation than they currently have. Even intoxicated patients may require significant sedation to enable the endotracheal tube to pass through the vocal cords and this is likely to impact on blood pressure and cerebral perfusion. Intubation also limits the ability to conduct a physical neurological assessment when the patient arrives at hospital. Other issues that should be considered with every intubation include:

- the consequences of a failed intubation
- the consequences of an unrecognised oesophageal intubation.

While these variables can appear confusing and vague, the solution is relatively simple. Where the oxygen saturation cannot be kept above 90–92% using oxygen and non-invasive airway support, the potential harm of widespread cerebral hypoxia outweighs the risks associated with advanced airway management. In Case study 1, the patient is not hypoxic and provided his airway can be maintained with positioning, he is unlikely to be intubated in the out-of-hospital setting or later on, in hospital. If the patient is hypoxic, refractory to non-invasive means of intubation should be considered.

managing specific overdoses or injuries. Before commencing specific management of overdose always ensure that any abnormalities of the following have been corrected.

- Hypoxia: ensure adequate rate and depth of ventilation and FiO_2.
- Hypercapnia: ensure adequate rate and depth of ventilation.
- Hypoglycaemia: ensure BSL > 4.0 mmol/L.
- Hypothermia: ensure temperature > 35°C.
- Hypotension: ensure adequate heart rate and blood pressure.

Airway

Posture (lateral) and jaw support are likely to be sufficient in this patient. Suctioning of excess saliva should be done with care in order to not provoke the gag reflex and vomiting. There is an increased risk of morbidity and mortality if an ethanol-intoxicated patient aspirates vomit into the lungs, but the risks associated with intubation outweigh the benefits if the airway can be controlled by position and support (see Box 27.7).

Breathing

Once the airway has been secured, it is necessary to ensure adequate breathing/ventilation. This patient's breathing is shallow so the tidal volume may be insufficient.

It would be unwise to assume that the cause of this patient's decreased GCS score is due to ethanol only. The normal breathing rate for an adult male is approximately 12–15 bpm. While this patient's rate is just below that, some would still consider it within the normal range. The depth of his respirations is a concern. It is essential that the paramedic assess for signs and symptoms of hypoxia including cyanosis of the buccal mucosa, tongue and lips.

Given the decrease in tidal volume, it would be worth commencing this patient on oxygen via a rebreather mask at 8 L/minute, despite his SpO_2 being relatively normal. This is unlikely to improve his conscious state but it will prevent rapid desaturation if the crew choose to intubate him. Gently assisting the depth of each ventilation using a bag valve mask (BVM) would also be recommended if hypoxia is suspected to be developing.

Circulation
This patient is borderline with regard to perfusion; IV fluids should be made ready but are not needed at this point. A bolus of 10 mL/kg would not be harmful and will provide a buffer, should the patient need to be sedated for intubation.

Other
An antiemetic such as ondansetron can be considered and given either IV or IM as part of treatment, especially if the patient has already vomited and is dry retching. Metoclopramide is a less desirable option as it may actually increase absorption of alcohol by promoting gastric emptying.

Glucose 10% IV can be considered and administered if the patient's BSL is low and requires correcting. If you give glucose (oral or IV) to a patient who has consumed alcohol, it is recommended that you notify the staff at triage about this so that they can include thiamine in their treatment.

4 EVALUATE

Evaluating the effect of any clinical management intervention can provide clues to the accuracy of the initial diagnosis. Some conditions respond rapidly to treatment so patients should be expected to improve if the diagnosis and treatment were appropriate. A failure to improve in this situation should trigger the clinician to reconsider the diagnosis.

The aim of out-of-hospital management of the acutely intoxicated patient is generally supportive and fits in the standard primary survey ABCDE of patient assessment. The patient with mild acute ethanol intoxication provides a dilemma. It is difficult to ascertain whether the patient's condition is going to worsen or not, as there is no way of knowing if their BAC is continuing to rise. If the patient refuses transport, this raises issues of autonomy and competence (see Ch 13). It is important to remember that this condition does not fall under the scope of mental health legislation, which allows involuntary admission of patients. The opportunity to engage such a patient in the health system relies on the paramedics' ability to convince the patient to accompany them to hospital. The patient in this case has severe ethanol intoxication and requires significant intervention and supportive care, and operating with implied consent is sufficient.

For more severe cases of ethanol intoxication where the conscious level is profoundly altered the focus becomes protection of the airway from vomit/secretions, especially in patients with severe CNS depression. Circulation may be compromised due to the vasodilation effects of ethanol and should be monitored and treated if necessary. Investigations and a thorough secondary survey should include searching for and treating other causes of a decreased GCS, such as hypoglycaemia, head injury or other types of overdose. All patients with severe CNS depression must be closely monitored in hospital. Mildly intoxicated patients may be supervised by a responsible adult who is not intoxicated if the patient is to remain at home.

Ongoing treatment

Treatment at hospital remains primarily supportive with repeated monitoring. Endotracheal intubation is avoided if possible as the patient's conscious state will start to improve within hours. Hypoglycaemia can develop but is usually responsive to treatment.

Investigations

If the patient is able to perform the test, the BAC is measured using a breathalyser; otherwise, it forms part of a blood analysis. Liver enzyme tests may be considered to assess chronic ethanol-related liver disease.

Hospital management

Provided the investigations do not reveal underlying disease and that the intoxication was not a deliberate attempt at self-harm, most patients will be discharged from the ED once they have achieved a GCS score of 15 and are cooperative, ambulant, eating and drinking fluids, and passing urine.

 CASE STUDY 2

Case 13423, 1030 hrs.

Dispatch details: A 36-year-old female who is unresponsive; caller states 'not breathing properly'.

Initial presentation: The crew find a 36-year-old female lying slumped on a couch. She has slow, shallow breathing.

---

1 ASSESS

1039 hrs Primary survey: The patient is in an altered conscious state. Her airway is clear with slow, shallow ventilations.

1041 hrs Vital signs survey: Perfusion status: HR 60 bpm, sinus; BP 105/80 mmHg; skin pale with cyanosed lips.

Respiratory status: RR 6 bpm, chest difficult to auscultate due to shallow ventilations; SpO$_2$ 85%.

Conscious state: GCS = 5 (E1, V1, M3), pupils 1 mm in size, unresponsive to light.

1045 hrs Pertinent Hx: The patient's boyfriend is present. He reports a history of daily intravenous heroin use. The patient has been more stressed recently and wanted to sleep to forget her problems and took a little extra heroin. She does not use any other drugs and has no other medical history apart from depression. She is not on any other medications.

2 CONFIRM

In many cases, paramedics are presented with a collection of signs and symptoms that do not appear to describe a particular condition. A critical step in determining a treatment plan in this situation is to consider what other conditions could explain the patient's presentation.

What else could it be?

Other drug overdose

For details regarding alcohols, see above. In this case there is no characteristic odour of ethanol, nor is there evidence of alcohol on the scene or from questioning the husband. The key to ruling out whether opioids are the cause of this patient's signs and symptoms is to give a challenge of naloxone and monitor

> **Consider!**
> - What naloxone dose should be used? If naloxone is used, the smallest dose possible to achieve adequate respiration is all that is needed.
> - Is there a possibility of opioid dependence and induction of the opioid withdrawal syndrome?

for a response. As naloxone is a competitive antagonist at opioid receptors, it will cease the action of opioids in the patient's system and her signs and symptoms will improve. If the patient does not respond to naloxone, then other drugs or causes for her symptoms must be considered.

Hypoglycaemia

Hypoglycaemic patients can present in a similar way to patients with an opioid overdose (see Ch 25). A simple BSL check will allow the paramedic to either detect and correct it or rule it out. A BGL should always be recorded for patients with an altered conscious state.

Hypoxia

Hypoxia (see Ch 2) is another condition that can be readily detected and corrected with oxygen therapy. This patient is definitely hypoxic as a result of respiratory depression. Correction of airway compromise, breathing assistance and oxygen should eventually rule out if hypoxia is the underlying cause of her decreased GCS but it may take several minutes before any improvement is noted. In this case it is unlikely that reversing the hypoxia will return the conscious state to normal but it must be provided immediately to reduce ongoing harm.

Head injury

In this case, the patient is on a couch so a recent head injury or trauma seems highly unlikely. However, the signs and symptoms may be the result of an injury sustained days earlier, so careful examination and questioning of the boyfriend regarding what the patient was doing prior to the paramedics' arrival and in the days preceding are essential. It is important to ascertain the last time the patient was seen behaving in her normal manner. A full secondary survey should be conducted.

Stroke

There is no way to perform a stroke assessment on this patient due to her low GCS. A quick look at the pupils will indicate whether they are equal in size and pinpoint. In severe stroke they may vary in size and may not react to light. If naloxone does not produce a response, then stroke could be a possibility.

Seizure

Seizure is a possible differential diagnosis and history such as abnormal movements, prior history of epilepsy and/or treatment with anti-epileptics is important. Signs such as tongue biting, urinary incontinence and confusion on waking can suggest a seizure; however, this is less likely in this instance.

Sepsis

Sepsis would be more likely to cause tachycardia in response to acidosis and hypotension, which is not seen in this case. An elevated respiration rate is one of the key signs and symptoms of sepsis signifying septic shock: this patient has respiratory depression. Once again, if a challenge of naloxone does not elicit a response, then sepsis should still be considered, despite the lack of typical signs.

③ TREAT

Opioid overdose is an emergency. Resuscitation must focus on airway, breathing and circulation, with naloxone an important but not essential adjunct. If there are sufficient resources at the scene and it does not delay treatment or transport, try to locate any empty medication containers that might indicate the extent of the overdose to assist hospital treatment.

1048 hrs: Manual support of the airway is combined with an oropharyngeal airway to maintain an open airway. Ventilations are supplemented with 12–16 bpm at 7 mL/kg IPPV using a BVM with oxygen at 15 L/minute to correct the effects of respiratory depression and hypoxia.

PRACTICE TIP

Suboxone is a combination of buprenorphine and naloxone and is used to treat opiate addiction. It is an oral medication and in this form buprenorphine alleviates withdrawal while producing very little euphoria; naloxone similarly has little effect when taken orally. Yet if suboxone were to be dissolved and injected it would be useless, as the naloxone will antagonise the opioid effect and, in some cases, can precipitate withdrawal.

Most local guidelines would direct paramedics to administer naloxone immediately to reverse the effects of an opioid overdose; however, caution is advised with the dose given. Giving a large dose of naloxone to a patient who is opioid dependent (as someone who uses intravenous heroin on a daily basis) could trigger the patient into sudden withdrawal (see Box 27.5). This situation requires small doses of naloxone, titrated to improve the patient's respiratory function, but this principle lies outside some existing paramedic guidelines, which direct large IM/IV doses until the patient is fully conscious. Provided the patient can be effectively ventilated and the hypoxia is reversed, there is time to consult with the receiving hospital or ambulance clinician regarding appropriate treatment for this patient.

4 EVALUATE

Evaluating the effect of any clinical management intervention can provide clues to the accuracy of the initial diagnosis. Some conditions respond rapidly to treatment so patients should be expected to improve if the diagnosis and treatment were appropriate. A failure to improve in this situation should trigger the clinician to reconsider the diagnosis.

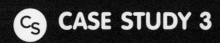

CASE STUDY 3

Case 19884, 1425 hrs.

Dispatch details: A 47-year-old female having a seizure.

Initial presentation: The paramedics arrive to find the patient's distraught husband gesturing them towards the bathroom. He hands them a packet of Endep (amitriptyline) (25 mg, 50 tablets) prescribed yesterday: all of them are missing. In the bathroom the paramedics find the patient lying fully clothed in an empty bathtub with her head supported by pillows.

---

1 ASSESS

1432 hrs Primary survey: The patient is unconscious but breathing.

1433 hrs Vital signs survey: Perfusion status: HR 118 bpm; sinus tachycardia; QRS = 0.14 sec; BP 80/52 mmHg; skin reddened, warm and dry; cyanosed around the lips. Respiratory status: RR 16 bpm, equal air entry bilaterally, normal tidal volume, SpO_2 94%. Conscious state: GCS = 4 (E1, V1, M2), pupils are dilated bilaterally. Other: Temperature 37.7°C; BSL 7.8 mmol/L.

1437 hrs Pertinent Hx: The patient's husband states that his wife seemed a little upset when he last spoke to her at lunchtime so he left work early and found her as she is. The patient has had clinical depression for 17 years and has been hospitalised three times for this condition. The last time was 2 months ago.

2 CONFIRM

In many cases paramedics are presented with a collection of signs and symptoms that do not appear to describe a particular condition. A critical step in

Ask!

- Has the patient attempted self-harm before?
- Are there any other drugs in the house (legal or not)?
- Is there any ethanol?
- Does the patient have any other illnesses (e.g. diabetes)?
- When was the last time anyone spoke to or saw the patient behaving 'normally'?
- What is the patient's weight, age, build?
- What is the patient's history in the days leading up to the event?

DIFFERENTIAL DIAGNOSIS

TCA overdose

Or

- Non-toxic seizure
- Other drug overdose
- Intracranial bleed
- Head injury

PRACTICE TIP ③

All patients with a suspected TCA overdose, whether symptomatic or not, must be transported to hospital because although they may initially present well, they can deteriorate rapidly to coma and death. Progression to coma occurs in the first few hours.

determining a treatment plan in this situation is to consider what other conditions could explain the patient's presentation.

What else could it be?

Other drug overdose

For details regarding alcohols see above. In this case there is no characteristic odour associated with ethanol, nor is there evidence of alcohol on the scene. Alcohol intoxication is not likely to present with the anticholinergic symptoms that this patient has. The lack of respiratory depression and the dilated pupils are not suggestive of opioid overdose.

Antihistamine overdose falls under the same toxidrome as TCA overdose (anticholinergic) but the presence of significant hypotension makes the diagnosis of antihistamine exposure less likely (Pierog et al., 2009). TCA overdose produces a distinctive ECG and this will help to confirm the diagnosis.

Sepsis

This patient is presenting with signs and symptoms that are similar to sepsis (tachycardia, hypotension and a slightly elevated respiration rate). Locating a causative factor for infection (e.g. urinary tract infection, chest infection) should be considered but an inability to find a locus of infection should not necessarily rule sepsis out. The patient's presentation is not consistent: the signs of sepsis are mild yet the conscious state is extremely poor. For sepsis to be the underlying cause of her unconsciousness we would expect her vital signs to be more deranged. The early signs of sepsis in this patient are suggestive that she may have already aspirated due to the overdose and is developing a chest infection. Auscultating her lungs reveals no adventitious sounds but on close inspection there is some vomit around her mouth.

Head injury

It is possible that collapse or seizure activity may have caused a head injury in this patient: a thorough head-to-toe examination would assist in ruling out traumatic head injury. As the patient appears to have set herself up in the bathtub with pillows it is unlikely that a fall/collapse was involved. Information at the scene and the incidents leading up to the presenting case can also provide vital clues.

TREAT

1440 hrs: Manual airway support, an oropharyngeal airway and IPPV via BVM are used to protect the patient's airway and provide non-invasive support. Should she not be able to maintain adequate oxygenation, advanced airway management strategies such as an endotracheal intubation may need to be employed.

Mild hyperventilation (20–24 bpm) is recommended in the intubated patient so that mild respiratory alkalosis is achieved (blood pH 7.50–7.55) to counter any effect of the TCA overdose. Acidosis caused by hypoxia (not the TCA overdose) has detrimental effects on the neurological and cardiac aspects of TCA overdose (sodium channel blockade) (Murray et al., 2015). Hyperventilation can be problematic in the non-intubated patient as air can be forced into the stomach. Care should be taken if this is the only option.

Intravenous access for drug administration and fluid administration should be provided as per local guidelines. Crystalloid fluids at 10–20 mL/kg are generally administered to support blood pressure.

An ECG should be obtained as soon as possible and patient monitoring should continue. IV sodium bicarbonate 100 mEq (2 mEq/kg) is indicated when there is a QRS duration >120 ms (see Fig 27.1). Sodium bicarbonate is considered an antidote for TCA overdose. Sodium bicarbonate provides sodium to counteract sodium channel blockade, and affects plasma pH, to prevent distribution of TCA to the CNS and cardiovascular system.

1446 hrs: The crew treat with 100 mL of sodium bicarbonate 8.4% administered IV over 3 minutes. Normal saline of 10 mL/kg is also administered. Generalised seizures are not uncommon in TCA overdose and multiple seizures are reported in up to 30% of cases, but they are usually brief. Preparation of benzodiazepines should be made up but not administered prophylactically.

(4) EVALUATE

Evaluating the effect of any clinical management intervention can provide clues to the accuracy of the initial diagnosis. Some conditions respond rapidly to treatment so patients should be expected to improve if the diagnosis and treatment were appropriate. A failure to improve in this situation should trigger the clinician to reconsider the diagnosis.

A failure to improve in patients who have overdosed is not unexpected as their condition is often complicated by the drugs ingested during the overdose attempt. The crew must now balance the complications of attempting endotracheal intubation in the field against the benefits of airway protection and control of ventilation. This will depend on the patient's anatomy, the likely presence of other drugs, the time to hospital and the ability to control hyperventilation using non-invasive means.

Future research

Patients who die following TCA overdose often do so due to cardiovascular toxicity. Future research is likely to focus on the role of new pharmacological therapy including inotropic agents, and mechanical support devices such as extracorporeal membrane oxygenation (ECMO).

Summary

Overdose can be accidental, recreational or intentional. In some cases, if intent cannot be determined or suicidal intent is volunteered by the patient or relatives, a psychiatric assessment is required. Supportive care is the mainstay of treatment with particular attention to airway in the setting of drugs that cause CNS depression. Antidotes may be required but should be used with caution as they are not benign in their own right. Poison information centres can be a useful resource and should be contacted where treating clinicians are unfamiliar or need additional advice regarding management. The main roles for the paramedic are recognition, supportive care, monitoring and initial management, while ensuring transport to hospital for definitive care.

References

Anderson, K., Alsina, M., Bensinger, W., Biermann, S., Cohen, A., Devine, S., Djulbegovic, B., Faber, E. A., Jr, Gasparetto, C., Hernandez-Illizaliturri, F., Huff, C. A., Kassim, A., Krishnan, A. Y., Liedtke, M., Meredith, R., Raje, N., Schriber, J., Singhal, S., Somlo, G., Stockerl-Goldstein, K., Treon, S. P., Weber, D., Yahalom. J., Yunus, F., Shead, D. A., & Kumar, R. (2013). Multiple myeloma, NCNN guidelines version 1. *Journal of the National Cancer Comprehensive Network, 11*(1).

Body, R., Bartram, T., Azam, F., & Mackway-Jones, K. (2011). Guidelines in Emergency Medicine Network (GEMNet): guideline for the management of tricyclic antidepressant overdose. *Emergency Medicine Journal, 28*, 347–368.

Braitberg, G., & Kerr, F. (2009). Central nervous system drugs. In P. Cameron, G. Jelinek, A. Kelly, L. Murray & A. Brown (Eds.), *Textbook of adult emergency medicine* (3rd ed.). Sydney: Elsevier.

Bryant, B., & Knights, K. (2011). *Pharmacology for health professionals* (3rd ed.). Sydney: Elsevier.

Burns, E. (2019). *Tricyclic overdose. Life in the Fast Lane.* 14 Sept. https://lifeinthefastlane.com/ecg-library/basics/tca-overdose/.

Cederbaum, A. I. (2012). Alcohol metabolism. *Clinics in Liver Disease, 16*(4), 667–685. http://doi.org/10.1016/j.cld.2012.08.002.

Darke, S., Kaye, S., & Duflou, J. (2017). Rates, characteristics and circumstances of methamphetamine-related death in Australia: a national 7-year study. *Addiction (Abingdon, England)*, *112*(12), 2191–2201. doi:10.1111/add.13897. Dec, [Epub 2017 Jul 11].

de Crespigny, C., Elliot, J., & Athanasos, P. (2011). Alcohol and other drug use. In K. Curtis, C. Ramsden & J. Friendship (Eds.), *Emergency and trauma nursing*. Mosby Elsevier.

Doyon, S. (2011). Opioids. In J. Tintinalli, S. Stapczynski, J. Ma, D. Cline, R. Cydulka & G. Meckler (Eds.), *Tintinalli's emergency medicine: a comprehensive study guide* (7th ed.). Sydney: McGraw-Hill.

Graudins, A., & Gunja, N. (2009). Antihistamine and anticholinergic poisoning. In P. Cameron, G. Jelinek, A. Kelly, L. Murray & A. Brown (Eds.), *Textbook of adult emergency medicine* (3rd ed.). Sydney: Elsevier.

Hawkins, D. J., & Unwin, P. (2008). Paradoxical and severe hypotension in response to adrenaline infusion in massive quetiapine overdose. *Critical Care and Resuscitation*, *10*(4), 320–322.

Lee, M., Silverman, S., Hansen, H., Patel, V., & Manchikanti, L. (2011). A comprehensive review of opioid-induced hyperalgesia. *Pain Physician*, *14*, 145–161.

Marx, J. A., Hockberger, R. S., & Walls, R. M. (2014). *Rosen's emergency medicine* (8th ed.). Elsevier.

Megarbane, B., Borron, S. W., & Baud, F. J. (2005). Current recommendations for treatment of severe toxic alcohol poisonings. *Clinical Toxicology*, *31*(2), 189–195. Feb, [Epub 2004 Dec 31].

Murray, L., Little, M., Pascu, O., & Hoggett, K. (2015). *Toxicology handbook*. Sydney: Elsevier.

Osborn, M., Horvath, N., & Bik To, L. (2009). New drugs for multiple myeloma. *Australian Prescriber*, *32*, 95–98.

Parkinson, S., Cadogan, M., Armstrong, J., & Nickson, C. (2011). Toxicological emergencies. In K. Curtis, C. Ramsden & B. Lord (Eds.), *Emergency and trauma care for nurses and paramedics*. Sydney: Elsevier.

Pierog, J. E., Kane, K. E., Kane, B. G., Donovan, J. W., & Helmick, T. (2009). Tricyclic antidepressant toxicity treated with massive sodium bicarbonate. *Am J Emerg Med*, 27(9), 1168.e3–1168.e7.

Pilgrim, J., Yafistham, S., Gaya, S., Saar, E., & Drummer, O. (2015). An update on oxycodone: lessons for death investigators in Australia. *Forensic Science, Medicine, and Pathology*, *11*, 3–12.

Roberts, D. M., Yates, C., Megarbane, B., Winchester, J. F., Maclaren, R., Gosselin, S., Nolin, T. D., Lavergne, V., Hoffman, R. S., & Ghannoum, M., EXTRIP Work Group. (2015). Recommendations for the role of extracorporeal treatments in the management of acute methanol poisoning: a systematic review and consensus statement. *Clinical Toxicology*, *43*(2), 461–472. doi:10.1097/CCM.0000000000000708. Feb.

CHAPTER 28

Anaphylaxis

By Ziad Nehme

OVERVIEW

- Anaphylaxis is a life-threatening condition that is commonly encountered in the out-of-hospital environment. Paramedics and clinicians providing emergency care in the field play an integral role in halting the pathophysiological cascade through the rapid assessment and early treatment of patients.
- Anaphylaxis is rapidly increasing in prevalence but is often underdiagnosed. Even when it is recognised, it can often be undertreated.
- Between 1997 and 2013, the Australian Bureau of Statistics (ABS) recorded an average of 20 cases of fatal anaphylaxis in Australia every year. Although iatrogenic causes (e.g. medications) are among the leading causes of fatal anaphylaxis, the trigger is unknown in the majority of deaths from anaphylaxis.
- Factors that increase the risk of fatal food-induced anaphylaxis include children and young adults, underlying peanut allergy, active asthma, ingestion of food prepared outside a known environment and delayed administration of adrenaline.
- Factors that increase the risk of fatal drug-induced anaphylaxis include older age, the presence of cardiovascular or respiratory comorbidities and antibiotic or anaesthetic agents.
- There was a 2.8-fold and a 4.0-fold increase in hospital admissions for all-cause anaphylaxis and food-related anaphylaxis in Australia between 1998–1999 and 2011–2012, respectively. Recent evidence also suggests that deaths from anaphylaxis are increasing in Australia by 6.2% annually.
- Intramuscular adrenaline is considered to be the first-line treatment.
- Fluids, H_1 and H_2 antihistamines and steroids are considered second-line treatments.
- The significant increase in the number of anaphylaxis presentations suggests that out-of-hospital personnel must remain vigilant in recognising and actively managing anaphylaxis to ensure that fatal anaphylaxis rates do not increase.
- Although the majority of patients with anaphylaxis present with typical clinical features involving two or more body systems, the diagnosis is not always obvious. In particular, skin features may be absent in 10–20% of anaphylaxis cases.
- Early recognition and management of the patient with anaphylaxis is essential to reduce morbidity and mortality.

Introduction

Anaphylaxis is an acute hypersensitivity reaction affecting multiple organ systems. The hypersensitivity reaction leads to a widespread release of inflammatory mediators which result in a systemic increase in capillary permeability, smooth-muscle contraction and peripheral vasodilation. The condition is characterised by flushing (erythema), hives, itching (pruritus), angio-oedema, stridor, wheezing or bronchospasm, vomiting, diarrhoea and cardiovascular compromise. If left untreated symptoms may progress to hypotension, respiratory arrest and death. Unlike allergic reactions, which are limited to a single body system, anaphylaxis produces systemic effects usually affecting two or more major body systems.

Pathophysiology

The term 'anaphylaxis' literally means 'against protection' and the potentially fatal condition results from an abnormal and exaggerated reaction of the body's normal immune response. In order to understand anaphylaxis, you first need to consider the body's normal immune system response. (For a complete description of the inflammatory response, see Ch 4.)

Allergen sensitisation

The purpose of the immune system is to protect the body from foreign substances (antigens) that are believed to be harmful. Certain antigens have the ability to evoke an allergic response, and these antigens are referred to as **allergens**. When an allergen enters the body for the first time—be it by ingestion, injection, absorption or inhalation—an immune response is triggered, resulting in the production of antigen-specific immunoglobulin antibodies by plasma cells in the blood. In the case of anaphylaxis, the process typically starts when an antigen stimulates the production of immunoglobulin E (IgE) antibodies, a specific subset of immunoglobulin that has evolved to target parasitic infections but sometimes reacts to antigens. Once formed, the IgE antibodies migrate to the surface of mast cells in the skin, gastrointestinal tract, respiratory system and peripheral blood basophils, which contain a range of potent chemicals that assist in the fight against invading allergens. The result is mast cells and basophils covered in antigen-specific immunoglobulins (antibodies; see Fig 28.1).

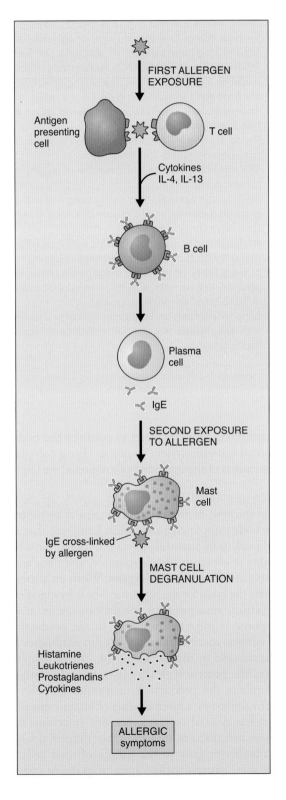

This initial exposure and response to an allergen is referred to as 'sensitisation'. The role of allergen sensitisation is to prepare the immune system for subsequent exposures to the allergen. It is therefore no surprise that mast cells populate in locations of the body where allergens are likely to enter, such as the connective tissues of the skin, lungs and gastrointestinal tract. Basophils, which are histologically very similar to mast cells, are also found in the bloodstream (Huether & McCance, 2016). In the absence of further exposure to the allergen, binding of IgE to mast cells and basophils produces no symptoms and goes unrecognised by the individual.

Mechanisms of anaphylaxis (IgE-dependent)

On subsequent exposure to the allergen the immune response is much quicker. The allergen binds to the IgE antibody, causing the mast cell or basophil membrane to rupture. The inflammatory mediators stored within these granulocytes are potent and are released within seconds, a process called degranulation (Huether & McCance, 2016). Although there is consensus that histamine is among the most significant of these inflammatory mediators, other mediators, such as prostaglandins, leukotrienes, bradykinin and cytokines, are also released and have synergistic effects on body systems. The fastest acting of these mediators is histamine and, together with the other inflammatory mediators released, it causes local blood vessels to dilate, bronchial smooth muscle to contract and capillary walls to become more permeable (Huether & McCance, 2016).

Although this process is typical of immune system responses and is designed to mobilise white blood cells (leucocytes) to fight the allergen, some individuals experience an abnormal escalation in

Figure 28.1
The immunological response in IgE-mediated anaphylaxis.
All allergies are the result of an excessive immune reaction. The process starts with a sensitisation phase where an antigen stimulates the production of immunoglobulin E, an immunoglobulin that has evolved to deal with large parasitic infections but sometimes reacts to other antigens. Immunoglobulin E attaches to mast cells to conclude the sensitisation stage. When the body is subsequently exposed to the antigen, it binds to the immunoglobulin E antibodies on the mast cells, triggering an uncontrolled release of histamine and other inflammatory mediators. These mediators cause symptoms that range from allergy to anaphylaxis. *Source: Castro & Kraft (2008), adapted from Novartis Pharmaceuticals.*

the inflammatory response. What should be a self-limiting process that results in nothing more than local swelling, redness and irritation (similar to the effects seen as a result of a mosquito bite) escalates into multi-system effects such as bronchoconstriction, systemic vasodilation and a widespread increase in capillary permeability. The reason for this abnormal reaction is not fully understood but it is thought to be due to genetic, infectious or environmental factors (Huether & McCance, 2016). This abnormal reaction can occur from within minutes to a few hours after exposure to the allergen and is known as an anaphylactic reaction or anaphylaxis.

In the case of anaphylaxis the actions of histamine are quickly replaced by the production of leuko-trienes, prostaglandins and other inflammatory mediators, which also exhibit potent effects on bronchial smooth-muscle and vascular permeability. In particular, these inflammatory mediators have a much longer effective life compared to histamine (Huether & McCance, 2016). There is also a complex set of interactions with components of the clotting system, cell membrane receptors and newly recognised chemicals such as interleukin-33 (IL-33) that may be responsible for propagating the reaction far from the site of the original allergen–antibody reaction.

This simple process of allergen sensitisation, IgE antibody production and subsequent inflammatory mediator release is the 'classic' anaphylactic pathway, and while it accounts for the majority of reactions, it is not the only cause of uncontrolled degranulation of mast cells and basophils (see Fig 28.2).

Mechanisms of anaphylaxis (IgE-independent, non-immunological and idiopathic)

There is a small group of immunological and non-immunological reactions that present identically to anaphylaxis but do not involve the usual IgE-mediated pathway. Previously termed anaphylactoid reactions, they are being increasingly referred to as *IgE-independent immunological anaphylaxis, non-immunological anaphylaxis* and *idiopathic anaphylaxis* (Simons et al., 2011). Some medications can trigger anaphylaxis through the activation of other immunological pathways, such IgG antibodies. In addition, non-immunological triggers such as exercise, cold environments and some medications (e.g. opioids) have been associated with direct activation of mast cells which do not require the usual antigen–antibody coupling. Finally, idiopathic anaphylaxis is diagnosed when no trigger can be identified despite a detailed history of the episode, allergen skin tests, measurement of serum IgE levels or other investigations (Simons et al., 2011). Given that the trigger allergen

of many reactions is never found, the ability to differentiate between the two types of anaphylaxis is not important in the emergency setting. However, it is vital to understand that a person doesn't need to have suffered a previous episode to be diagnosed with anaphylaxis.

Allergic reactions versus anaphylaxis

Although both allergic reactions and anaphylaxis share the same pathophysiological pathway (an exaggerated immune response to a trigger factor), the difference lies in the severity of the response. Allergic reactions are typically limited to a single body system (e.g. skin), while anaphylaxis produces systemic effects which are more severe and involve a combination of body systems, including respiratory, cardiovascular or gastrointestinal systems. For instance, an allergic response to an insect bite might result in a swollen and reddened arm far above the site of the bite, but unless the symptoms extend to include the respiratory, cardiovascular or gastrointestinal systems this is not an anaphylactic reaction.

Fatal anaphylaxis

Although anaphylaxis can vary in severity, fatal anaphylaxis is a rare occurrence. Between 1997 and 2013, the ABS recorded an average of 20 cases of fatal anaphylaxis in Australia every year (Mullins et al., 2016). In the out-of-hospital setting, there is limited data on the risk of cardiac arrest or death in patients presenting with anaphylaxis. A recent study from Victoria, Australia, showed that among 2137 cases of paediatric anaphylaxis presenting to paramedics, the rate of out-of-hospital cardiac arrest was 0.1% (Andrew et al., 2018). Investigations of fatal cases of anaphylaxis from Australia, the United States and the United Kingdom show that leading triggers were prescribed medication, insect venom and food (Turner & Campbell, 2016). Medication-related deaths from anaphylaxis are increasing in Australia and represent over half of all fatal cases of anaphylaxis.

There are a number of factors that influence the risk of fatal anaphylaxis which are relevant to paramedics and emergency health providers. Delayed or no administration of adrenaline as a result of misdiagnosis is a common theme in fatal cases of anaphylaxis (Simons et al., 2015). Good knowledge of the pathophysiology of anaphylaxis combined with thorough patient assessment is pivotal to its early recognition and treatment in the out-of-hospital setting. A sustained upright posture also increases the risk of cardiovascular collapse during anaphylaxis, and national guidelines recommend posturing victims in a sitting or supine position. A preexisting

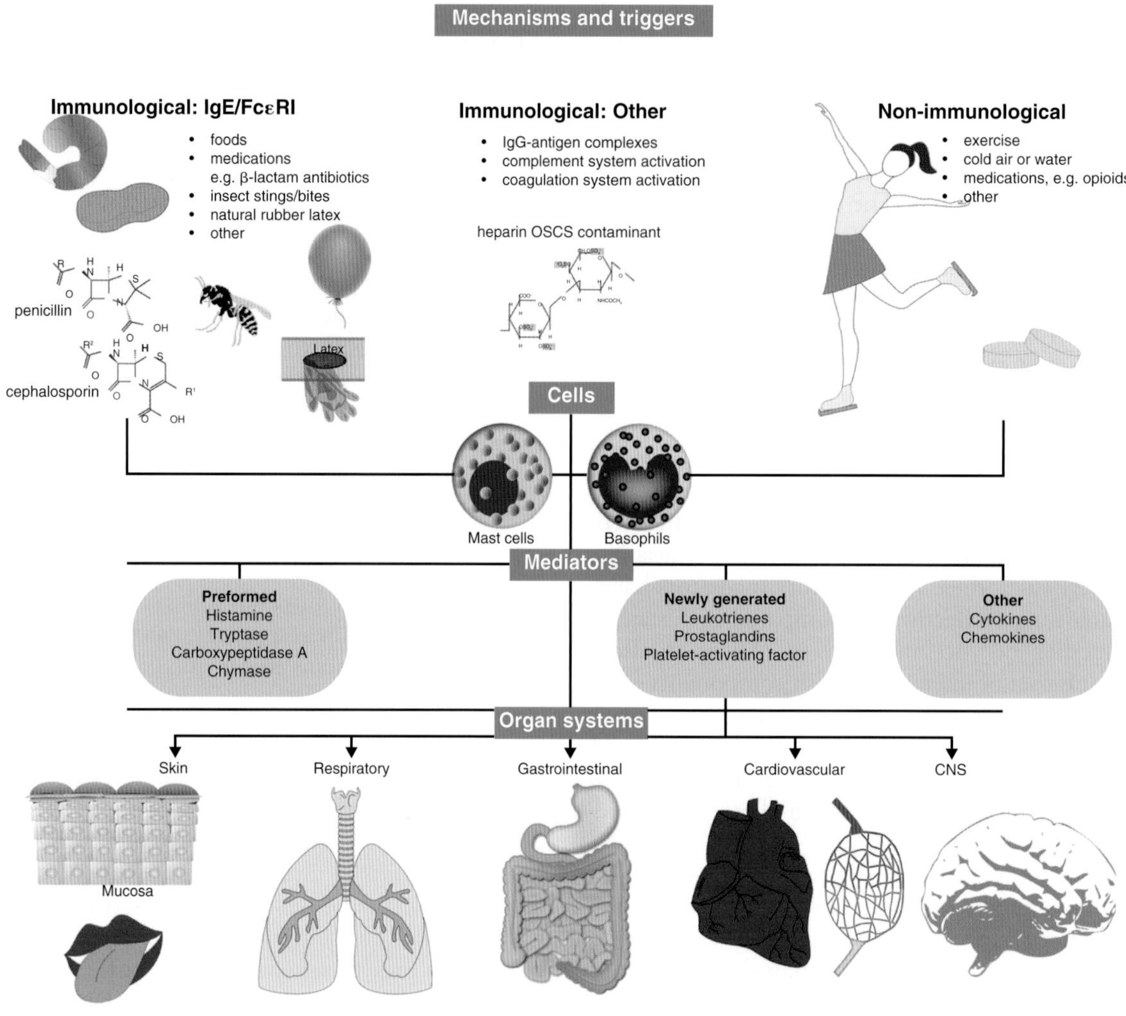

Figure 28.2
Mechanisms and triggers of anaphylaxis.
The classic anaphylactic mechanism involves exposure to an antigen that causes the body to produce IgE antibodies. On subsequent exposures to the allergen the IgE antibodies link with mast cells and basophils and cause the release of preformed inflammatory mediators (histamine) and the synthesis of other mediators (leukotrienes, prostaglandins, etc.). These mediators cause changes in the skin, mucosa, small airways, blood vessels and gastrointestinal system. Non-IgE-mediated responses are also possible, with IgG antibodies, exercise, heat and medications all potentially causing the uncontrolled release of inflammatory mediators.
Source: Estelle & Simons (2009).

history of asthma (especially if uncontrolled) and heart disease (particularly in older adults) are over-represented in fatal cases of anaphylaxis. Patients on anti-hypertensives and beta-blockers are also over-represented in fatal cases of anaphylaxis, but it is unclear if this is due to confounding from from other factors such as advanced age or underlying cardiovascular disease (Simons et al., 2015). Finally, systemic mastocytosis is a rare condition paramedics may be unfamiliar with. The condition is charac-terised by the production of an excessive number of mast cells which collect in various tissues and organs of the body. As a result, patients with systemic

mastocytosis are at high risk of recurrent and severe episodes of anaphylaxis which can be triggered idiopathically and may be difficult to diagnose (Gulen et al., 2014).

Definitions

The Australasian Society of Clinical Immunology and Allergy defines anaphylaxis as:

> *1. An acute onset illness with typical skin features (e.g. urticarial rash, flushing, and/or angioedema) plus the involvement of one or more of respiratory, cardiovascular or persistent severe gastrointestinal symptoms; or*

2. Any acute onset of hypotension or bronchospasm or upper airway obstruction where anaphylaxis is considered possible, even if typical skin features are not present.

(ASCIA, 2018)

The treatment recommendations provided in this chapter also follow the recommendations of the ASCIA.

 CASE STUDY 1

Case 10641, 2134 hrs.

Dispatch details: A 34-year-old female has had an allergic reaction to medication. She has been prescribed amoxicillin by her general practitioner for an upper respiratory tract infection, and has taken her first dose. She has a history of allergic reactions to penicillin as a child.

Initial presentation: The ambulance crew finds the patient sitting down. She is alert and acknowledges the crew as they enter the room. Her skin is flushed and she is complaining of itching and shortness of breath.

1 ASSESS

Patient history

The patient has provided the paramedics with several clues: she has taken a medication to which she knows she could be allergic (amoxicillin is a penicillin-based antibiotic). A short time later she is presenting with several signs of a systemic release of histamine and other inflammatory mediators, characterised by erythema and shortness of breath.

Given this history and the 'classic' presentation it is not difficult to see the connection, but too often the link between cause and effect is more difficult to ascertain (Turner & Campbell, 2016). As a consequence, a definitive cause for the reaction does not need to be made and it is the combination of abnormal vital signs and the paramedic's 'index of suspicion' that leads to the diagnosis.

Clinicians should be careful what they draw from a patient's past history of allergic reactions. Previous episodes of allergy or anaphylaxis should never be considered to be predictive or diagnostic for the severity of a reaction (Atkins & Bock, 2009). The immune system is never static and, while a previous allergic reaction indicates some degree of hypersensitivity, it is difficult to predict the severity of subsequent reactions. Accurately assessing the amount of allergen the patient has been exposed to, and the speed at which it is being absorbed, also make it difficult to predict outcomes based on history alone. There is perceived to be some relationship between the time of exposure and the speed and severity of symptoms, with the majority of fatal episodes displaying onset of symptoms within 30 minutes of exposure and death occurring before 60 minutes in just under half of these cases (Greenberger et al., 2007). But these timeframes would also be relevant for a vast number of non-fatal attacks, so this cannot be relied on as a particularly sensitive measure.

The relationship between onset of symptoms and severity of attack can also be distorted by the mechanism of exposure. Medications administered parenterally are more likely to provoke immediate reactions than those ingested

HISTORY

Ask!

- Have you had any previous episodes of allergy or anaphylaxis?
- Do you suffer from asthma?
- What time do you suspect you were exposed to the allergen?
- What was the first symptom you noticed?
- What other symptoms do you have? (What systems do they involve?)
- Are your symptoms getting better or worse?

BOX 28.1 Onset and severity

Drugs, latex and contrast media are among the most common cause of anaphylaxis in the hospital setting, while drugs, food (particularly nuts, shellfish, eggs and milk) and insect stings are the most common out-of-hospital causes (Turner & Campbell, 2016). Morphine can often cause a histamine release in the skin, leading to localised reactions at IV sites. An analysis of anaphylaxis fatalities in the United Kingdom found that the average time between onset of anaphylaxis symptoms and fatal cardiopulmonary arrest was 30 minutes for food reactions, 10–20 minutes for drug reactions, 15 minutes for insect stings and 5 minutes for iatrogenic reactions (Pumphrey, 2000). The average time taken for a reaction to develop after drugs were administered in hospital was only 5–10 minutes (Kaufman, 2003). Why is this less than the time taken for drug reactions in the community? It is probably because in-hospital administration is more likely to be intravenous and therefore have a quicker onset.

orally (Kaufman, 2003; see Box 28.1) but it may depend on the degree of sensitivity and dose as to how severely a reaction may ultimately evolve. Finally, approximately 5% of anaphylactic reactions are biphasic, with the second stage of the reaction being delayed for up to 72 hours and possibly being more severe than the initial reaction (Lee et al., 2015). This late-phase reaction, seen in both anaphylaxis and asthma, is very relevant when confronted with a patient who is feeling better and does not want to go to hospital.

What is significant and needs to be determined through history is the progression of the symptoms from one system to another. Symptoms related to the skin alone are less likely to progress towards a severe presentation than those events that include the respiratory and circulatory symptoms (Brown, 2007b). There is also a strong correlation between fatal reactions and respiratory symptoms that result from food sensitivity. Syncope and hypotension are the predictive signs of severity when the allergen is injected. Unfortunately, the causative agent cannot always be determined and the quickest mean time from onset of symptoms to cardiac or respiratory arrest occurs with iatrogenic reactions (Pumphrey, 2000).

While it is not always possible (or necessary) to identify the agent that triggered the reaction, this will need to be explored once the emergency phase of the treatment has concluded. Materials such as food or drug packaging that may be related to the reaction should be collected and transported with the patient.

Airway

Hypoxia caused by airway occlusion and severe bronchospasm contributes to the majority of deaths from anaphylaxis (Greenberger et al., 2007; Pumphrey, 2000). The combination of vasodilation and increased capillary permeability in the vascular tissues of the lips and tongue can cause them to swell. In addition to the swelling, the inflammatory mediators trigger increased glandular secretions and, combined with swelling of the upper airways, these secretions can cause a sudden and complete airway occlusion. The swelling can also present at the narrowest point of the airway—the larynx—which can affect the vocal cords.

Determine whether:
- the patient is having difficulty swallowing or feels a 'lump' in their throat
- the patient's tongue feels swollen
- the patient's voice sounds hoarse (a sign of high severity)
- there is evidence of stridor or tracheal tugging (a sign of high severity).

Remember, these signs are disproportionally represented in deaths from anaphylaxis.

Breathing

The effects of inflammatory mediators on the mucosa and smooth muscle of the lungs are identical to the hypersensitive reaction of asthma and so the diagnosis of anaphylaxis can easily be delayed in patients who have a past history of asthma. This delay may help explain why asthmatics are at a much higher risk of death from anaphylaxis (Turner et al., 2017). Many people would consider asthma and anaphylaxis as part of a continuum of allergic disease. Bronchoconstriction (leading to wheezing), hyperresponsive mucosal secretions, mucosal oedema and mucosal plugging are typical features of both asthma and anaphylaxis. However, evidence of respiratory symptoms combined with upper airway swelling, skin irritation, gastrointestinal symptoms or cardiovascular compromise (i.e. symptoms in other body systems) should immediately make paramedics suspicious of anaphylaxis.

Cardiovascular

Histamine and other inflammatory mediators have potentially potent effects on almost all of the cardiovascular system. They are potent dilators of both arterioles and veins, which can lead to distributive shock. They increase capillary permeability and can allow a fluid shift sufficient to cause hypovolaemic shock. They may even have a direct cardiac effect, creating arrhythmias and decreasing myocardial function to cause cardiogenic shock (Brown, 2007a). The severity of reaction and how each aspect contributes to the overall effect is difficult to predict, but in one United Kingdom study the resultant hypotension was the main cause of death in a quarter of fatal cases (Pumphrey, 2000, 2004).

The presentation of these effects needs to be carefully considered during paramedic assessment. Dilation of the small vessels leading into the capillary beds results in large amounts of blood pooling in the capillaries, particularly those near the skin. This erythema can make patients appear extremely flushed and they can radiate large amounts of heat. Increased capillary permeability allows a shift of fluid from the capillaries into the interstitial space and it is often first detected in the feet, hands, face (lips and eyelids) and upper airway (known as angio-oedema). Asking the patient to make a fist may detect whether their fingers are swollen, and asking family members if the patient's face and voice are normal can help detect facial and airway swelling.

Combined, the increased capillary permeability and pooling of blood in the veins and arterioles can cause a substantial drop in venous return. The standard physiological response to this is to increase sympathetic tone and this will present as a raised heart rate. Because paramedics tend to see anaphylactic patients soon after the onset of symptoms, this compensatory mechanism may still be in effect when they first assess the patient and the tachycardia can generate enough cardiac output to temporarily 'disguise' the loss of venous resistance and intravascular volume. In the early stages, the only sign of poor perfusion may be a persistent tachycardia. (For more on poor perfusion, see Ch 2.)

There remains considerable debate about the possible role of histamine on myocardial function and whether the inadequate perfusion often associated with anaphylaxis may also be associated with direct effects on cardiac tissue. The rare episodes of arrhythmias and cardiac dysfunction noted in some anaphylaxis patients may be secondary to prolonged poor perfusion of the myocardium rather than a direct effect of inflammatory mediators on the heart (Brown, 2007a).

Skin

Around 80–90% of anaphylactic reactions produce some form of skin irritation (Simons et al., 2011; see Fig 28.3). We have already described how the effects of histamine allow blood to pool in the capillaries leading to erythema (bright-red skin), and how increased capillary permeability can result in oedema. But

---

RESPIRATORY STATUS

Look for!
- Stridor
- Wheezes
- Increased work of breathing
- Symptoms in other body systems

Asthmatics are at a higher risk of fatal anaphylaxis!

PERFUSION STATUS

Ask!
- Is your tongue swollen?
- Do you have any swelling anywhere?
- Does your skin feel tight?
- Do you feel dizzy?
- Do you feel palpitations?

Also ask family members whether the patient's voice and face appear normal.

Look for!
- Tachycardia
- Hypotension: late sign
- Altered conscious state
- Erythema
- Pruritus
- Urticaria

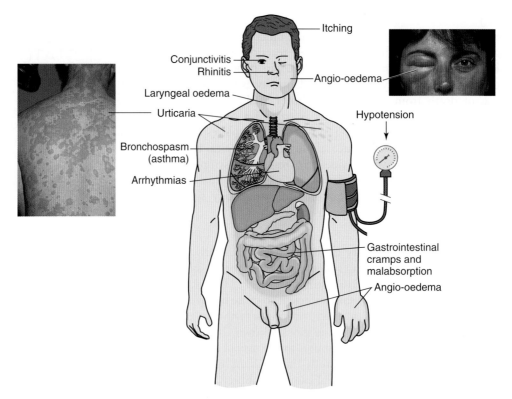

Figure 28.3
Signs and symptoms of anaphylaxis.
All the typical anaphylactic symptoms are the result of excessive inflammatory mediators. These mediators can cause any combination of the above conditions. While some, such as urticaria, may not appear life-threatening, they can indicate that other body systems may also be affected but are yet to fully reveal their involvement.
Source: McCance & Huether (2014); Male et al. (2013).

histamine and other inflammatory mediators have additional effects on the skin. The classic manifestation is urticaria (hives). These red, raised lesions are sometimes pale at their centre and can be any size and quite irregular in shape. They are almost always itchy but the irritation of histamine on nerve endings in the skin can also cause widespread itching without urticaria. This widespread itch is called **pruritus**. If the reaction is localised to the site of the cutaneous exposure (e.g. insect bite), it is less likely that there will be systemic manifestations.

Gastrointestinal system

As in the smooth muscle of the lungs, exposure to the inflammatory mediators of anaphylaxis causes intestinal smooth muscle to contract and become hyperactive. This often presents as intense abdominal cramping and profound nausea and may cause vomiting (emesis) and uncontrollable diarrhoea. Gastrointestinal symptoms occur in up to 45% of reactions (Simons et al., 2011; Brown, 2007b), are more commonly associated with ingested allergens and may have a later onset and more persistent presentation. (It may have occurred to you by now that all the body's responses in anaphylaxis are consistent with the body trying to 'remove' the allergen as well as trying to prevent any further contamination [i.e. bronchospasm and diarrhoea]).

Miscellaneous presentations

A number of other symptoms have been reported with anaphylaxis and while several (e.g. rhinitis, periorbital oedema and lacrimation) have obvious links to

GASTRO-INTESTINAL SYSTEM

Look for!
- Vomiting
- Diarrhoea
- Nausea
- Abdominal cramps

inflammation, the aetiology of others such as a 'sense of impending doom' are more difficult to explain. Anxiety and a sense of impending doom associated with anaphylaxis occur in a significant proportion of cases (Simons et al., 2011; Brown, 2007b) but it is difficult to assess whether they are caused directly by inflammatory mediators or by the symptoms (pain, shortness of breath, hypotension).

Initial assessment summary

Problem	The patient has ingested a drug (amoxicillin) that she is allergic to
Conscious state	Alert and oriented; GCS = 15
Position	Sitting upright in a chair, holding onto the arms of the chair
Heart rate	150 bpm, regular
Blood pressure	115/70 mmHg
Skin appearance	Within 5 minutes she is flushed and itchy all over
Speech pattern	Speaking in quick phrases
Respiratory rate	32 bpm
Respiratory rhythm	Regular, even cycles
Respiratory effort	Mild increase in the use of accessory muscles
Chest auscultation	Clear breath sounds, good bilateral air entry apices to bases
Pulse oximetry	99% on room air
Temperature	36.9°C
Motor/sensory function	Normal
History	She had a reaction to penicillin as a child but cannot remember any details

D: The source of the allergen has not been removed.
A: The patient is conscious with no current airway obstruction but needs frequent reassessment.
B: Respiratory function is currently normal but needs frequent reassessment. The respiratory rate is elevated but ventilation is normal.
C: Heart rate is elevated but there is a sufficient blood pressure.

The patient is displaying cutaneous, respiratory and cardiovascular symptoms of an allergic reaction. Therefore, there is sufficient evidence to suspect an anaphylactic reaction.

② CONFIRM

The essential part of the clinical reasoning process is to seek to confirm your initial hypothesis by finding clinical signs that should occur with your provisional diagnosis. You should also seek to challenge your diagnosis by exploring findings that do *not* fit your hypothesis: do not just ignore them because they do not fit.

Anaphylaxis is a clinical diagnosis, meaning that it is determined based on the patient's presentation rather than on laboratory results. This patient has presented with a known exposure to the allergen and a typical reaction has followed. Nonetheless, it is important to quickly consider what other conditions could be mimicking the patient's presentation and whether they can be excluded.

What else could it be?
Vasovagal syncope
Profound hypotension is common in severe anaphylaxis and distinguishing anaphylactic shock from other causes of hypotension can be difficult. The mechanism of neurally mediated syncope (e.g. vasovagal syncope) is not well understood but involves a simultaneous decrease in sympathetic tone with an increase in parasympathetic tone. The result is vasodilation without a tachycardic

DIFFERENTIAL DIAGNOSIS

Anaphylaxis
    Or
- Vasovagal syncope
- Arrhythmia
- Seizures
- Anxiety
- Asthma
- Airway obstruction
- Infection

response and this leads to a fall in blood pressure and subsequent collapse. Vasovagal reactions are an abnormal neural response to stimuli such as pain, fear or sudden changes of position, but they can also be caused by a shift of blood to the gastrointestinal vasculature (Satish, 2008). This means they can often occur during meals where prolonged sitting and eating combine to reduce venous return. Vasovagal syncope is usually relieved by recumbency and is associated with pallor and diaphoresis, but not with urticaria, respiratory symptoms or gastrointestinal symptoms (Simons et al., 2011).

Collapse due to hypotension is a strong indicator of severe anaphylaxis and paramedics need to avoid mistaking a vasovagal response for early anaphylactic shock. In this case, the differentiation between syncope and anaphylaxis is not difficult because urticaria, pruritus, tachycardia, angio-oedema and bronchospasm are not consistent with the presentation of syncope.

Arrhythmia

This patient's elevated heart rate and hypotension could be the result of a spontaneous arrhythmia such as supraventricular tachycardia. A careful examination of the ECG monitor should quickly exclude this arrhythmia, but again the presence of urticaria, pruritus, tachycardia, angio-oedema and bronchospasm are not consistent with a purely cardiac cause.

Seizures

Seizures can be caused by prolonged hypotension or hypoxia that causes inappropriate neural activity. Determining the cause of the seizure only becomes important or even possible once the activity has ceased. There can be many causes of hypoxia and/or hypotension in post-ictal patients, anaphylaxis being one of them.

Anxiety

Anxiety is one of the most difficult differentials to exclude in allergic and milder anaphylactic reactions. In this case the presence of urticaria, pruritus, tachycardia, angio-oedema and bronchospasm suggest the pathophysiology is more substantive than an emotional response.

Airway obstruction

Laryngeal oedema and the subsequent stridor associated with anaphylaxis can be difficult to distinguish from a sudden airway obstruction when the patient notices these symptoms while eating. A careful history, however, generally determines that the patient had effectively swallowed their food before the reaction. Airway obstructions caused by food are not likely to cause urticaria and pruritus.

Asthma

Because they share an inflammatory cause, asthma is a common anaphylactic mimic. A history of asthma is a strong risk factor in fatal anaphylactic reactions and this may be because patients and paramedics fail to differentiate between the two diseases and intervene quickly. As with all the above 'confounders', the diagnostic feature of anaphylaxis is not necessarily the speed of onset, the severity of symptoms or the known exposure to an allergen; rather, it is that the symptoms exist across more than one system.

Infection/sepsis

Depending on their location, infections can result in some similar symptoms to allergic reactions or even anaphylaxis. Erythema, pruritus, tachycardia, hypotension, altered level of consciousness and dyspnoea are all symptoms common to anaphylaxis and various types of infections. The ability to elicit a good patient history is important in differentiating between the two.

The clinical reasoning challenge in many cases is to differentiate between a severe allergic reaction and anaphylaxis. The key is to explore whether the reaction

CLINICAL COMMENT

The profound hypotension associated with anaphylaxis may lead to 'collapse' or 'fainting' and this may be the reason paramedics are dispatched. Allergies are not always suspected at first. See Case study 3.

has progressed beyond the 'system' from where it was introduced. Reactions that start with a sting (skin) and progress to a cardiovascular response indicate an uncontrolled systemic reaction. If the sting site swells more than normal but does not produce respiratory, cardiovascular or gastrointestinal symptoms, it 'fits' into the allergic spectrum of responses. Given that widespread reactions to the skin are the most common sign (80–90%), paramedics can use this to help build a differential diagnosis. Look for these changes and then assess cardiovascular and respiratory function. In summary, assess whether the patient is presenting with an acute-onset illness with typical skin features plus the involvement of one or more of respiratory, cardiovascular or persistent severe gastrointestinal symptoms. In this case, the patient provides strong evidence of two or more criteria, which supports the need for emergency treatment by the paramedic.

3 TREAT

Emergency management

Principles of management are outlined in Box 28.2.

Safety

If the allergen is known and can safely be removed (i.e. bee sting) or reduced, this should be undertaken. Moving the patient to a site where they will not suffer further envenomation should also be considered.

Position

The two factors most often associated with fatal anaphylaxis are hypotension and hypoxia (Greenberger et al., 2007; Pumphrey, 2000). While airway swelling and bronchospasm can make it uncomfortable for the patient to lie supine, there have been poor outcomes in hypotensive patients who have been managed seated or upright: patients should thus be managed in the recumbent or supine position provided it does not compromise their respiratory function (Simons et al., 2011).

Adrenaline

Fatalities from witnessed anaphylactic reactions are usually associated with the delayed administration of adrenaline (Lieberman et al., 2015). The overwhelming anecdotal evidence of adrenaline's effectiveness and the lack of alternative treatments have precluded any randomised controlled trials comparing adrenaline to other therapies in anaphylaxis (Sheikh et al., 2009). Although knowledge about the routes and timing of administration of adrenaline are well established, there is still some uncertainty about how adrenaline interacts with mast cells and basophils.

> **PRACTICE TIP**
>
> In the out-of-hospital setting it is important to look for the systemic effects of anaphylaxis to help reach your clinical decision.

BOX 28.2 Principles of management

Anaphylaxis
- Safety: Remove further exposure to allergen if possible.
- Adrenaline: Rapid administration of IM adrenaline. Repeat as required.
- Supportive: Management of other symptoms as required.
- Transport: For longer-acting medications and follow-up.

Adrenaline
- Injection into the quadriceps raises serum levels faster than using the deltoids.
- Dangerous arrhythmias are very uncommon with IM adrenaline.
- IV adrenaline should be reserved for patients at imminent risk of respiratory or cardiac arrest, or in severely hypotensive patients who have not responded to IM doses of adrenaline and IV fluid replacement.

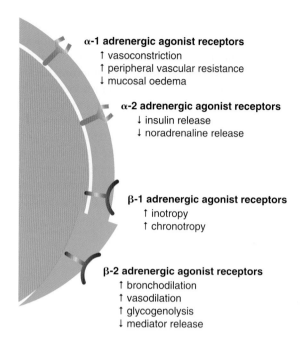

α-1 adrenergic agonist receptors
↑ vasoconstriction
↑ peripheral vascular resistance
↓ mucosal oedema

α-2 adrenergic agonist receptors
↓ insulin release
↓ noradrenaline release

β-1 adrenergic agonist receptors
↑ inotropy
↑ chronotropy

β-2 adrenergic agonist receptors
↑ bronchodilation
↑ vasodilation
↑ glycogenolysis
↓ mediator release

Figure 28.4
The effects of adrenaline.
With both alpha- and beta-agonist effects adrenaline has proved to be the most effective medication to manage anaphylaxis. Administered into a large muscle group it has been shown to reach therapeutic levels quickly and with no serious side effects. IV adrenaline should be reserved for patients at imminent risk of respiratory or cardiac arrest, or in severely hypotensive patients who have not responded to IM adrenaline.
Source: Estelle & Simons (2009).

On the surface, adrenaline's effectiveness in anaphylaxis is straightforward. Its alpha-agonist properties promote peripheral vasoconstriction and increase venous return, while its beta-receptor activity dilates the bronchial and gastrointestinal smooth muscle while increasing the force of myocardial contraction (Estelle & Simons, 2009; Kemp et al., 2008; see Fig 28.4). However, there are also beta-receptor sites on mast cells (and basophils) and, when bound with adrenaline, they trigger an increase in cyclic adenosine monophosphate (cAMP) production in the cells, which inhibits mediator release (Kemp et al., 2008). How much this mechanism impacts on the effectiveness of adrenaline remains unclear, but it may explain why adrenaline is more effective when given early.

Plasma adrenaline levels rise up to four times faster with IM administration compared with subcutaneous administration (Kemp et al., 2008). This is proportional to the size of the muscle into which it is injected and how well that muscle is perfused. The IM route has proven to be extremely safe and large reviews have not associated adrenaline administration with serious adverse events. Common side effects after a recommended dose of adrenaline include pallor, tremor, anxiety, palpitations, dizziness and headache. These symptoms indicate that a therapeutic dose has been given, and serious adverse effects such as ventricular arrhythmias, hypertensive crisis, and pulmonary oedema (which often concern health professionals) are uncommon (Simons et al., 2011). Because most of the serious adverse events from adrenaline have been associated with IV administration (Sheikh et al., 2009), the IV route should be reserved for patients who do not respond to repeat IM doses or where cardiac arrest is imminent (Simons et al., 2011). IV infusions appear safer than bolus doses and are often used for longer transport times when repeat IM injections will be problematic. Infusions of adrenaline can be commenced at a rate of 0.1 microgram/kg/min, and then titrated according to response (ASCIA, 2018).

For children aged 13 years and over and adults, the recommended IM dose is 0.5 mg repeated every 5 minutes as required (ASCIA, 2018). For children aged less than 13 years, the recommended IM dose is 0.01 mg/kg (10 microgram/kg) up to a maximum of 0.5 mg repeated every 5 minutes. IM doses are generally diluted 1:1000. Provided it is adequately absorbed the onset of adrenaline is relatively quick: patients often show improvement within 2 minutes and a complete resolution of symptoms is not unusual within 15 minutes. Unfortunately, symptoms can recur and repeat doses may be required. Nebulised adrenaline can assist in upper airway occlusion but studies show it fails to provide the serum levels of the IM route (Kemp et al., 2008). While it may be a useful adjunct to IM adrenaline if upper airway obstruction is present, it is not recommended as first-line therapy.

People who have suffered previous anaphylactic reactions often carry an adrenaline auto-injector with them: if it can be reached faster than you can draw up your own adrenaline, it is reasonable to use the patient's.

Oxygen therapy

Most international guidelines on anaphylaxis recommend the routine use of oxygen therapy in the early or critical stages of anaphylaxis, where hypotension or tissue hypoxia are commonly present (Simons et al., 2011; Lieberman et al., 2015; ASCIA, 2018). Although there is no direct evidence of benefit for oxygen supplementation in non-hypoxaemic patients, a significant number of deaths from anaphylaxis are secondary to hypoxia and upper airway obstruction. Local guidelines recommend the use of high-concentration oxygen in the early stages of treatment (via non-breather mask) followed by a target saturation of 92–96% once the patient's oxygen saturation can be measured reliably (Beasley et al., 2015). In this case, although there is little evidence of hypotension or hypoxia, it is reasonable to initiate oxygen therapy after adrenaline has been given. Oxygen should then be titrated once the condition has improved.

> **PRACTICE TIP**
>
> Encouraging the patient or a family member to administer the EpiPen under paramedic supervision will give them confidence to initiate this treatment for future occurrences before paramedics arrive.

(4) EVALUATE

Intubation of severely anaphylactic patients can be extremely difficult due to airway swelling and these patients can occlude quickly. While anaphylactic reactions generally respond to adrenaline treatment, do not underestimate the patients' ability to suddenly develop an airway occlusion or profound hypotension prior to their response to treatment. Patients who have required treatment with adrenaline should be assessed and transported with the highest level of care available within the ambulance service. A recurrence of symptoms is not uncommon.

Although the hypoxia and hypotension associated with anaphylaxis can provoke lethal arrhythmias in patients with preexisting coronary artery disease, the most likely arrest rhythm associated with the condition is pulseless electrical activity (PEA). Studies have shown the 'normal' appearance of this rhythm on ECGs is often the cause of delays in commencing CPR.

Is the patient:
- Improving after IM adrenaline?
  > Continue with the highest level of available care
- Deteriorating after IM adrenaline?
  > Continue with the highest level of available care
- Unconscious?
  > Start the primary survey
- Pulseless?
  > Assess the arrest rhythm on the monitor
  > Not VT or VF?
  > Commence CPR

Investigations

Although hundreds of chemical markers are released during anaphylaxis, laboratory investigations of anaphylaxis are limited in both scope and usefulness. Plasma histamine levels rise within 10 minutes of symptom onset but fall again within 60 minutes. Levels of tryptase, an enzyme released from mast cells during degranulation, also stay elevated for up to 3 hours after the onset of symptoms (Simons et al., 2011). However, both tests are not universally available in all emergency departments, are difficult to perform in the emergency setting and are often not specific to anaphylaxis. In addition, while serum tryptase levels could help support a clinical diagnosis of anaphylaxis from insect stings or injected medications, they are typically within normal levels in patients who experience food-induced anaphylaxis (Simons et al., 2011). Given that the symptoms demand urgent treatment, testing for either histamine or tryptase is of limited clinical usefulness and, for the moment at least, anaphylaxis remains diagnosed from its clinical presentation.

Ongoing management

Adrenaline is the drug of choice to manage anaphylaxis, but other second-line interventions can also be considered.

- *Corticosteroids.* There is a lack of evidence to support the routine use of corticosteroids in the management of anaphylaxis (Lieberman et al., 2015). Corticosteroids are traditionally given to suppress the production of inflammatory mediators at a cellular level. However, their onset time (generally 4–6 hours) is too long to support patients in the short term, and puts patients at risk of further deterioration. Although it is thought that suppressing the inflammatory response may reduce biphasic or prolonged reoccurrences of anaphylaxis, this is not supported by strong evidence (Lieberman et al., 2015).
- *Fluid replacement.* Intravenous fluid replacement with normal saline for patients with circulatory collapse and for patients who do not respond to adrenaline should be considered. Adrenaline should always be initiated first to reduce the increased vascular permeability, otherwise intravenous fluids could worsen oedema. Given patients' profound vasodilation and increased capillary permeability, it is highly unlikely that those suffering shock secondary to anaphylaxis could be resuscitated with fluid alone, and some case studies have demonstrated hypotension refractory to very large fluid infusions (Lieberman et al., 2015).

- *Beta-2 adrenergic agonists.* Asthmatic patients suffering anaphylaxis have been shown to exhibit bronchospasm and wheezing even after the majority of their symptoms have reduced. If bronchospasm persists after intramuscular adrenaline, the use of inhaled salbutamol, via either nebuliser or spacer, should be considered (Lieberman et al., 2015; Simons et al., 2011). The evidence supporting the use of salbutamol in anaphylaxis is largely extrapolated from studies involving asthma patients.
- *Antihistamines.* Antihistamines have no role in treating the respiratory or cardiovascular symptoms of anaphylaxis. Most of the evidence supporting their use is extrapolated from their use in other allergic conditions. Although their effectiveness is uncertain, they may be helpful in the relief of skin features such as urticaria or pruritus (Simons et al., 2011; Lieberman et al., 2015). Although antihistamines can be given orally or intravenously, some antihistamines can worsen hypotension when given intravenously.

Hospital admission

Patients who remain unstable after treatment in ED will be admitted to ICU. Patients who achieve successful resolution of symptoms are usually observed for at least 4–8 hours before discharge home. A recurrence of symptoms develops in about 5% of cases and can occur up to 72 hours after the initial event (Lee et al., 2015). The severity of the initial presentation does not correspond to the severity of the second presentation, and the symptoms can appear quickly or slowly, together or individually.

Some hospitals require overnight admission for paediatric patients, patients who have received more than one dose of adrenaline or any volume of fluid, patients who live alone or a significant distance from medical care, and those with comorbidities. Patients who have ingested their allergen tend to be kept in hospital longer than those whose contact was dermal or respiratory.

Post-discharge management

Prevention of future recurrences of anaphylaxis is a key strategy for reducing the burden of death and disability (see Fig 28.5). At the time of discharge, patients will be prescribed an EpiPen (or adrenaline auto-injector) and provided with education regarding the why, when and how to use an adrenaline auto-injector. Although there is no universally accepted management plan, individualised action plans should

ANAPHYLAXIS ON THE ROAD

Anaphylactic patients can go from appearing fit and well to being profoundly unwell within a matter of minutes. Left unmonitored and untreated, these patients have a real risk of death. But assessed quickly and accurately and treated with adrenaline they generally stabilise within minutes.

Like all health emergencies that occur in the community, paramedics have to balance a highly charged and emotional scene (remember, this person was probably in good health a few moments ago), which is often in a crowded place (anaphylaxis tends to occur in places where the patient isn't in control of the cooking—restaurants, parties), with the priorities of clinical decision-making. This is one of the cases where a standardised approach, good knowledge and good clinical skills will save a life.

be provided at the time of discharge which detail the importance of self-administration of adrenaline and timely access to emergency care (Simons et al., 2011). EpiPens are supplied in two fixed-dose forms: a green-labelled device containing 0.15 mg adrenaline for children 10–20 kg and a yellow-labelled device containing 0.3 mg adrenaline for children and adults over 20 kg.

Before discharge, anaphylaxis triggers suggested by the history of the acute episode can be evaluated in hospital by the measurement of allergen-specific IgE levels in serum. In addition, allergen skin tests can also be performed 3–4 weeks after the acute episode to determine possible triggers. Long-term management involves avoidance of known triggers, medication desensitisation (if the medication cannot be avoided) and stinging insect venom immunotherapy (Simons et al., 2011).

Anaphylaxis across the lifespan

Estimating the prevalence and severity of anaphylaxis is complicated by the lack of international consensus on a definition, the limited clinical tests to confirm the diagnosis and a reliance on hospital-based presentations (Turner & Campbell, 2016). Reactions to food represent the fastest-growing category but even non-food reactions presenting to hospitals are increasing by an average of 5–7% per year (Mullins et al., 2015). This aligns with the general consensus that allergic reactions are increasing in Western countries (Liew et al., 2009; Mullins et al., 2015). The number of hospital admissions for anaphylactic reactions in Australia is increasing at a similar rate to admissions in the United Kingdom and North America (Mullins et al., 2015). These presentations show specific age-related trends (see also Figs 28.6, 28.7 and 28.8).

- **0–4 years.** Although hospitalisations for anaphylaxis increased across all age groups in the 14 years prior to 2012, the increase was greatest in children aged 0–4 years (Mullins et al., 2015), up from 9 cases per 100,000 population in 1998/99 to 35 cases per 100,000 population in 2011/12. This was mainly the result of food-induced reactions. Allergies may appear in the toddler years and are usually associated with peanuts, eggs, milk and tree nuts (Liew et al., 2009). Fatalities in this age range remain relatively rare (Mullins et al., 2016).

- **5–14 years.** As children enter school they become exposed to a greater number of foods and other allergens: sensitivities to various nuts, fish and insects may emerge and presentations can be more serious. Risk of fatal episodes of anaphylaxis at this age is strongly associated with peanut allergies, asthma and previously unknown sensitivities. A study of 85 children who presented to ED found that cutaneous and respiratory manifestations were the most common symptoms (Bohlke et al., 2004). Insect stings are a more common presentation in this age group; about 10% of all deaths occur in this age group despite it contributing more than half of all presentations. Remember, it is difficult to predict with any accuracy the likely severity of a reaction based on a previous reaction. In this and the toddler age group, males are more likely to suffer from food-induced anaphylaxis, while females are at slightly higher risk of non-food-induced reactions (Poulos et al., 2007). Overall fatalities from food make up only a small proportion of deaths from anaphylaxis but it is important to remember that in as many as 60% of fatal cases of anaphylaxis the trigger is unknown (Mullins et al., 2016).

- **15–35 years.** This age group has fewer presentations than other age groups but has shown a similar growth rate in the number of presentations. This group—in particular 15–29-year-olds—shows a second peak in hospital admissions for food-related reactions but the lowest for drug-induced reactions. Crustacean and fish

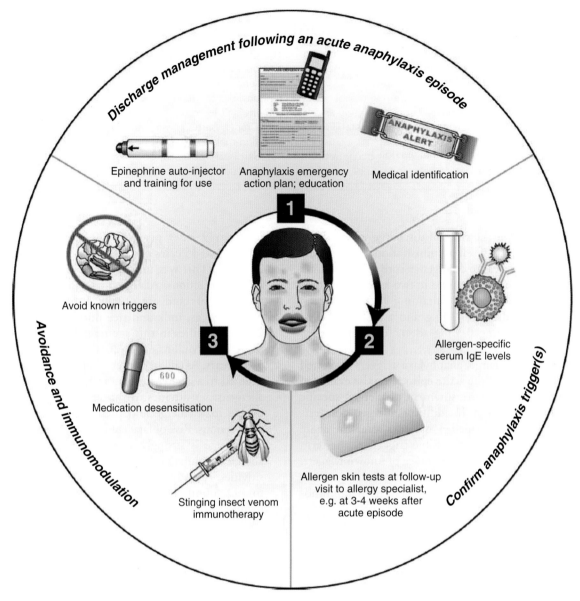

Figure 28.5
Discharge management and prevention of anaphylaxis.
Effective anaphylaxis management starts long before paramedics attend the scene. Panel 1 describes management at the time of discharge after treatment of an acute anaphylactic episode in a healthcare setting. Patients receive education on the use of an adrenaline auto-injector and an individualised action plan. Medical alert bracelets are also used to help identify individuals at risk. Panel 2 shows that anaphylaxis triggers suggested by the history of the acute episode should be confirmed by measurement of allergen-specific IgE levels and by allergen skin tests. Panel 3 summarises long-term risk reduction through avoidance of triggers and where relevant, immunomodulation to reduce medication or venom sensitivity.
Source: Simons et al. (2011).

allergies are added to the cohort of causes in this age group (Liew et al., 2009).

- **35+ years.** Although this age group is associated with the lowest incidence of anaphylaxis-related admissions, they account for the largest proportion of deaths from anaphylaxis (Liew et al., 2009; Mullins et al., 2015; Mullins et al., 2016).

In particular, a rise in deaths related to venom and medication-related anaphylaxis is seen in these ages. This is of course potentiated by the increasing number of medications and medical procedures that are administered with age and with comorbidities limiting the body's ability to resist the reaction.

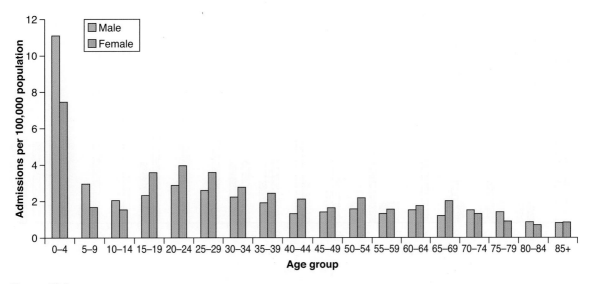

Figure 28.6
Anaphylaxis admissions to hospital, 1994–2005.
Young children make up the majority of hospital admissions but fatal episodes occur more frequently in adults (see Fig 28.8).
Source: Liew et al. (2009).

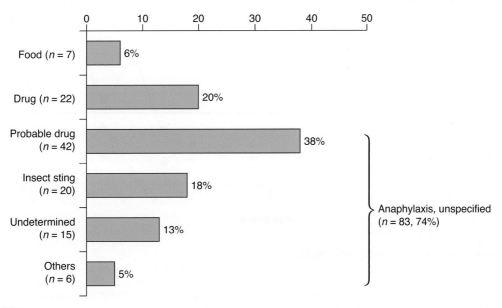

Figure 28.7
Fatal anaphylaxis triggers, 1994–2005.
Anaphylactic reactions to medications and insect stings make up the majority of fatal episodes. This is most likely to be because these instances often involve antigens being injected directly into tissues or the bloodstream.
Source: Liew et al. (2009).

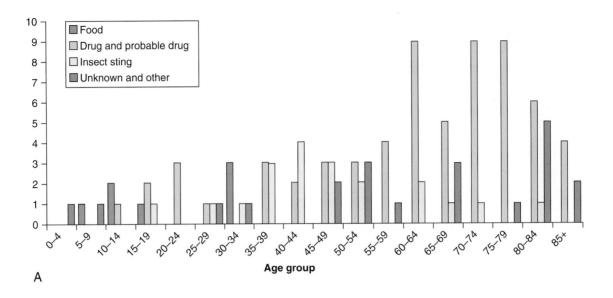

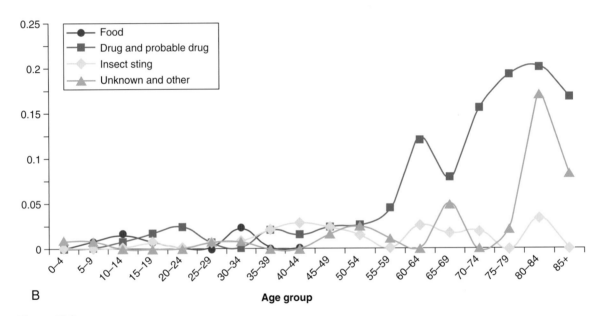

Figure 28.8
Anaphylaxis fatalities in Australia, 1994–2005.
A Absolute number of anaphylaxis deaths by cause and age group. **B** Anaphylaxis death rates by cause and age group. All but one food-induced anaphylaxis death occurred in people aged 10–35 years (1 death at 8 years), most insect sting–induced anaphylaxis deaths occurred in people aged 35–84 years and most drug-induced anaphylaxis deaths occurred in people aged 60–85 years.
Source: Liew et al. (2009).

CASE STUDY 2

Case 11441, 1520 hrs.

Dispatch details: A 21-year-old male with an allergic reaction to food. The patient has had a reaction to fish: he has a known allergy.

Initial presentation: The crew are led inside a private house and find the patient sitting on a chair in the kitchen.

1 ASSESS

1529 hrs Primary survey: The patient is conscious and talking.

Chief complaint: 'I ate some fish and now my lips are tingling and I'm itchy all over. I haven't eaten fish for years because I was allergic to it.' (For more about fish allergies, see Box 28.3.)

1530 hrs Vital signs survey: Perfusion status: HR 146 bpm, sinus tachycardia, BP 140/90 mmHg, skin warm and pink.

Respiratory status: RR 28 bpm, good air entry, L = R, mild expiratory wheeze across all fields, normal work of breathing, speaking in full sentences, denies shortness of breath, SpO_2 = 93%.

Conscious state: GCS = 15.

1531 hrs Pertinent hx: The patient is normally well and takes no medications. He hasn't eaten fish since he was a child because of an allergic reaction, but he can't remember how severe the reaction was. He took a bite of his friend's fish burger just to see how it tasted; he didn't think he was allergic anymore.

> ## PRACTICE TIP
>
> In the crowded and confusing world of emergency health in the community, the question 'Of all your symptoms, which is distressing you the most?' can be a great 'cut to the bone' question. Patients have many symptoms and they may want to explain them all to you. This lets you identify the most significant in the patient's eyes and also conveys empathy towards the patient.

> ## BOX 28.3 Fish allergies
>
> The majority of allergic reactions to fish are caused by a major protein called parvalbumin, which is present in most species of fish and other vertebrates. Although concentrations of parvalbumins vary according to the species of fish, the factors that determine an individual's reactivity to certain species is dependent on a range of factors and not only the concentration of parvalbumin proteins (Sharp & Lopata, 2014). Cross-sensitivity between fish species is common, but it varies according to how similar the two species are. Approximately 50% of individuals who describe sensitivity to fish will have cross-sensitivity to other fish species. Conversely, 75% of individuals who describe sensitivity to shellfish will experience cross-sensitivity to other shellfish species. Reactions to fish and shellfish are not only immune-system mediated as a result of allergies, but can also be caused by various toxins and parasites. The fish parasite *Anisakis simplex* is also a major allergen and can masquerade as a fish allergy. Although it is killed by freezing or cooking, *Anisakis* can still trigger reactions.

It's not uncommon for patients to think they no longer suffer from an illness because they have been good at avoiding triggers and maintaining treatments. The same can occur with patients with asthma and epilepsy.

'How long after eating the fish did the symptoms start?'

'The tingling in my mouth and lips started within about a minute and then I could feel my heart suddenly racing. My mate called the ambulance straight away.'
'Does your voice sound normal?'
'Yeah, I think so.'
(To the patient's friend) 'Is his face normal or swollen?'
'He may be a little puffy around the eyes.'

'If there is one thing I could fix for you right now, what would it be?'

'My lips feel like they're swelling but it's the itching that's driving me crazy. I'm itchy all over and I know if I start scratching I'll never stop.'

(2) CONFIRM

In many cases paramedics are presented with a collection of signs and symptoms that do not appear to describe a particular condition. A critical step in determining a treatment plan in this situation is to consider what other conditions could explain the patient's presentation.

What else could it be?
Anxiety
Anxiety rarely causes heart rates greater than 125 bpm and a sustained tachycardia of 143 bpm in a patient who is fit, sitting down, not short of breath and only mildly anxious is being driven by something significant. Tingling of the lips can be associated with the CO_2 imbalance caused by hyperventilation. It is possible that the patient is simply anxious after realising he has eaten fish and this has caused him to hyperventilate, resulting in the tingling. Look for other signs of the chemical imbalance caused by hyperventilation—that is, tetany (carpal spasm) of the fingers and forearms—then look at the patient: is he really that anxious?

Asthma
This patient has no history of asthma and it is unlikely that he has developed it at the same time as eating fish. The cutaneous signs are also inconsistent with asthma.

Scombridae food poisoning
Food poisoning rarely has such a sudden onset and this patient lacks the characteristic abdominal pain. However, one form of food poisoning should be considered: fish flesh contains the protein histidine and, if stored improperly, bacteria can metabolise this protein into large amounts of histamine. Once produced, the histamine is not destroyed by cooking. Mistakenly known as *Scombridae* fish poisoning it also affects fish outside the *Scombridae* family. Because patients ingest high levels of histamine the presentation is difficult to separate from anaphylaxis and symptoms typically include erythema, hot flushes, headache, nausea and vomiting (Feng et al., 2016). Definitive management is antihistamines but in the out-of-hospital setting the differentiation is too dangerous to make and treatment should be consistent with anaphylaxis. The only exception to this might occur when a group of people who have shared the meal all present with typical *Scombridae* symptoms.

(3) TREAT

This patient should be administered IM adrenaline 0.5 mg. The IM route (lateral thigh) is safe and has a short time of onset. Fear of increasing the heart

---

DIFFERENTIAL DIAGNOSIS

Food allergy/anaphylaxis
  Or
- Anxiety
- Asthma
- *Scombridae* food poisoning

PRACTICE TIP

If it's anaphylaxis, why isn't the patient hypotensive? Hypotension is a classic characteristic of anaphylaxis so why isn't this patient hypotensive? Paramedics tend to see patients early in their presentation when the full host of symptoms may not yet be present. Remember, hypotension is a late sign in all forms of shock.

rate and blood pressure are common barriers to the treatment of anaphylaxis by inexperienced paramedics. Remember, the cause of this patient's symptoms is the widespread and uncontrolled release of histamine leading to small vessel vasodilation, increased capillary permeability and smooth-muscle contraction. Adrenaline will reduce the histamine release and assist with both alpha and beta effects. Because it reduces the cause, you can expect the patient's heart rate to reduce after IM adrenaline. Similarly, you should not expect to see major changes in BP.

1535 hrs: The patient is given 0.5 mg of IM adrenaline into the right lateral thigh. Oxygen therapy is commenced using a non-rebreather mask. Upon administering the adrenaline the crew notice the patient becoming flushed and increasingly anxious about the itching.

1537 hrs: The symptoms start to subside and with 2 minutes the patient is calmer and says the itching and tingling have almost gone.

Perfusion status: HR 104 bpm, sinus tachycardia, BP 130/80 mmHg, skin warm and pink.

Respiratory status: RR 24 bpm, good air entry, L = R, normal work of breathing, speaking in full sentences, denies shortness of breath, SpO_2 = 100% on supplemental oxygen.

Conscious state: GCS = 15.

1541 hrs: The patient is loaded to the ambulance using a wheelchair. He is talkative and calm.

1545 hrs: One of the crew notices that the patient is rubbing his arms and asks whether the itching is returning. The patient confirms that it is. The recurrence of symptoms after 10–15 minutes is typical of moderate anaphylaxis.

Perfusion status: HR 120, sinus tachycardia, BP 110/80 mmHg, skin warm and pink.

Respiratory status: RR 28, good air entry, L = R, normal work of breathing, speaking in full sentences, denies shortness of breath.

Conscious state: GCS = 15

1546 hrs: The paramedic administers another 0.5 mg IM dose of adrenaline and the symptoms subside.

1559 hrs At hospital: Perfusion status: HR 104 bpm, sinus tachycardia, BP 130/80 mmHg, skin warm and pink.

Respiratory status: RR 24 bpm, good air entry, L = R, normal work of breathing, speaking in full sentences, denies shortness of breath. He is weaned from supplemental oxygen and his SpO_2 is 97% on room air.

Conscious state: GCS = 15.

④ EVALUATE

Evaluating the effect of any clinical management intervention can provide clues to the accuracy of the initial diagnosis. Some conditions respond rapidly to treatment so patients should be expected to improve if the diagnosis and treatment were appropriate. A failure to improve in this situation should trigger the clinician to reconsider the diagnosis.

In this case, it is likely that the patient will continue to receive short-term relief from IM adrenaline, but with the recurrence of symptoms once the adrenaline is metabolised.

CASE STUDY 3

Case 16532, 1940 hrs.

Dispatch details: A 29-year-old female has collapsed while playing netball. She is in an altered conscious state.

Initial presentation: The crew are met at the local netball stadium and led inside to find a female lying on her side. A doctor playing on the opposing team states that the patient was playing normally when she complained of 'feeling funny' to a team mate. She then collapsed, had a seizure that lasted a few seconds and vomited. She has remained on the ground since then.

 ASSESS

1950 hrs Primary survey: The patient is semi-conscious and moaning. There is no obvious injury.

1951 hrs Vital signs survey: Perfusion status: HR 115 bpm; sinus rhythm; BP 70/35; skin warm, pink, clammy.

Respiratory status: RR 18 bpm, good air entry, L = R, nil adventitious sounds, normal work of breathing, SpO_2 = 97% on room air.

Conscious state: GCS = 7; weak withdrawal, moans quietly (E 1, M 4, V 2).

1953 hrs Pertinent hx: The patient's medical history is not known to her team mates but they state she was playing normally until just before she collapsed. They say she did not strike her head when she collapsed.

1954 hrs Secondary survey: No obvious injuries. There is a small amount of vomit on the floor next to and under the patient's head and in her hair. Her team mates say she vomited after she collapsed.

 CONFIRM

In many cases paramedics are presented with a collection of signs and symptoms that do not appear to describe a particular condition. A critical step in determining a treatment plan in this situation is to consider what other conditions could explain the patient's presentation.

Patients who present in the field can be extremely difficult to diagnose. Sometimes the picture is clear (as in Case study 1) and it is easy to select and then confirm a hypothesis. But often the picture is incomplete and you need a method to help you sort the good information from the bad. The standardised clinical approach (see Ch 5) directs paramedics to ensure that the patient has a clear airway, is breathing and has circulation. It then sets out a path to obtain the relevant physiological information as quickly as possible. In this case the patient has an altered conscious state and is poorly perfused but has no obvious injuries. The cause is not clear and the crew need to contrast the information they have gained with their clinical knowledge. The DENT model is an effective problem-solving tool for difficult cases (see Ch 7).

Define

In this case the crew define the problem as extremely poor perfusion. It could be argued that the patient's altered conscious state is more significant; however, an altered level of consciousness has no physiological mechanism to cause hypotension.

Explore

The crew need to quickly explore the conditions that can cause profound and prolonged hypotension in an otherwise fit young woman. Hypoglycaemia or low blood sugar is a common cause of altered consciousness and the body tends to respond with an increased sympathetic output that causes tachycardia and clamminess but rarely hypotension. Nonetheless, it is worth considering.

Narrow

1956 hrs Blood glucose test: BGL 6.3 mmol/L.

Hypoglycaemia is eliminated. A quick check of the monitor reveals no arrhythmia and the patient moves all her limbs (albeit weakly and with a moan) to painful stimuli. Cardiac and spinal causes can be reasonably eliminated. What can be gained from the scene? A young female is lying on the ground with her face and hair spattered with her own vomit. This is not a voluntary position or 'place of comfort'. This patient is not well.

With no obvious cause the crew can still only define the problem as profound hypotension. Sometimes the out-of-hospital environment will not allow paramedics to 'pin' a more specific label on a patient and they have to start fixing the problem.

③ TREAT

2000 hrs: The crew place some folded clothing under the patient's legs to increase venous return. They keep the patient on her side in case she vomits again. Oxygen therapy is commenced using a non-rebreather mask.

2001 hrs: The crew insert an IV cannula and commence an infusion of an isotonic crystalloid (normal saline).

While they work to fix the defined problem they seek to further explore and narrow the cause of the patient's persistent hypotension. What are the causes of poor perfusion?

- *Hypoxia:* SaO$_2$ is good, no respiratory distress, lungs clear. *NO*
- *Hypovolaemia:* No external haemorrhage, lungs clear, abdomen soft. *NO*
- *Tension pneumothorax:* Good air entry, L = R, SaO$_2$ is good. *NO*
- *Spinal cord injury:* No trauma, the patient doesn't complain on spinal palpation, she is moving all limbs and is tachycardic. *NO*
- *Asthma:* Good air entry, SaO$_2$ is good, normal work of breathing. *NO*
- *Vasovagal:* Uncommon in the young, tachycardic. *NO*
- *Anaphylaxis:* By systematically analysing the presenting problem the crew have found a possible cause (anaphylaxis) they cannot eliminate. But can they confirm it? Is there evidence of a systemic hypersensitive immune response? The onset was rapid, the patient 'felt funny' before collapsing, she is extremely poorly perfused and has vomited. The lack of dermal symptoms is difficult to assess, and the patient was exercising and sweaty before she collapsed (see Box 28.4), but she is still tachycardic and flushed despite having been on the ground for more than 15 minutes.

2004 hrs: Perfusion status: HR 119 bpm; sinus tachycardia; BP 70/35; skin warm, pink, dry.

Respiratory status: RR 18 bpm, good air entry, L = R, nil adventitious sounds, normal work of breathing.

BOX 28.4 Exercise-induced anaphylaxis

Exercise-induced anaphylaxis is a relatively rare disorder in which anaphylaxis is triggered by physical activity (Lieberman et al., 2015). The symptoms are typical of other forms of anaphylaxis and their severity appears to be related to the intensity of the exercise but there seems to be a summative effect (Lieberman et al., 2015). This means that a combination of exercise along with certain foods and medications can create an anaphylactic response even when neither component causes symptoms in isolation. This has also been described as food-dependent exercise-induced anaphylaxis.

In this case a couple of hours before playing netball the patient ate a seafood pizza—a food she normally has no reaction to. A wide variety of foods have been linked to food-dependent exercise-induced anaphylaxis, including the triggers normally associated with other forms of anaphylaxis (shellfish, nuts, NSAIDs). Exercising in cold temperatures may also predispose the reaction. As with other triggers the response can fall along a continuum from pruritus and urticaria at one end to anaphylactic shock at the other. Milder symptoms generally resolve as exercise levels are reduced but, once triggered, there may be no way of reducing the severity of a full anaphylactic reaction.

The detailed pathophysiology of exercise-induced anaphylaxis and food-dependent exercise-induced anaphylaxis is not well understood. As with all forms of anaphylaxis, identifying a specific trigger is not required to diagnose the condition and the patient should be treated according to their clinical presentation.

Conscious state: GCS = 7; weak withdrawal, moans quietly (E 1, M 4, V 2).

2005 hrs: The patient is given 0.5 mg of IM adrenaline into the right vastus lateralis (lateral thigh). The fluid is continued.

2007 hrs: The patient's conscious status improves. Initially confused, she sits up and is horrified to find vomit in her hair. She recalls 'tingling' all over and feeling abdominal pain before collapsing. This has never happened before, and she has no history of allergies.

2009 hrs: Perfusion status: HR 104 bpm, sinus tachycardia, BP 105/75 mmHg, skin warm and pink.

Respiratory status: RR 18 bpm, good air entry, L = R, normal work of breathing, speaking in full sentences, denies shortness of breath.

Conscious state: GCS = 15.

 EVALUATE

Evaluating the effect of any clinical management intervention can provide clues to the accuracy of the initial diagnosis. Some conditions respond rapidly to treatment so patients should be expected to improve if the diagnosis and treatment were appropriate. A failure to improve in this situation should trigger the clinician to reconsider the diagnosis.

The patient is assisted onto the stretcher for transport. She is talkative and calm. No further treatment is required and she is discharged from ED the next morning.

CASE STUDY 4

Case 14718, 0740 hrs.

Dispatch details: A 79-year-old female is having an allergic reaction to an unknown substance. There is airway involvement.

Initial presentation: The crew arrive at a nearby nursing home and are directed to the patient, who is sitting up beside her bed. A nurse tells them that she noticed the patient had gross facial swelling when she came to shower her this morning before breakfast.

1 ASSESS

0750 hrs Primary survey: The patient is conscious and sitting upright. She has obvious facial swelling including periorbital oedema, which is restricting her vision. Her tongue is so swollen she cannot speak easily and she is drooling due to difficulty swallowing.

0751 hrs Vital signs survey: Perfusion status: HR 75 bpm, sinus rhythm, BP 140/90 mmHg; skin warm, pink and dry.

Respiratory status: RR 18 bpm, good air entry, L = R, no adventitious sounds, normal work of breathing, SpO_2 = 94% on room air.

Conscious state: GCS = 15.

0753 hrs Pertinent hx: The patient has a history of hypertension, angina, hyperlipidaemia, osteoporosis and bilateral knee replacements. She is normally well but requires assistance to shower and dress due to decreased mobility.

0754 hrs Secondary survey: Apart from the facial angio-oedema there are no other obvious signs or symptoms. Temperature: 36.8°C.

2 CONFIRM

In many cases paramedics are presented with a collection of signs and symptoms that do not appear to describe a particular condition. A critical step in determining a treatment plan in this situation is to consider what other conditions could explain the patient's presentation.

The crew are faced with a patient where the underlying cause is unclear. They need to use the DENT model (see Ch 7) as a problem-solving tool.

Define

A patient with no history of allergies is presenting with isolated angio-oedema without any obvious cause. The swelling is not producing hypoxia or a cardiovascular response.

Explore

Because they share a common pathophysiological pathway, differentiating between a severe allergic reaction and an anaphylactic reaction is one of the more challenging diagnostic tasks. The usual distinction lies in the involvement of secondary systems (i.e. cardiovascular, respiratory and gastrointestinal systems). But when the isolated symptoms are severe enough to potentially block the

BOX 28.5 Isolated angio-oedema

Non-pitting oedema of the face and neck and around the eyes is referred to as angio-oedema and it can extend to include the tongue and the floor of the mouth (Cicardi et al., 2014). Angio-oedema is usually classified into two major subtypes, including hereditary and non-hereditary (or acquired) causes. Hereditary angio-oedema is a rare condition caused by a hereditary gene mutation or deficiency. In comparison, non-hereditary angio-oedema is far more common, and is increasingly seen as a side effect to a particular group of medications. ACE inhibitors are a commonly prescribed antihypertensive medication that block the conversion of angiotensin I to angiotensin II and thus limit the amount of fluid reabsorbed by the kidneys. A side effect of this blocking action is an increase in an inflammatory mediator known as bradykinin. It is the same mediator that produces the chronic cough associated with ACE inhibitors. Although there is no direct evidence of the pathway, it is strongly suspected that this excess bradykinin invokes the localised reaction of angio-oedema in three patients per thousand taking ACE inhibitors (Cicardi et al., 2014). While the numbers may not seem significant at first, the millions of people who are prescribed ACE inhibitors every year can result in thousands of new cases of angio-oedema in the community. Interestingly, the bradykinin pathway may also explain reactions to non-steroidal anti-inflammatory drugs (NSAIDs).

Although the risk is low, patients taking ACE inhibitors account for the majority of all angio-oedema patients presenting to hospital. While not an anaphylactic reaction, it is likely that angio-oedema represents some form of an immunologically mediated hypersensitivity reaction and the crew in Case study 4 were not unreasonable in administering IM adrenaline. The mild response from adrenaline is typical of these cases and is usually safe. Although conventional treatments for angio-oedema are typically not available in the out-of-hospital setting, treatment with nebulised adrenaline (5 mg via nebuliser) could also be considered to alleviate signs of upper airway oedema (ASCIA, 2018). The action of adrenaline is localised and may reduce the swelling of the tongue and airway, but may not lead to a complete resolution of symptoms.

upper airway it can easily trigger paramedics to make a diagnosis of anaphylaxis even when it isn't supported by the evidence.

Narrow

Isolated oedema to a single body part anywhere in the body but the airway would not meet the criteria for anaphylaxis given the patient has no cardiovascular, respiratory or gastrointestinal symptoms (see Box 28.5). Epiglottitis is a bacterial infection of the epiglottis that causes it to swell and occlude the airway. Although commonly perceived as a disease of children, widespread vaccinations have virtually eradicated the disease in this cohort, but it is not unusual to see it in elderly people who have migrated from overseas. It is usually associated with a sore throat and fever, but it does not cause swelling of the tongue or face. In this case the crew elect to treat for anaphylaxis despite the presentation not completely supporting this diagnosis.

(3) TREAT

0800 hrs: The crew sit the patient upright to allow for better respiratory function.

0804 hrs: Concerned that the patient may occlude her airway the crew elect to treat with 0.5 mg of IM adrenaline into the right deltoid. Oxygen therapy is commenced using a face mask. They also request additional back-up in case intubation is required.

0808 hrs: Perfusion status: HR 78 bpm; sinus rhythm; BP 140/90 mmHg; skin warm, pink and dry.

Respiratory status: RR 18 bpm, good air entry, L = R, no adventitious sounds, normal work of breathing, SpO$_2$ 99% on supplemental oxygen.

Conscious state: GCS = 15.

0808 hrs: The patient nods when asked if she is feeling better and her angio-oedema appears to have improved slightly.

0812 hrs: Perfusion status: HR 78 bpm; sinus rhythm; BP 140/90 mmHg; skin warm, pink and dry.

Respiratory status: RR 18 bpm, good air entry, L = R, no adventitious sounds, normal work of breathing, SpO_2 99% on supplemental oxygen.

Conscious state: GCS = 15.

 ## EVALUATE

Evaluating the effect of any clinical management intervention can provide clues to the accuracy of the initial diagnosis. Some conditions respond rapidly to treatment so patients should be expected to improve if the diagnosis and treatment were appropriate. A failure to improve in this situation should trigger the clinician to reconsider the diagnosis.

The patient is assisted onto the stretcher for transport. She is calm and cooperative. The crew treat en route with a second dose of IM adrenaline, but the patient shows no improvement or deterioration.

REFLECTIVE BOX

1. Anaphylaxis is an acute systemic hypersensitivity reaction typically characterised by skin features and the involvement of at least one of three other body systems. Can you name them?
2. Approximately what proportion of patients with anaphylaxis present without typical skin features such as erythema, urticaria or pruritus?
3. What clinical features distinguish anaphylaxis from generalised allergic reactions?
4. What is the leading trigger for anaphylaxis in children?
5. What is the gold-standard first-line treatment of anaphylaxis? What route is it administered?

6. In what proportion of patients do biphasic reactions occur?
7. Preventable deaths from anaphylaxis are often the result of arrhythmias caused by adrenaline administration. True or false?
8. Adrenaline administration in anaphylactic patients with severe tachycardia (e.g. HR > 140) is contraindicated due to the risk of arrhythmia and further deterioration. True or false?
9. Fluid administration alone (without adrenaline) is useful in correcting hypotension associated with anaphylaxis. True or false?
10. The standard dose of an adrenaline auto-injector (EpiPen) is 0.3 mg for children and adults weighing over 20 kg. True or false?

Future research

A lack of universal diagnostic criteria for anaphylaxis has partly hindered the development of new clinical and epidemiological research. The International Consensus on Anaphylaxis (Simons et al., 2014) has proposed an international research agenda which targets areas of knowledge where there is little or no high-quality evidence to support the recommendations for the diagnosis, treatment or prevention of anaphylaxis. The agenda details the need for prospective studies assessing the incidence, epidemiology and triggers of anaphylaxis, the development and validation of anaphylaxis severity criteria, a deeper understanding of the various mechanisms of anaphylaxis and the development and validation of diagnostic criteria that can be used in the health-care setting. The agenda also highlights the need for further studies evaluating the effectiveness and safety of adrenaline, and second-line treatment options such as antihistamines and corticosteroids. Importantly, information on the epidemiology and treatment of anaphylaxis patients in the out-of-hospital setting is lacking (Andrew et al., 2018). This is particularly problematic given that the vast majority of patients will access emergency care via the ambulance service.

Summary

Anaphylaxis is a life-threatening medical emergency and paramedics are often the first healthcare professionals to assess these patients. Patients who exhibit the full gamut of manifestations of anaphylaxis may be readily diagnosed, but many patients present with only one or two features, thereby increasing diagnostic uncertainty and leading to delays in definitive treatment with adrenaline. Paramedics must be able to recognise anaphylaxis and implement treatment to prevent avoidable fatalities.

References

Andrew, E., Nehme, Z., Bernard, S., & Smith, K. (2018). Pediatric anaphylaxis in the prehospital setting: incidence, characteristics, and management. *Prehospital Emergency Care*, 1–7.

ASCIA. (2018). Anaphylaxis: emergency management for health professionals. *Australian Prescriber*, *41*, 54.

Atkins, D., & Bock, S. A. (2009). Fatal anaphylaxis to foods: epidemiology, recognition, and prevention. *Current Allergy and Asthma Reports*, *9*(3), 179–185.

Beasley, R., Chien, J., Douglas, J., Eastlake, L., Farah, C., King, G., Moore, R., Pilcher, J., Richards, M., Smith, S., & Walters, H. (2015). Thoracic Society of Australia and New Zealand oxygen guidelines for acute oxygen use in adults: 'Swimming between the flags'. *Respirology (Carlton, Vic.)*, *20*, 1182–1191.

Bohlke, K., Davis, R. L., DeStefano, F., Marcy, S. M., Braun, M. M., & Thompson, R. S. (2004). Epidemiology of anaphylaxis among children and adolescents enrolled in a health maintenance organization. *The Journal of Allergy and Clinical Immunology*, *113*(3), 536–542.

Brown, G. A. (2007a). The pathophysiology of shock in anaphylaxis. *Immunology and Allergy Clinics of North America*, *27*, 165–175.

Brown, S. (2007b). Clinical features and severity grading of anaphylaxis. *The Journal of Allergy and Clinical Immunology*, *114*(2), 371–376.

Castro, M., & Kraft, M. (2008). *Clinical asthma*. Philadelphia: Mosby.

Cicardi, M., Aberer, W., Banerji, A., Bas, M., Bernstein, J. A., Bork, K., Caballero, T., Farkas, H., Grumach, A., Kaplan, A. P., Riedl, M. A., Triggiani, M., Zanichelli, A., Zuraw, B., & Eaaci, H. U. T. P. O. (2014). Classification, diagnosis, and approach to treatment for angioedema: consensus report from the Hereditary Angioedema International Working Group. *Allergy*, *69*, 602–616.

Estelle, F., & Simons, R. (2009). Anaphylaxis: recent advances in assessment and treatment. *The Journal of Allergy and Clinical Immunology*, *124*, 625–636.

Feng, C., Teuber, S., & Gershwin, M. E. (2016). Histamine (scombroid) fish poisoning: a comprehensive review. *Clinical Reviews in Allergy and Immunology*, *50*, 64–69.

Greenberger, P. A., Rotskoff, B. D., & Lifschultz, B. (2007). Fatal anaphylaxis: postmortem findings and associated comorbid diseases. *Annals of Allergy, Asthma & Immunology*, *98*(3), 252–257.

Gulen, T., Hagglund, H., Dahlen, B., & Nilsson, G. (2014). High prevalence of anaphylaxis in patients with systemic mastocytosis—a single-centre experience. *Clinical and Experimental Allergy: Journal of the British Society for Allergy and Clinical Immunology*, *44*, 121–129.

Huether, S., & McCance, K. (2016). *Understanding pathophysiology* (6th ed.). St Louis: Mosby.

Kaufman, D. (2003). Risk of anaphylaxis in a hospital population in relation to the use of various drugs: an international study. *Pharmacoepidemiology and Drug Safety*, *12*, 195–202.

Kemp, S., Lockey, R., & Simons, F. (2008). Epinephrine: the drug of choice for anaphylaxis. A statement of the World Allergy Organization. *Allergy*, *63*, 1061–1070.

Lee, S., Bellolio, M. F., Hess, E. P., Erwin, P., Murad, M. H., & Campbell, R. L. (2015). Time of onset and predictors of biphasic anaphylactic reactions: a systematic review and meta-analysis. *The Journal of Allergy and Clinical Immunology. In Practice*, *3*, 408–416.e2.

Lieberman, P., Nicklas, R. A., Randolph, C., Oppenheimer, J., Bernstein, D., Bernstein, J., Ellis, A., Golden, D. B., Greenberger, P., Kemp, S., Khan, D., Ledford, D., Lieberman, J., Metcalfe, D., Nowak-Wegrzyn, A., Sicherer, S., Wallace, D., Blessing-Moore, J., Lang, D., Portnoy, J. M., Schuller, D., Spector, S., & Tilles, S. A. (2015). Anaphylaxis—a practice parameter update 2015. *Annals of Allergy, Asthma & Immunology*, *115*, 341–384.

Liew, W. K., Williamson, E., & Tang, M. L. (2009). Anaphylaxis fatalities and admissions in Australia. *The Journal of Allergy and Clinical Immunology*, *123*(2), 434–442.

Male, D., Brostoff, J., Roth, D., & Roitt, I. (2013). *Immunology* (8th ed.). St Louis: Mosby.

McCance, K., & Huether, S. (2014). *Pathophysiology: the biologic basis for disease in adults and children* (7th ed.). St Louis: Mosby.

Mullins, R. J., Dear, K. B., & Tang, M. L. (2015). Time trends in Australian hospital anaphylaxis admissions in 1998-1999 to 2011-2012. *The Journal of Allergy and Clinical Immunology*, *136*, 367–375.

Mullins, R. J., Wainstein, B. K., Barnes, E. H., Liew, W. K., & Campbell, D. E. (2016). Increases in anaphylaxis fatalities in Australia from 1997 to 2013. *Clinical and Experimental Allergy: Journal of the British Society for Allergy and Clinical Immunology*, *46*, 1099–1110.

Poulos, L. M., Waters, A.-M., Correll, P. K., Loblay, R. H., & Marks, G. B. (2007). Trends in hospitalizations for anaphylaxis, angioedema, and urticaria in Australia, 1993–1994 to 2004–2005. *The Journal of Allergy and Clinical Immunology, 120*(4), 878–884.

Pumphrey, R. S. (2000). Lessons for management of anaphylaxis from a study of fatal reactions. *Clinical and Experimental Allergy: Journal of the British Society for Allergy and Clinical Immunology, 30*, 1144–1150.

Pumphrey, R. S. (2004). Anaphylaxis: can we tell who is at risk of a fatal reaction? *Current Opinion in Allergy and Clinical Immunology, 4*, 285–290.

Satish, R. R. (2008). Is cardiac output the key to vasovagal syncope? A re-evaluation of putative pathophysiology. *Heart Rhythm, 5*(12), 1702–1703.

Sharp, M. F., & Lopata, A. L. (2014). Fish allergy: in review. *Clinical Reviews in Allergy and Immunology, 46*, 258–271.

Sheikh, A., Shehata, Y. A., Brown, S. G., & Simons, F. (2009). Adrenaline for the treatment of anaphylaxis: Cochrane systematic review. *Allergy, 64*, 204–212.

Simons, F. E., Ardusso, L. R., Bilo, M. B., El-Gamal, Y. M., Ledford, D. K., Ring, J., Sanchez-Borges, M., Senna, G. E., Sheikh, A., Thong, B. Y., for the World Allergy Organization. (2011). World Allergy Organization guidelines for the assessment and management of anaphylaxis. *The World Allergy Organization Journal, 4*, 13–37.

Simons, F. E., Ardusso, L. R., Bilo, M. B., Cardona, V., Ebisawa, M., El-Gamal, Y. M., Lieberman, P., Lockey, R. F., Muraro, A., Roberts, G., Sanchez-Borges, M., Sheikh, A., Shek, L. P., Wallace, D. V., & Worm, M. (2014). International consensus on (ICON) anaphylaxis. *The World Allergy Organization Journal, 7*, 9.

Simons, F. E., Ebisawa, M., Sanchez-Borges, M., Thong, B. Y., Worm, M., Tanno, L. K., Lockey, R. F., El-Gamal, Y. M., Brown, S. G., Park, H. S., & Sheikh, A. (2015). 2015 update of the evidence base: World Allergy Organization anaphylaxis guidelines. *The World Allergy Organization Journal, 8*, 32.

Turner, P. J., & Campbell, D. E. (2016). Epidemiology of severe anaphylaxis: can we use population-based data to understand anaphylaxis? *Current Opinion in Allergy and Clinical Immunology, 16*, 441–450.

Turner, P. J., Jerschow, E., Umasunthar, T., Lin, R., Campbell, D. E., & Boyle, R. J. (2017). Fatal anaphylaxis: mortality rate and risk factors. *The Journal of Allergy and Clinical Immunology. In Practice, 5*, 1169–1178.

CHAPTER 29

Seizures

By David Reid

OVERVIEW

- Seizures are a symptom of underlying instability of neuronal cell membranes.
- Seizures can represent the full extent of a disease, or develop as a result of infection, injury, cerebral ischaemia or lesions.
- Focal seizures produce neurological symptoms localised to discrete regions of the brain.
- Generalised seizures involve the whole brain and are associated with unconsciousness.

- New seizures and changes in seizure patterns are indicative of changes in the physiological environment, or in the use or effectiveness of medications, and require investigation.
- Emergency management of seizures is aimed at maintaining oxygenation and terminating the seizures, usually with benzodiazepines.
- Failure to terminate a seizure with benzodiazepines requires advanced airway management and circulatory support.

Introduction

A seizure is a sudden, uncontrolled electrical discharge in a group of brain cells (neurons). During a seizure neurons can fire up to 500 times a second—more than six times the normal rate—and for a brief period this can cause strange sensations, emotions and behaviour or convulsions and loss of consciousness (Epilepsy Foundation, 2019). Clinical signs may include alterations to sensation, movement, awareness or consciousness, behaviour and perception. Depending on the location of the seizure in the brain, seizures can produce clearly observable neurological symptoms, but in some cases the presentation can be subtle and may be missed by both the patient and observers.

The spectrum of seizure presentation extends from collapse with tonic–clonic movements (sometimes referred to as convulsions or fits) through to involuntary twitching of a particular muscle group while retaining full consciousness, to absences and visual disturbances. In general, seizure activity can occur in any individual in whom the normal neuronal depolarisation threshold is altered, but this usually requires either disease or injury to be present.

Seizures are generally self-resolving but some generalised seizures need intervention in the community setting; the use of benzodiazepines by paramedics has been shown to be safe and effective. A systematic review of the administration of benzodiazepines in response to seizure emergencies found that buccal, intranasal and intramuscular administration was more rapid compared to rectal and intravenous routes of administration. However, time

to seizure termination, seizure recurrence rates and adverse events were similar among all the routes of administration (Hautt et al., 2016).

Epilepsy is a condition encompassing a broad range of seizure disorders and is diagnosed in patients suffering recurrent seizures (Huff & Fountain, 2011). Epilepsy is one of the most common serious neurological dysfunctions (see Box 29.1). The incidence peaks in childhood, falls in the teenage age group and increases again in the over-60s. Epilepsy can affect anyone regardless of age, intelligence, gender, culture and background. It is a common neurological condition affecting up to 3% of the Australian population (Epilepsy Australia, 2019). Epileptic seizures are associated with frequent use of emergency departments (Girot et al., 2015).

Pathophysiology

Seizures are caused by synchronous, abnormal and excessive discharge of a population of neurons (Bazzigaluppi et al., 2017). Normal neuronal depolarisation occurs when positive ions (usually sodium) enter the neuron via channels in the cell membrane. These channels open (and close) according to the actions of neurotransmitters and adjacent cells, and the influx of positive sodium ions (Na^+) raises the resting membrane potential to a point where a threshold potential is reached. At this point further voltage-activated sodium channels open and allow more positive sodium ions to enter the cell and complete the depolarisation process. Repolarisation is achieved when positive potassium ions (K^+) leave the cell through voltage-regulated potassium channels following an ion gradient (see Fig 29.1). The ion

BOX 29.1 Epilepsy facts and figures

- Up to 10% of the world's population may have a seizure at some time in their life with 3–4% subsequently being diagnosed with epilepsy.
- Epilepsy is a common condition and can develop at any age, regardless of gender or ethnic group.
- In 50% of cases the cause of epilepsy is unknown.
- Approximately 70% of people diagnosed with epilepsy will have their seizure controlled with medication.

Source: Epilepsy Australia (2018).

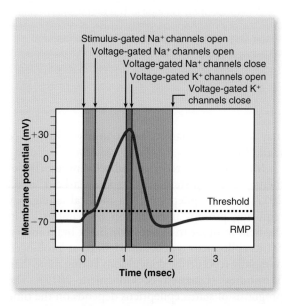

Figure 29.1
The action potential changes in membrane potential in a local area of a neuron's membrane result from changes in membrane permeability. RMP = resting membrane potential.
Source: Patton & Thibodeau (2010).

gradient is constantly maintained through the action of the sodium potassium ATP/ADP (adenosine triphosphate/adenosine diphosphate) pump (Guyton & Hall, 2006).

Individual neurons will depolarise once their threshold potential has been reached. A balance between excitatory neurotransmitters (allowing positive ions to enter the cell) and inhibitory neurotransmitters (allowing negative ions such as chloride to enter the cell) determines whether a neuron will depolarise. In the case of the brain it is the balance between excitatory and inhibitory that determines the level of brain function and it is closely related to consciousness (see Fig 29.2).

There are many neurotransmitters involved in the signalling and regulation of neuronal function, including acetylcholine, noradrenaline, dopamine, serotonin, histamine and various amino acids such as glutamate and gamma-aminobutyric acid (GABA). While most of these are excitatory, an important neurotransmitter responsible for inhibition is GABA, which binds to $GABA_A$ receptors allowing movement of chloride ions into the cell. This is an inhibitory process because it results in a decrease of the membrane potential, away from the threshold potential, preventing depolarisation. Increased release of excitatory neurotransmitters or decreased availability of GABA is associated with seizure activity, whereas increased GABA activity may result in sedation or coma. In the context of seizures, GABA chloride channels are important in the termination of seizure activity with benzodiazepines, which bind to the GABA chloride channel at a separate site, allowing negative chloride ions into the cell and lowering the resting membrane potential (Guyton & Hall, 2006). Bazzigaluppi and colleagues (2017) have also found that a malfunctioning sodium-potassium-ATPase, which is highly energy dependent, can be associated with neuronal hyperexcitability and thus lead to seizures.

Disruption to neuronal excitation-inhibition equilibrium or to normal ion homeostasis gives rise to a seizure if the resting membrane potential is too close to the threshold potential (see Table 29.1). Discharge of this neuron recruits surrounding susceptible neurons. In focal seizures the discharge is limited to a specific area, but in generalised seizures this discharge continues to spread across both hemispheres and subcortical structures such as the basal ganglia, thalamus and brainstem. Involvement of subcortical structures is responsible for alterations of consciousness. Disruption of neuronal excitation-inhibition equilibrium can occur as a result of changes to ions, neuronal cell receptors, neurotransmitters, cell networks or whole brain regions. The brain is particularly susceptible to the effects of hypoxia, hypoglycaemia, hyperthermia, hyponatraemia and sensory stimulation which may result in ictogenesis, the process of transition from interictal (normal) state to a seizure (Guyton & Hall, 2006). Seizures are generally self-limiting due to the loss of synchronous discharge and the impact of synaptic transmission fatigue, which occurs as excitatory neurotransmitters' supplies are exhausted, allowing the inhibitory effects of GABA to prevail (Chang & Lowenstein, 2003).

Excitation/inhibition balance

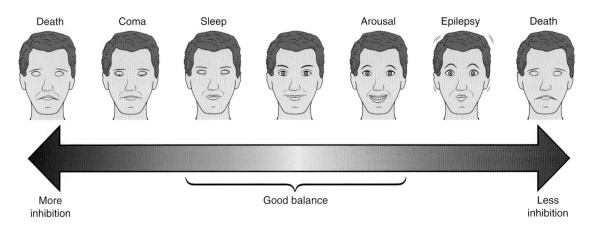

Figure 29.2
The spectrum of brain activity and consciousness.
Neuronal activity is complex and subject to various mechanisms that control the level of electrical activation. These mechanisms can act inside the cell, between the cells, in neighbouring cells or in the extracellular space. The neurotransmitter glutamate is the primary extracellular excitatory mechanism, while GABA is an inhibitory neurotransmitter that makes the cell interior more negative and less likely to reach threshold potential and depolarise. Both are intrinsically linked to seizure generation.
Source: Adapted from CC-BY, Arseny Khakhalin, http://khakhalin.blogspot.com.au/2012/08/excitation-inhibition-balance.html.

Table 29.1 Seizure generation

Excitation	Inhibition
Inward flow of sodium (+) and calcium (+) ions	Inward flow of chloride (–) and outward flow of potassium (+) ions
Triggered by glutamate	Triggered by GABA
Raises cell towards threshold potential	Makes the cell more negative, moving it away from threshold potential
Needs smaller stimulus to reach threshold	Needs larger stimulus to reach threshold

Seizure activity uses large amounts of ATP, the body's energy storage substrate, thus increasing oxygen and glucose consumption (Bazzigaluppi et al., 2017). The reflexive increase in cerebral blood flow, if accompanied by normal ventilation, will generally compensate for these changes with little lasting impact on brain function. Tachypnoea, tachycardia, hypertension and hyperglycaemia are normal clinical signs found in patients suffering seizures. In the absence of adequate ventilation, generally due to airway compromise, these people are at risk of hypoxia, hypercarbia and respiratory acidosis. Prolonged seizures can result in lactic acidosis, hyperthermia, hyperkalaemia and, rarely, rhabdomyolysis, and prolonged cerebral hypoxaemia

may lead to permanent brain injury (Guyton & Hall, 2006).

Most seizures are brief and self-limited (Betjemann & Lowenstein, 2015; Gainza-Lein et al., 2017). Status epilepticus is a medical emergency requiring prompt intervention by paramedics in the field in order to avoid permanent brain injury. Status epilepticus is generally defined as 'prolonged or rapidly reoccurring convulsions lasting more than 5 minutes' (Claassen & Goldstein, 2017). The prognosis of status epilepticus depends on the time between onset and the diagnosis and start of treatment (Requena et al., 2019). The definition of status epilepticus is being re-examined with a view to a focus on two critical timepoints. The first is the duration of the seizure and the second the time at which the prolonged seizure could lead to long-term consequences (Betjemann & Lowenstein, 2015).

Much of the pathophysiology of status epilepticus remains unclear, with animal studies leading to the most comprehensive understanding (Betjemann & Lowenstein, 2015). Failure of seizure-terminating processes (such as ATP depletion, acidosis or release of adenosine) or pro-seizure processes (such as breakdown of the blood–brain barrier and inflammation) or a combination of the two have been suggested as reasons why a seizure does not self-terminate. Prolonged convulsive seizures can lead to physiological compromise including hypotension, hypoxia and acidosis that contribute to neuronal damage (Walker, 2018). Irreversible neuronal injury is thought to commence sometime between 30 and 60 minutes after the start of the seizure due to excitotoxic cell injury, with further insult occurring due to the mismatch between the greatly increased metabolism of the seizing brain cell and declining blood flow and nutrient availability (Huff & Fountain, 2011). The research being undertaken into status epilepticus identified the importance of seizure cessation early on as the longer a seizure continues, the higher the incidence of pharmaco-resistance, in particular to benzodiazepines (Betjemann & Lowenstein, 2015). As such, it is recommended that pharmacological treatment of status epilepticus commence between 5 and 15 minutes after the onset of the seizure (Requena et al., 2019). Some guidelines indicate that pharmacological intervention for seizures with preeclampsia as an underlying cause commence within 2–3 minutes (Osborne et al., 2015).

PRACTICE TIP

- New seizures or changes in seizure pattern are significant.
- Seizure is a symptom of unstable neurons.
- Look for the cause of instability.

Seizure classification

Aetiology

The International League Against Epilepsy identifies that seizures are first categorised as having onset that is focal (initially engaging networks in one hemisphere), generalised (initially engaging bilateral networks) or unknown (Fisher, 2017). A seizure is classified as having impaired awareness if the awareness is impaired at any time during the seizure. Focal aware seizures roughly correspond to the old term 'simple partial seizures' and focal impaired awareness seizures to 'complex partial seizures' (Fisher, 2017).

Seizures occurring as a result of an identifiable cause can be referred to as provoked, reactive, secondary or acute symptomatic seizures. They can be due to a wide variety of causes (see Table 29.2) and do not recur once the cause is removed. The cause may be static (e.g. anatomical scarring), progressive (e.g. degenerative cortical disorders) or transient (e.g. acute electrolyte derangement). Other causes of seizures include trauma, drug ingestion and psychosis.

In some instances, a seizure may not resolve either spontaneously or with treatment and the condition is described as **status epilepticus**. Status epilepticus is generally defined as prolonged or rapidly recurring convulsions lasting more than 5 minutes (Claassen & Goldstein, 2017). In this case a seizure may represent a life-threatening emergency requiring further intervention that may not be available in the out-of-hospital setting. An emerging form of seizure is the **cluster seizure**, similar to status epilepticus but the patient returns to normal function between the seizures, which occur more frequently than the patient's normal seizure pattern (Zelano & Ben-Mencahem, 2016).

Febrile convulsions are the most common seizure type in young children. Febrile convulsions are defined as those occurring in children aged between 6 months and 5 years with a febrile illness (Joint Epilepsy Council Australia, 2009). The peak incidence is between 18 and 24 months of age. Fever is believed to lower the seizure threshold in susceptible children, but the exact pathophysiology of this lowered threshold is unknown; it may be related to either the peak temperature or the rate of temperature rise (Joint

Table 29.2 Common causes of provoked seizures

Drugs of abuse	Infectious/inflammatory
Alcohol	Meningitis
Stimulants	Cerebral abscess
Amphetamine/ methamphetamine	Cerebritis
Cocaine	Lyme disease
LSD (lysergic acid diethylamide)	Neurosyphilis
PCP (phencyclidine)	Lupus
Ecstasy	Encephalitis
Herbal products	Non-CNS infections
Guarana	Salmonella
	Rotavirus
Iatrogenic	**Metabolic disorders**
Antibiotics	Hypo/hyperglycaemia
Antiarrhythmic agents	Hypoxia
Pain medications	Hypo/hypernatraemia
Antidepressants	
Antipsychotics	
Lesions	**Systemic causes**
Tumours	Eclampsia
Intracranial haemorrhage	Extreme fever
Ischaemic stroke	Thyrotoxicosis
Trauma	

Source: Slattery & Pollack (2010).

ASK!

- What is the patient's history? (Ask a bystander/relative.)
- How did the seizure start?
- For how long has it been going on?
- Has it happened before?
- Is the patient on any regular treatment for it?
- Is there a known predisposing cause?

- Airway: is it clear and open?
- Breathing: is it adequate? What is the respiratory rate and SpO$_2$? Is the patient cyanosed?
- Circulation: is there evidence of perfusion?

Epilepsy Council Australia, 2009). These seizures may be categorised as simple or complex.

Simple febrile seizures are generalised, last less than 15 minutes and occur no more than once in 24 hours. They represent the majority of febrile seizures and carry few risks. *Complex febrile seizures* last longer than 15 minutes, occur more than once within 24 hours and may display a focal component (Eskandarifar et al., 2017).

Generally the child will be in a post-ictal state or have returned to a normal state prior to the paramedic arriving, but if the seizure is still occurring, treatment is the same as for other seizure types. There is no evidence that active cooling has a clinical impact on the risk of further seizures. Transport to ED for a first-time febrile seizure or a complex seizure is advised for comprehensive evaluation. Identifying the source of the fever is an important consideration even though the risk of bacterial infection in these children is the same as in children who present with seizure alone (Blumstein & Friedman, 2007).

Derangements of metabolism such as ischaemia, hypoxia and hypoglycaemia increase the concentrations of excitatory neurotransmitters such as glutamate, leading to an increased potential for seizure activity.

Seizure type

Seizures are commonly described in terms of their type based on an international classification system (see Box 29.2). The basic distinction is whether the seizure is partial or generalised.

Focal seizures generally involve only one hemisphere of the brain and originate from a particular cortical area of the brain. Awareness is used as a practical surrogate for consciousness, since consciousness comprises many aspects that can be difficult to assess. A seizure is classified as having impaired awareness if the awareness is impaired at any time during the seizure. Focal seizures can progress to generalised seizures.

Generalised seizures involve both hemispheres of the brain and do not originate from one cortical area. Generalised seizures always result in an alteration to consciousness. Generalised onset seizures are not characterised by level of awareness, because awareness is almost always impaired (Fisher, 2017).

BOX 29.2 Classification of clinical seizures

Focal onset (aware or impaired awareness)
Motor onsets
Automatisms
Atonic
Clonic
Epileptic spasms
Hyperkinetic
Myoclonic
Tonic

Non-motor onsets
Autonomic
Behaviour arrests
Cognitive
Emotional
Sensory
Focal to bilateral tonic–clonic

Generalised onset
Motor
Tonic–clonic
Clonic
Tonic
Myoclonic

Myoclonic–tonic–clonic
Atonic
Epileptic spasms

Non-motor
Typical
Atypical
Myoclonic
Eyelid myoclonic

Unknown onset
Motor
Tonic–clonic
Epileptic spasms

Non-motor
Behaviour arrest
Unclassified
Source: Fisher (2017).

An example of the unique electrical activity associated with each type of seizure can be seen in Figure 29.3.

Management

Emergency management of seizures should follow a systematic approach, including evaluation of ABCs (Osborne et al., 2015). Emergency management of seizures can be assisted by a classification system based on the clinical presentation (see Fig 29.4). This system considers whether the seizure involves an impairment of consciousness, whether it was provoked and whether it is simple or complex. The key operational decision is whether the patient requires active management with benzodiazepines now or may require it imminently.

Time-critical patients include those with major ABCD problems, serious head injury, status epilepticus following treatment, or underlying infection (Osborne et al., 2015). All patients having a seizure for the first time and those who have had serial seizures, difficulties in monitoring, infants under 1 year of age or children having a first febrile convulsion also require transport (Osborne et al., 2015). Patients who are still having a generalised seizure when the ambulance arrives warrant active intervention with an anticonvulsant medication to reduce the chance of neurological injury due to hypoxia (Silverman et al., 2017).

A large proportion of patients are transported to hospital after seizures, and there is little research into alternative care pathways (Osborne et al., 2015). One report from paramedics in London identified that known epileptic patients whose seizures self-resolve prior to arrival of an ambulance can pose a particular challenge. There is a lack of guidance on when to convey such patients, and clinicians largely relied on their own experience (Burrell et al., 2018). Another study identified that checklists may not accurately identify patients suitable for discharge at the scene (Tohira et al., 2016). Alternative care pathways may present opportunities for paramedics where such patients are haemodynamically stable, do not have any underlying co-morbidities and do not warrant immediate transport to an emergency department.

Advances in the delivery mechanisms for front-line medications for epilepsy and increased incidence

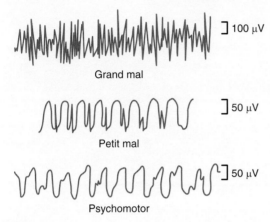

Figure 29.3
Electroencephalograms in different types of epilepsy.
Source: Hall (2010).

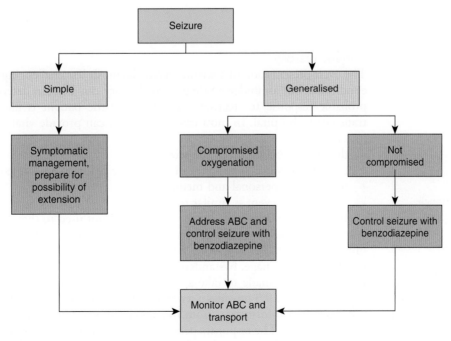

Figure 29.4
Basic treatment flowchart.

of community-administered medications through buccal and intranasal preparation is becoming more common. In this setting, research has shown buccal administration of diazepam to be as safe and as effective as rectal administration (Betjemann & Lowenstein, 2015). A further randomised trial showed that intranasal midazolam was as effective as intravenous diazepam when terminating febrile convulsions (Betjemann & Lowenstein, 2015) and this was confirmed in a review of the Cochrane Central Register of Controlled Trials (Brigo et al., 2015). Auto-injectors (in particular diazepam) may be available in some areas and seen in the community setting (Verrotti et al., 2015). Much of the research into seizure treatment medication has focused on the management of status epilepticus. The main advances have been in the use of alternatives for those patients resistant to benzodiazepines. These medications include valproate, levetiracetam and lacosamide (Zelano & Ben-Mencahem, 2016).

 ## CASE STUDY 1

Case 10994, 1006 hrs.

Dispatch details: A 42-year-old male was sitting at his office desk, when his colleague reports he heard a shrill cry and looked over to see the patient shaking violently on the floor. This lasted for 8 minutes and then the patient was unresponsive. His colleague placed him in the recovery position and called the ambulance.

Initial presentation: The paramedics find the patient in a lateral position. There is evidence of urinary incontinence. He is flushed and sweaty. He is responsive to pain, but appears confused and disoriented. There is evidence of haemorrhage around the corners of his mouth and a small laceration to his tongue.

 ## ASSESS

Patient history

The overt presentation of a seizure makes diagnosis less challenging than other conditions, but an understanding of the history can assist in determining the probable response to treatment and whether the patient is likely to resist transport to hospital. In most cases bystanders can provide vital information in terms of:

- the events leading up to the seizure
- the duration and appearance of the seizure before the paramedics arrived
- the patient's personal and medical history
- whether this event is similar to past events.

Bystanders are the 'eyes' for the event and if not used to their full capacity, correct diagnosis and subsequent management can become difficult. It is important to realise that while seizures may be a familiar presentation for paramedics to manage, bystanders can be stressed by such an event and every effort should be made to take a calm and reassuring approach when asking questions. Table 29.3 provides a series of questions as a framework for systematically soliciting information from bystanders to assist in the identification of the seizure type. The responses pertaining to the opening case study are noted.

In this case the paramedics also find a packet of valproate in the patient's belongings (see Box 29.3).

PRACTICE TIP

Some patients experience an aura prior to a seizure. This is a subjective symptom or sensation such as a smell or taste and represents a focal fit. The aura may provide information indicating where the generalised seizure began (Huff & Fountain, 2011).

Table 29.3 A framework for systematically soliciting information from bystanders

Question	Case study 1	
	Bystander response	Evidence
Did the patient make any noises just prior to the seizure?	Yes, loud shrill cry	Nil
Did the patient appear aware of their surroundings during the seizure?	No	AVPU remains decreased
Did the seizure affect only a limb, the face, speech or awareness?	No	Nil
Was the seizure violent with the whole body shaking violently?	Yes	Laceration to tongue; incontinence of urine; sweaty and flushed skin
For how long did the seizure last?	8 minutes	Compensation present for HR; RR and AVPU depressed still
Was there more than one seizure? If so, how long did it last?	No	Nil
When the patient started to wake up were they confused?	Yes	Nil
Is this the usual seizure for this patient?	No; has not had a seizure for years and recovered much faster last time	Change in disease process, medication may need reviewing and investigations for new/altered disease undertaken
Has the patient been ill, changed medications or had unusually stressful events recently?	Unusually late for work and disorganised, which is unusual	Work area appears very disorganised

AVPU = alert, voice, pain, unresponsive.

BOX 29.3 Common anti-epileptic drugs

Patients may have their chronic epilepsy controlled with drugs whose role is to stabilise the neuron cell membrane.

- Some work on sodium channels or sodium efflux.
  - Phenytoin
  - Lamotrigine
  - Valproate
  - Carbamazepine
  - Oxcarbazepine
- Some work on GABA (or like GABA) either on the channel or on the bioavailability of GABA.
  - Valproate
  - Gabapentin
  - Tiagabine
  - Pregabalin
  - Phenobarbitone
  - Clonazepam
  - Vigabatrin
  - Topiramate

Note that valproate appears in both lists.

Airway

The snoring suggests obstruction: consider either a foreign substance or the patient's tongue. Trismus (clenching of the jaw) and movement of the head and limbs can make it difficult to perform basic airway manoeuvres and the patient's jaw should not be forced open. The airway should be managed as circumstances allow without using invasive techniques. Vomiting is not common with seizures but excessive build-up of saliva may occur.

Breathing

Seizure-induced hypoxia can produce an elevated respiratory rate but spasm of the chest and abdominal muscles can concurrently reduce the patient's tidal volume. Aspiration of stomach contents into the lungs is possible and auscultation should occur once the seizure has resolved.

Cardiovascular

Seizure-induced hypoxia and the contraction of major muscles typically generate an elevated heart rate. Resolution of the acidosis caused by the seizure activity can take several minutes during which the respiratory rate and heart rate will remain elevated.

Initial assessment summary

Problem	Post-ictal
Conscious state	GCS = 9 (E 2, V 3, M 4)
Position	Lateral
Heart rate	95 bpm
Blood pressure	130/75 mmHg
Skin appearance	Sweaty and flushed
Speech pattern	Phrases
Respiratory rate	25 bpm
Respiratory rhythm	Even cycles
Respiratory effort	Normal effort
Chest auscultation	Snoring inspiratory sounds, clear chest bilaterally
Pulse oximetry	99% on room air
Temperature	37.2°C
Motor/sensory function	Appears normal
BGL	7.1 mmol/L
History	Seizure lasting 8 minutes The patient's colleague says that the patient has been very stressed at work recently. He has not had a seizure in several years and last time 'he recovered much faster and refused to go to hospital'.

D: The patient is now post-ictal and safe on the floor.
A: The patient is in an altered conscious state and is currently exhibiting signs of a partial airway obstruction (through the snoring).
B: Respiratory function is currently normal but needs frequent reassessment. The respiratory rate is elevated but ventilation is normal.
C: Heart rate is normal and there is sufficient blood pressure.

The patient appears to have suffered a generalised seizure that has resolved spontaneously and the patient is now presenting in a post-ictal state. The seizure is the first in several years and is not typical of previous episodes.

CONFIRM

The essential part of the clinical reasoning process is to seek to confirm your initial hypothesis by finding clinical signs that should occur with your provisional diagnosis. You should also seek to challenge your diagnosis by exploring findings that do not fit your hypothesis: don't just ignore them because they don't fit.

What else could it be?

Syncope

A sudden fall in blood pressure can cause temporary cerebral hypoxia, which in turn can cause a seizure, but this tends to be short-lived and the patient tends to either recover as perfusion returns or cease to have a seizure and

DIFFERENTIAL DIAGNOSIS

A seizure in the setting of long-term epilepsy
Or
- Syncope (neurocardiogenic, vasovagal, orthostatic, cardiac)
- Stroke/cerebrovascular accident
- Traumatic head injury
- Migraine with aura
- Movement disorder (e.g. dystonia, Parkinson's disease)
- Toxic or metabolic encephalopathy (hypoglycaemia, renal or liver dysfunction, recreational drug use)
- Sleep disorders
- Psychogenic

Table 29.4 Differentiation between cardiogenic syncope and generalised tonic–clonic seizure

Clinical feature	Cardiogenic syncope (vagal stimulus or arrhythmia)	Seizure
Loss of consciousness	Typical • With vagal reactions the patient usually regains some consciousness on becoming supine; confusion, if present, lasts only a few minutes • With arrhythmias, unconsciousness may persist after collapse	Typical: fatigue, confusion, agitation and headache can persist for more than 10 minutes
Length of event	Loss of consciousness usually resolves in seconds	Typically lasts for minutes
Prodromal events	May complain of warm flush, dizziness, nausea	Brief aura but often no warning; patient may moan loudly at start of event
Recollection of event	Nil or minimal	Nil
Ventilation	Normal with vagal events; cyanosis is atypical	
Inadequate with arrhythmias; cyanosis is common	Irregular during seizure; cyanosis is common	
Electrocardiographic (ECG) analysis	Bradycardia due to increased vagal tone is typical	Sinus tachycardia due to muscular exertion, but arrhythmias are rare

BOX 29.4 Sinister causes of hypotension and seizures

- Arrhythmias
- Atrial fibrillation
- Ventricular tachycardia
- Supraventricular tachycardia
- Third-degree heart block
- Sepsis
- Cardiogenic shock
- Hypovolaemia
- Acute coronary syndromes
- Anaphylaxis

become flaccid if this is the start of a cardiac arrest. In this case the seizure has been sustained so syncope is unlikely (see Table 29.4). Benign causes of hypotension are usually secondary to vasodilation from a hot environment and are common in elderly patients where their sympathetic response is not sufficient to maintain a cardiac output that supports cerebral perfusion. Hot showers, prolonged hot weather and newly prescribed drugs such as beta-blockers, calcium channel blockers or ACE inhibitors are all potential causes of benign transient hypotension. More sinister causes are listed in Box 29.4.

Stroke
A stroke may well present with either focal or generalised seizure activity, but it would be unlikely to leave the patient with no obvious neurological deficit once the seizure had ceased.

Traumatic head injury
Posttraumatic seizures (PTS) are a sequel to acute brain injury, and if occurring within 24 hours of injury are termed immediate PTS, but PTS may also occur later. The incidence of PTS is 2–2.5% in the civilian population, and increases with severe head injury (GCS < 9/15) to 10–15% in adults and 30–35% in children (Shorvon & Neligan, 2009). The occurrence of a seizure following a head injury has been associated with a higher likelihood of having an abnormal CT scan, and the approach to traumatic seizures follows the standard ABCDE primary survey to ensure that adequate oxygenated blood is supplied to the brain.

PRACTICE TIP

Traumatic head injury is an important known cause of epilepsy. The highest risk of epilepsy developing is within a few years of the head injury. Epilepsy associated with head injury is six times more common than familial epilepsy.

439

Migraine

Migraines can produce focal neurological symptoms, but they do not generally cause tonic–clonic seizure activity, nor would they leave the patient with no residual headache after the seizure.

Movement disorders

These could be mistaken for tonic–clonic epileptic activity but they tend to be long term, may resemble partial seizures rather than generalised seizures, and once again will not clear at the end of the seizure incident.

Toxic or metabolic encephalopathy

A low BGL is a common cause of seizures secondary to a lack of ATP in brain tissue, but this patient has a normal blood sugar, no history of diabetes and has returned to normal. Renal and liver dysfunction could both be contributing factors either upsetting the electrolyte balance in the case of renal dysfunction or failing to detoxify chemicals from the gut in liver dysfunction. Both of these could precipitate seizures in a susceptible individual and as the reason for a change in seizure pattern in this patient is yet to be ascertained, formal blood tests are indicated.

The use of stimulants could account for the change in seizure pattern for this patient. The stimulant could be a recreational drug (amphetamine or amphetamine-like class) or caffeine from coffee or an energy drink. Obtaining a more detailed history from this patient in a private setting will help with this assessment.

Sleep disorder

A sleep disorder creating fatigue may alter the patient's threshold to seizures and should be considered in the differential diagnosis.

Psychogenic

Pseudoseizures can look extremely like normal seizures (Avbersek & Sisodiya, 2010). This patient has a history of increased stress and a change in work pattern, which may raise the possibility of a psychogenic cause. In a pseudoseizure the patient will demonstrate clinical symptoms that mimic true seizures; however, the pseudoseizures are not associated with uncontrolled randomised depolarisation of neural tissue. It is important that this aetiology is explored carefully in the setting of the ED, as this is not a diagnosis that may be arrived at in the out-of-hospital environment.

Because focal epilepsy can present with the patient remaining conscious, evidence of the patient's conscious state cannot be taken as evidence of pseudoseizure. Hard evidence of a pseudoseizure would be the demonstration of the symptoms while recording a normal electroencephalogram. Other evidence could include the absence of raised levels of neurotransmitters in plasma following a prolonged seizure, but this is neither totally reliable nor available as a routine investigation.

 TREAT

Emergency management

Safety

A seizure can be a violent physical event. If the patient is still convulsing when the paramedics arrive, basic supportive measures should be applied to protect the patient from further injury. These include the following.

- Remove dangers from or around the patient, such as sharp objects and furniture. If this is not possible, consider moving the patient away from the danger.
- Pad the patient with pillows or blankets to prevent injury.

> ## BOX 29.5 Sudden unexpected death in epilepsy
>
> Over the past decade it has emerged that epileptics are at higher risk of death. The most likely mechanism for SUDEP is airway occlusion during the seizure and subsequent profound hypoxia that restricts the patient from waking after the seizure ceases (Thom, 2007). There is also emerging evidence that seizures can generate cardiac arrhythmias (cerebrogenic cardiac arrhythmias) or central respiratory depression. The arrhythmias may occur secondary to seizures, but this is difficult to diagnose without long-term ECG monitoring. The highest risk groups are males in their teens and young adults with convulsive seizures: those with a high frequency of seizures or who sleep unattended are most at risk. Fatality rates are higher if seizures occur unsupervised.

- Keep the area around the patient as quiet as possible. A hypoxic and acidotic brain is hypersensitive to noise.
  - Permit as few people as possible into the area.
  - Turn off appliances that make noise.
  - Turn down your portable radio or move away if communications are required.
- Remove animals as they often become frightened and may become aggressive.

Airway and breathing

Airway management in a patient who is having a simple or complex partial seizure is reasonably simple. The patient should be monitored and oxygen should be administered if necessary. Patients experiencing a generalised seizure move violently, usually have diaphragmatic and abdominal muscle spasms and are often sweaty. If the patient will tolerate a simple oropharyngeal airway, this should be used. If the patient is hypoxic, maintenance of positive end expiratory pressure (PEEP) via a bag valve mask (BVM) is ideal. However, this may be difficult to maintain due to the violent action of the seizure and the 'slipperiness' of the patient's sweaty face. Consideration should be given to placing the patient in the lateral position. Patients having seizures may have apnoea during seizures, however, and this has been implicated in sudden unexpected death in epilepsy (SUDEP; see Box 29.5). If a convulsing patient has a prolonged apnoea then BVM assistance providing intermittent positive pressure ventilation (IPPV) may be necessary, but great care has to be taken to avoid barotrauma and gastric inflation, which may lead to regurgitation and aspiration.

Where PEEP via BMV is difficult, common practice is to administer oxygen via a non-rebreather mask during the seizure. Once the seizure ceases, PEEP via BVM ventilation should be initiated (as the patient is usually hypoxic) in conjunction with an oropharyngeal airway and suction for foreign bodies (food, vomit, blood and sputum).

As the patient begins to re-establish normal breathing, they will correct their acid–base imbalance with long deep respirations. Oxygenation of the post-ictal patient is usually best decided by pulse oximetry, but patients with a rapidly increasing level of consciousness may not tolerate an oxygen mask.

Terminating the seizure

Terminating seizure activity is a primary management goal where the seizure has persisted for longer than 5 minutes. Clearly, in the out-of-hospital setting if a patient is still convulsing when the paramedics arrive, it is almost certain that this time has elapsed and the patient is therefore very likely to need seizure control. Benzodiazepines are the first-line medication for the emergency management of seizures and commonly used benzodiazepines include midazolam, diazepam and lorazepam.

Midazolam is generally the medication of choice for out-of-hospital management of active seizures: it can be administered intramuscularly, intranasally or intravenously; and it has a rapid onset of action and a relatively short duration of action (Duncan et al., 2006). Midazolam enhances the effects of GABA on neuronal inhibition by selectively binding to $GABA_A$ receptors, enhancing their affinity for GABA. This facilitates an increased opening frequency of GABA-activated chloride channels, resulting in a cellular Cl^- influx, and consequent hyperpolarisation reduces the high-frequency firing of neurons, leading to termination of the seizure.

Midazolam is capable of producing hypotension and respiratory depression, so the respiratory and cardiovascular status of patients receiving the drug should be monitored carefully post-administration. This is particularly the case in the presence of other CNS depressants such as alcohol or opioids. In addition, episodes of apnoea are more likely to occur following rapid intravenous administration. Finally, as the metabolic pathway for midazolam is susceptible to the effects of age and liver disease, its effects can be more pronounced in elderly patients.

Although midazolam enters the brain rapidly, it displays a slower effect-site equilibration time than other anticonvulsants—this is the interval between medication administration and subsequent measurable effect. As the measurable effects of midazolam take longer to manifest, repeat doses should be sufficiently delayed to allow observation of the dose peak clinical effect. Recommended doses for all routes of administration range from 0.1 to 0.2 mg/kg. Doses should be given 3–5 minutes apart with a maximum dose for adults of 10 mg. Midazolam is commonly administered via an intramuscular route but intravenous administration is faster and more effective if access is achievable, and intraosseous administration is becoming more routine. Intranasal administration is a viable alternative provided enough drug can be administered (intranasal volumes of absorption are limited to approximately 0.5 mL per nostril).

Communication and reassurance for patients, family and bystanders

Communication with the post-ictal patient can be challenging. Patients often exhibit repetitive questioning and have anterograde amnesia. The best way to communicate with patients who are having seizures or are post-ictal is in a calm, reassuring voice. Reducing surrounding noise can also be helpful. In terms of family or bystanders, the most effective reassurance is the performance of effective paramedic care, with a calm manner and regular provision of information.

Transport

Transport to hospital for the patient who has had a prolonged seizure, a first seizure or a change in seizure pattern (frequency or nature of seizure) is necessary to facilitate investigation of the cause.

(4) EVALUATE

Evaluating the effect of any clinical management intervention can provide clues to the accuracy of the initial diagnosis. Some conditions respond rapidly to treatment so patients should be expected to improve if the diagnosis and treatment were appropriate. A failure to improve in this situation should trigger the clinician to reconsider the diagnosis.

It is important to assess whether the patient is improving as would be expected given their history and their presentation. Post-ictal patients are often confused and non-compliant with any procedure performed, but this will

> ## PRACTICE TIP
>
> Midazolam only modulates the response of GABA receptors and requires the presence of GABA to exert an effect. Hydralazine poisoning inhibits GABA production and can result in midazolam being ineffective.

> ## PRACTICE TIP
>
> - Has the midazolam been effective?
> - Is the patient's ventilation adequate?
> - Are their oxygen saturations adequate?

usually improve with time. Once the seizure has ceased and the patient's level of consciousness is improving, it can be advantageous to allow the patient time and space before attempting to take vital signs and move them towards transport. Patients often recover consciousness to a large degree during transport, although they may experience retrograde amnesia following the event.

Ongoing management

Continuous or subsequent repeated seizure activity may be addressed with an extra dose of midazolam, but if after two doses the patient is still convulsing it is unlikely that further doses of benzodiazepines will have an effect. An alternative approach to controlling the seizure will then be necessary, such as phenytoin, which acts on sodium channels—however, this must be given slowly with continuous ECG monitoring, ideally in a controlled hospital setting.

Hospital admission

A patient who has a new seizure or a change in seizure pattern warrants a formal hospital assessment.

The components of this assessment include a detailed clinical examination for precipitating causes; blood tests to exclude electrolyte imbalance; investigations to exclude infection, tumour or cerebrovascular accident; drug screening and a detailed history to exclude toxins; and, if the patient is on routine anti-epileptic drugs, measurement of drug levels to see whether they are in the therapeutic range. Many adult patients experiencing their first seizure or a prolonged seizure or with any suspicion of trauma will receive a CT scan of the brain to rule out underlying lesions.

CASE STUDY 2

Case 13234, 1034 hrs.

Dispatch details: A 48-year-old female who has not been seen for 24 hours. The patient lives alone and uncharacteristically has not been seen since yesterday. The neighbour says there is a locked key box on the veranda.

Initial presentation: The paramedics find the patient on the kitchen floor; she shows no evidence of trauma. She is confused and her speech is slurred, which the neighbour confirms is not usual.

1 ASSESS

1054 hrs Primary survey: The patient is conscious and talking.

1055 hrs Chief complaint: The patient is confused and unable to answer questions appropriately. She is unable to explain why she is on the floor or identify how long she has been there.

1056 hrs Vital signs survey: Perfusion status: HR 122 bpm, sinus rhythm, BP 138/65 mmHg, skin cool and dry.

Respiratory status: RR 16 bpm, good, air entry bilaterally, normal work of breathing, SpO$_2$ 96% on room air.

Conscious state: GCS = 13 (E 4, V 4, M 5), PEARL (pupils equal and reacting to light).

Other: tympanic temperature 36.9°C; BGL 5.1 mmol/L.

1100 hrs Assessment: After 10 minutes, the patient becomes unconscious, begins to shake violently and is apnoeic with trismus. She quickly becomes centrally cyanosed and sweaty.

The initial presentation is a patient who appears to have signs and symptoms consistent with a stroke, then subsequently has a generalised tonic–clonic seizure in the paramedics' presence. The working hypothesis could be either stroke precipitating a generalised seizure or undisclosed epilepsy. Regardless, the seizure activity needs to be managed.

CONFIRM

In many cases paramedics are presented with a collection of signs and symptoms that do not appear to describe a particular condition. A critical step in determining a treatment plan in this situation is to consider what other conditions could explain the patient's presentation.

What else could it be?

Hypoglycaemia
The presentation of a decreased level of consciousness in a pale and sweaty patient who then proceeds to fit is entirely compatible with hypoglycaemia; however, in this patient this is excluded as she has a normal BGL.

Head injury/trauma
A head injury or other trauma could have occurred without leaving obvious signs, particularly if associated with intracranial bleeding, and could account for this patient's initial low GCS and subsequent seizure. A detailed clinical examination of the scalp may reveal evidence of a previously missed head injury, but this should not be performed until a full ABCDE primary survey has been completed and resuscitation commenced. A definitive investigation such as a CT scan is indicated (Roth & Drislane, 1998).

Toxins
There are a number of toxins including prescribed medications that could present with a decreased level of consciousness and then precipitate a seizure. An overdose of tricyclic antidepressants, sleeping tablets or even anti-epileptic medication is a possibility. Detailed examination of the patient's medicines would help but would not absolutely exclude this diagnosis.

Meningitis/encephalitis
Meningitis, encephalitis or another systemic infection could possibly present like this. This patient may have a reduced immune reaction to infection and therefore not be showing classic signs such as a high temperature, although this degree of reduction in immune reaction is more usual in an older person in their 80s. Blood tests might reveal raised inflammatory markers and raised white cell count, but once again this may be moderated by age. A lumbar puncture may be necessary, although a CT scan would normally be performed prior to this to exclude raised intracranial pressure from a space-occupying lesion or an intracranial bleed. Although unlikely, this diagnosis cannot be confidently excluded in the field.

Electrolyte abnormality
Electrolyte abnormalities can cause CNS changes and convulsions. A particularly common cause is a low-sodium diet, which may be associated with adrenal problems, or alternatively excessive water drinking. Blood tests for electrolytes and renal function will be necessary to exclude this.

Thermoregulation problems
Extremes of temperature could account for the patient's decreased level of consciousness and seizures are associated with hyperthermia. An assessment of both the environmental and the patient's temperature will be useful,

---

DIFFERENTIAL DIAGNOSIS ②

Seizure
Or
- Hypoglycaemia
- Head injury/trauma
- Toxins
- Meningitis/encephalitis
- Electrolyte abnormality
- Thermoregulatory problems

PRACTICE TIP

When to check for hypoglycaemia
Hypoglycaemia was found in one study to account for only 1.2% of seizure patients, and in each of those patients who were tested for hypoglycaemia first, benzodiazepine administration was delayed by up to 5.9 minutes. The authors concluded that it was more important to terminate the seizure before testing for hypoglycaemia (Beskind et al., 2014).

although caution should be used when interpreting non-invasive thermometer readings.

3 TREAT

The first priority is to protect the patient's airway while controlling the seizure: this patient is at risk of hypoxic brain injury unless the seizure can be controlled and normal ventilation re-established. Midazolam via the intramuscular route has been shown to be safe and effective and is easier to administer in patients suffering seizures than trying to gain IV access. IV, intraosseous and intranasal routes may be used according to local guidelines. IV access, if available, is potentially useful, as is pre-notification of the receiving hospital.

1102 hrs: The paramedics administer IM midazolam appropriate to the patient's age and weight. They also protect the patient's position and prepare oxygen and secondary doses of midazolam.

1105 hrs: The seizure activity is continuing.

Perfusion status: HR 104 bpm, sinus tachycardia, BP 160/85 mmHg, skin warm and pale.

Respiratory status: RR 10 bpm, clear chest bilaterally, irregular and uneven respirations, SpO_2 90%.

Conscious state: GCS = 3.

If the midazolam fails to control the seizure, a second dose is appropriate after 5 minutes. Multiple doses of midazolam have the potential to cause both hypotension and respiratory depression, but neither generally occurs to a significant degree in patients whose seizures resolve. More problematic is the patient who requires multiple doses and still does not regain full consciousness.

1111 hrs: The seizure activity has reduced but the patient still has increased muscle tone and remains unconscious.

Perfusion status: HR 114 bpm, sinus tachycardia, BP 150/85 mmHg, skin warm and pale.

Respiratory status: RR 10 bpm, clear chest bilaterally, irregular and uneven respirations, SpO_2 90%.

Conscious state: GCS = 3.

Most out-of-hospital guidelines allow up to 2.5 mg/kg of midazolam and this is usually more than sufficient to resolve most generalised seizures. There is, however, a small cohort of patients who are refractory to benzodiazepines and they present a unique clinical challenge in the out-of-hospital setting.

4 EVALUATE

Evaluating the effect of any clinical management intervention can provide clues to the accuracy of the initial diagnosis. Some conditions respond rapidly to treatment so patients should be expected to improve if the diagnosis and treatment were appropriate. A failure to improve in this situation should trigger the clinician to reconsider the diagnosis.

The first question to be asked is whether the seizure activity has actually ceased. The uncontrolled electrochemical activity of the brain that occurs with a seizure produces chaotic muscle contractions typical of a generalised seizure, but these movements can fatigue over time. This can be mistaken as the onset of the post-ictal period when in fact the seizure and its potential for brain injury continue. Increased muscle tone, nystagmus and irregular respirations are strong signs that seizure activity is continuing and needs to be managed. If these signs are not present, the patient's depressed conscious state may be a result of benzodiazepine administration. Either diagnosis requires intervention.

If the seizure activity has ceased and the patient is simply sedated from the benzodiazepine, they are likely to need both airway and circulatory support to counter the side effects of the midazolam. Non-invasive ventilation is usually adequate to prevent hypoxia, but in cases where the SpO_2 cannot be restored endotracheal intubation may be required. Fluid resuscitation with crystalloid fluids (up to 20 mL/kg) is usually adequate to counter the vasodilatory effects of midazolam.

If the seizure is determined to be ongoing (status epilepticus), consultation with the receiving hospital regarding further benzodiazepine is recommended—and may be required if the patient's movements and muscle tone make it impossible to move them safely from their environment. For patients in status epilepticus, hospital-based clinicians have a range of drug interventions such as sodium-channel blocking phenytoin or barbiturates that increase the sensitivity of the $GABA_A$ receptors, but these are rare in the out-of-hospital setting.

REFLECTIVE BOX

As a paramedic attending an out-of-hospital seizure think about the following questions.

- What aspects of the history of the incident will indicate the type of seizure being experienced by the patient?
- How will you differentiate between the different seizure types, and which ones require timely out-of-hospital pharmacological intervention?
- What are the important aspects of your systematic assessment, prior to administration of pharmacology for the actively convulsing patient?
- How will you select the most appropriate pharmacology intervention for different types of seizures?
- How will you manage the actively convulsing patient who is unresponsive to pharmacological intervention?
- How will you manage the post-ictal patient who may be combative or uncooperative? What underlying pathophysiologies cause such patient behaviour?
- What aspects of your patient assessment will indicate whether or not to refer the patient to healthcare facilities other than an emergency department?

Future research and trends

In line with the research already completed, and ongoing developments in community treatment of seizures, there are a number of avenues for out-of-hospital research:

- neurological effect of street drugs and the incidence of seizures after ingestion
- community administration of pharmacologies for status epilepticus via the intranasal route or IM auto-injector
- paramedic assessment of the post-ictal patient and referral to healthcare professionals other than emergency departments for those assessed as low risk or acuity.

Summary

Seizures can be life-threatening emergencies, not simply because of the physiological effects the patient is exposed to—other threats to the patient's life include the environment within which they have their seizure. For bystanders or first-aiders the primary treatment is to protect the person from harm. For healthcare professionals the aim of treatment is to stop the seizure activity to avoid the patient developing hypoxic brain injury.

The causes of seizures are broad. For some patients, seizures may be a part of their condition—such as epilepsy or hypoglycaemia. For others, seizure activity is not normal and further investigations should be undertaken at hospital.

References

Avbersek, A., & Sisodiya, S. (2010). Does the primary literature provide support for clinical signs used to distinguish psychogenic non-epileptic seizure from epileptic seizures? *Journal of Neurology, Neurosurgery, and Psychiatry, 81*, 719–725.

Bazzigaluppi, P., Amini, A., Weisspapir, I., Stefanovic, B., & Carlen, P. (2017). Hungry neurons: metabolic insights on seizure dynamics. *International Journal of Molecular Sciences, 18*, 2269.

Beskind, D., Rhodes, S., Stolz, U., Birrer, B., Mayfield, T., Bourn, S., & Denninghoff, K. (2014). When should you test for and treat hypoglycaemia in prehospital seizure patients? *Prehospital Emergency Care, 18*(3), 433–441.

Betjemann, J., & Lowenstein, D. (2015). Status epilepticus in adults. *The Lancet, 14*, 615–624.

Blumstein, M., & Friedman, M. (2007). Childhood seizures. *Emergency Medicine Clinics of North America, 25*(4), 1061–1086.

Brigo, F., Nardone, R., Tezzon, F., & Trinka, E. (2015). Nonintravenous midazolam versus intravenous or rectal diazepam for the treatment of early status epilepticus: a systematic review with meta-analysis. *Epilepsy and Behavior, 49*, 325–336.

Burrell, L., Noble, A., & Ridsdale, L. (2018). Decision-making by ambulance clinicians in London when managing patients with epilepsy: a qualitative study. *Emergency Medicine Journal, 30*, 236–240.

Chang, B. S., & Lowenstein, M. D. (2003). Epilepsy: mechanism of disease. *The New England Journal of Medicine, 349*, 1257–1266.

Claassen, J., & Goldstein, J. (2017). Emergency neurological life support: status epilepticus. *Neurocritical Care, 27*, 152–158.

Duncan, J. S., Sander, J. W., Sisodiya, S., & Walker, M. C. (2006). Adult epilepsy. *The Lancet, 367*(1).

Epilepsy Australia. (2018). *What is epilepsy?* Accessed 7 May 2018. Retrieved from http://www.epilepsyaustralia.net/epilepsy-explained/.

Epilepsy Australia. (2019). *Epilepsy facts*. Accessed 28 May 2019. Retrieved from https://www.epilepsy.org.au/wp-content/uploads/2017/08/Fact-Sheet-Epilepsy-Facts.pdf.

Epilepsy Foundation. (2019). *Understanding epilepsy*. Accessed 29 May 2019. Retrieved from https://www.epilepsyfoundation.org.au/understanding-epilepsy/.

Eskandarifar, A., Fatolahpor, A., Asadi, G., & Gaderi, I. (2017). The risk factors in children with simple and complex febrile seizures: an epidemiological study. *International Journal of Pediatrics, 5*(6), 5137–5144.

Fisher, R. (2017). An overview of the 2017 ILAE operational classification of seizure types. *Epilepsy and Behavior, 70*, 271–273.

Gainza-Lein, M., Benjamin, R., Stredny, C., McGurl, M., Kapur, K., & Loddenkemper, T. (2017). Rescue medications in epilepsy patients: a family perspective. *Seizure, 52*, 188–194.

Girot, M., Hubert, H., Richard, F., Chochoi, M., & Deplanque, D. (2015). Use of emergency departments by known epileptic patients: an underestimated problem? *Epilepsy Research, 113*, 1–4.

Guyton, A., & Hall, J. (2006). *Textbook of medical physiology*. St Louis: Elsevier Saunders.

Hall, J. (2010). *Guyton and Hall textbook of medical physiology* (12th ed.). St Louis: Saunders.

Hautt, S., Seinfeld, S., & Pellock, J. (2016). Benzodiazepine use in seizure emergencies: a systematic review. *Epilepsy and Behavior, 63*, 109–117.

Huff, J., & Fountain, N. (2011). Pathophysiology and definitions of seizures and status epilepticus. *Emergency Medicine Clinics of North America, 29*(1), 1–13.

Joint Epilepsy Council Australia. (2009). *A Fair Go for People Living with Epilepsy*. Australian Chapter for International Bureau for Epilepsy.

Osborne, A., Taylor, L., Reuber, M., Grunewald, R., Parkinson, M., & Dickson, J. (2015). Pre-hospital care after a seizure: evidence base and United Kingdom management guidelines. *Seizure, 24*, 82–87.

Patton, K. T., & Thibodeau, G. A. (2010). *Anatomy & physiology* (7th ed.). St Louis: Mosby.

Requena, M., Fonseca, E., Olivé, M., Quintana, A., Mazuela, G., Toledo, M., Salas-Puig, X., & Santamaria, E. (2019). The ADAN scale: a proposed scale for prehospital use to identify status epilepticus. *European Journal of Neurology, 26*, 760–765.

Roth, H. L., & Drislane, F. W. (1998). Neurologic clinics. *Seizures, 16*(2), 257–285.

Shorvon, S., & Neligan, A. (2009). Risk of epilepsy after head trauma. *The Lancet, 373*, 1060–1061.

Silverman, E., Sporer, K., Lemieux, J., Brown, J., Koenig, K., Gausche-Hill, M., Rudnick, E., Salvucci, A., & Gilbert, G. (2017). Prehospital care for the adult and pediatric seizure patient: current evidence-based recommendations. *The Western Journal of Emergency Medicine, 18*(3), 419–436.

Slattery, D., & Pollack, C. (2010). Seizures as a cause of altered mental status. *Emergency Medicine Clinics of North America, 28*, 517–534.

Thom, M. (2007). The autopsy in sudden unexpected adult death: epilepsy. *Current Diagnostic Pathology, 13*.

Tohira, H., Fatovich, D., Williams, T., Bremner, A., Arendts, G., Rogers, I., Celenza, A., Mountain, D., Cameron, P., Sprivulis, P., Ahern, T., & Finn, J. (2016). Paramedic checklists do not accurately identify post-ictal or hypoglycaemic patients suitable for discharge at the scene. *Prehospital and Disaster Medicine, 31*(3), 282–293.

Verrotti, A., Milioni, M., & Zaccara, G. (2015). Safety and efficacy of diazepam autoinjector for the management of epilepsy. *Expert Review of Neurotherapeutics, 15*(2), 127–133.

Walker, M. (2018). Pathophysiology of status epilepticus. *Neuroscience Letters, 667*, 84–91.

Zelano, J., & Ben-Mencahem, E. (2016). Treating epileptic emergencies—pharmacological advances. *Expert Opinion on Pharmacotherapy, 16*(16), 2227–2234.

CHAPTER 30

Pain

By Paul Jennings

OVERVIEW

- Pain is a common presenting symptom for emergency patients but it often remains undertreated. Approximately one-third of patients presenting to ambulance services complain of pain.
- The benefit of out-of-hospital analgesia goes well beyond the out-of-hospital phase of care.
- Early, effective pain management in both the out-of-hospital and the ED setting is critical in reducing the likelihood of chronic pain syndromes and pain-related anxiety and distress following the acute phase.
- Effective out-of-hospital analgesia facilitates the in-hospital diagnostic and therapeutic process and increases the likelihood of timely ED analgesia.

Introduction

Pain is defined as 'an unpleasant sensory and emotional experience associated with actual or potential tissue damage, or described in terms of such' (Merskey & Bogduk, 1994). It is well-established as a 'personal' and 'subjective' phenomenon, comprising many physical, psychological and experiential dimensions. For this reason, quantifying pain continues to be a challenge to both clinician and patient.

Acute pain is a common presentation to healthcare clinicians (Alonso-Serra et al., 2003; Hennes et al., 2005; McManus & Sallee, 2005; Jennings et al., 2011a; Friesgaard et al., 2018), is often associated with injury (Castillo et al., 2006) and is a significant contributor to disability many months, or years, following an injury. A study of a large Australian urban and rural ambulance service found that approximately one-third of patients presented complaining of pain. Their median age was 56 years and just under half were males (46%). The majority of patients had pain of a traumatic or medical aetiology (40% and 39%, respectively), while pain of a cardiac nature accounted for only 17% of presentations. Approximately half of patients presenting with pain received analgesia in the out-of-hospital setting, with opioid analgesics administered to 20% of patients reporting pain (Jennings et al., 2011a).

Patients presenting to ambulance services and the ED often do so with high-intensity pain. In one study 49% of patients complained of severe pain and 25% of these claimed the maximum possible pain intensity of 10 out of 10 (Todd et al., 2002). Another urban tertiary-care referral ED in North America found that 61% of presentations had a complaint of 'any pain' reported on their medical record: pain was documented as the patient's chief complaint in 85% of cases (Cordell et al., 2002).

A number of factors have been identified as predisposing people to clinically important pain reduction and these include age, pain aetiology and initial pain intensity (Jennings et al., 2011c). Age is associated with clinically important pain relief, with the 45–69-year age group less likely to achieve clinically important pain reduction than all other age groups. Pain aetiology is statistically associated with clinically important pain severity reduction, in that people presenting with pain of a traumatic origin are most likely to achieve effective pain reduction compared with people presenting with pain of a cardiac or medical aetiology. Initial pain severity is also a strong predictor of the likelihood of a patient achieving clinically important pain reduction: patients with moderate or severe pain are much more likely to achieve clinically important pain reduction than those who present with mild pain (Jennings et al., 2011c).

Pathophysiology

Pain is broadly classified into two categories: nociceptive pain and neuropathic pain. **Nociceptive pain** is caused by stimulation of the peripheral sensory nerve fibres responding to noxious stimuli (see Fig 30.1). **Neuropathic pain** is caused by damage or disease to the peripheral or central nervous system and results in abnormal processing of sensory signals. As an example the pain associated with a cut finger is initially nociceptive pain, while that associated with an inflamed nerve in shingles is neuropathic pain.

Highly specialised sensory fibres provide information about injurious or potentially injurious

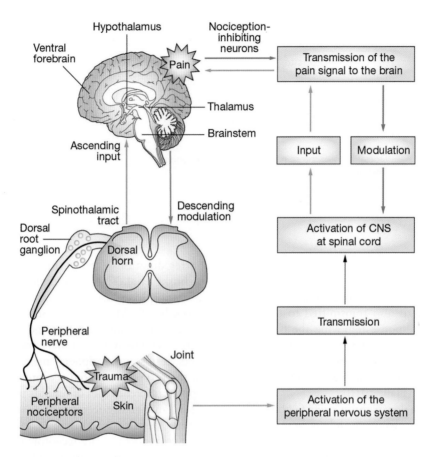

Figure 30.1
The nociceptive pain pathway.
Activation of peripheral pain receptors (nociceptors) by noxious stimuli generates signals that travel to the dorsal horn of the spinal cord via the dorsal root ganglion. From the dorsal horn, the signals are carried along the ascending pain pathway or the spinothalamic tract to the thalamus and the cortex. Pain can be controlled by pain-inhibiting and pain-facilitating neurons. Descending signals originating in supraspinal centres can modulate activity in the dorsal horn by controlling spinal pain transmission.
Source: Bingham et al. (2009).

stimuli, as well as environmental conditions such as warmth, cold or touch. **Nociceptors** are specialised sensory receptors that respond preferentially to noxious stimuli, providing information to the central nervous system regarding the location and intensity of noxious stimuli (Meyer et al., 2006). Injury results in a number of inflammatory mediators being released locally, including bradykinin, prostaglandins, leukotrienes, histamine and cytokines. Some of these agents directly activate nociceptors. Many of the chemical mediators released during inflammation can have a synergistic effect in potentiating nociceptor responses and therefore pain (Meyer et al., 2006). Endogenous opioids released locally, triggered by inflammatory mediators, appear to be part of an 'anti-nociceptive' system that reduces this pain. Opioid receptors have been identified on peripheral terminals of afferent fibres (Meyer et al., 2006). Different cortical regions may

be preferentially involved in the different aspects of the complex experience of pain. Somatosensory cortices are important for perception of sensory features. Limbic (emotional) regions are important for the emotional and motivational aspects of pain (Bushnell & Apkarian, 2006).

Pain has useful functions. A painful sensation will alert an individual to a hazard, causing them to react—removing their hand from a hotplate, for instance. This fast response to pain using the fast pain fibres (A fibres) produces a subconscious withdrawal reflex. This reflex is faster because the nerves involved in fast transmission are generally larger in diameter and have a thicker myelin sheath. The impulse travels to the spinal cord, which responds with an impulse sent to the motor neurons to remove the hand from the damaging hotplate, as well as an impulse sent to the muscles on the other side of the body to prepare for the shift in

Table 30.1: Receptor site, endogenous opioid and major effect of delta, kappa and mu receptors

Receptor type	Receptor site	Endogenous opioid	Major effect
δ (delta)	Limbic system	Encephalin	Analgesia
κ (kappa)	Hypothalamus	Dynorphin	Dysphoria Psychotomimetic effects Sedation Analgesia
μ (mu)	Dorsal horn of the spinal cord Thalamus	Beta-endorphin	Analgesia Respiratory depression Euphoria Nausea and vomiting Miosis

body weight. This transmission and motor response are done without the requirement for the impulse to travel to the brain, be processed and responded to. The impulse is also transmitted to the brain, but the motor response removing the hand from the stimulus will already have occurred. These fast pain pathways are generally stimulated by mechanical and thermal stimuli and are very localised in their pain perception (Hall, 2010).

There is also a slow pathway using C fibres. These fibres are small in diameter and are unmyelinated, producing a slow activation. They are stimulated by chemical, thermal and mechanical stimuli. Neurotransmitters involved in this pathway include substances that slowly build over time and linger, producing a delayed, less localised pain response. Because of the two types of pain transmission, the response to injury in this example is initially a sharp pain, provoking withdrawal, but then after a period of time with no further injury a pain remains. From a functional point of view the pain alerts the person to the danger and changes their behaviour.

It was once thought that due to the immaturity of the peripheral and central nervous systems in children and infants, they did not feel pain and therefore did not require analgesia. It is now widely accepted that infants can be exposed to considerable pain as the result of disease or injury, and that the adverse effects of this pain are both immediate and potentially long term, affecting future sensation and behaviour (Baccei & Fitzgerald, 2006).

Intravenous (IV) morphine has long been considered the gold standard for out-of-hospital care in Australia (Rickard et al., 2007) and other emergency medical systems internationally (Bruns et al., 1992). Intravenous fentanyl has recently gained favour as an analgesic agent in the out-of-hospital setting due to its rapid effect (even faster than morphine),

shorter duration of effect and equivalent efficacy (Galinski et al., 2005). Opioids, or 'drugs that have morphine-like actions, naturally occurring or synthetic' (MacIntyre & Schug, 2007), act as agonists on opioid receptors and are found in the central nervous system, urinary and gastrointestinal tracts, lungs and peripheral nerve endings. There are three types of opioid receptor: mu, delta and kappa. Different types of opioids produce different effects and analgesic efficacy as a result of their intrinsic activity (MacIntyre & Schug, 2007). The central effects of opiate receptors include analgesia and an alteration in both mood and the cognitive appreciation of pain. The peripheral effects allow opioids to imitate endogenous encephalins and endorphins, reducing the pain produced by the slow pain pathway. The analgesic effects of opioids are mediated predominantly by mu receptors, although delta and kappa receptors can also contribute to pain relief (see Table 30.1). Activation of opioid receptor sites and the subsequent effect on ion channel activities inhibit neuronal activity. Opioid receptor site activation, among other actions, opens potassium channels. This inhibits neurotransmitter release if the receptor is located on presynaptic terminals, and inhibits neuronal firing if the receptor is located postsynaptically on neural cell bodies (Dickenson & Kieffer, 2006). This therefore interrupts pain impulse transmission.

Association of acute pain and persistent pain

Early, effective pain management in both the out-of-hospital and the ED settings is likely to play a role in reducing the prospect of persistent pain and pain-related anxiety and distress following the acute phase (Buckenmaier et al., 2009; Thomas & Shewakramani, 2008; Turturro, 2002; Weisman et al., 1998). Common types of pain presenting in the acute setting are outlined in Box 30.1. Pain

BOX 30.1 Painful conditions frequently encountered in the out-of-hospital setting

Abdominal pain

- Provision of analgesia does not interfere with the diagnosis of acute abdominal pain (Schug et al., 2015).
- Acute abdominal pain may originate from visceral or somatic structures, may be referred or as a result of neuropathic pain states (Schug et al., 2015).
- Parenteral non-selective NSAIDs are as effective as parenteral opioids in the management of biliary colic (Schug et al., 2015).

Back pain (acute)

- Red flags that suggest a potentially serious condition include:
  › signs or symptoms of infection
  › history of trauma (including minor trauma in the elderly, patients with osteoporosis or those on corticosteroids)
  › history of malignancy or recent unexplained weight loss
  › neurological signs or cauda equina syndrome
  › age greater than 50 years (National Institute of Clinical Studies, 2011).

Burns

- Acute burn pain can be nociceptive and/or neuropathic in nature (Schug et al., 2015).
- Opioids are effective in burn pain and will most likely require titrated boluses (Schug et al., 2015).
- Opioid requirements will typically be higher for burns than for other emergency presentations (National Institute of Clinical Studies, 2011).
- Cool water is an effective analgesic if used for at least 20 minutes within 3 hours of the burn but hypothermia should be avoided (National Institute of Clinical Studies, 2011).

Cardiac pain

- Glyceryl trinitrate (GTN) is an effective and appropriate agent for the treatment of acute ischaemic chest pain (Schug et al., 2015).
- Morphine is an effective and appropriate analgesic for acute cardiac pain not responsive to GTN (Schug et al., 2015).

Fractures

- Immobilisation, ice and elevation of a suspected fracture are important in managing pain.
- Femoral nerve block and parenteral opioids are more effective than parenteral opioids alone for managing pain associated with a fractured neck of the femur (Schug et al., 2015).

Migraine/tension headache

- Acupuncture may be effective in the treatment of tension-type headache and migraine (Schug et al., 2015).
- Simple analgesics (i.e. aspirin, paracetamol, NSAIDs) either alone or in combination are effective in the treatment of episodic tension-type headache (Schug et al., 2015).
- Aspirin with metoclopramide is effective in migraine with mild symptoms and is the treatment of first choice (National Institute of Clinical Studies, 2011).
- Opioids are not recommended for the emergency treatment of migraine (British Association for the Study of Headache, 2010).
- IV metoclopramide administered with a litre of IV fluid is often effective in the treatment of migraine (Schug et al., 2015).
- Triptans are effective in the management of severe migraine (Schug et al., 2015).
- IV prochlorperazine, chlorpromazine or droperidol is effective in the treatment of migraine, especially in the ED (Schug et al., 2015)
- IV triptans or oxygen therapy are effective treatment for cluster headache (Schug et al., 2015).

Renal colic

- There is no difference in effectiveness between morphine and pethidine (an older synthetic opioid rapidly disappearing from practice) for renal colic (Schug et al., 2015).
- Non-selective NSAIDs and opioids provide effective analgesics for renal colic (National Institute of Clinical Studies, 2011).
- The onset of analgesia is faster with NSAIDs when administered intravenously, when compared with IM, oral or rectal administration (Schug et al., 2015).

lasting for more than 3 months (known as *persistent pain*) can be debilitating (Williamson et al., 2009) and it is becoming clear that unrelieved acute traumatic pain is a risk factor for the progression to persistent pain (Shipton & Tait, 2005). The prevalence of persistent pain following injury has been reported to be between 11% and 62% (Andrew et al., 2008; Moore & Leonardi-Bee, 2008; Rivara et al., 2008; Williamson et al., 2009). Persistent pain has a substantial impact on people's physical and mental health (Buckenmaier et al., 2009; Thomas & Shewakramani, 2008; Turturro, 2002; Weisman et al., 1998) and can delay functional recovery following traumatic injury (Castillo et al., 2006; Mkandawire et al., 2002). This phenomenon is also seen in surgery, where there is evidence that some early, focused anaesthetic/analgesic strategies reduce the incidence of persistent pain following surgery (Shipton & Tait, 2005).

Barriers to optimal acute pain management

Clinicians are often concerned with the legitimacy of a patient's complaint of pain, especially when the source of the pain is not visible, and pain often remains undertreated (Alonso-Serra et al., 2003; Luger et al., 2003; McLean et al., 2003; McManus & Sallee, 2005; Todd et al., 2002). The phenomenon of undertreating pain was so pronounced that it led to the term *oligoanalgesia*: 'oligos' from the Greek, meaning few or scanty; and 'analgesia' also from the Greek—'an', without, and 'algesis', sense of pain. There are many reasons for oligoanalgesia, most related to myths and biases held by healthcare providers brought about through education or culture (Hubert et al., 2009). Oligoanalgesia is a problem within the out-of-hospital and hospital settings (Rupp & Delaney, 2004).

The barriers to optimal acute pain management can be broken down into three main categories: (1) the caregiver's beliefs; (2) characteristics of pain management; and (3) systems barriers. The vast majority of these barriers to the provision of optimal analgesia in the out-of-hospital setting are myths and are not supported by evidence. Education aimed at dispelling the myths of pain management, pain assessment, use of guidelines and the importance of aggressive pain management regimens is critical to improving out-of-hospital provider practice (Hennes & Kim, 2006; Schug et al., 2015).

Caregiver's beliefs
- Analgesics may interfere with assessment of mental status in the patient with a head injury (Thomas & Shewakramani, 2008).
- Analgesics may interfere with general physical assessment (e.g. abdominal assessment) (Hubert et al., 2009; McManus & Sallee, 2005; Ricard-Hibon et al., 2008; Rupp & Delaney, 2004; Thomas & Shewakramani, 2008).
- Analgesics can cause haemodynamic or respiratory suppression (Thomas & Shewakramani, 2008) or result in unwanted side effects (Hennes & Kim, 2006; Hubert et al., 2009; Ricard-Hibon et al., 2008; Rupp & Delaney, 2004).
- Analgesics may preclude the ability to obtain informed consent for necessary procedures (Thomas & Shewakramani, 2008).
- Pain is inevitable in emergency situations (Hubert et al., 2009; Ricard-Hibon et al., 2008).
- Analgesia will be given immediately on arrival in ED (Hennes & Kim, 2006).
- The use of opioids in acute pain leads to addiction (McManus & Sallee, 2005; Rupp & Delaney, 2004; Turturro, 2002).
- Patients often overexaggerate pain (Hennes & Kim, 2006; McManus & Sallee, 2005; Rupp & Delaney, 2004).

Characteristics of pain management
- Insertion of intravenous cannula/intramuscular injection is painful in itself (Watkins, 2006).
- Children, females and those from lower socio-economic groups are less likely to receive adequate analgesia (Hennes, Kim & Pirrallo, 2005; Swor et al., 2005; Michael, Sporer & Youngblood, 2007).
- Patients are reluctant to report pain and to request analgesia (Duignan & Dunn, 2009; Thomas & Shewakramani, 2008).

Systems barriers
- Lack of educational emphasis placed on pain management for healthcare professionals (Hennes & Kim, 2006; Rupp & Delaney, 2004).
- Inadequate or non-existent clinical quality management programs (Rupp & Delaney, 2004).
- Some analgesics require intravenous access (Thomas & Shewakramani, 2008) and some crews are not trained in obtaining IV access.
- Evaluation of pain intensity (Hennes & Kim, 2006; Ricard-Hibon et al., 2008).
- A recent study identified that the clinical stability of patients with traumatic injury was associated with the standard of pain management provided en route to hospital and at trauma reception (Spilman et al., 2016). They reported that patients who were physiologically unstable were the least likely to receive a standardised pain assessment and to receive an opioid in the ED.

Tolerance, dependence and addiction

In considering analgesic agents and dosages, many clinicians are confused regarding the nature, identification and potential impact that tolerance, dependence and addiction can have on the management of acute pain. This can lead to inappropriate or suboptimal early management of pain and stigmatisation (Schug et al., 2015). *Tolerance* relates to a phenomenon whereby exposure to a drug results in a diminution of its effect or a larger dose is required in order to achieve an effect over time (Collett, 1998). Tolerance to a drug can occur as a result of pharmacokinetic or pharmacodynamic mechanisms, or it can be developed over time. Irrespective of the reason, tolerance, particularly relating to opioids, should be considered by the paramedic, especially in patients who have been receiving enteral or parenteral opioids on an ongoing basis, such as chronic cancer patients (Collett, 1998). Tolerance may be one explanation why some patients require larger doses of opioids than others with similar presentations.

Physical dependence is defined as the potential for withdrawal symptoms (abstinence syndrome) following abrupt discontinuation or reversal of the drug (Schug et al., 2015). The time it takes or the dose required to predispose a person to physical dependence is unknown (Collett, 1998). The prevention of unpleasant withdrawal symptoms is thought to be one motivation for people with physical dependence to seek drugs. Physical dependence should not influence clinical decision-making surrounding the management of pain.

Addiction is a type of physical dependence; it is a disease characterised by abnormal drug-seeking or maladaptive drug-taking behaviours, which may include cravings and compulsive drug taking despite the risks of physical, social and psychological harm (Schug et al., 2015). Identification of patients who are addicts or at risk of drug abuse can be difficult and effective treatment of the patient with an addiction disorder may be complex. Management of acute pain in this group should focus on the provision of effective analgesia, and this may require larger doses or administration of the drug for longer periods of time than for other patients. Pain management in patients with an addiction disorder can be challenging due to the patient's fear of being stigmatised, fear of the provision of inadequate analgesia based on their higher tolerance and history and past experiences and expectations (Schug et al., 2015).

CASE STUDY 1

Case 50614, 1715 hrs.

Dispatch details: A 25-year-old male cyclist has been struck by a car at low speed. The patient was riding home from his inner-city office when he was T-boned at an intersection.

Initial presentation: The paramedics find the patient lying on the ground supporting his right arm. His upper arm is obviously deformed and he is screaming in pain.

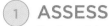

ASSESS

Patient history

The DOLOR or PQRST mnemonic can be used to elicit a thorough pain history from the patient (see Tables 30.2 and 30.3). Due to the subjective nature of pain, it can be very difficult for clinicians to quantify a patient's pain intensity and measure the qualitative characteristics of their pain experience. The pain severity perceived by the individual is dependent on a number of cognitive and experiential factors specific to the individual. For this reason,

Table 30.2: DOLOR pain assessment mnemonic

Description	'Can you describe the pain?'
Onset	'When did it start?' 'Did it come on suddenly or slowly?' 'What were you doing when it started?'
Location	'Can you point to the pain?'
Other signs and symptoms	'Apart from the pain, do you have any other problems you feel are connected with this?'
Relief	'Is there anything that makes the pain better or worse?'

Table 30.3: PQRST pain assessment mnemonic

Provocative, palliative factors	'What makes the pain better or worse?'
Quality of pain (i.e. burning, stabbing, heavy)	'What does the pain feel like?' 'Can you describe it to me?'
Region, radiation, referral	'Where does it hurt?' 'Does the pain move or travel?'
Severity (verbal numerical rating scale or adjective descriptive scale)	'Can you rate the pain according to this scale?' 'Could you sleep with the pain?' 'Is it worse than your previous worst experience with pain?'
Temporal factors (i.e. onset, duration)	'When did it start?' 'Is it constant and/or intermittent?' 'How long does it last?'

HISTORY

Ask!
Use an open approach along the lines of: 'I need to know if you have used or use morphine, heroin or other opioids regularly, so that I can increase your drug dose in order to get your pain under control'. Once the patient understands that you are interested in an accurate history so that you can increase the dose you plan to give them, they will be reassured and honest in their reporting.

assessment of pain should be based on the patient's perception of pain and not the clinician's.

When a patient is complaining of acute pain as a result of a traumatic injury (as is this case), it is quite easy for the clinician to link the complaint of pain with a physical injury. It is harder for the clinician to gain a sense of the intensity of the pain when it is related to a less obvious cause, such as ischaemic chest pain or generalised abdominal pain as a result of gastritis. To assist the clinician in assessing the patient's pain, it is important to gather some history of the patient's prior experience of pain relating to intensity and nature. This can provide clues as to the cause of the pain ('It's just like the pain I had when I had my heart attack back in January') or its relative intensity ('It's bad, really bad, even worse than when I had kidney stones last year').

Heart rate, blood pressure and respiratory rate can be affected by a number of factors beyond pain intensity, such as fever, anxiety and medications. Several studies have found poor correlation between the patient's reported pain intensity and vital signs including heart rate, blood pressure and respiratory rate (Bossart et al., 2007; Lord & Woollard, 2011; Marco et al., 2006). For this reason, vital signs cannot be used to validate pain intensity as reported by the patient (Lord & Woollard, 2011).

When gathering the patient history it is also important to establish any previous allergies, adverse experiences and exposure to potential analgesic agents. It is common for patients who have had unpleasant experiences or side effects to a drug—such as nausea, vomiting or disorientation—to describe these events as allergic reactions. In these situations the exact nature of the adverse event or side effect needs to be clarified and a distinction made between a side effect and a true drug allergy. This distinction is often important as it can limit the analgesic options available to the patient and risk suboptimal pain management in both the out-of-hospital and the ED settings.

Quantifying acute pain intensity

A reliable, objective pain measurement tool is particularly important as clinicians' perceptions have been shown to be inaccurate when used to quantify the intensity of pain being experienced by patients. Clinicians have a tendency to underestimate pain (Duignan & Dunn, 2008) and this underestimation becomes more pronounced with increasing clinical experience (Solomon, 2001). Several multidimensional measures exist and these aim to explore and measure the physical, psychological, social, cultural and spiritual components of pain. However, they are complex to administer, require specific training in their use and interpretation, are time-consuming and rely on the availability of assessment forms. For these reasons, their utility in the out-of-hospital setting is compromised.

The three most commonly used self-reported, unidimensional rating scales used for adults in the out-of-hospital setting are the verbal numerical rating scale (VNRS; Bijur et al., 2003; Cork et al., 2004; McLean et al., 2003), the visual analogue scale (VAS; Bijur et al., 2001; Ho et al., 1996; Lee, 2001; Price et al., 1994) and the adjective response scale (ARS; Maio et al., 2002). The two most commonly employed pain measurement tools for use in children are the faces pain scale and the Oucher scale.

The verbal numerical rating scale

The verbal numerical rating scale is commonly used in the out-of-hospital setting as it is valid and easily applied. The patient is asked to rate the intensity of their pain on an 11-point scale, where 0 is considered no pain and 10 is the worst possible pain. The benefits of the VNRS are that it is quick to administer and provides a quantitative rating of the patient's perceived pain intensity. It has been validated in patients aged 13 years and older (McLean et al., 2003; Gagliese et al., 2005). One potential barrier to its use is difficulty in translating instructions to patients if there is a language barrier (Bird, 2003).

The visual analogue scale

The visual analogue scale is commonly used for rapid assessment of pain severity and consists of a 100-millimetre horizontal or vertical line. The descriptors 'no pain' and 'worst pain ever' are placed at either end of the line (see Fig 30.2) and the patient is asked to place a mark on the line representative of their pain severity. The clinician then measures from the 'no pain' mark to the intersection of the mark drawn by the patient to find the pain intensity. This provides a pain rating score out of 10. The validity and reliability of this pain measure have been consistently demonstrated in a variety of settings (Bijur et al., 2001; Ho et al., 1996; Lee, 2001; Price et al., 1994).

Given the visual nature of this measure, reliability may be reduced when used by patients who are visually impaired. Likewise, cognitive impairment, lack of understanding of the task and an inability to follow instructions can impact on the accuracy of the measure (Bird, 2003). The VAS has been found to be less accurate in the elderly (Jensen et al., 1986) and young children (Shields et al., 2003). The measure relies on the immediate availability of the pain scale for patients to place their mark: Lord and Parsell (2003) reported that 26% of paramedics considered the VAS to be too cumbersome and said it was often lost or difficult to locate when required.

The VNRS has been found to be comparable in accuracy to the VAS (Bijur et al., 2003; Cork et al., 2004). Interestingly, while the VNRS has been found

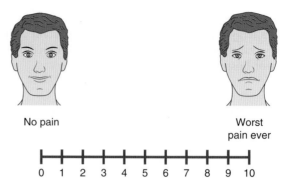

No pain

Worst
pain ever

0 1 2 3 4 5 6 7 8 9 10

Figure 30.2
Visual analogue scale.
Instruct the patient to point to the position on the line between the faces to indicate how much pain they are currently feeling. The far left end indicates 'no pain' and the far right end indicates 'worst pain ever'.

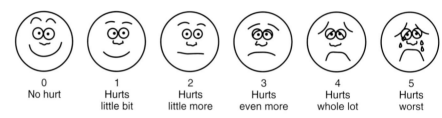

| 0 | 1 | 2 | 3 | 4 | 5 |
| No hurt | Hurts little bit | Hurts little more | Hurts even more | Hurts whole lot | Hurts worst |

Figure 30.3
The faces pain scale.
Explain to the child that each face is for a person who feels happy because they have no pain (no hurt) or sad because they have some or a lot of pain. Face 0 is very happy because they don't hurt at all. Face 1 hurts just a little bit. Face 2 hurts a little more. Face 3 hurts even more. Face 4 hurts a whole lot. Face 5 hurts as much as you can imagine, although you don't have to be crying to feel this bad. Ask the child to choose the face that best describes how they are feeling. The rating scale is recommended for children aged 3 years and older.
Source: Hockenberry & Wilson (2009).

to perform as well as the VAS in assessing changes to pain, patients consistently score their pain higher on the VNRS (Holdgate et al., 2003). One of the clear benefits of the VNRS is that it does not require any associated equipment, which is particularly beneficial in the out-of-hospital setting.

The adjective response scale

The adjective response scale consists of between three and five ranked verbal pain descriptors: 'none', 'slight', 'moderate', 'severe' and 'agonising'. The scale has been evaluated for its validity, reliability and ease of use, and strong correlations have been found between the ARS and the VAS. One of the limitations of the ARS is the relative lack of discrimination with a five-point scale. Also, like the VNRS, there are potential barriers around language and cross-cultural issues (Maio et al., 2002).

The faces pain scale

There are several versions of the faces pain scale that are predominantly used for assessing pain in children. Alternative measures are required as children have limited cognitive abilities and are unable to use most of the adult scales (McManus & Sallee, 2005). These scales use pictures of faces that illustrate steadily increasing intensities of pain or discomfort (see Fig 30.3).

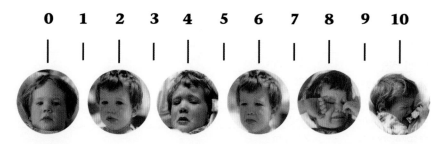

Figure 30.4
The Oucher scale.
'This picture shows no hurt [point to first picture]; this picture shows just a little bit of hurt [point to the second picture]; this picture shows a little more hurt [point to the third picture]; this picture shows even more hurt (point to the fourth picture]; this picture shows a lot of hurt [point to the fifth picture); and this picture shows the biggest hurt you could ever have [point to the last picture]. Can you point to the picture that shows how much hurt you are having right now?' The scale is available in various racial backgrounds.
Source: © The Caucasian version of the OUCHER was developed and copyrighted by Judith E. Beyer, PhD, RN, USA, 1983.

The Oucher scale

The Oucher scale (see Fig 30.4) is another pain scale used to measure pain in children and it combines pictures much like the faces pain scale with a vertical VAS. It has been previously validated in children 3–12 years of age (Maio et al., 2002). Although not yet validated in the emergency or out-of-hospital setting, the Oucher scale appears promising in the out-of-hospital environment warranting further research (Gausche-Hill et al., 2014).

Airway

This patient is screaming in pain, indicating there is no problem with his airway.

Breathing

The patient's breathing appears to be sufficient, given he has the tidal volume to scream. However, as he has just been hit by a car, his breathing should be monitored continuously. Trauma to the thoracic wall or damage to internal structures is a possibility and could potentially hinder the patient's breathing should it become worse.

Cardiovascular

For this patient, internal and external haemorrhages are a possibility. Also, while we have established that vital signs are not a particularly reliable indicator of pain severity, trends in the patient's condition can be tracked through cardiovascular vital signs.

Neurological

There are three aspects that need to be considered when undertaking a neurological assessment. First, were there any precipitating neurological events that led to the event? For example, in this case did the patient become dizzy and swerve in front of the car? Second, are there any neurological deficits as a result of the accident indicating a head injury? And thirdly, are there any sensory deficits distal to the site of injury—in this case, on the patient's arm? This patient had no precipitating neurological event before the accident and he has no neurological deficits following the accident, including those associated with injury to his arm.

> **SITUATIONAL AWARENESS**
>
> Individuals with drug tolerance and addiction may be influenced by prior contact with health service personnel who withheld opioids from them. Our sole focus as health professionals is improvement of our patients' pain; do not be judgmental about a patient's past use of opioids, whether prescribed or illegally obtained.

Initial assessment summary

Problem	Injury to upper right arm
Conscious state	GCS = 15; full recall of the event
Position	Supine, holding right arm
Heart rate	105 bpm
Blood pressure	120/80 mmHg
Skin appearance	Pink, warm, dry
Speech pattern	Sentences
Respiratory rate	24 bpm
Respiratory rhythm	Even cycles
Chest auscultation	Clear bilaterally
Pulse oximetry SpO$_2$	98%
Temperature	37.4°C
Capillary refill (seconds)	1 second
Pain score	10/10
Motor/sensory function	Normal sensory; patient can move fingers on right arm, but is reluctant to try anything else due to pain
Secondary survey	Deformity and swelling to right upper arm
History	The patient was T-boned by a vehicle at low speed. He fell between his bicycle and the front of the car (i.e. he was not thrown onto the bonnet of the car). He was wearing a helmet.

D: There is no danger to the ambulance crew or the patient.
A: The patient is conscious with no airway obstruction.
B: Respiratory rate is marginally elevated but this could be attributed to the pain.
C: Heart rate is elevated, but again this could be attributed to the pain. Blood pressure is within normal limits.

The patient is presenting with 10/10 pain and deformity and swelling to his upper right arm after being struck by a car while riding his bike. The secondary survey does not indicate any other injuries or involvement of other body systems.

2 CONFIRM

The essential part of the clinical reasoning process is to seek to confirm your initial hypothesis by finding clinical signs that should occur with your provisional diagnosis. You should also seek to challenge your diagnosis by exploring findings that do *not* fit your hypothesis: don't just ignore them because they don't fit.

What else could it be?
Referred cardiac chest pain
This scenario is unlikely in a patient of this age. However, when assessing patients involved in any sort of accident, it is important to determine any precipitating factors that may have led to the accident. For example, it is not uncommon for single-vehicle accidents to be caused by the driver losing consciousness due to experiencing a cardiac event. In this case, the patient is young and presumably fit and has a clear deformity to his right upper arm, and the pain is well localised to the site of the deformity.

Drug-seeking behaviour
The differential would be that the patient does not have pain, raising the possibility of drug-seeking behaviour or some other reason to report pain when in fact it does not exist. In this situation, there is a very obvious injury associated with the pain.

> DIFFERENTIAL DIAGNOSIS
>
> **Pain related to a fractured arm**
> Or
> - Referred cardiac chest pain
> - Drug-seeking behaviour

③ TREAT

Emergency management

In planning a pain management regimen, you should consider the appropriateness of both pharmacological and non-pharmacological approaches. The likely effectiveness of many non-pharmacological interventions is often underestimated or overlooked. As a minimum, techniques such as immobilisation and splinting of injured body parts and reassurance and temperature control to prevent shivering should be employed as first-line management.

Out-of-hospital analgesic options

Doses of analgesics should be based on locally approved clinical practice guidelines. Adjustments in dosing should be considered for the elderly, for those with diminished drug clearance such as renal or liver dysfunction (National Institute of Clinical Studies, 2011) and for those who may well have tolerance and thus potentially require much larger doses. Because a drug's clinical effectiveness is proportional to the logarithm of the drug concentration, you should be prepared to increase the dose if an earlier dose does not have an effect. In practice this means that if 2.5 mg of morphine has no effect, you need to either give subsequent doses rapidly or be prepared to give a larger dose. Some clinical guidelines are consistent with this pharmacodynamic principle, while others just rely on repeating the same dose.

Side effects and adverse events should be considered prior to administration and observed for following administration. A history of minor side effects may need to be weighed against the potential benefits of effective analgesia, and the incidence of adverse effects of opioids is commonly dose related (Schug et al., 2015). Ketamine as an analgesic has been found to be both effective and safe to use in the out-of-hospital setting (Jennings et al., 2011b), is superior to morphine alone for traumatic injury (Jennings et al., 2012) and is seeing a re-emergence of favour in the out-of-hospital, retrieval and emergency settings.

There is a need to have a range of analgesic agents that use various modes of administration. Table 30.4 summarises analgesic agents commonly available

Table 30.4: Analgesic agents commonly used in paramedic practice

Agent	Route of administration
Opioids	
Morphine sulphate	IV or IM
Fentanyl citrate	IV or IM or IN
Nalbuphine	IV or IM
Anaesthesia/analgesia	
Methoxyflurane	Inhalation
Nitrous oxide	Inhalation
Non-steroidal anti-inflammatory drugs (NSAIDs)	
Ketorolac	IV or IM
Parecoxib	IV
Other	
Ketamine	IV, IM or IN
Tramadol	IV
Paracetamol	IV

The incidence of nausea and vomiting following the administration of intravenous morphine for acute pain is low despite common misconceptions (Bradshaw & Sen, 2006). Furthermore, there is little evidence that prophylactic metoclopramide following administration of intravenous morphine for acute pain is beneficial—and, in fact, it may cause harm (Simpson et al., 2001).

in the out-of-hospital environment and their routes of administration. The oral route is often inappropriate to use due to poor absorption and gastric stasis in the critically ill (Borland et al., 2002) and the IV route is not always ideal or achievable. The IM route is not advised in patients with reduced perfusion and rarely has a role in acute emergencies due to variations in absorption in shock states and the difficulty of accurately titrating a good analgesic effect.

Inhalational agents have a rapid onset of action and are rapidly cleared via the lungs as soon as they are no longer applied. Nitrous oxide is still found in some ambulances around the world; however, studies have revealed that concentrations within this small confined space rise to many times the safety exposure limit unless a full scavenger system is operating. Methoxyflurane does not have this problem because it has a distinctive odour and so atmospheric concentrations are easy to detect. However, this odour can cause poor compliance among patients, so appropriate coaching is necessary for patients using methoxyflurane. The intranasal route is an important option for several out-of-hospital analgesic agents (Carr et al., 2004; Christensen et al., 2007; Rickard et al., 2007) and is particularly useful in managing paediatric pain (Borland et al., 2007) and in ambulance services where personnel are restricted in gaining IV access.

Non-pharmacological pain management options
While pharmacological analgesics and anaesthesia are considered the gold standard of pain management, non-pharmacological interventions are effective and should be considered as an adjunct to pharmacological agents to enhance pain management. Non-pharmacological interventions are divided into three broad categories (McManus & Sallee, 2005):
- cognitive—music, distraction, hypnosis, guided imagery
- behavioural—relaxation techniques, biofeedback exercises, breathing control
- physical—heat and cold (cryoanalgesia) application, massage or touch, position and comfort, temperature regulation, transcutaneous electrical nerve stimulation (TENS), acupuncture, chiropractic, immobilisation.

Unfortunately, many of these options are not available or feasible within the out-of-hospital environment. However, techniques such as talking and distraction, and parental presence for children, are easily implemented in the out-of-hospital setting and have been shown to be effective in reducing pain intensity (Hennes & Kim, 2006). They should be implemented where appropriate whether or not the patient is receiving pharmacological analgesics (Thomas & Shewakramani, 2008).

This patient will benefit from non-pharmacological measures of reassurance and splinting. An inhalational anaesthetic (methoxyflurane) may be very useful when preparing and applying the splint. Gaining IV access will allow the paramedics to administer opioids in small repeated doses, increasing as necessary until analgesia is achieved. If the paramedics plan to use morphine, it is important to remember that the maximum clinical effect of morphine is felt some 15 minutes after it is administered IV. Therefore, they should give the patient opioids until he tells them that his pain is significantly reduced but stop short of a target of zero pain because the effect will continue to increase for 15 minutes.

4 EVALUATE

Evaluating the effect of any clinical management intervention can provide clues to the accuracy of the initial diagnosis. Some conditions respond rapidly to treatment so patients should be expected to improve if the diagnosis and treatment were appropriate. A failure to improve in this situation should trigger the clinician to reconsider the diagnosis.

Regular reassessment of pain leads to improved acute pain management (Schug et al., 2015) and is important for several reasons. First, it provides the clinician with a sense of the *appropriateness* of the analgesic choice based on the response of the individual to the chosen treatment regimen. One opioid is not superior to other opioids; however, some opioids have better effects in some patients than others (Schug et al., 2015). Second, it allows the clinician to observe the trend of pain intensity improvement or otherwise much like a clinician observes trends in blood pressure, conscious state and heart rate. Pain intensity should be reassessed and documented regularly and form part of the routine vital signs assessment.

Ongoing management

Following the management of immediate life threats and the commencement of a pain management regimen, other injuries should be managed and other therapies initiated. It is important to remember that many interventions can increase the intensity of pain experienced by the patient. Pain associated with repositioning injured limbs, lifting and moving the patient and transporting them over rough terrain should be anticipated and taken into consideration when planning appropriate analgesia options and doses. Conversely, once a limb has been splinted and the pain sensation reduced, the opiate effect may be exaggerated and the patient may show signs of respiratory depression and sedation.

CASE STUDY 2

Case 11354, 0820 hrs.

Dispatch details: A 26-year-old female with a severe headache, not relieved by paracetamol.

Initial presentation: The paramedics are directed to the patient by her partner. She is lying in bed with her eyes closed.

1 ASSESS

0831 hrs Primary survey: The patient is conscious and talking.

0831 hrs Chief complaint: 'I've had a headache all night. Paracetamol has done nothing, and I think it's getting worse.'

0832 hrs Vital signs survey: Perfusion status: HR 90, sinus rhythm, BP 130/75 mmHg, skin warm and pink.
Respiratory status: RR 20 bpm, good air entry, L = R, normal work of breathing, speaking in full sentences, no complaint of dyspnoea.
Conscious state: GCS = 14 (E 3, V 5, M 6).

0834 hrs Pertinent hx: The patient is normally well and only takes the oral contraceptive pill. She says that she only occasionally gets headaches, generally thought to be due to 'stress', and they usually resolve within a few hours with paracetamol. She is nauseated but doesn't feel she is about to vomit. She rates her pain as 5/10.

The patient is presenting with a story of headache that is atypical for her and is not responding to simple analgesics. Although this could be a migraine it is not the classic presentation and is not following a well-established pattern and therefore needs formal evaluation and investigation in hospital. In the meantime, the paramedics should provide pain relief while they transport the patient.

(2) CONFIRM

In many cases paramedics are presented with a collection of signs and symptoms that do not appear to describe a particular condition. A critical step in determining a treatment plan in this situation is to consider what other conditions could explain the patient's presentation.

In this particular case, the fact that the patient has a headache is not in dispute. But the potential causes need to be considered. The issue here is how confident are the paramedics that this episode of pain is a benign headache?

What else could it be?
Subarachnoid haemorrhage
About 1–4% of patients who present to ED have subarachnoid haemorrhage (SAH). The incidence increases with age and is most common in the 40–60-year age group. Head trauma is the most common cause of SAH, while cerebral aneurysm is the most common non-traumatic cause. Headache is common in approximately 95% of SAH presentations and is typically sudden (within a few seconds in 75% of cases) and severe, often being the 'worst ever' headache. Up to half of patients with SAH describe a mild headache in the hours or days leading up to the major bleed. Nausea and vomiting are common in 75% of cases and brief or permanent loss of consciousness is common.

Intracerebral haemorrhage
Most commonly caused by chronic hypertension, intracerebral haemorrhage (ICH) typically presents clinically as a sudden onset of neurological deficit with associated headache and collapse. Patients often have a transient loss of consciousness, are hypertensive and vomit. About 20% of all strokes are attributed to ICH.

Ischaemic stroke
Ischaemic stroke is most commonly the result of thromboembolism arising from the cerebral vasculature, the heart or the aorta. Ischaemic stroke accounts for approximately 80% of all strokes. Signs and symptoms correspond to the area of the brain affected and imaging is performed to accurately identify whether the anterior or posterior circulation is affected and to definitively rule out haemorrhagic stroke.

Systemic viral infection
A number of systemic viral infections can cause headache. These are usually associated with other symptoms such as rhinitis, sinus congestion, cough, body aches and skin rash.

Rhinosinusitis
About half of the patients who present to ear, nose and throat specialists complain of severe headache. Headache is often present with rhinosinusitis, but may be aggravated with exertion, postural changes and coughing. Headaches associated with chronic sinusitis are usually mild and diffuse, becoming worse during the day.

DIFFERENTIAL DIAGNOSIS

Benign causes
Or
- Subarachnoid haemorrhage
- Intracerebral haemorrhage
- Ischaemic stroke
- Systemic viral infection
- Rhinosinusitis

PRACTICE TIP

Consider the following complaints when assessing a headache:
- subacute and/or progressive headache over months
- new or different headache
- 'worst headache ever'
- any headache of maximum severity at onset
- onset after the age of 50 years old
- symptoms of systemic illness
- seizures
- any neurological signs.

③ TREAT

For a simple primary (undiagnosed) headache, NSAIDs, paracetamol, prochlorperazine and opioids are all recommended. If the pain is severe, there is no contraindication to small doses of IV opioids. Some services restrict opioids for headaches due to the fear of generating an altered conscious state in the patient that may make hospital assessment difficult. Provided the medications are titrated carefully, this should not occur.

0836 hrs: The paramedics offer reassurance and encourage the patient to take her own oral medications if she has them.

0837 hrs: The paramedics administer IV fluids and metoclopramide.

④ EVALUATE

Evaluating the effect of any clinical management intervention can provide clues to the accuracy of the initial diagnosis. Some conditions respond rapidly to treatment so patients should be expected to improve if the diagnosis and treatment were appropriate. A failure to improve in this situation should trigger the clinician to reconsider the diagnosis.

This patient's vital signs have not changed but the nausea has subsided slightly. The crew administer 250 micrograms of fentanyl to reduce her pain and after 5 minutes she appears more comfortable. Small, titrated doses of opioids are suitable for undiagnosed headaches but large doses should be avoided. Any deterioration in the patient's neurological status would suggest some form of intracranial haemorrhage and the paramedics will need to notify the hospital of the change in her condition.

ⓒ CASE STUDY 3

Case 12067, 1020 hrs.

Dispatch details: A 58-year-old male with abdominal pain.

Initial presentation: The paramedics find the patient lying across the couch in his lounge room.

---

① ASSESS

1041 hrs Chief complaint: 'I've got a pain in my stomach.'

1043 hrs Vital signs survey: Perfusion status: HR 80, sinus rhythm, BP 160/90 mmHg, skin warm and pink.
Respiratory status: RR 20 bpm, good air entry, L = R, normal work of breathing, speaking in full sentences, no complaint of dyspnoea.
Conscious state: GCS = 15 (E 4, V 5, M 6).

1047 hrs Pertinent hx: The patient is moderately overweight and has a history of hypertension and hypercholesterolaemia. His current medications include an antihypertensive (ACE inhibitor) and lipid-lowering agent (statin). He states that he has not previously suffered from abdominal pain. He vomited three times this morning and is still nauseated. The pain is on his right side just under his ribs: it is intermittent and came on quickly about an hour ago. He rates the pain as 8/10.

CONFIRM

②

In many cases paramedics are presented with a collection of signs and symptoms that do not appear to describe a particular condition. A critical step in determining a treatment plan in this situation is to consider what other conditions could explain the patient's presentation.

This patient has diffuse abdominal pain associated with vomiting. The colicky history could be consistent with gallstones and cholecystitis but at this stage it is impossible to discern without further investigations. The key issue is that he needs pain relief before and during transportation.

What else could it be?

Peptic ulcer

Gastric or duodenal ulcer could present with pain. Usually the history is a little longer and often there is altered blood ('coffee grounds') in the vomit, which there is no history of in this case.

Abdominal aortic aneurysm

An aneurysm can present with diffuse abdominal pain, although classically one would expect more back pain and potentially groin pain. At this stage it remains a possibility, although unlikely. The absence of haemodynamic compromise is reassuring.

Mesenteric infarction

Mesenteric ischaemia or infarction can present with pain and vomiting but usually causes a metabolic acidosis that should be revealed because it causes a raised respiratory rate in an attempt to compensate. However, this may be difficult to differentiate in a patient with a raised sympathetic drive in response to pain. This raised sympathetic drive could also result in an increased respiratory rate. This is a possibility in this patient.

Acute myocardial infarction

Myocardial infarction can present with abdominal pain, particularly epigastric pain. Inferior myocardial infarction is more likely to present with nausea. This is certainly a diagnosis worth considering for this patient and he should be assessed using a 12-lead ECG.

Acute/chronic pancreatitis

Pancreatitis could present like this or it could present with the patient looking considerably sicker with signs of shock. Once again it is a diagnosis that will be considered and excluded with investigations in hospital.

Strangulated hernia

There is no history of a hernia but if there was and it had obstructed then a presentation with vomiting and pain is consistent.

Appendicitis

Appendicitis presents initially with nonspecific, non-localised pain. It can often occur with vomiting and as time passes the pain will localise to the right iliac fossa as the peritoneum becomes involved. Once again, although not the most likely diagnosis, it is possible in this case.

Inflammatory bowel syndrome

An exacerbation of an inflammatory bowel syndrome can present with pain, nausea and vomiting. The patient did not give a history that is consistent with this, but it is by no means excluded.

DIFFERENTIAL DIAGNOSIS

Gastroenteritis

Or

- Peptic ulcer
- Abdominal aortic aneurysm
- Mesenteric infarction
- Acute myocardial infarction
- Acute/chronic pancreatitis
- Strangulated hernia
- Appendicitis
- Inflammatory bowel syndrome

All of these possible explanations for this patient's abdominal pain could turn out to be correct; the issue at the moment is to arrange adequate analgesia. Confidently assessing the patient presenting with abdominal pain without the luxury of investigations or time to repeatedly observe the patient over a series of hours is extremely difficult and even the most experienced clinicians are often unable to make a confident diagnosis. The key is not to exclude any of the more serious diagnoses until proven otherwise.

3 TREAT

The patient requires adequate analgesia before being transported to hospital, bearing in mind that movement will exacerbate his pain. This exacerbation is particularly relevant to pain associated with conditions such as peritoneal inflammation. Inhalational anaesthetics (methoxyflurane) or intranasal opioids (such as fentanyl) are a good first step while also providing the patient with reassurance and undertaking further assessment. Once IV access has been established, IV opioids in repeated doses titrating the dose size to the effect will provide the best pain relief.

1050 hrs: The paramedics administer 250 micrograms of IN fentanyl to reduce the patient's pain and after 5 minutes he rates his pain as 5/10.

4 EVALUATE

Evaluating the effect of any clinical management intervention can provide clues to the accuracy of the initial diagnosis. Some conditions respond rapidly to treatment so patients should be expected to improve if the diagnosis and treatment were appropriate. A failure to improve in this situation should trigger the clinician to reconsider the diagnosis.

This patient's vital signs have not changed so the paramedics administer another 250 micrograms of IN fentanyl. With a quick onset and peak time, titrating fentanyl every 5 minutes should provide effective pain relief. Any signs of respiratory depression, poor perfusion or deterioration in the patient's conscious state indicate that the maximum safe dose has probably been exceeded.

Future research

Future research should focus on age- and case-specific interventions and aim to identify individual interventions, or combinations of interventions, which favourably impact on both pain intensity and short- and long-term quality of life. The role and utility of nerve blocks administered by paramedics in the out-of-hospital setting is worthy of investigation also. It is important that out-of-hospital studies of all analgesic interventions, both pharmacological and non-pharmacological, should utilise a rigorous experimental randomised design, include a control group and, where possible, be blinded to the patient and the paramedics.

The emerging link between acute and persistent pain also requires further investigation, and given that emergency medical services are responsible for the earliest phase of care, they are integral to studies focused on the link between acute pain management and the likelihood of future persistent pain. Providers of early trauma care are well placed to engage in preventive medicine and to contribute to significant reductions in the burden associated with traumatic pain.

Summary

Pain is a frequently encountered problem in the out-of-hospital setting. It affects some people and conditions more than others, but can be substantially improved with appropriate pharmacological and non-pharmacological agents. Factors associated with the likelihood of clinically important pain reduction include the patient's age, time criticality of the patient, pain aetiology, initial pain severity and the analgesic agent or combination administered to the patient. Knowledge of these characteristics associated with clinically important pain reduction is useful to clinicians, researchers, educators and policy makers and informs future practice.

References

Alonso-Serra, H. M., & Wesley, K., National Association of EMS Physicians. (2003). Prehospital pain management. *Prehospital Emergency Care, 7*(4), 482–488.

Andrew, N. E., Gabbe, B. J., Wolfe, R., Williamson, O. D., Richardson, M. D., Edwards, E. R., & Cameron, P. A. (2008). Twelve-month outcomes of serious orthopaedic sport and active recreation-related injuries admitted to level 1 trauma centers in Melbourne, Australia. *Clinical Journal of Sport Medicine, 18*(5), 387–393.

Baccei, M., & Fitzgerald, M. (2006). Development of pain pathways and mechanisms. In S. McMahon & M. Koltzenburg (Eds.), *Wall and Melzack's textbook of pain* (5th ed.). Philadelphia: Elsevier.

Bijur, P. E., Latimer, C. T., & Gallagher, E. J. (2003). Validation of a verbally administered numerical rating scale of acute pain for use in the emergency department. *Pain, 10*(4), 390–392.

Bijur, P. E., Silver, W., & Gallagher, J. (2001). Reliability of the visual analogue scale for measurement of acute pain. *Academic Emergency Medicine: Official Journal of the Society for Academic Emergency Medicine, 8*(12), 1153–1157.

Bingham, B., Ajit, S. K., Blake, D. R., & Samad, T. A. (2009). The molecular basis of pain and its clinical implications in rheumatology. *Nature Clinical Practice. Rheumatology, 5*, 28–37.

Bird, J. (2003). Selection of pain measurement tools. *Nursing Standard, 18*(13), 33–39.

Borland, M., Jacobs, I., King, B., & O'Brien, D. (2007). A randomized controlled trial comparing intranasal fentanyl to intravenous morphine for managing acute pain in children in the emergency department. *Annals of Emergency Medicine, 49*(3), 335–340.

Borland, M. L., Jacobs, I., & Rogers, I. R. (2002). Options in prehospital analgesia. *Emergency Medicine, 14*(1), 77–84.

Bossart, P., Fosnocht, D., & Swanson, E. (2007). Changes in heart rate do not correlate with changes in pain intensity in emergency department patients. *The Journal of Emergency Medicine, 32*(1), 19–22.

Bradshaw, M., & Sen, A. (2006). Use of a prophylactic antiemetic with morphine in acute pain: randomised controlled trial. *Emergency Medicine Journal, 23*(3), 210–213.

British Association for the Study of Headache. (2010). *Guidelines for all healthcare professionals in the diagnosis and management of migraine, tension-type headache, cluster headache and medication-overuse headache.* Retrieved from www.bash.org.uk. (Accessed 10 October 2012.)

Bruns, B. M., Dieckmann, R., Shagoury, C., Dingerson, A., & Swartzell, C. (1992). Safety of pre-hospital therapy with morphine sulphate. *The American Journal of Emergency Medicine, 10*(1), 53–57.

Buckenmaier, C. C., III, Rupprecht, C., McKnight, G., McMillan, B., White, R. L., Gallagher, R. M., & Polomano, R. (2009). Pain following battlefield injury and evacuation: a survey of 110 casualties from the wars in Iraq and Afghanistan. *Pain Medicine, 10*(8), 1487–1496.

Bushnell, M., & Apkarian, A. V. (2006). Representation of pain in the brain. In S. McMahon & M. Koltzenburg (Eds.), *Wall and Melzack's textbook of pain* (5th ed.). Philadelphia: Elsevier.

Carr, D. B., Goudas, L. C., Denman, W. T., Brookoff, D., Staats, P. S., Brennen, L., Green, G., Albin, R., Hamilton, D., Rogers, M. C., Firestone, L., Lavin, P. T., & Mermelstein, F. (2004). Safety and efficacy of intranasal ketamine for the treatment of breakthrough pain in patients with chronic pain: a randomized, double-blind, placebo-controlled, crossover study. *Pain, 108*, 17–27.

Castillo, R. C., MacKenzie, E. J., Wegener, S. T., Group, L. S., Castillo, R. C., & Bosse, M. J. (2006). Prevalence of chronic pain seven years following limb-threatening lower extremity trauma. *Pain, 124*(3), 321–329.

Christensen, K., Rogers, E., Green, G. A., Hamilton, D. A., Mermelstein, F., Liao, E., Wright, C., & Carr, D. B. (2007). Safety and efficacy of intranasal ketamine for acute postoperative pain. *Acute Pain, 9*, 183–192.

Collett, B. J. (1998). Opioid tolerance: the clinical perspective. *British Journal of Anaesthesia, 81*, 58–68.

Cordell, W. H., Keene, K. K., Giles, B. K., Jones, J. B., Jones, J. H., & Brizendine, E. J. (2002). The high prevalence of pain in emergency medical care. *The American Journal of Emergency Medicine, 20*, 165–169.

Cork, R. C., Isaac, I., Elsharydah, A., Saleemi, S., Zavisca, F., & Alexander, L. (2004). A comparison of the verbal rating scale and the visual analogue scale for pain assessment. *The Internet Journal of Anesthesiology, 8*(1).

Dickenson, A. H., & Kieffer, B. (2006). Opiates: basic mechanisms. In S. McMahon & M. Koltzenburg (Eds.), *Wall and Melzack's textbook of pain* (5th ed.). Philadelphia: Elsevier.

Duignan, M., & Dunn, V. (2008). Congruence of pain assessment between nurses and emergency department patients: a replication. *International Emergency Nursing, 16*, 23–28.

Duignan, M., & Dunn, V. (2009). Perceived barriers to pain management. *Emergency Nurse, 16*(9), 31.

Friesgaard, K. D., Riddervold, I. S., Kirkegaard, H., Christensen, E. F., & Nikolajsen, L. (2018). Acute pain in the prehospital setting: a register-based study of 41,241 patients. *Scandinavian Journal of Trauma, Resuscitation and Emergency Medicine, 26*(1), 53.

Gagliese, L., Weizblit, N., Ellis, W., & Chan, V. W. S. (2005). The measurement of postoperative pain: a comparison of intensity scales in younger and older surgical patients. *Pain, 117*, 412–420.

Galinski, M., Dolveck, F., Borron, S. W., Tual, L., Van Laer, V., Lardeur, J.-Y., Lapostolle, F., & Adnet, F. (2005).

A randomized, double-blind study comparing morphine with fentanyl in prehospital analgesia. *The American Journal of Emergency Medicine, 23*(2), 114–119.

Gausche-Hill, M., Brown, K. B., Oliver, Z. J., Sasson, C., Dayan, P. S., Eschmann, N. M., Weik, T. S., Lawner, B. J., Sahni, R., Falck-Ytter, Y., Wright, J. L., Todd, K., & Lang, E. S. (2014). An evidence-based guideline for prehospital analgesia in trauma. *Prehospital Emergency Care, 18*(Sup 1), 25–34.

Hall, J. E. (2010). *Guyton and Hall textbook of medical physiology* (12th ed.). Philadelphia: Elsevier.

Hennes, H., & Kim, M. (2006). Prehospital pain management: current status and future direction. *Clinical Pediatric Emergency Medicine, 7*, 25–30.

Hennes, H., Kim, M. K., & Pirrallo, R. G. (2005). Prehospital pain management: a comparison of providers' perceptions and practices. *Prehospital Emergency Care, 9*(1), 32–39.

Ho, K., Spence, J., & Murphy, M. F. (1996). Review of pain-measurement tools. *Annals of Emergency Medicine, 27*(4), 427–432.

Hockenberry, M. J., & Wilson, D. (2009). *Wong's essentials of pediatric nursing* (8th ed.). St Louis: Mosby.

Holdgate, A., Asha, S., Craig, J., & Thompson, J. (2003). Comparison of a verbal numeric rating scale with the visual analogue scale for the measurement of acute pain. *Emergency Medicine, 15*, 441–446.

Hubert, H., Guinhouya, C., Richard-Hibon, A., Wiel, E., Durocher, A., & Goldstein, P. (2009). Prehospital pain treatment: an economic productivity factor in emergency medicine? *Journal of Evaluation in Clinical Practice, 15*, 152–157.

Jennings, P. A., Cameron, P., & Bernard, S. (2011c). Determinants of clinically important pain severity reduction in the prehospital setting. *Emergency Medicine Journal, 29*(4). doi:10.1136/emj.2010.107094.

Jennings, P., Cameron, P., & Bernard, S. (2011a). Epidemiology of prehospital pain: an opportunity for improvement. *Emergency Medicine Journal, 28*, 530–531.

Jennings, P. A., Cameron, P., & Bernard, S. (2011b). Ketamine as an analgesic in the pre-hospital setting: a systematic review. *Acta Anaesthesiologica Scandinavica, 55*(6), 638–643.

Jennings, P. A., Cameron, P., Bernard, S., Walker, T., Jolley, D., Fitzgerald, M., & Masci, K. (2012). Morphine and ketamine is superior to morphine alone for out-of-hospital trauma analgesia: a randomized controlled trial. *Annals of Emergency Medicine, 59*(6), 497–503.

Jensen, P. M., Karoly, P., & Braver, S. (1986). The measurement of clinical pain intensity: a comparison of six methods. *Pain, 27*, 117–126.

Lee, J. S. (2001). Pain measurement: understanding existing tools and their application in the emergency department. *Emergency Medicine, 13*, 279–287.

Lord, B., & Woollard, M. (2011). The reliability of vital signs in estimating pain severity among adult patients treated by paramedics. *Emergency Medicine Journal, 28*, 147–150.

Lord, B. A., & Parsell, B. (2003). Measurement of pain in the prehospital setting using a visual analogue scale. *Prehospital and Disaster Medicine, 18*(4), 353–358. [Erratum appears in Prehospital & Disaster Medicine 2005, 20(1), v.].

Luger, T. J., Lederer, W., Gassner, M., Lockinger, A., Ulmer, H., & Lorenz, I. H. (2003). Acute pain is under-assessed in out-of-hospital emergencies. *Academic Emergency Medicine: Official Journal of the Society for Academic Emergency Medicine, 10*(6), 627–632.

MacIntyre, P. E., & Schug, S. A. (2007). *Acute pain management. A practical guide.* Philadelphia: Elsevier.

Maio, R. F., Garrison, H. G., Spaite, D. W., Desmond, J. S., Gregor, M. A., Stiell, I. G., & O'Malley, P. J. (2002). Emergency Medical Services Outcomes Project (EMSOP) IV: pain measurement in out-of-hospital outcomes research. *Annals of Emergency Medicine, 40*(2), 172–179.

Marco, C. A., Plewa, M. C., Buderer, N., Hymel, G., & Cooper, J. (2006). Self-reported pain scores in the emergency department: lack of association with vital signs. *Academic Emergency Medicine: Official Journal of the Society for Academic Emergency Medicine, 13*(9), 974–979.

McLean, S. A., Domeier, R. M., DeVore, H. K., Hill, E. M., Maio, R. F., & Frederiksen, S. M. (2003). The feasibility of pain assessment in the prehospital setting. *Prehospital Emergency Care, 8*, 155–161.

McManus, J. G., Jr, & Sallee, D. R., Jr. (2005). Pain management in the prehospital environment. *Emergency Medicine Clinics of North America, 23*(2), 415–431.

Merskey, H., & Bogduk, N. (1994). *Classification of chronic pain. IASP task force on taxonomy.* Seattle: IASP Press.

Meyer, R. A., Ringkamp, M., Campbell, J. N., & Raja, S. N. (2006). Peripheral mechanisms of cutaneous nociception. In S. McMahon & M. Koltzenburg (Eds.), *Wall and Melzack's textbook of pain* (5th ed.). Philadelphia: Elsevier.

Michael, G. E., Sporer, K. A., & Youngblood, G. M. (2007). Women are less likely than men to receive prehospital analgesia for isolated extremity injuries. *The American Journal of Emergency Medicine, 25*, 901–906.

Mkandawire, N. C., Boot, D. A., Braithwaite, I. J., & Patterson, M. (2002). Musculoskeletal recovery 5 years after severe injury: long-term problems are common. *Injury, 33*(2), 111–115.

Moore, C. M., & Leonardi-Bee, J. (2008). The prevalence of pain and disability one year post fracture of the distal radius in a UK population: a cross sectional survey. *BMC Musculoskeletal Disorders, 9*, 129.

National Institute of Clinical Studies. (2011). *Emergency care acute pain management manual.* Canberra: National Health and Medical Research Council.

Price, D., Bush, F., Long, S., & Harkins, S. (1994). A comparison of pain measurement characteristics of mechanical visual analogue and simple numerical rating scales. *Pain, 56*, 217–226.

Ricard-Hibon, A., Belpomme, V., Chollet, C., Devaud, M.-L., Adnet, F., Borron, S., & Marty, J. (2008). Compliance with a morphine protocol and effect on pain relief in out-of-hospital patients. *The Journal of Emergency Medicine, 34*(3), 305–310.

Rickard, C., O'Meara, P., McGrail, M., Garner, D., McLean, A., & Le Lievre, P. (2007). A randomised controlled trial of intranasal fentanyl vs intravenous morphine for analgesia in the prehospital setting. *The American Journal of Emergency Medicine, 25*, 911–917.

Rivara, F. P., Mackenzie, E. J., Jurkovich, G. J., Nathens, A. B., Wang, J., & Scharfstein, D. O. (2008). Prevalence of pain in patients 1 year after major trauma. *Archives of Surgery, 143*(3), 282–287, discussion 288.

Rupp, T., & Delaney, K. A. (2004). Inadequate analgesia in emergency medicine. *Annals of Emergency Medicine, 43*(4), 494–503.

Schug, S. A., Palmer, G. M., Scott, D. A., & Trinca, J., APM:SE Working Group of the Australian and New Zealand College of Anaesthetists and Faculty of Pain Medicine. (2015). *Acute pain management: scientific evidence* (4th ed.). Melbourne: ANZCA & FPM.

Shields, B. J., Cohen, D. M., Harbeck-Weber, C., Powers, J. D., & Smith, G. A. (2003). Pediatric pain measurement using a visual analogue scale: a comparison of two teaching methods. *Clinical Pediatrics, 42*(3), 227–234.

Shipton, E. A., & Tait, B. (2005). Flagging the pain: preventing the burden of chronic pain by identifying and treating risk factors in acute pain. *European Journal of Anaesthesiology, 22*, 405–412.

Simpson, P., Bendall, J., & Middleton, P. (2001). Prophylactic metoclopramide for patients receiving intravenous morphine in the emergency setting: a systematic review and meta-analysis of randomized controlled trials. *Emergency Medicine Australasia: EMA, 23*(4), 452–457.

Solomon, P. (2001). Congruence between health professionals' and patients' pain ratings: a review of the literature. *Scandinavian Journal of Caring Sciences, 15*(2), 174–180.

Spilman, S. K., Lechtenberg, G. T., Hahn, K. D., Fuchsen, E. A., Olson, S. D., Swegle, J. R., Vaudt, C. C., & Sahr, S. M. (2016). Is pain really undertreated? Challenges of addressing pain in trauma patients during prehospital transport and trauma resuscitation. *Injury, 47*(9), 2018–2024.

Swor, R., McEachin, C. M., Seguin, D., & Grall, K. H. (2005). Prehospital pain management in children suffering traumatic injury. *Prehospital Emergency Care, 9*(1), 40–43.

Thomas, S. H., & Shewakramani, S. (2008). Prehospital trauma analgesia. *The Journal of Emergency Medicine, 35*, 47–57.

Todd, K. H., Sloan, E. P., Chen, C., Eder, S., & Wamstad, K. (2002). Survey of pain etiology, management practices and patient satisfaction in two urban emergency departments. *CJEM, 4*, 252–256.

Turturro, M. A. (2002). Pain, priorities and prehospital care. *Prehospital Emergency Care, 6*(4), 486–488.

Watkins, N. (2006). Paediatric prehospital analgesia in Auckland. *Emergency Medicine Australasia: EMA, 18*(1), 51–56.

Weisman, S. J., Bernstein, B., & Schechter, N. L. (1998). Consequences of inadequate analgesia during painful procedures in children. *Archives of Pediatrics & Adolescent Medicine, 152*(2), 147–149.

Williamson, O. D., Gabbe, B. J., Cameron, P. A., Edwards, E. R., & Richardson, M. D. (2009). Predictors of moderate or severe pain 6 months after orthopaedic injury: a prospective cohort study. *Journal of Orthopaedic Trauma, 23*(2), 139–144.

CHAPTER 31

Acute Abdominal Pain

By Alexander Olaussen

OVERVIEW

- Abdominal pain is a common presentation in out-of-hospital emergency care, and the commonest cause for ED presentations (Bhuiya et al., 2010).
- The causes of abdominal pain range from minor and self-resolving to serious and life-threatening.
- The severity of the pain and its location are unreliable indicators of seriousness.
- As diagnoses can become clearer with time, the aim is not necessarily to identify the cause, but rather provide safe symptomatic treatment and identify patients who may progress to a worse condition.

- Out-of-hospital management is usually supportive rather than definitive and may consist only of transport based on an awareness of the possible diagnosis.
- Early identification of serious causes for abdominal pain requires a high degree of clinical suspicion as there is no reliable out-of-hospital test.
- In-hospital assessment includes blood tests, urine testing and imaging (e.g. CT and ultrasound). Some patients may also proceed to a diagnostic or curative surgical operation.

Introduction

The abdomen extends superiorly from the xiphoid process, inferiorly to the pelvis and laterally to the flanks, contains many organs and is often difficult to interrogate and diagnose due to its concealed nature.

Abdominal pain, nausea and vomiting can be very distressing for patients and the causes of the symptoms can range from relatively minor and self-resolving to life-threatening. Being able to determine the cause can be extremely difficult in the out-of-hospital setting. In fact, in many cases the diagnostic challenges persist after the patient arrives at hospital and many patients will not be diagnosed until hours after admission or until surgery with a substantial proportion never receiving a diagnosis on their first visit. Discharge from ED, or the out-of-hospital setting, should include advice on representation if the pain worsens, vomiting starts or does not settle, there is fever, or if the pain persists (Macaluso & McNamara, 2012).

Paramedic management of specific abdominal conditions is also limited but early assessment of abdominal pain is essential in order to avoid the life-threatening end-stage of a number of causes of abdominal pain: an acute abdomen. The term 'acute abdomen' describes a clinical syndrome rather than suggesting a specific aetiology and is the physiological result of intraabdominal haemorrhage, organ inflammation, organ perforation/rupture or intestinal obstruction. Unfortunately, the early symptoms of these conditions can be vague, variable and seemingly transient. Cases of a fully evolved acute abdomen

usually require urgent surgery (Doherty, 2010; Matthews & Hodin, 2011).

Pathophysiology

Anatomy

The abdomen contains a tightly packed set of organs that differ remarkably in structure and function to each another (Fig 31.1).

The abdomen contains the digestive system (including bowels, pancreas, liver, gall bladder and appendix), vessels (including aorta and vena cava) and genitourinary organs. Each of the digestive organs is surrounded by a visceral pleura that is poorly innervated for sensation, while the abdominal space itself is lined by the peritoneal pleura, which is much more sensitive to irritation.

The function of some organs (such as the bowel) makes them more likely to present with specific symptoms (e.g. diarrhoea), while the structure (hollow versus solid) can influence the type of pain that disease will generate (Fig 31.2).

A detailed understanding of the abdominal anatomy is essential for making safe clinical decisions when confronted with patients with abdominal symptoms. The contents of the hollow organs of the abdomen will, if they are able to escape the confines of the organs, irritate the parietal peritoneum and cause a well localised pain. They are also likely to damage nearby tissues and lead to infection and ultimately sepsis. The sudden escape of contents is unlikely, and in most cases disease of the organ wall has to have existed for days or more before it

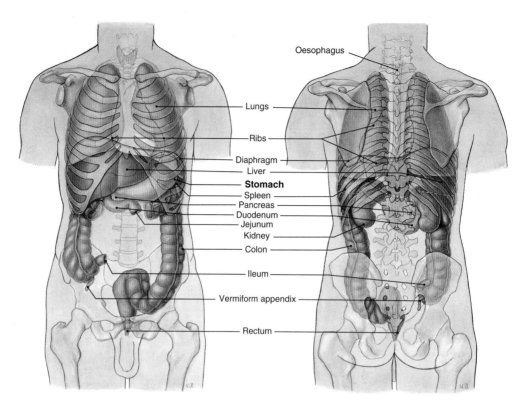

Figure 31.1
Location of the digestive organs.
Source: Paulsen (2013).

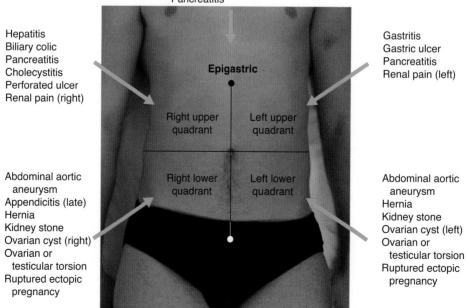

Figure 31.2
Location of abdominal pain and possible origins.
Source: Adapted from Talley & O'Connor (2013); image courtesy of Glenn McCulloch.

ruptures and spills its contents. It is during this time that the source and seriousness of the pain can be difficult to identify.

In reality, an acute abdomen as defined by severe pain and shock is not difficult to diagnose: it is determining whether abdominal pain in its early stages is likely to progress to an acute abdomen that challenges most clinicians. Acute abdominal emergencies presenting with pain but adequate perfusion could represent the early stages of conditions that will evolve into an acute abdomen or may be associated with conditions unlikely to produce shock. Paramedic assessment of a patient with an acute abdominal emergency involves assessing and managing the patient's pain and any associated cardiovascular or respiratory compromise, as well as considering the aetiologies of the abdominal emergency.

Clinicians also have to consider pathologies outside of the abdomen that may present with abdominal pain, such as myocardial infarction and pneumonia. Further challenges to assessment and management include the relatively short timeframe that paramedics have to observe the changes and development of a clinical condition, plus the fact that they may be assessing the patient early in the clinical development before some signs become more obvious.

Reassuringly, it is not absolutely necessary to reach a definitive diagnosis in the emergency setting. Rather, the emphasis is on recognising a wide range of possibilities and formulating a safe management plan that covers all of the possible clinical risks. Definitive treatment, which requires a definitive diagnosis, occurs with the benefit of time, repeated observations and specific investigations.

Abdominal pain

Abdominal pain is a common symptom and patients with complaints of abdominal pain represent a high percentage of presentations in the out-of-hospital and hospital settings (Niska et al., 2010). Just as understanding the function and location of organs is essential for managing acute abdominal pain, so too is a basic understanding of how the abdominal organs generate pain and how the pain is perceived by patients.

The organs of the abdomen are innervated by a complex arrangement of afferent neuroreceptors that are involved in the normal subconscious regulation of gastrointestinal (GI) system activities and the perception of abnormal noxious stimuli. Such stimuli include the mechanical changes of organ distension, torsion or contraction; chemical changes associated with inflammatory mediators; and

ischaemia (Farquhar-Smith, 2008). Stimuli such as lacerations or crushing do not tend to invoke pain as there are no neuroreceptors for these kinds of stimuli within the abdomen (Millham, 2010).

There are two types of neuroreceptors involved in nociception: unmyelinated C fibres and thinly myelinated A-delta fibres. Due to a lack of myelin, C fibres have a slow conduction velocity and when stimulated mediate diffuse, dull, burning and poorly localised pain. In contrast, A-delta fibres have a rapid conduction velocity and mediate brief, sharp and well-localised pain (Farquhar-Smith, 2008). The nerve fibres responsible for the sensation of visceral pain are predominantly C fibres (Knowles & Aziz, 2009) while the peritoneum is innervated by A-delta fibres (Minter & Mulholland, 2008).

Visceral pain
Anatomical basis for visceral pain
C and A-delta fibres are spinal visceral afferent fibres that synapse in dorsal root ganglia of the spinal cord. The level at which these fibres enter the spinal cord for a particular organ are not well established as the cell bodies of visceral afferent fibres for a particular organ are not confined to a specific level(s) of the spinal cord. Instead, they have a broadly distributed overlapping pattern across a range of dorsal root ganglia. It is thought that this broad distribution in the spinal cord, the small number of spinal visceral afferent fibres available for nociception and the dominance of C fibres all contribute to the experience of visceral pain as diffuse, dull, burning and poorly localised (Knowles & Aziz, 2009). The diffuse and poorly localised aspects of visceral pain are experienced within the central abdominal regions; for example, the midline in the epigastric region or lower abdomen, or around the umbilicus (periumbilical). This centralisation of abdominal pain is thought to be due to the bilateral innervation of abdominal organs; that is, the spinal visceral afferent fibres transmit impulses to both the right and left sides of the spinal cord (Flasar & Goldberg, 2006). Ischaemia, stretching, inflammation and spasm are all typical causes of visceral pain.

Parietal pain
Parts of all the abdominal organs lie against parts of the parietal peritoneum and when a disease affecting an organ extends to the surface of the organ, the parietal peritoneum can also be affected. The parietal peritoneum is innervated by A-delta fibres, which are branches of somatic afferent fibres supplying the skin and muscle of the abdominal wall. As a consequence, when the peritoneum is irritated, parietal pain is sharp and well localised

and can result in local reflex muscle spasm over the area of irritation (Millham, 2010). Because pain associated with peritoneal inflammation transmitted by the A-delta fibres is well localised, this explains the perception that the site of pain moves as inflammation moves from being purely visceral to involving the peritoneum. Parietal pain is made worse by anything that causes stretch of the peritoneum, such as coughing, moving in bed or walking (Glasgow & Mulvihill, 2003). Hence, patients with abdominal pain with parietal involvement are likely to lie still in bed, avoid moving and lie with their legs bent rather than stretched out straight.

Referred pain

Visceral pain can be associated with pain sensation in another part of the body; for example, patients with pancreatitis can experience referred pain in the epigastrium and upper back. The anatomical basis for referred pain lies in the common pathways taken by somatic and visceral afferent fibres as they transmit impulses into the spinal cord. The higher levels of the brain interpret the sensations from the visceral afferent fibres as coming from the somatic fibres, because of 'mnemonic trace', the functional unit of memory. The frequent experience of somatic sensation compared to visceral sensation over a person's lifespan contributes to the interpretation of stimuli arising from a somatic rather than a visceral source and pain is experienced at the somatic site (Giamberardino et al., 2010) (see Figs 31.3 and 31.4).

Associated symptoms: autonomic influences

Visceral pain can be accompanied by nausea and vomiting, pallor, sweatiness and increases in blood pressure and heart rate. As visceral pathways lie close to the autonomic outflow tracts, it is generally accepted that the autonomic nervous system modulates the body's response to pain, particularly with respect to heart rate and blood pressure, but the mechanisms are still unclear (Bantel & Trapp, 2011). The mechanism underlying the association of pain with nausea and vomiting is also unclear. It is known that stimulation of vagal afferent fibres can cause nausea and that visceral afferents share the same neural pathways as vagal afferents; however, shared pathways may not explain the phenomenon, as nausea can still exist in patients with vagotomy. This finding could mean that the visceral afferents are mediators of nausea (Andrews & Horn, 2006). However, other theories suggest a potential neuroendocrine mechanism as nausea has been associated with high levels of adrenaline mediated by sympathetic outflow (Andrews & Horn, 2006). Further research is required to explain the associated symptoms of visceral pain.

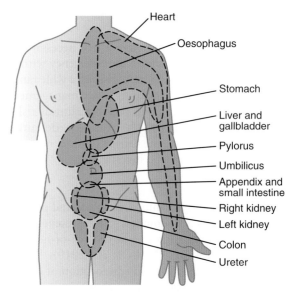

Figure 31.4
Surface areas of referred pain from different visceral organs.
When visceral pain is referred to the surface of the body, the person generally localises it in the dermatomal segment from which the visceral organ originated in the embryo, not necessarily where the visceral organ now lies. For instance, the heart originates in the neck and upper thorax, so the heart's visceral pain fibres pass upwards along the sympathetic sensory nerves and enter the spinal cord between segments T1 and T5.
Source: Hall (2012).

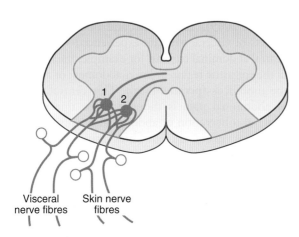

Figure 31.3
Mechanism of referred pain from visceral origins.
Branches of visceral pain fibres are shown to synapse in the spinal cord on the same neurons (1 and 2) that receive pain signals from the skin. When the visceral pain fibres are stimulated, pain signals from the viscera are conducted through at least some of the same neurons that conduct pain signals from the skin and can lead to the sensation of referred pain.
Source: Hall (2012).

Specific conditions

Differential diagnoses

A thorough and working knowledge of the differential diagnoses for abdominal pain is essential. There are numerous benign, self-limiting and non-emergency causes of abdominal pain for which the reader is referred to other texts. Important differential diagnoses can be broken down into different categories:

- Inflammatory/infectious
  - Appendicitis
  - Pancreatitis
  - Cholecystitis
  - Diverticulitis
  - Peritonitis
  - Gastroenteritis
  - Inflammatory bowel disease (Crohn's disease and ulcerative colitis)
- Vascular
  - Abdominal aortic aneurysm
  - Embolic/thrombotic events
  - Ectopic pregnancy
- Perforation
  - Perforated viscus
- Obstruction
  - Intestinal obstruction
  - Renal stones
  - Urinary retention
- Pressure
  - Ascites
  - Hernia

Inflammatory/infectious

Appendicitis

Anatomy

The vermiform appendix is a short, narrow, hollow tube variably described as being between 2 and 20 cm long (Gray, 2000). This blind-ended tube is attached to the posteromedial surface of the caecum of the large intestine, approximately 3 cm from the ileocaecal valve (Horn & Ufberg, 2011; Wolfe & Henneman, 2010) with a great deal of variability. It is surrounded by a fold of peritoneum that supports the arterial supply to the appendix (Gray, 2000).

Pathology

'Acute appendicitis' is the term used to describe the inflammation and infection of the vermiform appendix (Melloni et al., 2003; Stedman, 2006). Appendicitis may present in many different ways, for two main reasons. First, the position of the appendix causes a lack of certain signs and presence of others. Second, the characteristics of the pain differ at the evolving stages of appendicitis, spanning early on from anorexia, nausea and vague pain, to

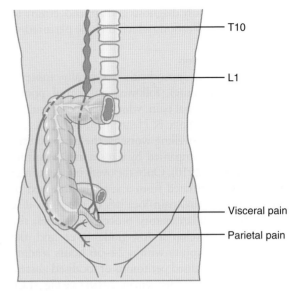

Figure 31.5
Visceral and parietal transmission of pain signals from the appendix.
Pain impulses pass first from the appendix through visceral pain fibres located within sympathetic nerve bundles and then into the spinal cord at about T10 or T11; this pain is referred to an area around the umbilicus and is of the aching, cramping type. Pain impulses also often originate in the parietal peritoneum where the inflamed appendix touches or is adherent to the abdominal wall. These cause pain of the sharp type directly over the irritated peritoneum in the right lower quadrant of the abdomen.
Source: Hall (2012).

peritonitis and a rigid abdomen following perforation. Most cases of acute appendicitis are due to lumen obstruction, typically by a faecalith (i.e. hard and impacted faeces). Other obstructing causes include a calculus, foreign body, tumour, adhesions, enlarged lymph nodes or parasites such as intestinal worms. After blockage, hyperperistalsis follows, which is aimed at overcoming the obstruction. This may be unsuccessful and then distension of the appendix follows. This triggers vague and poorly localised visceral pain referred to the periumbilical region (see Fig 31.5), because the appendix is located in the midgut. As the obstruction continues, the congestion worsens and the organ swells, progressing towards the dangerous complication of perforation (Jaffe & Berger, 2010).

Epidemiology/significance

Appendicitis most commonly occurs in young patients (7–35 years old) and is common, with an annual crude incidence rate of 8.9 per 10,000 (Ceresoli et al., 2016). Males are slightly more likely to get acute appendicitis than females (Ceresoli et al., 2016). The significance of appendicitis lies in the importance of early diagnosis and appendectomy to avoid late complications which include perforation and peritonitis.

Clinical presentation

The first sign of appendicitis is typically anorexia (i.e. loss of appetite), followed by central poorly described abdominal pain, which may be a result of hyperperistalsis (Wolfe & Henneman, 2010). As the obstruction and swelling worsens, the pain worsens and may be accompanied by nausea and vomiting (Jaffe & Berger, 2010). Once the overlying peritoneal wall becomes irritated from a severely inflamed or infarcted appendix, pain localises to the right iliac fossa. As the inflammatory process continues, the patient can develop a low-grade fever and the appendix can rupture within 24–36 hours leading to either a generalised peritonitis or localised abscess formation (Wolfe & Henneman, 2010) (see Fig 31.6). The perforation rate of acute appendicitis may be up to 20% (Andersson et al., 1992; Horn & Ufberg, 2011). The morbidity of acute appendicitis is low except when complicated by perforation, which is more common in the very young and the elderly. Of all age groups, diagnostic accuracy is the lowest and perforation incidence is the highest in children under 5 years of age and in adults over 65 years of age (Korner et al., 2001). Early suspicion and diagnosis is thus required necessitating early transport to hospital to aid the diagnosis. There are a number of 'atypical presentations' of appendicitis, relating to the anatomical position of the appendix, the patient's age and whether or not the patient is pregnant.

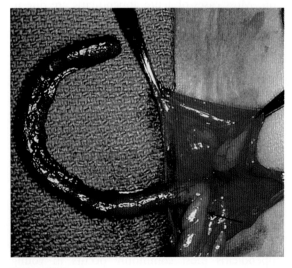

Figure 31.6
Acute appendicitis.
Note the arrow showing inflamed tissue surrounding the base of a gangrenous appendix (which appears black).
Source: Craft et al. (2011).

A retrocaecal appendix is one that lies behind the caecum. This position, being away from the anterior abdominal wall, limits typical findings. Complaints of blunted abdominal pain, flank pain or back pain are suggestive features (Jaffe & Berger, 2010). The psoas sign (i.e. a sharp increase in pain on flexing the hip in a straight leg raise) may be positive as the psoas muscle lies under the site of inflammation. In young children presentations of appendicitis are nonspecific and can be confused with other conditions that cause nausea and vomiting, such as urinary tract infection and gastroenteritis. The thinner appendiceal wall in children increases the risk of perforation (Horn & Ufberg, 2011; Wolfe & Henneman, 2010). Elderly patients also tend to present atypically, as there is a change in pain nociceptors. Mortality from appendicitis in patients over 70 years of age may be as high as 1 in 3 (Horn & Ufberg, 2011). The rate of appendicitis in pregnant women is slightly higher than in the general population. Diagnostic challenges stem from nausea and vomiting being common in early pregnancy, and abdominal pain being mistaken for onset of labour in late pregnancy. The gravid uterus can cause displacement of the appendix from its normal position away from the abdominal wall, leading to atypical signs and symptoms and causing delay in diagnosis. Appendicitis in pregnancy is associated with an increased risk of premature labour, and risk of fetal mortality if perforated (Horn & Ufberg, 2011; Wolfe & Henneman, 2010).

Treatment

The treatment of appendicitis in the out-of-hospital setting is aimed at symptom control and transport to hospital. Analgesia should be adequate and should not be withheld based on the notion that it will hinder in-hospital diagnosis (Noble et al., 2010). Nausea and emesis is probably best treated with ondansetron, rather than metoclopramide (given the prokinetic properties of metoclopramide). Sniffing an isopropyl alcohol wipe is also a simple, quick and safe novel evidence-based treatment for nausea. The definitive in-hospital treatment is surgical removal. Although there is increasing evidence comparing antibiotic therapy and appendectomy (Salminen et al., 2015), these patients often require CT imaging before starting on antibiotics, and as such should be transported to hospital, rather than referred to a GP.

Pancreatitis

Anatomy/pathology

The pancreas, an endocrine and exocrine organ located in the upper abdomen partly retroperitoneally, is vital in digestion. When inflamed (i.e. pancreatitis), pancreatic enzymes spill out, causing auto-digestion and local damage. The two commonest causes of pancreatitis are excessive alcohol ingestion (for unclear reasons; Chowdhury & Gupta, 2006) and gallstones (due to blockage of the release of pancreatic enzymes). Chronic pancreatitis on the other hand is a progressive fibroinflammatory disease often due to a complex mix of environmental and genetic factors (Braganza et al., 2011). If the pancreatic digestive enzymes erode through major blood vessels, haemorrhagic pancreatitis—a surgical emergency—is present.

Epidemiology/significance
Patients with pancreatitis can get unwell rapidly. In-hospital monitoring and observation is required. There is a risk of cyst formation or haemorrhagic transformation.

Clinical presentation
The typical pain from pancreatitis is situated in the epigastrium. It onsets fairly suddenly, is dull and constant in nature and radiates to the back.

Treatment
Out-of-hospital treatment includes symptomatic relief and transport. Analgesia should be given, but avoid morphine (as that may cause sphincter of Oddi spasm) (Sheehy et al., 2013) and thus worsening the pancreatitis. In-hospital treatment involves fluid and electrolyte replacement. Sepsis is closely monitored for and treated with antibiotics if present.

Cholecystitis
Anatomy/pathology
The gallbladder rests under the liver and stores bile (which the liver produces) and spits that bile into the GI system to help digestion of fats. Gallstones may form inside the gallbladder giving rise to biliary colic pain (i.e. cholelithiasis). The gallbladder may get inflamed/infected (i.e. cholecystitis) if a gall stone gets stuck in the neck of the gall bladder, or occasionally in the absence of gallstones. If the stone gets stuck further down in the biliary tree (e.g. common bile duct), then pain (i.e. choledocholithiasis) or infection (i.e. cholangitis) may occur.

Epidemiology/significance
Gallstones are common and many patients have the gallbladder electively removed after a few symptomatic attacks. The significance of cholecystitis is that the infection may get severe and/or be in the common bile duct (i.e. cholangitis), the common bile duct may get obstructed or the gallbladder may become gangrenous (Tintinalli et al., 2016).

Clinical presentation
The typical presentation and risk factors of a patient with cholelithiasis is often summarised by a number of 'Fs'. Classically a fat, fair (Caucasian), fertile (or pregnant) female in her forties with family history

of gall stones is present. The pain from cholecystitis is situated in the right upper quadrant (RUQ) and occasionally radiates to the back/tip of the scapula, it onsets suddenly post a fatty meal, is dull and is colicky in nature before the stone gets stuck and the gallbladder infected (when the pain becomes constant). It is associated with nausea and vomiting and sometimes fever if the infection is severe. Murphy's sign (i.e. the patient is unable to complete a full breath due to pain upon pressure of the inflamed gallbladder, in the RUQ [Yokoe et al., 2013]) has a strong diagnostic specificity, meaning when the sign is elicited the diagnosis is likely. Charcot's triad (i.e. jaundice, fever and RUQ pain) is suggestive of cholangitis, while Reynold's pentad (i.e. Charcot's triad plus altered mental status and hypotension) is even more severe for cholangitis.

Treatment
Out-of-hospital treatment includes symptomatic relief and transport. In-hospital treatment includes delayed or urgent cholecystectomy or endoscopic retrograde cholangiopancreatography (ERCP) depending on the presence and location of the gall stones as seen on ultrasound.

Diverticulitis
Anatomy/pathology
The colon, most often the sigmoid and descending colon, can develop outpouchings (diverticulae) causing the disease (diverticulosis). If these diverticulae get inflamed or infected (diverticulitis) there is a risk of focal necrosis, abscess formation or perforation (Sheehy et al., 2013).

Epidemiology/significance
The incidence of diverticular disease increases with age, being present in half of patients above 70 years of age. Risk factors for the development of diverticula relate to constipation, obesity and a low-fibre diet (through increased intraluminal pressure). Simple diverticulitis (i.e. without abscess formation or perforation and clinical mildly symptomatic) is often treated by GPs in the community with or without antibiotics and a clear fluid diet (Sheehy et al., 2013). However, the evidence suggests that antibiotics do not improve recovery time nor lessens complications or the recurrence rate (Chabok et al., 2012). Potential complications include perforation, abscess formation, fistula formation and bowel obstruction (Tintinalli et al., 2016) which mandates urgent in-hospital investigation and management.

Clinical presentation
The typical presentation is unilateral left iliac fossa or left flank pain, constitutional symptoms of anorexia, nausea/vomiting and bowel changes including rectal bleeding.

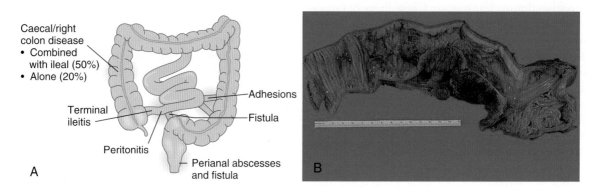

Figure 31.7
Crohn's disease.
A The disease is localised to the terminal ileum, ascending colon and transverse colon in most cases.
B A segment of colon that has a thickened wall and in which the mucosa has lost the regular folds, indicative of Crohn's disease.
Source: Craft et al. (2011).

Treatment

Out-of-hospital treatment includes symptomatic relief and transport. In-hospital treatment includes IV hydration, antibiotics and surgery emergently if perforated, or electively if recurrent attacks of diverticulitis is deemed more troublesome than the risk of the operation.

Peritonitis

Peritonitis is inflammation of the peritoneum. It can be caused by bacterial invasion or chemical irritation (Turner, 2009). Perforation of the appendix can result in generalised peritonitis and an acute abdomen. The infective and inflammatory processes involving the peritoneal membrane result in fluid exudate accumulating in the abdominal cavity. Depending on the size of the area affected, fluid losses can effectively render the patient hypovolaemic. The bowel's ability to function is inhibited and a paralytic ileus results. Patients with generalised peritonitis may therefore exhibit acute global abdominal pain, elevated temperature, nausea and vomiting, tachycardia and hypotension.

Gastroenteritis

Gastroenteritis is an acute inflammation of the GI tract that occurs suddenly in patients who are otherwise well. It is due to direct invasion of the GI tract by bacteria, bacterial toxins, viruses or parasites. It is associated with any combination of pain, nausea, vomiting and diarrhoea (Craig & Zich, 2010; Getto et al., 2011). Diarrhoea is defined as a change in bowel habit with stools increasing in frequency (more than three times a day) and more liquid in content. Diarrhoea is considered

acute when it lasts less than 14 days (Getto et al., 2011).

Crohn's disease

Crohn's disease is an autoimmune disease resulting in inflammation of the wall of the GI tract (see Fig 31.7).

It is a disease characterised by periods of relapses and remissions. It is most commonly seen in the distal small bowel and proximal colon, but is not limited to the small and large intestines; it can affect all parts of the GI tract including the mouth and rectum (Sands & Siegel, 2010). In Crohn's disease, susceptible individuals have an abnormal immune response to the bacteria normally found in the bowel. The pathophysiology is complex and not entirely clear. A number of factors are thought to contribute to the development of the disease.

Crohn's disease is characterised by areas of focal inflammation—(i.e. areas of inflamed bowel surrounded by normal bowel). Early stages of the disease are characterised by small mucosal ulcers (less than 3 mm in size) called aphthous ulcers, which are surrounded by areas of inflamed tissue; and granulomas (nodules of inflammatory tissue), which are frequently but not always present. Ultimately, as the disease progresses ulceration of the intestinal wall and extension of inflammation to the outer serosal layer of the bowel can result in abscess and fistula formation and adherence of loops of bowel, which can cause bowel obstruction. The chronic inflammation of the walls of the intestine associated with Crohn's disease also leads to the development of fibrous tissue, scarring and thickening of the intestinal wall, which predisposes the development of strictures and lumen obstruction (Sands & Siegel, 2010).

Diarrhoea in Crohn's disease can be caused by changes in motility and decreased absorptive capacity due to inflammation, as well as loss into the gut lumen of inflammatory exudates and red blood cells (Sands & Siegel, 2010).

The long-term effect of Crohn's disease on the patient is variable and depends on the severity. As a general statement, the relapse rate for an individual in the first 2 years of diagnosis tends to set the pattern for the following 5 years. Studies of patients over 4 years show that patients are likely to follow one of three courses: remission, active disease or a combination of active and inactive disease (Sands & Siegel, 2010). While the cause of Crohn's disease is complex and multifactorial, patients who stop smoking are compliant with their medications, avoid non-steroidal anti-inflammatory drugs (NSAIDs) and implement techniques and strategies to reduce stress in their lives can reduce the potential for relapse (Sands & Siegel, 2010).

Treatment includes symptom relief (avoiding NSAIDs) and transport to hospital for disease severity assessment and medication review.

Vascular
Abdominal aortic aneurysm
Anatomy/pathology
An arterial aneurysm is a localised dilation of the arterial wall that occurs as a consequence of vessel wall weakness or high sustained pressure. Aneurysms can be due to congenital abnormalities or pathological causes, the most common of which are atherosclerosis and hypertension (Mitchell & Schoen, 2009). An abdominal aortic aneurysm (AAA) is variably defined as a dilation of the abdominal aorta that is greater than half the normal diameter of the aorta (i.e. aortic width greater than 1.5 times normal, measured at the level of the renal arteries (Siddiqi, 2012) or where the minimal anteroposterior diameter is 3 cm (Bessen, 2010). The most common site for an aneurysm is the abdominal aorta between the renal arteries and the aortic bifurcation (see Fig 31.8) (Lewiss et al., 2011).

An aortic dissection occurs when blood enters the tunica media through a damaged intimal wall and then tracks up the medial layer, effectively dissecting the artery (Bessen, 2010). Aneurysm formation is related to alterations in the composition of the medial and adventitious layers of the aortic wall, which in the past was thought to be due to atherosclerosis. Changes in the aortic wall in early aneurysm formation reflect a reduction in the density

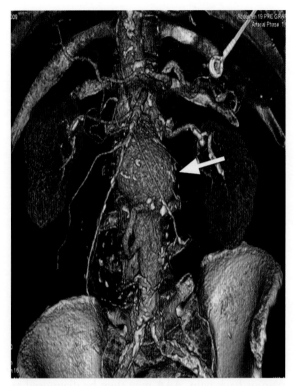

Figure 31.8
Three-dimensional reconstruction of a CT scan in a patient with an infra-renal abdominal aortic aneurysm (arrow).
Source: Bonow et al. (2011).

of smooth muscle cells in the tunica media due to degenerative changes and loss of elastin in this layer. The progressive weakening of the aortic wall and increase in size of an AAA ultimately results in rupture of the aortic wall. Degradation of collagen in the adventitia is thought to contribute to the progression to rupture (Bessen, 2010; Lewiss et al., 2011). These changes appear to be caused by processes other than atherosclerosis. The presence of raised levels of cytokines and macrophages in aneurysm tissue points to inflammatory processes being involved.

Epidemiology/significance
AAA most commonly occurs in elderly males with a smoking history and atherosclerotic disease, as well as a family history of AAA (Hirsch et al., 2006). Men are more than four times likely to develop AAA than women and the incidence increases with age (Singh et al., 2001). For men, the average age at diagnosis is between 65 and 70 years and autopsy findings show that nearly 6% of men aged between 80 and 85 years have an AAA (Hirsch et al., 2006). The significance of AAA is that it may one day dissect and hence it is referred to as a ticking bomb

in the abdomen. Prophylactic surgery is favoured when the aneurysm is large enough (> 5.5 cm). Once developed, the AAA will progressively enlarge until it ruptures the aortic wall. The most important predictor of rupture is the size of the aneurysm. Aneurysms that measure at least 6 cm are associated with a rupture risk of 40%, while those that are larger than 7 cm have a rupture risk of 50% (Hirsch et al., 2006). Only 50% of patients who have a ruptured AAA will survive to hospital (Lewiss et al., 2011). The overall survival rate of a ruptured AAA is 18% (Sakalihasan et al., 2005).

Clinical presentation
Patients with retroperitoneal rupture of AAA may occasionally have a small tear and bleed, which is contained as an extra-aortic haematoma. This haematoma can exist for weeks or months, but the patient is at risk of rupture at any time. Clinically the patient may present with acute abdominal or flank pain that diminishes but develops into a chronic pain pattern. Although AAA is usually asymptomatic, on occasion patients may present with gradual onset of vague abdominal pain, flank pain or back pain. AAA may then be diagnosed as an incidental finding. Subtle clinical signs to suggest a ruptured AAA include a delay in radial-radial or radial-femoral pulsation, depending on where in the aorta the rupture is. This is appreciated by simultaneously palpating both radial arteries followed by palpation of the right radial artery plus the femoral artery.

Diagnosis
Bedside point-of-care ultrasound (POCUS) can identify the size of the aorta and the presence of free fluid. Contrast CT scan with dedicated viewing of the vessels is definitively diagnostic.

Treatment
Out-of-hospital treatment includes transport to hospital and perfusion treatment. No delays in transport should occur in the setting of a suspected ruptured AAA, and some services accept a carotid pulse to emphasise the importance of load and go. Fluid therapy should be minimal to avoid coagulopathy and to avoid the disruption of clot formation. Treat pain, being aware of morphine's hypotensive side effects. In-hospital treatment includes large-bore access (if not already achieved out of hospital), blood transfusions and urgent surgical intervention.

Embolic and thrombotic disease
Portal venous thrombus, a blood clot in the portal venous system, may occur in patients with clotting risk factors who are generally not on anticoagulation or antiplatelet treatment. Mesenteric arterial ischaemia is a potential complication of atrial fibrillation and often presents with severe pain out of proportion to clinical findings.

(Ruptured) ectopic pregnancy
Anatomy/pathology
An ectopic pregnancy is a pregnancy that is outside the uterus. Given the vascular innervation of any fetus, because an ectopic pregnancy cannot be maintained the entire gestation, it will at some point rupture. This has the likely potential for causing severe internal haemorrhage.

Epidemiology/significance
Ectopic pregnancies typically present 6–8 weeks after the last menstrual period (LMP), but can be later, depending on the location of the ectopic pregnancy.

Clinical presentations
Vaginal bleeding and abdominal pain are the commonest symptom. Up to 18% of vaginal bleeds in first trimester are ectopic (Casanova et al., 2009).

Diagnosis
Work-up in ED includes serum beta hCG levels and ultrasound.

Treatment
Treatment includes transport, pain relief and fluid resuscitation.

Perforation
Perforated viscus
Anatomy/pathology
A hollow viscus has the potential to perforate, which allows bacteria to enter the sterile peritoneal cavity, causing peritonitis.

Epidemiology/significance
Most perforated organs require antibiotics and operative intervention.

Clinical presentations
Patients with a perforation will often be symptomatic, with sudden severe pain and peritoneal irritation. Risk factors (e.g. GI instrumentation, foreign body ingestion, peptic/gastric ulcer disease and medication such as NSAIDs and steroids) are often present.

Diagnosis
Work-up in ED includes erect chest x-ray to look for free air under the diaphragm (indicative of a perforation) and CT imaging to locate the source and extent.

Treatment
Treatment involves transport and symptom relief. Metoclopramide is contraindicated as stimulation of the bowel can worsen the perforation.

Obstruction
Bowel obstruction
Bowel obstruction is the partial or complete blockage of the lumen of the small or large intestine, which impedes the flow of intestinal contents. Obstruction

may be due to mechanical or neurogenic causes. Mechanical obstruction can be a simple or closed-loop obstruction. Closed-loop obstruction is more sinister as the bowel is obstructed at two points causing a loop, such as if it twists on itself or is caught in the opening of a hernia. This type of obstruction can potentially result in compromised blood flow and subsequent ischaemia of the bowel, which is commonly referred to as strangulation (Torrey & Henneman, 2010). Neurogenic bowel obstruction, also known as adynamic ileus, is obstruction that occurs as a consequence of disturbance of gut motility. In neurogenic obstruction, the flow of intestinal contents is impeded because of a failure of peristalsis rather than a physical blockage (Torrey & Henneman, 2010).

Mechanical bowel obstruction occurs as a consequence of adhesions that often act as a tethering point to allow twisting and hence obstruction. Mechanical bowel obstruction can also occur with bowel cancer, causing a progressive stricture. Entrapment of the bowel within a hernia is a common cause of bowel obstruction. Less common causes include inflammatory diseases like Crohn's and intussusception, where the bowel is folded in on itself. Many of these conditions are more likely in elderly patients, hence the extreme caution when assessing an elderly patient with some abdominal pain and an alteration in bowel habit of any sort.

Complete obstruction to the lumen of the bowel prevents the onward passage of the contents of the bowel proximal to the obstruction. Early in the course of the disease, normal GI activities take place and the lumen of the bowel proximal to the obstruction fills with secretions and swallowed air. Distension of the lumen results and peristalsis above and below the obstruction is stimulated, so frequent loose bowel motions may accompany bowel obstruction in the early stages (Torrey & Henneman, 2010). Peristaltic activity becomes more intense and frequent in an attempt to overcome the obstruction; this gives rise to colicky abdominal pain. As the bowel becomes fatigued, peristaltic activity ultimately decreases and stops.

Distension of the lumen also triggers the normal GI response that occurs when distension is due to food (i.e. secretion of intestinal juices, electrolytes and fluids), which serves to increase the volume of fluid in the lumen (Hayanga et al., 2005). A point is ultimately reached where the hydrostatic pressure within the lumen of the gut is greater than that in the mucosal lymphatics, with resultant obstruction to lymph flow and swelling of the bowel wall. The changes in pressure in the lumen and walls of the bowel alter the reabsorptive capacity of the mucous membrane and the fluid dynamics of the capillaries in the gut. Movement of proteins and fluids across the capillaries into the gut lumen ensues. Such 'third space' losses of fluid from the circulating volume into the gut can be extensive and lead to hypovolaemic shock (Hayanga et al., 2005).

Intestinal stasis occurs as a consequence of obstruction. This leads to the proliferation of intestinal bacteria and an increase in intestinal gas and other products of fermentation, which worsen luminal distension (Cappell & Batke, 2008). As intraluminal pressure continues to rise, the arterial supply to the gut ultimately becomes compromised and ischaemia can ensue, leading to necrosis, bowel perforation, peritonitis and sepsis. More commonly this occurs because of interruption to the mesenteric supply of blood to part of the distended bowel, which has become so large it twists on itself and causes strangulation (Hayanga et al., 2005).

Treatment
Do not give metoclopramide, as stimulation of the bowel in this setting is dangerous.

Renal stones
Renal colic produces severe intermittent, wave-like (i.e. colic) pain in the back, flank or abdomen. Blood in the urine is another diagnostic clue, although it is often only microscopic. Management includes adequate analgesia and transfer to hospital for definitive diagnosis and ruling out associated complications such as infection and renal impairment.

Urinary retention
Urinary retention, typically due to prostate enlargement or a blocked catheter, can cause severe lower abdominal pain and agitation. Urgent relief from insertion, or clearing of preexisting, catheter is required.

Pressure
Ascites
Ascites is a condition where there is a pathological accumulation of fluid in the abdominal cavity. In 85% of cases, liver cirrhosis is the underlying cause (Cesario et al., 2010; Kalia et al., 2012). Ascites develop in patients secondary to the development of portal hypertension—an increase in blood pressure in the portal vein (see Fig 31.9).

In the normal liver, hepatic vessel diameter, and hence blood flow within the liver, is balanced between the effects of nitric oxide (NO), which promotes vasodilation, and endothelin-1 (ET-1), which promotes vasoconstriction. In cirrhosis, the liver becomes nodular and fibrotic and production of these substances is affected: for unknown reasons, levels of NO decrease and levels of ET-1 increase.

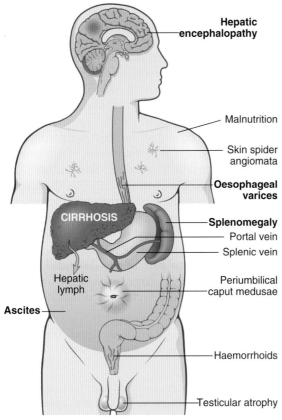

Figure 31.9
Major clinical consequences of portal hypertension due to cirrhosis. In women, oligomenorrhoea, amenorrhoea and sterility are frequent, as a result of hypogonadism.
Source: Kumar et al. (2009).

The net effect is marked vasoconstriction of hepatic vessels and increased hepatic resistance to blood flow. Other vasoactive mediators such as angiotensin and thromboxane, which are elevated in cirrhosis, are also thought to contribute to increased hepatic resistance. In addition, cirrhosis affects the architecture of the hepatic vessels causing a reduction in vessel diameter and compounding the effects of vasoactive mediators (Shah & Kamath, 2010).

In cirrhosis, the high vascular resistance creates portal hypertension. Ultimately, this leads to leakage of hepatic lymphatic fluid from the surface of the liver into the abdominal cavity. This fluid then becomes known as ascites fluid (Arroyo & Navasa, 2007). Once formed, the ascites fluid is in dynamic exchange with capillaries in the visceral peritoneum and dependent on the continued process of sodium and water retention (Garcia-Tsao, 2011).

This patient appears to be suffering from ascites. Patients with alcoholic liver cirrhosis will provide a history of chronic alcohol use over decades. Men who consume 40–80 g of alcohol (4–8 standard drinks) per day over 10–12 years are at significant risk of developing alcoholic liver disease. Other factors that compound this risk are smoking and obesity (Carithers & McClain, 2010). Patients suffering from chronic ascites are often on spironolactone. Spironolactone is a potassium-sparing diuretic that promotes sodium loss from the body by blocking the effect of aldosterone (secreted by the adrenal cortex) on the distal renal tubules and collecting ducts.

At least 1500 mL of ascetic fluid must be in the abdomen for it to be detected on abdominal examination (Kalia et al., 2012). This patient's large, bulging abdomen indicates that a much larger volume will be present. Umbilical hernias develop in 20% of patients with ascites due to intraabdominal pressure (Garcia-Tsao, 2011).

Hernias

Hernias can present in several spots in the abdominal and groin area. Reduction (i.e. pushing the lump back in) should be done if the obstruction has not been going on for too long (i.e. < 4 hours). Reduction can be facilitated by laying the patient flat, or even in the Trendelenburg position. Failure to reduce the hernia requires urgent transport to hospital for further attempts or surgical management to avoid ischaemia of the content of the hernia.

A key part of the out-of-hospital management of patients with abdominal pain is symptomatic relief with analgesia and antiemetics. Considering the potential aetiologies for the patient's presentation is necessary in order to provide safe and effective treatment. Table 31.1 provides an overview of commonly used analgesics and antiemetics, their dosing and considerations.

Table 31.1 Overview of commonly used analgesics and antiemetics

Symptom	Delivery	Typical dose	Contraindications	Comments
Pain				
Methoxyflurane	Inhaled	3 mL × 2	Renal disease; tetracycline antibiotics; susceptibility to MH; muscular dystrophy	Pain relief onset after 6–10 breaths; analgesia lasts for several minutes after stopping
Paracetamol	PO/IV	500 mg × 2	Na⁺ restrictions (because paracetamol contains large amounts of sodium); phenylketonuria (because paracetamol may contain aspartame)	There is no evidence to caution against the use of paracetamol in patients with liver failure
Morphine	IV/IM/ subcutaneous	2.5–10 mg	Renal impairment (because active metabolites accumulate and may cause respiratory depression and delirium); severe hepatic impairment (because it may cause excessive sedation); late second stage of labour	Avoid in pancreatitis (due to spasm of sphincter of Oddi); reduce dose in renal impairment (due to accumulation); be aware of the drop in BP and respiration
Fentanyl	IN/IV	25–200 microgram	Late second stage of labour (as it may cause respiratory depression in the newborn)	Avoid the IN route in those with facial trauma or an unclear nostril (e.g. rhinitis)
Nausea/vomiting				
Metoclopramide	PO/IV	10 mg TDS	Any conditions where increased GI motility may be harmful (e.g. GI haemorrhage, obstruction, perforation); < 20 years old and renal impairment (because there is an increased risk of extrapyramidal side effects); phaeochromocytoma	Due to the risks associated with metoclopramide, some ambulance services have chosen to no longer carry any
Ondansetron	PO/IV	4–8 mg TDS	Phenylketonuria (as it contains aspartame); prolonged QTc interval or conditions potentially causing prolonged QTc (e.g. hypokalaemia and hypomagnesaemia); concurrent apomorphine use (as the combination may cause profound hypotension)	Avoid in first trimester of pregnancy
Prochlorperazine	PO/IV/IM	PO 10–20 mg IM/IV 12.5 mg	CNS depression and Parkinson's disease; children (< 2 years old)	IV administration of prochlorperazine (i.e. Stemetil) is generally avoided and if necessary done slowly over at least 2 minutes
Isopropyl alcohol	Sniff	1–2 alcohol wipes	Patients in which alcohol administration is contraindicated (e.g. cephalosporin antibiotics, disulfiram and metronidazole)	Aromatherapy with isopropyl alcohol provides greater nausea relief than oral ondansetron alone

NSAIDs = nonsteroidal anti-inflammatory drugs; PO = oral; IM = intramuscular; IV = intravenous; IN = intranasal; TDS = three times a day; BP = blood pressure; MH = malignant hyperthermia.

Source: April et al. (2018) and Australian Medicines Handbook (2020).

CASE STUDY 1

Case: 11064, 2134 hrs.

Dispatch details: A 25-year-old female with abdominal pain and vomiting for 36 hours, now in severe pain.

Initial presentation: The ambulance crew arrive to find the patient slightly flushed, lying quietly on her side in bed with her legs bent, covered by a duvet. A damp washcloth and empty bowl are beside the bed.

 ASSESS

Patient history

The patient states the pain came on yesterday morning in the middle of the tummy shortly after she arrived at work. She had had a light breakfast of cereal and a single episode of vomiting. She remained at work but lost her appetite. She came home, took some paracetamol, had a warm shower and went straight to bed. She woke this morning with the worse pain migrating towards the lower abdomen on the right side. Throughout the day she has developed chills and as her analgesia is no longer working, she phoned for an ambulance.

Regarding the pain, question using the SOCRATES acronym (site, onset, character, radiation, associated symptoms, time course, exacerbating/alleviating factors and severity). Ask about similar previous episodes, bowel changes and past medical history (including abdominal surgery suggesting presence of adhesions) (Avunduk, 2008). This patient has no past medical history. Ask about the presence of infective symptoms such as fevers, chills or rigors. Ask about the time of the LMP (with concern for pregnancy/ectopic pregnancy if inexplicably overdue, or for gynaecological pathology particularly midcycle). This patient had a normal menstrual period 10 days ago. Ask about drug and alcohol use (with consideration for pancreatitis or liver disease) (Poston, 2005), which this patient denies. Recent travel may be helpful diagnostically if the patient presents with fever or diarrhoea (Flasar & Goldberg, 2006). This patient has not travelled recently. Ask about urinary tract infection (UTI) symptoms (e.g. dysuria, frequency, urgency) to rule out a likely differential diagnosis. She denies UTI symptoms.

General appearance

The patient lies in a curled position and is minimising movement—a behaviour consistent with peritonitis.

Airway/breathing/circulation

A: The patient is fully conscious and managing her own airway.

B: She takes shallow breaths and has a slightly elevated respiratory rate of 24 bpm. Auscultation of her chest reveals no abnormal or adventitious sounds. Pneumonia of the lower lobes of the lungs can lead to inflammation of the diaphragm and progression of this inflammation to the organs in the upper quadrants of the abdomen. The location of the abdominal pain (central and lower) and the absence of abnormal breath sounds exclude an obvious respiratory cause for her abdominal pain.

PRACTICE TIP

A change in vital signs in a patient with abdominal pain is indicative of serious pathology (Flasar & Goldberg, 2006; McNamara & Dean, 2011).

C: Vital signs assessment of the patient indicates a sinus tachycardia of 115 bpm (confirmed with cardiac monitor) and a blood pressure of 125/65 mmHg. Her temperature is 38.5°C, suggesting an infective process is present. Appendicitis can be associated initially with low-grade fever that becomes more elevated as the pathology worsens but it is important not to confirm links prematurely. Fever is also associated with gastroenteritis and UTI. Rigors are more commonly present with urinary and biliary infections (Platt et al., 2008) and, along with painful or offensive-smelling urine, is a worthwhile symptom to explore.

GI system

Observation of the patient's abdomen reveals no old scars (which might indicate past surgery and risk for obstruction). A tense abdomen that is not moving normally with respiration is consistent with peritonitis as is the patient bracing the abdomen to avoid pain with respiratory movement. This patient indicates that her whole abdomen is tender and that pressure anywhere on her abdomen produces pain, although it is sharpest over the right iliac fossa even when the pressure is in the left lower quadrant (i.e. Rovsing's sign). Identification of the duration and volume of diarrhoea and vomiting, including a description of the vomitus, is important to potentially exclude bowel obstruction and to quantify degree of dehydration. In surgical conditions, such as appendicitis, vomiting usually occurs after the onset of pain and is not pronounced (McNamara & Dean, 2011). Vomiting is associated with appendicitis in 75% of cases (Jaffe & Berger, 2010). A change in frequency and consistency of bowel motions can provide useful information: constipation is associated with bowel obstruction and diarrhoea with gastroenteritis. With appendicitis, constipation is more frequently reported than diarrhoea (Jaffe & Berger, 2010).

Gynaecological system

A gynaecological history must be taken when assessing females presenting with abdominal pain (Soon & Hardy, 2002). For women of childbearing age, identify the date of their LMP and ascertain the possibility of pregnancy. In pregnant women the differential diagnosis should include ectopic pregnancy, threatened abortion, endometriosis and ovarian cysts (see Table 31.2 for the characteristics of abdominal pain of a gynaecological cause). In this patient a history of a normal menstrual period 10 days ago with no subsequent bleeding excludes the potential for pregnancy as a cause of abdominal pain and is a little early for mid-cycle pain associated with follicular rupture. The severity of the pain with no previous abdominal discomfort is not typical of ovarian disease or endometriosis, but neither can be ruled out conclusively at this stage.

Pain

The onset of vague abdominal pain 36 hours previously, gradually getting worse, is a typical progression of appendicitis. Worsening of the pain and migration to the right iliac fossa is indicative of peritoneal involvement and the generalised spread suggests appendiceal rupture and generalised peritonitis.

Initial assessment summary

Problem	Generalised abdominal pain
Conscious state	GCS 15
Position	Lying on her side with her knees up
Heart rate	115 bpm
Blood pressure	125/65 mmHg
Skin appearance	Pale, hot, dry
Speech pattern	Speaks in sentences

> ## PRACTICE TIP
>
> Performing a full abdominal examination including percussion and auscultation takes time and may cause the patient significant pain. Although the examination provides valuable information, in a metropolitan setting it is unlikely to change the paramedic's course of action. However, in a rural setting where the decision to transport can involve prolonged timeframes (and significant expense), extra time spent on the examination may be worthwhile.

Table 31.2 Typical presentations of gynaecological pain

Condition	Onset	Quality	Location	Radiation/symptoms	Vaginal discharge	Menstrual cycle
Ruptured ectopic pregnancy	Rapid	Constant	Unilateral (can become diffuse with time)	Shoulder tip (may indicate intraperitoneal bleeding) Syncope	Bleeding in most cases, may be severe	Typically overdue (≥ 6 weeks since last period)
Dysmenorrhoea	Gradual	Sharp to crampy	Diffuse, central to bilateral	Nil	Usually precedes bleeding	Due within 36 hours
Endometriosis	Gradual	Sharp to crampy	Diffuse, central to bilateral	Nil Dyspareunia	Some bleeding	Usually during
Pelvic inflammatory disease (PID)	Gradual	Steady ache	Diffuse, bilateral	Right upper quadrant Fever, malaise	Mucopurulent	Typically 5–7 days after period
Ruptured ovarian cyst	Sudden; peaks early and may subside	May be sharp initially then constant	Unilateral (can become diffuse with time)	Shoulder tip (may indicate intraperitoneal bleeding)	Some bleeding likely	Typically 5–7 days before period
Spontaneous abortion	Sudden to gradual	Crampy to constant	Central, diffuse, may radiate to back	Nil Fever, nausea	May occur, typically prior to pain	Typically overdue (≥ 6 weeks since last period)

Source: Adapted from Sanders (2007).

Respiratory rate	24 bpm
Respiratory rhythm	Even cycles
Chest auscultation	Good air entry bilaterally
Pulse oximetry	98%
Temperature	38.5°C
Motor/sensory function	Normal
Pain	7/10
History	Onset 36 hours ago. Started as mild central before moving to the right iliac fossa and now has become generalised. Associated with vomiting and fever and no bowel actions since the onset of the pain.
Physical assessment	The patient is guarding her abdomen; very tender abdomen on palpation.

The patient's presentation is consistent with perforated appendicitis, now causing generalised peritonitis. Abnormal vital signs (tachycardia and fever) suggest a condition that is likely to deteriorate further.

 CONFIRM

The essential part of the clinical reasoning process is to seek to confirm your initial hypothesis by finding clinical signs that should occur with your provisional diagnosis. You should also seek to challenge your diagnosis by exploring findings that do not fit your hypothesis.

What else could it be?

Revisiting the list of differentials is worthwhile after a suspicion of peritonitis is present.

Differential diagnoses
- Most likely
  - › Peritonitis (given the widespread peritoneal pain) from appendicitis (given the typical history and absence of other features)
- Most serious not to miss
  - › Ruptured ectopic pregnancy
    - ■ Unlikely given the recent normal menstrual cycle and the presence of fever
  - › Anaphylaxis
    - ■ Although patients with anaphylaxis can present with profound nausea and possible vomiting, intense abdominal cramping and diarrhoea, anaphylaxis is not supported in this patient as there are no skin or other systemic signs, no respiratory wheeze, no history of previous allergy, no presence of allergens and no hypotension.
- Other potential serious causes
  - › Acute myocardial infarction (AMI)
    - ■ Patients with AMI, particularly inferior wall AMI leading to irritation of the diaphragm, can present with epigastric or less commonly lower abdominal pain. In all patients with abdominal pain, careful history taking is required to rule out AMI, particularly in patients at high risk of cardiac disease. In this case study, the patient's age, sex and pain history all support a non-cardiac cause for her abdominal pain. The patient also presents with signs of peritoneal irritation and warm dry skin, which support an abdominal pathology as the cause of her symptoms. However, despite this she should be monitored and if there is any possibility of a cardiac cause a 12-lead ECG is indicated. Cardiac complications from the inflammatory process of appendicitis need to be considered as well as a primary cardiac condition. Atrial fibrillation and acute ischaemia have both been observed in young patients with appendicitis, though rare.
  - › Diabetic ketoacidosis (DKA)
    - ■ Patients with DKA can present with symptoms that include abdominal pain. Abdominal pain can be due to abdominal pathologies and actually precipitate DKA, or it can be part of the symptomatology of DKA itself with the severity of the pain correlating directly with the level of acidosis (Laine et al., 2010). This patient's symptoms have developed slightly more rapidly than expected for DKA. She also does not have a ketotic (sweet) smelling breath and no Kussmaul breaths. If there is doubt, a normal random blood sugar test will be diagnostic.
  - › Pneumonia
    - ■ Patients with lower lobe pneumonia can present with epigastric, and sometimes lower abdominal, pain due to irritation of the diaphragm. This patient is slightly febrile which would go together with chest infection, but with a clear chest and no productive cough a respiratory infection is not supported.

> **PRACTICE TIP**
>
> In the out-of-hospital setting, the critical aspect of clinical judgment in patients with abdominal pain is to ensure that life-threatening conditions from other body systems are considered and either included or excluded as the cause of the pain.

(3) TREAT

Emergency management

This patient is at risk of her condition worsening as her peritonitis progresses and she is in need of immediate surgery. Although she is normotensive, her tachycardia, fever, vomiting and absence of food for 36 hours makes underlying or pending dehydration likely. She should therefore be given fluid resuscitation. Additionally, she should get symptom relief and urgent transport.

The priorities of emergency management are outlined in Box 31.1.

> ## BOX 31.1 Principles of management of the acute abdomen
>
> - Fluid resuscitation
> - Pain relief
> - Relief of other symptoms, but avoid prokinetics (e.g. metoclopramide)
> - Transport for diagnosis and definitive care with pre-notification

Fluid resuscitation

The inflammatory process of peritonitis will precipitate a general vasodilation and loss of fluid from the capillaries, as well as exudate accumulation in the abdomen. If indicated by assessment, fluid resuscitation may be needed.

Pain relief

Administration of narcotic analgesics to patients with abdominal pain before definitive diagnosis has been controversial for many years, but it is now clear that use of narcotic analgesics for patients with acute abdominal pain 'does not increase the risk of diagnosis error or the risk of error in making decisions regarding treatment' (Manterola et al., 2011) and that narcotics 'can safely be given before full assessment and diagnosis in acute abdominal pain (Level 1 evidence)' (National Institute of Clinical Studies, 2008).

Relief of other symptoms

This patient has experienced nausea and vomiting and requires surgery. The effect of peritoneal irritation will be the development of a paralytic ileus, so making the patient 'nil by mouth' is required to minimise the risk of vomiting and reduce the risk of aspiration of stomach contents during induction of anaesthesia. Use of intravenous antiemetics is indicated for the patient's nausea. Ondansetron or prochlorperazine can be considered according to local guidelines. Metoclopramide is contraindicated in cases of perforation, or other situations where bowel stimulations can be dangerous. Sniffing an alcohol wipe (isopropyl) is increasingly evidenced as effective (April et al., 2018).

Transport

The patient needs to be transported to hospital for further investigation and surgery. Presence of peritonitis warrants urgent transport. One issue to consider is that movement will exacerbate the peritoneal irritation and therefore increase the pain. In fact, pain worsening when travelling over speed bumps is also a diagnostic clue towards appendicitis (perforated or not), with a positive predictive value of ~60% (Ashdown et al., 2012).

 ## EVALUATE

The expected response to the emergency management of this patient is a slight improvement in hydration status and comfort. Her central venous pressure as observed by neck veins and dilated veins on the dorsum of her hands will act as feedback. Her pain management needs to be assessed during transport, noting that once she stops moving she will have much less stimulus. The ideal endpoint for pain relief should be just short of complete analgesia because once stimulation is reduced the analgesia will be more effective.

Ongoing management in hospital

Following initial emergency management, the key decision will be to confirm whether the patient requires surgery and the possible approach to that surgery. Radiographic studies, blood studies and serial physical examination will be carried out in this instance. Serial physical examination in such patients has not been associated with any increase in perforation rate (Wolfe & Henneman, 2010) and one of the advantages of admitting patients to hospital is the ability to perform serial observations over a period of time if there is any doubt about the need for immediate surgery. Patients managed by observation will take one of two courses: 1. diagnosis of appendicitis or another condition requiring surgery; or 2. discharge home in the reliable care of family or friends with a follow-up medical appointment, instructions about what to do if symptoms worsen and guidance on gradual resumption of normal dietary intake (Wolfe & Henneman, 2010).

Hospital admission

These patients will undergo further assessment at hospital. Surgical intervention is likely if they have peritonitis. For uncomplicated CT-proven simple appendicitis, some centres are moving towards antibiotic therapy alone (Salminen et al., 2015).

CASE STUDY 2

Case 14064, 1523 hrs.

Dispatch details: A 45-year-old male with abdominal pain, vomiting and diarrhoea.

Initial presentation: The ambulance crew arrive to find the patient curled up in bed, shivering and covered by blankets.

ASSESS

The patient explains that he has colicky abdominal pain and has been suffering from vomiting and frequent diarrhoea, with small amounts of blood in it, which started a few hours after a buffet lunch at work. He says that he has no significant previous medical history. He has not travelled overseas nor been in contact with anyone else that has been unwell.

Initial assessment summary

Problem	Abdominal pain, vomiting, diarrhoea
Conscious state	GCS 15
Position	Curled up in bed
Heart rate	98 bpm
Blood pressure	135/77 mmHg
Skin appearance	Warm and dry
Speech pattern	Speaks in sentences
Respiratory rate	20 bpm
Respiratory rhythm	Even cycles, good air entry bilaterally
Temperature	37.3°C
Physical assessment	Heart and lungs clear; abdomen soft not tender

CONFIRM

In many cases paramedics are presented with a collection of signs and symptoms that do not appear to describe a particular condition. A critical step in determining a treatment plan in this situation is to consider what other conditions could explain the patient's presentation.

What else could it be?
Differential diagnoses

- Most likely
  - › Gastroenteritis
    - Given the exposure to a potential food source, and vomiting plus diarrhoea plus colicky abdominal pain
- Most serious not to miss
  - › Ruptured AAA
    - Unlikely given the absence of other vascular risk factors (e.g. hypertension or hypercholesterolaemia) as well as haemodynamically not compromised. Vomiting from pain secondary to AAA is possible, but diarrhoea would not occur.
  - › Appendicitis
    - Unlikely as appendicitis is typically paraumbilical pain which later localises to the right iliac fossa. Although the central colicky abdominal pain the patient is experiencing could be early appendicitis, diarrhoea is unusual unless the patient's appendix is located behind the ileum or protrudes into the pelvic cavity. Vomiting is a late sign in appendicitis. A key defining feature of gastroenteritis as compared to appendicitis is the pain pattern. This patient's pain is colicky and generalised across the abdomen. Also, blood in the diarrhoea is not usually associated with appendicitis.
  - › Intestinal obstruction
    - Unlikely as this patient does not have any previous abdominal surgery. In the presence of intestinal obstruction there would also be signs of distension and complaints of bloating. Bloody diarrhoea is not consistent with intestinal obstruction.
  - › Inflammatory bowel disease
    - Gastroenteritis and inflammatory bowel disease (i.e. Crohn's disease and ulcerative colitis) share some common clinical features, but with no previous history of inflammatory bowel disease it is unlikely. The presence of mucus in addition to blood might suggest inflammatory bowel disease. Extra-intestinal manifestations (e.g. finger clubbing) may be present, but is of minimal diagnostic aid in the out-of-hospital field.

 TREAT

Emergency management

The emergency management of this patient is rehydration, correction of electrolyte abnormalities and symptom relief. If the patient can drink, this is achieved with oral fluids, electrolyte solution and oral analgesia. This patient may require IV fluids and antiemetic; IV opiates are not usually needed.

Fluid resuscitation

Fluid resuscitation can be achieved by intravenous or oral intake, depending on the severity of vomiting and degree of hypovolaemia. However, if there is any doubt about the diagnosis, and a surgical cause is a possibility, then it is safest to avoid the oral route and keep the patient nil by mouth (NBM).

Pain relief

Administration of analgesics to patients with gastroenteritis is reasonable, but should rarely require opioids. Buscopan (hyoscine butylbromide), which the patient might have at home, can aid in relieving abdominal cramps.

Relief of other symptoms

Nausea and vomiting may be treated with ondansetron, metoclopramide or sniffing an alcohol wipe (isopropyl).

Transport

Most severely symptomatic gastroenteritis patients need transportation to hospital for further investigation. However, it must be remembered that acute gastroenteritis carries infectious control needs.

(4) EVALUATE

Evaluating the effect of any clinical management intervention can provide clues to the accuracy of the initial diagnosis. Some conditions respond rapidly to treatment so patients should be expected to improve if the diagnosis and treatment were appropriate, whereas other conditions are unlikely to respond in the timeframes normally associated with ambulance transport times. In such cases, a failure to improve should not be considered an indication of a misdiagnosis.

In this case pain relief should be effective, although the reduction in nausea and vomiting from antiemetic administration can be variable. Intravenous fluids should maintain or slightly improve the patient's perfusion status but the effect is likely to be minimal.

Priorities for ongoing management are focused on rehydration and correction of electrolyte abnormalities, management of symptoms and potential complications, prevention of the spread of infection and consideration of public health measures (see Box 31.2). Most cases of gastroenteritis are short-lived and self-limiting and few patients are admitted to hospital from the emergency department, unless there is significant co-morbidity or need for lengthy correction of imbalances.

BOX 31.2 Public health issues: acute gastroenteritis

The public health issues relating to acute gastroenteritis comprise containing and preventing the spread of infection. For this reason, paramedics should determine whether the patient absolutely requires transport to hospital or can be managed at home. Key messages relating to proper food preparation, storage and reheating, and personal hygiene (with an emphasis on handwashing) are the responsibility of all healthcare professionals.

Out-of-hospital awareness of the importance of preventing the spread of infection means seeking information about family members and friends who have been in contact with the patient. Close contacts can either transmit the infection or become infected themselves, and paramedics may need to recommend that they seek medical attention. Simple public health measures such as handwashing and using hand sanitiser do a great deal to limit the spread of gastroenteritis to those who may not have the immune capacity to respond to it.

CASE STUDY 3

Case 12064, 2134 hrs.

Dispatch details: A 63-year-old male with increasing abdominal pain and shortness of breath.

Initial presentation: The ambulance crew finds a middle-aged man with sallow complexion sitting back in his lounge chair. His abdomen appears very large.

 ASSESS

The patient states he has had this pain before, but that it has got worse in the last few days. The patient admits to have been drinking heavily and that there are some liver issues, but he does not take any regular medications.

Initial assessment summary

Problem	Vomiting and abdominal pain
Conscious state	GCS 15
Position	Sitting slumped in chair
Heart rate	98 bpm
Blood pressure	145/95 mmHg
Skin appearance	Cool and dry
Speech pattern	Speaks in sentences
Respiratory rate	28 bpm
Respiratory rhythm	Shallow respiration, good air entry bilaterally Sats 94% on room air
Temperature	36.9°C
Physical assessment	Shallow complexion. Tense large abdomen with a protruding umbilical hernia.

 CONFIRM

The presentation appears to suggest ascites (intraabdominal fluid associated with cirrhosis of the liver) that is causing pain and respiratory embarrassment because of the pressure effect of the large volume of fluid in the abdomen.

What else could it be?

Revisiting the list of differentials is worthwhile after a suspicion of ascites is present.

Differential diagnoses
- Most likely
  - Ascites, from alcoholic cirrhosis
- Most serious not to miss
  - Ruptured AAA
    - Must be considered in elderly men with abdominal pain, but the separation of the muscular media from the elastic outer external wall of the abdominal aorta typically causes a sharp, sudden and 'tearing' abdominal pain. If the externa ruptures, the patient will quickly

exsanguinate with the blood loss accumulating in the abdominal cavity. The initial pain is often associated with a brief syncopal episode as the initial aneurysm triggers a fall in blood pressure. This patient has indeed risk factors for AAA, but the presentation is not consistent, and the perfusion status does not reflect a ruptured AAA pathology.

> Anaphylaxis
  - It is always good to consider anaphylaxis when dealing with abdominal pain, especially when accompanied by shortness of breath. But absence of hypotension, wheeze, rash and acute onset makes it unlikely.

- Other potential serious causes
> AMI
  - Can present as abdominal pain and shortness of breath. However, an AMI will often be accompanied by some degree of chest pain, nausea or diaphoresis. Twelve-lead ECG is not unreasonable. Treatment with aspirin based on presumed cardiac cause needs to be weighed up against the most likely cause and the potential damage aspirin might have if the presentation is more consistent with a bleeding pathology.
> Pneumonia
  - Lower lobe pneumonia can present with abdominal pain. The shortness of breath is another supportive factor. But absence of cough, fever and the presence of a clear chest makes it unlikely.
> Congestive cardiac failure
  - Congestive cardiac failure due to alcoholic cardiomyopathy is the cause of ascites in less than 5% of patients with ascites (Runyon, 2010). This patient has no history of cardiac disease and on physical examination his chest is clear. Congestive cardiac failure is an unlikely cause for his ascites.

③ TREAT

This patient presents with acute abdominal pain and shortness of breath due to ascites secondary to alcoholic cirrhosis. The priorities of emergency management are symptom relief and transport.

An opiate such as morphine is usually used for analgesia, but morphine is primarily metabolised in the liver and so its effect will be prolonged in this case. As a result, adjustments will need to be made to this patient's morphine regimen.

As this patient is experiencing shortness of breath due to the large volume of ascites fluid in his abdomen, he should be supported in a position of comfort.

④ EVALUATE

Evaluating the effect of any clinical management intervention can provide clues to the accuracy of the initial diagnosis. Some conditions respond rapidly to treatment so patients should be expected to improve if the diagnosis and treatment were appropriate, whereas other conditions are unlikely to respond in the timeframes normally associated with ambulance transport times. In such cases, a failure to improve should not be considered an indication of a misdiagnosis.

In this case pain relief should be effective, although the primary improvements will come from positioning the patient to allow for normal diaphragmatic movement. Ambulance stretchers are not suited to this, so transporting the patient in a seated position may be more effective. Supplemental oxygen will assist in reducing the dyspnoea. Provided the patient is well-positioned, the paramedics should expect to see a slight improvement in this patient during transport.

Priorities for ongoing management are focused on relief of symptoms and control of the ascites. Blood will need to be drawn for normal analysis of liver and kidney function markers. A priority for this patient is to perform abdominal paracentesis (drainage of some of the ascetic fluid) and withdraw ascites fluid to relieve his respiratory and abdominal symptoms (Runyon, 2010; Garcia-Tsao, 2011). Paracentesis is a safe procedure, with a complication rate of less than 1% (Cesario et al., 2010). Serial paracentesis may be required.

 CASE STUDY 4

Case 12064, 2134 hrs.

Dispatch details: A 76-year-old male with sudden onset of lower back and groin pain.

Initial presentation: The ambulance crew arrive to find a pale, overweight elderly man lying on the couch. He appears distressed.

 ASSESS

The patient states that he has not had this pain before. It started suddenly in the lumbar back and the general abdomen while he was just seated. He is now feeling faint. To direct questioning, he admits to having high blood pressure and a small myocardial infarction 6 years ago. He used to smoke, but quit after he had his heart attack. The pain is described as sharp, severe and constant.

Initial assessment summary

Problem	Back pain and abdominal pain
Conscious state	GCS 14 (confused to time)
Position	Lying on couch
Heart rate	115 bpm
Blood pressure	105/70 mmHg
Skin appearance	Cool and clammy
Speech pattern	Speaks in sentences
Respiratory rate	24 bpm
Respiratory rhythm	Shallow respiration, clear and good air entry bilaterally
Temperature	36.9°C
Physical assessment	Pale appearance; pulsating mass is felt in the abdomen

 CONFIRM

The presentation appears to suggest an AAA (given the risk factors) and that it has ruptured (given the sudden onset and the now haemodynamic compromise). It is important to appreciate that a systolic blood pressure of 105 mmHg is not reassuring in the elderly—and certainly not in the patient with preexisting hypertension.

What else could it be?

Revisiting the list of differentials is worthwhile after a suspicion of AAA is present. However, there are no more urgent causes that need ruling in or out

PRACTICE TIP

The presence of neurological signs (e.g. syncope) and back pain/abdominal pain should prompt the clinician to consider AAA.

in the out-of-hospital setting. Absence of trauma and onset at rest excludes musculoskeletal causes. Renal colic can present suddenly, but will typically be colicky as the stone migrates down the urinary system.

3 TREAT

Patients with a suspected ruptured AAA may survive the initial rupture but further bleeding will follow and haemodynamic deterioration will ultimately ensue if the patient is not diagnosed and treated promptly. Urgent transport to hospital is mandatory. It is important to remember that any preexisting coronary vascular disease (which patients at risk of AAA often have) might cause cardiac ischaemia from blood loss and hypovolaemia.

Fluid resuscitation

Two large-bore intravenous cannulae should be inserted, one in each of the patient's arms, but transport should not be delayed. Actual fluid administration should be cautious, giving only enough fluid to maintain a palpable pulse (carotid) and the patient's consciousness level. Permissive hypotension should be maintained until the operating theatre, when haemorrhage can be directly controlled. The therapeutic aim should be to achieve a blood pressure that is sufficient to maintain perfusion of the vital organs. Although this varies from patient to patient, a target of 80–100 mmHg systolic is suggested (Bessen, 2010).

Pain relief

While provision of analgesia is humane, this patient may well lose his blood pressure if opiates are used. This is one situation where analgesia should be used very cautiously, or not at all. Keep the patient nil by mouth in anticipation of surgery.

4 EVALUATE

Evaluating the effect of any clinical management intervention can provide clues to the accuracy of the initial diagnosis. Some conditions respond rapidly to treatment so patients should be expected to improve if the diagnosis and treatment were appropriate, whereas other conditions are unlikely to respond in the timeframes normally associated with ambulance transport times.

In such cases, a failure to improve should not be considered an indication of a misdiagnosis. In this case, the lack of effective treatment options available to paramedics means that the crew should not expect any improvement in the patient's condition during transport. In fact, depending on the extent of the bleeding, the patient may continue to deteriorate during transport as the blood pressure reduces.

Ongoing management

On arrival in ED the clinical priority will be to continue resuscitative efforts, confirm a diagnosis of a ruptured AAA and prepare the patient for urgent surgical haemostasis and repair of the defect. Bedside ultrasonography can be performed quickly and is reliably able to confirm or exclude a ruptured AAA (Bessen, 2010). Urgent consultation by a vascular surgeon is required to assess the patient and the potential for surgical repair.

CASE STUDY 5

Case 13064, 1009 hrs.

Dispatch details: A 58-year-old female with severe colicky abdominal pain over some hours associated with severe vomiting that is not abating.

Initial presentation: The ambulance crew arrive to find the patient sitting on the edge of her bed in the process of vomiting.

 ASSESS

The patient states she has never had this kind of pain before. She had surgery for an ovarian cyst 12 months ago and does not suffer from any other past medical conditions.

Initial assessment summary

Problem	Vomiting and abdominal pain
Conscious state	GCS 15
Position	Sitting on bed
Heart rate	110 bpm
Blood pressure	140/80 mmHg
Skin appearance	Warm and dry
Speech pattern	Speaks in sentences
Respiratory rate	20 bpm
Respiratory rhythm	Even cycles, good air entry bilaterally
Temperature	37.1°C
Physical assessment	Abdominal scars related to previous surgery; old striae from previous pregnancies; no umbilical hernia is seen; tense-appearing abdomen which is mildly distended. Bowel sounds are heard: they are rushing, high-pitched and tinkling. Mild tenderness on palpation is noted. The patient's vomitus is bile-stained. She has not had a bowel motion for two days (which is unusual for her), but she is passing flatus.

 CONFIRM

In many cases paramedics are presented with a collection of signs and symptoms that do not appear to describe a particular condition. Even though this presentation is consistent with bowel obstruction (given the risk factor of previous abdominal surgery and bilious vomit combined with constipation), it is good practice to consider differential diagnoses for the patient's presentation.

What else could be the cause?

Differential diagnoses

- Most likely
  - Bowel obstruction, secondary to adhesions from the ovarian cyst surgery last year
- Most serious not to miss
  - Renal or biliary colic
  - Appendicitis
  - Gastroenteritis

Renal or biliary colic

The pattern of pain in renal colic often presents in the back and to one side, but it can radiate across the back. The presentation is not typical of renal colic but it cannot be totally excluded at this stage. Biliary colic most often presents with pain under the right costal margin radiating around to the back. Classically, the pain is worse after eating. This does not seem to fit this patient's presentation and hence is unlikely.

Appendicitis

Appendicitis is classically associated with paraumbilical pain localising later on to the right iliac fossa, anorexia, nausea and vomiting. It cannot be totally excluded, but the patient's pain has not followed this pattern and she is vomiting bile.

Gastroenteritis

Gastroenteritis tends to present with some degree of diarrhoea.

3 TREAT

Patients with bowel obstruction are at risk of becoming hypovolaemic and developing complications such as ischaemia of the bowel or perforation. This patient's vital signs do not indicate that she is hypovolaemic, but she is likely to be dehydrated from the loss of fluid into the bowel. The priorities of emergency management for this patient are:

- fluid resuscitation
- pain relief
- transport.

Some fluid resuscitation will be needed as the patient has been vomiting and is unable to drink. Management of abdominal pain should be with narcotics. A smooth and gentle drive to hospital will reduce the chance of the patient vomiting and inhaling the vomit. She will probably be most comfortable in a sitting position, allowing her to lean forwards and vomit if necessary. Do not give metoclopramide to patients with suspected bowel obstruction. Good antiemetic alternatives include ondansetron and sniffed isopropyl.

4 EVALUATE

Evaluating the effect of any clinical management intervention can provide clues to the accuracy of the initial diagnosis. Some conditions respond rapidly to treatment so patients should be expected to improve if the diagnosis and treatment were appropriate, whereas other conditions are unlikely to respond in the timeframes normally associated with ambulance transport times. In such cases, a failure to improve should not be considered an indication of a misdiagnosis.

In this case, pain relief should be effective and, with IV fluids, the patient's pulse and blood pressure figures should improve slightly. The reduction in nausea and vomiting from antiemetic administration can be variable. A significant deterioration in the patient's vital signs would strongly suggest that the obstruction may have ruptured.

Ongoing management

Following initial emergency management, priorities for management of patients with large or small bowel obstruction are volume resuscitation, correction of electrolyte abnormalities, pain relief, bowel decompression and surgical consultation (Torrey & Henneman, 2010). Nasogastric tube insertion to empty the stomach, decompress the bowel and prevent aspiration pneumonia is also indicated. Diagnosis is aided with radiography. Plain abdominal films, both erect and supine, are useful to identify the presence of obstruction. On x-ray, distended loops of bowel can be seen and fluid levels may be evident on erect films.

Bowel obstruction across the lifespan

Small bowel obstruction can occur in adults at any age and in 50% of cases is caused by adhesions, particularly following abdominal or gynaecological surgery or surgery for peritonitis or major abdominal trauma (Hayden & Sprouse, 2011; Torrey & Henneman, 2010). Hernias and neoplasms account for the next largest cause of small bowel obstruction, accounting for 15% of cases (Torrey & Henneman, 2010). In children, the most common cause of small bowel obstruction in infancy and early childhood is intussusception (Torrey & Henneman, 2010).

Large bowel obstruction is more common in the elderly and is associated with an in-hospital mortality of 10%. It is caused by conditions likely to affect older populations such as carcinoma of the bowel, which is the cause in approximately 60% of cases of large bowel obstruction (Hayden & Sprouse, 2011; Peterson, 2010). Other causes include faecal impaction (typically after new or increased opioid analgesia) and sigmoid colon volvulus, which is thought to be contributed to by immobility, debility and poor diet and is frequently seen in institutionalised elderly people. Strictures and abscesses arising from chronic diverticulitis account for 10% of cases (Hayden & Sprouse, 2011).

Summary

Any visceral pathology will initially present as diffuse poorly localised pain; localisation occurs only when there is peritoneal involvement. The aim of out-of-hospital assessment is not to reach a final diagnosis, but facilitate symptom relief and transport. Recognition of severely ill patients, from either peritonitis or vascular catastrophe such as AAA, is needed as it demands urgent transport. Most symptom relief is safe, but avoid NSAIDs where bleeding is a concern and metoclopramide where bowel stimulation is a concern.

References

Andersson, R. E., Hugander, A., & Thulin, A. J. (1992). Diagnostic accuracy and perforation rate in appendicitis: association with age and sex of the patient and with appendicectomy rate. *The European Journal of Surgery, 158*, 37–41.

Andrews, P., & Horn, C. (2006). Signals for nausea and emesis: implications for models of upper gastrointestinal diseases. *Autonomic Neuroscience: Basic and Clinical, 125*, 100–115.

April, M. D., Oliver, J. J., Davis, W. T., Ong, D., Simon, E. M., Ng, P. C., & Hunter, C. J. (2018). Aromatherapy versus oral ondansetron for antiemetic therapy among adult emergency department patients: a randomized controlled trial. *Annals of Emergency Medicine, 72*(2), 184–193.

Arroyo, V., & Navasa, M. (2007). Ascites and spontaneous bacterial peritonitis. In E. Schiff, M. Sorrell & W. Maddrey (Eds.), *Schiff's diseases of the liver* (10th ed.). Philadelphia: Lippincott Williams & Wilkins.

Ashdown, H. F., D'Souza, N., Karim, D., Stevens, R. J., Huang, A., & Harnden, A. (2012). Pain over speed bumps in diagnosis of acute appendicitis: diagnostic accuracy study. *British Medical Journal, 345*, e8012.

Australian Medicines Handbook. (2020). *Internet*. Retrieved from https://amhonline.amh.net.au.acs.hcn.com.au. (Accessed 8 July 2020).

Avunduk, C. (2008). *Manual of gastroenterology: diagnosis and therapy*. Philadelphia: Lippincott Williams & Wilkins.

Bantel, C., & Trapp, S. (2011). The role of the autonomic nervous system in acute surgical pain processing: what do we know? *Anaesthesia, 66*, 541–544.

Bessen, H. (2010). Abdominal aortic aneurysm. In J. Marx, R. Hockberger, R. Walls & J. Adams (Eds.), *Rosen's emergency medicine* (7th ed.). Philadelphia: Mosby.

Bhuiya, F. A., Pitts, S. R., & McCaig, L. F. (2010). Emergency department visits for chest pain and abdominal pain: United States, 1999-2008. *NCHS Data Brief*, 1–8.

Bonow, R. O., Mann, D., Zipes, D., & Libby, P. (2011). *Braunwald's heart disease: a textbook of cardiovascular medicine* (9th ed.). Philadelphia: Saunders.

Braganza, J. M., Lee, S. H., McCloy, R. F., & McMahon, M. J. (2011). Chronic pancreatitis. *The Lancet, 377*, 1184–1197.

Cappell, M. S., & Batke, M. (2008). Mechanical obstruction of the small bowel and colon. *Medical Clinics of North America, 92*, 575–597.

Carithers, R., Jr, & McClain, C. (2010). Alcoholic liver disease. In M. Feldman, L. Friedman & L. Brandt (Eds.), *Sleisenger and Fordtran's gastrointestinal and liver disease* (9th ed.). Philadelphia: Saunders.

Casanova, B. C., Sammel, M. D., Chittams, J., Timbers, K., Kulp, J. L., & Barnhart, K. T. (2009). Prediction of outcome in women with symptomatic first-trimester pregnancy: focus on intrauterine rather than ectopic gestation. *Journal of Women's Health, 18*, 195–200.

Ceresoli, M., Zucchi, A., Allievi, N., Harbi, A., Pisano, M., Montori, G., Heyer, A., Nita, G. E., Ansaloni, L., & Coccolini, F. (2016). Acute appendicitis: epidemiology, treatment and outcomes-analysis of 16544 consecutive cases. *World Journal of Gastrointestinal Surgery, 8*, 693.

Cesario, K., Choure, A., & Carey, W. (2010). Complications of cirrhosis: ascites, hepatic encephalopathy and variceal haemorrhage. In W. Carey (Ed.), *Cleveland clinic: current clinical medicine* (2nd ed.). Philadelphia: Saunders.

Chabok, A., Påhlman, L., Hjern, F., Haapaniemi, S., Smedh, K., & AVOD Study Group. (2012). Randomized clinical trial of antibiotics in acute uncomplicated diverticulitis. *British Journal of Surgery, 99*, 532–539.

Chowdhury, P., & Gupta, P. (2006). Pathophysiology of alcoholic pancreatitis: an overview. *World Journal of Gastroenterology, 12*, 7421.

Craft, J., Gordon, C., & Tiziani, A. (2011). *Understanding pathophysiology*. Sydney: Elsevier.

Craig, S., & Zich, D. (2010). Gastroenteritis. In J. Marx, R. Hockberger, R. Walls & J. Adams (Eds.), *Rosen's emergency medicine* (7th ed.). Philadelphia: Mosby.

Doherty, G. (2010). The acute abdomen: introduction. In G. Doherty & L. Way (Eds.), *Current diagnosis & treatment: surgery* (13th ed.). New York: Lange Medical Books/McGraw-Hill.

Farquhar-Smith, W. (2008). Anatomy, physiology and pharmacology of pain. *Anaesthesia and Intensive Care Medicine, 9*, 3–7.

Flasar, M., & Goldberg, E. (2006). Acute abdominal pain. *The Medical Clinics of North America, 90*, 481–503.

Garcia-Tsao, G. (2011). Ascites. In J. Dooley, A. Lock, A. Burroughs & E. Heathcote (Eds.), *Sherlock's diseases of the liver and biliary system* (12th ed.). Chichester: Wiley-Blackwell.

Getto, L., Zeserson, E., & Breyer, M. (2011). Vomiting, diarrhea, constipation and gastroenteritis. *Emergency Medicine Clinics of North America, 29*, 211–237.

Giamberardino, M., Affaitati, G., & Costantini, R. (2010). Visceral referred pain. *Journal of Musculoskeletal Pain, 18*, 403–410.

Glasgow, R., & Mulvihill, S. (2003). Abdominal pain, including the acute abdomen. In M. Feldman, L. Friedman & M. Sleisenger (Eds.), *Sleisenger and Fordtran's gastrointestinal and liver disease* (7th ed.). Philadelphia: Saunders.

Gray, H. 2000. Anatomy of the human body. *New York*, Bartleby.com.

Hall, J. (2012). *Guyton and Hall textbook of medical physiology* (12th ed.). St Louis: Saunders.

Hayanga, A., Bass-Wilkins, K., & Bulkley, G. (2005). Current management of small-bowel obstruction. *Advances in Surgery, 39*, 1–33.

Hayden, G., & Sprouse, K. (2011). Bowel obstruction and hernia. *Emergency Medicine Clinics of North America, 29*, 319–345.

Hirsch, A., Haskel, Z., Hertzer, N., Bakal, C., Creager, M., Halperin, J., Halperin, J. L., Hiratzka, L. F., Murphy, W. R. C., Olin, J. W., Puschett, J. B., Rosenfield, K. A., Sacks, D., Stanley, J. C., Taylor, L. M., White, C. J., White, J., & White, R. A. (2006). ACC/AHA 2005 practice guidelines for the management of patients with peripheral arterial disease (lower extremity, renal, mesenteric, and abdominal aortic): a collaborative report from the American Association for Vascular Surgery/Society for Vascular Surgery, Society for Cardiovascular Angiography and Interventions, Society for Vascular Medicine and Biology, Society of Interventional Radiology, and the ACC/AHA Task Force on Practice Guidelines (Writing Committee to Develop Guidelines for the Management of Patients with Peripheral Arterial Disease). *Circulation, 113*, e463–e654.

Horn, A., & Ufberg, J. (2011). Appendicitis, diverticulitis and colitis. *Emergency Medicine Clinics of North America, 29*, 347–368.

Jaffe, B., & Berger, D. (2010). The appendix. In F. Brunicardi, D. Andersen, T. Biliar, D. Dunn, J. Hunger, J. Matthews & R. Pollock (Eds.), *Schwartz's principles of surgery* (9th ed.). New York: McGraw-Hill.

Kalia, H., Grewal, P., & Martin, P. (2012). Cirrhosis. In E. Bope & R. Kellerman (Eds.), *Conn's current therapy*. Philadelphia: Saunders.

Knowles, C., & Aziz, Q. (2009). Basic and clinical aspects of gastrointestinal pain. *Pain, 141*, 191–209.

Korner, H., Soreide, J., Pedersen, E., Bru, T., Sondenaa, K., & Vatten, L. (2001). Stability in incidence of acute appendicitis. *Digestive Surgery, 18*, 61–66.

Kumar, V., Abbas, A., Fausto, N., & Aster, J. (2009). *Robbins and Cotran pathologic basis of disease* (8th ed.). Philadelphia: Saunders.

Laine, C., Williams, S., Turner, B., & Wilson, J. (2010). Diabetic ketoacidosis. *Annals of Internal Medicine, 152*, 1–16.

Lewiss, R., Egan, D., & Shreves, A. (2011). Vascular abdominal emergencies. *Emergency Medicine Clinics of North America, 29*, 253–272.

Macaluso, C. R., & McNamara, R. M. (2012). Evaluation and management of acute abdominal pain in the emergency department. *International Journal of General Medicine, 5*, 789.

Manterola, C., Vial, M., Moraga, J., & Astudillo, P. (2011). Analgesia in patients with acute abdominal pain (Review). *The Cochrane Database of Systematic Reviews*, (1), CD005660.

Matthews, J., & Hodin, R. (2011). Acute abdomen and appendix. In M. Mulholland, K. Lillemoe, G. Doherty, R. Maier, D. Simeone & G. Upchurch Jr (Eds.), *Greenfield's surgery scientific principles and practice* (5th ed.). Philadelphia: Lippincott Williams & Wilkins.

McNamara, R., & Dean, A. (2011). Approach to acute abdominal pain. *Emergency Medicine Clinics of North America*, 29, 159–173.

Melloni, J., Dox, I., Melloni, B., & Eisner, G. (2003). *Melloni's pocket medical dictionary: illustrated.* Taylor & Francis.

Millham, F. (2010). Acute abdominal pain. In M. Feldman, L. Friedman & L. Brandt (Eds.), *Sleisenger and Fordtran's gastrointestinal and liver disease* (9th ed.). Philadelphia: Saunders.

Minter, R., & Mulholland, M. (2008). Approach to the patient with acute abdomen. In T. Yamada, D. Alpers, A. Kalloo, N. Kaplowitz, C. Owyand & D. Powell (Eds.), *Principles of clinical gastroenterology*. Chichester: Wiley-Blackwell.

Mitchell, R., & Schoen, F. (2009). Blood vessels. In V. Kumar, A. Abbas, N. Fausto & J. Aster (Eds.), *Robbins and Cotran pathological basis of disease* (8th ed.). Philadelphia: Saunders.

National Institute of Clinical Studies. (2008). *Pain medication for acute abdominal pain*. Canberra: National Health and Medical Research Council.

Niska, R., Bhuiya, F., & Xu, J. (2010). *National Hospital Ambulatory Medical Care Survey: 2007 Emergency Department Summary.: National Health Statistics Reports*.

Noble, V. E., Liteplo, A. S., Nelson, B. P., & Thomas, S. H. (2010). The impact of analgesia on the diagnostic accuracy of the sonographic Murphy's sign. *European Journal of Emergency Medicine*, 17, 80–83.

Paulsen, F. (2013). *Sobotta atlas of human anatomy* (15th ed., Vol. 2). Munich: Elsevier.

Peterson, M. (2010). Disorders of the large intestine. In J. Marx, R. Hockberger, R. Walls & J. Adams (Eds.), *Rosen's emergency medicine* (7th ed.). Philadelphia: Elsevier.

Platt, M., Doshi, S., & Telfer, E. (2008). Abdominal pain. In C. Stone & R. Humphries (Eds.), *Current diagnosis and treatment: emergency medicine* (6th ed.). New York: McGraw-Hill.

Poston, G. (2005). The acute abdomen: assessment, diagnosis and pitfalls. *Clinical Risk*, 11, 159–165.

Runyon, B. (2010). Ascites and spontaneous bacterial peritonitis. In M. Feldman, L. Friedman & L. Brandt (Eds.), *Sleisenger and Fordtran's gastrointestinal and liver disease* (9th ed.). Philadelphia: Saunders.

Sakalihasan, N., Limet, R., & Defawe, O. (2005). Abdominal aortic aneurysm. *Lancet*, 365, 1577–1589.

Salminen, P., Paajanen, H., Rautio, T., Nordström, P., Aarnio, M., Rantanen, T., Tuominen, R., Hurme, S., Virtanen, J., & Mecklin, J.-P. (2015). Antibiotic therapy vs appendectomy for treatment of uncomplicated acute appendicitis: the APPAC randomized clinical trial. *JAMA: The Journal of the American Medical Association*, 313, 2340–2348.

Sanders, M. J. (2007). *Mosby's paramedic textbook*. St Louis: Mosby.

Sands, B., & Siegel, C. (2010). Crohn's disease. In M. Feldman, L. Friedman & L. Brandt (Eds.), *Sleisenger and Fordtran's gastrointestinal and liver disease* (9th ed.). Philadelphia: Saunders.

Shah, V., & Kamath, P. (2010). Portal hypertension and gastrointestinal bleeding. In M. Feldman, L. Friedman & L. Brandt (Eds.), *Sleisenger and Fordtran's gastrointestinal and liver disease* (9th ed.). Philadelphia: Saunders.

Sheehy, S. B., Hammond, B. B., & Zimmermann, P. G., Emergency Nurses Association. (2013). *Sheehy's manual of emergency care*. St Louis: Elsevier/Mosby.

Siddiqi, N. (2012). Aneurysm, abdominal aorta. In F. Ferri (Ed.), *Ferri's clinical advisor*. Philadelphia: Elsevier.

Singh, K., Bonaa, K., Jacobsen, G., Bjork, L., & Solberg, S. (2001). Prevalence of and risk factors for abdominal aortic aneurysms in a population-based study: the Tromsø study. *American Journal of Epidemiology*, 154, 236–244.

Soon, Y., & Hardy, R. (2002). Acute abdomen. *Surgery (Oxford)*, 20, 169–172.

Stedman, T. (2006). *Stedman's medical dictionary*. Baltimore: Lippincott Williams & Wilkins.

Talley, N., & O'Connor, S. (2013). *Clinical examination* (7th ed.). Sydney: Churchill Livingstone.

Tintinalli, J. E., Stapczynski, J. S., Ma, O. J., Cline, D., Meckler, G. D., & Yealy, D. M., McGraw-Hill Companies. (2016). *Tintinalli's emergency medicine : a comprehensive study guide* (8th ed.). New York: McGraw-Hill.

Torrey, S., & Henneman, P. (2010). Disorders of the small intestine. In J. Marx, R. Hockberger, R. Walls & J. Adams (Eds.), *Rosen's emergency medicine* (7th ed.). Philadelphia: Mosby.

Turner, J. (2009). The gastrointestinal tract. In V. Kumar, A. Abbas, N. Fausto & J. Aster (Eds.), *Robbins and Cotran pathological basis of disease* (8th ed.). Philadelphia: Saunders.

Wolfe, J., & Henneman, P. (2010). Acute appendicitis. In J. Marx, R. Hockberger, R. Walls & J. Adams (Eds.), *Rosen's emergency medicine* (7th ed.). Philadelphia: Mosby.

Yokoe, M., Takada, T., Strasberg, S. M., Solomkin, J. S., Mayumi, T., Gomi, H., Pitt, H. A., Garden, O. J., Kiriyama, S., & Hata, J. (2013). TG13 diagnostic criteria and severity grading of acute cholecystitis (with videos). *Journal of Hepato-Biliary-Pancreatic Sciences*, 20, 35–46.

CHAPTER 32

Sepsis

By Daniel Cudini and Ben Meadley

OVERVIEW

- Sepsis and its associated syndromes are life-threatening conditions that are frequently encountered in the out-of-hospital environment.
- Early recognition and treatment of the patient with sepsis is essential to reduce morbidity and mortality.
- The early signs of sepsis can be triaged as low acuity and the symptoms can be insidious, so often the diagnosis is not obvious.
- Paramedics and other clinicians providing emergency care in the field play an integral role in recognising the pathophysiological process using

thorough assessment and adhering to current evidence-based sepsis identification criteria.
- Fluid resuscitation +/− inotropes, blood culture and antibiotic administration are considered the main paramedic treatments; however, they are associated with limitations in the out-of-hospital setting.
- More research is needed focusing on out-of-hospital sepsis identification criteria, the role of point-of-care blood lactate and paramedic administered blood culture collection/empiric antibiotic administration.

Introduction

Sepsis is one of the most frequent causes of emergency department (ED) attendance worldwide, with an annual incidence in adults of 300 cases per 100,000 (Angus et al., 2001; Gaieski et al., 2013; Jawad et al., 2012; Kaukonen et al., 2014). It is recognised by the World Health Organization as a global health priority and has a reported in-hospital mortality of 20% to 50% (Reinhart et al., 2017; NSW Government Clinical Excellence Commission, 2018; Peake and ARISE Investigators, 2007). This greatly exceeds that seen in acute myocardial infarction (AMI), stroke or traumatic injury (NSW Government Clinical Excellence Commission, 2018; Peake and ARISE Investigators, 2007). Sepsis mortality in the paediatric population is also high (ranging from 10–35%) and infected children < 1 year of age have been identified as a risk factor for developing septic shock (Angus et al., 2001; Gaieski et al., 2013; Gaines et al., 2012). In Australia and New Zealand, the annual incidence of sepsis is > 17,000 episodes; interestingly, in-hospital mortality rates have been declining in both the adult and the paediatric settings since 2002. In adults, absolute mortality in sepsis decreased from 35.0% to 18.4% (2002–2012) and in children mortality from septic shock reduced to 17% (2002–2013) (Schlapbach et al., 2015; Kaukonen et al., 2014). This reduction in mortality has been largely attributed to the implementation of the Surviving Sepsis Campaign recommendations (first published in 2004) which have been supported/implemented by prominent national and international intensive care societies

over the past 15 years (Dellinger et al., 2004). In Australia and New Zealand significant focus has been placed on early sepsis recognition, resuscitation with rapid IV fluids, antibiotics within the first hour of recognition of sepsis and referral to the appropriate tertiary hospitals/specialty medical teams (NSW Government Clinical Excellence Commission, 2018). Out-of-hospital care plays an integral role in extending point-of-care medicine from the in-hospital to the out-of-hospital setting. Improving out-of-hospital sepsis care may lead to significant decreases in mortality and morbidity similar to the established paramedic interventions for stroke, AMI and major trauma.

Definitions

The definition of sepsis has evolved significantly over the past 15 years and is formally referred to as a four-part physiological process: **systemic inflammatory response syndrome (SIRS)**, **sepsis**, **severe sepsis** and **septic shock** (Dellinger et al., 2013; ACCP/SCCM Consensus Conference, 1992). In 2016, the Third International Consensus Definitions for Sepsis and Septic Shock (Sepsis-3 Task Force) was published forming a contemporary definition highlighting only two categories: **sepsis** and **septic shock**.

- **Sepsis** is now defined as a life-threatening organ dysfunction caused by a dysregulated host response to infection (Singer et al., 2016).
- **Septic shock** is a subset of sepsis in which underlying circulatory and cellular/metabolic abnormalities are profound enough to substantially

increase mortality. It can be identified in patients with a clinical finding of sepsis with refractory hypotension to fluid therapy requiring inotropes/vasopressors to maintain MAP ≥ 65 mmHg or in the out-of-hospital environment, a systolic BP ≥ 100 mmHg, and a serum lactate level > 2 mmol/L despite adequate volume. When these criteria are present, hospital mortality is in excess of 40% (Singer et al., 2016).

The use of the categories 'SIRS' and 'Severe sepsis' were unanimously considered to be unhelpful by the Sepsis-3 Task Force and removed from the previous definitions. The SIRS criteria were found to not necessarily indicate a dysregulated, life-threatening response and are often present in many hospitalised patients, including those who never develop infection and never incur adverse outcomes (Singer et al., 2016).

Organ dysfunction is assessed by an acute change of ≥ 2 points in the sequential organ failure assessment score (SOFA). The SOFA score is a common in-hospital organ failure assessment tool which reviews components of partial pressure of oxygen in arterial blood/fractional inspired oxygen (PaO_2/FiO_2) ratio, Glasgow coma scale, mean arterial pressure, inotrope/vasopressor use, serum creatinine or urine output, bilirubin and platelet count. A higher SOFA score is associated with an increased probability of mortality (Gotts & Matthay, 2016).

Pathophysiology

Sepsis and its associated syndromes are potentially fatal conditions that result from an infective pathogen and the body's dysregulated host response to that infection. The most common sites of infection that may lead to sepsis are the skin (e.g. cellulitis, invasive medical devices), genitourinary tract (e.g. urinary tract infection), respiratory tract (e.g. pneumonia) and gastrointestinal tract (e.g. parasites, viruses).

Sepsis is commonly caused by bacterial organisms, although viral infections, fungi and parasites can cause sepsis; in addition, some cases have an unknown cause (see Box 32.1; ACCP/SCCM Consensus Conference, 1992; Ebby, 2005; Tintinalli, 2016). Once an organism has infiltrated the bloodstream, the body recognises that it has been invaded by a foreign substance and initiates the *immune response*, and in particular the *inflammatory response* (see Fig 32.1 and Ch 4). One of the main inflammatory mediators released in response to a sustained infection in the bloodstream is cytokines. Cytokines can be divided into two distinct subgroups: pro-inflammatory and anti-inflammatory.

As the body's immune/inflammatory response combats the invading pathogen, it may destroy it and, over time, rid the body of any organism or endotoxins from the destroyed organism that act as the triggers for the immune response. However, if the serum levels of the organism continue to accumulate, the inflammatory response will proceed and anti-inflammatory cytokines will continue to fight the disease. With this comes a paradoxical pro-inflammatory cytokine response and, importantly, the additional release of nitric oxide (Rangel-Frausto et al., 1995; Kellum et al., 2007). The abundance of pro-inflammatory cytokines and nitric oxide, as well a multitude of other factors involved in the complex process of inflammation, lead to significant physiological consequences.

As inflammation progresses, the process of sepsis interferes with the normal function of the vascular endothelium, causing an increase in capillary permeability (Tintinalli, 2016). Endothelial involvement often leads to the release of a number of harmful substances, the most important being tissue factor, which depresses the inhibition of coagulation and interferes with intrinsic fibrinolysis. Inhibition of the exceptionally complex coagulation cascade leads to widespread disseminated intravascular coagulopathy (DIC). Combined with the affected intrinsic fibrinolysis, diffuse microvascular clotting leads to poor blood flow, especially to vital organs. This may lead to organ ischaemia and, if unabated, infarction and organ death.

In severe cases of septic shock, multiple organs may be affected, leading to multiple organ dysfunction syndrome (MODS), which carries a high mortality.

The responses to widespread inflammation are numerous and complex and beyond the scope of this text. However, the pathophysiological response to continued systemic inflammation can be summarised as:
- widespread peripheral vasodilation
- increased capillary permeability
- complex coagulopathy (abnormal clotting processes)
- depressed myocardial function (Latto, 2008).

> ## BOX 32.1 Common pathogens that may lead to sepsis
> - Bacteria such as *Streptococcus pneumoniae* and *Neisseria meningitidis*
> - Viruses such as influenza and rhinovirus
> - Fungi such as *Histoplasma capsulatum*
> - Parasites such as *Toxoplasma gondii*

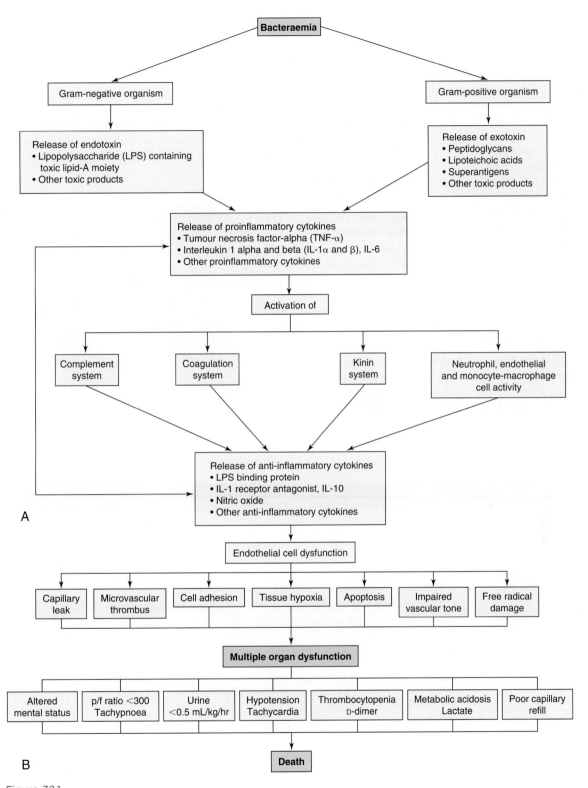

Figure 32.1
Summary of sepsis pathology.
*Source: **A** Larson & Barke (1999). **B** Copyright © 2003, Eli Lilly and Company. All rights reserved. Reprinted with permission from Eli Lilly and Company.*

Sepsis-associated syndromes

Common yet complex sepsis-associated syndromes include:

- SIRS
- MODS
- acute lung injury/acute respiratory distress syndrome
- disseminated intravascular coagulation.

Systemic inflammatory response syndrome

SIRS describes the presence of a pathophysiological continuum of deranged physiological values with or without the presence of an identifiable source of infection (ACCP/SCCM Consensus Conference, 1992). It may occur as a result of non-infective insults, including but not limited to acute pancreatitis, severe burns, shock or major trauma. Thus, a patient may have SIRS but not sepsis; however, sepsis will eventually manifest as SIRS if not managed effectively (see Fig 32.2). It is imperative

to understand that meeting SIRS criteria *and* identifying an infective source are important in distinguishing between isolated SIRS, a severe infection and actual sepsis (see Figure 32.3).

Pathophysiology of the SIRS criteria

Temperature > 38.5°C or < 35.0°C

Fever occurs for numerous reasons. In SIRS and sepsis the mechanism is pro-inflammatory cytokines. Cytokines directly stimulate the hypothalamus and

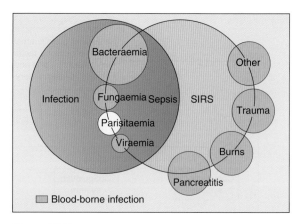

Figure 32.2
Conditions associated with SIRS.
Source: Cohen & Powderly (2010).

Category	Definition
PREVIOUS DEFINITIONS	
SIRS (systemic inflammatory response syndrome)	Two of the following: • Temperature > 38°C or < 35°C • Heart rate > 90 beats/min • Respiratory rate > 20 breaths/min or arterial carbon dioxide pressure < 32 mmHg • White blood cell count > 12×10^9/L or < 4×10^9/L
Sepsis	SIRS with infection (presumed or proven)
Severe sepsis	Sepsis with evidence of acute organ dysfunction (hypotension, lactic acidosis, reduced urine output, reduced PaO_2/FiO_2 ratio, raised creatinine or bilirubin, thrombocytopenia, raised international normalized ratio)
Septic shock	Sepsis with persistent hypotension after fluid resuscitation
REVISED DEFINITIONS	
Sepsis	Life-threatening organ dysfunction caused by a dysregulated host response to infection
Septic shock	Sepsis and vasopressor therapy needed to increase mean arterial pressure to ≥ 65 mmHg and lactate to > 2 mmol/L despite adequate fluid resuscitation

Figure 32.3
Previous and recently revised definitions of sepsis and related syndromes.
Source: Gotts & Matthay (2016).

cause prostaglandin secretion, resulting in a 'resetting' of the hypothalamic thermostat. The hypothesised physiological purpose of this is inhibition of bacterial growth. However, it is widely accepted that low-grade fever may be tolerated, but higher temperatures can lead to denaturing of proteins and potential neuronal damage and therefore should be managed (Marieb & Hoehn, 2007).

In patients whose temperature is < 35°C, the mechanism for this is failure of thermoregulation. The 'cold sepsis' patient is likely to have progressed down the inflammatory process to a point where widespread cytokine and nitric oxide activity has caused continued peripheral vasodilation and increased capillary permeability. The sympathetic nervous system will have activated and attempted to maintain normal organ perfusion; however, these mechanisms may have begun to fail. Peripheral vasoconstriction secondary to noradrenaline and adrenaline release results in cool extremities. Global vasodilation and loss of vascular integrity may persist to varying degrees and decompensation will occur if the response is inadequate. Due to this loss of vascular tone, much of the intravascular volume will move to the interstitium and blood circulating through major organs will be low, therefore core temperature drops. 'Cold sepsis' and SIRS patients will be critically unwell (Kellum et al., 2007).

Heart rate > 90 bpm
As a result of falling systemic vascular resistance (due to peripheral vasodilation and increased capillary permeability), HR must increase to maintain cardiac output (CO). Recall: 1. blood pressure (BP) is a function of CO and systemic vascular resistance (SVR); and 2.:

$$CO = HR \times stroke\ volume\ (SV)$$

Thus, if SVR decreases, so too will BP. By increasing the sympathetic response to this drop in SVR, as sensed by baroreceptors, adrenaline and noradrenaline released from the adrenal medulla into the bloodstream will:

- increase vascular tone (SVR)
- increase myocardial contractility (SV)
- increase HR—thus the body attempts to maintain normal BP.

Patients with SIRS can be expected to demonstrate higher-than-normal heart rates, and although 90 is used as the lower limit in the SIRS criteria, patients will often be quite tachycardic.

Respiratory rate > 20 bpm or PaCO₂ < 32 mmHg
A respiratory compensation for the metabolic acidosis that has occurred secondary to poor perfusion (lactic acidosis) leads to a raised respiratory rate and low CO_2. Another contributor to the metabolic acidosis

is a raised temperature, which increases the metabolic rate and oxygen demand in a patient with poor perfusion. Many sepsis patients can be hypoxic for varying reasons, including respiratory tract infection or lung injury secondary to cytokine activity. The combination of increased demand and reduced oxygen supply trigger anaerobic production of ATP and lactate is a byproduct of anaerobic metabolism. Eventually, serum lactic acid levels increase, as do levels of hydrogen ion concentration. Recall the bicarbonate buffering equation:

$$H^+ + HCO_3^- \leftrightarrow H_2CO_3 \leftrightarrow H_2O + CO_2$$

As hydrogen ion concentrations increase, the sensitivity of the respiratory centre to CO_2 increases. The respiratory rate increases expiring CO_2, effectively reducing the total hydrogen ion concentration by pulling this equation to the right. Thus, by breathing faster and lowering the $PaCO_2$, the hydrogen ion concentration is lowered also.

Although the respiratory rate is included in the SIRS criteria and is easily assessed in the out-of-hospital setting, $PaCO_2$ is still a valuable measure in both patients who are conscious and spontaneously breathing and those who are unconscious and ventilated. $PaCO_2$ can be estimated by attaching an electronic capnograph or capnometer to a standard face mask, proprietary nasal prongs, endotracheal tube or supraglottic airway. However, if there is a barrier to adequate gas exchange as in respiratory or cardiovascular pathology, end-tidal CO_2 ($EtCO_2$) measured by capnography or capnometry may not be an accurate predictor of $PaCO_2$. The relationship of $PaCO_2$ to end-tidal CO_2 is most accurate in healthy individuals and least accurate in those patients with significant cardiovascular or respiratory compromise. Therefore, it is unlikely that an $EtCO_2$ reading in a patient with sepsis will correlate accurately to the arterial CO_2 reading.

Multiple organ dysfunction syndrome
Multiple organ dysfunction syndrome (MODS) has been established as the natural progression of SIRS if it is left untreated or if treatment is ineffective. It is defined as the failure of two or more organs in critical illness, where homeostasis is unable to be maintained without medical intervention. MODS can occur as sepsis progresses; however, it may also occur secondary to other pathophysiological processes such as prolonged hypovolaemia or burns (Tintinalli, 2016; Cunha & Bronze, 2012). Although the intricate pathophysiology of MODS is not completely understood, it is suggested that widespread continued inflammation and microvascular clotting lead to progressive organ failure, which, if

left untreated, progresses to failure of the organism and death. MODS is recognised as a complex and difficult-to-manage progression of sepsis that carries a high mortality.

Acute lung injury/acute respiratory distress syndrome

Acute lung injury (ALI) and acute respiratory distress syndrome (ARDS) are two descriptions of the range of serious lung complications associated with ongoing systemic inflammation. Although they can occur in non-sepsis illness, SIRS and sepsis often progress to involve the respiratory system. Continued pro-inflammatory cytokine activity causes significant damage to the alveolar/capillary endothelial membrane (Latto, 2008). Initially, this inflammation can cause impairment in oxygenation and ventilation, as well as decreasing overall lung compliance. This disrupts normal ventilation mechanics and physiology and can make mechanical ventilation problematic.

If the alveolar-capillary membrane continues to become inflamed, it becomes more damaged. Progressive alveolar damage promotes further cytokine release and lung injury is worsened. As this occurs, large proteins that normally would not cross the semi-permeable respiratory membrane are able to pass from the respiratory capillary network into the alveoli. This leads to movement of fluid from the capillaries to the alveoli, causing non-cardiogenic pulmonary oedema. When pulmonary oedema decreased lung compliance and hypoxaemia are present, ALI is diagnosed. The basic difference between ARDS and ALI: ARDS is unresolved hypoxaemia despite high-flow, high-concentration supplemental oxygen (Latto, 2008).

Disseminated intravascular coagulation

Disseminated intravascular coagulation is a complication of refractory sepsis. It is most commonly seen in meningococcal septicaemia and manifests as the classic non-blanching purpuric rash. DIC is exceptionally complicated, but can be summarised as an imbalance between clotting and endogenous fibrinolysis (see Fig 32.4), or clot breakdown, resulting in the consumption of clotting factors so that clotting is impaired (Tintinalli, 2016; Amaral et al., 2004).

As tissue factor is secreted from the vascular endothelium in response to continued inflammation, clotting continues. However, the body reacts to these multiple microvascular clots by attempting to 'lyse' or break them down, primarily by secreting fibrinolytic plasmin. However, there is not an endless supply of clotting factors, plasmin or other endogenous fibrinolytics. Therefore, as time progresses, either clotting or bleeding will dominate as the clotting and lysis factors are consumed. In the vast majority

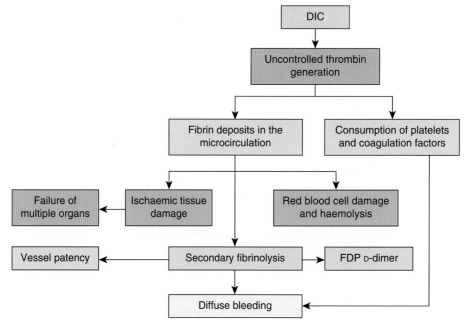

Figure 32.4
The process of DIC.
Source: Longo et al. (2011).

of cases, it is thought that the clotting factors, including fibrinogen and fibrin, are consumed more than plasmin, which continues its function, so DIC patients suffer widespread microvascular bleeding (Tintinalli, 2016; Amaral et al., 2004). These patients often bleed from the eyes, mucosa, intravenous access sites and genitals. The purpuric rash in meningococcal sepsis is subcutaneous microvascular haemorrhage. However, in a few cases, microvascular clotting dominates, resulting in widespread tissue ischaemia and infarction (Tintinalli, 2016; Amaral et al., 2004).

Meningococcal septicaemia

Meningococcal septicaemia is a type of sepsis that can often manifest as septic shock and rapidly progress to DIC, MODS and cardiac arrest. If a patient progresses rapidly from being mildly unwell to critically ill with impending cardiovascular collapse, the process is termed *fulminant meningococcal sepsis*. Although widely reported in the media due to its rapid onset, spectacular deterioration and high morbidity/mortality, meningococcal septicaemia is not common. In Australia, the national incidence of meningococcal disease is low at approximately 1.3 per 100,000 population (Australian Government Department of Health, 2018). However, it is a life-threatening condition that can be catastrophic for the patient. If recognised or suspected and treated early, meningococcal sepsis can be managed and its progression slowed.

Neisseria meningitides is almost always the offending organism. About 5–10% of the population are asymptomatic carriers of this organism, but this can increase to 60–80% in closed populations such as the military or long-term camps. The organism lives in the nasopharynx, anus and genitourinary tract and is usually benign unless it enters the bloodstream. It is transmitted through respiratory droplets and is prevalent in populations such as

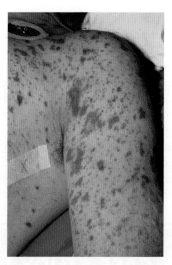

Figure 32.5
Characteristic purpura with petechiae and ecchymoses in a patient who has severe sepsis and meningitis due to *Neisseria meningitidis*.
Source: Courtesy of Professor W. Zimmerli, University of Basel, Switzerland. From Cohen & Powderly (2010).

adolescents and young adults who may kiss, share cigarettes and drinks or congregate in large numbers (Tintinalli, 2016). When *Neisseria meningitides* enters the circulation, the immune response can be overwhelming, with rapid onset of sepsis and progression to DIC. This manifests as a non-blanching, purpuric rash (see Fig 32.5).

In children and adults, consider a diagnosis of meningococcal disease if signs and symptoms include (Victorian Government, Australia. Department of Health, 2018):

- fever, pallor, rigors, sweats
- headache, neck stiffness, photophobia, backache, cranial nerve palsy
- vomiting and/or nausea, and diarrhoea
- lethargy, drowsiness, irritability, confusion, agitation, seizures or altered conscious state
- moaning, unintelligible speech
- painful or swollen joints, myalgia or difficulty walking.

The key clinical features of meningococcal septicaemia are:

- non-blanching purpuric rash
- fever, rigor, joint and muscle pain
- cold hands and feet
- SIRS criteria.

Note: The absence of a rash does not exclude meningococcal disease, and haemorrhagic rash (particularly of a pinprick, petechial or purpuric appearance) should be a clinical flag (Victorian Government, Australia. Department of Health, 2018).

Meningeal signs such as photophobia and neck stiffness may be present but do not need to be involved to diagnose meningococcal septicaemia. If the patient appears to have signs of meningococcal septicaemia, especially the non-blanching purpuric rash, empirical antibiotic therapy should be administered immediately according to local guidelines. Meningococcal septicaemia is a life-threatening medical emergency and is the one form of sepsis where paramedics should institute antibiotic therapy as soon as it is recognised. This will most likely be ceftriaxone at 50 mg/kg up to 2 g IV/IM (adults/children) and if ceftriaxone is not available, benzylpenicillin 60 mg/kg to a maximum of 3 g in

adults (max 2.4 g in children). Penicillin should only be withheld in people who have a definite history of penicillin-associated anaphylaxis. If any doubt exists the paramedic should consult with the receiving ED (Victorian Government, Australia. Department of Health, 2018; Royal Children's Hospital, Melbourne, Australia, 2018). Historical evidence has highlighted an approximate 5–10% cross-reactivity rate among penicillin and third-generation cephalosporins (ceftriaxone); however, current evidence now supports this to be < 1% (Romano et al., 2010, 2015).

 CASE STUDY 1

Case 10433, 1218 hrs.

Dispatch details: An 82-year-old male with a long, complicated medical history is a resident of a low-level aged care facility. The staff at the facility called an ambulance as the man has been feeling generally unwell.

Initial presentation: The crew arrive and find the patient sitting in a chair; his skin is flushed and he appears lethargic.

 ASSESS

Patient history

The staff state that the patient has had a fever for a few days, a productive cough and increased frequency of urination. He has been complaining of dizziness and shortness of breath. His GP prescribed paracetamol as required and antibiotics. However, the patient has not improved and today he is quite lethargic and confused, which is unusual for him.

Collectively, the patient and staff highlight a combination of signs and symptoms that point to an active infection and likely source. Before progressing to the next stage of assessment, given this history and the patient's age, the paramedics should explore other facets of the presentation, which may include the following:

- establishing whether the patient is feeling better since he started the medications
- asking for more detail about the patient's urinary habits, including actual frequency or any discomfort while urinating
- ascertaining from the staff the patient's normal conscious state and comparing that to how he presents today
- investigating the complaint of 'feeling hot', such as chills, rigor or diaphoresis.

There are many other pertinent questions that should be asked of all patients with suspected infection. These questions include, but are not limited to, the following.

- Have you travelled overseas or to areas with known infectious disease outbreaks recently (i.e. potential exposure to various influenza strains)?

- Have you been exposed to someone who has travelled overseas or to areas with known infectious disease outbreaks recently?
- Have you been exposed to people with known infectious illness (e.g. gastroenteritis)?
- Have you eaten food you suspected of being contaminated (i.e. salmonella)?

Probing further into the patient's recent history may uncover an obvious underlying cause for the presenting clinical picture.

Airway

Airway intervention is sometimes required in patients with sepsis; however, this will most likely occur late in the clinical course when inadequate cerebral perfusion and respiratory distress are leading to airway compromise (Tintinalli, 2016). Coma, although uncommon, is possible in acute sepsis due to profound cerebral hypoperfusion. In patients with suspected sepsis, the airway should be rapidly assessed and, if compromised, basic airway management instituted.

Breathing

Respiratory assessment in sepsis can be challenging. If the initial suspicion is of a respiratory source (e.g. pneumonia), crepitations and wheezes may be prevalent upon auscultation. Alternatively, if sepsis is not of a respiratory source and the patient has progressed some way down the clinical path, then ARDS or ALI may develop. On auscultation, it may be difficult to distinguish between respiratory tract infection and ARDS or ALI, as the breath sounds are not dissimilar. This is even more pertinent in the out-of-hospital setting, where ambient noise and movement can complicate chest auscultation. Despite this, if there exists a barrier to gas exchange, the patient may experience dyspnoea, hyperventilation or hypoventilation late in the clinical course. Poor oxygen saturation may be present and supplemental oxygen may be required. Severe respiratory tract infection and ARDS or ALI may lead to respiratory failure, lactic acidosis, which in turn is a reflection of poor cellular perfusion. Therefore, a patient with sepsis may have a raised respiratory rate due to metabolic acidosis or a gas exchange problem. This might be the primary source of the infection necessitating assisted ventilation and/or endotracheal intubation.

Cardiovascular and skin

Ongoing inflammation that is associated with infection leads to widespread peripheral vasodilation. SVR is decreased and CO will increase to maintain normal BP and organ perfusion. In conjunction with vasodilation, there is myocardial depression, which decreases CO further contributing to the decrease in BP. Key diagnostic criteria of sepsis include tachycardia and hypotension (Dellinger et al., 2013; Rhodes et al., 2016). These signs should be expected in patients with sepsis. As peripheral vasodilation and increased capillary permeability progress, the skin may initially appear flushed in early infection. This can also be attributed to blood flow being diverted to the peripheries in the presence of fever. As sepsis progresses, widespread catecholamine release will lead to peripheral vasoconstriction in an effort to increase SVR. Therefore, the patient may develop poor perfusion in the peripheries and become pale and mottled with cool skin. In addition, myocardial contractility and HR will increase in response to the high circulating levels of adrenaline, and tachycardia may increase further.

Increased capillary permeability allows a shift of fluid from the capillaries to the interstitial space and although angio-oedema is not classically described in sepsis, it certainly can be present, but not to the degree seen in syndromes such as anaphylaxis.

Arrhythmias are common in sepsis, most commonly supraventricular tachyarrhythmias including atrial fibrillation. There is no clear understanding of the mechanisms; causes may include preexisting arrhythmia, inadequate

HISTORY

Ask!

- Do you have a history of infection?
- Have you been prescribed any medications, especially antibiotics, immunosuppressants or antifungals?
- If so, do you think the medications are working?
- Is there a chance you might have been exposed to an infectious disease?
- What was the first symptom you noticed?
- Are the symptoms getting better or worse?

RESPIRATORY STATUS

Look for!

- Scattered, coarse crackles
- Unilateral or bilateral
- Bronchial breath sounds
- Increased work of breathing/increased respiratory rate
- Hypoventilation and impending respiratory failure

PERFUSION STATUS

Look for!

- Tachycardia
- Hypotension
- Weak peripheral pulses
- Altered conscious state
- Pallor
- Cool peripheries
- Mottled skin (especially paediatrics)

Ask!

- Do you feel cold or hot?
- Do you feel dizzy?
- Do you feel thirsty?

coronary perfusion and sepsis-induced cardiomyopathy (Heinz, 1999). The paramedic should ensure that a thorough history is taken to establish the presence of preexisting arrhythmia. Bradycardia is also common, especially in patients suffering sepsis secondary to fungal infections (Heinz, 1999).

Gastrointestinal system

Gastrointestinal assessment can also prove difficult. Systemic effects of sepsis can cause inadequate perfusion to the gastrointestinal tract, leading to abdominal cramping and diarrhoea (Tintinalli, 2016). Alternatively, the cause of sepsis may be intraabdominal, such as bowel obstruction, bowel perforation or appendicitis (Cunha & Bronze, 2012).

Genitourinary

One of the most common causes of sepsis in the elderly is urinary tract infection. Renal perfusion is a key indicator of vital organ perfusion and urine output should be in the vicinity or 1–2 mL/kg/hour. As a minimum, 0.5 mL/kg/hour is ideal in critically unwell patients (Tintinalli, 2016). In sepsis patients, a reduction in urine output is a sign of poor perfusion and a low central venous pressure (CVP). Recent urine output should be determined and if catheterised, this output should be measured or cross-referenced with the carer's medical documentation.

Initial assessment summary

Problem	Generally unwell
Weight	84 kg
Conscious state	Altered GCS = 13; E 3, V 4, M 6
Position	Sitting in a chair
Heart rate	116 bpm
Blood pressure	105/70 mmHg
Skin appearance	Flushed and hot
Speech pattern	Phrases
Respiratory rate	28 bpm
Respiratory rhythm	Even cycles
Chest auscultation	Clear chest sounds bilaterally
Pulse oximetry	93% on room air
Temperature	38.8°C
Motor/sensory function	Appears normal
Pain	No pain
History	Fever for a few days, a productive cough, dizziness, dyspnoea and increased frequency of urination
Physical assessment	No abnormalities detected

D: There is no immediate danger.
A: The patient is conscious with no current airway obstruction, but requires frequent reassessment.
B: Respiratory function is currently adequate; however, this requires frequent reassessment. The respiratory rate is elevated but no work of breathing is evident.
C: HR is elevated and the BP is labile.

Out-of-hospital sepsis assessment criteria

Out-of-hospital assessment of sepsis can be significantly challenging for paramedics, and currently much focus has been placed on early identification and intervention. Several out-of-hospital sepsis screening tools and criteria exist and are associated with varying degrees of sensitivity and specificity. The Sepsis 3 taskforce recommended the use of the qSOFA (quick SOFA), which is an abbreviation of the SOFA assessment but less robust. The qSOFA incorporates the following criteria: altered mentation, systolic BP of 100 mmHg or less and respiratory rate of 22 bpm or greater. It is intended to provide simple point-of-care criteria to identify adult patients who present with suspected infection and are at risk of a poor outcome (Singer et al., 2016). If the patient presents with two or more qSOFA criteria, this should then guide the clinician to further consider the presence of organ dysfunction (SOFA assessment) and escalate clinical care or referral to the appropriate specialty. Interestingly, the Sepsis 3 Task Force recommended the use of the qSOFA assessment in the out-of-hospital environment; however, as a screening tool its sensitivity and specificity has undergone very little out-of-hospital scrutiny or validation.

Recently in Switzerland, Tusgul and colleagues (2017) undertook a retrospective study of 886 patients transported by emergency medical services (EMS) to the ED over a 12-month period. The out-of-hospital qSOFA score, SIRS criteria and sepsis definition were retrospectively analysed and also at ED triage as predictors of ICU admission, stay and mortality. In the out-of-hospital setting, the sensitivity of qSOFA reached 36% for ICU admission and 68% for 48-hour mortality. The sensitivity of SIRS criteria was higher for ICU admission (68%); however, 48-hour mortality was slightly less (64%). Of note, the out-of-hospital sensitivity of the sepsis definition did not reach 60% for any outcome. Conversely, at ED triage the sensitivity of qSOFA was less than that of the out-of-hospital finding (ED triage; 31% for ICU admission and 60% for 48-hour mortality). Of note, the ED triage sensitivity of SIRS criteria was found to be associated with an 80% 48-hour mortality.

These findings highlight that the qSOFA score, SIRS criteria and sepsis definition have a low identification sensitivity in determining out-of-hospital sepsis patients. This is comparable with other study findings which found SIRS criteria were not reliable predictors of sepsis or mortality in the ward setting and therefore not applicable to the out-of-hospital setting (Churpek et al., 2015; Kaukonen et al., 2015; Vincent et al., 2013; Smyth et al., 2016a, 2016b). Furthermore, Raith and colleagues (2017) found that the more comprehensive SOFA assessment was more accurate in predicting in-hospital mortality than both SIRS and qSOFA criteria and the qSOFA score had little additional predictive value over the SIRS criteria among patients admitted to the ICU with suspected infection.

More evidence-based evaluation of out-of-hospital sepsis screening tools is needed with greater focus on validating the inclusion of more organ dysfunction criteria and also non-SIRS criteria such as point-of-care blood lactate, blood glucose and BP (Smyth et al., 2016a, 2016b; Raith et al., 2017).

Interestingly, The UK Sepsis Trust has developed one of the most relevant and comprehensive out-of-hospital sepsis screening tools (UKSTPHSS) using an algorithmic approach which incorporates infective history, physiological criteria suggestive of organ dysfunction and at-risk patient groups. The UKST-PHSS is an amalgamation of expanded SIRS criteria (the NEWS score) and the Robson and BAS 90-30-90 sepsis screening tools which has been endorsed by the National Institute for Health Care and Excellence (NICE) and the United Kingdom's National Health Service (NHS) and Royal College of Physicians (Tusgul et al., 2017; Robson et al., 2009; Swedish Society of Infectious Disease, 2012; Royal College of Physicians, National Early Warning Score [NEWS] 2, 2017) (see Fig 32.6).

② CONFIRM

An essential component of clinical assessment is confirming clinical signs that should be present in support of your provisional diagnosis. You should also

SEPSIS SCREENING TOOL PREHOSPITAL | AGE 12+

01 START THIS CHART IF THE PATIENT LOOKS UNWELL OR NEWS2 IS 5 OR ABOVE

RISK FACTORS FOR SEPSIS INCLUDE:

- ☐ Age > 75
- ☐ Impaired immunity (e.g. diabetes, steroids, chemotherapy)
- ☐ Recent trauma / surgery / invasive procedure
- ☐ Indwelling lines / IVDU / broken skin

02 COULD THIS BE DUE TO AN INFECTION? — YES

LIKELY SOURCE:

- ☐ Respiratory
- ☐ Brain
- ☐ Urine
- ☐ Surgical
- ☐ Skin / joint / wound
- ☐ Other
- ☐ Indwelling device

NO → **SEPSIS UNLIKELY, CONSIDER OTHER DIAGNOSIS**

03 ANY RED FLAG PRESENT? — YES

- ☐ Objective evidence of new or altered mental state
- ☐ Systolic BP ≤ 90 mmHg (or drop of >40 from normal)
- ☐ Heart rate ≥ 130 per minute
- ☐ Respiratory rate ≥ 25 per minute
- ☐ Needs O_2 to keep SpO_2 ≥ 92% (88% in COPD)
- ☐ Non-blanching rash / mottled / ashen / cyanotic
- ☐ Lactate ≥ 2 mmol/l
- ☐ Recent chemotherapy
- ☐ Not passed urine in 18 hours (<0.5ml/kg/hr if catheterised)

YES → **RED FLAG SEPSIS START PH BUNDLE**

04 ANY AMBER FLAG PRESENT? — NO

IF UNDER 17 & IMMUNITY IMPAIRED TREAT AS RED FLAG SEPSIS

- ☐ Relatives concerned about mental status
- ☐ Acute deterioration in functional ability
- ☐ Immunosuppressed
- ☐ Trauma / surgery / procedure in last 8 weeks
- ☐ Respiratory rate 21-24
- ☐ Systolic BP 91-100 mmHg
- ☐ Heart rate 91-130 or new dysrhythmia
- ☐ Temperature <36°C
- ☐ Clinical signs of wound infection

YES → **FURTHER INFORMATION AND REVIEW REQUIRED:**

- TRANSFER TO DESIGNATED DESTINATION
- COMMUNICATE POTENTIAL OF SEPSIS AT HANDOVER

NO AMBER FLAGS OR UNLIKELY SEPSIS: ROUTINE CARE - CONSIDER OTHER DIAGNOSIS - SAFETY-NET & SIGNPOST AS PER LOCAL GUIDANCE

PREHOSPITAL SEPSIS BUNDLE*:

RESUSCITATION:
Oxygen to maintain saturations of >94% (88% in COPD)
Measure lactate if available
250ml boluses of Sodium Chloride: max 250mls if normotensive, max 2000ml if hypotensive OR lactate >2 mmol/l

COMMUNICATION:
Pre-alert receiving hospital.
Divert to ED (or other agreed destination)
Handover presence of Red Flag Sepsis

*NICE recommends rapid transfer to hospital is the priority rather than a prehospital bundle

THE UK SEPSIS TRUST

UKST 2019 3.2 PAGE 1 OF 1
UKST, REGISTERED CHARITY 1158843

Figure 32.6
Prehospital Sepsis Screening and Action Tool.
Source: Reproduced with permission of UK Sepsis Trust 2020, available online at https://sepsistrust.org/wp-content/uploads/2019/12/Sepsis-Prehospital-12-231219.pdf

seek to challenge your provisional diagnosis by exploring findings that do not fit your hypothesis: don't just ignore them because they don't fit.

What else could it be?

Mild infection

Context is an important part of any assessment and this is certainly the case with patients who may have sepsis. Early signs of infection are varied, including tachycardia, fever and feeling generally unwell. It is prudent not to 'jump' to the conclusion that the patient is septic. If the patient presents with SIRS criteria in conjunction with a history that suggests sepsis, then erring on the side of the more serious diagnosis is safe. However, if the patient has only early signs of infection, does not meet SIRS criteria or the history doesn't 'gel' with the presenting symptoms, the paramedic should be cautious of a diagnosis of sepsis.

Anaphylaxis

Patients with anaphylaxis share similar symptoms to patients with sepsis, including hypotension, tachycardia and respiratory distress. As such, differentiation between the two may be challenging. The key difference is the history. In anaphylaxis, the patient may obviously have been exposed to an allergen, although this will not always be the case. In sepsis, the prodromal period will often occur over hours to days or even weeks. Even if there has been no obvious exposure to an allergen, anaphylaxis usually demonstrates relatively rapid physiological manifestations and deterioration. Excluding fulminant meningococcal septicaemia, the progression of most manifestations of sepsis may be relatively slower.

Physically, anaphylaxis patients typically demonstrate one or more of the following symptoms: urticaria, erythema, angio-oedema and pruritus (Tintinalli, 2016). These symptoms are not typical of sepsis, especially the 'cherry-red' erythema and urticaria often seen in anaphylaxis. For paramedics confronted with a patient with an ambiguous history, hypotension, tachycardia and a mild fever, the approach should be to look for dermal signs that would sway the diagnosis towards anaphylaxis, and appropriate management should be commenced promptly.

Acute myocardial infarction and cardiogenic shock

Similar to anaphylaxis, patients with AMI may exhibit tachycardia and hypotension. Similar to sepsis, patients with AMI may be pale secondary to peripheral vasoconstriction, irritable, mildly warm or cold and have respiratory distress (Tintinalli, 2016). The patient may have 'classic' AMI symptoms such as chest pain, nausea, shortness of breath and sweating, although often these symptoms do not occur (Tintinalli, 2016). The key to differentiating between AMI and sepsis is the history. It is vital to establish any important comorbidities such as hypercholesterolaemia, hypertension and diabetes mellitus. Although these coexisting illnesses do not preclude a diagnosis of sepsis, they are strongly associated with AMI risk, and in conjunction with the patient's ECG, history and presenting complaints should be considered to differentiate AMI from sepsis or SIRS.

As AMI progresses to cardiogenic shock, the haemodynamic status may deteriorate further, where vital organ perfusion is compromised. Again, history will be vital. The patient suffering from cardiogenic shock can mimic sepsis closely; therefore, the paramedic should be vigilant in assessing the ECG and recent history, ruling out AMI as a cause of inadequate perfusion if possible and managing the patient accordingly.

Acute pulmonary oedema

Signs of right and left heart failure such as increased jugular venous pressure, peripheral oedema and a productive cough with pink, frothy sputum may point towards acute pulmonary oedema as opposed to a respiratory tract infection

DIFFERENTIAL DIAGNOSIS

Sepsis
Or
- Mild infection
- Anaphylaxis
- Acute myocardial infarction
- Cardiogenic shock
- Acute pulmonary oedema
- Pulmonary embolism (PE)

PRACTICE TIP

SIRS and/or sepsis are clinical diagnoses in the out-of-hospital setting, meaning that the diagnosis is determined on the patient's presentation rather than laboratory results. This patient has the hallmarks of sepsis; however, it is important not to discount other causes. A clinical problem-solving approach should be adopted to systematically explore and eliminate other diagnoses.

(Tintinalli, 2016). The clinical assessment challenge is to differentiate between infection as a root cause of inadequate perfusion, altered consciousness and/or respiratory distress and a multitude of other usual cardiac causes. This may require repeated observations over time to establish patterns and response to treatment.

③ TREAT
Emergency management
Safety

The patient may be infectious, so standard personal protective equipment (PPE) including gloves, glasses and possibly protective face mask may be appropriate.

Positioning

Patients who are haemodynamically compromised will benefit from supine posturing in order to assist venous return to the heart, thereby increasing CO (Marieb & Hoehn, 2007). However, in cases of respiratory distress or primary respiratory tract infection, supine posturing may worsen the respiratory distress. In such cases, the patient should be placed in a semi-recumbent position, where respiratory distress is minimised and venous return minimally opposed.

Antibiotics

Ideally, broad-spectrum antibiotics should be administered early in the course of sepsis (Kumar et al., 2006; Leibovici et al., 1998; Rhodes et al., 2016). This is of particular importance in fulminant meningococcal septicaemia, where early administration of antibiotics such as ceftriaxone or benzyl penicillin may halt the progression of sepsis and prevent serious morbidity and/or mortality (Hart et al., 1993; Schwartz et al., 1988).

However, the international standard for sepsis care, the Surviving Sepsis Guidelines, states that ideally blood cultures should be obtained before administering antibiotics (Rhodes et al., 2016). The rationale is that if the organism causing sepsis can be identified, antibiotic therapy can be specifically targeted. As a result, empirical broad-spectrum antibiotic therapy is not currently largely supported in the out-of-hospital setting, as it may make identification of the pathogen difficult. The exception to this is suspected meningococcal sepsis; it is possible to identify the organism using polymerase chain reaction technology even after the organism has been killed. Current research in this area may lead to a change in out-of-hospital practice resulting in blood culture collection and subsequent broad-spectrum antibiotic administration in identified sepsis patients.

In some circumstances, where broad-spectrum antibiotics are available in ambulances, it is prudent to consult with the receiving hospital regarding the appropriate administration of antibiotics. If the transport time is prolonged, or the patient is critically unwell, and the receiving doctor deems it appropriate for antibiotics to be administered without blood cultures, then paramedics may administer the medication. This is a decision based on weighing the pros and cons of early treatment versus the difficulty of identifying the organism and its sensitivities. A further complication of administering IV antibiotics prior to the ED is that massive bacterial lysis may precipitate an anaphylactoid reaction (otherwise described as a 'septic shower' or 'endotoxin shower'), releasing large volumes of endotoxins into the circulation and reducing the BP further. If out-of-hospital antibiotics are administered, this possible reaction should be considered and large-bore IV access obtained while preparing inotropes if necessary.

Serum lactate

Serum lactate should be measured in patients with suspected SIRS and sepsis as soon as is practicable if the technology to do so is available (Van Beest et al., 2009; Mikkelsen et al., 2009). In the presence of the SIRS criteria and an elevated serum lactate of greater than 4 mmol/L, fluid therapy should be instituted immediately. Even if the BP is normal to borderline, the presence of elevated serum lactate secondary to widespread anaerobic metabolism is a strong indicator of inadequate tissue perfusion (shock) (Van Beest et al., 2009; Mikkelsen et al., 2009). Note: despite the association between rising lactate, hypotension and mortality, elevated lactate can be present in other conditions and is therefore not specific to sepsis and should be considered in conjunction with clinical judgment (Tintinalli, 2016; Trzeciak et al., 2007; Shapiro et al., 2005).

Fluids

Sepsis is characterised by widespread peripheral vasodilation and increased capillary permeability. Often aggressive fluid therapy is indicated in the out-of-hospital phase to increase intravascular volume and venous return. The minimum starting point is 20 mL/kg of crystalloid fluid, either normal saline or compound sodium lactate (Hartmann's solution) depending on local guidelines (Tintinalli, 2016; Mikkelsen et al., 2009). However, fluid challenges should be administered and titrated when haemodynamic response occurs and/or BP improves (Rhodes et al., 2016).

Patients suffering sepsis can require large volumes of fluid (Dellinger et al., 2008), hence the advisability of considering inotropes/vasopressors early in the process. Depending on the length of the out-of-hospital phase, it may not be unusual to administer 40–60 mL/kg of fluid. Fluid therapy should ideally be titrated to urine output (> 0.5 mL/kg/hour) and serum lactate (Dellinger et al., 2008); however, if these measures are not available, then skin perfusion, BP, HR and conscious state may be used to guide management.

Once 20 mL/kg crystalloid fluid has been administered, a comprehensive reassessment of the patient's haemodynamic status and organ perfusion should be performed (Tintinalli, 2016; Dellinger et al., 2008). If there is little or no improvement in organ perfusion or haemodynamics, inotropes/vasopressors are indicated. In the absence of intensive care paramedic services or local guidelines to manage patients with IV sympathomimetics, fluid therapy should continue, titrated to response (Tintinalli, 2016; Dellinger et al., 2008) and transport to an appropriate facility where inotropes/vasopressors can be commenced.

Vasopressors/inotropes

The use of inotropes/vasopressors is indicated in patients where 20 mL/kg of fluid has achieved an optimum preload (10–15 cm of water positive) and has not led to an improvement in vital organ perfusion. In patients who would now be classed as in septic shock, the aim is to maintain a mean arterial BP (MABP) of > 65 mmHg (Rhodes et al., 2016; Singer et al., 2016). The use of vasopressors or inotropes is limited to intensive care paramedic services or in-hospital use. The choice of agent is important: the Surviving Sepsis Guidelines indicate that noradrenaline or dopamine is the agent of choice (Rhodes et al., 2016; Mikkelsen et al., 2009). The reality is that most out-of-hospital services in Australasia do not routinely carry these medications as part of their standard stock, although in cases of inter-facility transfer they may be available. Noradrenaline is by far the more commonly used agent in Australasia.

Noradrenaline is an alpha-adrenergic receptor agonist and its primary mechanism is peripheral vasoconstriction. It has limited cardiac (beta$_1$) effects and has rapid onset and offset. Its significant limitation is that if extravasation of the drug occurs, there is a real risk of tissue ischaemia and necrosis that can threaten limbs (Martin et al., 1993). As such, use of noradrenaline through a peripheral IV cannula should be reserved for secure, patent and reliable access points; administration through a central venous catheter is preferred and should be instituted as soon as is practical. This will be reserved for inter-facility transport or in-hospital use (Dellinger et al., 2008).

In most out-of-hospital services, intensive care paramedics will have access to bolus IV adrenaline or adrenaline by infusion. Adrenaline is not the drug of choice in sepsis, but can be used in the absence of noradrenaline for short-term therapy (Dellinger et al., 2008). Adrenaline is not ideal as it can reduce splanchnic blood flow and alter tissue oxygen delivery. Additionally, the beta$_1$ adrenergic effects increase HR and myocardial oxygen consumption and potentially worsen acidosis (Dellinger et al., 2008; Rhodes et al., 2016). If adrenaline must be administered, it should be titrated to BP and, importantly, fluid therapy must continue to ensure that intravascular volume is maintained with a view to improvement.

If infusion of adrenaline or noradrenaline is not possible, bolus adrenaline may be used at a dose of between 10 and 25 micrograms, starting with lower doses and titrated to effect being mindful of cardiac arrhythmia. Alternatively, metaraminol 500 micrograms IV bolus as required may be used in initial resuscitation efforts. Due to its extreme potency, noradrenaline *must not* be administered as a bolus and must only be delivered using a controlled delivery device such as an electronic syringe driver (Tintinalli, 2016; Dellinger et al., 2008).

Summary of therapeutic goals
- High-flow oxygen
- IV fluid therapy, titrate to haemodynamic response
- Consider consultation for IV empiric antibiotic therapy if significant out-of-hospital transport time exists
- Consideration given to inotrope if refractory to fluid therapy
- Transport to appropriate tertiary ED

(4) EVALUATE

Evaluating the effect of any clinical intervention can provide clues to the accuracy of the initial diagnosis. Some conditions respond rapidly to treatment so patients should be expected to improve if the diagnosis and treatment were appropriate. In this case the patient is unlikely to improve significantly during the short time he is in ambulance care. His SpO$_2$ should improve to > 96%; however, his HR and BP pressure are unlikely to improve significantly unless the paramedics administer an inotrope. A failure to improve should trigger the paramedics to reconsider the diagnosis.

Is the patient:
- Improving after IV crystalloid fluids?
  - Continue with the highest level of available care.
- Deteriorating or unchanged after IV fluids?
  - Continue with the highest level of available care.
- Now unconscious?
  - Start the primary survey.
- Now pulseless?
  - Check the monitor. Not VT or VF? Commence CPR!

Ongoing management

Corticosteroids

There is a lack of research to support the use of IV corticosteroids in the acute management stage of sepsis. Previously, corticosteroids were indicated early in the management algorithm; however, the Surviving Sepsis Guidelines now support only low-dose hydrocortisone therapy in patients with a poor response to fluid therapy *and* vasopressor therapy (Tintinalli, 2016; Rhodes et al., 2016; Venkatesh et al., 2018). Corticosteroids are therefore no longer recommended for administration in the out-of-hospital phase of care and are generally strictly reserved for patients in the intensive care unit. In cases of prolonged transport time or inter-facility transfer, consultation with the receiving hospital for the administration of hydrocortisone may be appropriate, depending on the clinical context.

Mechanical ventilation and airway management

Although ventilatory support and airway management are uncommon in the out-of-hospital setting, they may be required, especially in patients with sepsis and respiratory failure. Assisted ventilation should be provided when oxygen saturation cannot be maintained > 90% on high-flow oxygen or when respiratory failure is imminent (Tintinalli, 2016). Non-invasive ventilation (CPAP or BiPAP) may be considered if expertise and equipment are available; however, hypotension secondary to positive end-expiratory pressure should be anticipated. If drug-facilitated endotracheal intubation is required, the need for vasopressors/inotropes post-intubation should be anticipated due to a significant decrease in venous return secondary to positive pressure ventilation. The intricacies of managing the non-invasively or invasively ventilated sepsis patient are beyond the scope of this text.

Transport

The patient with sepsis should be placed in the context of their likely outcome. For example, a very frail and elderly patient with septic shock who is living in a high-level aged care facility is unlikely to have a positive outcome; this is probably a terminal event (Finfer et al., 2004). These patients may have advance care directives in place that guides clinical care in this difficult circumstance. Conversely, a middle-aged patient with sepsis pneumonia will have a greater chance of survival, and consideration should be given to transporting this patient to an appropriate facility. If a higher level of care is within a reasonable transport distance, this should be considered over a closer smaller regional hospital, thus negating the need for secondary transfer. Similar to major trauma patients, patients with sepsis can benefit from being delivered to the appropriate facility in a timely fashion.

Sepsis across the lifespan

Sepsis varies in cause and pathophysiology characteristics across the lifespan. The most at-risk patients are the very young and the very old (Tintinalli, 2016).

- **0–14 years.** The paediatric population, especially the very young, are at high risk of sepsis, primarily due to immature immune function. Infants and neonates have 10 times the risk of sepsis than older children. Boys are more likely to suffer sepsis up to the age of 10. In children < 1 year, sepsis is the fourth-leading cause of death, and in those aged 1–14 it is the second most common cause (Watson & Carcillo, 2005).
- **15–35 years.** This age group shows a decrease in the incidence of sepsis, probably due to the immune system being at the height of its function. Although this group can be at risk, especially if significant comorbidities are present, the late teens and early 20s have the lowest incidence, at a rate of about 0.2–0.5% of the population (Angus et al., 2001).
- **65+ years.** Sepsis in the elderly is a major concern for Western countries as their populations age. US data shows that nearly 60% of patients admitted to hospital for sepsis are older than 65 years of age. In addition, these patients carry a much higher mortality rate than other age groups, approaching an average of 40% (Destarac & Ely, 2002).

CASE STUDY 2

Case 11412, 0932 hrs.

Dispatch details: A 19-year-old female at a campsite is generally feeling unwell. Her estimated weight is 75 kgs.

Initial presentation: The crew arrive and are led inside a large tent. The patient is lying on a camp bed, surrounded by multiple friends of the same age. She seems oblivious to her surroundings. Her friends deny that she has ingested any alcohol or drugs and have been encouraging her to drink large volumes of water.

PRACTICE TIP

If the only available antibiotic is penicillin and the patient has a stated penicillin allergy, the paramedics will have to decide whether to administer penicillin. Factors to be considered include distance from hospital (for an alternative antibiotic), confidence in the diagnosis (and thus the urgency) and the exact history of any previous allergic reactions if known. If the paramedics decide to administer penicillin, they should first prepare to manage a potential anaphylactic reaction.

DIFFERENTIAL DIAGNOSIS

Meningococcal septicaemia
Or
- Flu-like illness
- Drug effects
- Dehydration
- Diabetic ketoacidosis

ASSESS

1007 hrs Primary survey: The patient is drowsy and agitated although rousing to pain.

1010 hrs Chief complaint: The patient refuses to talk and open her eyes. She feels hot. Her friends explain that she has had the flu for the last 3 days and won't stop complaining about a headache.

1015 hrs Vital signs survey: Perfusion status: HR 120 bpm, sinus tachycardia, BP 80/40 mmHg, skin mottled and dry, temperature 39.2°C.
Respiratory status: RR 24 bpm, good air entry bilaterally, increased work of breathing, SpO_2 95% on room air.
Conscious state: GCS = 12; eyes open to voice, confused, localises to pain. BGL: 6.6 mmol/L.

1020 hrs Pertinent hx: The patient has a history of flu-like symptoms for the last 3 days. She takes no medications and is allergic to penicillin.

1024 hrs Secondary survey: Spotty, purple rash to lower legs and arms. The cardinal sign of meningococcal septicaemia is a non-blanching purpuric rash. The paramedics perform the 'glass test', which involves rolling a clear glass over the rash to see whether it disappears when compressed: it does not.

CONFIRM

This patient is exhibiting some very concerning signs suggestive of meningococcal septicaemia: photophobia, headache, hypotension, tachycardia at rest, an odd-looking rash, increased respiratory rate and fever. However, in many cases paramedics are presented with a collection of signs and symptoms that do not appear to describe a particular condition. A critical step in determining a treatment plan in this situation is to consider what other conditions could explain the patient's presentation.

What else could it be?
Flu-like illness
Health professionals occasionally dismiss nonspecific symptoms such as these as simply being a viral illness and the secondary survey (i.e. physical examination of the patient in the medical setting) is often neglected: it has become routine in trauma patients and should not be left out of *any* comprehensive assessment. This patient's symptoms are too significant to dismiss without further investigation and comprehensive assessment combined with thorough history taking suggests that this is more than just the flu.

Drug effects
Given the social situation of a large gathering of young adults where the intent is probably to have some fun, it would be easy to assume that drugs and/or alcohol may play a part in the patient's presentation. However, if history taking is thorough, it should be easy to discount this, as in this case. Her friends have explicitly told the paramedics that although the patient normally drinks alcohol, she has not in this instance. Thus, probing further into the history and clinical presentation is essential.

Dehydration
It is very common for dehydration to manifest in signs and symptoms similar to those of meningeal irritation (i.e. headache, photophobia, irritability and fatigue). Hydration can be assessed by investigating signs such as skin turgor, mucosal membrane moisture and urine output. Sepsis patients will have signs of dehydration. Also, the friends have explicitly said that she has been consuming large volumes of water, so dehydration can be ruled out for this patient.

Diabetic ketoacidosis

Polydipsia, or insatiable thirst, is a hallmark of diabetic ketoacidosis and hyperglycaemia. To rule this out as a diagnosis, a simple blood glucose level will answer the question. All patients with a GCS of 14 or less should have a blood glucose level taken to rule out hypo- or hyperglycaemia as a cause of their symptoms. This patient's blood glucose is 6.6 mmol/L so hyperglycaemia can be eliminated as a cause.

The most likely diagnosis is meningococcal septicaemia and the patient should be treated for this.

③ TREAT

1031 hrs: The paramedics place the patient in the semi-recumbent position and give high-flow oxygen. They also establish IV access and administer 2 g of ceftriaxone and 20 mL/kg normal saline. Given the patient's history of an allergic reaction to penicillin, the paramedics closely monitor for signs of anaphylaxis; however, the slight chance of a reaction to the ceftriaxone is outweighed by the need to treat the meningococcal septicaemia. Remember the cross-reactivity rate among penicillin and third-generation cephalosporins (ceftriaxone) is < 1% (Romano et al., 2010, 2015).

1040 hrs: The patient's oxygen saturations improve to 99% on 8 L.
Perfusion status: HR 110 bpm, sinus tachycardia, BP 90/60 mmHg, skin colour improving slightly.
Respiratory status: RR 20 bpm, good air entry, L = R, increased work of breathing, speaking in short sentences, patient states no shortness of breath.
Conscious state: GCS = 14; confused.

1043 hrs: The paramedics administer 20 mL/kg of normal saline for ongoing fluid resuscitation, even after antibiotics have been given.

Summary of therapeutic goals
- High-flow oxygen
- IV fluid therapy
- IV empiric antibiotic therapy
- Consideration given to inotrope if refractory to fluid therapy
- Transport to appropriate tertiary ED

④ EVALUATE

Evaluating the effect of any clinical management intervention can provide clues to the accuracy of the initial diagnosis. Some conditions respond rapidly to treatment so patients should be expected to improve if the diagnosis and treatment were appropriate, whereas other conditions are unlikely to respond in the timeframes normally associated with ambulance transport times. In such cases, a failure to improve should not be considered an indication of a misdiagnosis.

Responses to the treatment of meningococcal septicaemia with ceftriaxone can be unpredictable, ranging from no response to a slight improvement but also to a sudden deterioration. In severe cases, the action of ceftriaxone to break down the bacterial walls can trigger an immune response that worsens the shock.

Future research

Sepsis management is one of the most researched and funded areas in medicine. Research is primarily focused on determining how and why the immune response occurs in sepsis and ways to modulate this response. Some studies include the use of novel drugs to support BP and promote organ perfusion. Antibiotic resistance is also a significant concern and researchers are looking into enhanced antimicrobial agents to combat the ever-growing number of medication-resistant pathogens.

Out-of-hospital assessment of serum lactate has been proposed as an effective tool in measuring the degree of anaerobic metabolism and acidosis and the effectiveness of early therapy. Van Beest and colleagues (2009) found that by measuring the serum lactate level of out-of-hospital sepsis patients and then managing those patients who showed signs of septic shock based on the lactate level spent less time in ICU and had improved long-term outcomes. In addition, the value of blood lactate as a risk stratification tool in sepsis is an established evidence-based in-hospital practice. Elevated blood lactate has been shown to be a strong predictor of mortality in infection and critical care populations (Boland et al., 2016; Chippendale et al., 2017; Jansen et al., 2008). However, the worth of out-of-hospital point-of-care blood lactate assessment (POCBLA) as a risk stratification tool in identifying sepsis still requires further research.

Many feasibility studies exist, although very little out-of-hospital research has focused on POCBLA and its ability to enhance paramedic sepsis identification/treatment (Chippendale et al., 2017). Shiuh and colleagues (2012) reported in conjunction with using an out-of-hospital sepsis protocol (which included POCBLA) clinicians correctly identified 76.7% of sepsis presentations. In addition, Boland and colleagues (2016) reported that patients with elevated out-of-hospital lactate were more likely to be admitted to the ICU (23% versus 15%) and to have been diagnosed with sepsis (38% versus 22%) than those with normal lactate levels; however, these differences were not statistically significant. In a recent study, Swan and colleagues (2018) compared paramedic POCBLA with in-hospital lactate levels and found that when the time between measurements was less than 60 minutes, normal out-of-hospital lactate predicted normal in-hospital lactate levels with 100% accuracy (false-positive rate of 18.2%). Furthermore, other studies (Hokanson et al., 2012; Shiuh et al., 2012; Guerra et al., 2013) all reported a strong correlation between out-of-hospital lactate levels and ED lactate levels. These findings certainly give weight to POCBLA assisting

in out-of-hospital sepsis identification, especially if further research confirms no difference in the accuracy of blood lactate assessed in the out-of-hospital setting when compared to the ED setting.

POCBLA may also have significant implications for identifying and treating occult sepsis or cryptic sepsis. Interestingly, some out-of-hospital sepsis patients can present with cryptic sepsis and maintain normal BP but will manifest hypoxia indicated by a lactate level > 4 mmol/L (Puskarich et al., 2010; NSW Government Clinical Excellence Commission, 2018). Puskarich and colleagues (2010) undertook a secondary analysis of multicentre ED-based randomised controlled trial of early sepsis resuscitation. They found that cryptic sepsis (cryptic sepsis = SIRS criteria, blood lactate ≥ 4 mmol/L and normotension) carries a mortality rate not significantly different from that of overt septic shock (overt septic shock = SIRS criteria, blood lactate ≥ 4 mmol/L and hypotension). Cryptic sepsis was associated with an in-hospital mortality of 20%, highlighting a 1% difference compared to overt septic shock (19%). These findings were similar in an Australian sepsis population ($n = 3851$) which reported a mortality rate of 13% in the cryptic sepsis group (NSW Government Clinical Excellence Commission, 2018). Although further research is needed, out-of-hospital POCBLA may be a useful tool to assist paramedics with identifying/treating sepsis patients. Devices and consumables used to measure serum lactate are affordable and readily available. As such, this cheap yet effective assay is likely to become a common out-of-hospital assessment in the near future.

Paramedic administration of antibiotics in the out-of-hospital setting is a contentious intervention which receives much debate among the emergency medicine community. The issues relate to accuracy of sepsis identification leading to inappropriate antibiotic administration, the inability to obtain blood culture prior to antibiotic administration and impact on antibiotic resistance. It has been postulated that early intervention by paramedics prior to arrival at the ED may lead to improved outcomes among sepsis patients (Smyth et al., 2016a, 2016b). Furthermore, the opportunity to improve out-of-hospital sepsis care could produce outcomes far greater than other out-of-hospital time-critical conditions that are life-threatening such as AMI, stroke and major trauma (Smyth et al., 2016a, 2016b; Abdullah et al., 2008; American College of Emergency Physicians, 2012; Kumar et al., 2006; NSW Government Clinical Excellence Commission, 2018).

Paramedics may play a key role in the management of sepsis via reduction in time to antibiotic treatment through out-of-hospital administration of antibiotics. Evidence from observational studies have found that the time between the onset of hypotension to administration of antibiotics has a significant impact on mortality in patients with acute sepsis (Kumar et al., 2006; Ferrer et al., 2014; Burrell et al., 2016). In a landmark study, Kumar and colleagues (2006) found that initiation of effective antimicrobial therapy within the first hour following onset of hypotension related to septic shock was associated with 79.9% survival to hospital discharge. As a result, mortality increased by 7.6% for every hour of delay in starting antibiotic therapy after the onset of hypotension.

Some EMS, through the use of local guidelines, allow paramedics to obtain blood cultures and administer broad-spectrum antibiotics in identified sepsis patients. Interestingly, Chippendale and colleagues (2017) undertook a prospective feasibility study where paramedics were trained/educated to collect blood cultures and administer broad-spectrum antibiotics to 'red flag' sepsis patients. Of the patients that were identified as 'red flag' sepsis, 93% received a hospital diagnosis of infection and 7.14% of blood cultures were reported contaminated compared to 8.48% of those taken in ED. In 2017, the first large out-of-hospital randomised controlled trial was publish in *The Lancet*. This study aimed to determine the impact of out-of-hospital blood culture collection and subsequent antibiotic administration on survival. The intervention group received antibiotics a median of 26 minutes before arriving at the ED, whereas the usual care group median time to antibiotics after arriving at the emergency department was 70 minutes (Phantasi et al., 2018). Phantasi and colleagues (2018) concluded that EMS personnel training improved early sepsis recognition and overall care; however, administering antibiotics in the out-of-hospital setting did not lead to improved survival (28-day mortality; 8% of patients had died in the intervention group and 8% had died in the usual care group). The methodology of

this study has received much debate among the critical care research community, largely due to using only SIRS criteria to enrol patients regardless of illness severity. This certainly warrants a need for further out-of-hospital RCTs with more sensitive/specific enrolment criteria to validate or disprove the above findings.

An evidence-based change in the out-of-hospital treatment for patients with severe community-acquired sepsis to enable out-of-hospital antibiotic administration could result in a significant reduction in mortality. If proven to have a mortality benefit, this intervention would highlight the integral role that ambulance services play in extending point-of-care medicine from the in-hospital to the out-of-hospital setting and influencing general medical care on a national/international scale.

Summary

Sepsis is a progressive disorder that begins with bacterial, viral, parasitic or fungal infection. If the infection is not able to be managed by the body or by first-line medical care, it may progress to sepsis, as identified by widespread inflammatory response (i.e. SIRS). If sepsis progresses, inflammation abounds, vascular integrity is compromised, myocardial function is suppressed, respiratory function may be compromised and progressive clotting and/or endogenous fibrinolysis may lead to multi-organ failure and death. Sepsis is a life-threatening medical emergency and paramedics are often the first healthcare professionals to assess/treat these patients. Patients meeting SIRS criteria in the presence of a suspected or confirmed infection may be readily diagnosed, but some signs and symptoms may be discreet, so thorough assessment and history taking are vital. It is important to manage these patients aggressively and early, even in the case of diagnostic uncertainty. As such, paramedics must be able to recognise sepsis and institute early treatment to minimise morbidity and mortality.

References

Abdullah, A. R., Smith, E. E., Biddinger, P. D., Kalenderian, D., & Schwamm, L. H. (2008). Advance hospital notification by EMS in acute stroke is associated with shorter door-to-computed tomography time and increased likelihood of administration of tissue-plasminogen activator. *Journal of Prehospital Emergency Care, 12*(4), 426–431.

Amaral, A., Opal, S., & Vincent, J. (2004). Coagulation in sepsis. *Intensive Care Medicine, 30*(6), 1032–1040.

American College of Chest Physicians/Society of Critical Care Medicine (ACCP/SCCM) Consensus Conference. (1992). Definitions for sepsis and organ failure and

guidelines for the use of innovative therapies in sepsis. *Critical Care Medicine, 20*, 864–874.

American College of Emergency Physicians. (2012). Trauma care systems development, evaluation, and funding. Policy statement. *Annals Emergency Medicine, 60*(2), 249–250.

Angus, D., Linde-Zwirble, W. T., Lidicker, J., Clermont, G., Carcillo, J., & Pinsky, M. R. (2001). Epidemiology of severe sepsis in the United States: analysis of incidence, outcome, and associated costs of care. *Critical Care Medicine, 29*(7).

Australian Government Department of Health (2018). *Meningococcal disease in Australia*. Retrieved from http://www.health.gov.au/internet/main/publishing.nsf/Content/ohp-meningococcal-W.htm.

Boland, L. L., Hokanson, J. S., Fernstrom, K. M., Kinzy, T. G., Lick, C. J., Satterlee, P. A., & LaCroix, B. K. (2016). Prehospital lactate measurement by emergency medical services in patients meeting sepsis criteria. *Western Journal of Emergency Medicine*, *17*(5), 648–655.

Burrell, A. R., McLaws, M. L., Fullick, M., Sullivan, R. B., & Sindhusake, D. (2016). Sepsis kills: early intervention saves lives. *The Medical Journal of Australia*, *204*(2), 73.

Chippendale, J., Lloyd, A., Payne, T., Dunmore, S., & Stoddart, B. (2017). A pilot study to assess the feasibility of paramedics delivering antibiotic treatment to 'red flag' sepsis patients. *Emergency Medicine Journal*, *34*, 695.

Churpek, M. M., Zadravecz, F. J., Winslow, C., Howell, M. D., & Edelson, D. P. (2015). Incidence and prognostic value of the systemic inflammatory response syndrome and organ dysfunctions in ward patients. *American Journal of Respiratory and Critical Care Medicine*, *192*(8), 958–964.

Cohen, J., & Powderly, W. G. (2010). *Infectious diseases* (3rd ed.). Philadelphia: Elsevier.

Cunha, B., & Bronze, M. (2012). *Bacterial sepsis*. Accessed 21 January 2012. Retrieved from http://emedicine.medscape.com/article/234587-overview.

Dellinger, R., Levy, M., Carlet, J., Bion, J., Parker, M. M., Jaeschke, R., Reinhart, K., Angus, D. C., Brun-Buisson, C., Beale, R., Calandra, T., Dhainaut, J.-F., Gerlach, H., Harvey, M., Marini, J. J., Marshall, J., Ranieri, M., Ramsay, G., Sevransky, J., Thompson, B. T., Townsend, S., Vender, J. S., Zimmerman, J. L., Vincent, J.-L., International Surviving Sepsis Campaign Guidelines Committee; American Association of Critical-Care Nurses; American College of Chest Physicians; American College of Emergency Physicians; Canadian Critical Care Society; European Society of Clinical Microbiology and Infectious Diseases; European Society of Intensive Care Medicine; European Respiratory Society; International Sepsis Forum; Japanese Association for Acute Medicine; Japanese Society of Intensive Care Medicine; Society of Critical Care Medicine; Society of Hospital Medicine; Surgical Infection Society; World Federation of Societies of Intensive and Critical Care Medicine. (2008). Surviving Sepsis Campaign: international guidelines for the management of severe sepsis and septic shock. *Critical Care Medicine*, *36*, 296–327.

Dellinger, R. P., Carlet, J. M., Masur, H., Gerlach, H., Calandra, T., Cohen, J., Gea-Banacloche, J., Keh, D., Marshall, J. C., Parker, M. M., Ramsay, G., Zimmerman, J. L., Vincent, J. L., & Levy, M. M. (2004). Surviving sepsis campaign management guidelines committee. Surviving sepsis campaign guidelines for management of severe sepsis and septic shock. *Journal of Critical Care Medicine*, *32*(3), 858–873.

Dellinger, R. P., Levy, M. M., Rhodes, A., Annane, D., Gerlach, H., Opal, S. M., Sevransky, J. E., Sprung, C. L., Douglas, I. S., Jaeschke, R., Osborn, T. M., Nunnally, M. E., Townsend, S. R., Reinhart, K., Kleinpell, R. M.,

Angus, D. C., Deutschman, C. S., Machado, F. R., Rubenfeld, G. D., Webb, S., Beale, R. J., Vincent, J. L., & Moreno, R. (2013). Surviving sepsis campaign guidelines committee including the pediatric subgroup. Surviving sepsis campaign: international guidelines for management of severe sepsis and septic shock. *Journal of Intensive Care Medicine*, *39*(2), 165–228.

Destarac, L., & Ely, E. (2002). Sepsis in older patients: an emerging concern in critical care. *Advances in Sepsis*, *2*(1).

Ebby, O. (2005). Community-acquired pneumonia: from common pathogens to emerging resistance. *Emergency Medicine Practice*, *7*(12).

Ferrer, R., Martin-Loeches, I., Phillips, G., Osborn, T., Townsend, S., Dellinger, R. P., Artigas, A., Schorr, C., & Levy, M. (2014). Empiric antibiotic treatment reduces mortality in severe sepsis and septic shock from the first hour: results from a guideline-based performance improvement program. *Journal of Critical Care Medicine*, *42*, 1749–1755.

Finfer, S., Bellomo, R., Lipman, J., French, C., Dobb, G., & Myburgh, J. (2004). Adult-population incidence of severe sepsis in Australian and New Zealand intensive care units. *Intensive Care Medicine*, *30*(4), 589–596.

Gaieski, D. F., Edwards, J. M., Kallan, M. J., & Carr, B. G. (2013). Benchmarking the incidence and mortality of severe sepsis in the United States. *Journal of Critical Care Medicine*, *41*(5), 1167–1174.

Gaines, N. N., Patel, B., Williams, E. A., & Cruz, A. T. (2012). Etiologies of septic shock in a pediatric emergency department population. *The Pediatric Infectious Disease Journal*, *31*(11), 1203–1205.

Gotts, J. E., & Matthay, M. A. (2016). Sepsis: pathophysiology and clinical management. *British Medical Journal*, *353*, i1585.

Guerra, W. F., Mayfield, T. R., Meyers, M. S., Clouatre, A. E., & Riccio, J. C. (2013). Early detection and treatment of patients with severe sepsis by prehospital personnel. *Journal of Emergency Medicine*, *44*(6), 1116–1125.

Hart, C. A., Cuevas, L. E., Marzouk, O., Thomson, A. P., & Sills, J. (1993). Management of bacterial meningitis. *The Journal of Antimicrobial Chemotherapy*, *32*(Suppl.A), 49–59.

Heinz, G. (1999). Infection, sepsis and cardiac arrhythmia. *Wiener klinische Wochenschrift Gesellschaft der Ärzte in Wien*, *111*(21), 868–875.

Hokanson, J., Boland, L., Olson, T., Fernstrom, K., & Lick, C. (2012). Use of lactate meters and temporal artery thermometers by paramedics to aid in the Out-of-Hospital recognition of sepsis: a pilot. *Study Annals of Emergency Medicine*, *60*(4), S43.

Jansen, T. C., van Bommel, J., Mulder, P. G., Rommes, J. H., Schieveld, S. J., & Bakker, J. (2008). The prognostic value of blood lactate levels relative to that of vital signs in the pre-hospital setting: a pilot study. *Journal of Critical Care*, *12*(6), R160.

Jawad, I., Luksic, I., & Rafnsson, S. B. (2012). Assessing available information on the burden of sepsis: global estimates of incidence, prevalence and mortality. *Journal of Global Health*, *2*(1), 010404.

Kaukonen, K. M., Bailey, M., Pilcher, D., Cooper, J., & Bellomo, R. (2015). Systemic inflammatory response syndrome criteria in defining severe sepsis. *The New England Journal of Medicine*, *372*, 1629–1638.

Kaukonen, K. M., Bailey, M., Suzuki, S., Pilcher, D., & Bellomo, R. (2014). Mortality related to severe sepsis and septic shock among critically ill patients in Australia and New Zealand, 2000-2012. *JAMA*, *311*(13), 1308–1316.

Kellum, J., Lan, K., Fink, M., Weissfeld, L. A., Yealy, D. M., Pinsky, M. R., Fine, J., Krichevsky, A., Delude, R. L., Angus, D. C., & GenIMS Investigators. (2007). Understanding the inflammatory cytokine response in pneumonia and sepsis. *Archives of Internal Medicine*, *167*(15), 1655–1663.

Kumar, A., Roberts, D., Wood, K. E., Light, B., Parrillo, J. E., Sharma, S., Suppes, R., Feinstein, D., Zanotti, S., Taiberg, L., Gurka, D., Kumar, A., & Cheang, M. (2006). Duration of hypotension before initiation of effective antimicrobial therapy is the critical determinant of survival in human septic shock. *Journal of Critical Care Medicine*, *34*(6), 1589–1596.

Larson, V., & Barke, R. A. (1999). Gram-negative bacterial sepsis and the sepsis syndrome. *The Urologic Clinics of North America*, *26*(4), 687.

Latto, C. (2008). An overview of sepsis. *Dimensions of Critical Care Nursing*, *27*(5), 195–200.

Leibovici, L., Shraga, I., Drucker, M., Konigsberger, H., Samra, Z., & Pitlik, S. D. (1998). The benefit of appropriate empirical antibiotic treatment in patients with bloodstream infection. *Journal of Internal Medicine*, *244*, 379–386.

Longo, D., Fauci, A. S., Kasper, D. L., & Hauser, S. L. (2011). *Harrison's principles of internal medicine* (18th ed., *Vol. 1 and 2*). New York: McGraw-Hill Professional.

Marieb, E., & Hoehn, K. (2007). *Human anatomy and physiology* (7th ed.). Redwood City, CA: Pearson Benjamin Cummings.

Martin, C., Papazian, L., Perrin, G., Saux, P., & Gouin, F. (1993). Norepinephrine or dopamine for the treatment of hyperdynamic septic shock? *Chest*, *103*, 1826–1831.

Mikkelsen, M., Miltiades, A., Gaieski, D., Goyal, M., Fuchs, B. D., Shah, C. V., Bellamy, S. L., & Christie, J. D. (2009). Serum lactate is associated with mortality in severe sepsis independent of organ failure and shock. *Critical Care Medicine*, *37*, 1–8.

NSW Government Clinical Excellence Commission (2018). *Sepsis Kills Program*. Retrieved from http://www.cec.health.nsw.gov.au/patient-safety-programs/adult-patient-safety/sepsis-kills.

Peake, S., for the ARISE Investigators. (2007). The outcome of sepsis and septic shock presenting to the Emergency Department in Australia and New Zealand. *Journal of Critical Care*, *11*(2), 73.

Phantasi, A. N., Oskam, E., Stassen, P. M., Exter, P. V., van de Ven, P. M., Haak, H. R., Holleman, F., Zanten, A. V., Leeuwen-Nguyen, H. V., Bon, V., Duineveld, B. A. M., Nannan Panday, R. S., Kramer, M. H. H., & Nanayakkara, P. W. B., PHANTASi Trial Investigators and the ORCA (Onderzoeks Consortium Acute Geneeskunde) Research Consortium the Netherlands. (2018). Prehospital antibiotics in the ambulance for sepsis: a multicentre, open label, randomised trial. *The Lancet. Respiratory Medicine*, *6*(1), 40–50.

Puskarich, M., Trzeciak, S., Shapiro, N., & Kline, J. (2010). Outcomes of cryptic septic shock compared with overt septic shock. *Annals of Emergency Medicine*, *56*(3), S44.

Raith, E. P., Udy, A. A., Bailey, M., McGloughlin, S., MacIsaac, C., Bellomo, R., & Pilcher, D. V., Australian and New Zealand Intensive Care Society (ANZICS) Centre for Outcomes and Resource Evaluation (CORE). (2017). Prognostic accuracy of the SOFA score, SIRS criteria, and qSOFA score for In-Hospital mortality among adults with suspected infection admitted to the intensive care unit. *Journal of American Medical Association*, *317*(3), 290–300.

Rangel-Frausto, M., Pittet, D., Costigan, M., Hwang, T., Davis, C., & Wenzel, R. (1995). The natural history of the systemic inflammatory response syndrome (SIRS): a prospective study. *JAMA*, *273*, 117–123.

Reinhart, K., Daniels, R., Kissoon, N., Machado, F. R., Schachter, R. D., & Finfer, S. (2017). Recognizing sepsis as a global health priority—A WHO resolution. *The New England Journal of Medicine*, *377*(5), 414–417.

Rhodes, A., Evans, L. E., Alhazzani, W., Levy, M. M., Antonelli, M., Ferrer, R., Kumar, A., Sevransky, J. E., Sprung, C. L., Nunnally, M. E., Rochwerg, B., Rubenfeld, G. D., Angus, D. C., Annane, D., Beale, R. J., Bellinghan, G. J., Bernard, G. R., Chiche, J. D., Coopersmith, C., De Backer, D. P., French, C. J., Fujishima, S., Gerlach, H., Hidalgo, J. L., Hollenberg, S. M., Jones, A. E., Karnad, D. R., Kleinpell, R. M., Koh, Y., Lisboa, T. C., Machado, F. R., Marini, J. J., Marshall, J. C., Mazuski, J. E., McIntyre, L. A., McLean, A. S., Mehta, S., Moreno, R. P., Myburgh, J., Navalesi, P., Nishida, O., Osborn, T. M., Perner, A., Plunkett, C. M., Ranieri, M., Schorr, C. A., Seckel, M. A., Seymour, C. W., Shieh, L., Shukri, K. A., Simpson, S. Q., Singer, M., Thompson, B. T., Townsend, S. R., Van der Poll, T., Vincent, J. L., Wiersinga, W. J., Zimmerman, J. L., & Dellinger, R. P. (2016). Surviving sepsis campaign: international guidelines for management of sepsis and septic shock. *Journal of Intensive Care Medicine*, *43*(3), 304–377.

Robson, W., Nutbeam, T., & Daniels, R. (2009). Sepsis: a need for prehospital intervention? *Journal of Emergency Medicine*, *26*, 535–538.

Romano, A., Gaeta, F., Valluzzi, R. L., Caruso, C., Rumi, G., & Bousquet, P. J. (2010). IgE-mediated hypersensitivity to cephalosporins: cross-reactivity and tolerability of penicillins, monobactams, and carbanems. *Journal of Allergy Clinical Immunology*, *126*(5), 994–999.

Romano, A., Gaeta, F., Valluzzi, R. L., Maggioletti, M., Zaffiro, A., Caruso, C., & Quaratino, D. (2015). IgE-mediated hypersensitivity to cephalosporins: cross-reactivity and tolerability of alternative cephalosporins. *Journal of Allergy Clinical Immunology*, *136*(3), 685–691.

Royal Children's Hospital, Melbourne, Australia (2018). *Clinical Practice Guidelines—Acute meningococcal disease*. Retrieved from https://www.rch.org.au/clinicalguide/guideline_index/Acute_meningococcal_disease/.

Royal College of Physicians. National Early Warning Score (NEWS) 2 (2017). *Standardising the assessment of acute illness severity in the NHS*. Retrieved from https://www.rcplondon.ac.uk/projects/outputs/national-early-warning-score-news-2.

Schlapbach, L. J., Straney, L., Alexander, J., MacLaren, G., Festa, M., Schibler, A., & Slater, A., ANZICS Paediatric Study Group. (2015). Mortality related to invasive infections, sepsis, and septic shock in critically ill children in Australia and New Zealand, 2002-13: a multicentre retrospective cohort study. *The Lancet Infectious Diseases Journal*, *15*(1), 46–54.

Schwartz, B., Al-Tobaiqi, A., Al-Ruwais, A., Fontaine, R. E., A'ashi, J., Hightower, A. W., Broome, C. V., & Music, S. I. (1988). Comparative efficacy of ceftriaxone and rifampicin in eradicating pharyngeal carriage of group A Neisseria meningitidis. *The Lancet*, *1*(8597), 1239–1242.

Shapiro, N. I., Howell, M. D., Talmor, D., Nathanson, L. A., Lisbon, A., Wolfe, R. E., & Weiss, J. W. (2005). Serum lactate as a predictor of mortality in emergency department patients with infection. *Annals of Emergency Medicine*, *45*(5), 524–528.

Shiuh, T., Sweeney, T., Rupp, R., Davis, B., & Reed, J. (2012). An emergency medical services protocol with Point-of-Care lactate accurately identifies Out-of-Hospital patients with severe infection and sepsis. *Annals of Emergency Medicine*, *60*(4), S44.

Singer, M., Deutschman, C. S., Seymour, C. W., Shankar-Hari, M., Annane, D., Bauer, M., Bellomo, R., Bernard, G. R., Chiche, J. D., Coopersmith, C. M., Hotchkiss, R. S., Levy, M. M., Marshall, J. C., Martin, G. S., Opal, S. M., Rubenfeld, G. D., van der Poll, T., Vincent, J. L., & Angus, D. C. (2016). The third international consensus definitions for sepsis and septic shock (Sepsis-3). *JAMA*, *315*(8), 801–810.

Smyth, M. A., Brace-McDonnell, S. J., & Perkins, G. D. (2016a). Identification of adults with sepsis in the prehospital environment: a systematic review. *British Medical Journal*, *6*(8), e011218.

Smyth, M. A., Brace-McDonnell, S. J., & Perkins, G. D. (2016b). Impact of prehospital care on outcomes in sepsis: a systematic review. *Journal of Emergency Medicine*, *17*(4), 427–437.

Swan, K. L., Keene, T., & Avard, B. J. (2018). A 12-Month clinical audit comparing Point-of-Care lactate measurements tested by paramedics with In-Hospital serum lactate measurements. *Journal of Prehospital Disaster Medicine*, *33*(1), 36–42.

Swedish Society of Infectious Disease (2012). *Guidelines for treatment of severe sepsis and septic shock – early recognition and initial management*. Retrieved from www.infektion.net/vardprogram.

Tintinalli, J. (2016). *Emergency medicine: a comprehensive study guide* (8th ed.). New York: McGraw-Hill.

Trzeciak, S., Dellinger, R. P., Chansky, M. E., Arnold, R. C., Schorr, C., Milcarek, B., Hollenberg, S. M., & Parrillo, J. E. (2007). Serum lactate as a predictor of mortality in patients with infection. *Journal of Intensive Care Medicine*, *6*, 970–977.

Tusgul, S., Carron, P. N., Yersin, B., Calandra, T., & Dami, F. (2017). Low sensitivity of qSOFA, SIRS criteria and sepsis definition to identify infected patients at risk of complication in the prehospital setting and at the emergency department triage. *Scandinavian Journal of Trauma, Resuscitation and Emergency Medicine*, *25*(1), 108.

Van Beest, P., Mulder, P. J., Oetomo, S. B., van den Broek, B., Kuiper, M. A., & Spronk, P. E. (2009). Measurement of lactate in a prehospital setting is related to outcome. *European Journal of Emergency Medicine*, *16*(6), 318–322.

Venkatesh, B., Finfer, S., Cohen, J., Rajbhandari, D., Arabi, Y., Bellomo, R., Billot, L., Correa, M., Glass, P., Harward, M., Joyce, C., Li, Q., McArthur, C., Perner, A., Rhodes, A., Thompson, K., Webb, S., & Myburgh, J., ADRENAL Trial Investigators and the Australian–New Zealand Intensive Care Society Clinical Trials Group. (2018). Adjunctive glucocorticoid therapy in patients with septic shock. *The New England Journal of Medicine*, *378*(9), 797–808.

Victorian Government, Australia. Department of Health (2018). *Meningococcal disease*. Retrieved from: https://www2.health.vic.gov.au/public-health/infectious-diseases/disease-information-advice/meningococcal-disease.

Vincent, J. L., Opal, S. M., Marshall, J. C., & Tracey, K. J. (2013). Sepsis definitions: time for change. *The Lancet*, *381*, 774–775.

Watson, S., & Carcillo, J. (2005). Scope and epidemiology of pediatric sepsis. *Pediatric and Critical Care Medicine*, *6*(3).

Bleeding From the Gastrointestinal and Urinary Tract

By Alexander Olaussen

OVERVIEW

- Bleeding from the gastrointestinal (GI) tract can be gradual or rapid, chronic or acute.
- Bleeding from the urinary tract tends to be gradual.
- Rapid bleeding may lead to haemodynamic instability and require resuscitation.
- Gradual bleeding can be a sign of malignancy or other sinister pathologies and requires investigation and observation.

- Haematuria and melaena can be extremely distressing and confronting for patients.
- Upper GI bleeding has a 28-day mortality rate of 13–20% depending on whether or not it is due to varices (Crooks et al., 2011).
- It may be difficult to accurately diagnose the site of bleeding solely from external clinical observation.

Introduction

Acute gastrointestinal (GI) bleeding can be a medical emergency if the blood loss is significant. Measuring blood loss from the bowel can be difficult (even a small amount can stain toilet water bright red) so out-of-hospital assessment and management should focus on identifying patients with life-threatening haemodynamic compromise and rapidly initiating appropriate resuscitation. The mortality rate of patients admitted to hospital with acute GI bleeding can be predicted with several scoring systems (Stanley et al., 2017). Elderly patients (> 65 years old) who are hypotensive (≤ 90 mmHg) and confused, and have abnormal liver and coagulation studies have a more than 30% risk of in-hospital mortality (Thandassery et al., 2015).

From an anatomical definitional point of view, upper GI bleeding (UGIB) originates proximal to the ligament of Treitz (i.e. in the oesophagus, stomach or duodenum), while lower GI bleeding (LGIB) originates distal to the ligament (i.e. jejunum, ilium, small bowel, colon or anus) (Benevides & dos Santos, 2016).

GI haemorrhage may be chronic or acute, with acute haemorrhages ranging from minor to life-threatening catastrophic bleeds. UGIB is four times more common than LGIB (Pezzulo & Kruger, 2014), with a small proportion of patients in ED with GI bleed having both UGIB and LGIB (Scottish Intercollegiate Guidelines Network [SIGN], 2008).

Acute upper GI tract bleeding generally has a worse prognosis than lower GI tract bleeding, and the prognosis is significantly worse for older, comorbid patients. Factors associated with poor outcomes have been studied and several scoring systems exist, such as AIMS65 (Saltzman et al., 2011) and the Glasgow-Blatchford Bleeding Score (Blatchford et al., 2000).

The major causes of upper GI haemorrhage include the following.

- Peptic (stomach) ulcer disease is the most common cause of UGIB, accounting for approximately half of all acute cases (British Society of Gastroenterology, 2007).
- Oesophageal ulcers, erosions or malignancies are a common cause of mild UGIB, but they rarely cause clinically significant acute haemorrhage.
- Mallory-Weiss Syndrome (MWS) describes bleeding from a tear in the mucosal surface of the gastro-oesophageal junction. It may account for up to 14% of UGIB. It classically presents as haematemesis after forceful vomiting, but can also occur post severe coughing, status asthmaticus, convulsions and hiccups (Brown, 2015).
- A rupture of oesophageal varices (dilated veins) is likely to result in catastrophic haemorrhage. Oesophageal varices are generally associated with portal hypertension and cirrhosis. The mortality rate of patients presenting with variceal haemorrhage is 14%.
- Gastric malignancies may also bleed, but this is generally chronic or minor bleeding (Cappell & Friedel, 2008).
- Duodenal ulcers can produce GI haemorrhage in the same way as gastric ulcers.
- For approximately 20% of patients presenting with UGIB no cause is identified (Cappell & Friedel, 2008).

Acute lower GI tract bleeding occurs most often in the elderly. As with UGIB, the presence of comorbidities or shock increases the mortality rate. Patients taking aspirin or non-steroidal anti-inflammatory drugs (NSAIDs) are at increased risk of severe, acute lower GI haemorrhage (Velayos et al., 2004). The causes of acute LGIB vary with age, the most common being:

- diverticular disease—this is the most frequent cause of rectal bleeding in patients aged over 50 years (23–48% of acute lower GI haemorrhages)
- colorectal neoplasms
- ischaemic colitis
- colorectal polyps
- inflammatory bowel disease (IBD)/ulcerative colitis such as Crohn's disease
- congenital vascular malformations (angio-dysplasia)
- damage to the intestinal epithelium from radiation treatment (radiation enteropathy)
- ruptured haemorrhoids and anal fissures—these are the most common causes of rectal bleeding in patients younger than 50 (Cameron et al., 2009).

Loss of blood into the urinary tract can originate at any site between the kidneys and the urethra but unlike bleeding into the GI tract the volume of blood involved is rarely sufficient to present as an acute emergency. For patients unused to the sight of blood in their urine, however, a toilet bowl stained bright red can be extremely confronting and upsetting.

Pathophysiology

Upper GI bleeds

Bleeding from the oesophagus usually results in clinically subacute bleeding as most of the blood is swallowed. In small amounts this blood passes into the lower GI tract and through the bowel with food, resulting in dark stools. But in larger volumes the blood acts as an emetic and can trigger vomiting. Blood that has been mixed with gastric acid becomes clumped and dark and once vomited appears as 'coffee grounds'. If the bleeding is prolonged and undetected, the patient can become anaemic with symptoms of blood loss (e.g. shortness of breath, lethargy, dizziness early on and syncope, confusion, angina and palpitations later on).

The most catastrophic UGIB occurs when an oesophageal varix ruptures. Oesophageal varices are dilated superficial veins located in the lower third of the oesophagus. These veins drain into the portal system via the left gastric vein. If they develop an obstruction of portal blood flow (often associated with liver cirrhosis), blood 'backs up' in the oesophageal veins. Normally, the pressure in the portal vein is approximately 4 mmHg, allowing adequate return of venous blood to the heart. If damage or scarring in the liver increases this pressure to greater than 10 mmHg, venous return is slowed and oesophageal varices often form (Grow & Chapman, 2001). Rupture of an oesophageal varix may cause a dramatic haemorrhage with a large amount of blood rapidly entering the stomach. The patient will often vomit before the action of gastric acid has had a chance to change the appearance of the blood (haematemesis). Blood that is not vomited progresses through the bowel and exits as dark, sticky altered blood or faeces (melaena). Sometimes the rate of bleeding is so rapid that blood from the upper GI tract (oesophageal varices or ulcers) can appear relatively unchanged at the lower end of the GI tract and bright-red blood may be passed through the rectum (haematochezia). It is estimated that up to 15% of rectal bleeding originates in the upper GI tract (Pezzulo & Kruger, 2014). The complications of bleeding oesophageal varices include:

- massive hypovolaemia and hypovolaemic shock
- possible aspiration and aspiration pneumonia associated with a decreased conscious level and vomiting
- exacerbation of hepatic encephalopathy.

The mortality from bleeding oesophageal varices is 50% and if bleeding is stopped, 50% will bleed again within a week (Grow & Chapman, 2001). Oesophageal varices are the most common cause of death associated with GI bleeding (Klebi et al., 2005).

Out-of-hospital management of a ruptured oesophageal varix is limited to management of the associated haemodynamic instability or shock and concurrent management of any airway compromise. Definitive treatment requires urgent surgical or endoscopic intervention. In-hospital emergency treatment pivots on immediate control of bleeding with sclerosis (Palmer, 2007), banding of the oesophageal varices via endoscopy or, for refractory haemorrhage, direct pressure using an inflatable oesophageal balloon (Klebi et al., 2005). Pressor drugs, generally terlipressin, somatostatin and octreotide, are used to induce splanchnic vasoconstriction. Longer-term measures to reduce portal pressure include portocaval shunts and drugs to lower portal vein pressure, beta-blockers or nitrates and, in some cases, liver transplant.

Mallory-Weiss tears in the mucosa at the gastro-oesophageal junction may produce bleeding, usually evident as frank red blood in the vomit. Causes

Table 33.1 Common causes of haematemesis and melaena

Oesophageal	Reflux oesophagitis
	Oesophageal varix (portal hypertension)
	Oesophageal tumour
	Mallory-Weiss mucosal tear
Gastric	Gastric ulcer (usually benign)
	Haemorrhagic gastritis
	Gastric varix
	Gastric cancer
	Delafoy lesion
Duodenum	Duodenal ulcer
	Duodenitis

include violent or sustained vomiting, retching, coughing or hiccupping. Most patients diagnosed with significant bleeding from a Mallory-Weiss tear will have other mucosal abnormalities associated with portal hypertension or liver disease. In one study patients presenting to ED with Mallory-Weiss–associated bleeding had a 20% incidence of shock; a similar case series reported a mortality rate of 10% (Akhtar & Padda, 2011).

GI ulcers are found most commonly in the stomach or duodenum. When these ulcers erode, the result is a low-volume chronic blood loss. The patient generally presents with anaemia and dark stools that test positive for occult blood. GI ulcers that damage larger blood vessels may produce significant haematemesis (see Table 33.1). Of the ulcers that erode into larger blood vessels, 30% produce haematemesis or 'coffee-ground' vomit (Cappell & Friedel, 2008). Elderly patients, patients taking aspirin or NSAIDs and patients with comorbidities are at increased risk of developing gastric ulcers. Infection with *Helicobacter pylori* is associated with an increased risk of bleeding from gastric ulcers (Hopper & Sanders, 2011), as is taking antiplatelet medications (Henriksen et al., 2008).

Lower GI bleeds

Bleeding from the lower GI tract will resolve spontaneously without treatment in 80–85% of patients; however, 10% of patients presenting with gross rectal bleeding (haematochezia) will require active fluid resuscitation and/or immediate surgical intervention (Pfeifer, 2011). The most frequent source of bleeding in patients presenting to hospital with severe haematochezia is diverticulitis (40% of presentations); however, bleeding from a colorectal malignancy should always be considered, especially in patients with a history of weight loss and pain. Colorectal malignancies account for approximately 10% of cases of acute rectal bleeding.

Bleeding directly from the anus can be associated with haemorrhoids, an anal fissure or, rarely, an anal malignancy. In this situation, a small amount of bright-red blood is seen on the toilet paper and sustained significant haemorrhage does not usually occur. However, the patient will be concerned and should have the problem formally investigated. The patient can be reassured that the majority of anal bleeding is benign and easily treated. The possibility of local trauma due to the insertion of a foreign body or anal sex should be considered.

> **CLINICAL COMMENT**
> - Chronic low-grade blood loss into the intestinal tract causes anaemia and should always be investigated urgently (within days).
> - Acute high-volume GI blood loss often leads to haemodynamic instability requiring active resuscitation.

Urinary tract bleeds

Bleeding from the urinary tract can present as blood-stained urine (haematuria) or, less frequently, frank blood clots in the urine. The more common causes include urinary tract, prostate or kidney infection; kidney, bladder or prostate cancer; kidney or bladder stones; post-prostate surgery; and trauma. A cause cannot be determined for more than 60% of patients presenting with haematuria (Khadra et al., 2000). Urinary tract bleeding is rarely life-threatening, generally causing chronic bleeding and anaemia. However, in patients with an impaired clotting ability (medication-induced or pathological) haematuria may present as an acute medical emergency. Bleeding into the bladder may lead to the formation of clots that can obstruct urinary outflow through the urethra or through a urinary catheter. The resultant urinary obstruction causes pain and distress, autonomic nervous system stimulation and pressure on the kidneys. Unless the paramedic is trained and equipped to perform catheterisation, the management of this is outside the realm of paramedic practice.

Specific conditions
Differential diagnoses

A thorough and working knowledge of the differential diagnoses for GI/GU bleeding is important, but the main focus is on supportive treatment and transport. Important differential diagnoses can be broken down into different categories.

CASE STUDY 1

Case 10466, 0735 hrs.

Dispatch details: A 70-year-old male with diarrhoea and vomiting.

Initial presentation: When the paramedics arrive, they find a pale, diaphoretic male sitting on the toilet and holding a bucket. He is conscious and alert and seems to be breathing normally.

 ASSESS

Ask!

Ask specifically about:
- previous history (many people with gastric ulcer disease re-bleed)
- use of NSAIDs, aspirin or steroids
- a comprehensive history leading up to the event
- progress of symptoms (increasing shortness of breath, dizziness and tachycardia)
- alcohol use and previous illnesses—anything suggesting cirrhosis?

Patient history

The patient's wife states that he has been complaining of abdominal pain for the past week and that the vomiting and diarrhoea started abruptly at about 3 am. She adds that both the vomit and the diarrhoea are 'dark and smelly'. The patient has a past history of hyperlipidaemia and hypertension. His medications include aspirin. He also drinks two standard drinks per day and gave up smoking 10 years ago.

Airway

The patient is currently managing his own airway. However, if his conscious level decreases, his repeated episodes of vomiting put him at high risk of a compromised airway.

Breathing

Hypovolaemia causing poor tissue oxygenation and lactic acid production has caused increased stimulation of this patient's respiratory centre. Both of these factors (hypoxaemia and acidosis) increase his sensitivity to CO_2, increasing his respiratory drive. A raised respiratory rate is an indicator of prolonged poor perfusion.

Circulation

The patient's cardiovascular observations confirm that he is currently hypotensive despite a sympathetic response, generating a tachycardia and pale, sweaty skin. His cardiovascular observations are consistent with either an acute, rapid loss of blood volume or a longer episode of gradual bleeding resulting in a prolonged period of poor perfusion. A raised respiratory rate would indicate that he has been poorly perfused for a longer period of time because he is now showing compensatory signs to metabolic acidosis. It is also a possibility that without appropriate intervention, he will progress to a generalised inflammatory response and irreversible shock due to the prolonged period of poor perfusion and poor tissue oxygenation.

Abdomen

Examining the abdomen can be of limited diagnostic use as it is likely that the gastric ulcer will produce some tenderness. The presence of a large amount of blood within the bowel may also produce tenderness and if the ulcer has eroded through the gastric wall, allowing gastric acid into the peritoneal space, peritonitis may have developed.

Vomiting and diarrhoea

The patient is holding a bucket that contains about 800 mL of a brown, 'grainy' liquid with some fresh blood, which his wife says he has vomited over the last couple of hours. The toilet contains a very dark and odorous liquid. The coffee-ground blood in the vomitus with fresh blood streaks in it indicates that although a lot of the blood has been altered by gastric acid, the rate of bleeding is brisk enough that some is being vomited up unchanged. He is also passing melaena, which the patient has described as diarrhoea. It is clear that he has a haemorrhage from the GI tract and that it is significant enough to cause hypovolaemia. He is not passing frank blood per rectum (haematochezia), so the rate of bleeding has not been catastrophic. This positive sign should be interpreted cautiously, as there may be a delay between significant bleeding onset and haematochezia.

Initial assessment summary

Problem	Diarrhoea and vomiting
Conscious state	GCS = 15
Position	Sitting
Heart rate	110 bpm
Blood pressure	90/70 mmHg
Skin appearance	Pale, cool, diaphoresis
Speech pattern	Normal
Respiratory rate	22 bpm
Respiratory rhythm	Even cycles
Chest auscultation	Good breath sounds bilaterally
Pulse oximetry	95%
Temperature	37.1°C
Motor/sensory function	Normal
Pain	4/10 upper left quadrant abdominal pain
History	The patient's wife states that he has been complaining of abdominal pain for the past week and that the vomiting and diarrhoea started abruptly at about 3 am

The patient is displaying the cardiovascular symptoms of acute hypovolaemia. The history of this incident is consistent with a gastric or duodenal ulcer causing ongoing abdominal pain and eventually eroding a blood vessel, precipitating an acute haemorrhage. This could be exacerbated by use of aspirin. This patient also has tachycardia, hypotension and a raised respiratory rate associated with the metabolic acidosis of poor perfusion. These signs indicate that he has lost a significant amount of blood.

2 CONFIRM

The essential part of the clinical reasoning process is to seek to confirm your initial hypothesis by finding clinical signs that should occur with your provisional diagnosis. You should also seek to challenge your diagnosis by exploring findings that do not fit your hypothesis: don't just ignore them because they don't fit. Estimation of blood loss is difficult and of limited value. It is more important to determine the perfusion status.

What could it be?

Revisiting the list of differentials is worthwhile after a suspicion of ulcer bleeding is present.

PERFUSION STATUS

Look for!
- Raised respiratory rate and depth
- Tachycardia
- Skin colour (capillary refill time)
- Hypotension: late sign
- Altered conscious state

Differential diagnoses

- Most likely
  › Gastric or duodenal ulcer with significant bleed
- Most serious not to miss
  › MWS, but there is no history of multiple forceful vomits
- Other potential serious causes
  › Oesophageal variceal rupture

Mallory-Weiss syndrome

Not all Mallory-Weiss bleeding is associated with a clear history of vomiting. This is not as unlikely as traditionally thought but does not alter the immediate management.

Oesophageal variceal rupture

This patient has no history of cirrhosis or liver disease so is not likely to have portal hypertension. The extent of his haemorrhage could be consistent with bleeding from an oesophageal varix. Bleeding from oesophageal varices can be catastrophic, which is one of the reasons they are associated with the highest mortality of any GI haemorrhage. Other reasons behind the high mortality rate include the high rate of re-bleed, the underlying hepatic pathology and the associated problems of encephalopathy and aspiration. This patient may still have bleeding oesophageal varices despite the lack of history and any clinically obvious signs of cirrhosis. In the out-of-hospital setting, management of bleeding from oesophageal varices is the same as for bleeding from a gastric ulcer. The immediate concern is fluid resuscitation and protection of his airway, which is at risk if his conscious level falls.

 TREAT

Emergency management

This patient is showing signs of hypovolaemia and his respiratory response indicates a metabolic acidosis due to sustained poor perfusion. His immediate need is for volume replacement. Venous access should be established immediately and cautious fluid resuscitation commenced. Crystalloid fluids should be administered at a rate sufficient to maintain a palpable peripheral pulse, which will generally correspond to a systolic blood pressure of approximately 80 mmHg. Attempting to reach a 'normal' blood pressure with IV fluids risks increasing the rate of haemorrhage.

At the moment the patient presents no challenges in terms of maintaining his airway but as his bleeding is ongoing, it would be wise to be prepared for a decrease in his conscious level necessitating ventilatory and airway support. Should he become unconscious, endotracheal intubation is the best way to prevent aspiration of blood or vomit.

As this patient has a pain score of 4/10, appropriate pain relief should also be administered, in line with local protocols.

Not least of the patient's immediate needs is urgent transfer to a place of definitive care for active fluid resuscitation. A clear and timely prior notification will assist in ensuring an efficient reception.

 EVALUATE

The paramedics' out-of-hospital goals were to support this patient's circulating volume to maintain a base level of perfusion and safely transfer him to definitive care. Monitoring trends in his respiratory rate, skin colour, cardiovascular observations and conscious state will give some indication of either further bleeding or response to volume replacement if needed. A sustained improvement following IV fluid administration would indicate either minimal or no further bleeding, while a transient improvement may indicate continued bleeding. No improvement would indicate either catastrophic haemorrhage or some other cause of poor perfusion. Obvious external haemorrhage, either haematemesis or haematochezia, may not reflect current bleeding and is therefore of dubious value in ongoing patient monitoring.

Ongoing management

These patients require ongoing fluid resuscitation, potentially including a massive transfusion of fresh frozen plasma, platelets and whole blood. Gastroscopic assessment will reveal the site of bleeding, allowing further management to be planned. Approximately 80% of upper GI bleeds resolve spontaneously; the other 20% that re-bleed require endoscopic haemostasis or surgery. Drugs to reduce gastric acid production (proton pump inhibitors and H_2-receptor antihistamines) are used for non-variceal bleeding.

GI/urinary tract haemorrhage in the field

Minor presentations of GI and urinary tract haemorrhage do not require emergency treatment. There is a risk that the paramedic's reassurance that the situation is not critical may be interpreted as confirmation that any subsequent investigation is unnecessary. Significant painless haematuria is the classical clinical sign of bladder cancer and an early investigation may make the difference between cure and palliation. It should be a reminder of the importance of carefully choosing words when reassuring patients.

GI haemorrhage can be a trap for the unwary in that the initial presentation may not appear to be significant blood loss but it may progress to continued and/or accelerated haemorrhage causing significant hypovolaemia. Transport to hospital for evaluation and further investigation is prudent for all patients presenting with GI haemorrhage. Cases of urinary tract haemorrhage still require investigation and unless a guaranteed efficient alternative investigation plan can be devised, a similar approach is wise.

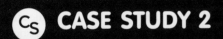

CASE STUDY 2

Case 11054, 1142 hrs

Dispatch details: A 62-year-old female with rectal bleeding.

Initial presentation: The paramedics find the patient sitting in her lounge room in her dressing gown, looking anxious. Her husband and daughter are present and are also concerned.

1 ASSESS

1205 hrs Primary survey: The patient is conscious and alert.

1206 hrs Chief complaint: The patient is complaining of passing a large amount of blood and blood clots when she used her bowels about an hour ago.

1209 hrs Vital signs survey: Perfusion status: HR 82 bpm, strong and regular; BP 130/85 mmHg; skin pink and dry; temperature 37.0°C; capillary refill 2 seconds.

Respiratory status: RR 14 bpm; good, clear air entry bilaterally; SpO_2 99% on room air.

Conscious state: GCS = 15.

1212 hrs Pertinent hx: The patient explains that when she went to the toilet about an hour ago, she noticed a large amount of blood and blood clots in the toilet bowl. This has not happened before and she has no pain or discomfort in her abdomen. She called for an ambulance as the amount of blood made her quite anxious. She is postmenopausal. She had an appendicectomy as a child. She takes fish oil daily and NSAIDs occasionally for headaches. The patient's presentation is consistent with LGIB.

② CONFIRM

In many cases paramedics are presented with a collection of signs and symptoms that do not appear to describe a particular condition. A critical step in determining a treatment plan in this situation is to consider what other conditions could explain the patient's presentation.

What could it be?

Revisiting the list of differentials is worthwhile after a suspicion of lower GI bleed is present.

Differential diagnoses
- Most likely
  › Lower GI bleed, due to a number of causes (e.g. haemorrhoids, anal fissure, colorectal neoplasm/polyps, diverticular disease, IBD, angiodysplasia)
- Other potential serious causes
  › Bleeding from the genital tract

Haemorrhoids

A haemorrhoid is a dilated vein that may be forced through the anus with straining, causing pain and bleeding. Haemorrhoids are commonly associated with constipation and may also be associated with raised portal venous pressure—the haemorrhoids are formed between the portal and systemic circulatory systems in a similar fashion to oesophageal varices. Bleeding associated with haemorrhoids is generally minimal and short-lived and is usually seen as blood on the toilet paper or a few drops in the toilet bowl. Haemorrhoids are the most common cause of rectal bleeding in patients younger than age 50. The volume of blood passed makes this diagnosis seem unlikely.

Anal fissure

An anal fissure is a split in the mucosa of the anus, usually associated with constipation or trauma. Anal fissures can bleed a minimal amount after passing stool and present as a smear of blood on the toilet paper. The volume of blood passed makes this diagnosis seem unlikely.

Colorectal neoplasm/polyp

Bleeding from a polyp or neoplasm in the rectum or colon generally results in the expulsion of blood from the rectum. The blood loss may be significant enough to provide a dramatic appearance, including clots of blood. This could well be the source of bleeding in this case.

Diverticular disease

Bleeding from diverticulitis is arterial, acute and painless and can be alarming in volume. Diverticula (outpouches of large bowel wall caused by straining against constipation) are the source of bleeding in up to 60% of cases in adults over the age of 50 (Cameron et al., 2009). Patients with diverticulitis often have a history of abdominal pain and changed bowel habits (Yang & Chen, 2005).

Inflammatory bowel disease/ulcerative colitis
Bleeding from ulcerative colitis generally presents as small amounts of blood mixed with stool. Patients are generally young and have pre-diagnosed and widespread disease.

Congenital vascular malformations (angiodysplasia)
Angiodysplastic lesions account for up to 12% of cases of rectal bleeding in adults. Blood loss is generally chronic; very rarely, a patient may present with an acute haemorrhage.

Bleeding from the genital tract
In this patient, there is a possibility that the bleeding may originate from the genital tract and in a postmenopausal patient it could be a sign of a neoplasm of either the cervix or the uterus.

The presenting history and the patient's age suggest that the most likely cause of the bleeding is a colorectal polyp or neoplasm.

③ TREAT

The patient is not showing signs of significant hypovolaemia and so at this stage IV fluid infusion is not seen as a priority. However, compensatory mechanisms may sustain vital signs at near-normal levels despite a loss of up to 15% of total blood volume. Also, the patient may progress to more rapid bleeding or a catastrophic re-bleed. She requires careful observation and continual reassessment of her vital signs. If possible, establishing early venous access would be prudent.

④ EVALUATE

Evaluating the effect of any clinical management intervention can provide clues to the accuracy of the initial diagnosis. Some conditions respond rapidly to treatment so patients should be expected to improve if the diagnosis and treatment were appropriate, whereas other conditions are unlikely to respond in the timeframes normally associated with ambulance transport times. In such cases, a failure to improve should not be considered an indication of a misdiagnosis. In this case, there should be no change to the patient's condition during transport.

 CASE STUDY 3

Case 10983, 2230 hrs.

Dispatch details: A 45-year-old male has collapsed. He has been vomiting blood.

Initial presentation: The paramedics arrive at a private house and are led to the bathroom by the patient's wife. The patient is lying on the floor near the toilet.

① **ASSESS**

2243 hrs Chief complaint: There is a large amount of frank blood in the toilet and on the floor and walls around the toilet. The patient has blood on his face and in his mouth. He is lying on his side, breathing quietly. He does not respond to anyone speaking to him and only groans in response to one of the paramedics squeezing his trapezium.

2245 hrs Vital signs survey: Perfusion status: HR 140 bpm, weak; BP 80/50 mmHg; skin pale, diaphoretic, jaundiced; temperature 37.0°C.

Respiratory status: RR 18 bpm, clear air entry bilaterally, SpO$_2$ 97%.

Conscious state: GCS = 7; eye opening to pain, groaning and withdrawing.

BGL: 3.9 mmol/L.

2248 hrs Pertinent hx: His wife and one teenage child are present and they give a history of the patient feeling sick, going to the bathroom and vomiting copiously. Then they heard him collapse. His wife says that he is a chronic alcoholic and has been drinking all evening. He has had alcohol-induced cirrhosis for the past 10 years, as well as type 2 diabetes mellitus, and he is a heavy smoker.

2249 hrs Secondary survey: The paramedics find abdominal ascites and distended abdominal veins.

The patient is not responsive and appears to be suffering from profound hypovolaemic shock. Considering his current presentation and medical history, the most likely cause is haemorrhage from ruptured oesophageal varices (see Fig 33.1). The dilated veins around the patient's umbilicus are a result of portal

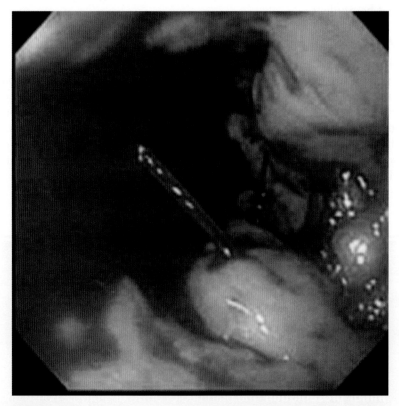

Figure 33.1
Actively bleeding varices.
Source: Courtesy of David L. Carr-Locke, MD, Brigham and Women's Hospital.

hypertension causing a backflow of blood from the left portal vein through the paraumbilical veins and into the periumbilical systemic veins in the abdominal wall. The patient's distended abdomen is a late complication of cirrhosis. Cirrhosis causes systemic vasodilation, effectively decreasing arterial blood pressure. Compensatory activation of the renin-angiotensin-aldosterone system and the sympathetic nervous system and the release of antidiuretic hormone lead to renal retention of sodium and water. Fluid leaks through the abnormally permeable splanchnic vasculature into the peritoneal space, resulting in ascites (Kashani et al., 2008). The patient's decreased conscious level is most likely the result of impaired cerebral perfusion from hypovolaemic shock, but hepatic encephalopathy may also contribute. In hepatic encephalopathy, a cirrhotic liver fails to remove some neurotoxic by-products of digestion, including ammonia and manganese. These neurotoxins cause morphological changes within the brain and have been shown to cause raised intracranial pressure, coma and death. The cirrhosis will also impair the functioning of his clotting factors, exacerbating any bleeding.

② CONFIRM

In many cases paramedics are presented with a collection of signs and symptoms that do not appear to describe a particular condition. A critical step in determining a treatment plan in this situation is to consider what other conditions could explain the patient's presentation.

Differential diagnoses
- Most likely
  - › Ruptured oesophageal varices, because of the background history and the profound haemorrhagic shock
- Most serious not to miss
  - › Rectal bleed
    - ▪ Unlikely, as the paramedics find no evidence of rectal bleeding, indicating that no blood has transited through the gut. The patient has collapsed, indicating that he has lost a significant amount of blood in a short space of time. The blood that he has vomited is bright red and has not been contained within the stomach for long enough to be chemically altered by gastric acid.
  - › Gastric ulcer
    - ▪ In a patient with cirrhosis and decreased clotting factors bleeding from a gastric ulcer may be more marked than usual. Up to 40% of patients with cirrhosis and GI bleeding have gastric erosions as the source of haemorrhage (Cameron et al., 2009).
  - › MWS
    - ▪ Mallory-Weiss tear can potentially cause significant haemorrhage, especially in the context of repeated vomiting, as seen in this patient. The treatment is the same.

Although the history and examination indicate oesophageal varices as the most probable source of haemorrhage for this patient, this needs to be confirmed by gastroscopy, as the definitive treatment of these conditions differs significantly. Gastroscopy also offers strategies such as sclerosing and banding to reduce or control haemorrhage. The out-of-hospital treatment for this patient is the same for all potential causes.

③ TREAT

The immediate treatment for this patient is fluid with a target of raising perfusion sufficiently to improve his conscious state and to enable him to protect his own airway. If his conscious state does not improve with treatment, endotracheal intubation will need to be considered as the optimal way to maintain a safe airway. If intubation is not possible due to scope of practice, the patient will have to be managed on his side at all times, as he is at high risk of aspirating blood. If he needs respiratory support and is not intubated, considerable care will have to be taken not to inflate his stomach, potentially precipitating vomiting and aspiration.

Two large-bore IV cannulae should be established and IV fluid should be administered until an improvement in the patient's conscious state is witnessed: this often coincides with a palpable brachial or carotid pulse. At this stage it would be prudent to titrate the fluid administration to his conscious state and pulse, as continued bleeding from the oesophageal varices combined with excessive fluid administration may result in overdilution of haemoglobin, platelets and clotting factors.

A nasogastric tube to decompress the stomach and drain free blood will not only reduce the volume in the stomach and the risk of aspiration but also indicate whether bleeding is continuing. This may be replaced with an oesophageal balloon tube in hospital as a last resort.

Rapid transfer to a hospital resuscitation unit with the capacity to manage massive transfusions is indicated.

 EVALUATE

Evaluating the effect of any clinical management intervention can provide clues to the accuracy of the initial diagnosis. Some conditions respond rapidly to treatment so patients should be expected to improve if the diagnosis and treatment were appropriate, whereas other conditions are unlikely to respond in the timeframes normally associated with ambulance transport times. In such cases, a failure to improve should not be considered an indication of a misdiagnosis.

In this case, the paramedics cannot directly manage the underlying cause and can provide only symptomatic treatment while expediting rapid transport to definitive care. The patient's response will depend on the extent of the ongoing bleed and the paramedics' ability to maintain a patent airway. If the bleed remains uncontrolled, the patient is likely to progress to a pulseless electrical activity (PEA) arrest.

Despite the relatively young age of this patient, his presentation of dramatic collapse and massive bleeding from oesophageal varices does not carry a particularly optimistic prognosis. Given the long-term and chronic nature of alcoholic cirrhosis, family may appear less distressed than expected.

Hospital management

Hospital management will include replacement of blood volume, platelets and clotting factors using a massive transfusion protocol. Drugs to promote splanchnic vasoconstriction may reduce portal pressure and haemorrhage rate. Banding of the oesophageal varices will often control haemorrhage, as will injecting inflammatory chemicals to promote sclerosis in and around the varix. In refractory bleeding, a modified orogastric tube containing a large balloon or an oesophageal balloon inflated within the oesophagus can function as a tamponade (see Fig 33.2).

Surgical and intravascular procedures to create a shunt from the portal system directly to the systemic system will reduce the pressure on the portal veins and thus the pressure on the oesophageal varices. While these shunts control pressure, allowing blood to effectively bypass the liver may exacerbate hepatic encephalopathy. A liver transplant is also an option, dependent on the patient's eligibility and the availability of a suitable donor.

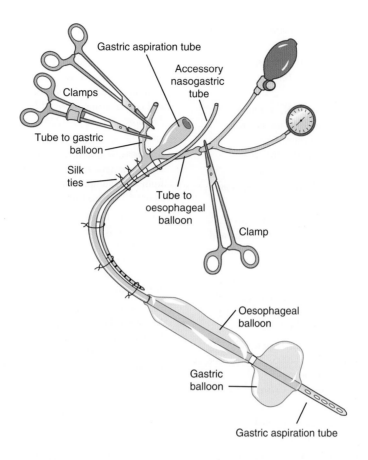

Figure 33.2
The modified Sengstaken-Blakemore tube. Note the accessory nasogastric tube for suctioning of secretions above the oesophageal balloon and the two clamps, one secured with tape, to prevent inadvertent decompression of the gastric balloon.
Source: Rikkers (1981).

Summary

Significant GI haemorrhage is a life-threatening emergency and may occur following a less significant initial haemorrhage. Out-of-hospital assessment and management of patients with GI tract bleeding should focus on identifying those patients with life-threatening haemodynamic compromise and on initiating appropriate resuscitation. Out-of-hospital management should maintain fluid administration to a level that ensures essential organ perfusion, while limiting delays in transferring the patient to definitive care.

References

Akhtar, A., & Padda, M. (2011). Natural history of Mallory-Weiss tear in African-American and Hispanic patients. *Journal of the National Medical Association, 103,* 412–415.

Benevides, I. B. D. S., & dos Santos, C. H. M. (2016). Colonoscopy in the diagnosis of acute lower gastrointestinal bleeding. *Journal of Coloproctology, 36,* 185–188.

Blatchford, O., Murray, W. R., & Blatchford, M. (2000). A risk score to predict need for treatment for upper gastrointestinal haemorrhage. *The Lancet, 356,* 1318–1321.

British Society of Gastroenterology. (2007). *UK comparative audit of upper gastrointestinal bleeding and the use of blood.* Retrieved from www.bsg.org.uk/pdf_word_docs. (Accessed 27 February 2013).

Brown, J. D. (2015). Hiccups: an unappreciated cause of the Mallory-Weiss syndrome. *The American Journal of Medicine, 128,* e19–e20.

Cameron, P., Jelinek, G., Kelly, A.-M., Murray, L., & Brown, A. F. T. (Eds.), (2009). *Textbook of adult emergency medicine.* Sydney: Elsevier.

Cappell, M. S., & Friedel, D. (2008). Initial management of acute upper gastrointestinal bleeding: from initial evaluation up to gastrointestinal endoscopy. *Medical Clinics of North America, 92,* 491–509.

Crooks, C., Card, T., & West, J. (2011). Reductions in 28-day mortality following hospital admission for upper gastrointestinal hemorrhage. *Gastroenterology, 141,* 62–70.

Grow, P. J., & Chapman, R. W. (2001). Modern management of oesophageal varices. *Postgraduate Medicine Journal, 77,* 75–81.

Henriksen, P. A., Palmer, K., & Boon, N. A. (2008). Management of upper gastrointestinal haemorrhage complicating dual anti-platelet therapy. *QJM: An International Journal of Medicine, 101,* 261–267.

Hopper, A. D., & Sanders, D. S. (2011). Upper GI bleeding requires prompt investigation. *The Practitioner, 255,* 15–19.

Kashani, A., Landaverde, C., Medici, V., & Rossaro, L. (2008). Fluid retention in ascites: pathophysiology and management. *QJM: An International Journal of Medicine, 101,* 71–85.

Khadra, M. H., Pickard, R. S., Charlton, M., Powell, P. H., & Neal, D. E. (2000). A prospective analysis of 1930 patients with hematuria to evaluate current diagnostic practice. *Journal of Urology, 163,* 524–527.

Klebi, F. H., Bregenzer, N., Schöfer, L., Tamme, W., Langgartner, J., & Schölmerich, J. (2005). Comparison of inpatient and outpatient upper gastrointestinal haemorrhage. *International Journal of Colorectal Disease, 20,* 368–375.

Palmer, K. (2007). Acute upper gastrointestinal haemorrhage. *British Medical Bulletin, 283,* 307–324.

Pezzulo, G., & Kruger, D. (2014). Assessing upper gastrointestinal bleeding in adults. *Journal of the American Academy of PAs, 27,* 19–25.

Pfeifer, J. (2011). Surgical management of lower gastrointestinal bleeding. *European Journal of Trauma and Emergency Surgery, 37,* 365–372.

Rikkers, L. F. (1981). Portal hypertension. In H. Goldsmith (Ed.), *Practice of surgery.* Philadelphia: Harper & Row.

Saltzman, J. R., Tabak, Y. P., Hyett, B. H., Sun, X., Travis, A. C., & Johannes, R. S. (2011). A simple risk score accurately predicts in-hospital mortality, length of stay, and cost in acute upper GI bleeding. *Gastrointestinal Endoscopy, 74,* 1215–1224.

Scottish Intercollegiate Guidelines Network (SIGN). (2008). *Management of acute upper and lower gastrointestinal bleeding a national clinical guideline [Online].* Retrieved from www.yumpu.com/en/document/read/29737848/sign105 [Accessed July 2020].

Stanley, A. J., Laine, L., Dalton, H. R., Ngu, J. H., Schultz, M., Abazi, R., Zakko, L., Thornton, S., Wilkinson, K., & Khor, C. J. (2017). Comparison of risk scoring systems for patients presenting with upper gastrointestinal bleeding: international multicentre prospective study. *British Medical Journal, 356,* i6432.

Thandassery, R. B., Sharma, M., John, A. K., Al-Ejji, K. M., Wani, H., Sultan, K., Al-Mohannadi, M., Yakoob, R., Derbala, M., & Al-Dweik, N. (2015). Clinical application of AIMS65 scores to predict outcomes in patients with upper gastrointestinal hemorrhage. *Clinical Endoscopy, 48,* 380.

Velayos, F. S., Williamson, A., Sousa, K. H., Lung, E., Bostrom, A., & Weber, E. J. (2004). Early predictors of severe lower gastrointestinal bleeding and adverse outcomes: a prospective study. *Clinical Gastroenterology and Hepatology, 2,* 485–490.

Yang, P.-M., & Chen, D.-S. (2005). Caput medusae. *The New England Journal of Medicine, 353,* e19.

SECTION 12:
The Paramedic Approach to the Trauma Patient

In this section:

The clinical challenges associated with the patient who has suffered traumatic injuries epitomise the paramedic work environment: the scene is usually highly emotional and there may be confusion about where the scene boundaries are and how many patients are affected. The body's ability to compensate for internal injuries can also distract paramedics away from those patients most in need of transport to those with obvious but often not life-threatening injuries.

The need to accurately assess and manage traumatic injuries in the minutes after they occur, with limited diagnostic equipment, is a clinical challenge unparalleled in healthcare. Having a structured approach to trauma assessment that recognises and compensates for these challenges is an essential component of the paramedic's skillset. Because the need for a structured approach is so important, this section commences with a specific clinical approach to trauma assessment that builds on the medical assessment strategy described in Section 8. Subsequent chapters then explore common traumatic injuries and the principles of management for each one—based on the assessment approach outlined in Chapter 14.

CHAPTER 34

Head Injuries

By Tim Andrews

OVERVIEW

- The term 'head injury' is a broad classification that includes injuries to the face, scalp, skull or brain. Facial and scalp injuries can be painful and distressing but brain injuries have the greatest potential for mortality and morbidity.
- Early recognition and management of traumatic brain injuries (TBIs) can reduce mortality and morbidity.
- TBIs are usually the result of direct trauma to the head but can also occur as a result of severe acceleration or deceleration without head strike. TBI is the leading cause of death and disability in young adults (Shum, 2007).
- Primary TBI occurs at the time of impact due to direct neuronal damage (Dunn et al., 2015) and describes the destruction of neurons and vascular structures by the mechanical forces of impact or deceleration (Atkinson & Wilberger, 2003).
- Secondary TBI evolves as a result of the body's inability to maintain normal brain perfusion following the primary injury. Inflammation, haemorrhage, oedema, blood pressure and hypoxaemia all contribute to the development of a secondary injury. Unlike the primary injury, the degree of secondary injury is subject to paramedic management.
- TBIs are classified as mild (Glasgow Coma Scale score [GCS] 13–15), moderate (GCS 9–12) or severe (GCS < 9), but a GCS score obtained early in the clinical course is not a strong predictor of severity of injury (Reith et al., 2017).
- National statistics for the incidence of TBI are lacking, but in New South Wales (NSW) the rates of all TBI are 99.1:100,000 (Pozzato et al., 2019), while in Victoria, incidence of *severe TBI* are 4.2:100,000 (Beck et al., 2016).
- Overall mortality from TBI is 5.9:100,000 (Pozzato et al., 2019), while for severe TBI, there was a 42.5% rate of mortality (Beck et al., 2016).
- Males outrate females in TBI at a rate of 2.9:1 (Pozzato et al., 2019).
- Indigenous Australians suffer TBI at three times the rate of non-Indigenous Australians (Farrell & Dempsey, 2016), while in NSW, Indigenous Australians suffered TBI at a rate of 1.7 times that of the state populace (Pozzato et al., 2019).
- The elderly are overrepresented for head injuries sustained from falls. Those aged > 65 years are overrepresented in both high and low (> 1 m or < 1 m) falls.
- Head injury from child abuse is common and is estimated to represent up to 66% of TBI cases in children (Marx et al., 2017), and children of low socioeconomic status families are more likely to suffer head injuries than children of higher socioeconomic status families (Trefan et al., 2016).
- While survival rates from TBI in Australia and New Zealand are not readily available as a national sample, in NSW TBI resulted in death 5.3% of the time (Pozzato et al., 2019), while that number increases to 42.5% of severe TBI resulting in death, and further increases to 78% death for severe TBI if the patient is over 64 years old (Beck et al., 2016).
- Falls were the greatest cause of death when assessing all levels of head injury, with 67.9% of all deaths in NSW fall related (Pozzato et al., 2019). This means falls with low mechanism can result in death, especially in the over-65 age group.
- The accepted signs of brain injury (unequal pupils, hypertension, bradycardia, irregular respirations) are very late signs of severe injury and as such do not act as a diagnostic tool for mild to moderate injuries that may subsequently evolve into more serious injuries.

Introduction

The term **head injury** usually refers to traumatic brain injury (TBI) but in a broader sense it can refer to any injury to structures above the neck, involving scalp and skull (Pushkarna et al., 2010). These injuries can be divided into two basic categories: those involving injuries to the brain (craniocerebral) and those involving injuries to the face or scalp (craniomaxillofacial). While facial injuries can be painful, confronting and dangerous, this chapter is primarily concerned with injuries where the force applied to the skull is transmitted through to the cranium and damages the soft tissues of the brain. The anatomical structure of the skull and brain are such that severe brain injuries can evolve from relatively minor events and with little sign of external injury. The ability to assess, triage and manage TBIs poses a number of clinical reasoning challenges and so this chapter focuses on these types of injuries.

Hospital management of TBIs has undergone significant changes in the past decade and these changes are now flowing out into the out-of-hospital environment. For example, rapid sequence intubation (RSI) by paramedics is now well established in several Australian states but requires significant training and support if the clinical benefits of this complex procedure are to be realised. Some of these recent changes to TBI management also contradict longstanding out-of-hospital practices and may be difficult to integrate without organisational support and ongoing training and education.

Statistics regarding the type and causes of head injuries may be limited or incomplete as they are not likely to include patients who die at the scene (or those who decline health services). However, in most developed countries there has been a decline in mortality and morbidity from TBIs over the past two decades due to a systematic approach to trauma care, which includes safety strategies such as seatbelt legislation, drink-driving legislation and bicycle helmet use (Cameron et al., 2014).

Anatomy

In order to understand the presentation and evolution of head and brain injuries, paramedics must have an understanding of the anatomy of the skull and the soft tissues that surround and are contained within it. Functionally and structurally, the skull can be divided into two distinct areas: the cranium and the face. The cranium can be described as a vault made up of flat bones that contain the brain: frontal, temporal, parietal, occipital, sphenoid and ethmoid (Mandavia et al., 2011; see Figs 34.1–34.4). The bones are 2–6 mm thick and are at their thinnest in the temporal region and at the base of the skull. Communication between the cranium and the rest of the body occurs through the foramina located beneath the cranium.

The bones that make up the face (maxilla, mandible, zygoma, lacrimal) attach to the anterior-inferior surface of the cranium and encompass the sensory organs and airways. Some bones such as the sphenoid are part of both the cranium and the face. The bones of the cranium are flat and thickened by a cancellous (spongy) middle layer where they are exposed to the external environment, while the bones of the face tend to be thinner, more delicate and complex.

Text continued on page 544

DEFINITIONS

- *Acquired brain injury (ABI):* any acquired damage to the brain. The damage may occur before, during or after birth. ABI before or during birth may be caused by many of the same events that cause injuries after birth, such as infection, hypoxia, trauma, drugs and alcohol, and stroke (Brain Injury Australia, 2012). ABI is diagnosed in approximately 1 in every 45 people, with the vast majority (75%) of these patients being under 65 years of age. Stroke is the most common cause of ABI, sustained by approximately 394,000 people per year having a stroke, with 40% of these patients having ongoing brain injury and disability. The second most common cause of ABI is trauma resulting from a force applied to the head (TBI; Brain Injury Australia, 2012).
- *Traumatic brain injury (TBI):* impairment of brain function as a result of mechanical force. This dysfunction can be temporary or permanent, mild (e.g. dazed) or profound (e.g. unresponsive or comatose; Tintinalli et al., 2016). It has been described as progressive, so early intervention can impact outcomes (Bernard, 2006; Tintinalli et al., 2016). Such injuries can be further defined as primary or secondary; and mild, moderate or severe.
  - › *Primary brain injury (PBI):* injury that occurs at the time of impact due to direct neuronal

  damage (Dunn et al., 2015) and describes the destruction of neurons and vascular structures by the mechanical forces of impact or deceleration (Atkinson & Wilberger, 2003).
  - › *Secondary brain injury (SBI):* injury that evolves as a result of the body's inability to maintain normal brain perfusion following the primary injury. Inflammation, haemorrhage, oedema and blood pressure all contribute to the development of a secondary injury. Unlike the primary injury, the degree of secondary injury is subject to paramedic management.
  - › *Mild brain injury:* injury that may have a brief period of unconsciousness and present initially with a GCS of 13–15; can have long-lasting sequelae (Rajajee, 2018a, 2018b).
  - › *Moderate brain injury:* injury defined by a wide variety of clinical presentations such as GCS of 9–12, commonly with a change in level of consciousness at the time of injury. May be followed by seizures, amnesia and vomiting and person can be confused or somnolent (Rajajee, 2018a, 2018b).
  - › *Severe brain injury:* injury defined by GCS of < 9 at presentation (Rajajee, 2018a, 2018b).

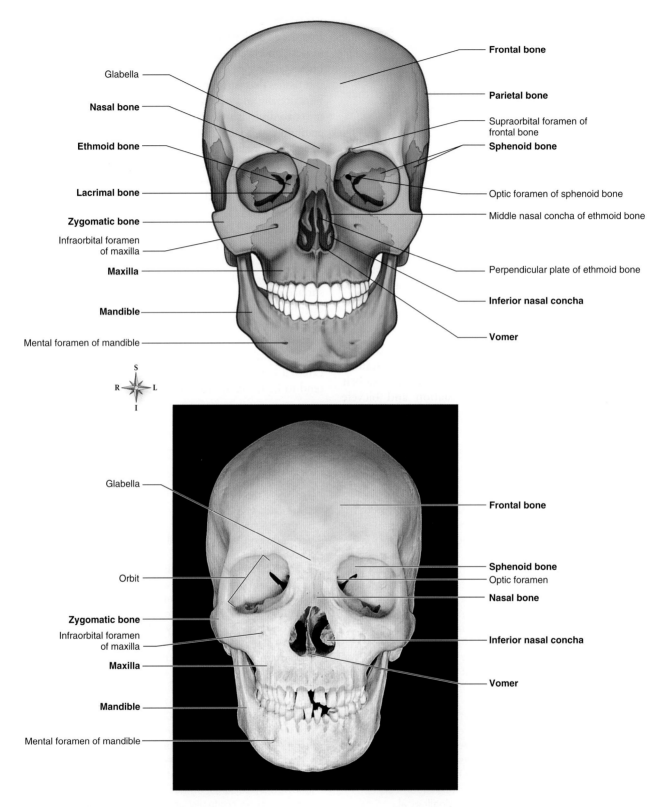

Figure 34.1
Anterior view of the skull.
Source: Patton & Thibodeau (2019).

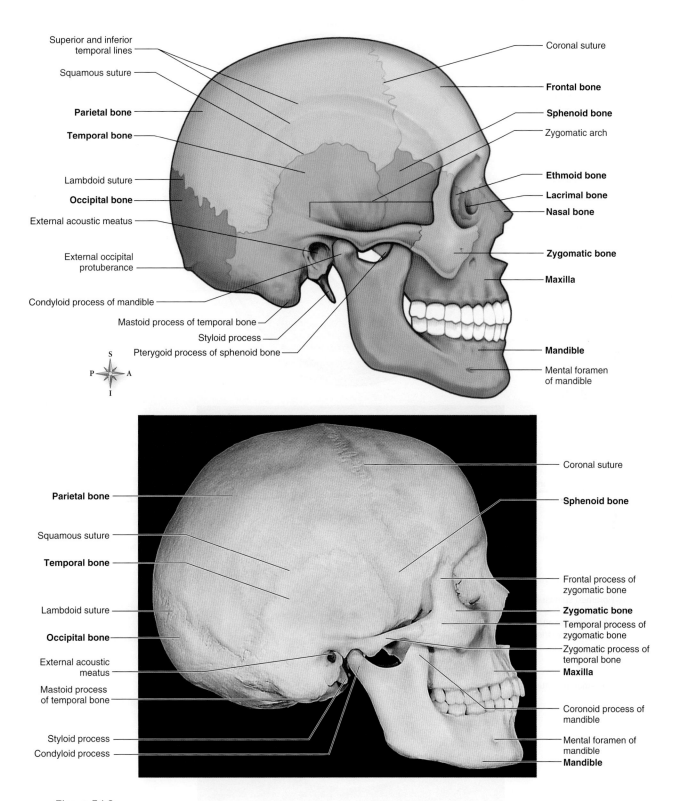

Figure 34.2
Right view of the skull.
Source: Patton & Thibodeau (2019).

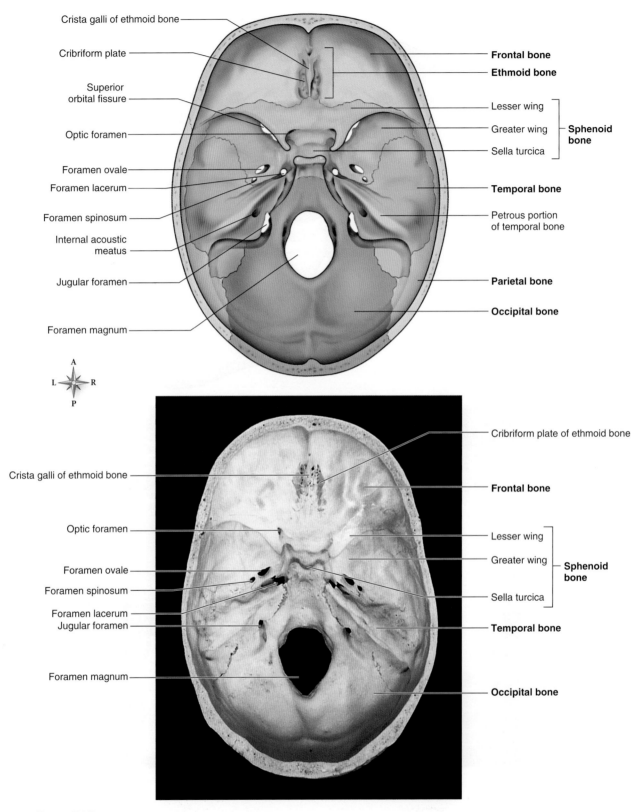

Crista galli of ethmoid bone
Cribriform plate
Superior orbital fissure
Optic foramen
Foramen ovale
Foramen lacerum
Foramen spinosum
Internal acoustic meatus
Jugular foramen
Foramen magnum

Frontal bone
Ethmoid bone
Lesser wing
Greater wing
Sella turcica
Sphenoid bone
Temporal bone
Petrous portion of temporal bone
Parietal bone
Occipital bone

Cribriform plate of ethmoid bone
Crista galli of ethmoid bone
Optic foramen
Foramen ovale
Foramen spinosum
Foramen lacerum
Jugular foramen
Foramen magnum

Frontal bone
Lesser wing
Greater wing
Sphenoid bone
Sella turcica
Temporal bone
Occipital bone

Figure 34.3
Floor of the cranial cavity viewed from above.
Source: Patton & Thibodeau (2019).

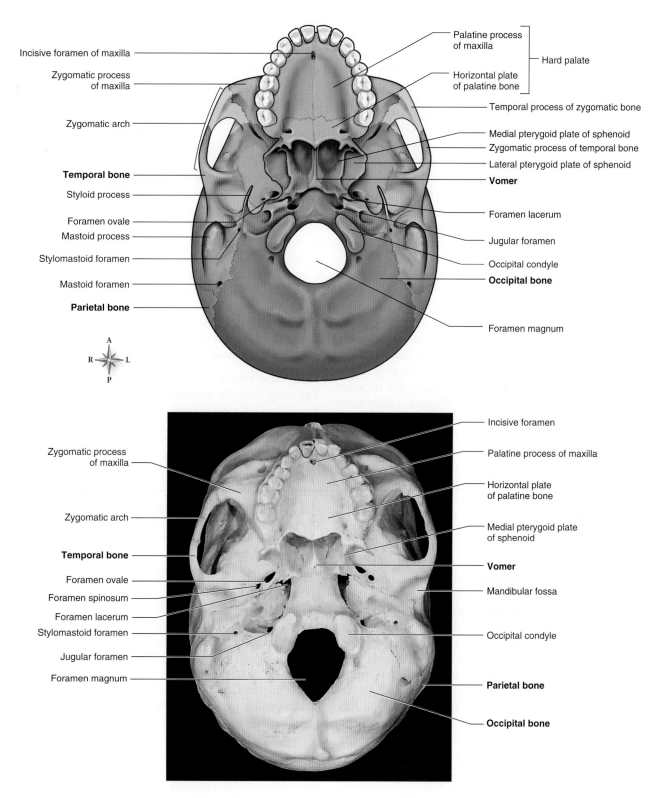

Incisive foramen of maxilla

Zygomatic process
of maxilla

Zygomatic arch

Temporal bone

Styloid process

Foramen ovale

Mastoid process

Stylomastoid foramen

Mastoid foramen

Parietal bone

Palatine process
of maxilla

Hard palate

Horizontal plate
of palatine bone

Temporal process of zygomatic bone

Medial pterygoid plate of sphenoid

Zygomatic process of temporal bone

Lateral pterygoid plate of sphenoid

Vomer

Foramen lacerum

Jugular foramen

Occipital condyle

Occipital bone

Foramen magnum

Zygomatic process
of maxilla

Zygomatic arch

Temporal bone

Foramen ovale

Foramen spinosum

Foramen lacerum

Stylomastoid foramen

Jugular foramen

Foramen magnum

Incisive foramen

Palatine process of maxilla

Horizontal plate
of palatine bone

Medial pterygoid plate
of sphenoid

Vomer

Mandibular fossa

Occipital condyle

Parietal bone

Occipital bone

Figure 34.4
Skull viewed from below.
Source: Patton & Thibodeau (2019).

543

Severe injuries to the face can pose issues of airway patency (obstruction from teeth, blood, etc.) or require specialist care (e.g. eyes, teeth, jaw). If the mechanism of injury is blunt force, paramedics should always consider the potential for brain injury, even when the primary presenting injury is to the face.

Essential to an understanding of both primary and secondary brain injuries is the knowledge that the bones of the cranium protect the brain in a structure that does not allow for expansion or contraction. Within the cranium three meningeal layers and cerebrospinal fluid (CSF) further protect the brain. Understanding the placement and structure of the meninges can provide clues to the type of injury a patient has suffered and how the injury may evolve.

The innermost meningeal layer is the *pia mater* and it is attached to the external surface of the brain, the cerebral cortex (see Fig 34.5). The thin and transparent pia mater provides support to the network of blood vessels on the surface of the brain and follows the brain's surface into its sulci. Moving out, the delicate, web-like *arachnoid mater* is actually attached to the *dura mater*, the outermost meningeal layer. The space between the pia mater and the arachnoid mater is filled with CSF and is described as the subarachnoid space. The arachnoid mater actually extends small villi through the dura into the venous sinus to allow CSF to exit the subarachnoid space and return to the bloodstream. The dura mater (literally, tough mother) is a white, fibrous layer that is tightly bound to the inside of the skull bones. Importantly, the dura extends three strong and large folds between the right and left sides of the brain (falx cerebri), the right and left side of the cerebellum (falx cerebelli), and the cerebellum and the cerebral hemispheres (tentorium cerebelli). These folds anchor the brain within the skull as the head turns or nods. They also provide support for the thin-walled venous sinuses that drain blood from the brain, which is returned to the heart via the superior sagittal sinus. CSF is constantly being produced: it is exuded from capillaries lining the ventricles of the brain and returns to the bloodstream via the arachnoid villi. The normal amount of CSF in an adult is approximately 140 mL: 23 mL is contained in the ventricles of the brain and the remainder is contained in the subarachnoid space and the spinal cord (see Fig 34.6). Together, the meninges and CSF provide blood, hydration and physical protection to the brain.

Pathophysiology
Primary brain injury
Primary brain injury (PBI) occurs at the time of trauma and can be the result of direct impact, rapid acceleration/deceleration, penetrating injury or blast waves: in essence any mechanism where external forces or energy is transferred to brain tissue, resulting in injury (Abdelmalik et al., 2019). In most cases it is a result of direct trauma to the head and usually involves tissue damage to the scalp and skull. While the presence of scalp and skull injuries can indicate that PBI has occurred, the absence of external head injuries does not preclude PBI. The difficulty in detecting mild PBI in the field requires paramedics and other primary responders to understand the types of external and internal injuries that can occur as a result of direct head trauma. These include:

- scalp lacerations
- skull fractures
- brain contusions
- epidural haematomas
- subdural haematomas
- subarachnoid haemorrhage
- intracerebral haemorrhage
- diffuse axonal injury
- penetrating head injuries.

Scalp lacerations
The scalp is tough, mobile and multilayered and is the thickest layer of skin in the body, with underlying subcutaneous tissue containing hair follicles and the rich blood supply for the scalp (Mandavia et al., 2011). It is highly vascular and the vessels fixed within the scalp are unable to retract and constrict when lacerated. This is why they bleed profusely and can result in haemorrhagic shock (Mandavia et al., 2011). Direct pressure is usually sufficient to control bleeding but the pressure may need to be prolonged. Close examination of any wound (visual and tactile) should indicate any underlying bony injury.

Skull fractures
Fractures to the external bones of the cranium are usually caused by localised trauma against sharp or hard objects. Fractures are described as linear, depressed, basilar or open.

Linear fractures
Linear fractures (which appear straight in x-rays) make up 80% of all skull fractures (Mandavia et al., 2011). Motor vehicle crashes cause the majority of skull fractures, and 85% of these occur in males (Mandavia et al., 2011). Seatbelts, airbags and motorcycle helmets have contributed to a decrease in frequency of fractures. Other causes of linear fractures include falls and assaults. Provided they are not depressed or open, these fractures are not prone to complications, but they do indicate that significant force has been applied to the cranium, some of which will have been transmitted to the brain.

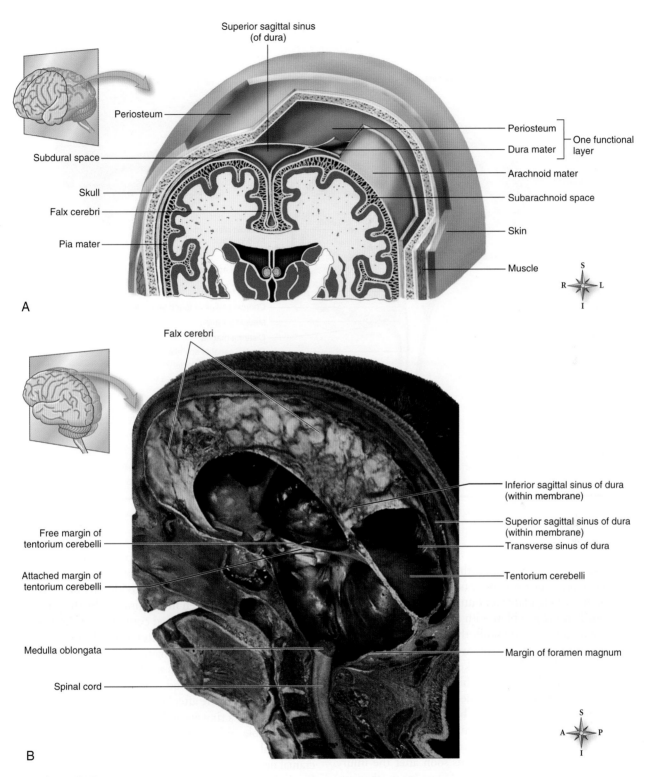

Figure 34.5
Coverings of the brain.
A Frontal section of the superior portion of the head, as viewed from the front. Both the bony and the membranous coverings of the brain can be seen. **B** Sagittal section of the skull, viewed from the left. The dura mater has been retained in this specimen to show how it lines the inner roof of the cranium and the falx cerebri extending inwards.
Source: Patton & Thibodeau (2019).

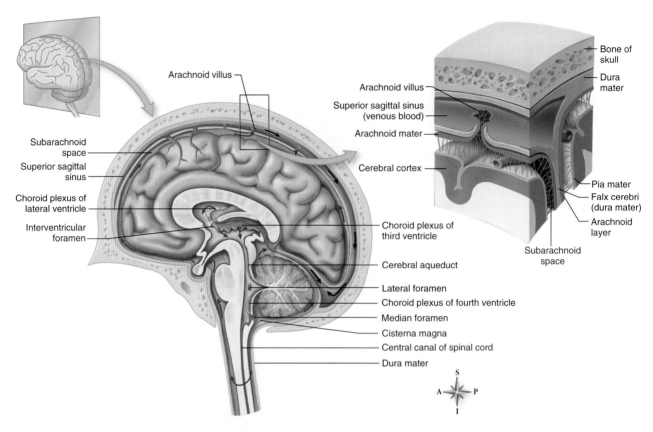

Figure 34.6
Flow of cerebrospinal fluid.
The fluid produced by filtration of blood by the choroid plexus of each ventricle flows inferiorly through the lateral ventricles, interventricular foramen, third ventricle, cerebral aqueduct, fourth ventricle and subarachnoid space and to the blood.
Source: Patton & Thibodeau (2019).

Depressed fractures

Depressed fractures describe the inward displacement of a fractured portion of bone (see Fig 34.7). This usually occurs when a large amount of force is applied to a small area (e.g. a blow with a hammer). On physical examination of the skull, the fracture is commonly not palpable because of swelling of the soft tissue. The displaced bone is likely to cause underlying brain tissue damage: one-third of depressed fractures cause a haematoma or tissue contusion. If the area of depression is small and not badly displaced, the actual amount of brain tissue damaged can be quite small: patients with this type of injury may not have any significant neurological signs soon after the injury. However, the total amount of force (or mechanism) will assist in determining whether a widespread brain injury is likely to have occurred.

Basilar fractures

Basilar fractures to the base of the skull are usually associated with high mechanisms of injury and major trauma. They can occur because the mandible has been forced superiorly and posteriorly, fracturing

the base of skull, or due to an upward force from the spinal column causing a linear fracture. These fractures are notoriously difficult to identify on x-ray and the diagnosis is often made clinically by the presence of CSF mixed with blood coming from the ears (haemotympanum), or ecchymosis beneath both eyes (raccoon eyes) or above the mastoid processes (Battle's sign; see Fig 34.8). CSF leaks are difficult to diagnose if the fluid is mixed with blood. The classically described 'bulls-eye' sign, where after being absorbed by a cloth the CSF leaves a ring around the central blood stain, is not reliable and testing for CSF can be conducted at hospital. Treatment is generally conservative unless cranial nerve injury mandates surgical decompression. Signs of infection or meningitis are closely monitored. A persistent CSF leak beyond 2 weeks may require operative repair with a dural patch (Mandavia et al., 2011).

Open fractures

Open fractures describe wounds where there is direct communication between a scalp laceration and brain

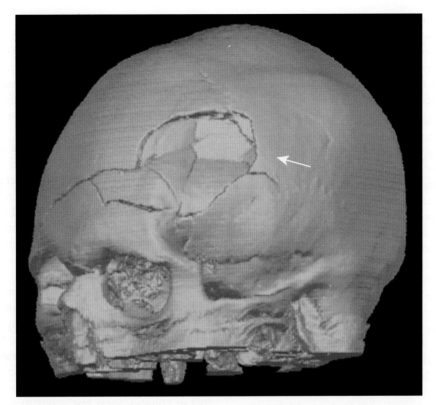

Figure 34.7
CT scan showing a depressed skull fracture.
Source: Parrillo & Dellinger (2019).

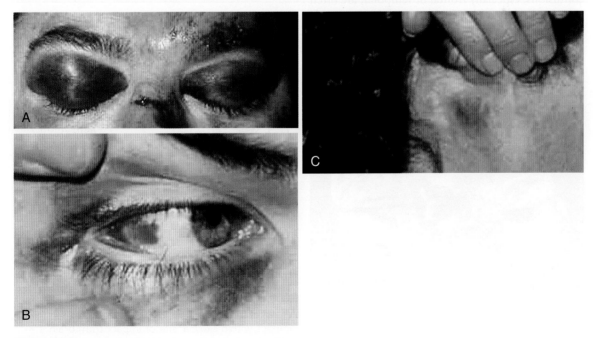

Figure 34.8
Signs of skull base fracture.
A Periorbital bruising ('raccoon' or 'panda' eyes). **B** Subconjunctival haemorrhage. **C** Battle's sign. Note these signs may not appear until several hours or even days after the injury.
Source: Douglas et al. (2018).

tissue. These are usually associated with significant mechanisms or injury (high-speed motor vehicle crashes, gunshot wounds) and a high mortality rate. Open fractures require surgical debridement and repair and in the field efforts should be made to limit further contamination of the wound.

Brain contusions

Cerebral contusion occurs when the brain parenchyma strikes fixed portions of the skull during acceleration or deceleration. The forces of compression or shearing can damage the cells and vasculature of the brain and effectively cause bruising of the brain tissue (see Fig 34.9).

While the skull is smooth on the outer surface, within the cranial vault there are many protrusions and ridges, particularly on the base of the vault, which can generate high levels of compression or shearing when brain tissue is forced against them. Flexion and extension of the neck can result in contusions on the opposite side to where the force was originally applied (contrecoup; see Fig 34.10).

The frontal lobe striking the frontal bone and the temporal lobe striking the sphenoid bone are the two most common locations for cerebral contusions (Mandavia et al., 2011). Frontal lobe contusions are typically characterised by agitation, confusion, repetitive questioning, impaired short-term memory and aggressiveness that often requires physical and chemical restraint. These cerebral contusions, especially frontal or temporal, are often characterised by a high incidence of posttraumatic seizures and neurosurgeons often recommend routine prophylactic treatment with anticonvulsants for approximately 7 days post-injury (Mandavia et al., 2011).

Epidural haematomas

Epidural haematomas (EDHs) occur in about 2.7–4% of head injuries (Bullock et al., 2006a) and are characterised by blood collecting between the dura mater and the skull bone. EDH is most commonly due to the rupture of the middle meningeal artery, often the result of trauma to the skull (Bullock et al., 2006a).

In more than 90% of EDHs this occurs due to a fracture of the skull near the temple, as the pterion is the weakest part of the skull. Branches of the middle meningeal artery often lie in bony canals in this region and fracture will lead to rupture of the artery. These types of fractures most commonly occur following motor vehicle crashes, including with pedestrians, and sports injuries (Mandavia et al., 2011).

Because the dura is tightly adhered to the skull, EDHs can develop slowly as blood under systemic arterial pressure slowly forces its way between the dura and the bone (see Fig 34.11). EDHs represent the difficulties of assessing head injuries in the field: the force required to fracture the skull in this region is often sufficient to cause a brief loss of consciousness but is not sufficient to cause widespread primary injury. As a result, the patient will often have recovered from their initial loss of consciousness and be lucid upon presentation to clinicians; however, as the haematoma continues to increase in size, the patient's clinical progression

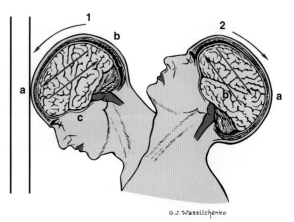

Figure 34.10
Coup and contrecoup brain injury following blunt trauma.
1 Coup injury: impact against object; **a**, site of impact and direct trauma to brain; **b**, shearing of subdural veins; **c**, trauma to base of brain. **2** Contrecoup injury: impact within skull, **a**, site of impact from brain hitting opposite side of skull; **b**, shearing forces through brain. These injuries occur in one continuous motion—the head strikes the wall (coup) and then rebounds (contrecoup).
Source: McCance & Huether (2018); Rudy (1984).

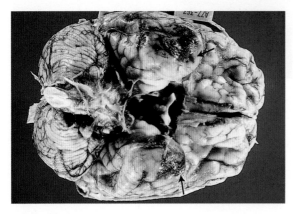

Figure 34.9
The temporal poles are discoloured by areas of haemorrhage (arrows). Such lesions represent 'bruises' on the surface of the brain caused by violent contact between the delicate brain parenchyma and the hard inner surface of the skull.
Source: Kumar et al. (2017).

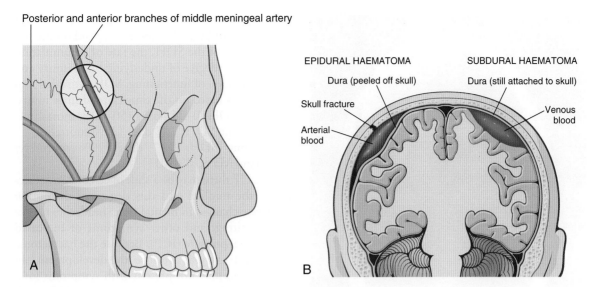

Posterior and anterior branches of middle meningeal artery

A

EPIDURAL HAEMATOMA

SUBDURAL HAEMATOMA

Dura (peeled off skull)

Dura (still attached to skull)

Skull fracture

Venous blood

Arterial blood

B

Figure 34.11
A The middle meningeal artery is injured in epidural haematomas. The blue circle is over the pterion.
B Comparison between epidural and subdural haematomas. Note that because the dura is so firmly adherent to the skull at the suture lines, epidural haematomas are not strong enough to peel the dura off the sutures and therefore cannot cross suture lines. However, subdural haematomas are under the dura (hence, subdural) and therefore can cross suture lines.
Source: FitzGerald et al. (2011).

Table 34.1: Comparison of intracranial injuries

	Type of patient	Anatomical location	CT findings	Common cause	Classic symptoms
Epidural haematomas	Young, rare in elderly and those aged < 2	Potential space between skull and dura mater	Biconvex football-shaped haematoma	Skull fracture with tear of middle meningeal artery	Immediate loss of consciousness, with lucid period prior to deterioration (20% of patients)
Subdural haematomas	Higher risk in elderly and alcoholic patients	Space between dura mater and arachnoid	Crescent or sickle-shaped haematoma	Acceleration/ deceleration with tearing of the bridging veins	Acute: rapid loss of consciousness Chronic: altered mental state, gradual decrease in consciousness
Subarachnoid haematomas	Any age group after blunt trauma	Subarachnoid	Blood in the basilar cisterns, hemispheric sulci and fissures	Acceleration/ deceleration with tearing of the subarachnoid vessels	Mild, moderate or severe injury and meningeal symptoms
Contusion/ intracerebral haematoma	Any age group after blunt trauma	Usually anterior temporal or posterior frontal lobe	May be normal initially, delayed bleed	Severe or penetrating trauma, shaken baby syndrome	Symptoms range from normal to loss of consciousness

Source: Adapted from Tintinalli et al. (2016).

will continue, with symptoms of headache, lethargy and confusion likely, as well as potentially seizure activity and hemiparesis, the result of an expanding haematoma compressing underlying brain tissue (see Table 34.1). The speed of this clinical progression can vary, depending on the blood vessel which has ruptured, and whether the bleed is arterial (faster progression) or venous (slower progression). However, this pattern of unconscious, lucid period and then unconscious is only reported in 47% of

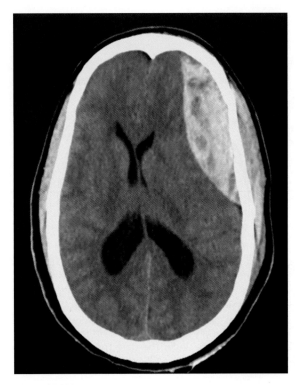

Figure 34.12
CT scan showing an epidural haematoma.
Source: DeCuypere & Klimo (2012).

cases, and the overall mortality for EDH is around 10% (Bullock et al., 2006a).

Definitive diagnosis is based on CT but the typical 'biconvex lens-like' presentation may not occur early if the amount of bleeding is small (see Fig 34.12). In adults the haematoma will not cross suture lines because the dura is tightly adhered at the sutures, but this is not the case in children and the haematoma can extend across a wide area (Mandavia et al., 2011). Approximately 8% of EDHs are detected after a significant delay. Patients who are not in a coma at the time of presentation usually recover very well as there is often little underlying brain damage.

Subdural haematomas

Subdural haematoma (SDH) describes the presence of blood between the dura mater and the brain (see Fig 34.11). This most often occurs due to movement of the brain inside the skull tearing the thin-walled venous sinuses that cross this space. Deceleration with or without head strike is a common cause and those whose brain has decreased in size (e.g. due to age, alcoholism) are at greater risk as the degree of movement is potentially greater. Reports show that SDH occurs in approximately 21% of all head injuries and occurs in all age groups (Bullock

et al., 2006b). Unlike EDH, skull fractures are not common with SDH. Symptoms depend on the size and location of the SDH, the rate of accumulation of blood, the degree of underlying brain injury and premorbid level of functioning. SDH is divided into three phases based on the time elapsed since injury.

- Acute SDH: 0–24 hours (50–80% mortality)
- Sub-acute SDH: 1–7 days (25% mortality)
- Chronic SDH: > 7 days (20% mortality) (Mandavia et al., 2011)

On CT there may be a shift of cerebral structures across the midline and this degree of disruption can cause changes in mental state, headache, nausea and vomiting, and other symptoms of increased intracranial pressure (ICP). Because the haematoma forms under venous pressure, the development can be slow and may not present with symptoms for a number of days after the primary injury. Patients who are on anticoagulant medications are at higher risk (also because of age and increased likelihood of falls) and changes in mental state can be difficult to detect if confusion, disorientation, lethargy and depression are already present (Mandavia et al., 2011).

SDH can develop from head trauma that may have been relatively minor and forgotten by the patient. Treatment for large SDH in the acute or subacute phases is via craniotomy. Small haematomas are managed conservatively with close neurological observation. Decisions on chronic SDH depend on premorbid function, the size of the haematoma and the presence or absence of symptoms (Mandavia et al., 2011).

Subarachnoid haemorrhage

Subarachnoid haemorrhage (SAH) describes bleeding between the arachnoid membrane and the pia mater: the space normally occupied by CSF. This may occur spontaneously as a result of a cerebral aneurysm (see Ch 26) but is more commonly associated with head trauma (Parrillo & Dellinger, 2019). The vessels most often involved are those arteries that contribute to the circle of Willis at the base of the brain, but other vessels may be involved. Determining the relationship between SAH and trauma can be difficult as patients who suffer a spontaneous SAH and subsequent loss of consciousness while operating a vehicle are likely to present to paramedics and emergency responders following some sort of collision. Similarly, the altered level of consciousness following a collapse from a SAH can be difficult to separate from a headstrike unless the patient complained of symptoms prior to collapsing. Outcomes from SAH are dependent on the extent of the haemorrhage.

Intracerebral haemorrhage

The compressive and shearing forces that occur when the brain collides with the skull can cause bleeding in the brain parenchyma. Intracerebral haemorrhages describe collections of more than 5 mL of blood in the brain tissue. Symptoms depend on the size and location of the haematoma and also the cause. Low-velocity penetrating wounds (e.g. from knives) may produce a localised haematoma without significant surrounding tissue damage, while high-velocity wounds from gun shots can produce small haematomas with extensive surrounding tissue damage.

Diffuse axonal injury

Diffuse axonal injury (DAI) is the widespread damage to axons in the brain, particularly the brain neural tracts, corpus callosum and brainstem, and its diagnosis is an independent factor in increased mortality. DAI can exist without any external trauma being evident, and is more often associated with high-energy trauma such as traffic crashes or non-accidental injury in infants. Importantly, motor-cyclists are at an increased risk of DAI because while the helmet worn may prevent visible skull damage, the acceleration/deceleration forces that occur during a motorcycle crash may lead to axonal injury. DAI can be clinically diagnosed by coma lasting greater than 6 hours, after excluding swelling or brain lesions, and it is commonly associated with loss of brain function and persistent vegetative states. Studies have shown that over time, return to normal, or near-normal, cognitive function can occur; however, 25% of patients with DAI will die. The globalised swelling and inflammation, caused by axonal damage, leads to increased ICP, which in turn can inhibit brain perfusion, which further worsens inflammation and swelling.

Penetrating head injuries

Penetrating head injuries involving gunshot wounds frequently result in death or profound disability. When a bullet enters the skull it produces multiple, high-velocity fragments from both bullet fragmentation and skull fragmentation (Mandavia et al., 2011). As the projectile enters the brain, it can produce a cavity up to four times larger than the bullet, transferring a large amount of kinetic energy which leads to the majority of brain destruction. The initial GCS can be a reliable predictor of outcome in gunshot wounds to the brain, with a GCS < 5 having a 100% mortality rate; however, patients with a GCS of 9 or higher *and* reactive pupils only have a mortality rate of 25% (Tintinalli et al., 2016).

Penetrating injuries from knives usually have less kinetic energy and therefore a better prognosis (Tintinalli et al., 2016). Small penetrating wounds can be missed because they are covered with matted hair, and blades may be broken off and embedded in the cranium. Patients with exposed brain matter, gunshot wounds that cross the midline of the brain, severe coagulopathy or early transtentorial herniation invariably die of their injuries but can still be considered as potential organ donors (Mandavia et al., 2011).

Concussion

The term 'concussion' is often used to describe mild TBI. The traditional definition usually includes the phrases 'fully reversible brain injury' and 'lack of abnormalities on radiological examination'. These criteria are now being challenged as the frequency of long-term symptoms from apparently minor brain injuries becomes more widely understood. The term 'post-concussion syndrome' (PCS) is often applied to these patients (Brown & Edwards, 2014), but which symptoms are included, their severity and duration are not widely agreed upon (Rees, 2003).

Concussion typically refers to the disruption of higher cortical functions for a short period that resolves without treatment. The short loss or altera-tion of consciousness occurs when the forces acting to compress or shear brain tissue interrupt the function of the reticular activating system. This usually returns quickly but the widespread effects of the forces persist and develop.

The clinical indicators for concussion have been narrowed down to the following four criteria (Carney et al., 2014):

1. observed and documented disorientation and confusion immediately after the event
2. impaired balance within 1 day after injury
3. slower reaction time within 2 days after injury
4. impaired verbal learning and memory within two days after injury.

The pathophysiology of concussion is not unlike that of DAI; however, the severity is significantly reduced. Concussion is often the result of sporting injury, and the range of symptoms present can vary depending on the patient and the force which has occurred. Symptoms can include cognitive impair-ment, impairment of balance as well as emotional symptoms. This can result in clinical presentations such as:

- delayed verbal responses or an inability to focus or maintain attention
- headache, nausea and blurred vision
- retrograde or anterograde amnesia, especially repeat questioning after the event
- disproportionate emotional responses (crying over seemingly small issues)

seizure activity has been reported in only approximately 5% of all patients with concussion; of those 5%, it is estimated that 25% will have a seizure in the first hour post-injury and 50% will have a seizure within 24 hours (Evans & Whitlow, 2019).

The presence of these signs and symptoms is not definitive as there is still no definitive test for concussion; however, these clinical signs and symptoms will result in the patient being deemed likely to have sustained a concussion (Carney et al., 2014). Equally as important is to recognise possible signs and symptoms that do *not* correlate with concussion, including focal limb weakness, hemiparesis, pupillary abnormalities or Horner syndrome (Evans & Whitlow, 2019).

Adequate assessment and testing of patients with concussion is essential in the out-of-hospital setting, with a number of validated tests for concussion available. The majority of these tests rely on a baseline being established prior to the event, and while paramedics and other healthcare professionals may not have these baseline readings available to them, the format and symptoms assessed can help the clinician to perform repeatable and comparable tests to assess the patient's clinical trajectory.

- Standardised Assessment for Concussion: This was developed to be a standardised tool for assessment of concussion, and assesses areas including orientation, immediate memory, concentration, delayed recall, neurological screening and exertional manoeuvres (McCrea et al., 1997).
- Westmead Post-Traumatic Amnesia Scale: This test has been shown to be an easy, repeatable and rapid (reportedly less than 1 minute) test for concussion. It has a good correlation to more detailed neuropsychological testing and was found to be more valid than the GCS when predicting patients with concussion (Shores et al., 2008).

Secondary brain injury

The injury caused by PBI is determined by a number of factors including patient age and mechanism of injury. Clinicians, especially in the out-of-hospital setting, can affect the degree to which secondary brain injury (SBI) occurs and reduce SBI through effective management and goal-directed therapies. Following the initial impact injury, there are a number of unavoidable clinical and biochemical responses that, if not managed, can escalate a survivable primary injury into a fatal event. SBI should be considered an injury that evolves as a result of the body's inability to maintain normal brain function following the primary injury. Management of SBI relies on the maintenance of homeostasis, in particular maintaining ventilation and perfusion.

Avoid secondary brain injury by preventing the following:

- hypocapnia or hypercapnia by maintaining CO_2 levels within the range of 30–35 mmHg
- hypoxia, maintaining $SpO_2 > 90\%$
- hypotension—targeting blood pressures over 100 mmHg; similarly, exceedingly high blood pressures should also be avoided
- hyperthermia—targeting normothermia and prevention of fevers
- hypoglycaemia, ensuring blood glucose readings are > 4 mmol/L
- seizure management—seizure activity is high in oxygen and glucose demand; prompt seizure management is essential.

Paramedics have a crucial role in the prevention of SBI. While procedures such as RSI show improved outcomes for patients with TBI (Bernard, 2006), timely and holistic care should be the cornerstone of all management.

Hypoxic-ischaemic brain injury

The brain is metabolically extremely active and, despite contributing less than 5% of total body mass, it requires 20% of the body's total oxygen requirements and 15% of total cardiac output (Tintinalli et al., 2016). Hypoxia ($PaO_2 < 40$ mmHg) within the first 24 hours significantly increases the risk of death in patients with TBI (Ó Briain et al., 2018); therefore, maintenance of $SpO_2 > 90\%$ is crucial.

Unlike muscle tissue, the integrity of brain cell membranes is limited and even a short period of poor perfusion can cause increased permeability, swelling (see Box 34.1) and apoptosis. Brain tissue is also unique because, being enclosed in a bony vault, any increase in volume within the skull causes a corresponding increase in pressure and a subsequent decrease in the perfusion of brain tissue.

The release of blood or cellular contents into the interstitial space as a result of the primary injury

BOX 34.1 Brain swelling

There are two forms of brain swelling: congestive oedema and cerebral oedema. Congestive oedema describes an increase in intravascular blood volume that can occur from vasodilation. Cerebral oedema describes the shift of fluid into (and subsequent swelling of) the brain cells (Marx et al., 2017). Typically, congestive oedema develops before cerebral oedema, but in the out-of-hospital setting it is impossible to distinguish between the two and in trauma cases it is likely that both will exist to some degree.

triggers a typical inflammatory response (see Ch 4). This results in vasodilation and tissue oedema at the site of the injury. This increase in cerebral volume increases the ICP and forces some of the CSF surrounding the brain out of the cranial vault. If the degree of swelling exceeds the amount of CSF that can be transferred out of the skull, pressure in the intracranial space will start to rise beyond the normal limit of 10–15 mmHg. Normal ICP is the pressure that blood must overcome if it is to enter the cranial vault and perfuse the brain. Cerebral blood flow is largely dependent on cerebral perfusion pressure (CPP), which can be calculated as mean arterial pressure (MAP) less ICP (Cameron et al., 2014).

$$CPP = MAP - ICP$$

The body's ability to autoregulate cerebral perfusion (by means of heart rate, vasoconstriction and vasodilation) usually ensures that the brain receives an adequate supply of blood, even when MAP ranges from 50 to 150 mmHg. To maintain CPP when ICP rises, MAP must also rise. In the case of severe head injury, the swelling that occurs (from bleeding and inflammation) after the primary injury may raise the ICP beyond the point at which the body can raise the MAP and maintain cerebral perfusion. Injured brain tissue and the release of inflammatory mediators can also limit the brain's ability to control local flow and perfusion can be inadequate despite extremely high systolic and diastolic pressures. Cerebral autoregulation has been shown to become impaired in one-third of all patients with a severe TBI (Rajajee, 2018a, 2018b), therefore maintaining systolic blood pressure over 100 mmHg for patients 50–69 years of age, and a systolic of > 110 mmHg for patients 15–49 years or over 70 years is recommended to ameliorate this possible impact on autoregulation (Carney et al., 2016). While future research may develop medications that limit the inflammatory response and/or the resistance to damage of individual brain cells, the only current strategy to limit secondary head injury is to maintain cerebral perfusion in the period after injury.

Although the mechanism of moderate to severe primary head injuries can vary, understanding the physiological stages that contribute to the secondary injury can assist paramedics in identifying patients who are likely to deteriorate or who are deteriorating. The potential for apnoea in the critical phase is the opportunity to stop a survivable injury progressing to a fatal event.

- *Critical phase.* This commences at the time of injury and extends for up to 10 minutes. A traumatic loss of consciousness usually invokes some degree of apnoea (Atkinson & Wilberger, 2003). If this persists, cerebral hypoxia can become severe and generate a widespread inflammatory response regardless of the severity of the primary injury. A loss of consciousness can also allow for positional occlusion of the airway that will generate hypoxia even if the ventilatory reflex returns. Manually maintaining a patent airway and assisting ventilations during this period are essential to limit the evolution of a secondary injury. Cerebral hypoxia will generate a sympathetic response that increases both heart rate and blood pressure (see Ch 3), but the degree of sympathetic response in head injury exceeds that usually associated with hypoxia or hypercarbia and it is likely there is a direct mechanism between brain injury and the sudden release of catecholamines (Atkinson & Wilberger, 2003). The surge can cause blood pressure to rise sufficiently to cause neurogenic pulmonary oedema.
- *Exponential phase.* Extending for up to 24 hours, the secondary injury becomes established during this phase as the inflammatory cascade provokes vasodilation and fluid to shift from the intravascular space. Tissue that was ischaemic from the primary injury becomes necrotic and previously uninjured tissue experiences ischaemia as the brain swells and ICP rises.
- *Plateau phase.* After 24 hours ICP should be stabilised but may still be raised. While the acute inflammatory cascade has subsided, the necrotic tissue is still evolving and can cause further bleeding. Up to 75% of deaths from head injury in hospitalised patients occur during this phase.
- *Resolution phase.* In this phase maximally swollen necrotic tissue begins to resolve but cerebral oedema is still present. There is a continued risk of intracerebral haemorrhage (Atkinson & Wilberger, 2003). This phase can extend for weeks but the long-term sequelae may persist for months or years.

It is vital at this point to reinforce the variability of head injuries. An isolated epidural haematoma under a linear fracture may appear dramatic and can restrict perfusion to a portion of the brain, but the amount of tissue damage may not be sufficient to cause the cascade of inflammatory mediators that leads to widespread brain swelling and extensive secondary injury. The factors that influence the development of secondary injury are highly individual, with the degree of injury, the location of bleeding and the extent of the inflammatory response all contributing.

The most important factor in reducing SBI is to maintain adequate perfusion and oxygenation:

brain cells exposed to prolonged ischaemia will swell or rupture, contributing to both oedema and the inflammatory process. Even short periods of systemic hypoxia (PaO_2, 40 mmHg) or hypotension (systolic BP, 100/110 mmHg) increase the likelihood of a poor outcome (Carney et al., 2016). The combination of both hypotension and hypoxia, for a little as 5 minutes, can result in poorer outcomes (Stein et al., 2010).

 CASE STUDY 1

Case 12215, 1530 hrs.

Dispatch details: A 20-year-old male has collided with another male during a game of football (head vs knee). The patient was unconscious, now conscious.

Initial presentation: The ambulance crew find the patient sitting on the bench at the football ground being attended to by the club doctor. The patient is pale, confused and slightly agitated and complaining of a headache. There is an obvious haematoma above his left eyebrow. He doesn't want to 'let the team down' and insists on returning to the field to take his position. The coach states that he was unconscious for about 1 to 2 minutes after the collision. Vital signs: heart rate 110, regular; BP 130/70 mmHg; respiratory rate 26; pupils equal and reactive to light (PEARL); GCS 14.

 ## ASSESS

The variety of mechanisms and patterns of head injury, the heterogeneity of responses and the unpredictable evolution of SBI create significant diagnostic challenges for paramedics when confronted with patients who have suffered a head injury. While the traditional division of mild, moderate and severe head injuries appears to offer a degree of initial classification, the diagnostic challenge for paramedics who encounter patients shortly after their primary injury is to identify which patients are likely to progress from mild to a more severe injury.

Patient history

Determining the mechanism of injury contextualises decision-making and planning in all traumatic injuries and should always be the starting point of the assessment. Obtaining a detailed history of the traumatic event is an ideal starting point when assessing patients with head injury. While the force of a fist or knee to the head in a game of football is not comparable to the large impact of a motor vehicle collision, the area of impact and immediate effects should be taken into consideration. Such an injury is unlikely to cause massive secondary injuries, but this should be considered a possibility in the minutes following the impact.

As detailed in the history, this patient suffered a brief loss of consciousness, which is indicative of a primary head injury, and based on his GCS of 14, his head injury can be categorised as mild (Evans & Whitlow, 2019). However, there are no keys as to whether or not this patient will develop an SBI based on mechanism or GCS alone.

Longer periods of loss of consciousness are associated with greater severity of injury but, importantly, a TBI can also occur without loss of consciousness. Brief tonic–clonic seizures ('concussive convulsions') are also not uncommon immediately following loss of consciousness, but similarly there is a lack of evidence as to whether they are predictive of injury severity. Where a patient is involved in a contact sport there is the possibility that the current injury is not the only TBI to have occurred recently and this must be considered. Second impact syndrome (SIS) describes the sudden development of an SBI following a relatively minor impact in a patient whose brain is still recovering from an earlier injury (McCrory et al., 2012).

Posttraumatic amnesia or confusion can complicate gaining a specific and general medical history. Recent alcohol and drug use are also complicating factors, but any alteration in consciousness following trauma should be considered as a brain injury and not the result of alcohol or illicit drug use.

Airway, breathing and circulation

Apnoea and loss of the gag reflex may follow the primary injury but a conscious and talking patient indicates these are no longer an issue. Nonetheless, a baseline set of vital signs should always be established.

Neurological exam

Conscious state

A number of tools can be used to assess the patient's level of consciousness and severity of TBI. The GCS score (see Box 34.2 and Table 34.2) is by far the most common and it offers a widely understood tool that allows serial measurements of the patient's conscious state. The GCS is not without its limitations as it was originally designed for non-traumatic injuries, clinicians are notoriously poor at calculating scores and the three categories were never intended to be added together and are less accurate as a sum than when considered individually (Green, 2011). Despite the GCS authors advising against using the scale to predict severity or outcome of TBI (Teasdale & Jennett, 1978), it has become the standard tool to separate mild, moderate and severe TBI. A wide variety of clinical presentations occur with moderate head injury, but an important clinical scenario in the spectrum of moderate head injury is that of the 'talk and deteriorate' patient. These patients have a GCS of ≥ 13 on presentation but deteriorate to a GCS of ≤ 8 within 48 hours (Marx et al., 2017). A GCS score < 9 is an indication for advanced airway management in some regions, but possibly the greatest utility of the GCS in the out-of-hospital setting is that it sets a reproducible baseline and a deterioration of 2 points or more should be considered significant (NZGG, 2006). Any GCS score should be considered a reliable indicator of TBI only after hypotension, hypoxia, hypoglycaemia and hypercapnia have been corrected.

HISTORY

Ask!

- What was the mechanism of injury and the type of impact?
- Was the patient unconscious? If so, for how long?
- Did the patient have any seizure activity? If so, how long did it last? What did it look like?
- Did the patient have any amnesia, retrograde and/or anterograde? If so, how long did it last?
- Does the patient have any recent history of TBI in the last 4 weeks?

BOX 34.2 The Glasgow Coma Scale

Despite its limitations, the GCS is the principal clinical method for grading TBI severity. The 15-point scale is scored on the patient's ability to interact with their environment (Tintinalli et al., 2016) and assesses the patient's best eye, verbal and motor responsiveness (see Table 34.2). It should be considered accurate for head injury only in patients who are haemodynamically stable and adequately oxygenated and have normal blood glucose levels. Hypoxia, hypotension and intoxication can falsely lower the GCS score and fractured limbs or occult spinal injuries may interfere with the motor examination (Marx et al., 2017). The GCS has become a standard acute measure of neurological function because of its inter-rater reliability, reliance on objective clinical data and ease of application (Marx et al., 2017). It is useful for categorising patients in terms of the severity of their head injuries but it is not sufficient to determine the presence or absence of neurological injury as it does not assess subtle changes in mentation, cranial nerve injury, skull fractures or pupils.

Table 34.2: The Glasgow Coma Scale score

	Criteria	Description	Score
Eye response (E)	Eyes opening spontaneously		4
	Eye opening to speech	Not to be confused with the awakening of a sleeping person; such patients receive a score of 4, not 3	3
	Eye opening in response to pain stimulus	A peripheral pain stimulus, such as squeezing the lunula area of the patient's fingernail, is more effective than a central stimulus such as a trapezius squeeze, due to a grimacing effect	2
	No eye opening		1
Verbal response (V)	Oriented	Responds coherently and appropriately to questions such as their name and age, where they are and why, the year, month, etc.	5
	Confused	Responds to questions coherently but there is some disorientation and confusion	4
	Inappropriate words	Random or exclamatory articulated speech, but no conversational exchange	3
	Incomprehensible sounds	Moaning but no words	2
	No verbal response		1
Motor response (M)	Obeys commands	Does simple things as asked	6
	Localises to pain	Purposeful movements towards painful stimuli (e.g. hand crosses midline and gets above clavicle when supraorbital pressure applied)	5
	Flexion/withdrawal to pain	Flexion of elbow, supination of forearm, flexion of wrist when supraorbital pressure applied; pulls part of body away when nail bed pinched	4
	Abnormal flexion to pain (see Fig 34.13)	Flexor posturing: adduction of arm, internal rotation of shoulder, pronation of forearm, flexion of wrist, decorticate response	3
	Extension to pain (see Fig 34.13)	Extensor posturing: abduction of arm, external rotation of shoulder, supination of forearm, extension of wrist, decerebrate response	2
	No motor response		1

There are a number of validated tests for concussion available that aren't simply the GCS. The majority of these tests rely on a baseline being established prior to the event, and while paramedics and other healthcare professionals may not have these baseline readings available to them, the format and symptoms assessed can help the clinician to perform repeatable and comparable tests to assess the patient's clinical trajectory.

A negative result on any one of the following questions is considered a positive test for cognitive impairment after a head injury.

- What is your name?
- What is the name of this place?
- Why are you here?
- What month are we in?
- What year are we in?
- What town/suburb are you in?
- How old are you?
- What is your date of birth?
- What time of day is it (morning/afternoon/night)?

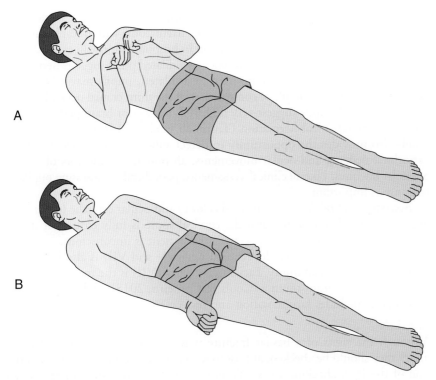

Figure 34.13
A Abnormal flexion (decorticate posturing). **B** Abnormal extension (decerebrate posturing).
Source: Carroll (2010).

Table 34.3: Normal pupil presentation

Asymmetrical pupils	Differ more than 1 mm in size
Dilated pupils	Greater than or equal to 4 mm in adults
Fixed pupils	Less than 1 mm change in response to bright light

Posttraumatic amnesia

An inability to recall events leading up to a head injury is referred to as retrograde amnesia, while memory loss following the event is differentiated as antegrade amnesia. The presence of these symptoms is important to ascertain during patient assessment and can be assessed easily through standardised, repeatable questioning. These symptoms may also be self-evident by the patient repeatedly asking the same questions of healthcare clinicians.

Cranial nerve assessment

A neurological examination of a patient with TBI requires the assessment of cranial nerve function; particularly nerves III to VII (Evans & Whitlow, 2019). Changes to pupil size, reactivity and response to light are all signs of TBI (Tintinalli et al., 2016) but they are a result of significant brain swelling and rarely occur in patients with a high GCS. As such they are rarely predictive of a developing injury, but can indicate TBI in a patient who is found unconscious. While drugs can influence pupil presentation, this usually occurs symmetrically and one-sided changes in an unconscious patient who is not hypoxic, hypotensive or hypoglycaemic strongly suggest TBI.

While there is no out-of-hospital clinical intervention derived directly from pupil asymmetry, early assessment against normal values (see Table 34.3) will act as a baseline for deterioration. In an unresponsive patient, a single fixed and dilated pupil may indicate an intracranial haematoma with uncal herniation that requires rapid operative decompression in hospital (Tintinalli et al., 2016). Pupillary asymmetry, loss of the light reflex or a dilated pupil suggests herniation of the brain. Before they become fixed and dilated, pupils may take on an ovaloid appearance as a result of compression of the third cranial nerve. Bilateral fixed and dilated pupils suggest very high ICP with poor brain perfusion and possibly bilateral uncal herniation (Tintinalli et al., 2016). Checking of the pupils also provides the opportunity to detect subconjunctival haemorrhage, periorbital oedema and ocular movements: all potential indicators of orbital or basilar fractures. Like all clinical assessments, periodically re-assessing pupillary response is important.

Assessment of oculovestibular (cold caloric) and ocular cephalic (doll's eyes) responses should not occur until the cervical spine is fully cleared of injury and this will not happen at the scene if the patient is unconscious.

Assessment of facial muscles (cranial nerves V and VII) is also important in patients with a head injury. Facial nerve palsy (VII) is the most commonly affected nerve in blunt trauma (Cools & Carneiro, 2018), and assessment of these nerves includes face sensation and movement.

Physical exam

Although the signs of a basilar fracture may not appear for hours after an injury they should be checked, at least to set a baseline. Widening the examination of the face, checking for swelling, pain and misalignment of teeth, can indicate facial fractures (see Fig 34.14). Similarly, examining the scalp for lacerations or fractures should be mandatory.

In addition to vital signs, a blood glucose level measurement should be standard for all patients presenting in an altered conscious state.

Initial assessment summary

Problem	The patient is confused and complaining of a global headache
Conscious state	Alert but confused; GCS = 14
Position	Sitting upright on a bench
Heart rate	112 bpm, regular
Blood pressure	130/70 mmHg
Skin appearance	Pale, cool
Speech pattern	Speaking freely
Respiratory rate	26 bpm

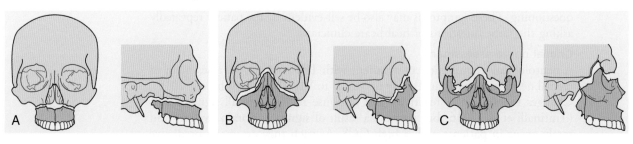

Figure 34.14
A Le Fort I facial fractures (lateral and frontal views). **B** Le Fort II fractures (lateral and frontal views). **C** Le Fort III fractures (lateral and frontal views). These fractures represent the separation of portions of the face from the cranium (craniofacial dislocation). The associated pain and bleeding can make management difficult, or they can be relatively symptomatic. Significantly, Le Fort II and III fractures can suggest a basilar fracture. Elongation of the face, pulling of the lower eyelids and epistaxis are common signs.
Source: Curran (2008).

Respiratory rhythm	Regular even cycles
Respiratory effort	Normal
Chest auscultation	Clear breath sounds, good bilateral air entry apices to bases
Pulse oximetry	99% on room air
Temperature	36.9°C
BGL	6.4 mmol/L
Motor/sensory function	Normal
Neuro exam	Pupils are equal, round, reactive Patient cannot recall incident or leaving the field
History	Nil medical history

D: There is no danger to the patient or crew.
A: The patient is conscious with no current airway obstruction.
B: Respiratory function is currently normal.
C: Heart rate is slightly elevated but consistent with recent activity. There is a sufficient blood pressure.

The patient has suffered a traumatic head injury with a brief loss of consciousness and now presents with signs consistent with a mild TBI. He is well perfused, and neither hypoxic nor hypoglycaemic.

2 CONFIRM

The essential part of the clinical reasoning process is to seek to confirm your initial hypothesis by finding clinical signs that should occur with your provisional diagnosis. You should also seek to challenge your diagnosis by exploring findings that do not fit your hypothesis: don't just ignore them because they don't fit.

Mild TBI is typically described as a GCS of ≥ 13 following head trauma that may or may not include a brief loss of consciousness (see Table 34.4). While this patient clearly fits that category, paramedics are often required to assess patients only minutes after the trauma and before a secondary injury has time to evolve.

In reality a significant range of presentations fit within the mild category and they can assist in determining the severity and likelihood of an evolving secondary injury. Patients who present with a GCS of ≥ 13 usually lose points

> **DIFFERENTIAL DIAGNOSIS**
> **Mild TBI**
> Or
> - Moderate TBI

Table 34.4: Signs and symptoms associated with mild TBI

Cognitive symptoms	Physical signs and symptoms	Behavioural changes
Attention difficulties	Headaches	Irritability
Concentration problems	Dizziness	Depression
Amnesia and perseveration	Insomnia	Anxiety
Short-term and long-term memory problems	Fatigue	Sleep disturbances
Orientation problems	Uneven gait	Emotional lability
Altered processing speed	Nausea, vomiting	Loss of initiative
Altered reaction time	Blurred vision	Loneliness and helplessness
Calculation difficulties and problems with executive function	Seizures	Problems related to job, relationship, home or school management

Source: Tintinalli et al. (2016).

Table 34.5: Criteria for classifying the severity of TBI

Definitions of the severity of TBI vary across organisations and the literature. The most commonly used measures are the GCS and any loss of consciousness.

Severity of TBI	GCS on initial assessment	Duration of posttraumatic amnesia	Loss of consciousness
Mild	13–15	< 24 hours	Nil
Moderate	9–12	1–6 days	Brief (< 5 min)
Severe	3–8	> 7 days	> 5 min

Source: Reith et al., 2017

BOX 34.3 Principles of management

Mild TBI
- Avoid hypoxia
- Avoid hypotension
- Monitor for signs of neurological disturbances

---

due to either confusion and/or drowsiness (i.e. the motor responses are rarely altered). One of the limitations of the GCS is that there are degrees of both drowsiness and confusion but they are all scored equally. A patient who quickly opens their eyes to voice and then interacts (even if confused) is neurologically quite different from a patient who requires a firm direction to open their eyes and then returns quickly to a 'sleeping' presentation. Patients who are persistently drowsy may fit the mild category but should be treated with suspicion and, depending on local transport times and resources, it can be worth treating them as if they fit the moderate category. The 'disproportionate' step between a GCS of 13 and a GCS of 14 is reflected in a number of agencies expanding the moderate criteria to include a GCS of 13.

The presence of a persistent global headache in this patient is a reason for concern and if any other neurological signs such as vomiting or photophobia were to develop they should be considered as deterioration, even if the GCS score remains unchanged (see Table 34.5).

In this case the patient is not drowsy, is talking freely and shows no signs of agitation. For the moment the condition can be described as mild TBI.

③ TREAT

Emergency management
Principles of management for mild TBI are outlined in Box 34.3.

Safety
There is no danger to patient or crew at this point.

Reducing secondary brain injury
Hypoxia and hypotension are the two major external factors that contribute to an SBI. Avoiding systemic hypoxia or hypotension is essential but supplemental oxygen or fluids is not required while the patient presents with mild symptoms and remains stable.

Cervical spine care
Cervical spine injury may be associated with blunt head trauma, especially when high forces are involved, but it is rare for spinal injuries to present asymptomatically following trauma (Sanchez et al., 2005). In many ambulance

> ## BOX 34.4 Cervical spine clearance criteria
>
> Mechanism alone is not a strong predictor of spinal injury and cervical collars and spinal immobilisation are not without risk. To reduce the routine application of collars, some services direct paramedics to consider a patient's cervical spine to be clear of injury if the following preconditions are met.
> - The patient is fully alert and oriented.
> - The patient has not consumed drugs or alcohol.
> - The patient has no neck pain.
> - The patient has no abnormal neurology.
> - The patient has no significant other 'distracting' injury (an injury that may 'distract' the patient from complaining about a possible spinal injury). Provided these preconditions are met, the patient's neck may be examined. If there is no bruising or deformity, no tenderness and a pain-free range of *active* movements, the cervical spine can be cleared.

services, cervical spine immobilisation using a stiff collar remains a routine component of managing any head injury. However, questions regarding both the efficacy and the safety of cervical collars with and without full spinal immobilisation (Sundstrøm et al., 2013; Theodore et al., 2013) have led to a number of services introducing spinal injury clearance procedures to reduce the routine application of collars to asymptomatic patients (see Box 34.4). In this case, the patient meets the clearance criteria and no collar is applied.

Positioning
Head injuries have traditionally been managed with the head slightly elevated. There is a lack of strong evidence to support this practice, but it remains common when cervical collars and spinal immobilisation are not applied. Vomiting is a symptom of head injury and is one of the reasons why full spinal immobilisation is not favoured by all clinicians in the setting of isolated head injury. Although having the head raised may have no impact on reducing ICP, it will allow for adequate venous draining from the head, and in the non-intubated patient, will allow the patient better airway patency if vomiting occurs.

Prophylactic antiemetics
There is a significant decrease in the rates of nausea experienced by trauma patients, regardless if they are experiencing symptoms of nausea to begin with when routinely treated with antiemetics. Prophylactic antiemetics decreased the rates of nausea from 61% (no antiemetic given) to 5% (antiemetic given) (Easton et al., 2012). In patients who are spinally immobilised, the use of antiemetics is important to reduce the risk of aspiration.

Pain relief
Headache is a common symptom that may be associated with either primary or secondary injury due to raised ICP. Certain opiate based analgesic medications present a risk of sedating and mimicking the extension of the brain injury (NZGG, 2006). In mild TBI the use of oral analgesics such as paracetamol may be appropriate. If narcotic analgesia is used, it should be administered conservatively and titrated carefully.

Steroids
The role that inflammation plays in the evolution of SBI has led to a number of trials of anti-inflammatory medications during the acute phase of injury. While glucocorticoids were considered a mainstay of treatment for TBI, more recent studies have shown no benefit, and in some cases harm. Methylprednisolone has been shown to increase mortality for patients with TBI and increased ICP (Carney et al., 2016).

Table 34.6: Sample guidelines for the transport of patients with isolated TBI

Urgent ambulance transport to ED	ED assessment needed but ambulance not a requirement	Assessment at hospital not required
• LOC > 5 min • Deterioration of GCS • Irritability/photophobia • Seizure • High mechanism of injury • Suspected cervical injury • Cranial fracture or penetrating injury	• LOC < 5 min but now fully resolved • Amnesia • Single episode of vomiting • Persistent mild headache • Patient is on anticoagulant medications • Patient is older than 65	• Low mechanism of injury • No LOC • No factors from higher categories

Source: Adapted from ACC (2007).

PRACTICE TIP

Any head injury is associated with a low but increased risk of developing an intracranial complication, such as an expanding haematoma and as such should be transported for possible CT scan (Borg et al., 2004).

Transport

If the patient is conscious, has no neurological symptoms, neck pain or nausea, and requires only oral analgesia, the necessity to transport the patient to hospital is often raised by patients, their family and even ambulance crews. The unpredictability of head injuries usually dictates a conservative approach and transport under clinical supervision, but in rural areas with limited resources there may be guidelines that suggest alternative pathways (see Table 34.6). In this instance, a prolonged period of unconsciousness (> 1 minute) and alterations to the patient's mental status, even without abnormal neurological findings, mean this patient should be transported to hospital for observation and possible imaging (Evans & Whitlow, 2019). Additionally, hospital assessment at the time of injury may allow the patient and carers to be educated about possible symptoms and their subsequent management.

 EVALUATE

Evaluating the effect of any clinical management intervention can provide clues to the accuracy of the initial diagnosis. Some conditions respond rapidly to treatment so patients should be expected to improve if the diagnosis and treatment were appropriate. A failure to improve in this situation should trigger the clinician to reconsider the diagnosis.

Excluding hypoxia, hypoglycaemia and hypotension, the out-of-hospital management of mild traumatic head injuries can only act to limit the progression of an SBI. While this is essential in the long term, it means that patients will show little improvement during transport to hospital. Any deterioration must be considered to indicate a rapid extension of the injury, and ensuring hypoxia and hypotension do not occur is essential. Isolated head injuries in adults do not have the potential to cause hypovolaemia and the development of hypotension after a traumatic head injury should trigger suspicion that an uncontrolled haemorrhage is present in another area.

Ongoing management

Unless the patient deteriorates, ongoing management of mild TBI is conservative pain relief and regular observations (30 min to 4-hourly) to monitor for deterioration. In cases where the patient has a GCS of 15 and no loss of consciousness or amnesia, this could be conducted in the waiting room at hospital or under supervision at home. Observation for 24 hours is recommended in all cases of mild TBI, and any deterioration of symptoms can prompt further neurological examination (Evans & Whitlow, 2019).

Investigations

Diagnostic studies of head injuries are aimed at identifying the cause and the potential for progression of brain trauma. Magnetic resonance imaging (MRI) and particularly CT have revolutionised the assessment of head injuries and are integral to selecting management pathways. The specific criteria that direct patients towards CT or MRI may vary between centres.

While CT scans in patients with mild TBI are often normal, they are recommended as there is a small subgroup in which abnormalities will be revealed, making the examination worthwhile for the broader patient population. There is an estimated prevalence of 5% abnormal CT findings in mild TBI patients with a GCS of 15, and up to 30% of patients with a GCS of 13 (Borg et al., 2004).

A patient with a moderate or severe TBI will have an early CT as the preferential imaging modality as this can identify skull fractures, cerebral oedema as well as intracranial hematomas (Rajajee, 2018a, 2018b) and these scans can help determine specific management requirements such as depressive craniotomy.

Posttraumatic seizures, open or depressed skull fractures, basilar fractures, acute deterioration, loss of consciousness, amnesia and a high mechanism of injury are common indicators for CT investigation. Adults with head injuries who are over the age of 65 and/or who are on anticoagulant medications are required to have a CT scan in some centres (Tintinalli et al., 2016).

Skull x-rays are no longer routinely performed as they lack sensitivity for fractures, do not reveal soft-tissue damage and expose injured tissue to unnecessary radiation. Skull radiography should be performed only if CT is not available, and a negative finding may provide a false sense of security.

The insertion of probes to monitor ICP in severe TBI remains a standard practice in many advanced trauma centres and is a strong recommendation from the Brain Trauma Foundation (Carney et al., 2016). Probes can be inserted into the ventricles, the parenchyma or the subarachnoid or extradural spaces. The most invasive intraventricular probes are also the most accurate and enable drainage of CSF to lower pressure, but they carry the highest risk of infection and bleeding. The insertion of ICP monitoring will help monitor rises in ICP, and alterations to CPP, allowing intensivists to ameliorate these changes and ensure brain perfusion is maintained at all stages of treatment.

Other tests that may be used include cerebral electro-encephalogram (EEG), transcranial Doppler studies and infrared spectroscopy for region cerebral oxygenation. Positron emission tomography (PET) is also used to diagnose the cause of increased ICP (Brown & Edwards, 2014). Lumbar puncture is not performed with increased ICP, due to the risk of cerebral herniation with a sudden release of pressure in the skull from the area above the lumbar puncture (Brown & Edwards, 2014).

Hospital admission

The following criteria are associated with hospital admission after assessment:
- GCS ≤ 13
- abnormalities on CT (e.g. any intracranial haematoma, mass effector midline shift)
- seizures
- neurological deficit
- ongoing emesis
- abnormal bleeding parameters from underlying bleeding diathesis or oral anticoagulation (Evans & Whitlow, 2019).

Hospital discharge

After presentation at the hospital the following criteria are associated with safe discharge:
- 6 hours of observations or vital signs in the normal range, or 4 hours if discharged into the care of a responsible third party
- normal clinical examination
- no vomiting
- not intoxicated
- suitable adult assistance available at home
- monitoring of older people for declining neurological function, as they recover more slowly
- instructions on the avoidance of agents with any platelet effects (e.g. aspirin, NSAIDs)
- avoidance of contact sports for at least 1 week
- instructions for carers about possible complications
- appropriate follow-up (Dunn et al., 2015).

Head injuries across the lifespan
Paediatric patients

The size and mass of a child's head in relation to its body is greater than in adults. They are therefore commonly thrust forwards or fall head-first, and the impact is often to the head (Mandavia et al., 2011). Children are also vulnerable to TBI following assaults from adults, especially the injury known as shaken baby syndrome. In one study from the United Kingdom, the most common cause of head injury in children was related to low falls (< 1 m or < 5 stairs) and accounted for 32.1% of all presentations, which was greater than all sporting injuries combined (13.7%) (Trefan et al., 2016). There was also a noted positive correlation with socioeconomic status; children who presented to an ED with head injuries were more likely to have come from a poor socioeconomic status household (55.1 per 100,000) compared to the highest socioeconomic status household (39.7 per 100,000) (Trefan et al., 2016).

The child's skull is more compliant than an adult's, yet skull fractures are relatively common in children and cerebral contusion and SDH are common injuries. EDH is relatively rare in young children because of the tight adherence of the dura to the skull. Another injury that occurs almost exclusively in children with head trauma is transient cortical blindness (Mandavia et al., 2011). The incidence is unknown, but is thought to be a secondary phase of spasm induced by trauma. This occurs most often in children younger than 1 year.

In infant concussion syndrome, patients present with a broad range of symptoms from nonspecific complaints to seizure or coma. Classic findings include retinal haemorrhages, subdural haematomas, subarachnoid blood and no signs of external trauma (Mandavia et al., 2011). Children with cerebral concussion often present differently from adults. The infant concussion syndrome consists of transient appearance of pallor, diaphoresis, vomiting, tachycardia and somnolence and weakness, often occurring from minor head trauma such as falling off a change table. Usually the diagnosis is made by CT scan. Children may also present with lethargy, irritability, seizures, vomiting, poor feeding and periods of apnoea (Tintinalli et al., 2016). All these symptoms should raise the suspicion of a more serious head injury. It is important when assessing the child that you allow them time to adapt and become comfortable with your presence and if the child is sleeping they should be gently woken.

In infants, linear skull fractures often extend from one suture to another and result in the development of a cephalohaematoma. Other key points when assessing children with head injury include the following.

- Children are more likely to experience cerebral oedema than adults.
- Conducting a neurological assessment in children can be difficult due to their limited language skills.
- Children have an increased incidence of posttraumatic seizures after severe head injuries.
- Child abuse must be considered in all children with unexplained injuries, or injuries not consistent with the history provided.
- Child abuse must be suspected in the case of intracerebral injury or skull fracture in infants or children.

- Until the cranial sutures close, children's skulls are more distendable than those of adults and young children may sustain a lower increase in ICP after head trauma than adults with comparable mechanisms of injury.
- Very young children (< 1 year) have a higher mortality after head trauma than older children with the same level of injury. Many factors contribute to this. Medical attention is often delayed in children with non-accidental injuries because of limited language and comprehension, and accurate formal neurological examination in young children is difficult. Medical personnel are often reluctant to initiate invasive procedures such as IV access for sedation in CT scanning. The GCS is difficult to apply to children younger than 5 years of age. Modified scales have been developed but none has been rigorously validated.
- Children with severe or moderate head injuries are clinically similar to adults although with increased incidents of posttraumatic seizure after severe head injury. Children who sustain minor head injuries often have more pronounced physical signs than adults despite apparently trivial trauma: children may appear pale and lethargic, vomit and complain of headaches and dizziness.
- Many children experience a brief impact seizure at the time of a relatively minor head injury; by the time the child is evaluated, they have returned to baseline neurological function.
- There is a close association between SDH and child abuse and they are often associated with rib and long bone fractures. Approximately 10% of SDH cases are not accidental. Shaken babies have a reduced sucking reflex, a bulging anterior fontanelle, asymmetrical motor function and reflex responses, seizures, apnoea, bradycardia or vomiting. Shaken babies show no, or few, external signs of trauma and retinal haemorrhages.

Older patients

Elderly people are at an increased risk of falls and subsequent TBI. Falls account for 85% of TBI in patients over 65 and mortality rates increased dramatically the older the patients are over 65 years of age (Hawley et al., 2017). Altered mental status, seizures and focal neurological deficits should not be ascribed to intoxication, dementia or other chronic conditions if there is a history or evidence of head trauma. Patients taking anticoagulant medications should be considered at high risk of developing a secondary head injury. Atrophy of brain tissue provides a larger space for brain swelling to occur before compression starts to limit perfusion: signs of raised ICP in the elderly may take longer to develop.

CASE STUDY 2

Case 11437, 1525 hrs.

Dispatch details: You are responding to a 19-year-old male motorcyclist who has collided with a vehicle and has been thrown from his bike. The patient is reported to be unconscious.

Initial presentation: As the crew arrive the patient is supine on the roadside, bystanders aiding him. The patient appears to be talking.

1 ASSESS

1529 hrs Safety: The crew position their vehicle to provide protection from traffic.

1529 hrs Primary survey: The patient is conscious and talking but appears confused. His speech is delayed and at times he uses inappropriate words. The patient's motorbike helmet is still in situ.

1530 hrs Pertinent hx: Bystanders state that the patient was riding his motorbike, weaving in and out of traffic. He was looking over his shoulder at the traffic when a car merged out from a side road. He swerved just before impact but his front wheel hit the bonnet of the car and he landed on the road, approximately 15–20 m away. He appeared unconscious for up to a minute. He woke up just before the crew arrived and appeared confused and unable to move.

The patient appears sweaty and confused. He is wearing jeans and a leather riding jacket. His motorcycle helmet has damage to the right side where it appears to have hit the road. The helmet is safely removed while maintaining in-line neck stabilisation. He has no other obvious injuries.

The patient is loaded onto the stretcher via spine board and is taken to the ambulance to continue the assessment.

1532 hrs Vital signs survey: Conscious state: Eyes open, appears alert = 4; inappropriate verbal response = 3; localises to pain = 5: GCS = 12.

Perfusion status: HR 126 bpm; sinus tachycardia; BP 150/90 mmHg; skin cool, pale, clammy.

Respiratory status: RR 22 bpm, good air entry, L = R, no adventitious sounds, normal work of breathing, mumbling constantly; SpO_2 98% on room air.

Medical hx: The patient does not answer the crew's questions but is not aggressive or obstructive: he simply does not respond. He is not wearing a medical bracelet. A police member has made contact with the patient's family by phone and inform the crew that the patient has asthma but no allergies.

1535 hrs Secondary survey: The patient has abrasions to his right elbow and shoulder, and a haematoma over his right forehead but no obvious underlying bony damage. The skin is red and haemorrhaging slightly.

Neuro exam: Pupils are equal, round and reactive. Spontaneous movement of all limbs. No obvious facial palsy or altered sensation.

1539 hrs: The patient starts to vomit and the crew maintain in-line alignment and roll the ensure airway patency.

1540 hrs: The patient is now unresponsive to the crew. His GCS is as follows: Eyes open but catatonic = 1, verbal incomprehensible (when painful stimuli is applied the patient groans) = 2, motor withdraws both hands when painful stimuli is applied = 4, GCS = 7.

Despite this rapid decline in conscious state, the patient's HR, BP and SpO$_2$ remain as per above.

2 CONFIRM

In many cases paramedics are presented with a collection of signs and symptoms that do not appear to describe a particular condition. A critical step in determining a treatment plan in this situation is to consider what other conditions could explain the patient's presentation.

What else could it be?

Drugs/alcohol
The patient's behaviour prior to the incident combined with his risk-taking behaviour (weaving in and out of traffic at speed) suggests that he may possibly be affected by drugs or alcohol. However, his neuro observations (pupils) and vital signs (hypertensive and tachycardic) are not consistent with this, and in the setting of trauma any altered conscious state should be considered to be a TBI.

Hypoglycaemia
Hypoglycaemia could explain both his behaviour prior to the accident and his confusion following. It is also consistent with an overt sympathetic response (pale, cool, clammy, tachycardic). His BGL is tested and it is 8.0 mmol/L.

Hyperthermia
Profound heat stress can produce confusion and hyponatraemia, which can lead to cerebral oedema and subsequently reduced perfusion. The day is cool and the patient's tympanic temperature is already decreasing to 35.2. Ensuring the patient remains normothermic in the setting of trauma is a key component of good holistic trauma care.

Seizure activity/post-ictal
Seizures are possible after a head strike and may result in changes to a patient's conscious state, including periods of unconsciousness afterwards, followed by a gradual return to normal GCS. However, in this case, witnesses did not describe any overt seizure activity.

Mental illness
Mental illness should be considered only when other causes of altered consciousness can be eliminated.

Cerebral haemorrhage
The three phases of this clinical journey—unconscious, lucid and unconscious again—could suggest a progressive intracranial haemorrhage, in particular an epidural haematoma.

3 TREAT

As bleeding into the fixed space of the cranium continues, it raises ICP. Whether due to direct insult or in response to poor cerebral perfusion, a profound sympathetic response often occurs shortly after the primary injury, producing a rise in both heart rate and blood pressure (Atkinson & Wilberger, 2003). The primary aim of TBI management is to limit any rise in ICP and minimise any SBI, but ensure homeostasis. Unfortunately, the maximal physical exertions

DIFFERENTIAL DIAGNOSIS

TBI
Or
- Drugs/alcohol
- Hypoglycaemia
- Hyperthermia
- Complex partial seizure
- Mental illness
- Cerebral irritation

BOX 34.5 Out-of-hospital paramedic intubation of patients with severe TBI

Recent literature has challenged the benefits of out-of-hospital intubation (Lafferty & Adler, 2011), although some earlier international studies indicated limited success using standing orders and supervision by a medical director telephone debrief immediately post-procedure (Ochs et al., 2002). Unsuccessful attempts at intubation at the scene may delay transport and increase the risk of aspiration and hypoxia (Marx et al., 2017). In a review of the literature on current Australian practice by Bernard (2006), it was reported that most ambulance services do not allow the use of appropriate drugs to facilitate intubation. Bernard found evidence from the trauma registries that intubation without appropriate drugs had a worse outcome than no intubation. He recommended that RSI should be limited to appropriate clinical trials and patients transported by helicopter. Any patient who has been intubated should be transported with waveform capnography.

that can occur with cerebral irritation directly raise ICP and also increase oxygen and glucose consumption.

In the hospital setting treatment involves administering sedation and a muscle relaxant and maintaining the patient's ventilation by inserting an endotracheal tube. This treatment has been proven to reduce the extent of secondary injury and improve patient outcomes, but the combination of a sedative and a muscle relaxant can have potentially severe consequences if the clinician is not able to intubate and adequately ventilate the patient. Until recently paramedics in some areas used repeated doses of sedatives (benzodiazepines) and analgesic agents (opioids) to lower the patient's level of consciousness in order to achieve intubation. Unfortunately, the combination of activating the gag reflex during laryngoscopy (raising ICP) and the vasodilatory effects of the drugs (lowering MAP) had the net effect of lowering cerebral perfusion and led to poor patient outcomes regardless of whether endotracheal tube insertion was successful (Bernard, 2006; see Box 34.5). A number of states have subsequently trained paramedics to adopt the in-hospital practice of administering a small dose of sedation followed immediately by a rapid-acting muscle relaxant (suxamethonium, rocuronium) that acts to temporarily paralyse the patient. This procedure enables intubation to be achieved without the gag reflex causing a rise in ICP or the induction agents causing a significant fall in blood pressure. Short-acting paralysis also allows a better airway view during laryngoscopy, increasing intubation success rates. IV fluid administration and maintaining paralysis and sedation after intubation ensures hypoxia and hypotension are avoided.

The administration of benzodiazepines during the intubation process may reduce the likelihood of post-injury seizures, but there is no evidence that treating seizures prophylactically in head-injured patients improves their outcomes (see Box 34.6). Inversely, the avoidance of large doses of benzodiazepines during the induction process may prevent decreases in blood pressure. The use of anaesthetic agents, such as ketamine, afford clinicians a safer induction process, less impact on perfusion and increased maintenance of the patient's own airway tone.

RSI allows for the safe and effective management of patients with head injuries who would otherwise be 'wrestled' to hospital, putting both themselves and the crew in danger. The process of RSI is potentially dangerous, as the

BOX 34.6 Seizure prophylaxis management

Seizure activity following TBI can extend SBI and is linked to poor outcomes (Schierhout & Roberts, 2001). Seizures increase secondary injury by increasing cerebral metabolic demand (increases ischaemia), raising ICP and releasing excess neurotransmitters. The safety and effectiveness of prophylactically managing seizures in patients with head injuries remains unclear. Although seizures following trauma are associated with poor outcomes, they are not common and the routine administration of barbiturates has been shown to be harmful to TBI patients (Ghajar, 2000). Other studies using different agents have shown the incidence of seizures can be reduced by prophylactic management but it makes no difference to patient outcomes (Schierhout & Roberts, 2001). There is insufficient data to support the use of benzodiazepines in this role and their potential to reduce blood pressure and airway control suggests they should be used with extreme care. Seizures that do occur should be managed according to local guidelines as, once manifested, they need to be controlled.

PRACTICE TIP

The goal of TBI management is to prevent secondary injuries to the brain from hypoxia, hyperglycaemia, hypotension, hyperthermia and hypercarbia. Patients are typically not fasted and are at risk of aspiration of oral and gastric secretions (Mandavia et al., 2011). Consequently, securing an airway and ensuring adequate ventilation are of the highest priority.

PRACTICE TIP

There is no place for 'permissive hypotension' in patients with head injuries as has been advocated in selected cases of penetrating trauma (Bersten & Soni, 2018).

patient can become hypoxic during the procedure as the short-term neuro-muscular blockade removes the ability to breathe. The intent to avoid hypoxia (through endotracheal intubation) can in fact cause hypoxia if the crew are not adequately trained and prepared.

The administration of sedation alone (usually a benzodiazepine) to transport the patient is also likely to risk both hypoxia and hypotension as the drug suppresses conscious state, respiratory drive and vasomotor tone. For patients with TBI and agitation/cerebral irritation, judicious analgesia is desirable over benzodiazepines, remembering that the brain injury suffered will also be painful.

Long delays to definitive care may require remote area doctors to perform urgent craniotomy or burr holes in patients with head injuries to evacuate an expanding mass lesion such as EDH or SDH. This may be required in remote communities where patients have clinical signs of intracranial herniation or witnessed deterioration and surgical evacuation may be lifesaving. The indications are a deteriorating neurological state and an inability to access neurosurgical assistance within 2 hours; pupillary dilation must be present and the site of the extradural collection is often indicated by bogginess over the scalp fracture. Approximately 75% of extradural haematomas are temporal; the landmarks are above the midpoint of the zygomatic arch and two fingers' breadth anterior to the external auditory canal (Dunn et al., 2015). Mannitol creates an osmotic draw of fluid from the interstitial space into the vascular space and may be used to reduce ICP. It can temporarily improve cerebral blood flow, CPP and brain metabolism (Tintinalli et al., 2016).

1545 hrs: The patient is now extending to painful stimuli and his verbal responses are incomprehensible.

Conscious state: Eyes open but catatonic = 1; incomprehensible verbal response = 2; extends abnormally to pain = 2: GCS = 5.

Perfusion status: HR 126 bpm; sinus tachycardia; BP 160/90 mmHg; skin cool, pale, clammy.

Respiratory status: RR 24 bpm, good air entry, L = R, no adventitious sounds, normal work of breathing, SpO_2 98% on room air.

The crew consider transporting the patient without RSI but transport time exceeds 40 minutes. They request a second crew to assist in RSI.

1547 hrs: The crew insert an IV line and commence 10 mL/kg crystalloid for hydration.

Despite this patient's high blood pressure, his head injury has led to poor cerebral perfusion, and the administration of any sedation is likely to lower blood pressure and reduce cerebral perfusion further. Infusing 10 mL/kg prior to intubation will protect against transient hypotension.

1549 hrs: The crew commence oxygen therapy via a bag valve mask.

Although the patient is not currently hypoxic, replacing the atmospheric nitrogen in the lungs with oxygen will delay any desaturation that will start the moment the muscle relaxant stops the patient ventilating. It is important that the patient is on 100% oxygen for at least 3 minutes prior to RSI to completely denitrogenate their lungs. The addition of nasal cannula will assist in apnoeic oxygenation of the patient, further limiting the risk of hypoxia (Weingart, 2010).

1552 hrs: The crew undertake RSI, using a combination anaesthetic/analgesic combined with a short-term neuromuscular blockade.

1555 hrs: Post RSI care is important in minimising or preventing SBI, ensuring the patient's $EtCO_2$ remains in the range 30–35 mmHg, $SpO_2 > 95\%$ and BP 120 mmHg. Timely transport to hospital is also critical, so undertaking care while moving is important.

(4) EVALUATE

Evaluating the effect of any clinical management intervention can provide clues to the accuracy of the initial diagnosis. Some conditions respond rapidly to treatment so patients should be expected to improve if the diagnosis and treatment were appropriate. A failure to improve in this situation should trigger the clinician to reconsider the diagnosis.

As the paramedics are not treating the underlying cause of the patient's condition there should be no improvement in his condition. In fact, the primary aim of evaluation here is to maintain sufficient levels of sedation, muscle relaxants, ventilation and fluid support to ensure that there is no change.

The crew intubate the patient and perform post intubation checks to ensure tube placement is confirmed. Waveform capnography is the only absolute confirmation that can be used to confirm tube placement (DAS, 2015). Once tube placement is confirmed and the endotracheal tube is secured, commencement of ongoing sedation and long-term paralysis is important to reduce noxious stimuli which can increase ICP.

Close measurement of vital signs is the key to limiting SBI in this patient.

- Ventilation parameters need to be set, targeting $EtCO_2$ levels in the range 30–35 mmHg, and oxygen levels above 95%. Often in the out-of-hospital setting an FiO_2 of 1.0 is utilised.
- Perfusion maintenance should be over 100 mmHg, most often through fluid administration. The use of pressor therapy is controversial in TBI.
- Holistic patient care involves ensuring the patient remains warm and is postured appropriately (slight head elevation in patients without a spinal injury not only helps venous draining from the cranial vault but also allows for better lung oxygenation and perfusion). Periodic measurement of blood glucose and temperature is required.
- It is important that transport to hospital is always forefront in the mind of out-of-hospital clinicians, and limiting any delays that occur will ensure the patient is taken to the appropriate hospital for definitive care.

Future research

The most effective treatment for TBI is prevention. Driver and passenger airbags and age-appropriate child restraints have reduced the number of deaths from TBI, as have helmets for motorcyclists, cyclists and other sportspeople. Long-term recovery can be improved by investigating patients shortly after their injury: early brain imaging might enable accurate prediction of the severity of the injury for the benefit of the patient's family, the community and funding agencies.

Attempts using medications to reduce the inflammatory response and provide a form of neuroprotection have not proved successful but there are a number of trials in which TBI patients are aggressively cooled after intubation. Therapeutic hypothermia has been demonstrated to provide some cerebral benefit post cardiac arrest (Bernard et al., 2002) but the studies involving the process in TBI are yet to prove conclusive (Sandestig et al., 2014).

Hyperglycaemia may be caused by the post-injury surge of catecholamines and therefore can occur in patients who normally maintain good glucose control (i.e. non-diabetics; Atkinson & Wilberger, 2003). A high BGL is associated with poorer outcomes, and the next stage of out-of-hospital treatment of TBI may be restoration of normal BGL. This will require care and training, as patients who have been sedated and intubated may not show overt signs of hypoglycaemia following treatment.

TBIs that are apparently similar in mechanism and severity can produce vastly different outcomes between individuals and this may be partially explained by recent research that has identified the apolipoprotein E gene as directing at least part of the pathological response to neural injury (Sun & Jiang, 2008).

Summary

'Head injury' is a broad term that includes injuries to the scalp and face but is used clinically to describe a TBI. The injury caused at the time that the force is applied will result in tissue damage that, if sufficiently severe and widespread, can cause a cascade of responses that lead to poor cerebral perfusion. If not corrected this SBI can cause profound morbidity and death. Recognition of the mechanism of injury, a detailed neurological examination and monitoring for deterioration are key in identifying the progression of a secondary injury. Hypoxia and hypotension increase the development of an SBI and must be actively managed if they are present.

References

Abdelmalik, P. A., Draghic, N., & Ling, G. S. F. (2019). Management of moderate and severe traumatic brain injury. *Transfusion, 59*(S2), 1529–1538. doi:10.1111/trf.15171.

Accident Compensation Corporation (ACC). (2007). *Traumatic brain injury: diagnosis, acute management and rehabilitation. Evidence-based best practice guideline.* Wellington: ACC.

Atkinson, D. J., & Wilberger, J. E. (2003). Multiple organ system injuries resulting from and critical care of isolated severe central nervous system trauma. In A. J. Layon, A. Gabrielli & W. A. Friedman (Eds.), *Textbook of neurointensive care.* Philadelphia: Saunders.

Beck, B., Bray, J., Cameron, P. A., Cooper, D. J., & Gabbe, B. J. (2016). Trends in severe traumatic brain injury in Victoria, 2006-2014. *The Medical Journal of Australia, 204*(11).

Bernard, S. (2006). Paramedic intubation of patients with severe head injury: a review of current Australian practice and recommendations for change. *Emergency Medicine Australasia: EMA, 18,* 221–228. doi:10.1111/j.1742-6723.2006.00850.x.

Bernard, S., Gray, T. W., Buist, M. D., Jones, B. M., Silvester, W., Gutteridge, G., & Smith, K. (2002). Treatment of comatose survivors of out-of-hospital cardiac arrest with induced hypothermia. *The New England Journal of Medicine, 346.*

Bersten, A. D., & Soni, N. (2018). *Oh's intensive care manual* (8th ed.). China: Butterworth–Heinemann.

Borg, J., Holm, L., Cassidy, J. D., Peloso, P. M., Carroll, L. J., von Holst, H., & Ericson, K. (2004). WHO Collaborating Centre Task Force on Mild Traumatic Brain Injury, Diagnostic procedures in mild traumatic brain injury: results of the WHO Collaborating Centre Task Force on Mild Traumatic Brain. *Journal of Rehabilitation Medicine, 43*(Suppl.), 6175.

Brain Injury Australia. (2012). *About acquired brain injury.* Retrieved from www.bia.net.au/index.php?option=com_content&view=article&id=2&Itemid=3. (Accessed 8 April 2012.)

Brown, D., & Edwards, H. (2014). *Lewis's medical-surgical nursing: assessment and management of clinical problems* (4th ed.). Sydney: Elsevier.

Bullock, M., Chesnut, R., Ghajar, J., Gordon, D., Hartl, R., Newell, D. W., Servadei, F., Walters, B. C., Wilberger, J. E., & Surgical Management of Traumatic Brain Injury Author Group. (2006a). Surgical management of acute epidural hematomas. *Neurosurgery, 58*(3).

Bullock, M., Chesnut, R., Ghajar, J., Gordon, D., Hartl, R., Newell, D. W., Servadei, F., Walters, B. C., Wilberger, J.

E., & Surgical Management of Traumatic Brain Injury Author Group. (2006b). Surgical management of acute subdural hematomas. *Neurosurgery, 58*(3).

Cameron, P., Jelinek, G., Kelly, A., Murray, L., & Brown, A. (Eds.), (2014). *Textbook of adult emergency medicine* (4th ed.). Elsevier.

Carney, N., Totten, A., O'Reilly, C., Ullman, J. S., Hawryluk, G. W. J., Bell, M. J., Bratton, S. L., Chesnut, R., Harris, O. A., Kissoon, N., Rubiano, A. M., Shutter, L., Tasker, R. C., Vavilala, M. S., Wilberger, J., Wright, D. W., & Ghajar, J. (2016). *Guidelines for the management of severe traumatic brain injury* (4th ed.). Brain Trauma Foundation.

Carney, N., Ghajar, J., Jagoda, A., Bedrick, S., Davis-O'Reilly, C., du Coudray, H., Hack, D., Helfand, N., Huddleston, A., Nettleton, T., & Riggio, S. (2014). Concussion guidelines step 1. *Neurosurgery, 75*(3).

Carroll, R. G. (2010). *Problem-based physiology.* Philadelphia: Saunders.

Cools, M., & Carneiro, K. (2018). Facial nerve palsy following mild mastoid trauma on trampoline. *The American Journal of Emergency Medicine, 36.*

Curran, J. E. (2008). Anaesthesia for facial trauma. *Anaesthesia and Intensive Care Medicine, 9*(8), 338–343.

DeCuypere, M., & Klimo, P. (2012). Spectrum of traumatic brain injury from mild to severe. *The Surgical Clinics of North America, 92*(4), 939–957.

Difficult Airway Society. (2015). *Difficult intubation guidelines.* London: DAS.

Douglas, G., Nicol, F., & Robertson, C. (2018). *Macleod's clinical examination* (14th ed.). Philadelphia: Elsevier.

Dunn, R., Dilley, S., Brookes, J., Leach, D., MacLean, A., & Borland, M. (2015). *The emergency medicine manual* (6th ed., Vol. 2). Tennyson, South Australia: Venom Publishing.

Easton, R., Bendinelli, C., Sisak, K., Enninghorst, N., & Balogh, Z. (2012). Prehospital nausea and vomiting after trauma: prevalence, risk factors, and development of a predictive scoring system. *The Journal of Trauma and Acute Care Surgery, 72*(5).

Evans, R., & Whitlow, C. (2019). Acute mild traumatic brain injury (concussion) in adults. *BMJ UpToDate.*

Farrell, M., & Dempsey, J. (2016). *Smeltzer & Bare's textbook of medical-surgical nursing* (4th ed.). Sydney: Lippincott Williams & Wilkins.

FitzGerald, M. J. T., Gruener, G., & Mtui, E. (2011). *Clinical neuroanatomy and neuroscience* (6th ed.). Philadelphia: Saunders.

Ghajar, J. (2000). Traumatic brain injury. *The Lancet, 356*(9233).

Green, S. M. (2011). Cheerio, laddie! Bidding farewell to the Glasgow Coma Scale. *Annals of Emergency Medicine, 58*, 5.

Hawley, C., Sakr, M., Scapinello, S., Salvo, J., & Wrenn, P. (2017). Traumatic brain injury in older adults—6 years of

data for on UK trauma centre: retrospective analysis of prospectively collected data. *Emergency Medicine Journal, 34.*

Kumar, V., Cotran, R. S., & Robbins, S. L. (2017). *Robbins basic pathology* (10th ed.). Philadelphia: Saunders.

Lafferty, K. A., & Adler, J. (2011). Rapid sequence intubation. *Medscape.* Retrieved from http://emedicine.medscape.com/article/80222-overview. (Accessed 9 November 2013.)

Mandavia, D. P., Newton, E. J., & Demetriades, D. (2011). *Colour atlas of emergency trauma.* Cambridge, UK: Cambridge University Press.

Marx, J. A., Hockberger, R. S., & Walls, R. M. (2017). *Rosen's emergency medicine: concepts and clinical practice* (9th ed.). St Louis: Mosby.

McCance, K., & Huether, S. (2018). *Pathophysiology: the biologic basis for disease in adults and children* (8th ed.). Philadelphia: Mosby.

McCrea, M., Kelly, J. P., Kluge, J., Ackley, B., & Randolph, C. (1997). Standardized assessment of concussion in football players. *Neurology, 48*(3).

McCrory, P., Davis, G., & Makdissi, M. (2012). Second impact syndrome or cerebral swelling after sporting head injury. *Current Sports Medicine Reports, 11*(1), 21–23.

NZGG. (2006). *Traumatic brain injury: diagnosis, acute management and rehabilitation. Evidence-based best practice guideline.* Wellington: NZGG.

Ó Briain, D., Nickson, C., Pilcher, D., & Udy, A. (2018). Early hyperoxia in patients with traumatic brain injury admitted to intensive care in Australia and New Zealand: a retrospective multicenter cohort study. *Neurocritical Care.*

Ochs, M., Davis, D., Hoyt, D., Baily, D., Marshall, L., & Rosen, P. (2002). Paramedic-performed rapid sequence intubation of patients with severe head injuries. *Annals of Emergency Medicine, 40*(2).

Parrillo, J. E., & Dellinger, R. P. (2019). *Critical care medicine: principles of diagnosis and management in the adult* (5th ed.). Philadelphia: Mosby.

Patton, K. T., & Thibodeau, G. A. (2019). *Anatomy and physiology* (10th ed.). St Louis: Mosby.

Pozzato, I., Tate, R., Rosenkoetter, U., & Cameron, I. (2019). Epidemiology of hospitalized traumatic brain injury in the state of New South Wales, Australia: a population-based study. *Australian and New Zealand Journal of Public Health.*

Pushkarna, A., Bhatoe, H. S., & Sudambrekar, S. M. (2010). Head injuries. *Medical Journal, Armed Forces India, 66*(4).

Rajajee, V. (2018a). Management of acute severe traumatic brain injury. *BMJ UpToDate.*

Rajajee, V. (2018b). Traumatic brain injury: epidemiology, classification and pathophysiology. *BMJ UpToDate.*

Rees, P. M. (2003). Contemporary issues in mild traumatic brain injury. *Archives of Physical Medicine and Rehabilitation, 84*(12).

Reith, F., Lingsma, H., Gabbe, B., Lecky, F. E., Roberts, I., & Maas, A. I. R. (2017). Differential effects of the Glasgow Coma Scale Score and its components: an analysis of 54, 069 patients with traumatic brain injury. *Injury, 48.*

Rudy, E. B. (1984). *Advanced neurological and neurosurgical nursing.* St Louis: Mosby.

Sanchez, B., Waxman, K., Jones, T., Conner, S., Chung, R., & Becerra, S. (2005). Cervical spine clearance in blunt trauma: evaluation of a computed tomography–based protocol. *The Journal of Trauma, 59*(1).

Sandestig, A., Romner, B., & Grände, P. (2014). Therapeutic hypothermia in children and adults with severe traumatic brain injury. *Therapeutic Hypothermia and Temperature Management, 4*(1), 10–20.

Schierhout, G., & Roberts, I. (2001). Antiepileptic drugs for preventing seizures following acute traumatic brain injury. *The Cochrane Database of Systematic Reviews*, (4), CD000173.

Shores, E. A., Lammel, A., Hullick, C., Sheedy, J., Flynn, M., Levick, W., & Batchelor, J. (2008). The diagnostic accuracy of the Revised Westmead PTA Scale as an adjunct to the Glasgow Coma Scale in the early identification of cognitive impairment in patients with mild traumatic brain injury. *Journal of Neurology, Neurosurgery, and Psychiatry, 79*(10), 1100–1106.

Shum, D. (2007). *Evaluation of Rehabilitation after Traumatic Brain Injury.* NHMRC. Retrieved from http://nhmrc.gov.au/news/snapshots/descriptions/shum.htm.

Stein, S. C., Georgoff, P., Meghan, S., Mirza, K. L., & El Falaky, O. M. (2010). Relationship of aggressive monitoring and treatment to improved outcomes in severe traumatic brain injury. *Journal of Neurosurgery, 112*(5), 1105–1112. doi:10.3171/2009.8.JNS09738.

Sun, X. C., & Jiang, Y. (2008). Genetic susceptibility to traumatic brain injury and apolipoprotein E gene. *Chinese Journal of Traumatology, 11*(4).

Sundstrøm, T., Asbjørnsen, H., Habiba, S., Sunde, G. A., & Wester, K. (2013). Prehospital use of cervical collars in trauma patients: a critical review. *Journal of Neurotrauma, 15*(6), 31.

Teasdale, G., & Jennett, B. (1978). Assessment of coma and severity of brain damage. *Anesthesiology, 49.*

Theodore, N., Hadley, M., Aarabi, B., Dhall, S. S., Gelb, D. E., Hurlbert, R. J., Rozzelle, C. J., Ryken, T. C., & Walters, B. C. (2013). Prehospital cervical spinal immobilization after trauma. *Neurosurgery, 72*(Suppl 2), 22–34.

Tintinalli, J. E., Wright, D. W., Merck, L. H., Stapczynski, J. S., Ma, O. J., Cline, D. M., Cydulka, R. K., & Meckler, G. D. (2016). *Tintinalli's emergency medicine: a comprehensive study guide* (8th ed.). Boston: McGraw-Hill.

Trefan, L., Houston, R., Pearson, G., Edwards, R., Hyde, P., Maconochie, I., Parslow, R. C., & Kemp, A. (2016). Epidemiology of children with head injury: a national overview. *British Medical Journal, 101*(6), 527–532.

Weingart, S. D. (2010). Preoxygenation, Reoxygenation and delayed sequence intubation in the emergency department. *The Journal of Emergency Medicine, 40*(6), 661–667.

CHAPTER 35

Chest Injuries

By Shaun Whitmore

OVERVIEW

- Simple rib fractures and chest wall contusions as the result of direct trauma are common injuries and require adequate analgesia to be properly assessed.
- Forces that cause injuries to the chest wall can be transmitted to the underlying lungs and cause serious injury.
- Pulmonary contusions can impede respiration, resulting in poor oxygen saturation despite treatment.
- Damage to the lung via traumatic means can allow tension pneumothorax to develop.
- Untreated lung injury can result in preventable out-of-hospital death.
- Open pneumothoraces require novel dressing application.
- Tamponade and tension pneumothorax are associated with reduced cardiac output when the preload pressure is exceeded.

- Moderate to severe chest injuries are generally multifactorial. Where a serious injury to the chest is identified, there is a strong possibility that other injuries will be present. Chest injuries often occur in combination with other severe injuries such as injuries to the extremities, head, brain and abdomen (Richter & Rageller, 2011).
- Analgesia, procedural intervention and recognition of potential occult injury combined with expedient transport are the key to minimising morbidity and mortality in serious chest injury.
- Increased access to procedures such as ultrasound improves the diagnostic capability of serious chest injury in the out-of-hospital environment.

Introduction

Chest trauma is any injury to the chest wall (skin, ribs, muscles and vessels) or its contents, including the heart, lungs, trachea/bronchi, great vessels, oesophagus and diaphragm (see Table 35.1). As a result, chest trauma can result in problems of ventilation, respiration and perfusion (or any combination of these). In Australia, chest trauma is the most frequent presentation associated with road/pedestrian trauma and assaults (NSW ITIM, 2012), with approximately 25% of severely injured patients dying as a result of their chest injuries (CDC, 2010). Where the traumatic injuries are isolated to the chest, the mortality rate is between 5 and 8% (Richter & Rageller, 2011).

The physiological consequences of chest trauma may occur almost immediately after the application of force or they may develop over hours, and the ability to effectively manage these injuries in the field is not necessarily proportional to the speed of onset (see Table 35.2). In the out-of-hospital environment it can be difficult to accurately assess the extent of underlying chest injuries, with the mechanism of injury and the vital signs survey providing the majority of the diagnostic information. The paramedic role in chest-injured patients should include aggressive analgesic administration, application of

appropriate procedures such as thoracostomy and recognition of serious underlying injury requiring expedient surgical intervention.

Pathophysiology

Such is the complexity and variability of chest injuries that the ability to effectively triage and treat patients with a chest injury is based on a detailed understanding of chest anatomy and the mechanics of ventilation, respiration and perfusion.

Impairment of ventilation and/or perfusion

The chest wall is defined superiorly, laterally, posteriorly and anteriorly by the ribs and their connection with the spine and the sternum. The diaphragm forms the inferior wall of the chest cavity (see Fig 35.1). All the ribs posteriorly articulate onto two adjacent vertebrae. Anteriorly, ribs I–VII articulate with the sternum by a less flexible cartilaginous joint, while ribs VIII–X articulate with the costal cartilages of the ribs above. Ribs XI and XII are floating ribs and do not articulate anteriorly. In combination the ribs, joints and muscles that comprise the thoracic cavity provide a compromise between offering protection to the underlying structures and allowing enough movement for ventilation of the lungs to occur.

The movement of air in and out of the lungs of the healthy individual depends on the ability of the muscles of the thoracic cavity (and those that attach to it) to expand the volume of the chest wall. During inspiration contraction of the diaphragm flattens the dome-shaped resting state of the muscle, while the inspiratory muscles pull the ribs into a more horizontal position. Both these actions increase the volume of the chest cavity, creating an area of low pressure inside the chest, which atmospheric air moves in to equalise. Relaxation of the inspiratory muscles allows the elasticity of the chest wall and diaphragm to reduce the volume of the chest, forcing air out into the atmosphere (see Figs 35.2 and 35.3).

The lungs and chest wall are separated by two layers of pleura and a small amount of lubricating fluid (see Fig 35.4 and Ch 20). The parietal layer of the pleura lines the inner thoracic wall, and the visceral layer lines the lung itself. Between these two layers there is a potential space referred to as the pleural space, which contains a small amount of serous fluid that reduces friction between the lungs and the thoracic wall during ventilation. The intrapleural pressure (P_{IP}) is often referred to as being 'lower' than either atmospheric or alveolar pressure (Jantz & Pierson, 1994) but as the space is only a 'potential' space this concept can be confusing. A more accurate way to describe the negative pressure is to understand that the elasticity of lung tissue wants to draw the lungs smaller than they are, even at rest. Simultaneously, the structures of

Table 35.1 Injuries from chest trauma

	Type of injury
Musculoskeletal	Rib fractures Sternal fractures Spinal fractures Scapular and clavicle fractures Intercostal muscle injuries
Heart and vessel injuries	Aortic dissection Cardiac contusion Pericardial tamponade Cardiac rupture/infarction
Lung injury	Pneumothorax Haemothorax Pulmonary contusion Tracheobronchial injury
Diaphragm	Rupture/enterothorax Bleeding

Source: Adapted from Richter & Rageller (2011).

Table 35.2 Common chest injuries from trauma: symptoms and management

Injury	Definition	Clinical manifestations	Emergency management
Pneumothorax	Air in pleural space	Dyspnoea, decreased movement of involved chest wall, diminished or absent breath sounds on the affected side, hyperresonance to percussion	Chest tube insertion with chest drainage system
Haemothorax	Blood in the pleural space, usually occurs in conjunction with pneumothorax	Dyspnoea, diminished or absent breath sounds, dullness to percussion, shock	Chest tube insertion with chest drainage system; autotransfusion of collected blood, treatment of hypovolaemia as necessary
Tension pneumothorax	Air in pleural space that does not escape; continued increase in amount of air shifts intrathoracic organs and increases intrathoracic pressure	Tachycardia, tachypnoea, severe respiratory distress, hypotension, decreased or absent breath sounds, subcutaneous emphysema, neck vein distension	Medical emergency: needle decompression followed by chest tube insertion with chest drainage system
Flail chest	Fracture of two or more adjacent ribs in two or more places with loss of chest wall stability	Paradoxical movement of chest wall, respiratory distress, associated haemothorax, pneumothorax, pulmonary contusion	Stabilise flail segment with intubation in some patients; taping in others; oxygen therapy; treat associated injuries; analgesia
Cardiac tamponade	Blood rapidly collects in pericardial sac, compresses myocardium because the pericardium does not stretch and prevents heart from pumping effectively	Muffled, distant heart sounds, hypotension, neck vein distension, increased central venous pressure	Medical emergency: pericardiocentesis with surgical repair as appropriate

Source: Brown & Edwards (2012).

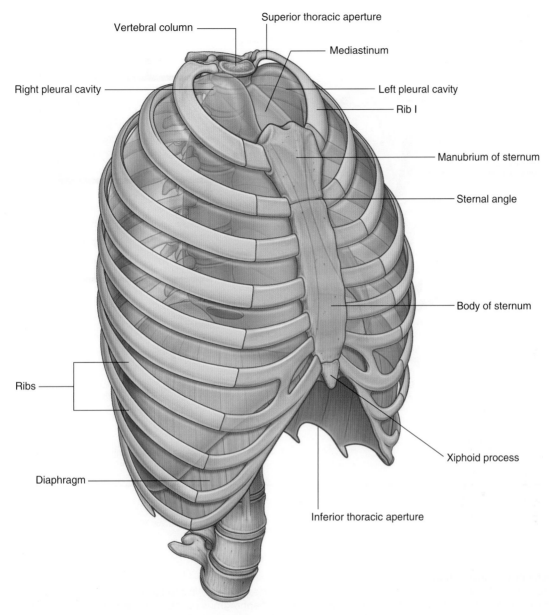

Figure 35.1
The thoracic cavity is a flexible space and consists of the vertebrae, ribs, muscles and sternum. Inferiorly, the thoracic cavity is enclosed by the diaphragm. Overall the cavity can be divided into a left and a right pleural cavity (each surrounding a lung) and the mediastinum, which contains the heart, great vessels and oesophagus. Of these structures the aorta, inferior vena cava and oesophagus pass through the diaphragm into the abdominal cavity.
Source: Drake et al. (2009).

the chest wall want to expand the chest wall larger than it is at rest. As a result there is a constant 'tension' between the chest wall and the lungs, with each trying to pull away from the other. The lungs' natural elasticity is constantly trying to contract the organs; the ribs and muscles of the chest wall would 'rest' at an expanded state if it weren't for the inward pull of the lungs. Any separation is prevented, as there is no air or fluid to fill the potential space. If, however, the seal between the chest wall and the lungs is somehow broken the 'tension' between the two structures will be realised and the lungs will be able to collapse away from the chest wall. This can lead to air or blood entering the space between the two pleura and disturbing the ability to ventilate the lungs when chest wall movement is normal.

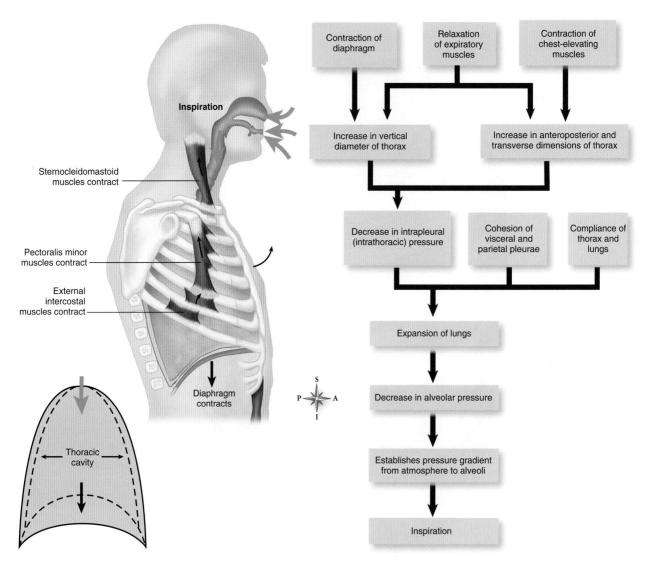

Figure 35.2
Mechanism of inspiration.
Increasing the volume of the thoracic cavity, which decreases pressure in the lungs and thus draws air inwards, requires muscular contraction. At rest, contraction of the diaphragm is usually sufficient, but when greater volumes are required use of the accessory muscles (pectoralis major and minor) and external intercostals raises the ribs and increases the anterior-posterior volume of the cavity.
Source: Patton & Thibodeau (2012).

The following injuries can impair ventilation:

- rib fractures
- closed pneumothorax
- open pneumothorax
- tension pneumothorax
- haemothorax
- tracheobronchial injury
- diaphragmatic injury
- spinal cord injury.

Rib fractures
While pneumothorax and haemothorax are the most dramatic forms of injuries that impair ventilation, simple or complex rib fractures can also reduce effective ventilation (Richter & Rageller, 2011). Rib fractures are one of the most common injuries in patients with chest trauma (Sirmali et al., 2003). The pain from a simple rib fracture can be sufficient to cause substantial symptomatic respiratory embarrassment due to incapacity to properly ventilate. Two consecutive ribs fractured in two places can create a free-floating segment known as a *flail segment* (see Fig 35.5). Having lost their bony connection to the rest of the chest wall, flail segments move independently of the chest wall and will move inwards (drawn in by the negative pressure inside

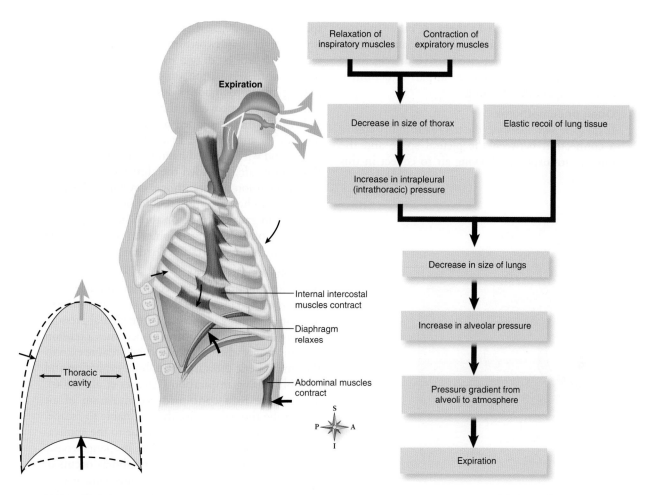

Figure 35.3
Mechanism of expiration.
Relaxing the muscles of inspiration allows the natural elasticity of the chest wall to reduce the size of the thoracic cavity, increasing the air pressure within the lungs and forcing air out. Compared with inspiration, this is a passive process unless changes to airway resistance require contraction of the accessory muscles of expiration (abdominal muscles and internal intercostals).
Source: Patton & Thibodeau (2012).

the thoracic cavity) during inspiration and outwards during expiration. This 'paradoxical movement' decreases the amount of air that enters and leaves the lungs for the degree of chest wall movement, but any hypoxia is most likely to be due to contusions impairing gas exchange in the underlying lung tissue and pain limiting respiratory movement (see the discussion on pulmonary contusion below; Trinkle et al., 1975).

Closed pneumothorax

The accumulation of air in the pleural space is referred to as a pneumothorax and it can occur as the consequence of disease or trauma. In the setting of trauma, air gains access to the pleural cavity because there has been a rupture of either the chest wall or the lung wall (or both). On some occasions the rupture allows a one-time movement of air into the space and creates a *simple pneumothorax*: a stable volume of air in the pleural space. On other occasions the breach acts as a one-way valve allowing air to enter the space with each breath but not to escape. This development of a *tension pneumothorax* affects ventilation, respiration and perfusion and is a life-threatening condition (see below).

A simple closed pneumothorax (see Fig 20.3) occurs when air accumulates between the visceral and parietal pleura. In chest trauma, this is generally as a result of blunt pulmonary tissue injury, laceration of the lung (usually from a fractured rib), alveolar rupture or a penetrating injury. Healthy individuals have large reserve capacities of both circulation and ventilation and a closed pneumothorax is not life-threatening unless it occupies more than

40% of the hemithorax or there are other injuries impacting perfusion (Sanders, 2007). A simple closed pneumothorax may not need active management in the field but can be drained as part of definitive care, re-expanding the lung.

Open pneumothorax

In an *open pneumothorax*, the traumatic injury creates a connection between the pleural space and the outside atmosphere, allowing air to collect in this

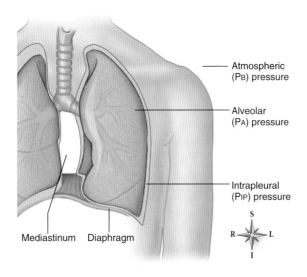

Figure 35.4
Pressure in the chest cavity.
Source: Patton & Thibodeau (2012).

space (see Fig 20.2). If the opening in the chest wall is larger than two-thirds of the tracheal cross-section, air will be drawn in and out through the wound with ventilation, impairing the efficiency of lung inflation on both sides (see Box 35.1). This can be treated by covering the opening on the chest wall with a dressing taped on three sides to allow one side for air to escape. In an emergency, covering the wound with a gloved hand will improve ventilation and is safe, provided the clinician is watching in case a tension pneumothorax develops. All suspicious open chest wounds should be covered with petrolatum gauze secured on three sides to prevent the entry of air during inspiration and allow the exit of air during expiration (Arthurs et al., 2017).

Tension pneumothorax

A tension pneumothorax occurs when air leaking from an injured lung into the pleural space is unable to escape, resulting in increased intrapleural pressure (see Fig 20.4). A pneumothorax becomes a tension pneumothorax when the intrapleural pressure exceeds the atmospheric pressure throughout expiration and possibly during inspiration (Greaves et al., 2006). This is due to a continued accumulation of air within the thoracic cavity that is unable to escape. In apnoeic patients this is often due to the application of positive pressure ventilation. In spontaneously breathing patients tension pneumothorax occurs in the presence of a one-way valve mechanism (e.g. tissue flap or lung tissue acting as a pressure valve in association with penetrating chest wound, lower

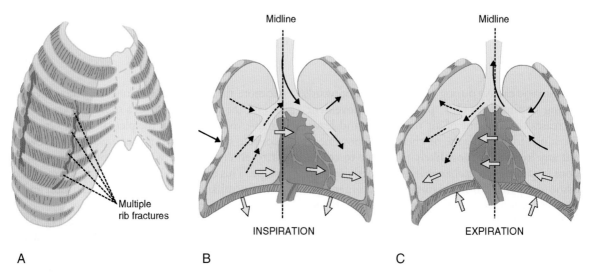

Figure 35.5
Flail chest.
A Flail chest. **B** Flail chest during inspiration. While the diaphragm flattens and the ribs are raised during inspiration the negative intrathoracic pressure draws the flail segment inwards. **C** During expiration the high intrathoracic pressure pushes the flail segment out.
Source: Black & Hawks (2009).

BOX 35.1 Sucking chest wounds

Penetrating trauma can cause a constant communication between the atmosphere and the pleural space. With air entering the pleural space with each inspiration a 'sucking' sound may be heard. Manage the patient as follows:

1. Close the chest wound. This can be done by applying a sterile plastic dressing and securing it with tape. Medical direction may advise that only three sides of the dressing be taped (see Fig 35.6). This provides a venting mechanism (or one-way valve). It also allows spontaneous decompression of a developing tension pneumothorax. Closely monitor for the development of a tension pneumothorax if the patient's dressing does not provide a venting mechanism.
2. Provide ventilatory support with high-concentration oxygen. Airway management includes assisting ventilations with a bag-mask device and intubation.
3. Treat the patient for shock by administering judicious crystalloid fluid per local guidelines to maintain palpable carotid pulse.
4. Rapidly transport the patient to an appropriate medical facility.

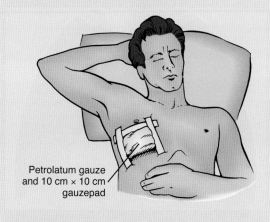

Petrolatum gauze and 10 cm × 10 cm gauzepad

Figure 35.6
Sucking chest wound.
Source: Auerbach (2012).

BOX 35.2 Signs of tension pneumothorax

Signs of a tension pneumothorax include the signs of a pneumothorax as well as:
- hypoperfusion (pale, hypotensive)
- tachycardia (likely)
- dyspnoea and tachypnoea (likely)
- ipsilateral or bilateral decrease in breath sounds
- hyperresonance
- decreasing conscious state
- surgical emphysema
- increase in jugular venous pressure (late/unreliable)
- tracheal deviation due to a shift of the mediastinum to the unaffected side (late/unreliable).

Note: Most of these signs could be the result of trauma to any region and could simply be the result of bleeding or pain, while others are late signs. Maintaining a high index of suspicion of tension pneumothorax in patients who have suffered chest trauma is the key to making an effective clinical decision. If other causes have been treated (i.e. pain, perfusion) and the symptoms remain, suspect tension pneumothorax.

As this accumulation of air increases, intrathoracic pressure increases, placing pressure on the mediastinum and the low-pressure vessels returning blood to the heart. This impedes venous return to the heart. The decreased venous return results in reduced cardiac output and hypotension. As the tension pneumothorax extends, the unaffected lung is compressed, resulting in a rapid and catastrophic deterioration of the patient's respiratory function. Tension pneumothorax is a life-threatening condition of both the cardiovascular and the respiratory systems. However, the classic physical examination findings of tracheal deviation and distended neck veins are poorly sensitive in the diagnosis of tension pneumothorax (Inocencio et al., 2017). The definitive warning signs include rapidly deteriorating respiratory, cardiovascular function and conscious state (see Box 35.2 with Fig 35.6; Greaves et al., 2006). This situation of increasing respiratory distress with decreasing blood pressure and conscious state in the setting of chest trauma requires urgent decompression of the affected side using a standard large-bore IV cannula, a commercially available device such as the Arrow or ARS, or finger thoracostomy. Finger thoracostomy was identified as an

airway narrowing in asthma, or application of an occlusive dressing to a wound associated with open pneumothorax). In either case, air enters the pleural space during inspiration, but does not exit during exhalation, leading to an increasing accumulation of air in the pleural space (Greaves et al., 2006).

intervention which may have improved outcomes in 17 of 113 out-of-hospital trauma deaths in a Victorian study, whereas thoracotomy was not considered to be potentially lifesaving in the same study group (Beck et al., 2019). Triggers for intervention in most ambulance systems generally include cardiovascular and CNS compromise. Limitations of the use of IV cannulae are well documented and should be recognised, but should not preclude their use in the absence of other devices. It has now been shown that 25% of patients experiencing a tension pneumothorax have a chest wall thickness at the second intercostal space in the mid-clavicular line of greater than 5 cm (Givens et al., 2004).

Haemothorax

A haemothorax is a collection of blood in the pleural cavity (see Fig 35.7). It can occur as a result of and in tandem with similar injuries that result in pneumothorax. Patients with a large haemothorax may present with profound hypovolaemic shock and respiratory compromise. Other key clinical signs include dullness to percussion over the haemothorax and absent breath sounds on the affected side.

Tracheobronchial injuries

Injuries to the major airways are usually associated with major trauma and patients rarely survive to hospital (Richter & Rageller, 2011). Most injuries to the lower portion of the major airways occur within 3 cm of the carina and the high energy associated with these injuries can lead to complete transection of the bronchus. Haemoptysis, subcutaneous emphysema and recurrent pneumothorax are signs, but it is very difficult to definitively diagnose these injuries in the field. Major tracheobronchial injury in trauma is rare but when present is associated with an 80% mortality in the field (Platz et al., 2017).

Diaphragmatic injuries

The application of blunt force to the chest can cause sufficient pressure for the diaphragm to rupture. The structure of the lungs means that they rarely protrude into the abdominal cavity but the reverse does not apply and force to the abdomen can rupture the diaphragm and force bowel into the chest cavity (see Fig 35.8). Signs and symptoms of a ruptured diaphragm include abdominal pain, shortness of breath and decreased breath sounds (Sanders, 2007). Decreased breath sounds in the base of the affected side may also occur. Out-of-hospital treatment is limited, but positioning the patient semi-recumbent rather than supine will assist in maximising ventilation.

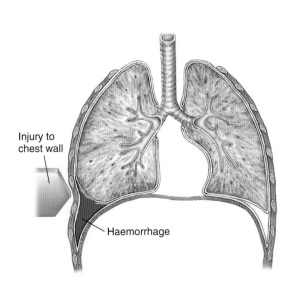

Figure 35.7
Haemothorax.
The accumulation of blood in the pleural spaces is usually associated with damage to the lung parenchyma or major blood vessels. Where major vessels are involved the volume can be extensive, leading to both hypovolaemia and significantly impaired ventilation and a critically ill patient.
Source: Wilson & Giddens (2013).

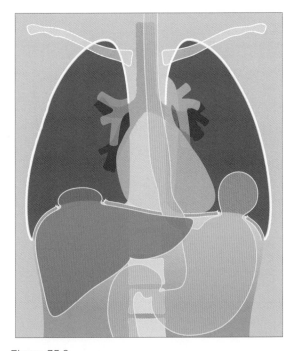

Figure 35.8
Diaphragmatic rupture.
Sudden compression of the abdomen may increase intraabdominal pressure, causing the abdominal contents to rupture through the thin diaphragmatic wall and enter the chest cavity.
Source: de Lacey et al. (2008).

Spinal cord injury

The final type of chest injury that can impair ventilation is any spinal injury that damages the nerves that innervate the muscles of inspiration. The diaphragm is innervated by the phrenic nerves, which leave the spinal column at the mid-cervical level (C3–C5), while the intercostal nerves originate from T1 to T11. Injuries to any of these spinal segments can limit the amount of muscle contraction and subsequently inspiration. Abdominal/paradoxical respiration movement may also occur.

> ## PRACTICE TIP
>
> Air escaping from the lungs into the tissues can result in subcutaneous emphysema. This can occur when the visceral pleura has been penetrated allowing air into the fascial layer. The patient will present with swelling, which when palpated feels like bubbles under the skin. Subcutaneous emphysema is generally found in the upper chest and can extend to the neck and face.

> ## PRACTICE TIP
>
> On chest auscultation sometimes bowel sounds may be heard in the chest, which is a strong indication of a ruptured diaphragm.

Impairment of respiration

The following injury can impair respiration:

- pulmonary contusion (intra-parenchymal haemorrhage)
- aspiration.

Pulmonary contusion

Pulmonary contusions are contusions (or bruising) of the lung parenchyma, and are literally blood pneumonia. They often occur in blunt trauma and are generally associated with fractured ribs and bruising of the overlying chest wall, but they can occur without any obvious chest wall trauma (see Fig 35.9). Lung tissue is damaged and over the next 24 hours bleeding drains into the alveoli, effectively occluding them. This results in decreased gas exchange, increased pulmonary vascular resistance and a reduction in lung compliance. The blood products in the lungs cause an inflammatory response producing mucus and oedematous fluid, exacerbating the decrease in respiratory function and potentially causing acute respiratory distress syndrome (ARDS). The inflamed pleural surfaces may eventually cause pain with ventilation. Haemoptysis is not common with the early stages of pulmonary contusions and chest trauma patients with this sign are more likely to have torn a blood vessel in the lungs or upper bronchial tree. If this blood accumulates in the alveoli, it will directly impair gas exchange but could also trigger an inflammatory response that will lead to mucosal oedema and bronchospasm.

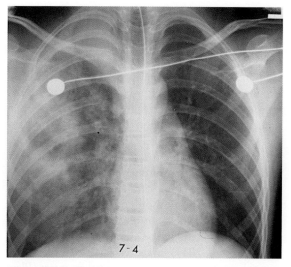

Figure 35.9
Pulmonary contusion.
Bruising of the lung tissue (opacity in upper right lung) impairs gas exchange in the area. The development of the contusion can be insidious with no obvious chest wall trauma or abnormal breath sounds for several hours.
Source: Townsend et al. (2012).

Aspiration

In the setting of major injury mechanism aspiration may also be present, where loss of consciousness has occurred. Differentiation from contusion is difficult, but both may result in the presence of crackles on chest auscultation. Long-term sequelae similar to contusion may occur due to associated inflammatory processes and hypoxia. An increased alveolar permeability leads to diffuse alveolar infiltration with the development of an interstitial pulmonary oedema. As a consequence, the lung compliance decreases and a mismatch of ventilation and perfusion occurs (Janda et al., 2006). In the out-of-hospital setting either contusion or aspiration are serious complications of chest injury which are difficult to treat.

Impairment of perfusion

The following injuries can impair perfusion:

- tension pneumothorax
- myocardial contusion
- pericardial tamponade
- rupture of major vessels.

Tension pneumothorax

The development of a tension pneumothorax that may restrict blood flow back to the heart should be the first consideration in any patient who presents with inadequate perfusion in the setting of chest trauma. Tension pneumothorax is a life-threatening condition; however, it is reversible in the out-of-hospital setting.

Myocardial contusion

Myocardial contusion following blunt chest trauma occurs as a result of either direct pressure on the myocardium or indirect effects secondary to increased intrathoracic pressures with shearing stresses experienced in high-velocity impacts such as motor vehicle crashes and falls. The dense myocardial tissue absorbs more kinetic energy than pulmonary tissue and is therefore likely to sustain more damage as a result of the same force. Myocardial contusion leads to myocardial inflammation, which may reduce contractility and thus cardiac output. The right ventricle is most commonly injured because of its position behind the sternum; however, myocardial injury often occurs in the absence of external signs (Fallouh et al., 2017). Seventy-six per cent of cardiac contusions are associated with sternal fractures (Platz et al., 2017).

Cardiac output can fall even without direct left ventricular injury because of reduced left atrial preload. The resultant drop in cardiac output after severe myocardial contusion may be up to 40% (Kaye & O'Sullivan, 2002). An ECG may show cardiac injury patterns similar to those seen in ischaemia. However, as ECGs largely reflect atrial and left ventricular activity, they are not sensitive in the diagnosis of right ventricular myocardial contusion. Also, similar ECG changes may occur as a reflection of a number of metabolic abnormalities associated with significant trauma (Roxburgh, 1996). Severe myocardial contusion can result in cardiogenic shock, and very rarely a direct blow over the heart can result in a lethal arrhythmia (*commotio cordis*).

Pericardial tamponade

Pericardial tamponade is a collection of blood or exudate in the pericardial space surrounding the heart. Pericardial tamponade is generally a result of non-traumatic infections and malignancies, but blood filling the pericardial space as a result of either myocardial contusion or traumatic penetration of the heart or pericardium may cause an acute pericardial tamponade. The fibrous pericardium is a relatively inflexible sac and a sudden increase in volume in the pericardial space will increase pressure on the heart, subsequently inhibiting the filling capacity of the ventricles. Due to the poor compliance of the pericardium, as little as 50 mL of blood can lead to tamponade. Beck's triad may be a manifestation of cardiac tamponade, with hypotension, increased jugular venous distension and muffled heart sounds. Though considered standard symptoms, all three are only present concurrently 15% of the time and individually are too vague to be accurately predictive (Platz et al., 2017).

Differentiation from tension pneumothorax in the out-of-hospital setting is difficult without point-of-care ultrasound (POCUS). The increased use of ultrasound in the emergency room has helped to alleviate some of the ambiguity in diagnosis, with a sensitivity of 96% and a specificity of 98% in detection (Platz et al., 2017). Increased use of POCUS in paramedic-based ambulance systems is continuing to rise. Paramedic interpretation in most studies was confirmed by ultrasound experts (Meadley et al., 2017).

Definitive management of tamponade requires evacuation of the blood or fluid from the pericardial space via a needle (pericardiocentesis) or a direct surgical incision (pericardiotomy), neither of which are routine out-of-hospital interventions. The use of IV fluid to increase preload may be implemented in the short term out of hospital prior to surgical intervention.

Rupture of major vessels

Aortic tears from blunt chest injury usually occur from forces such as those seen in rapid deceleration where acute shearing forces cause a rupture in the aortic wall. The proximal descending aorta, around the ligamentum arteriosum, is the most common site of injury, as this is the transition point at which the relatively mobile aortic arch becomes the fixed descending aorta. If there is a complete transection of the aorta, catastrophic haemorrhage is caused and the patient rapidly exsanguinates. If, however, the tear is partial thickness, the blood may be contained and further bleeding is often controlled by localised tamponade. The patient may show some signs of shock, complain of pain in the chest and back and have a widened mediastinum on imaging. These patients are often well perfused and do not appear to have serious injury. However, if left untreated, the in-hospital mortality rate approaches 70% (Arthurs et al., 2017). Out-of-hospital diagnosis of traumatic aortic dissection is near-impossible, and treatment consists of support of breathing, oxygenation, treatment of shock and rapid transportation for surgical management. Pulmonary vessel or vena caval tears may result in similar presentation.

Mechanism of injury

Trauma to the chest is generally described as either blunt or penetrating, although both can occur concurrently. Blunt trauma can result in compression injuries (from direct transmission of force to the chest wall) or distraction injuries (caused by shearing forces from the rapid acceleration/deceleration of heavy organs suspended by fixed vessels and

SITUATIONAL AWARENESS

Once the ambulance crew's safety has been assured, patients with penetrating chest trauma should be transported to a definitive trauma centre as rapidly as possible. Stabilisation should be undertaken during transit, as surgery is often the only way to stop bleeding.

Penetrating trauma

Penetrating trauma to the chest can occur with any sharp object or ballistic missile and results in direct trauma to structures in the track of the wound. Penetrating trauma is uncommon in Australia and New Zealand, comprising less than 10% of all trauma admissions (Civil, 2015). There has been a dramatic increase in the use of knives in murder and a more gradual increase in relation to attempted murder, while their use has remained relatively constant for the other three offence types (sexual assault, kidnapping, robbery) (Bartels, 2011). Any penetrating injury to the central chest must be assumed to have damaged the heart and all major vessels until proven otherwise. The assumed trajectory may give an indication of the likely damage, but is difficult to assess. Penetrating wounds to the heart most commonly injure the right ventricle, followed by the right atria, as these two chambers are anterior when the heart is lying in its normal

ligaments). Penetrating trauma results from a sharp object/projectile traversing the chest wall and causing direct injury to the thoracic wall viscera or vessels. While well accepted, the division of injuries into the categories of blunt and penetrating can oversimplify the types of injuries and both can be present depending on what event the patient has suffered.

position. A lateral blow from the left will penetrate the left ventricle first, but such injuries are rare. If a patient still has a penetrating object within the heart, the external part of the object may be observed moving synchronously with the heart rhythm. The object should be left in situ until the patient is in the operating theatre. Penetrating trauma can also cause injury to the lungs and result in pneumothorax, tension pneumothorax or haemothorax.

Ballistic trauma

Firearm deaths in Australia and New Zealand are relatively uncommon, as noted in the preceding section. In Australia 79% (166 cases) of deaths resulted from intentional self-harm (suicide) and 17% (36 cases) resulted from assault (homicide) (AIHW, 2017). These figures differ markedly from other parts of the world such as the United States and South Africa where penetrating trauma is more prevalent. Ballistic chest trauma causes local damage along the inter-thoracic trajectory of the missile. The pressure wave from high-velocity missiles will temporarily expand tissue around the track of the missile, causing a much larger secondary cavitation injury. High-velocity missiles are often associated with small entry wounds and massive exit wounds as the bullet tumbles and deforms while transferring kinetic energy to thoracic structures. Gunshot wounds to the lung are often less severe than those to muscles (including myocardium), as the lung parenchyma is not as dense and absorbs less kinetic energy from the missile. At close range shotgun pellets are some of the most devastating missiles because all of the kinetic energy is transferred to the victim, with none of the pellets leaving the body.

 CASE STUDY 1

Case 93518, 1130 hrs.

Dispatch details: A 17-year-old male has fallen from his mountain bike while trying to ride at low speed along a log lying on the ground. He is conscious but short of breath.

Initial presentation: The paramedics find the patient in obvious pain holding the left side of his chest. He speaks in single words and short phrases. He and his friend state that his wheels slipped and he landed on the log on his left side when he fell from his bike. He did not strike his head or lose consciousness, but he became increasingly short of breath over the next few minutes.

ASSESS

Patient history

Determining the mechanism of injury contextualises decision-making and planning. The low speed of impact and lack of head strike in this case suggest only minor injuries, so any significant alterations of vital signs should not be ignored. Early identification of any history related to the main presenting symptom (dyspnoea) can also assist in reaching an accurate diagnosis.

Airway

The patient is conscious and there is no obvious airway compromise. There is no blood in the sputum.

Breathing

Injuries to the chest wall can impede ventilation from pain alone but can also affect respiration. Pneumothorax can also impede respiration. Other factors that must be considered in poor ventilatory effort or respiration outcome in chest injuries include the various types of pneumothorax, tracheal or bronchial rupture, pulmonary contusions and localised areas of atelectasis. Any trauma to the lung parenchyma can result in air or blood escaping and causing increased intrathoracic pressures or reduced space for the lungs, ultimately affecting ventilation and respiration.

Cardiovascular

Significant chest injuries can directly injure the heart or vessels within the thorax. The patient's vital signs will indicate early signs of deterioration. Be aware: the cardiovascular system will naturally respond to pain and the patient's respiratory compromise, potentially resulting in elevated values. A reduction in blood pressure, however, must be considered seriously, as increasing intra-thoracic pressure can easily overcome the low pressures associated with the venous system and the right side of the heart.

Physical examination

Skin and chest wall contusions at the site of impact are a good indication of potential further injury. Compression of the chest wall at a distance from the tender area may be used to clinically identify a fractured rib. If the patient complains of pain at the impact point when the chest wall is compressed at a point distant from the impact point, the pain is probably being created by movement of an unstable fracture. Crepitus at the site of pain is likely to be definitive of a fracture but of little actual value to management and may cause the patient significant discomfort. Observing the chest wall for normal movement is likely to be a more sensitive test for a severe injury.

Subcutaneous emphysema is another sign to actively seek when examining the skin. This is an indicator that the pleura, bronchi or trachea have been breached and the patient must be closely monitored to ensure that they do not progress to a tension pneumothorax.

Initial assessment summary

Problem	The patient fell off his mountain bike and is now complaining of pain
Conscious state	Alert and oriented; GCS = 15
Position	Sitting upright, holding left side ribs with his right hand
Heart rate	96 bpm
Blood pressure	120/85 mmHg
Skin appearance	Normal; developing contusion at the site of impact
Speech pattern	Speaking in quick phrases
Respiratory rate	28 bpm

HISTORY

Ask!
- What was the speed of the impact?
- Do you have any history of dyspnoea? Asthma?

RESPIRATORY STATUS

Look for!
- Increased respiratory effort
- Uneven chest wall movement
- Skin signs of hypoxia
- Subcutaneous emphysema

PERFUSION STATUS

Look for!
- Hypotension
- Tachycardia
- Poor skin perfusion

SKIN STATUS

Look for!
- Contusions (external)
- Subcutaneous emphysema
- Protruding structures (ribs)
- Uneven chest wall symmetry
- Pallor/sweating

Respiratory rhythm	Even cycles
Respiratory effort	Shallow
Chest auscultation	Poor sounds due to shallow ventilations but air entry can be heard bilaterally
Pulse oximetry	95% on room air
Temperature	36.9°C
Motor/sensory function	Normal
History	No other significant history

D: The source of the injury is not a threat.

A: The patient's airway is not compromised.

B: Respiratory function is currently compensating. The respiratory rate is elevated as the patient has altered his mechanical ventilation to manage his pain. Despite his elevated respiratory rate his oxygen saturations are slightly lower than would be expected, indicating there may be ventilation/perfusion (V/Q) alterations developing.

C: Heart rate and blood pressure are currently within normal limits, but the heart rate is higher than it should be at rest. It is difficult to determine if this is in response to pain or a challenge to perfusion. The normal blood pressure and skin suggest pain is the more likely cause.

This patient has a raised respiratory rate, rapid shallow ventilation and decreased oxygen saturation. The origin of his pain is likely to be chest wall contusions and probable fractured rib/ribs, and this pain is contributing to his inability to ventilate effectively. The most likely diagnosis for this patient is fractured ribs with underlying chest wall contusion.

 CONFIRM

The essential part of the clinical reasoning process is to seek to confirm your initial hypothesis by finding clinical signs that should occur with your provisional diagnosis. You should also seek to challenge your diagnosis by exploring findings that do not fit your hypothesis: don't just ignore them because they don't fit.

What else could it be?

Pneumothorax

The patient's impact with the log could have fractured a rib, the sharp end of which could have lacerated his pleura or lung. Alternatively, the sudden compression of his chest wall could have caused a spike in intrathoracic pressure that has torn his lung tissue and pushed air into the pleural cavity (barotrauma). The clinical signs of a pneumothorax (hyperresonance and decreased ipsilateral breath sounds) may be difficult to pick up in this setting and the presence of a simple pneumothorax will not change immediate management. The presence of a pneumothorax would increase the likelihood of a tension pneumothorax developing, but the patient's adequate perfusion at this point suggest this is not occurring. Small, simple pneumothoraces are often left untreated in hospital and unless this fully conscious and well-perfused patient shows signs of developing a tension pneumothorax (increasing respiratory distress, decreasing blood pressure) it is acceptable to closely monitor him in case of deterioration (associated with a tension pneumothorax, for instance), even if a simple pneumothorax is suspected.

Haemothorax

Bleeding into the pleural cavity can be associated with fractured ribs, but the signs can be difficult to detect in the field (dulled resonance and altered ipsilateral breath sounds). In this setting it is unlikely the bleed is substantial given the mechanism of injury. The oxygen saturations and perfusion suggest he does not appear to be suffering from a clinically significant haemothorax.

PRACTICE TIP

Remember, the patient's pain may be only one factor affecting his ventilation and respiration effectiveness. Pain is something that can be addressed in the field, as is a tension pneumothorax, but most of the other causes of altered ventilation and respiration cannot be treated by paramedics.

DIFFERENTIAL DIAGNOSIS

Rib fracture

Or

- Pneumothorax (simple or tension)
- Haemothorax
- Pulmonary contusion

Pulmonary contusion

Pulmonary contusion is quite likely to be associated with the blow and some of the decreased gas exchange may be attributable to local pulmonary contusion. Clinical signs of pulmonary contusion such as localised inspiratory/expiratory crackles will continue to develop over the next 24 hours.

In reality, it is possible that all these diagnoses are present in this patient and that he may deteriorate as the pulmonary contusion becomes established, the haemothorax accumulates or the pneumothorax extends.

 ## TREAT

Emergency management

Position

This patient has a peripheral oxygen saturation of 95%, which is slightly low and could probably be rectified by oxygen supplementation via a rebreather mask. However, as this is primarily due to a ventilation problem, the focus should be on improving the patient's tidal volume. Generally, patients complaining of any sort of dyspnoea will position themselves in such a way that their ventilation is maximised. This should be supported where possible: this patient is sitting upright splinting his ribs with his upper arm and he should be left that way until adequate pain relief is administered (vital).

Oxygen

Increasing the fraction of inspired oxygen via a rebreather mask may help to rectify the saturation level but in reality this is not critical at this point and oxygen should not take priority over pain relief or positioning.

Analgesia

Inhaled analgesics such as methoxyflurane have the advantage of being rapid and simple to administer, but their delivery via the lungs requires adequate ventilation and with this patient that may mean that the drug fails to reach therapeutic levels. Establishing IV access and administering opioids will provide effective, controlled pain relief. Routine monitoring of all haemodynamic parameters is essential during the administration of opiates such as morphine. Other agents such as ketamine may also be introduced in conjunction with opiates to provide effective analgesia. Opiate infusions are also effective once initial analgesia is obtained.

Wound dressing

Splinting of fractured ribs using strapping is not recommended, as it reduces respiratory movement and this patient's most critical requirement is increased respiratory volume. Patients may voluntarily splint their chest wall using their hand, and if this increases their respiratory volume it should be encouraged. Only open wounds that need haemorrhage or infection control should be dressed in this setting.

 ## EVALUATE

Evaluating the effect of any clinical management intervention can provide clues to the accuracy of the initial diagnosis. Some conditions respond rapidly to treatment so patients should be expected to improve if the diagnosis and treatment were appropriate. A failure to improve in this situation should trigger the clinician to reconsider the diagnosis.

If this patient has fractured ribs and suffered only minor pulmonary contusion or a simple pneumothorax it would be expected that, once provided with adequate pain relief, he should become more comfortable and his vital signs should return approximately to normal within 10–15 minutes. Administering

> ## PRACTICE TIP
>
> Sometimes pain and distress can result in a reduction in vital signs such as blood pressure. Appropriate analgesia and splinting must be the first step in managing traumatic injuries before considering other causes of hypotension.

high-flow oxygen will make his oxygen saturation reading less sensitive to deterioration as the increased partial pressure of oxygen will compensate for reduced effective ventilation for some time. Any deterioration in his perfusion status (pulse, blood pressure, skin, consciousness) should be considered as indicating a developing tension pneumothorax and treated accordingly.

Is the patient:
- Improving after analgesia and positioning?
  › Continue with highest level of available care
- Deteriorating despite analgesia and positioning?
  › Continue with highest level of available care
  › Consider other causes for poor ventilation
- Now unconscious?
  › Start primary survey
  › Check for tension pneumothorax
- Now pulseless?
  › Check monitor
- Now VT/VF/PEA?
  › Commence CPR

Ongoing management

In hospital this patient will undergo routine imaging to exclude a pneumothorax. This may also identify a haemothorax and provide evidence of any consolidation associated with pulmonary contusion. Fractured ribs are often difficult to identify on x-ray, so failure to see them does not exclude the diagnosis. Specific views are often required—taken from different angles—in order to see fractures in curved bones but they rarely change the management plan and are not usually ordered.

Investigations

Patients presenting to the ED with chest injuries will undergo various investigations to determine the extent of their injuries. Some of these investigations will include x-ray, CT and blood gases.

Hospital admission

Depending on the injury the patient may or may not be admitted to hospital or undergo surgical procedures. If a significant haemothorax or pneumothorax is present, a chest tube thoracostomy may be done to drain the air and/or blood. If both are present, two tubes may be inserted in different positions to aid the removal or the air and blood (see Fig 35.10). In conscious patients the insertion site is injected first with a local anaesthetic before a small incision is made and the tube guided into the pleural space. The catheter can be placed in the second intercostal space to remove air while a posterior insertion between the eighth and ninth ribs can be used to drain fluid and blood. In most cases the tube is inserted anterior to the mid-axillary line in the fourth or fifth intercostal space as there is less superficial muscle. Once inserted the tubes are sutured to the chest wall and the wound is covered with a dressing. After the tubes are in place, they are connected to an underwater seal drainage system that stops air or fluid moving back into the space. If the tube is correctly placed, the drainage system will rise and fall slightly with each ventilation. This 'swing' reflects the changes in pressure that occur with ventilation. An appropriate analgesia regimen must be established that allows continued deep ventilation and coughing, as this will markedly decrease a patient's chances of developing a chest infection. This is particularly critical for elderly patients and those with lung conditions (smokers).

Long-term role

The ability of young, fit individuals to compensate for traumatic injuries can mask the severity of their injuries in the first few hours. While it is true that chest x-rays are rarely taken to confirm fractured ribs and that most patients will not require the insertion of chest tubes for a simple pneumothorax, this patient is yet to reveal the full extent of his injuries. Transport to hospital for what is effectively observation will reduce the likelihood of complications.

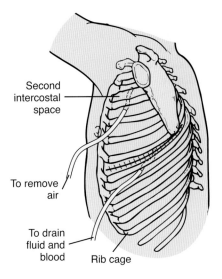
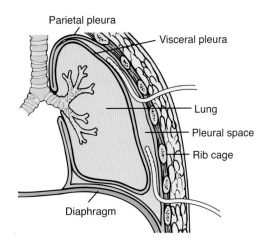

Figure 35.10
Placement of chest tubes.
Source: Brown & Edwards (2012).

Chest trauma across the lifespan

Fractured ribs are more common in elderly people with osteoporosis and less common in children, who have relatively compliant rib cages. A child with a rib fracture has a high probability of concomitant and significant intrathoracic organ damage, due to the large forces necessary to cause a fracture. Children can also present with internal injuries without rib fractures due to the higher rib cage compliance. Elderly patients with preexisting chest pathology are more likely to suffer from complications of chest trauma and are also more likely to develop chest infections from simple fractured ribs. Elderly patients generally sustain blunt chest trauma as a result of falls. When chest trauma complicates other injuries, it is associated with a worse patient outcome, generally due to the associated difficulties with ventilation and oxygenation.

 CASE STUDY 2

Case 10210, 1539 hrs.

Dispatch details: A 40-year-old male has fallen 4 m from a haystack. He lost his footing while standing on top of the haystack and landed on the left side of his chest on some farming machinery.

Initial presentation: The patient is conscious, with abnormal breathing.

 ASSESS

1550 hrs Chief complaint: The patient is complaining of chest pain following the fall.

1551 hrs Vital signs survey: Perfusion status: HR 135 bpm, thready carotid and femoral pulse (unable to palpate radial or brachial pulse), sinus tachycardia, BP 70/55 mmHg, skin pale and sweaty.

Respiratory status: RR 35 bpm, poor tidal volume, even breath cycles. Unable to obtain oxygen saturations due to poor peripheral perfusion. The patient is anxious.

Conscious state: GCS = 15; however, the patient is unable to speak.

Other signs and symptoms: The patient has extensive bruising to his left chest wall and distended neck veins. Examination of his chest reveals a flail segment on the left side with subcutaneous emphysema palpable under the skin. Percussion of his chest reveals left-sided hyperresonance, and tracheal deviation towards his right side is identified through suprasternal palpation.

1552 hrs Pertinent hx: The patient is normally well and takes no medications.

'Why did you fall? Were you dizzy or short of breath or did you have any chest pain prior to falling?'

The patient is not able to answer but a bystander explains that he lost his footing and fell.

'Why can't you speak? Is it because of your breathing?'

The patient nods.

'Which is worse, your breathing or your pain?'

The patient gives a 'thumbs up' on the word 'breathing'.

② CONFIRM

In many cases paramedics are presented with a collection of signs and symptoms that do not appear to describe a particular condition. A critical step in determining a treatment plan in this situation is to consider what other conditions could explain the patient's presentation.

What else could it be?
Pneumothorax
This patient does have a pneumothorax, but it appears to have extended to the point where the pressure within his chest is now putting tension on other structures within the thorax. That is, it is now presenting as a tension pneumothorax.

Haemothorax
While this is a possibility there is no dullness upon percussion over the dependent area of the left chest wall.

Pulmonary contusion
Massive pulmonary contusion is quite likely to be present with this degree of chest trauma, but it is difficult to diagnose and assess in the field. The clinical impact of the contusion will progress over the subsequent hours.

Myocardial contusion
Myocardial contusion could well have occurred following this injury and would result in markedly decreased cardiac output, which is consistent with the clinical signs of dilated neck veins and poor perfusion. An ECG monitor may show ST-segment changes and ectopic beats indicative of myocardial contusion. However, the paramedics should ascertain whether he has underlying ischaemic heart disease, as stress-related ischaemic ECG changes may be also present.

Pericardial tamponade
Pericardial tamponade occurring due to either traumatic injury from the fractured rib or effusion associated with myocardial contusion would prevent ventricular

---

DIFFERENTIAL DIAGNOSIS

Tension pneumothorax
Or
- Pneumothorax
- Haemothorax
- Pulmonary contusion
- Myocardial contusion
- Pericardial tamponade

filling, leading to dilated neck veins and poor perfusion. Although tamponade is associated with muffled heart sounds, it is unlikely that these can be confidently assessed in this setting.

③ TREAT

This patient should be treated with decompression of the affected side of the chest, in the second intercostal space in the midclavicular line. A simple needle (14- or 16-gauge IV cannula) can be used, as a valve is not required with a small-gauge cannula—the cannula bore is very much smaller than the cross-sectional area of the trachea and air will preferentially flow to the unaffected lung (see Fig 35.11). The intention is not to reinflate the lung but merely to remove the pressure and allow venous return to the heart. If a commercially produced set with a needle and valve is available, this may be used.

Even if decompression produces a dramatic improvement in haemodynamic status, the patient will still need to have two large-bore IV lines inserted and fluid resuscitation titrated to a palpable peripheral pulse. An improvement in conscious state will also provide evidence of improving perfusion. Two large-bore

> **PRACTICE TIP**
>
> The patient's condition should be reassessed continually, as needle thoracostomies are prone to blockage and being dislodged, potentially causing a relieved tension pneumothorax to re-tension.

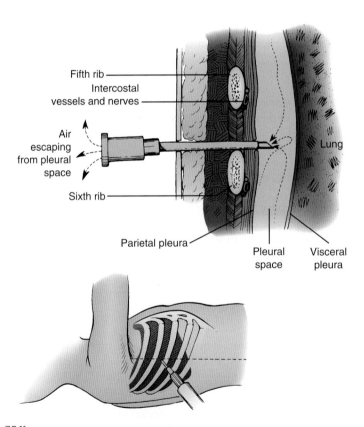

Figure 35.11
Needle decompression.
A 50-mm or longer 14- or 16-gauge hollow needle or catheter is inserted into the affected pleural space. The needle is usually placed in the second intercostal space in the midclavicular line, but some trauma teams position the needle in the mid-axillary line as shown. After insertion of the needle, an audible rush of air may be noted as pressure escapes from the pleural space, but is not always obvious. The catheter is secured in place with Opsite tape. Care is taken to prevent re-entry of air into the pleural space. The patient's respiratory status is monitored carefully.
Source: Auerbach (2012).

IV lines should be routinely established in trauma cases to ensure that a functioning line is always available should rapid fluid/blood infusion be required.

1554 hrs: One of the paramedics immediately locates the second intercostal space in the midclavicular line on the left side of the patient's chest and marks the location. After cleansing the site, she uses a large-bore, long cannula and inserts it at 90° to the patient's chest wall, angling towards the vertebral column. She notices a small amount of blood bubbling at the insertion site and hears air escaping from the cannula once the needle is removed. She then administers 8 L of oxygen via a Hudson mask.

1556 hrs: The patient's dyspnoea significantly reduces, along with his anxiety.

Perfusion status: HR 104 bpm; sinus tachycardia; BP 95/55 mmHg; skin warm, pink and dry.

Respiratory status: RR 24 bpm, good air entry on R side, dull over L lung field. Patient is able to speak in phrases, breathing in even cycles. Oxygen saturations 88%.

Conscious state: GCS = 15.

The paramedic notices the patient is still splinting his left ribs with his right hand and has a slightly reduced tidal volume. The patient rates his pain as 8/10.

1558 hrs: The paramedic inserts an IV line into the patient's forearm and administers IV analgesia.

1602 hrs: The patient offers to walk to the ambulance but the paramedics move him in a wheelchair.

4️⃣ EVALUATE

Evaluating the effect of any clinical management intervention can provide clues to the accuracy of the initial diagnosis. Some conditions respond rapidly to treatment so patients should be expected to improve if the diagnosis and treatment were appropriate. A failure to improve in this situation should trigger the clinician to reconsider the diagnosis.

The primary concern is that the damaged lung can re-tension, but in this case the patient's blood pressure and pulse are not indicative of intrapleural pressure rising again. However, providing sufficient pain relief to allow normal chest excursion is essential.

1604 hrs: Perfusion status: HR 98 bpm; sinus rhythm; BP 105/60 mmHg; skin warm, dry and pink.

Respiratory status: RR 24 bpm, reduced tidal volume due to pain.

Conscious state: GCS = 15.

Pain: 7/10.

The paramedics administer another IV dose of analgesia and continue incremental doses until the patient's pain has reduced, allowing for a more productive ventilation cycle.

At hospital: Perfusion status: HR 84 bpm; sinus rhythm; BP 115/65 mmHg; skin warm, dry and pink.

Respiratory status: RR 18 bpm, speaking in full sentences, denies shortness of breath.

Conscious state: GCS = 15.

Pain: 2/10; the patient is still splinting his chest with his hand.

> **PRACTICE TIP**
>
> The patient will need careful cardiac monitoring because of the risk of myocardial contusion and subsequent arrhythmias.

CASE STUDY 3

Case 14891, 1715 hrs.

Dispatch details: A middle-aged man has been stabbed multiple times in the chest and is now in an altered conscious state.

Initial presentation: When the paramedics arrive the police are already on the scene. The paramedics are directed to a back bedroom of a suburban house. The patient is sitting on the floor leaning against the wall and there is a large amount of blood on the floor.

Look for!
- Patient's posterior trunk for further stab wounds
- Patency of thoracostomy needle (may require flushing with normal saline if patency is lost)
- Improvement in respiratory and cardiovascular status post needle insertion

DIFFERENTIAL DIAGNOSIS

Exsanguination
Or
- Tension pneumothorax
- Haemothorax
- Hypoxia

1 ASSESS

1725 hrs Primary survey: The patient's airway is clear. He is taking rapid, shallow breaths and is extremely pale and sweaty. He has no palpable peripheral pulse but has a central pulse.

1726 hrs Vital signs survey: Perfusion status: HR 145 bpm, BP 50/P (palpation), skin pale and sweaty.

Respiratory status: RR 36 bpm, bilateral air entry, SPO$_2$ unable to sense, extremely anxious.

Conscious state: GCS = 12; eye opening, saying only 'help me' and localising to stimuli; combative.

Other signs and symptoms: The patient has obvious severe respiratory distress and there are at least four stab wounds to the anterior chest wall.

2 CONFIRM

In many cases paramedics are presented with a collection of signs and symptoms that do not appear to describe a particular condition. A critical step in determining a treatment plan in this situation is to consider what other conditions could explain the patient's presentation.

What else could it be?
- Tension pneumothorax
- Haemothorax
- Other causes of unconsciousness

Define

This patient's problem (aside from the stab wounds) is extremely poor perfusion. He is pre-arrest and action needs to be taken quickly. It is likely that his altered level of consciousness is the result of his perfusion problems, rather than the other way around, so this must be the paramedics' focus.

Explore

The blood around the patient and the stab wounds are a good indication that his perfusion problems may be due to hypovolaemia. However, a clinical sign of dilated neck veins in the presence of profound shock is not consistent with hypovolaemia. Despite the fact that the patient has four stabs wounds to his chest and pleural space (which could potentially enable any increasing intrapleural pressure to vent), a tension pneumothorax is a potential cause. The paramedics must also consider the mediastinum in their exploration of the problem. Has the knife pierced the patient's pericardium, myocardium or any vessels within his chest?

1729 hrs Bilateral chest decompression: There is no notable release of pressure. His neck veins remain distended and his observations do not change. There is no escape of blood.

Tension pneumothorax is eliminated. What is left? The sound of bilateral air entry and no blood escaping following decompression indicate that ventilation may be occurring throughout most of the lung fields, meaning that a massive haemothorax is unlikely to be causing this patient's problems. The paramedics must now turn their attention to the mediastinum. If any of the great vessels had been severely compromised by the stabbing, the patient would most likely have exsanguinated by now. The crew request back up from an intensive care unit.

Sometimes the out-of-hospital environment does not allow paramedics to 'pin' a more specific label on a patient and they just have to start fixing the problems they find. Don't forget to evaluate the effect of these treatments.

3 TREAT

1733 hrs: The crew attempt to lie the patient down, but he becomes increasingly more combative and tries to sit up. This causes his wounds to haemorrhage and his breathing to become more erratic.

1734 hrs: The paramedics gain IV access with a large-bore cannula in each arm. They attempt to put an oxygen mask on the patient's face but he quickly removes it. They do not agitate the patient by attempting to readminister it.

1736 hrs: Perfusion status: HR 148 bpm, sinus tachycardia with premature ventricular contractions, BP 50/P, skin pale and sweaty.

Respiratory status: RR 36 bpm, bilateral air entry.

Conscious state: GCS = 12; eye opening, saying only 'help me' and localising to stimuli; combative.

4 EVALUATE

Evaluating the effect of any clinical management intervention can provide clues to the accuracy of the initial diagnosis. Some conditions respond rapidly to treatment so patients should be expected to improve if the diagnosis and treatment were appropriate. A failure to improve in this situation should trigger the clinician to reconsider the diagnosis.

With no response to the chest decompression, this patient is almost certainly bleeding internally from a large vessel and any response to out-of-hospital treatment is unlikely to be significant. Cardiac tamponade must also be considered.

The patient is in an altered conscious state and treatment so far has not improved his vital signs. He requires urgent surgical intervention and needs to be transported to receive the highest level of trauma care.

With the help of the police the paramedics lift the patient onto the stretcher, disrupting the patient as little as possible. This patient is in an extremely fragile state: his vital signs are already strained and any exertion could result in cardiac arrest.

Future research

Current research into traumatic thoracic injury is largely driven by military organisations, primarily due to increased Western military activity. Less-invasive techniques and minimal incision approaches are increasingly being developed in the treatment of thoracic trauma. Use of POCUS in the out-of-hospital setting is now becoming more common in many EMS systems to better evaluate the presence of pneumothoraces. Use of strong analgesic agents such as ketamine and infusion-based analgesia is increasing. Implementation of these strategies results in better out-of-hospital management of trauma. Several studies have demonstrated that adequate pain control has a benefit on ventilation, as well as risk of pulmonary complications (Bouzat et al., 2017). Interventional radiological techniques can safely treat many patients with intrathoracic vascular injuries and have been successfully used to retrieve intracardiac missiles (Popper & Gifford, 2010), and traumatic aortic injuries have been treated with stenting. Currently, however, traditional approaches and techniques are the mainstay of the treatment of critically injured, haemodynamically unstable patients, with newer approaches currently used only for stable patients. The increased use of POCUS in the field is currently occurring to improve out-of-hospital diagnostics and treatment. Chest ultrasonography has a great potential for increasing the sensitivity of the initial diagnostic assessment concerning pneumothorax and haemothorax in trauma patients (Staub et al., 2018). Out-of-hospital sonography was identified as an adjunct assessment which may have improved outcomes in 17 of 113 potentially preventable deaths in a Victorian out-of-hospital trauma study (Beck et al., 2019).

Summary

Chest injuries can range from minor soft tissue injury to life-threatening catastrophic vessel and organ injury. The focus of out-of-hospital assessment and treatment should focus on analgesia, implementation of available procedures such as thoracostomy, awareness of potential occult injury and transport to the highest level of trauma care available for continuing management. Strong focus on analgesic management is a major component of the paramedic role in improving a patient's ventilation and respiration. Diligent out-of-hospital management and further introduction of novel interventions in chest injury can contribute to improved outcomes in this patient group.

References

Arthurs, Z. M., Starnes, B. W., Sohn, V. Y., Singh, N., Martin, M. J., & Andersen, C. A. (2017). Thoracic trauma. Functional and survival outcomes in traumatic blunt thoracic aortic injuries: an analysis of the National Trauma Databank. *Journal of Vascular Surgery 2009, 49,* 988.

Auerbach, P. S. (2012). *Wilderness medicine* (6th ed.). Philadelphia: Mosby.

Australian Institute of Health and Welfare (AIHW). (2017). *Firearm injuries and deaths fact sheet. Cat. no. INJCAT 187.* Canberra: AIHW.

Bartels, L. (2011). *'Knife crime' in Australia: incidence, aetiology and responses. Technical and background paper series no. 45.* Canberra: Australian Institute of Criminology. https://aic.gov.au/publications/tbp/tbp045.

Beck, B., Smith, K., Mercier, E., Bernard, S., Jones, C., Meadley, B., St Clair, T., Jennings, P. A., Nehme, Z., Burke, M., Bassed, R., Fitzgerald, M., Judson, R., Teague, W., Mitra, B., Mathew, J., Buck, A., Varma, D., Gabbe, B., Bray, J., McLellan, S., Ford, J., Siedenburg, J., & Cameron, P. (2019). Potentially preventable trauma deaths: a retrospective review. *Injury, International Journal of the Care of the Injured, 50*(2019), 1009–1016.

Black, J. M., & Hawks, J. A. (2009). *Medical-surgical nursing* (8th ed.). St Louis: Saunders.

Bouzat, P., Raux, M., David, J. S., Tazarourte, K., Galinski, M., Desmettre, T., Garrigue, D., Ducros, L., Michelet, P., Expert's group; Freysz, M., Savary, D., Rayeh-Pelardy, F., Laplace, C., Duponq, R., Monnin Bares, V., D'Journo, X. B., Boddaert, G., Boutonnet, M., Pierre, S., Léone, M., Honnart, D., Biais, M., & Vardon, F. (2017). Chest trauma: first 48 hours management. *Anaesthesia Critical Care & Pain Medicine, 36*(2), 135–145. April.

Brown, D., & Edwards, H. (2012). *Lewis's Medical-surgical nursing: assessment and management of clinical problems* (2nd ed.). Sydney: Elsevier.

Centers for Disease Control and Prevention (CDC). (2010). *Injury prevention and control: data and statistics (WISQARS).* Retrieved from www.cdc.gov/injury/wisqars/index.html.

Civil, I. (2015). *Rich's Vascular Trauma, Third Edition Section 5 International Perspectives.*

de Lacey, G., Morley, S., & Berman, L. (2008). *The Chest X-Ray: a survival guide.* Edinburgh: Saunders.

Drake, R., Vogl, A., & Mitchell, A. (2009). *Gray's anatomy for students* (2nd ed.). Philadelphia: Elsevier.

Fallouh, H., Dattani-Patel, R., & Rathinam, S. (2017). Blunt thoracic trauma. *Cardiothoracic Surgery II, 35*(5), 262–268.

Givens, M., Ayotte, K., & Manifold, C. (2004). Needle Thoracostomy: implications of computed tomography chest wall thickness. *Academic Emergency Medicine: Official Journal of the Society for Academic Emergency Medicine, 11*(2), 211–213.

Greaves, I., Porter, K., Hodgetts, T., & Woollard, M. (2006). *Emergency care: a textbook for paramedics.* London: Elsevier.

Inocencio, M., Childs, J., Chilstrom, M. L., & Berona, K. (2017). Ultrasound findings in tension pneumothorax: a case report. *The Journal of Emergency Medicine, 52*(6), e217–e220. June.

Janda, M., Scheeren, T. W., & Nöldge-Schomburg, G. F. (2006). Management of pulmonary aspiration. *Best Practice and Research. Clinical Anaesthesiology, 20*(3), 409–427.

Jantz, M. A., & Pierson, D. J. (1994). Pneumothorax and barotrauma. *Clinics in Chest Medicine, 15,* 75–91.

Kaye, P., & O'Sullivan, I. (2002). Myocardial contusion: emergency investigations and diagnosis. *Emergency Medicine Journal, 19,* 8–10.

Meadley, B., Olaussen, A., Delorenzo, A., Roder, N., Martin, C., St Clair, T., Burns, A., Stam, E., & Williams, B. (2017). Educational standards for training paramedics in ultrasound: a scoping review. *BMC Emergency Medicine, 17,* 18. https://doi.org/10.1186/s12873-017-0131-8.

New South Wales Institute of Trauma and Injury Management (NSW ITIM). (2012). *The NSW trauma registry profile of serious to critical injuries: 2009.* Sydney: NSW Health.

Patton, K. T., & Thibodeau, G. A. (2012). *Anatomy and physiology* (7th ed.). St Louis: Mosby.

Platz, J. J., Fabricant, L., & Norotsky, M. (2017). Thoracic trauma: injuries, evaluation, and treatment. *The Surgical Clinics of North America, 97*(4), 783–799. 2017 Aug.

Popper, B. W., & Gifford, S. M. (2010). Wartime thoracic injury: perspectives in modern warfare. *Annals of Thoracic Surgery, 89,* 1032–1036.

Richter, T., & Rageller, M. (2011). Ventilation in chest trauma. *Journal of Emergencies, Trauma, and Shock, 4*(2).

Roxburgh, J. C. (1996). Myocardial contusion: a review. *Injury, 27,* 603–605.

Sanders, M. J. (2007). *Mosby's paramedic textbook (rev* 3rd ed.). St Louis: Mosby.

Sirmali, M., Turut, H., Topcu, S., Gülhan, E., Yazici, U., Kaya, S., & Taştepe, I. (2003). A comprehensive analysis of traumatic rib fractures: morbidity, mortality and management. *European Journal of Cardio-Thoracic Surgery, 24,* 133–138.

Staub, L. J., Biscaro, R. R. M., Kaszubowski, E., & Maurici, R. (2018). Chest ultrasonography for the emergency diagnosis of traumatic pneumothorax and haemothorax: a systematic review and meta-analysis. *Injury, 49*(3), 457–466. Mar.

Townsend, C. M., Beauchamp, R. D., Evers, B. M., & Mattox, K. L. (2012). *Sabiston textbook of surgery: the biological basis of modern surgical practice* (19th ed.). Philadelphia: Saunders.

Trinkle, J., Richardson, J., Franz, J., Grover, F. L.,, Arom, K. V., & Holmstrom, F. M. (1975). Management of flail chest without mechanical ventilation. *Annals of Thoracic Surgery, 19*(4), 355–363.

Wilson, S., & Giddens, J. (2013). *Health assessment for nursing practice* (5th ed.). St Louis: Mosby.

CHAPTER 36

Musculoskeletal Injuries

By Dianne Inglis and Jeff Kenneally

OVERVIEW

- Musculoskeletal injuries are common and regularly account for emergency presentations.
- Musculoskeletal injuries include soft-tissue and bony-tissue injuries.
- Soft-tissue injuries include bruising/haematoma, sprains, strains and dislocations. They may be in isolation or accompany other injuries.
- Bony injuries include fractures, from simple to complicated, and may include damage to the surrounding muscle, blood vessels, nerves or skin.
- Pain is usually associated with these injuries and can be severe: adequate analgesia is an important consideration in patient management.

- Basic first aid including appropriate bandaging, splinting and immobilisation is effective and can reduce complications significantly.
- Recovery from a musculoskeletal injury may take many months and require ongoing rehabilitation.
- Complications may be perfusion-related and include hypovolaemia and ischaemia; deformity and loss of function; and impairment of activities of daily living.
- Fatalities can occur as a result of musculoskeletal injuries; this may be due to the primary injury or to complications that develop as a result of the injuries.
- Definitive out-of-hospital diagnosis is difficult.

Introduction

Musculoskeletal injuries (MSIs) include damage to the muscular or skeletal systems and related tissue including muscle, bone, joints, tendons and ligaments. Associated tissues such as skin, blood vessels and nerves may also be damaged as a result of the traumatic event. The injuries may occur in isolation but more commonly also involve nearby structures to varying degrees (Orchard & Best, 2002).

Pathophysiology

The nature of MSI dictates there will be marked variation in pathophysiology with the differing tissues, traumatic mechanisms involved, varying ages and underlying health. Injuries may be minor and isolated or numerous, life-threatening or in conjunction with other severe injuries. The traumatic event may be the primary mechanism, accidental or intentional, or may follow a medical event such as stroke or arrhythmia. MSI may occur in sport, during high-risk activities, in the workplace, in the home and even during sedentary activities where repetitive or overuse injuries can occur.

The role of the musculoskeletal system is principally to provide for movement and support of the body structure. The key components are:

- bones that form the skeleton
- articulations or joints between the bones and the cartilage or ligaments that support them

- muscles that produce the movement
- tendons that attach the muscles to the bones.

MSIs affect one in four adults of European descent and are the most common cause of severe long-term pain and physical disability (Woolf et al., 2012). Australian workers compensation figures for 2012/2013 showed 45% of serious claims were for traumatic joint/ligament and muscle/tendon injury (Safe Work Australia, 2014) and the most common 'serious' workplace injury between 2004 and 2014 (Lane et al., 2016). Between 2004 and 2010 Australian lower limb sporting injuries rates increased by 26%, costing the community over $110 million (Finch et al., 2015). Paramedics and health workers suffer relatively high MSI rates, making this a major focus of workplace strategies to minimise (Gray & Collie, 2017; Paul & Hoy, 2015; Roberts et al., 2015). Though the majority of MSIs occur in the workplace or during sport, motor vehicle crashes and the home account for a significant proportion (ABS, 2006).

Musculoskeletal injuries

MSIs are common and account for a large number of emergency department (ED) and local medical centre presentations for assessment and treatment. Injuries can be divided into two broad groups:

- *soft-tissue injuries* include sprains, strains, muscular damage, joint injury, subluxation and dislocation

- *bony injuries* include simple or complicated fractures and traumatic amputation.

Soft-tissue injuries

Soft-tissue injuries include bruising and haematoma, strain, subluxation, dislocation and sprain and are most common among the 25–34-year age group (ABS, 2006).

Bruising and haematoma

Bruising, also called **contusion**, is minor superficial closed bleeding into soft tissue. It ranges from small and harmless to involving extensive muscle and other body tissue. Larger bleeding in deeper tissue is called **haematoma**. Finding bruising or haematoma can suggest more significant underlying injury, particularly on the head, chest or abdomen.

Blunt trauma is the most common cause, with likelihood increasing with trauma severity. Bruising can be classified as mild, moderate or severe depending on functional impairment (Maffulli et al., 2015). Where bruising or haematoma is more severe or unexpected, it may suggest an underlying medical disorder or be from medications including antiplatelet drugs and anticoagulants increasing bleeding likelihood.

Bruising patterns and characteristics can indicate abuse, particularly of children (Kemp et al., 2014; Pierce, 2017; Pierce et al., 2010) and the elderly (Berzlanovich et al., 2018), often underappreciated for what it can suggest. Alternatively, bruising in children and the elderly can easily occur from simple falls or bumps.

Pain and tenderness may be caused by these injuries along with some movement difficulty. Management of bruising and haematoma is similar to other soft-tissue injuries provided it is considered in the context of its origin and potential underlying injuries.

Strain

A **strain** is damage to muscles or tendons by overstressing them beyond their functional capacity. Damaged muscle cells release cellular content into surrounding tissue. Histamine and protein release causes vasodilation and increased osmotic pressure causing oedema, in turn impacting flow of blood and lymph. The oedema obstructs muscle contraction and places pressure on nerves, causing pain.

Strain injuries can be graded on severity ranging from mild to severe. Mild injuries have no great loss of limb function and may only be realised after the injury. Moderate injury has partial muscle tear of the muscle and some function loss. Severe injury has complete tear and will be recognised immediately, probably with considerable pain. Strains can be distinguished by muscular location as proximal, middle or distal and whether the injury is muscle alone or involves fascia and tendon (Chan et al., 2012; Pollock et al., 2014).

Strains are common sporting injuries (Dönmez et al., 2015; Tonino & Sinclair, 2011), particularly in the leg muscles. Strains may be from acute injury or of a more chronic nature caused by overuse and repetitive movements.

Overuse injuries

A commonly referred to strain injury is **repetitive strain injury (RSI)**. Variously referred to as overuse syndrome or repetitive motion syndrome, this is usually associated with a workplace or sometimes a recreational activity. Injury is not caused by an acute event but develops over time through tiresome repetition of the same motion or prolonged maintenance of poor posture. Damaged tendon and muscle can tear, contract and scar. Most commonly affected are the upper limbs, particularly from elbows to the hands, although shoulders, knees, ankles and even the spine can be affected. It can involve tendons, muscles and peripheral nerves. Examples of RSI include tendonitis, bursitis and carpal tunnel syndrome.

RSI can present with pain, inflammation, altered sensation such as numbness and tingling and alterations in function including weakness or reduced movement. Assessment is usually made on physical examination, presenting history and magnetic resonance imaging (MRI).

Once diagnosis is made, treatment can involve anti-inflammatory medication, rest of the affected part, occupational therapy or physiotherapy and steroids or muscle relaxants. Most treatments are varied and questionable in effect. Occasionally surgery may be indicated if everything else is ineffective. Ultimately the curative solution is to avoid the activity or modify it sufficiently to avoid the injurious mechanism.

Sprains

Sprains result from traumatic injury to the ligaments and muscles surrounding a joint. Sprains are graded based on severity, ranging from minimal injury with little sign, medium injury with some loss of function and swelling, to severe injury with complete tear, pain and swelling. In the latter, the joint is unstable and can even include associated bone fracture.

Symptoms of sprain are typically pain, swelling, loss of function and bruising around the joint.

> ## DEFINITIONS
>
> - *Bruising:* superficial bleeding under the skin.
> - *Haematoma:* deeper bleeding into muscle or tissue.

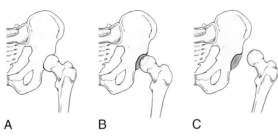

Figure 36.1
Soft-tissue injury of the hip. A Normal. **B** Subluxation (partial dislocation). **C** Dislocation.
Source: Brown & Edwards (2012).

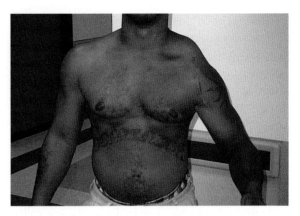

Figure 36.2
Dislocation of the left shoulder. The most obvious clinical manifestation of a dislocation is deformity. The complications of a dislocated joint include *avascular necrosis* (bone cell death as a result of inadequate blood supply) and damage to nerve tissue.
Source: Roberts (2009).

DEFINITIONS

- *Strain:* overstressed muscle or tendon.
- *Sprain:* ligament and muscle injury surrounding a joint.

Obvious deformity is suggestive of fracture, dislocation or combination of the two; absence does not exclude fracture. Severe pain and swelling at a joint with inability to bear weight requires further investigation to exclude structural damage. Patients may report hearing a loud 'snap' or 'crack' at the time of the injury and mistakenly believe they have sustained a fracture.

Knees are the most commonly injured joint among adolescent athletes (Gage et al., 2012), particularly among female athletes, possibly due to the nature of popular sports such as netball. Incidence varies with the sport, player contact and impact direction on the joint (Swenson et al., 2013). Ankle injuries are spread evenly across the genders with no particular injury risk factors.

Subluxation and dislocation
Joints are supported by muscles and ligaments allowing for varying but limited ranges of movement.

DEFINITIONS

- *Subluxation:* the bones of a joint move incompletely out of alignment.
- *Dislocation:* the bones of a joint remain out of alignment.

When a joint is forced beyond normal movement range ligaments can stretch or rupture allowing the bone ends to move out of normal alignment. **Dislocation** occurs when the respective bones are not fractured but the head of one bone remains out of alignment from the joint after the force (see Fig 36.1). If the force results in partial misalignment, the term **subluxation** is used.

Ligament damage can occur with either subluxation or dislocation. Swelling, loss of function and

BOX 36.1 Types of fracture

- Comminuted: two or more bone fragments.
- Segmented fracture: at least two fracture lines and a free-floating segment.
- Transverse: occurs at right angles to the long axis of the bone.
- Oblique: runs obliquely to the long axis.
- Fracture dislocation: also involves joint disruption.
- Greenstick: incomplete fracture where the bone is bent but fractured on the outer arc of the bend; particularly likely in children.

pain are typical. Visible deformity is usually obvious, particularly when compared to the non-affected limb (see Fig 36.2). Usually there will be some trauma mechanism leading to the injury. Previous injury or congenitally deformed joints may require comparatively less trauma and result in less pain.

Bony injuries
Fractures
A **fracture** occurs when force is applied to a bone that exceeds its strength, creating a break in the bone continuity. The type and amount of damage to the bones depends on the amount of force applied (see Box 36.1). Fractures may be difficult to differentiate from other MSIs with similar presenting features, such as loss of function, swelling, tenderness, pain and irregularity. Deformity and unnatural

movement are more associated with fractures and dislocations, with crepitus suggestive of fracture.

Types of fractures

Fractures may be in the middle or end of bones. They can range from hairline, where the bone integrity remains continuous, to displaced, where it does not. The bone may splinter into multiple pieces or even fragments and the fracture may extend into joints or be combined with a dislocation (see Fig 36.3).

Classification of fractures

Fractures may be classified as open or closed.

- If the skin is intact over the fracture it is a **closed fracture**. Injury to the surrounding muscle, nerve and blood vessels will vary.
- If the fracture is exposed to the outside environment it is considered an **open fracture** (see Fig 36.4). The fracture may be obviously open with gross skin and muscle damage or with bony ends protruding. It may also be as obscure as a

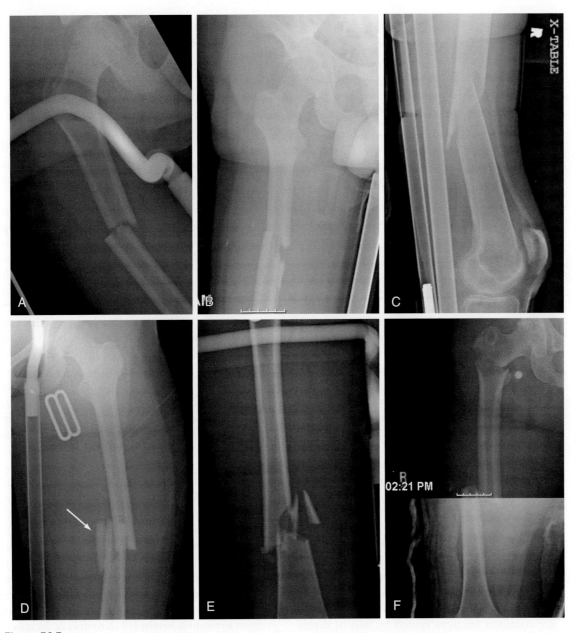

Figure 36.3
The range of femoral shaft fractures. A Transverse midshaft fracture. **B** Short oblique fracture. **C** Long oblique fracture. **D** Butterfly (or wedge) fragment in a midshaft femoral fracture. **E** Segmental fracture. **F** Comminuted fracture.
Source: Townsend et al. (2012).

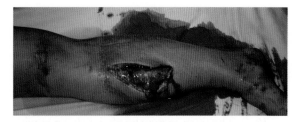

Figure 36.4
Open type IIIB: tibial fracture with vascular injury.
Source: Canale & Beaty (2007).

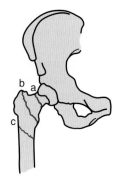

Figure 36.5
Fractures of the proximal femur: neck (a);
intertrochanteric (b); subtrochanteric (c).
Source: Pfenninger & Fowler (2010).

Table 36.1 Grades of open fracture

Grade I	Less than 1 cm long; clean with minimal soft-tissue injury
Grade II	Laceration up to 5 cm; mild–moderate contamination; mild–moderate soft-tissue injury
Grade III A Involves extensive soft-tissue stripping of bone	Contamination with severe soft-tissue injury
B Periosteal stripping has occurred	Contamination requiring soft-tissue reconstruction
C Major vascular injury present	Contamination with soft-tissue and vascular injury

Source: Gustilo, Merkow & Templeman (1990); Sinha & Anand (2010).

small puncture wound or laceration over the injured area. Include suspicion if skin integrity has been disrupted but the cause is unknown and manage as an open fracture. Open fractures are more difficult to manage and are at risk of infection. They are graded according to severity (see Table 36.1).

Specific fractures

- *Clavicle:* The clavicle, or collarbone, is most commonly fractured following a direct blow or a fall onto an outstretched hand where the force is transmitted up the arm.
- *Scapula:* The flat posterior bone that forms part of the shoulder joint is more difficult to fracture and usually requires a direct blow to break it.
- *Humerus:* The upper arm can break at the humeral neck, midshaft or elbow. A neck or elbow fracture can also involve dislocation. These are common fractures caused by falls or direct force. In younger people a significant amount of force may be required to break the humerus.
- *Forearm fractures:* The lower arm can similarly break at the elbow, midshaft or wrist. The fracture

may include the radius and/or the ulna. These are common in falls, particularly among children and the elderly.

- *Carpal and phalange fractures:* The hands and fingers are a complexity of smaller bones that can break when playing sport or from direct force.
- *Hip fractures:* The most common types of hip fractures involve the neck of the femur (see Fig 36.5). These injuries occur most frequently in the home. Women are represented almost three times more than males of the same age with around 14% of women having a hip fracture in their lifetime (Sanford et al., 2018). The elderly are most at risk with frailty, bone and muscle mass loss and increased fall likelihood (Sanford et al., 2018), and increased morbidity and mortality. The age group afflicted is predominantly over-65 years, with a large proportion over 80 years (Kreisfeld & Newson, 2006). Likelihood of death is 3.5 times more likely once injured (Lystad et al., 2017). Death rates following hip fracture are 10% at 10 days post-injury rising to 36% at 1 year, even following standing-height falls (Australian Institute of Health and Welfare [AIHW], 2010; Abrahamsen et al., 2009; Asplin et al., 2017; LeBlanc et al., 2011; Roberts et al., 2017; Sanford et al., 2018). Complications of immobility are chiefly to blame including deep vein thrombosis, pulmonary emboli, pressure areas and pulmonary infection. Early surgical intervention can improve outcomes (Sanford et al., 2018). This fracture can occur from a standing-height fall (Kreisfeld & Newson, 2006) and is the most common reason for orthopaedic ward admission (AIHW, 2010). Hip fracture care includes initial hospitalisation and rehabilitation (Kreisfeld & Newson, 2006;

AIHW, 2010). Following hip fracture, patient lifestyle commonly becomes sedentary and restricted (Zusman et al., 2017). The fracture classically presents with the injured leg slightly shorter than the other and externally rotated with the foot pointing outwards. Hip fracture in younger people is usually associated with substantial trauma.

- *Femur fractures:* The femur is usually a strong bone requiring considerable force to fracture, such as motor vehicle crashes. This force suggests likelihood of other injuries. Pathological fractures can be caused by lesser force. The femur is highly vascular and is surrounded by considerable soft tissue and major blood vessels, so appreciable blood loss can accompany a femur fracture.

   Femur fracture brings potential complications of neurovascular injury, fat embolism and requirement for more complex surgical procedures to heal. Where the fracture is open, the large muscle mass surrounding dictates specific management involving reduction, immobilisation and traction. Femoral fractures in small children (< 2 years of age) can occur but, like bruising, can raise suspicion of abusive origin (Volkman, 2016).

- *Knee/patella fractures:* The patella, distal femur or proximal tibia can be fractured following direct trauma from a fall or strike such as from the dashboard strike in motor vehicle trauma. These are relatively uncommon fractures (Schmal et al., 2010).

- *Tibia/fibula fractures:* These can occur together or in isolation as with the forearm. They usually follow direct trauma. Fibula fractures alone are less common and problematic as the bone is non-weightbearing. The tibia is a major long bone and, like the femur, usually takes considerable force to fracture.

- *Ankle fractures:* The ankle is a complex joint that can be broken by twisting or by direct trauma. Injuries to the ankle may involve the distal tibia and fibula that make up part of the ankle joint.

- *Talus/calcaneus (heel)/tarsal/metatarsal fractures:* Even more complex than the hand, the feet and toes are comprised of multiple small bones. Many of these fractures are less common injuries and are associated with particular activities or mechanisms such as a fall landing on the feet or direct trauma to the area.

- *Spinal fractures:* Although part of the musculo-skeletal system these fractures are covered in Chapter 37.

Many fractures in isolation have no major long-term consequences and are in themselves not life-threatening. However, where there are multiple long bone fractures, such as the femur and the tibia, this can change. These injuries suggest major force, potential for other body system trauma and increased bleeding risk and are a significant finding.

Pathological fractures

Increasingly, long bone fractures, including of the femur, associated with less trauma, largely due to the prevalence of osteoporosis in the elderly (AIHW, 2010). Pathological fractures differ from other fractures being based on underlying disease causing predisposing bone weakness. The most common intrinsic factors are osteoporosis, although cancer is frequently associated (Clout et al., 2016; Edwards et al., 2016; Ota et al., 2017). Extrinsic factors include surgical interventions such as previous fracture repair or effects of radiotherapy (Davies, 2008). A traumatic mechanism is still required to cause injury, although the force involved may be comparatively slight, including normal activities. The force will not usually be enough to fracture an otherwise healthy bone (Davies, 2008).

Fracture management principles remain the same. Surgical procedures must consider other patient therapies current, such as chemotherapy or radiotherapy (Edwards et al., 2016; Offluoglu et al., 2009). Healing can still occur even where the cancerous lesion remains active and under treatment (Moradi et al., 2010). The injury may affect patient outcome, as can its management (Papagelopoulos et al., 2008; Ruggieri et al., 2010).

Stress fractures

Stress fractures are commonly caused by activities such as running where repeated stress is applied to the bones. As bone is living tissue growing and replacing itself, continued stress can interfere with cortical resorption, healing and growing, predisposing to fracture development (Dhingra et al., 2017; Matcuk et al., 2016). Stress fractures occur throughout the limbs, with the most common being the lower leg and feet accounting for up to 20% of all MSIs in runners (Changstrom et al., 2015; Wright et al., 2015). They can also occur from normal bone loading where the bone itself is previously weakened such as by cancer or osteoporosis (Dhingra et al., 2017).

This fracture will be incomplete and difficult to detect, requiring radiography, particularly MRI (Matcuk et al., 2016) and perhaps scintigraphy. Often, pain is present only during the causative exercise. Symptoms in athletes should raise suspicion (Mayer et al., 2014) with this requiring surgical repair if it doesn't heal with rest (Patel et al., 2011). Previous injury and females are at greater risk (Wright et al., 2015).

DEFINITIONS

- *Greenstick fracture:* bones of children can fracture like a green tree branch, splitting but maintaining alignment.
- *Epiphyseal plate:* fractures involving the bony end growth plates present particular challenges for repair and management.

Fractures in children

MSI in children differs significantly from in adults. Fractures are typically more common for boys than girls. The bones of children have two major differences to adults. First, they have not completed the process of calcification and have immature collagen enzymatic cross linking, making them comparably softer and more flexible. This introduces **greenstick fracture** allowing forces to be transmitted to underlying and surrounding tissue without bony injury being as apparent. The bones of children can 'plastically deform' in a manner that adult bones cannot and require greater energy to break (Anisha et al., 2011; Berteau et al., 2015). Second, younger bone has **epiphyseal plates** or growth plates. These are essentially cartilage from where longitudinal bone growth occurs (Mirtz et al., 2011). Injury to these plates causes difficulties for medical repair of young fractured bones. Where the plate is not correctly aligned there could be complications for limb development and use (Eastwood & de Gheldere, 2011; Nau et al., 2015). Though many fractures result from accident and playful activities, some result from abuse. Suspicions can be heightened where the explanation for fracture changes, seems inadequate or other injuries are not consistent with one causative mechanism (Ryznar et al., 2015).

Traumatic amputation

Amputations range from comparatively minor, involving a finger or toe, through to major loss of one or more limbs. Blunt trauma, motor vehicle crashes and machinery accidents are the most common mechanisms for major loss. Traumatic amputation involves bony and soft-tissue injury (nervous, vascular, ligament, tendon, skin) with varying tissue destruction depending on forces involved. Management of the patient and the amputated part is necessary.

Assess!

A traumatic amputation is often described as a 'distracting injury'. The overt and distressing nature of the injury can mean other potentially life-threatening, but less obvious, injuries are overlooked. A thorough assessment is necessary.

CASE STUDY 1

Case 12364, 1430 hrs.

Dispatch details: A 19-year-old male has an ankle injury after playing in a local football match.

Initial presentation: The crew find the patient conscious and alert in the changing rooms with the club trainer in attendance. The trainer is holding an ice pack on the patient's left ankle. The patient gives a slight wave as the paramedics enter. A number of witnesses, including the trainer, describe how the patient was attempting to mark the ball when he was bumped heavily by another player. He fell to the ground, immediately clutching at his ankle.

 ASSESS

Patient history

What happened to the patient during the trauma provides clues to aid injury identification. Mechanisms of injury that can cause MSI are diverse and range from simple running or falls to industrial accidents and high-impact events such as motor vehicle crashes. Injury mechanism carries greater risk if the patient is aged/elderly, a child, pregnant woman or has significant comorbidities. Pattern of injury assessment and history taking allows logical processing of information. This considers trauma force and its actual impact on the body providing clues to what injuries might be found. For example, simple falls are likely to result in injuries to limbs when attempts are made to break the fall. Force transmitted directly up an arm can cause injury to the shoulder. Front seat vehicle occupants can slide forwards in frontal impact, striking knees on the dashboard. If this force is great enough, it can be transmitted along the upper leg damaging thigh, hip and pelvis. When forces are applied from multiple directions, such as vehicle rollover, pattern of injury is more difficult to apply.

A traumatic event might occur secondary to a primary medical event including syncope or seizure, particularly likely in elderly people. Consider any precipitating event when assessing a traumatic event; for example, a single vehicle crash where the car ran off the road without explanation or a patient complaining of dizziness or cardiovascular symptoms prior to a fall. Questions to explore include preceding symptoms such as palpitations, pain or weakness. Witnesses should be asked to describe any signs or complaints observed or made by the patient. Trauma patient assessment might also include medical assessment. Conversely, medical patient assessment, such as a person found lying on the floor suffering apparent stroke, might require trauma assessment to uncover any injuries sustained.

The patient in Case study 1 had no prodrome with his injury, determinable from witness information and the patient himself. He has suffered direct force to his lower leg from the awkward landing, transmitted directly to his foot and joint. Look for other incidental traumatic injury, such as his head hitting the ground.

Past medical history

Previous similar injury can predispose to repeat dislocations, sprains and strains. Some risk factors increase fall and injury risk. The elderly are more predisposed to both, with even standing-height falls potentially leading to major injuries and mortality. Unstable gait and chronic alterations in conscious state, such as dementia, increase risk. Medications that modify cardiovascular responses increase risk, particularly combinations. These can adversely impact on postural changes predisposing to syncope, light-headedness and falls or exacerbate injury once occurred. Osteoporosis or neuromuscular disease increases MSI risk.

Physical assessment

Begin patient assessment by identifying and addressing any hazards present first then dealing with life-threatening complications. Address airway, breathing and circulation as well as controlling major external haemorrhage. For major trauma patients, musculoskeletal trauma may not be the major injury and be subordinate to more pressing urgencies.

Assessment for MSI is part of secondary examination and includes physical examination and detailed history taking. Look for visible injuries, complaint of pain and detectable tenderness or abnormality. Progressively move from head to toes. The mnemonic PILSDUCT is a useful tool for assessing MSI. Even where only one minor injury is suspected or reported, follow a systematic approach to ensure nothing is overlooked. This may necessitate acknowledging to the patient their injury and a return to it as soon as practicable. MSI can cause distraction during assessment. This includes patient inability to provide reliable assessment due to overwhelming pain. It also includes assessor distraction where a gross or serious injury becomes the primary focus before establishing other injuries. An open femur fracture, for example, might obscure blunt

HISTORY

Ask!
- Where is the pain?
- Do you have any significant medical history?

Look for!
- Pattern of injury
- Mechanism of injury
- Modifying factors
- Factors contributing to the event
- Factors that might lead to greater injuries

ASSESSMENT

Look for!
Pain
Irregularity
Loss of function
Swelling
Deformity
Unnatural position
Crepitus
Tenderness

abdominal trauma hiding a more serious injury. Skin visualisation is important and must be balanced against environmental factors, privacy and injury aggravation where clothing is removed.

Examination of this patient can occur in the position as found. Sometimes this may not be possible if there is a pressing safety or environmental threat. Patient assessment on hot road surfaces, in cold, wet or windy ambient air or in full public view might be unacceptable in many cases. The patient in Case study 1 has been safely removed to the changing room already, allowing unnecessary people to be ushered away. Continue the progressive 'top to toe' secondary survey looking for other injuries; having already identified the limb injury, acknowledge it with the promise of early return to its management.

In this case there is uncertainty whether there is ankle fracture or soft tissue only. Minimise movement to decrease further muscle, skin, nerves and ligaments irritation and decrease pain.

Pain
Pain is usually the most distinctive feature of MSI. The skin and musculoskeletal system components are well supplied with receptors so MSI is likely to produce pain that can be severe and easy for the patient to locate.

Irregularity
Not all fractures involve displacement of fractured bone portions making this a non-essential finding. When bone irregularity is observed it can indicate fracture. Irregularity near joints are more difficult to differentiate from dislocation. Indeed, both may be present at joints increasing injury complexity and difficulty managing.

Loss of function
This is an easy sign of MSI to understand. Integrity of muscles, bones, joints and other components is important for effective movement. If integrity is damaged, movement is likely to be impaired. Loss of function is not specifically diagnostic as it may account for dislocation, sprain, nerve or vascular injury or fracture. Ability to continue to move an injured body part does not preclude MSI.

Swelling
Swelling is a general term for inflammation from a variety of causes including injury or infection. It frequently accompanies MSI although it is not a reliable predictor of injury severity or fracture likelihood.

Deformity
Deformity differs from irregularity. Substantial fractures including spiral, comminuted and segmented can all result in limb angulation. Deformity may appear as limb shortening caused by surrounding muscle spasm and pulling an overlapping bone along itself. It can also be found with injuries other than fractures, particularly dislocations.

Unnatural position
Gross deformation following a fracture is not common but limb fractures can cause the limb to be in an unnatural position compared to the other limb and to what would normally be expected to be found.

Crepitus
Crepitus is felt and heard when injured bone ends rub together. If a hand is placed gently over the injured area this can often be felt. It can be described as grating of the bone ends. Detecting crepitus means moving the limb, invariably resulting in pain and risking further injury. Crepitus should not be intentionally looked for during examination, but may be subsequently noted where necessary alignment or movement during splinting occurs.

Tenderness

Like irregularity, tenderness is detectable on injury site palpation. This should be gentle and brief. Tenderness is a common injury sign and associated not only with MSI. It has been surmised that damaged tissue that can produce pain via the nociceptive system can also lead to localised neuronal hypersensitivity. This hypersensitivity can extend to surrounding tissue, making tenderness unreliable for identifying injury location (Siegenthaler et al., 2010).

Neurological assessment

Injuries to joints or bones have potential to damage surrounding tissues. Upper limbs are most commonly involved and the damage can be transient or cause permanent changes including loss of sensation, weakness and numbness. Key nerves are the radial and ulnar. Lower limbs are also vulnerable, in particular the femoral, sciatic, peroneal and tibial. In the lower leg, nerve injuries with hip and knee dislocations are most common (Immerman et al., 2014). Peripheral nerves are least injured if simply lacerated and more difficult to repair if crushed, compressed or stretched. Occasionally injury can occur during treatment such as incorrect traction (Immerman et al., 2014). Emergency assessment includes determining any peripheral neurological abnormalities distal to the MSI including peripheral motor function using light and sharp touch (Immerman et al., 2014; Moore et al., 2015). Abnormal findings must be differentiated from central nervous system injury. Delayed nerve abnormality indicates evolving complication such as haematoma. Increasing ongoing pain could suggest compartment syndrome. Treatment for nerve injury varies considerably from simple observation to complex surgical intervention (Immerman et al., 2014).

> **Look for!**
> - Peripheral pulse
> - Pallor of the limb
> - Paraesthesia
> - Pain of the limb compartment
> - Capillary refill

Vascular assessment

Just as nerves can be compromised in MSI, so can blood vessels. Vascular injuries are significant for: 1. the associated blood loss, internal and external; 2. compromised blood supply distal to any injury; 3. bleeding into the confined space of a limb can lead to compartment syndrome; and 4. compromised perfusion can lead to cellular death within the limb. At particular risk are the shoulder, elbow and knee where, respectively, the axillary and brachial, femoral and popliteal arteries all closely pass.

Before applying any splint or compressive bandaging it is important to assess the limb peripheral to the injury. Is the skin pink and warm or pale and cool? (Take into account any ice packs in situ.) What is the capillary refill like? When blanched, does skin colour return within seconds or does it remain pale? If the affected limb is a foot, as for this footballer patient, is sensation in the foot and toes 'normal'? Is there a readily palpable distal pulse? Compare with the non-injured limb to determine any anomalies.

Duration of circulation compromise is important; the longer the period, the more likely irreversible tissue damage will occur. Not all vascular injury is concealed. Major open fracture or amputation can cause significant external haemorrhage that can be life-threatening. This is more likely in blast or ballistic trauma such as experienced in combat, but can be seen in industrial and heavy vehicle accidents. Controlling major haemorrhage is a priority and must precede MSI management.

Haemorrhage

All MSIs have potential for bleeding. Large muscle strains can bleed within tissue. Open fractures have greater potential for blood loss than closed fractures. The bleeding source is the rich vascular supply to the bone itself, as well as damaged surrounding soft tissue. Bleeding may be highly visible or seen as major swelling or bruising/haematoma. It may occur unseen in a cavity, such as a fractured pelvis, or in a large muscle such as the quadriceps. Significant

Table 36.2 Estimated blood loss from fracture

Fracture site	Estimated blood loss (L)
Humerus	0.25–0.5
Tibia	0.5–1.0
Femur	1.0–2.0
Pelvis	1.0 (or extensive if bleeding into abdominal cavity)

drops in haemoglobin have been shown between time of injury and surgery, contributing to anaemia and mortality (Smith et al., 2011).

Although pelvic fractures are the fractures most often associated with high mortality rates, these are declining with improved fracture management (Black et al., 2016; Cheng et al., 2015; Hermans et al., 2018; White et al., 2009; Yoshihara & Yoneoka, 2014). Long bone fractures may be associated with major blood loss (see Table 36.2). Despite fractures being capable of causing significant blood loss, consideration should always be given to more significant truncal sources of blood loss as an accompanying cause.

It is logical that more significant injuries such as head, chest, abdomen, pelvis and penetrating injuries receive priority consideration. That said, MSI should always be managed, no matter how minor. Poorly managed injuries have increased likelihood of complications that interfere with later recovery. Out-of-hospital care should allow concurrent or in-transit MSI management with other major injuries.

Assessing the paediatric patient

Children are more difficult to assess. Their response to pain, injury and traumatic events may cause them to become distressed or very quiet. Such variation from 'normal' may be a vital clue that something is wrong. Asking a parent their opinion of their child's presentation is useful. Younger children may be unable to effectively communicate verbally, so interpreting pain expressions is necessary. Consider using tools such as toys or dolls (to point to painful areas) or a paediatric pain scale. Lack of exposure to paediatric patients can lead to natural paramedic trepidation. A calm and inclusive approach is important when assessing children including introduction, parents and explanation before examination.

Initial assessment summary

Problem	Painful left ankle
Conscious state	GCS = 15
Position	Lying on a bench in the changing rooms, with the trainer holding an ice pack to his ankle
Heart rate	96 bpm
Blood pressure	110/60 mmHg
Skin appearance	Pink, warm dry
Speech pattern	Normal
Respiratory rate	14 bpm
Respiratory rhythm	Even cycles
Chest auscultation	Good breath sounds bilaterally
Pulse oximetry	99%
Temperature	37.2°C

Motor/sensory function	Too painful to move toes, the ankle is swollen and pale; he has sensation distal to the injury
Pain	9/10
History	The injury was sustained when the patient landed awkwardly after going for a mark. He is unable to stand on his left leg due to significant pain in his ankle. He reports hearing a loud cracking noise as he landed.
Physical assessment	The ankle is swollen and pale, although there is no obvious deformity.

D: There are no dangers to the patient or crew.

A: The patient is conscious with no current airway obstruction.

B: Respiratory function is currently normal.

C: Heart rate and blood pressure are within normal limits.

Once in the change room, the trainer unlaced the player's boot, removed it then cut off the sock to allow assessment. The patient's ankle is noticeably swollen and appears laterally deformed. The ankle does not appear at an abnormal or unnatural angle. The patient complains of significant pain but he can slightly move his foot and toes with normal sensation, warmth and foot colour. There is no evidence of irregularity or crepitus, the latter not intentionally assessed for. The provisional diagnosis is a severe ankle sprain injury.

2 CONFIRM

The essential part of the clinical reasoning process is to seek to confirm your initial hypothesis by finding clinical signs that should occur with your provisional diagnosis. Challenge the diagnosis by exploring findings that do not fit your hypothesis: don't just ignore them because they don't fit.

Unlike medical cases where a number of possible causes need to be excluded, the mechanism of injury is often more obvious in trauma. However, the most obvious injury is not always the most serious and visually dramatic and painful injuries can distract both the patient and the paramedic from other possibilities.

The history and presentation may not be sufficient to differentiate between some MSIs.

What else could it be?

Fracture

The patient reported hearing a loud cracking noise at the time of injury. Fractures and sprains share a number of symptoms: pain, tenderness, loss of function and discolouration of the skin over the injured area. Fractures may also present with irregularity and deformity, as well as crepitus. Fractures can occur simultaneously with softer tissue injuries so are not mutually exclusive.

Dislocation

Deformity is usually obvious, loss of function is absolute and pain generally significant. The ankle joint here appears intact and the patient is able to move his foot up and down, albeit restricted by pain. Dislocation does not seem likely.

> ### DIFFERENTIAL DIAGNOSIS
>
> **Sprain**
> Or
> - Fracture
> - Dislocation

3 TREAT

Principles of management of MSI are outlined in Box 36.2.

Emergency management

Safety

MSI usually follows trauma and some events may create hazards. Paramedics should assess the scene on approach and consider how the injury occurred.

> ## BOX 36.2 Principles of management
>
> **Musculoskeletal injuries**
> - Safety: patient and rescuers
> - Airway care
> - Respiratory support
> - Circulation support
> - Haemorrhage control
> - Fluid volume replacement
> - Cervical care
> - RICE (Rest, Ice, Compression, Elevation)
> - Splinting
> - Careful handling
> - Manage other injuries

> ## BOX 36.3 Shock
>
> Shock is a term used in both a medical and a non-medical sense. Medically, shock describes the physiological sequelae of events resulting in an inadequacy of the cardiovascular system to meet the body's cellular needs at the time. Shock is a serious condition that may result in death if not identified and managed. This is quite significantly different to the layperson's diagnosis of shock, which generally relates to an emotional response. As a health professional, use this term in the medical sense rather than the colloquial one.

Access and egress should be considered from the outset and extra resources requested early to assist as required.

In this case the patient was injured on the football field and is now in the changing rooms. Access and egress may be complicated by crowd and vehicle traffic. Unruly crowds and the effects of alcohol should not be underestimated.

Haemorrhage

MSI and limb injuries are not usually in themselves acutely life-threatening, but this can change when associated with significant blood loss and other injuries. Address external bleeding as part of initial care.

Rarely, external bleeding cannot be controlled. This is more common with penetrating trauma and amputation, frequently in the military setting or with high-impact trauma. Arterial tourniquets have been shown to be effective in such life-threatening haemorrhage circumstances without adverse outcomes (Scerbo et al., 2017; Teixeira et al., 2018; Perkins et al., 2012). Tourniquet use accompanying direct pressure is best applied before physiological shock occurs (see Box 36.3) to provide temporary opportunity for a more substantial haemorrhage control option (Sinha & Anand, 2010). A tourniquet should be broad, well-padded, placed as distally as possible and at sufficient pressure to occlude arterial supply.

Realignment, immobilisation and splinting of a limb decreases bleeding in several ways. Realigning fractured ends to a more natural position reduces the size of the cavity and acts to tamponade the bleeding site. Immobilisation reduces movement of the bony ends, limiting ongoing soft-tissue damage. This also facilitates clot formation and physiological attempts to control bleeding.

Wound management

Wounds associated with fractures should be dressed as any other wound, mindful not to introduce any infection source. More severe wound

> ## BOX 36.4 RICE
>
> Rest. Avoid activities that exacerbate the pain. A sling or crutches may be required.
>
> Ice. Apply for 15–20 minutes each hour and continue for 48 hours.
>
> Compression. Apply a crepe or an elastic bandage. A finger should be able to be inserted beneath the bandage.
>
> Elevation. Aim heart level or higher. Elevate limb on a pillow or apply a hand/arm sling with hand/arm elevated.

contamination, such as dirt, gravel or other foreign material, should be irrigated first with copious sterile water or normal saline to clean it. Irrigate when an open fracture will have traction applied to minimise deeper tissue contamination.

Management of soft-tissue injuries

Regional swelling after injury is common with severe swelling thought to slow the healing process. The most accepted practice for acute MSI management is described by the mnemonic Rest, Ice, Compression, Elevation (RICE) (see also Box 36.4).

- *Rest.* Rest the limb and avoid activities that cause significant pain. A sling or crutches may be required. Severe injuries may require immobilisation with a cast or splint. Muscle injuries can benefit from moderate exercise and stretching over the few days following injury. Rest can reduce haematoma and swelling (Maffulli et al., 2015).
- *Ice.* Ice causes localised vasoconstriction and decreases oedema. This lowers injured tissue temperature, lowering metabolic rate and secondary hypoxic injury (Bleakley et al., 2007; Maffulli et al., 2015). Recommended application times vary, typically 15–20 minutes each hour when awake for the first 48 hours post-injury. Intermittent ice applications can have an analgesic effect by inhibiting pain receptors (Bleakley et al., 2007; Maffulli et al., 2015; Malanga et al., 2015).
- *Compression.* Compression applies external pressure over the injury to reduce oedema development. It inhibits fluid build-up and leaking from damaged tissue that leads to oedema. It may also improve the cooling effect by improving contact with the ice and reducing inflow of warm blood flow. Compression works well when combined with cold therapy (Maffulli et al., 2015).
- *Elevation.* Historically, the injured limb has been raised above the level of the heart to slow blood delivery to the injured area and to facilitate drainage from the limb. This may require elevating a leg onto several pillows or applying a sling. More recently it has been shown the extent of elevation is not critical provided the limb is not left in a gravity-dependent position (Gillette et al., 2017).

To these can be added an initial letter P for *Protection*. This includes splinting, immobilisation or other physical support including boots making the mnemonic *PRICE* (Maffulli et al., 2015).

These principles, modified where appropriate, can be applied to suspected fracture. Compression may increase pain, but certainly rest (splinting and immobilisation), elevation (once splinted, elevate the limb onto a pillow) and ice (may prove difficult but worth it—although not at the expense of the previous points) may offer some relief (Black & Becker, 2009).

In the case study, the patient has had ice applied to his ankle and, given probability of fracture or dislocation, this is likely to offer some benefit.

Pain relief/analgesia

Pain from MSI can be significant, particularly dislocations and fractures. Analgesia should be provided as per local clinical practice guidelines and depending on pain severity until comfort is achieved. Mild-to-moderate pain may be managed differently from severe pain. Furthermore, severe pain that is difficult to relieve may require further interventions.

Analgesia can be administered variously including oral, inhaled, intranasal and intravenous. The most appropriate analgesia route considers:

- the likely requirement for ongoing analgesia
- the likelihood the pain will subside spontaneously
- the nature of the injury sustained
- other interventions that may help alleviate the pain, including splinting, RICE, immobilisation.

The last point is significant as these three therapies make a major contribution to pain relief. Generally, intent of analgesia is to follow effective splinting and address residual pain. In practice there is often need to move patients or affected limbs during MSI management and analgesia may be required beforehand to enable this.

There are a variety of pain management strategies with varying effectiveness. Many biases impact on analgesia provision, including racial and cultural stereotyping; pain undertreatment is common. Children are often the least well-managed given assessment difficulties and concern with side effects. The most common substantial out-of-hospital pharmacological analgesia options are opioids including morphine and fentanyl administered intravenously or intramuscularly. Fentanyl can be administered intranasally using a suitable presentation. Other options include inhaled options including methoxyflurane and nitrous oxide, with comparative advantages of quick onset and short half-life. Analgesics such as paracetamol and codeine have a place in the out-of-hospital setting for less severe MSI pain.

Manage pain as necessary. Less subjective systems of allocating a patient's pain score may assist (see Chapter 30) as can subjective evaluation for grimacing or discomfort signs (Hogan, 2011). For pain intractable to initial therapies consider more substantial options such as intravenous ketamine, the muscle relaxant midazolam or local nerve block.

Our footballer patient has a significantly painful injury. Assess the RICE benefit and whether pain continues sufficiently to warrant further analgesia. Splinting may also help.

Realignment

As a general principle, MSI including fractures are managed in the position found. Occasionally limb realignment may be required before splinting or immobilisation can be performed, particularly where gross deformity is evident. Transfer with an unsplinted limb should not occur. When limb deformity compromises distal perfusion, alignment may be particularly indicated, and where prolonged out-of-hospital times are anticipated or where it may prove impractical to transport the patient.

Realignment can decrease pain and minimise soft-tissue and neurovascular damage. Femur fractures are often associated with muscle spasm that can increase pain and delay treatment until resolved. Early realignment and splinting helps avoid this. Realignment can be achieved by supporting under the limb just above the fracture with one hand and grasping the distal limb with the other. If the fracture is too high, have an assistant provide the upper support. Gently pull distally along the line of the limb until the muscle spasm begins to relax; this may take more than a minute of gentle traction. When the muscle spasm has relaxed and length is achieved, readjust the limb back to its normal position. In practice, if done slowly and gently the bones tend to align themselves, as the relative opposing muscle group tension balances again. The force required to reduce a fracture dislocation of an ankle is only that which can be applied with a gentle one-handed pull. It should be possible to maintain this pull for several minutes without any effort. This will undoubtedly cause trepidation and probably transient pain. Adequate analgesia must accompany or precede realignment.

Dislocations that cause anatomical deformity are a completely different problem and should not be realigned without prior medical assessment and a thorough understanding of appropriate techniques to such injuries. Joint anatomy predisposes for nerve and vascular injury if dislocation reduction is not performed properly. Some dislocations, notably knee and shoulder, can be reduced where there is previous history of the same injury, no prospect of fracture or complicating injury and the correct reduction method is understood. Out-of-hospital management should frequently centre on good splinting and immobilisation rather than manipulation methods.

Fortunately, our footballer patient does not have any gross deformity evident so does not require any manipulation or relocation.

Splinting and immobilisation

Splinting and immobilisation are important to consider in MSI to minimise pain and swelling and reduce ongoing injury or damage to surrounding tissue (Sinha & Anand, 2010). Soft-tissue injuries are often confused with fractures and on most occasions require radiographic investigations if the diagnosis suggests fracture. Patients often report hearing or feeling a crack/snap/pop at the time of the injury in fracture, sprain and strain injuries. If in doubt, treat as though fractured and splint accordingly.

Splinting was once taught in a very precise manner, with different splints prescribed for different fractures. Current out-of-hospital splinting is less precise with greater reliance on the general principle of simply immobilising limb and joints above and below the fracture site. Splinting may involve purpose-built devices (see Fig 36.6) or may be improvised using pillows, cardboard or magazines (see Fig 36.7). Do not compress soft tissue so much that it occludes local blood supply. Take care when using inflatable splints that air pressure exerted does not cause local ischaemia. Inflatable splints can place indiscriminate pressure over the injury, potentially increasing pain.

Splinted and immobilised lower arm injuries are usually best supported using a sling. Upper arm fractures may benefit from anatomical splinting to the chest. Leg injuries can be anatomically splinted to the other leg. Midshaft femur fractures and fractures of the upper two-thirds of the lower leg may benefit from traction splinting given propensity for large muscle spasm. A traction splint can decrease pain, bleeding, pulmonary complications and risk of injury worsening (Hoppe et al., 2015). Despite this, out-of-hospital traction splint application is often not applied when indicated (Maqungo et al., 2015; Nackenson et al., 2017). Traction should not be applied where any joints are involved for risk of further injuring the joints, nerves or vascular supply. Once applied, traction should be continuous until ED handover.

The patient in the case study has an injury mechanism, pain and swelling suggesting ankle MSI. Splinting in the position as found is preferred. A formable splint, manufactured lower leg splint or improvised splint such as a pillow wrapped around the limb could prove effective as long as it provides stability and immobilisation. Ice can be applied simultaneously.

Intravenous fluid therapy

IV fluid administration will only be required if external bleeding is controlled and blood loss has been severe. Blood loss from long bone fractures or external

MANAGEMENT DILEMMA

Most patients with a fractured limb usually find a position of comfort they are reluctant to change, even to allow splinting. Is it adequate to allow a patient to anatomically splint a fractured forearm by holding their arm to their chest, or should more formal splinting be applied? Consider all options and provide the most suitable and effective splinting and immobilisation.

PRACTICE TIP

Manage life-threatening external haemorrhage before commencing IV fluids.

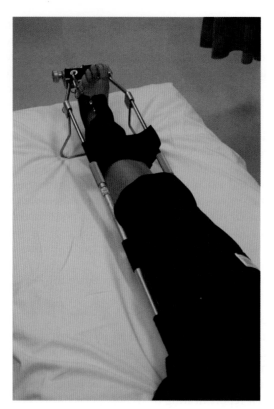

Figure 36.6
Traction splint applied to a lower leg.
Source: Marx et al. (2010).

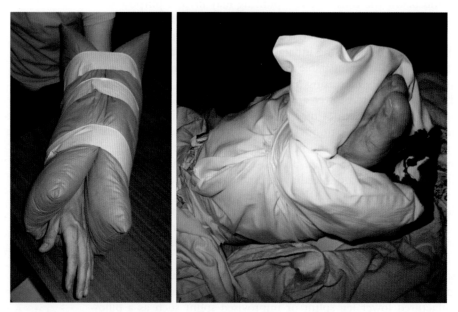

Figure 36.7
A pillow folded as an improvised splint.
Source: Auerbach (2011).

bleeding can result in inadequate perfusion requiring fluid therapy. Patients with a soft-tissue injury presenting with inadequate perfusion should prompt paramedics to consider the following.

- The injury is more significant than first thought.
- There are other injuries causing inadequate perfusion.
- The patient is in pain.

Of these, significant concealed injury should always be considered uppermost. Address all basic management concurrently including analgesia, splinting/immobilisation and patient warmth.

Amputated limb management

Amputated limb management is important for survival and for maximising body part salvation. Patients still trapped by limb remnants must be managed on a case-specific basis with urgency of release dictated by presentation. Where time permits, disassembling machinery in which the patient is trapped may be appropriate, but if the patient is time-critical, infield amputation may be the only option. In reality, such incidence is extremely rare. Amputation should be performed by a medical practitioner if possible, although where minimal soft tissue is all that remains a paramedic may be compelled to intervene. Address uncontrolled haemorrhage. Surgical techniques allow a great chance of salvage, although contamination and crush damage reduce success.

Amputated part care

Locate the amputated part if possible and treat as potentially salvageable. Little evidence exists for best method of caring for the amputated part. The overriding principles include the following.

- Apply a sterile normal-saline soaked dressing to the exposed tissue and bone limb ends.
- Protect the entire amputated limb with a waterproof covering (such as a plastic bag).
- Keep the limb cool but not frozen. This can use whatever resources are at hand, including ice packs, frozen products or ice. Any ice should not be in direct limb contact, as extreme cooling can lead to tissue damage, reducing viability. Consider wrapping the limb or ice packs in sheets/towels, or place ice in water to provide a cold medium to surround the limb. Small tissue fragments found with the amputated part should be kept as well, as they may be of use during surgery.

(4) EVALUATE

Evaluating clinical intervention effect can provide clues to accuracy of initial diagnosis. Some conditions respond rapidly to treatment so patients should be expected to improve if the diagnosis and treatment were appropriate. Failure to improve should trigger reconsidering the diagnosis.

Ongoing management

Out-of-hospital management revolves around preventing any worsening of the injury and providing symptomatic relief. Initially, staff in the ED will extend this and initiate definitive diagnosis and management.

Pain relief

Patients may still have persistent significant pain on arrival in the ED or require ongoing analgesia for several hours. This can include pharmacotherapy options of analgesia, sedation, nerve block or alterations in splinting or alignment.

Sedation

Out-of-hospital sedation is controversial given the potential impacts on the patient's conscious state and perfusion for uncertain benefit. In the ED, however, sedation may be a very useful adjunct. Typically, short-term sedation is administered to enable procedures such as simple reductions of fractures or dislocations.

Nerve block

Nerve block involves local anaesthetic injection into the immediate vicinity of a nerve. The anaesthetic effect is produced by impeding movement of sodium ions across the nerve cell membrane, interfering with nerve impulse transmission. Nerve blocks can produce effective pain reductions allowing procedures to be performed. They can reduce but not remove need for opioids and minimise their side effects (Hartmann et al., 2017; Kassam et al., 2018; Singh et al., 2016; Üzümcügil et al., 2015). There is clearly skill in determining the optimal injection site, sometimes requiring ultrasound to improve identification (Bendtsen et al., 2011). Nerve blocks are not without risk of nerve injury or adverse reaction (Sharma et al., 2010), contributing to their restricted out-of-hospital use.

Interim splinting or alignment

Out-of-hospital splinting may be absent, adequate or improvised. Even correctly applied splinting may become loose and less effective due to movement and patient position change. The original splint may be removed to enable full examination of the injury. Not all MSIs lend well to out-of-hospital management, with some relocation too risky or painful. Patients may have splinting options reapplied or temporary alternative splints applied. In some cases urgent realignment or reduction of any injury may be required to assist with pain or compromised peripheral perfusion.

Wound management

Depending on the original traumatic event, foreign material including dirt, chemicals or gravel can enter the wound and interfere with wound healing. Wounds can be irrigated and, within the limits, antiseptic added. The optimal wound management time is unclear and may vary according to the urgency of other injuries. The standard, once within 6 hours of injury, is now within 24 hours with suitable prior antibiotic administration (Perkins et al., 2012). Surgical debridement and wound cleaning include wound irrigation and close inspection and removal of foreign material and blood clots. Non-salvageable tissue is removed until the wound appears clean. Larger bone fragments may be kept for fracture repair (Sinha & Anand, 2010).

Optimal wound closure time is also unclear. A typical care regimen has the wound left open for several days. This allows potential for nosocomial infection. Around 4–7 days post-injury the wound can be inspected and, if clean, closed over (Fulkerson & Egol, 2009).

Temporary reduction or fixation

Although injury repair may be indicated there may be reasons for providing temporary therapies rather than definitive options. Patients may have life-threatening or more urgent priorities. Physiological stabilisation might increase survival chances following surgery (Pape et al., 2009). Optimal time for substantive injury repair depends on many variables. Many injuries are managed non-surgically. Timing of surgical interventions remains unclear and varies with injury though earlier rather than later is associated with fewer complications (Byrne et al., 2017; Siebenbürger et al., 2015; Vallier et al., 2015).

Investigations

X-ray

The x-ray has long been the mainstay of assessment and diagnosis for MSI, particularly fractures. Multiple X-rays maximise view and diagnostic capacity. As the x-ray is a form of radiation, there are limitations to the allowable exposure with some at increased risk, including children and pregnant women.

Computed tomography and MRI

Computed tomography (CT) and MRI can be used to assess musculoskeletal trauma and are widely accepted for diagnostic procedures. CT takes multiple x-ray images, providing a two-dimensional MSI view, improving diagnostic ability. MRI uses radiofrequency waves to create three-dimensional views. MRI has become a mainstay of sports injury assessment. Both CT and MRI can be used to assess strain injuries, with MRI more useful. They can also be used to help localise injuries to a single muscle within a group and highlight features such as atrophy and fibrosis.

Ultrasound

Ultrasound is useful in identifying greenstick fractures in children (Pountos et al., 2010) and in some cases as a substitute for x-ray when not immediately available (Farahmand et al., 2017; Weinberg et al., 2010). Ultrasound is useful for assessing strain injuries, early stress fractures and to assess blood flow distal to an injury where circulation may be impaired (Rao et al., 2017). Ultrasound is comparatively easy to perform even in acute situations and avoids radiation exposure (Ko et al., 2019; Schmid et al., 2017; Sharma et al., 2017; Woodhouse & McNally, 2011).

Scintigraphy

Scintigraphy, or radionuclide bone scanning, can detect abnormalities not found by radiography, including child and stress fractures (Drubach, 2017;

Leffers & Collins, 2009; Nadel, 2010). It is less commonly used, limited in the injury type it can assess and vulnerable to misinterpretation (Gnana-segaran et al., 2009; Leffers & Collins, 2009). It can detect metabolic activity increases from injury healing and can be useful in stress fracture diagnosis (Dhingra et al., 2017). It is not effective in the acute stage of injury and is typically used several days post-injury.

Ongoing management of uncomplicated injuries

Most patients with MSI have a short and unremark-able medical requirement. Mild-to-moderate strains and sprains can be managed with little more than the basic out-of-hospital care and ongoing oral analgesia or anti-inflammatory medication. Strains and sprains may benefit from continued RICE for the first few hours, with ice then used intermittently for the next 24–72 hours depending on injury severity. The acute inflammatory phase may last up to a week, replaced with a period of tissue removal, new growth and repair. Immobilisation in the initial period allows this repair to occur and limits con-nective scar-tissue growth within soft-tissue injuries. Prolonged immobilisation is not usually advocated for most MSI following the acute period; recom-mencing mobilisation varies with injury type. Methods used frequently commence within a few days of injury and involve targeted and specifically controlled movements and stretching exercises. Where injury is more substantial, such as fracture or ligament tear, greater immobilisation is required and potentially surgical repair.

Torn muscle repair

Most muscle strains and tears heal within a few weeks without major intervention and require only rehabilitation (Tonino & Sinclair, 2011). MRI is not commonly necessary in assessing injury. It may be useful delineating severity and appropriate management as it can reveal muscle regeneration within scar tissue even after clinical signs of injury have dissipated and activity returned (Moen et al., 2014). Non-steroidal anti-inflammatory medications may reduce initial pain and strength loss but may limit long-term repair (Mackey et al., 2012; Morelli et al., 2018; Schoenfeld, 2018).

Dislocation reduction

Dislocations with no fracture can usually be repaired by closed reduction or manipulation of the bone back into correct position. This may be achieved by traction to overcome muscle spasm or by manipulation to push the bone back into position.

If injury has occurred previously, laxity may develop in the joint in either the capsule or the supporting ligaments or muscles. Surgery may be required to repair the joint capsule, ligaments or muscles. First-time episodes are typically treated with limited movement, or even immobilisation, for up to 6 weeks, followed by rehabilitation.

Fracture reduction

Closed fracture reduction is performed when a fracture is returned to its desired position for healing without skin incision required. In contrast, open reduction requires skin incision and is typically used where open fractures have occurred or where internal fixation is required. Bone healing follows a predict-able pathway, commencing with initial inflammatory phase after the injury, followed by development of a soft callus at the injury site that progressively converts to hard callus (rigid bone). Bone rejoining is completed by reshaping to complete healing. The goal of fracture reduction and fixation is to hold the injured bone in place to enable healing and eventual return of normal mobility. The option selected depends on injury extent and the best method of providing stability.

Closed reduction methods

Closed reduction is more traditional and conservative comprising reduction and realignment of bone back to its normal position without any skin opening at the injury site. Splinting or stabilisation maintains position until healed.

Casting

Arguably the most stereotypical management of fractures is the simple cast (see Fig 36.8). Casts are commonly made from wet plaster of Paris and cotton padding that dry hard after application, but other materials such as woven fibreglass or plastic have recently found popularity. The simple cast can be moulded to suit a great number of injuries, from simple distal limb injuries covering the wrist or

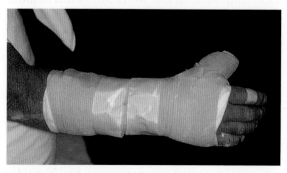

Figure 36.8
Forearm in a plaster cast.
Source: Roberts (2009).

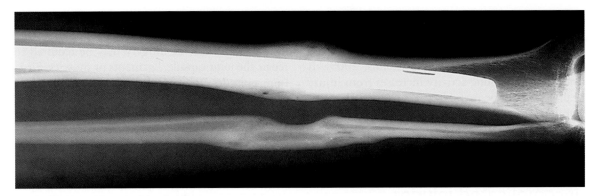

Figure 36.9
X-ray of fractured tibia with internal intramedullary nail.
Source: Resnick & Kransdorf (2005).

ankle and a small portion of limb either side of the injury to the more extensive hip spica that immobilises hips and one or both lower legs. Shoulder spicas may be used following shoulder surgery.

The cast is not suited to all fractures and is not without complications, including pressure sores, skin irritation, inability to use the muscle and joints and, potentially, compartment syndrome. In situations where fresh and progressive swelling is occurring, the cast can be applied so that it is not fully circumferential (back slab) but rather provides support on one side only. This is particularly useful for wrist injuries (Wik et al., 2009). These are commonly not reliably applied (Jayaraman et al., 2016).

A displaced fracture is often returned to a better position under mild sedation or a general anaesthetic. It is then maintained in position using a plaster back slab, which can be made up into a full plaster once the swelling has ceased.

Open reduction methods
Although practised in early forms as far back as the 19th century, open reduction is comparatively new and involves various surgical methods for realignment and stabilisation. More substantial injuries brought about by blast and gunshot trauma, particularly military or industrial activity related, use advanced methods of fracture repair.

Internal fixation
Internal fixation has numerous forms including placement of a long intramedullary nail through the length of the bone (see Fig 36.9), use of wires around the injury and joint or plates that sit across a fracture and are screwed into healthy bone on either side. The optimal choice depends on injury type and extent, and underlying patient health. Variables including extent of open wound and underlying bone strength are important choice factors.

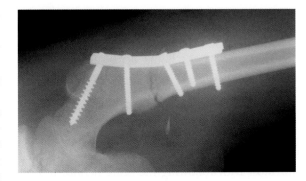

Figure 36.10
X-ray of fractured femur with internal plate and screw fixation.
Source: Green & Swiontkowski (2009).

Typically, nails or plates are used on long bone fractures of the humerus, femur and tibia. An intramedullary nail is removed 1 or 2 years post-surgery. Screws used in fixation must be able to be inserted into bone strong enough to hold them from being pulled out (see Fig 36.10). When using internal methods, the potential for injury to surrounding soft and neurovascular tissue and the bone itself must be considered. Screws that are too long may cause injury through too deep penetration. Localised ongoing pain can be a problem, with eventual device removal the solution. Other complications include pulmonary embolism, wound infection and the subsequent need for amputation (SooHoo et al., 2009; Berglund & Messer, 2009; Berkes et al., 2010; Chen et al., 2010; Kleweno et al., 2011).

External fixation
With external fixation, part of the splinting and stabilising device remains outside of the body tissue (see Fig 36.11). Typically external fixation involves

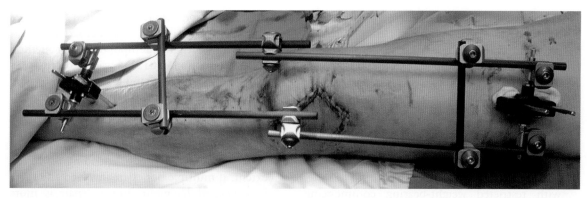

Figure 36.11
External limb fixation
Source: Canale & Beaty (2007).

realigning the fractured bone, placing screws or wires into the bone beyond the injury site and attaching these to a rigid device or frame to provide stabilisation. Infection prevention where the skin is penetrated is extremely important. External fixation is indicated where an open fracture wound is substantial or in children to avoid the growth plate. External fixation has the advantage of being faster and causing less blood loss than internal fixation (Sinha & Anand, 2010). In addition, flexibility of control is possible during the healing process.

Traction splinting

Traction, as typically applied to proximal femur and hip fractures, can be useful preoperatively and may provide some adjunct to pain relief. It can be applied as skin traction using tapes applied to the skin or as skeletal traction through the use of pins though there is limited evidence supporting any particular method (Handoll et al., 2011; Matullo et al., 2016). Where closed reduction does not provide a successful result, wires can be inserted through a wound site near the fracture, passed along the length of the bone and buried into soft tissue. Bends in the wire can then have gentle traction applied along the length. The most common fractures requiring this method are the femur and humerus and distal fractures of the arm and leg.

Management of specific fractures

- *Clavicle:* This injury usually heals with little more than adequate splinting and light exercise to keep the shoulder joint mobile. It requires surgical repair only if the bone will not heal or if there is injury to the shoulder joint as well.
- *Scapula:* Healing is very similar to the clavicle, with limited intervention required unless the shoulder joint is involved.

- *Humerus:* Management can vary considerably from conservative sling immobilisation to surgical repair. Injury repair is more complex if wound debridement is required or there is nerve involvement. Healing and rehabilitation differs if the shoulder is immobilised with a cast compared to use of a fixation device where earlier movement is possible.
- *Forearm fractures:* Depending on location, a cast may be suitable. Surgical repair may be required if the injury is in the joint. Compartment syndrome is associated with these fractures. Wrist injuries may require surgical fixation and can be problematic in the long term for arthritis and joint stiffness.
- *Carpal and phalange fractures:* Management may be as simple as a cast following manual manipulation or may involve specialist surgical repair including plate insertion. Full movement return may be difficult, particularly where there is tendon injury. These injuries may take as little as 6 weeks or as much as 12 weeks to heal.
- *Hip fractures:* Hip fractures present variously, all involving femoral head, neck and trochanter injury and is usually diagnosed on x-ray or occasionally MRI or CT. Depending on location, injury severity and underlying bone health, internal fixation is usually required, sometimes with entire replacement of the femoral head. Avascular necrosis is among a range of complications including deep vein thrombosis (DVT), pulmonary embolism and pneumonia. Hospital discharge may be comparatively quick (as little as 5 days) if the patient can ambulate, but typically takes several weeks (Sund et al., 2009; Kondo et al., 2010). Ongoing rehabilitation may take 3–6 months before return to full activity with as many as 40–60% never fully achieving this (Dyer et al., 2017; Roberts et al., 2017).

Discharge is typically to a nursing home for up to 90 days, although longer periods are not uncommon (Asplin et al., 2017; Bentler et al., 2009). Integrated team rehabilitation is necessary for maximum rehabilitation (Dyer et al., 2017; Roberts et al., 2017).

- *Femur fractures:* The most common method of managing midshaft femur fracture is with intramedullary nail insertion (Parkes et al., 2017; Wild et al., 2010). This is a very significant injury and typically takes 3–4 months for full healing, with restricted weight-bearing commencing within a few days of internal fixation. Repair for most isolated paediatric femur fractures remains the simple cast with or without traction. There is an increasing use of intramedullary rods (Khazzam et al., 2009), although the hip spica remains common for younger children. External fixation is useful for more complex injuries (Allison et al., 2011; McKeon et al., 2010). The optimal time for surgical repair is unclear but delay beyond 12 hours in the presence of other major trauma can increase complications including fat embolus and adult respiratory distress syndrome and increase mortality (Morshed et al., 2009).

- *Knee/patella fractures:* Surgery is not always necessary for these fractures; when required, repair can include internal fixation of wire placement through the patella or screw fixation (Schmal et al., 2010). These injuries are typically complicated by ligament injury that may require further surgery to repair and provide long-term joint stability. Recovery can follow cast or brace immobilisation for up to 6 weeks. Patella injury can result in injury to the soft tissue beneath it and increase arthritis risk. Rehabilitation usually commences as soon as possible to return joint function, with movement and weight-bearing dependent on underlying injury (Melvin & Mehta, 2011). Knee injuries such as caused by twisting motion during sports can damage ligaments, destabilising the joint. In particular, the anterior cruciate ligament with its major responsibility for knee stabilisation may not heal without intervention. Surgical repair (knee reconstruction) of the ligament involves removing the damaged ligament and attaching a new graft in its place. This procedure usually involves a minimal hospital period with rehabilitation commencing soon afterwards.

- *Tibia/fibula fractures:* Depending on injury extent, a fractured tibia/fibula can be managed using a simple cast. If the fracture is more complex and unstable, internal fixation may be performed. Repeated surgery may be required to remove screws or pins originally inserted. External fixation is an alternative temporary repair method (Beck & Benson, 2012). Healing occurs over 8–12 weeks, with rehabilitation and return to normal activity taking a similar timeframe. Complications for tibia fractures include compartment syndrome, fat embolism and DVT.

- *Ankle fractures:* The ankle can be complicated to repair, with outcomes depending on injury extent. If multiple bones are involved and there is associated ligament injury, repair is more complex with longer healing. Simpler stable fractures involving only one bone and no complex features can heal over up to 6 weeks using a brace cast. Where this is not so, open reduction and internal fixation using plates and/or screws may be required along with any ligament repair. Although most ankle injuries heal uneventfully within a few months, reduction in joint mobility may be noted for many months. Arthritis may remain an ongoing problem following joint injury. Subsequent removal of the internal fixation is not usual though can be necessary to reduce ongoing pain or increase joint movement (Jung et al., 2016; Williams et al., 2017).

- *Talus/heel/tarsal/metatarsal fractures:* Some of the bones involved have a rich vascular supply and any interruption can lead to avascular necrosis. Depending on the injury extent, either closed or open reduction may be required. It can be difficult to differentiate these from ankle injuries, or they may occur concurrently. Arthritis and ongoing joint stiffness are common regardless of repair method. Healing usually takes 2–3 months, although rehabilitation programs to re-establish normal walking can be prolonged. Metatarsal fractures are probably the least complicated and uneventful of these injuries.

Complications of MSIs

Infection

Infection is the most common and one of the most severe open fracture complications. Early and effective wound cleaning and antibiotic therapy are important in managing infection.

Nerve injury

Nerve injury can occur directly from the trauma or follow subsequent complications including compartment syndrome. Neuropraxia is nerve contusion that disrupts nervous impulse, usually transiently with slight sensory loss, with normal nerve function returning over weeks to months. Axonotmesis is more significant including nerve injury within their sheaths. Nerve repair is possible but usually very slow, taking many months. Neurotmesis is complete nerve severing and generally requires surgical repair. Table 36.3 shows nerve injuries associated with particular fractures.

Vascular injury

Acute artery obstruction can directly threaten any limb and must be managed expeditiously. Out-of-hospital care includes recognition, considering limb-saving realignment and hospital notification. Unnecessary transport delays should be avoided as permanent injury can occur in < 6 hours. Compromise to limb circulation can be managed using temporary shunts. Angiography can be used to assess vascular compromise, although the Doppler stethoscope can be useful to detect blood flow.

Table 36.3 Nerve injuries commonly associated with fractures

Orthopaedic injury	Nerve injury
Elbow injury	Median or ulnar
Shoulder dislocation	Axillary
Acetabulum fracture	Sciatic
Femoral shaft fracture	Peroneal nerve
Knee dislocation	Tibial or peroneal
Lateral tibial plateau fracture	Peroneal
Hip dislocation	Femoral nerve

Compartment syndrome

Bleeding or oedema in an enclosed compartment causes increased pressure and tissue damage if not managed. **Compartment syndrome** typically involves the lower leg or forearm (Sinha & Anand, 2010; Via et al., 2015; Von Keudell et al., 2015) where the space is bound by bone, muscle and membrane and expansive capacity is limited. However, compartment syndrome can develop anywhere skeletal muscle is surrounded by substantial fascia, including the buttock and thigh. Increased pressure within the confined fascial compartment can cause circulation impairment and ischaemia (Via et al., 2015) and further injury to muscle, nerves and limb vasculature (see Fig 36.12). A large compartment syndrome can cause tissue necrosis leading to loss of the limb distal to the compression, renal failure (as commonly as one in four cases) and even death with mortality as high as 47% when it occurs in the thigh (Via et al., 2015).

Compartment syndromes can follow severe or minor injuries. It can be classified as acute or chronic, depending on the cause of the increased pressure and symptom duration. Acute compartment syndromes are a surgical emergency (Via et al., 2015). The most common causes of acute compartment syndrome are fractures, soft-tissue trauma, arterial injury, limb compression during altered consciousness and burns. Chronic compartment syndrome is caused by recurrence of increased pressure, most often in the anterior or deep posterior compartment

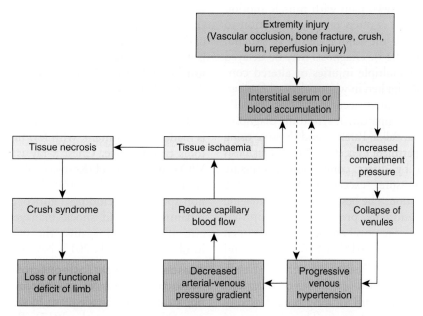

Figure 36.12
Pathophysiological evolution of compartment syndrome.
Source: Cameron (2010).

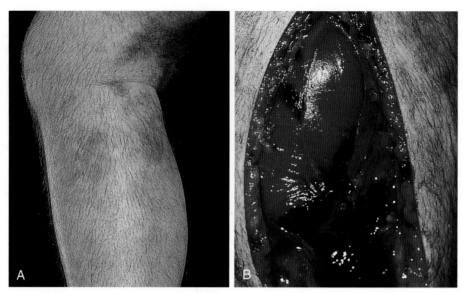

Figure 36.13
Compartment syndrome. A Severe calf swelling due to anterior and posterior compartment syndromes after ischaemia-reperfusion. B Appearance after emergency fasciotomy. Note oedematous muscle and haematoma.
Source: Courtesy Michael J. Allen, FRCS, Leicester, UK.

of the leg but also elsewhere, including paediatric humerus fracture (Robertson et al., 2018) and forearms in weightlifters. Exercise can increase muscle volume by 20%, causing increase in pressure in a noncompliant compartment. Exertional compartment syndrome is most common in long-distance runners and military recruits pushed past normal limits of functional tolerance.

Signs of acute compartment syndrome include compartment tightness, pain with muscle motion and weakness. Pain is often out of proportion to that expected with the injury (Sinha & Anand, 2010; Via et al., 2015). Diagnosis may be delayed in patients with multiple injuries or altered consciousness and in children in whom physical findings cannot be documented accurately. The five 'P's commonly assist compartment syndrome diagnosis: Pain, Paraesthesia, Pallor, Paralysis and Pressure rising within the compartment (Via et al., 2015). Diagnosis may be aided by direct compartment pressure monitoring: pressures exceeding 35–40 mmHg warrant intervention. The best method of managing compartment syndrome, provided simple options such as plaster cast removal are ineffective, is open fasciotomy (Via et al., 2015), where the skin and fascia are incised to release pressure (see Fig 36.13).

Fat embolism
Fat embolism occurs with all long bone fractures but is uncommonly problematic. There is increased risk post-intramedullary nail insertion (Shaikh, 2009). Fat embolus involves bone marrow entering the circulation, where fat globules lodge in capillaries. Inflammatory and thrombotic responses can follow intramedullary exposure of blood to fat cells leading to clot embolism (Kosova et al., 2015).

Signs and symptoms of fat embolism are not immediate and usually take > 24 hours to present (Kosova et al., 2015; Shaikh, 2009). Severity ranges from gradual hypoxaemia onset, neurological symptoms, fever and petechial rash to acute presentation of respiratory distress/failure leading to death (Rozema et al., 2018). The classical combination of dermatological, pulmonary and neurological signs is fat embolism syndrome. Pulmonary signs are usually evident first including hypoxaemia (Shaikh, 2009). Neurological signs of confusion, headache and even convulsions may follow (Kosova et al., 2015; Rozema et al., 2018). The clinical diagnosis is made on assessment, with few further diagnostic tools confirmative. Chest x-ray is supportive and V/Q scanning useful (Kosova et al., 2015; Newbigin et al., 2016; Shaikh, 2009). Treatment is typically non-specific including anticoagulation, anti-inflammatory and shock management strategies critically weighed against the original traumatic insult (Kosova et al., 2015; Newbigin et al., 2016).

Avascular necrosis (osteonecrosis)
Avascular necrosis or osteonecrosis is death of bone caused by inadequate blood supply to the area (Narayanan et al., 2017). Bone is often an end organ and is very dependent on blood supply without collateral circulation (Orban et al., 2009).

Most commonly affected are the epiphyses of long bones including femoral and humeral heads, but other smaller bones such as the talus are also affected (Tofferi & Gilliland, 2009). A common cause is severe trauma causing vascular occlusion and interrupted extraosseous blood supply (Tofferi & Gilliland, 2009).

Symptoms are not acutely evident. CT or MRI may be required in diagnosis. Avascular necrosis causes bone infarction and joint collapse (Barbhaiya et al., 2017). As many as one-third of young patients with neck of femur fractures have this complication, with urgent need for early fixation to improve blood flow (Fulkerson & Egol, 2009). Conservative therapies include physical therapy and anti-inflammatories, while surgical options include removal of some inner bone core to relieve pressure or bone reshaping (Orban et al., 2009).

Rehabilitation

Rehabilitation is essentially returning strength and flexibility while maintaining the patient's underlying health and endurance. It may involve drug therapies such as anti-inflammatories and steroids, muscle relaxants and analgesics. Initial MSI management, particularly where there is immobilisation or surgical intervention, dictates how soon rehabilitation can commence. The period of rehabilitation may be comparatively short or it may take months and depends on the severity of injury.

To maintain functional tissues, remobilisation is included in rehabilitation. Management of strain injuries, including those requiring surgical repair, benefit from early mobilisation to increase revascularisation and restore muscle growth replacing connective scar tissue (Jarvinen et al., 2000). Muscle strength is lost without early mobilisation. Bed rest is associated with major reduction in muscle mass and strength in as little as 4–6 weeks and reduction in bone strength may not be regained for many months once exercise is resumed (Bloomfield, 1997). Exercise and weight-bearing encourage growth plate development in children and are important in injury repair (Mirtz et al., 2011).

Long-term impact

Recovery from severe MSI can take months or years and often requires ongoing rehabilitation and other costly therapies. Where rehabilitation is inadequate, there is an increased risk of recurrence of injury. For athletes attempting to return to sport, absence of appropriate rehabilitation must be balanced against recurrence risk and even longer absence from the sport.

CASE STUDY 2

Case 11050, 0720 hrs.

Dispatch: A 69-year-old female found in the hallway by her daughter after falling. She has no obvious injuries, and is conscious and breathing.

Initial presentation: The paramedics are met at the front door by the patient's daughter and follow her into the hallway. The patient is lying on her right side with a pillow under her head.

1 ASSESS

0758 hrs Primary survey: The patient is conscious and responsive. There are no immediate life-threatening problems.

0805 hrs Vital signs survey: Perfusion status: HR 86; sinus rhythm; BP 105/80 mmHg; skin cool, pale and dry. Tympanic temperature 36°C.

Respiratory status: RR 18 bpm, shallow respirations, no adventitious sounds, normal pattern, air entry L = R.

Conscious state: GCS = 15 (E4, V5, M6); pupils equal and reactive.

0810 hrs Pertinent hx: The patient is still lying on the floor wearing only her nightie but with a blanket over her. She has good recall of the event and loss of consciousness is not suspected. She is a reliable historian. While getting out of bed to go to the toilet she remembers tripping on a fold in the carpet and falling to the floor. She felt pain in her hip from where she landed and could not get up again. Her family heard the fall and attended to her immediately.

0815 hrs Secondary survey: The patient is complaining of pain in her groin on the right side. Her right leg appears slightly shorter than her left and her foot is externally rotated away from her hip. There is a small graze to her right elbow that is not currently bleeding. No other abnormalities are found.

0820 hrs Past hx: The patient is normally well and takes antihypertensive medications.

② CONFIRM

The shortening and rotation associated with right-sided hip pain and a mechanism of a fall in an elderly patient indicates this patient possibly has a fractured right neck of femur (see Fig 36.14).

What else could it be?

Cardiovascular cause

It is important when questioning anyone about a fall to ascertain the precipitating event. Cardiovascular clues include past history and new complaints of chest pain, palpitations or breathlessness. A cardiac monitor and vital signs may help identify an ongoing issue, but it will not exclude an arrhythmia now

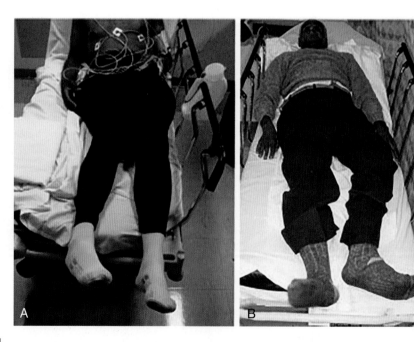

Figure 36.14
Rotation deformity typical of hip fractures. A Posterior hip dislocation in a patient with a hip prosthesis. The right leg is adducted, flexed at the knee, shortened and internally rotated. B The much less common anterior dislocation. The left leg is shortened, abducted, flexed at the knee and externally rotated, similar to the appearance of a hip fracture.
Source: Roberts (2013).

resolved (such as ventricular tachycardia or a bradycardic episode). This patient identified the reason for her fall as tripping over a fold in the carpet.

Neurological cause

In addition to establishing the precipitating event, paramedics must ensure that the patient has a full recall of the events surrounding the incident, both before and after, to establish absence of neurological symptoms before or after the event. This can be difficult as transient neurological symptoms are not always obvious to the patient.

Medical cause

Medical causes such as infection or hypoglycaemia must be considered when assessing someone who has fallen. Both can be readily excluded with history taking and assessment.

Complicating factors

Not everything to consider will occur before or during any fall or collapse. Some findings can unfold after the event. If the patient is left for long enough, pressure areas can develop. If this involves compromise to a sufficiently large area, such as a leg, this could lead to unwanted rhabdomyolysis. Exposure and immobility can cause body temperature loss, with the elderly and frail commonly unable to generate sufficient heat to avoid hypothermia. Dehydration can follow if unable to drink and urinary incontinence occurs.

3 TREAT

0840 hrs: The paramedics gain IV access and administer opioids to manage the patient's pain, taking into account her age, weight and other medications when deciding on the dose. This is provided prior to moving her limbs given the pain this is likely to cause.

4 EVALUATE

Using a short-acting analgesic such as methoxyflurane during transfer from the floor can reduce total opioid required for pain relief; providing comfort remains the aim of treatment. The paramedics align and immobilise her legs by anatomically splinting them together using triangular bandages. They pad between her bony knee and ankle prominences and incorporate slight knee flexion to relax the thigh muscles. They transfer her to the stretcher ready to administer ongoing analgesia if required. During transport they assess her feet for adequate perfusion and sensation.

CASE STUDY 3

Case 19453, 1015 hrs.

Dispatch details: A 19-year-old male has been involved in a dirt-bike accident approximately 2 hours ago. He has sustained an injury to his leg. He is being carried out of the bush to the main road. No other details are available.

Initial presentation: The paramedics meet a rescue team at a predetermined clearing site where the patient is lying on a stretcher. He is supine and in good spirits despite complaining of great pain in his leg. He was wearing suitable trail bike body armour that has been removed. He has had some rudimentary anatomical splinting applied to his left leg.

 ASSESS

1118 hrs Primary survey: The patient is conscious and responsive. There are no immediate life-threatening injuries noted, although he has a blood-soaked gauze applied over his left leg that is of concern.

1119 hrs Vital signs survey: Perfusion status: HR 116; sinus tachycardia; BP 85/50 mmHg; skin cool, pale and clammy.

Respiratory status: RR 20 bpm, normal respiration effort, no adventitious sounds, air entry L = R. SpO$_2$ 99% on air.

Conscious state: GCS = 15 (E4, V5, M6); pupils equal and reactive.

The patient rates his pain as 9 out of 10.

1121 hrs Pertinent hx: The patient is a fit and healthy young man who recalls losing control of his bike after jumping over a fallen tree without realising there was a 3-metre ditch on the other side. When he landed his bike came down heavily on his left leg. He has not walked since and his helmet has been removed. Loss of consciousness is not suspected.

1123 hrs Secondary survey: No helmet damage is noted. The patient has abrasions extending from his lower left chest to his upper abdomen. Some tenderness is felt on gentle palpation and his abdomen is soft on palpation. He is complaining of severe pain at the mid-thigh level of his left leg. A loose-fitting dressing has been placed over an open wound at the site, which has a slow continuous bleed. His left thigh is significantly swollen compared to the other side. No other abnormalities are found.

1124 hrs Past history: The patient is normally well and takes no medications.

 CONFIRM

In many cases paramedics are presented with a collection of signs and symptoms that do not appear to describe a particular condition. A critical step in determining a treatment plan in this situation is to consider what other conditions could explain the patient's presentation.

This patient has an obvious open fracture of his left femur. One of the concerns with an injury as identifiable as this is the distraction it creates and the possibility that other injuries may be missed. A full secondary survey has identified abrasions across his chest and abdomen.

What else could it be?

Soft-tissue injury only

The patient has obvious associated soft-tissue injury, although the deformity, loss of function, irregularity and pain suggest injury more likely to be fracture. The thigh wound suggests open fracture rather than soft-tissue injury alone. Assessment also reveals tenderness over the patient's upper abdomen and lower chest, indicating blunt trauma with potential for underlying ribs, lungs, liver or mesentery damage.

Major musculoskeletal trauma

Suspected femur fracture is certainly major skeletal trauma. The force required to break this strong bone is significant and should always prompt suspicion of other injuries. This injury is not in isolation and all injuries must be identified to establish a true and accurate injury profile. In this case there is also blunt truncal trauma and compromise of perfusion.

Major time-critical trauma

The patient has a major skeletal injury and can be described as a multi and time-critical trauma. This patient is in actual physiological distress with tachycardia of 116 bpm and blood pressure of 85/50 mmHg. There is evidence of a long bone fracture and a pattern of blunt trauma to his chest and abdomen, all contributing to the inadequate perfusion. This blunt truncal trauma could cause injuries including rib fractures, pulmonary contusions or haemothorax/pneumothorax. Although the patient's respiratory rate is 20, his normal pulse oximetry suggests normal lung function. Blunt abdominal trauma can result in major injuries to organs or blood vessels and is easily concealed, particularly in the presence of major distracting injury.

③ TREAT

The paramedics control the external haemorrhage with a dressing and direct pressure. They apply a precautionary cervical collar and cover the patient with blankets to minimise heat loss. IV access is obtained and opioid analgesia and fluids administered according to local guidelines.

④ EVALUATE

After 5 minutes this patient's pain remains 9/10 and his vital signs are HR 116 bpm, BP 85/50 mmHg and RR 20 bpm. The paramedics apply a traction splint and clean the wound, but do not irrigate it.

The patient remains poorly perfused and in severe pain. Further IV analgesia is titrated to reduce pain. The continuing poor perfusion is concerning. They administer further crystalloids as per local guidelines. Consideration moves to more substantial pain relief, such as IV ketamine, if adequate pain relief cannot be achieved.

> ## DIFFERENTIAL DIAGNOSIS
>
> **Isolated open fractured left femur**
> Or
> - Soft-tissue injury only
> - Major musculoskeletal injury
> - Major time-critical trauma

> ## Planning!
> - Is this patient time-critical?
> - Is this patient transport-critical?
> - What other assessments do you need to consider?
> - Have you got enough history and scene assessment?
> - What management regimens you are considering?

Future research

Future MSI research should focus on refining and improving current methods while continuing to explore new advances:

- improving understanding of what occurs to different tissues during trauma
- improving healing methods, tissue repair and regeneration
- understanding effects of ageing and disease in contributing to MSI, prevention and management
- comparing effectiveness and contributions of new medical interventions including surgical

techniques and alternatives such as pharmacological agents, prostheses, conservative therapies and rehabilitation
- optimal methods for diagnosing and timing to perform procedures.

Summary

There is a vast array of musculoskeletal injuries. Many injuries are simply managed without hospital treatment. Some require surgical intervention followed by extensive and prolonged rehabilitation. Complications can present occasionally as life-threatening or more commonly cause ongoing issues for the rest of the patient's life. Age impacts on MSIs and must be factored into assessments of patterns and mechanisms of injuries. Out-of-hospital care is a major factor in patient outcomes, with paramedics able to make positive contributions with regard to neurovascular outcomes, pain management, infection avoidance and transport to the most suitable destination. Appropriate out-of-hospital management is imperative, even where there is significant other illness or major trauma. MSIs present far more commonly than many other medical paramedic callouts such as stroke, acute coronary syndrome or asthma and must be well understood for recognition and management.

References

Abrahamsen, B., van Staa, T., Ariely, R., Olson, M., & Cooper, C. (2009). Excess mortality following hip fracture: a systematic epidemiological review. *Osteoporosis International, 20*(10), 1633–1650.

Allison, P., Dahan-Oliel, N., Jando, V. T., Yang, S. S., & Hamdy, R. C. (2011). Open fractures of the femur in children: analysis of various treatment methods. *Journal of Children's Orthopaedics, 5*(2), 101–108.

Anisha, S., Swischuk, L., & Siddharth, J. (2011). Plastic bending fractures in children. *Contemporary Diagnostic Radiology, 34*(20), 1–6.

Asplin, G., Carlsson, G., Zidén, L., & Kjellby-Wendt, G. (2017). Early coordinated rehabilitation in acute phase after hip fracture–a model for increased patient participation. *BMC Geriatrics, 17*(1), 240.

Auerbach, P. S. (2011). *Wilderness medicine* (6th ed.). St Louis: Mosby.

Australian Bureau of Statistics (ABS). (2006). *Musculoskeletal Conditions in Australia: A Snapshot, 2004–2005.* Cat. no. 4823.0.55.001. Canberra: ABS.

Australian Institute of Health and Welfare (AIHW). (2010). *The Problem of Osteoporotic Hip Fracture in Australia.* Cat. no. AUS 121. Canberra: AIHW.

Barbhaiya, M., Dong, Y., Sparks, J. A., Losina, E., Costenbader, K. H., & Katz, J. N. (2017). Administrative algorithms to identify avascular necrosis of bone among patients undergoing upper or lower extremity magnetic resonance imaging: a validation study. *BMC Musculoskeletal Disorders, 18*(1), 268.

Beck, D., & Benson, C. D. (2012). External fixation of long bones. In D. Seligson, et al. (Eds.), *External fixation in orthopedic traumatology.* USA: Springer.

Bendtsen, T. F., Nielsen, T. D., Rohde, C. V., Kibak, K., & Linde, F. (2011). Ultrasound guidance improves a continuous popliteal sciatic nerve block when compared with nerve stimulation. *Regional Anesthesia and Pain Medicine, 36*(2), 181–184.

Bentler, S. E., Liu, L., Obrizan, M., Cook, E. A., Wright, K. B., Geweke, J. F., Chrischiles, E. A., Pavlik, C. E., Wallace, R. B., Ohsfeldt, R. L., Jones, M. P., Rosenthal, G. E., & Wolinsky, F. D. (2009). The aftermath of hip fracture: discharge placement, functional status change and mortality. *American Journal of Epidemiology, 170*(10), 1290–1299.

Berglund, L. M., & Messer, T. M. (2009). Complications of volar plate fixation for managing distal radius fractures. *Journal of the American Academy of Orthopaedic Surgeons, 17*(6), 369–377.

Berkes, M., Obremskey, W. T., Scannell, B., Kent Ellington, J., Hymes, R. A., & Bosse, M. (2010). Maintenance of hardware after early postoperative infection following fracture internal fixation. *Journal of Bone and Joint Surgery, 92*, 823–828.

Berteau, J. P., Gineyts, E., Pithioux, M., Baron, C., Boivin, G., Lasaygues, P., Chabrand, P., & Follet, H. (2015). Ratio between mature and immature enzymatic cross-links correlates with post-yield cortical bone behavior: an insight into greenstick fractures of the child fibula. *Bone, 79*, 190–195.

Berzlanovich, A., Schleicher, B., & Rásky, É. (2018). Abuse and neglect of the elderly. In *Perspectives on elderly crime and victimization* (pp. 173–180). Champaign, IL: Springer.

Black, S. R., Sathy, A. K., Jo, C., Wiley, M. R., Minei, J. P., & Starr, A. J. (2016). Improved survival after pelvic fracture: 13-year experience at a single trauma center using a multidisciplinary institutional protocol. *Journal of Orthopaedic Trauma, 30*(1), 22–28.

Black, W. S., & Becker, J. A. (2009). Common forearm fractures in adults. *American Family Physician, 80*(10), 1096–1102.

Bleakley, C. M., O'Connor, S., Tully, M. A., Rocke, L. G., MacAuley, D. C., & McDonough, S. M. (2007). The PRICE Study: design of randomised controlled trial comparing standard versus cryokinetic ice applications in the management of acute ankle sprain. *BMC Musculoskeletal Disorders*, 8, 125.

Bloomfield, S. A. (1997). Changes in musculoskeletal structure and function with prolonged bed rest. *Medicine & Science in Sports & Exercise*, 2(2), 197–206.

Brown, D., & Edwards, H. (2012). *Lewis's Medical-surgical nursing: assessment and management of clinical problems* (2nd ed.). Sydney: Elsevier.

Byrne, J. P., Nathens, A. B., Gomez, D., Pincus, D., & Jenkinson, R. J. (2017). Timing of femoral shaft fracture fixation following major trauma: a retrospective cohort study of United States trauma centers. *PLoS Medicine*, 14(7), e1002336.

Cameron, J. L. (2010). *Current surgical therapy* (10th ed.). Philadelphia: Elsevier.

Canale, S. T., & Beaty, J. H. (2007). *Campbell's operative orthopaedics* (11th ed.). Philadelphia: Elsevier.

Chan, O., Del Buono, A., Best, T. M., & Maffulli, N. (2012). Acute muscle strain injuries: a proposed new classification system. *Knee Surgery, Sports Traumatology, Arthroscopy*, 20(11), 2356–2362.

Changstrom, B. G., Brou, L., Khodaee, M., Braund, C., & Comstock, R. D. (2015). Epidemiology of stress fracture injuries among US high school athletes, 2005-2006 through 2012-2013. *The American Journal of Sports Medicine*, 43(1), 26–33.

Chen, R. C., Harris, D. J., Leduc, S., Borelli, J. J., Tornetta, P., & Ricci, W. M. (2010). Is ulnar nerve transposition beneficial during open reduction internal fixation of distal humerus fractures? *Journal of Orthopaedic Trauma*, 24(7), 391–394.

Cheng, M., Cheung, M. T., Lee, K. Y., Lee, K. B., Chan, S. C. H., Wu, A. C. Y., Chow, Y. F., Chang, A. M. L., Ho, H. F., & Yau, K. K. W. (2015). Improvement in institutional protocols leads to decreased mortality in patients with haemodynamically unstable pelvic fractures. *Emergency Medicine Journal*, 32(3), 214–220.

Clout, A., Narayanasamy, N., & Harris, I. (2016). Trends in the incidence of atypical femoral fractures and bisphosphonate therapy. *Journal of Orthopaedic Surgery*, 24(1), 36–40.

Davies, A. M. (2008). Pathological fractures in the immature skeleton. *Imaging in Pediatric Skeletal Trauma*, 2, 337–355.

Dhingra, M., Dhingra, V. K., & Moga, A. (2017). Rapid diagnosis of "Fatigue" stress fractures using bone scintigraphy: a practical approach. *International Journal of Orthopaedics*, 3(2), 710–713.

Dönmez, G., Diliçıkık, U., Aydoğ, S. T., Evrenos, M. K., Tetik, O., Demirel, M., & Doral, M. N. (2015). *Muscle Injuries: Strains, Contusions, and Ruptures. Sports Injuries: Prevention, Diagnosis, Treatment and Rehabilitation*, pp.1-18.

Drubach, L. A. (2017). Nuclear medicine techniques in pediatric bone imaging. In *Seminars in nuclear medicine* (Vol. 47, pp. 190–203). Elsevier.

Dyer, S., Diong, J., Crotty, M., & Sherrington, C. (2017). Rehabilitation following hip fracture. In *Orthogeriatrics* (pp. 145–163). Champaign, IL: Springer.

Eastwood, D. M., & de Gheldere, A. (2011). Physeal injuries in children. *Surgery*, 29(4), 146–152.

Edwards, B. J., Sun, M., West, D. P., Guindani, M., Lin, Y. H., Lu, H., Hu, M., Barcenas, C., Bird, J., Feng, C., & Saraykar, S. (2016). Incidence of atypical femur fractures in cancer patients: the MD Anderson Cancer Center experience. *Journal of Bone and Mineral Research*, 31(8), 1569–1576.

Farahmand, S., Arshadi, A., Bagheri-Hariri, S., Shahriarian, S., Arbab, M., & Sedaghat, M. (2017). Extremity fracture diagnosis using bedside ultrasound in pediatric trauma patients referring to emergency department; a diagnostic study. *International Journal of Pediatrics*, 5(10), 5959–5964.

Finch, C. F., Kemp, J. L., & Clapperton, A. J. (2015). The incidence and burden of hospital-treated sports-related injury in people aged 15+ years in Victoria, Australia, 2004–2010: a future epidemic of osteoarthritis? *Osteoarthritis and Cartilage*, 23(7), 1138–1143.

Fulkerson, E. W., & Egol, K. A. (2009). Timing issues in fracture management. *Bulletin of the NYU Hospital for Joint Diseases*, 67(1), 58–67.

Gage, B. E., McIlvain, N. M., Collins, C. L., Fields, S. K., & Dawn Comstock, R. (2012). Epidemiology of 6.6 million knee injuries presenting to United States emergency departments from 1999 through 2008. *Academic Emergency Medicine: Official Journal of the Society for Academic Emergency Medicine*, 19(4), 378–385.

Gillette, C. M., Doberstein, S. T., DeSerano, D. L., & Linnell, E. J. (2017). The effect of elevation on volumetric measurements of the lower extremity. *International Journal of Kinesiology and Sports Science*, 5(3), 1–5.

Gnanasegaran, G., Cook, G., Adamson, K., & Fogelman, I. (2009). Patterns, variants, artefacts and pitfalls in conventional radionuclide bone imaging and SPECT/CT. *Seminars in Nuclear Medicine*, 39(6), 380–395.

Gray, S. E., & Collie, A. (2017). The nature and burden of occupational injury among first responder occupations: a retrospective cohort study in Australian workers. *Injury*, 48(11), 2470–2477.

Green, N. E., & Swiontkowski, M. F. (2009). *Skeletal trauma in children* (4th ed.). Philadelphia: Elsevier.

Gustilo, R. B., Merkow, R. L., & Templeman, D. (1990). The management of open fractures. *Journal of Bone and Joint Surgery*, 72, 299–304.

Handoll, H. H. G., Queally, J. M., & Parker, M. J. (2011). Pre-operative traction for hip fractures in adults. *The Cochrane Database of Systematic Reviews*, (12), CD000168.

Hartmann, F. V. G., Novaes, M. R. C. G., & de Carvalho, M. R. (2017). Femoral nerve block versus intravenous fentanyl in adult patients with hip fractures–a systematic review. *Brazilian Journal of Anesthesiology (English Edition)*, *67*(1), 67–71.

Hermans, E., Edwards, M. J. R., Goslings, J. C., & Biert, J. (2018). Open pelvic fracture: the killing fracture? *Journal of Orthopaedic Surgery and Research*, *13*(1), 83.

Hogan, C. J. (2011). Pain control in trauma patients. *Trauma Reports*, *12*(5), 1–12.

Hoppe, S., Keel, M. J. B., Rueff, N., Rhoma, I., Roche, S., & Maqungo, S. (2015). Early versus delayed application of Thomas splints in patients with isolated femur shaft fractures: the benefits quantified. *Injury*, *46*(12), 2410–2412.

Immerman, I., Price, A. E., Alfonso, I., & Grossman, J. A. (2014). Lower extremity nerve trauma. *Bulletin (Hospital for Joint Diseases (New York, N.Y.))*, *72*(1), 43–52.

Jarvinen, T. A. H., Kaariainen, M., Jarvinen, M., & Kalimo, H. (2000). Muscle strain injuries. *Current Opinion in Rheumatology*, *12*(2), 155–161.

Jayaraman, S., Haque, S., & Ellis, D. (2016). Audit on adequacy of back-slab application for ankle fracture. *The Online Journal of Clinical Audits*, *8*(4).

Jung, H. G., Kim, J. I., Park, J. Y., Park, J. T., Eom, J. S., & Lee, D. O. (2016). Is Hardware removal recommended after ankle fracture repair? *BioMed Research International*, *2016*.

Kassam, A. A. M., Gough, A. T., Davies, J., & Yarlagadda, R. (2018). Can we reduce morphine use in elderly, proximal femoral fracture patients using a fascia iliac block? *Geriatric Nursing*, *39*(1), 84–87.

Kemp, A. M., Maguire, S. A., Nuttall, D., Collins, P., & Dunstan, F. (2014). Bruising in children who are assessed for suspected physical abuse. *Archives of Disease in Childhood*, *99*(2), 108–113.

Khazzam, M., Tassone, C., Liu, X. C., Lyon, R., Freeto, B., Schwab, J., & Thometz, J. (2009). Fixation in treating femur fractures in children. *American Journal of Orthopedics*, *38*(3), E49–E55.

Kleweno, C. P., Jawa, A., Wells, J. H., O'Brien, T. G., Higgins, L. D., Harris, M. B., & Warner, J. P. (2011). Midshaft clavicular fractures: comparison of intramedullary pin and plate fixation. *Journal of Shoulder and Elbow Surgery*, *20*(7), 1114–1117.

Ko, C., Baird, M., Close, M., & Cassas, K. J. (2019). The diagnostic accuracy of ultrasound in detecting distal radius fractures in a pediatric population. *Clinical Journal of Sport Medicine: Official Journal of the Canadian Academy of Sport Medicine*, *29*(5), 426–429.

Kondo, A., Zierler, B. K., Isokawa, Y., Hagino, H., Ito, Y., & Richerson, M. (2010). Comparison of lengths of hospital stay after surgery and mortality in elderly hip fracture patients between Japan and the United States: the relationship between the lengths of hospital stay after surgery and mortality. *Disability and Rehabilitation*, *32*(10), 826–835.

Kosova, E., Bergmark, B., & Piazza, G. (2015). Fat embolism syndrome. *Circulation*, *131*(3), 317–320.

Kreisfeld, R., & Newson, R. (2006). *Hip Fracture Injuries. Briefing no. 8*. South Australia: AIHW National Injury Surveillance Unit, Research Centre for Injury Studies, Flinders University.

Lane, T. J., Collie, A., & Hassani-Mahmooei, B. (2016). *Work-related injury and illness in Australia, 2004 to 2014*. AU: Melbourne.

LeBlanc, E. S., Hillier, T. A., Pedula, K. L., Rizzo, J. H., Cawthon, P. M., Fink, H. A., Cauley, J. A., Bauer, D. C., Black, D. M., Cunnings, S. R., & Browner, W. S. (2011). Hip fracture and increased short term but not long term mortality in healthy older women. *Archives of Internal Medicine*, *171*(20), 1831–1837.

Leffers, D., & Collins, L. (2009). An overview of the use of bone scintigraphy in sports medicine. *Sports Medicine and Arthroscopy Review*, *17*(1), 21–24.

Lystad, R. P., Cameron, C. M., & Mitchell, R. J. (2017). Mortality risk among older Australians hospitalised with hip fracture: a population-based matched cohort study. *Archives of Osteoporosis*, *12*(1), 67.

Mackey, A. L., Mikkelsen, U. R., Magnusson, S. P., & Kjaer, M. (2012). Rehabilitation of muscle after injury: the role of anti-inflammatory drugs. *Scandinavian Journal of Medicine and Science in Sports*, *22*(4).

Maffulli, N., Del Buono, A., Oliva, F., Via, A. G., Frizziero, A., Barazzuol, M., Brancaccio, P., Freschi, M., Galletti, S., Lisitano, G., & Melegati, G. (2015). Muscle injuries: a brief guide to classification and management. *Translational Medicine @ UniSa*, *12*, 14.

Malanga, G. A., Yan, N., & Stark, J. (2015). Mechanisms and efficacy of heat and cold therapies for musculoskeletal injury. *Postgraduate Medicine*, *127*(1), 57–65.

Marx, J., Hockberger, R., & Walls, R. (2010). *Rosen's emergency medicine* (7th ed.). St Louis: Mosby.

Maqungo, S., Allen, J., Carrara, H., Roche, S., & Rueff, N. (2015). Early application of the Thomas splint for femur shaft fractures in a Level 1 Trauma Unit. *SA Orthopaedic Journal*, *14*(3), 75–79.

Matcuk, G. R., Jr, Mahanty, S. R., Skalski, M. R., Patel, D. B., White, E. A., & Gottsegen, C. J. (2016). Stress fractures: pathophysiology, clinical presentation, imaging features, and treatment options. *Emergency Radiology*, *23*(4), 365–375. doi:10.1007/s10140-016-1390-5.

Matullo, K. S., Gangavalli, A., & Nwachuku, C. (2016). Review of lower extremity traction in current orthopaedic trauma. *JAAOS-Journal of the American Academy of Orthopaedic Surgeons*, *24*(9), 600–606.

Mayer, S. W., Joyner, P. W., Almekinders, L. C., & Parekh, S. G. (2014). Stress fractures of the foot and ankle in athletes. *Sports Health*, *6*(6), 481–491.

McKeon, K., O'Donnell, J. C., & Gordon, J. E. (2010). Pediatric femoral shaft fractures: current and future treatment. *International Journal of Clinical Rheumatology*, *5*(6), 687–697.

Melvin, J. S., & Mehta, S. (2011). Patellar fractures in adults. *Journal of the American Academy of Orthopaedic Surgeons*, *19*(4), 198–207.

Mirtz, T. A., Chandler, J. P., & Eyers, C. M. (2011). The effects of physical activity on the epiphyseal growth plates: a review of the literature on normal physiology and clinical implications. *Journal of Clinical Medicine Research*, *3*(1), 1–7.

Moen, M. H., Reurink, G., Weir, A., Tol, J. L., Maas, M., & Goudswaard, G. J. (2014). Predicting return to play after hamstring injuries. *British Journal of Sports Medicine*, *48*.

Moore, A. M., Wagner, I. J., & Fox, I. K. (2015). Principles of nerve repair in complex wounds of the upper extremity. In *Seminars in plastic surgery* (Vol. 29, p. 40). Thieme Medical Publishers.

Moradi, B., Zahlten-Hinguranage, A., Lehner, B., & Zeifang, F. (2010). The impact of pathological fractures on therapy outcome in patients with primary malignant bone tumours. *International Orthopaedics*, *34*(7), 1017–1023.

Morelli, K. M., Brown, L. B., & Warren, G. L. (2018). Effect of NSAIDs on recovery from acute skeletal muscle injury: a systematic review and Meta-analysis. *The American Journal of Sports Medicine*, *46*(1), 224–233. doi:10.1177/0363546517697957.

Morshed, S., Miclau, T., Bembon, O., Cohen, M., Knudson, M. M., & Colford, J. M. (2009). Delayed internal fixation of femoral shaft fracture reduces mortality among patients with multisystem trauma. *Journal of Bone and Joint Surgery*, *91*(1), 3–13.

Nackenson, J., Baez, A. A., & Meizoso, J. P. (2017). A descriptive analysis of traction splint utilization and IV analgesia by Emergency Medical Services. *Prehospital and Disaster Medicine*, *32*(6), 631–635.

Nadel, H. R. (2010). Pediatric bone scintigraphy update. *Seminars in Nuclear Medicine*, *40*(1), 31–40.

Narayanan, A., Khanchandani, P., Borkar, R. M., Ambati, C. R., Roy, A., Han, X., Bhoskar, R. N., Ragampeta, S., Gannon, F., Mysorekar, V., & Karanam, B. (2017). Avascular necrosis of femoral head: a metabolomic, biophysical, biochemical, electron microscopic and histopathological characterization. *Scientific Reports*, *7*(1), 10721.

Nau, C., Marzi, I., Ziebarth, K., & Berger, S. (2015). Fractures in children and adolescents. In *Intramedullary nailing* (pp. 395–417). London: Springer.

Newbigin, K., Souza, C. A., Torres, C., Marchiori, E., Gupta, A., Inacio, J., Armstrong, M., & Peña, E. (2016). Fat embolism syndrome: state-of-the-art review focused on pulmonary imaging findings. *Respiratory Medicine*, *113*, 93–100.

Offluoglu, O., Erol, B., Ozgen, Z., & Yildiz, M. (2009). Minimally invasive treatment of pathological fractures of the humeral shaft. *International Orthopaedics*, *33*(3), 707–712.

Orban, H. B., Cristescu, V., & Dragusanu, M. (2009). Avascular necrosis of the femoral head. *MEDICA: A Journal of Clinical Medicine*, *1*, 26–34.

Orchard, J., & Best, T. (2002). The management of muscle strain injuries: an early return versus the risk of recurrence. *Clinical Journal of Sport Medicine*, *12*(1), 3–5.

Ota, S., Inoue, R., Shiozaki, T., Yamamoto, Y., Hashimoto, N., Takeda, O., Yoshikawa, K., Ito, J., & Ishibashi, Y. (2017). Atypical femoral fracture after receiving antiresorptive drugs in breast cancer patients with bone metastasis. *Breast Cancer (Tokyo, Japan)*, *24*(4), 601–607.

Papagelopoulos, P. J., Mavrogenis, A. F., Savvidou, O. D., Benetos, I. S., Galanis, E. C., & Soucacos, P. N. (2008). Pathological fractures in primary bone sarcomas. *Injury*, *39*(4), 395–403.

Pape, H.-C., Tornetta, P., Tarkin, I., Tzioupis, C., Sabeson, V., & Olson, S. A. (2009). Timing of fracture fixation in multitrauma patients: the role of early total care and damage control surgery. *Journal of the American Academy of Orthopaedic Surgeons*, *17*(9), 541–549.

Parkes, R. J., Parkes, G., & James, K. (2017). A systematic review of cost-effectiveness, comparing traction to intramedullary nailing of femoral shaft fractures, in the less economically developed context. *BMJ Global Health*, *2*(3), e000313.

Patel, D. S., Roth, M., & Kapil, N. (2011). Stress fractures: diagnosis, treatment and prevention. *American Family Physician*, *83*(1), 39–46.

Paul, G., & Hoy, B. (2015). An exploratory ergonomic study of musculoskeletal disorder prevention in the Queensland Ambulance Service. *Journal of Health, Safety and Environment*, *31*(3), 1–13.

Perkins, Z. B., De'Ath, H. D., Sharp, G., & Tai, R. M. (2012). Factors affecting outcome after traumatic limb amputation. *British Journal of Surgery*, *99*(S1), 75–86.

Pfenninger, J. L., & Fowler, G. C. (2010). *Pfenninger and Fowler's procedures for primary care* (3rd ed.). Philadelphia: Saunders.

Pierce, M. C. (2017). *Bruising characteristics from unintentional injuries in children: the 'green flag' study*.

Pierce, M. C., Kaczor, K., Aldridge, S., O'Flynn, J., & Lorenz, D. J. (2010). Bruising characteristics discriminating physical child abuse from accidental trauma. *Pediatrics*, *125*(1), 67–74.

Pollock, N., James, S. L., Lee, J. C., & Chakraverty, R. (2014). British athletics muscle injury classification: a new grading system. *British Journal of Sports Medicine*, pp.bjsports-2013.

Pountos, I., Clegg, J., & Siddiqui, A. (2010). Diagnosis and treatment of greenstick and torus fractures of the distal radius in children: a prospective randomised single blind study. *Journal of Children's Orthopaedics*, *4*, 321–326.

Rao, A., Pimpalwar, Y., Sahdev, R., Sinha, S., & Yadu, N. (2017). Diagnostic ultrasound: an effective tool for early detection of stress fractures of tibia. *Journal of Archives in Military Medicine*, *5*(2).

Resnick, D., & Kransdorf, M. (2005). *Bone and joint imaging* (3rd ed.). Philadelphia: Elsevier.

Roberts, D. (2009). *Clinical procedures in emergency medicine* (5th ed.). St Louis: Elsevier.

Roberts, J. L., Din, N. U., Williams, M., Hawkes, C. A., Charles, J. M., Hoare, Z., Morrison, V., Alexander, S., Lemmey, A., Sackley, C., & Logan, P. (2017). Development of an evidence-based complex intervention for community rehabilitation of patients with hip fracture using realist review, survey and focus groups. *BMJ Open*, *7*(10), e014362.

Roberts, J. R. (2013). *Roberts and Hedges' clinical procedures in emergency medicine* (6th ed.). Philadelphia: Saunders.

Roberts, M. H., Sim, M. R., Black, O., & Smith, P. (2015). Occupational injury risk among ambulance officers and paramedics compared with other healthcare workers in Victoria, Australia: analysis of workers' compensation claims from 2003 to 2012. *Occupational and Environmental Medicine*, pp.oemed-2014.

Robertson, A. K., Snow, E., Browne, T. S., Inneh, I., & Hill, J. F. (2018). Who gets compartment syndrome?: a retrospective analysis of the national and local incidence of compartment syndrome in patients with supracondylar humerus fractures. *Journal of Pediatric Orthopaedics*, *38*(5), e252–e256.

Rozema, R., El, M. M., Boonstra, E. A., Jacobs, B., & Poos, H. P. A. M. (2018). Challenges in the diagnostic management of fat embolism syndrome—from divergence in clinical presentation to diagnosis. *Nederlands Tijdschrift Voor Geneeskunde*, *162*, D2259.

Ruggieri, P., Mavrogenis, A. F., Casadei, R., Errani, C., Angelini, A., Calabro, T., Pala, E., & Mercuri, M. (2010). Protocol of surgical treatment of long bone pathological fractures. *Injury*, *41*(11), 1161–1167.

Ryznar, E., Rosado, N., & Flaherty, E. G. (2015). Understanding forearm fractures in young children: abuse or not abuse? *Child Abuse & Neglect*, *47*, 132–139.

Safe Work Australia. (2014). *Australian workers' compensation statistics, 2012–13*. Canberra, Australia: Safe Work Australia.

Sanford, A. M., Morley, J. E., & McKee, A. (2018). *Orthogeriatrics and Hip Fractures*.

Scerbo, M. H., Holcomb, J. B., Taub, E., Gates, K., Love, J. D., Wade, C. E., & Cotton, B. A. (2017). The trauma center is too late: major limb trauma without a pre-hospital tourniquet has increased death from hemorrhagic shock. *The Journal of Trauma and Acute Care Surgery*, *83*(6), 1165–1172.

Schmal, H., Strohm, P. C., Niemeyer, P., Reising, K., Kuminack, K., & Sudkamp, N. P. (2010). Fractures of the patella in children and adolescents. *Acta Orthopædica Belgica*, *76*, 644–650.

Schmid, G. L., Lippmann, S., Unverzagt, S., Hofmann, C., Deutsch, T., & Frese, T. (2017). The investigation of suspected fracture—a comparison of ultrasound with conventional imaging: systematic review and meta-analysis. *Deutsches Ärzteblatt International*, *114*(45), 757.

Schoenfeld, B. J. (2018). Non-steroidal anti-inflammatory drugs may blunt more than pain. *Acta Physiologica*, *222*(2), e12990.

Shaikh, N. (2009). Emergency management of fat embolism syndrome. *Journal of Emergencies, Trauma, and Shock*, *2*(1), 29–33.

Sharma, S., Iorio, R., Specht, L. M., Davies-Lepie, S., & Healy, W. L. (2010). Complications of femoral nerve block for total knee arthroplasty. *Clinical Orthopaedics and Related Research*, *468*, 135–140.

Sharma, S., Ohri, P., Singh, H., & Singh, S. (2017). Comparison between Ultrasonography and Conventional Radiography in the Detection of Bony Fractures. *Indian J Appl Radiol*, *3*(1), 112.

Siebenbürger, G., Van Delden, D., Helfen, T., Haasters, F., Böcker, W., & Ockert, B. (2015). Timing of surgery for open reduction and internal fixation of displaced proximal humeral fractures. *Injury*, *46*, S58–S62.

Siegenthaler, A., Eichenberger, U., Schmidlin, K., Arendt-Nielsen, L., & Curatolo, M. (2010). What does local tenderness say about the origin of pain? An investigation of cervical zygapophysial joint pain. *Anaesthesia and Analgesia*, *110*(3), 923–927.

Singh, A. P., Kohli, V., & Bajwa, S. J. S. (2016). Intravenous analgesia with opioids versus femoral nerve block with 0.2% ropivacaine as preemptive analgesic for fracture femur: a randomized comparative study. *Anesthesia, Essays and Researches*, *10*(2), 338.

Sinha, V. K., & Anand, S. (2010). Extremity and orthopaedic injuries. *Medical Journal Armed Forces India*, *66*, 342–346.

Smith, G. H., Tsang, J., Molyneux, S. G., & White, T. O. (2011). The hidden blood loss after hip fracture. *Injury*, *42*(2), 133–135.

SooHoo, N. F., Krenek, L., Eagan, M. J., Gurbani, B., Ko, C. Y., & Zingmond, D. S. (2009). Complication rates following open reduction and internal fixation of ankle fractures. *Journal of Bone and Joint Surgery*, *91*, 1042–1049.

Sund, R., Riihimaki, J., Makela, M., Vehtari, A., Luthje, P., Huusko, T., & Hakkinen, U. (2009). Modelling the length of the care episode after hip fracture: does the type of fracture matter? *Scandinavian Journal of Surgery*, *98*(3), 169–174.

Swenson, D. M., Collins, C. L., Best, T. M., Flanigan, D. C., Fields, S. K., & Comstock, R. D. (2013). Epidemiology of knee injuries among US high school athletes, 2005/06–2010/11. *Medicine and Science in Sports and Exercise*, *45*(3), 462.

Teixeira, P. G., Brown, C. V., Emigh, B., Long, M., Foreman, M., Eastridge, B., Gale, S., Truitt, M. S., Dissanaike, S., Duane, T., Holcomb, J., Eastman, A., Regner, J., & Texas Tourniquet Study Group. (2018). Civilian prehospital tourniquet use is associated with improved survival in patients with peripheral vascular injury. *Journal of the American College of Surgeons*, *226*(5), 769–776.e1.

Tofferi, J. K., & Gilliland, W. (2009). *Avascular necrosis.* Retrieved from http://emedicine.medscape.com/article/333364-overview.

Tonino, P. M., & Sinclair, M. K. (2011). Pathophysiology of muscle injuries. *Orthopaedic Journal of Sports Medicine, 1,* 31–40.

Townsend, C. M., Beauchamp, R. D., Evers, B. M., & Mattox, K. L. (2012). *Sabiston textbook of surgery: the biological basis of modern surgical practice* (19th ed.). Philadelphia: Saunders.

Üzümcügil, F., Saricaoglu, F., & Aypar, Ü. (2015). *Anesthesia managements for Sports-Related musculoskeletal injuries.* (pp. 1–13). Sports Injuries: Prevention, Diagnosis, Treatment and Rehabilitation.

Vallier, H. A., Moore, T. A., Como, J. J., Wilczewski, P. A., Steinmetz, M. P., Wagner, K. G., Smith, C. E., Wang, X. F., & Dolenc, A. J. (2015). Complications are reduced with a protocol to standardize timing of fixation based on response to resuscitation. *Journal of Orthopaedic Surgery and Research, 10*(1), 155.

Via, A. G., Oliva, F., Spoliti, M., & Maffulli, N. (2015). Acute compartment syndrome. *Muscles, Ligaments and Tendons Journal, 5*(1), 18.

Volkman, T. (2016). Femoral fractures in children under 2 years of age in Western Australia: how common is inflicted injury and what are the risk factors? *European Journal of Pediatrics, 175*(11), 1861–1862.

Von Keudell, A. G., Weaver, M. J., Appleton, P. T., Bae, D. S., Dyer, G. S., Heng, M., Jupiter, J. B., & Vrahas, M. S. (2015). Diagnosis and treatment of acute extremity compartment syndrome. *The Lancet, 386*(10000), 1299–1310.

Weinberg, E. R., Tunik, M. G., & Tsung, J. W. (2010). Accuracy of clinical performed point of care ultrasound for the diagnosis of fractures in children and young adults. *Injury, 41*(8), 862–868.

White, C. E., Hsu, J. R., & Holcomb, J. B. (2009). Haemodynamically unstable pelvic fractures. *Injury, 40*(10), 1023–1030.

Wik, T. S., Aurstad, A. T., & Finsen, V. (2009). Colles' fracture: dorsal splint or complete cast during the first 10 days? *Injury, 40*(4), 400–404.

Wild, M., Gehrmann, S., Jungbluth, P., Hakami, M., Thelen, S., Betsch, M., Windolf, J., & Wenda, K. (2010). Treatment strategies for intramedullary nailing of femoral shaft fractures. *Orthopaedics, 33*(10), 726.

Williams, B., Chau, M., McCreary, D., Cunningham, B., Peña, F., & Swiontkowski, M. (2017). Does Hardware removal improve function following ankle open reduction and internal fixation? *Foot & Ankle Orthopaedics,* doi: doi.org/10.1177/2473011417S000409.

Woodhouse, J. B., & McNally, E. G. (2011). Ultrasound of skeletal muscle injury: an update. *Seminars in Ultrasound, CT and MRI, 32*(2), 91–100.

Woolf, A. D., Erwin, J., & March, L. (2012). The need to address the burden of musculoskeletal conditions. *Best Practice & Research Clinical Rheumatology, 26*(2), 183–224.

Wright, A. A., Taylor, J. B., Ford, K. R., Siska, L., & Smoliga, J. M. (2015). Risk factors associated with lower extremity stress fractures in runners: a systematic review with meta-analysis. *British Journal of Sports Medicine, 49*(23), 1517–1523.

Yoshihara, H., & Yoneoka, D. (2014). Demographic epidemiology of unstable pelvic fracture in the United States from 2000 to 2009: trends and in-hospital mortality. *The Journal of Trauma and Acute Care Surgery, 76*(2), 380–385.

Zusman, E. Z., Dawes, M. G., Edwards, N., & Ashe, M. C. (2017). A systematic review of evidence for older adults' sedentary behavior and physical activity after hip fracture. *Clinical Rehabilitation,* doi: doi.org/10.1177/0269215517741665.

CHAPTER 37

Traumatic Spinal Injuries

By Dianne Inglis and Jeff Kenneally

OVERVIEW

- Spinal injuries can be divided into two major types: spinal column injuries and spinal cord injuries (SCIs).
- SCI may be caused by primary mechanisms at the time of the trauma or develop with inflammatory response to injury.
- Moving an SCI patient requires specialised equipment and teamwork.
- In the out-of-hospital setting it is often impossible to provide the degree of spinal care recommended in specialist spinal care wards.
- SCI may be the major presenting problem or part of a greater range of traumatic injuries.
- Spinal injuries may present with a full suite of classic symptoms or some combination of them.
- The primary out-of-hospital aim is SCI recognition and protection against further injury.
- Close patient observation is important, as changes to respiration, pulse, blood pressure, body tem-

perature and motor and sensory function are all possible with SCI.
- Victims of major trauma should be treated as potential SCI patients.
- Some victims of lesser trauma may be successfully cleared of spinal injury in the out-of-hospital setting provided defined criteria can be satisfied.
- Children, particularly under 8 years of age, can suffer SCI without vertebral structure injury making them difficult to clear of spinal injury in the out-of-hospital setting.
- The elderly may injure the spinal column from comparatively minor trauma.
- Despite crippling disabilities caused by SCI, cost to the community and the typical patient being a young adult, there have been few advances in rehabilitation of damaged spinal cord tissue.

Introduction

Spinal injuries can be divided into two major types: spinal column injuries and spinal cord injuries. **Spinal column injuries** involve any of the vertebral structural components of the spine—muscles, ligaments and bones—and result in sprains, strains, fractures and dislocations. Characterised by pain and localised tenderness, spinal column injuries can occur in isolation or include cord injury. **Spinal cord injuries** are less common but far more debilitating, characterised by cord function alterations including motor and sensation. In some instances, SCI can be sustained without associated column injury.

Pathophysiology

The spinal column

The spinal column performs three disparate roles. It must provide sufficient strength and structure to support the upper body (see Fig 37.1), allow upper body mobility and flexibility, and provide spinal cord protection. Each of these functions can compromise the others. Vertebral bodies are relatively dense 'blocks' of bone joined by flexible fibrous

discs to provide a strong column. Extending from each vertebral body posterior is a bony arch with articular surfaces that guide movement of each vertebra. Bony processes extending from the arch provide areas for muscle attachment. The spinal cord resides within the arch, protected by bone and with nerve roots exiting at each vertebral segment (see Fig 37.2).

The spinal column is classified by regions: the first seven vertebrae form the cervical region (C1–C7), the next 12 the thoracic region (T1–T12), the next five the lumbar region (L1–L5), the next five are essentially fused to form the sacrum and the final four form the coccyx. Thoracic vertebrae have ribs articulating between two vertebral lamina and the transverse process. The sacrum forms the posterior pelvis and together with the lumbar vertebrae is substantially weight-bearing. The coccyx is considered a legacy of evolution. When viewed posteriorly, the normal spinal column appears straight. However, from the lateral view the spinal column has a number of curves (kyphosis) including anterior cervical curve, posterior thoracic curve before a final lumbar anterior curve. This has implications for patient handling and immobilisation.

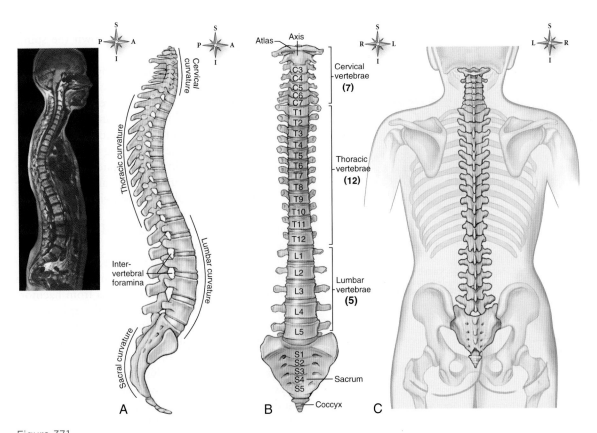

Figure 37.1
The vertebral column.
A Right lateral view. **B** Anterior view. **C** Posterior view. The photo inset shows a midline sagittal MRI of the vertebral column.
Source: Patton & Thibodeau (2012).

Vertebral injuries may involve the vertebral body, lamina or the processes. Potential for cord involvement depends on injury type and extent of damage to vertebrae and surrounding tissues and vessels.

The spinal cord

The spinal cord and brain comprise the central nervous system (CNS). The spinal cord runs from the medulla oblongata in the brainstem down to around the second lumbar vertebra. It transmits nervous impulses up and down its length, including those of sensory feedback and motor function. It also provides reflex arcs. Within the cord are multiple columns or tracts, each with a differing transmission function. Injury can result in complete cord transection, or more commonly incomplete. Partial cord injury can produce differing dysfunction depending on tract(s) affected. Some continued function may be noted, important in rehabilitation and ongoing quality of life (Rowland et al., 2008).

At each spinal segment between vertebrae, a pair of spinal nerves arises from the cord. These provide sensory (receptor) and motor (effector) nerves and are part of the peripheral nervous system. From the lower thoracic segment onwards spinal nerves may travel downwards or join soon after arising from the cord. This is a hugely important feature in SCI assessment. Injury to the spinal cord can also affect cardiovascular and respiratory systems, bladder and bowel control and, importantly, temperature control.

Spinal injury is frequently traumatic following mechanisms including falls, diving accidents, sporting collisions and motor vehicle crashes. Some may be non-traumatic, including following degenerative vertebrae disease or secondary to oncological causes allowing increased injury likelihood and severity from lesser trauma (AIHW: Tovell, 2018).

Spinal cord injury

In Australia in 2012–2013, 241 people (< 15 years of age) suffered SCI from traumatic causes of which 227 were discharged from hospital alive; 79% were male. Prevalence is greatest in the 15–24 age group, with 26% of injuries reported. Land transport crashes accounted for 46% of injuries followed by falls 34%, water related 8% and horse and football related 2% each. One third were associated with sporting/leisure

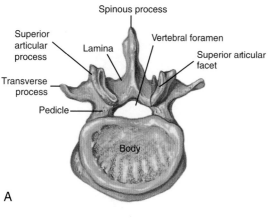

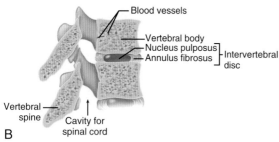

Figure 37.2
A Lumbar vertebra, superior view;
B Intervertebral disc.
Source: McCance & Huether (2014).

activities. 37% of the land crashes were on quad bikes. Most commonly the cervical spine was involved (55% of all injuries), frequently at C4–C5 (62%), followed by thoracic spine (31%), lumbar (14%) while 68% of injuries were incomplete (AIHW: Tovell, 2018). In the United States, more than a quarter of a million people live with SCI with 17,000 new cases annually, 80% male. Two-thirds are caused by vehicle accidents and falls (White & Black, 2016). Globally, injury rates are rising in developing countries due to vehicle accidents; rates from elderly falls are rising in developed nations (Lee et al., 2014).

Primary SCI mechanisms

Primary SCI is nerve and vascular damage caused by the initial mechanism and sustained pressure from subsequent vertebra displacement. Classification can be subdivided depending on the direction of trauma to the spine.

- Pushing the spine backwards causing *hyperextension* may compress the posterior spine. This injury is typical of the head being pushed backwards when struck from the front.
- Pushing the spine forwards causing *hyperflexion* may compress the anterior spine. This injury is typically caused by force to the back, bending the person forwards.

- Pushing the spine downwards causing *compression* may cause generalised injury down the spinal column.
- Pulling the spine along its length causes *over-stretching*. This typically results from the head being held and the body weight producing a pulling force down the spine, as occurs in accidental or intentional hanging.
- *Rotation* of the spine in differing directions causes vertebrae to move in opposite directions. Typically this arises in high tumbling falls and motor vehicle trauma such as rollover or side-impact collision.

Significant energy is required to injure spinal vertebrae, decreasing with age and bone disease.

Causes of secondary SCI

After the initial mechanical injury, a secondary injury can follow. Within 2 hours of injury, detectable changes become apparent. Oedema from haemorrhage and inflammation around the spinal cord cause ischaemia or cell death. This ischaemia can extend over multiple spinal segments worsening with accompanying hypotension. Injury progression leads to cell membrane dysfunction and electrolyte dysregulation, particularly influxes of calcium and sodium. This produces an inflammatory response period of excitotoxicity and exaggerated stimulation, contributing to cell death (Anwar et al., 2016; Witiw & Fehlings, 2015; Rowland et al., 2008). Mitochondrial failure from calcium influx leads to increased reactive oxygen species production that in turn damages cell structures and functions including proteins (Fatima et al., 2015).

Mishandling unstable spinal injuries can precipitate new or further SCI. Any patient with potential SCI, even without acute neurological abnormalities, should be managed with spinal care. This is particularly relevant for patients who report transient alteration in neurology post-injury—either movement or sensation—but whose symptoms have seemingly resolved.

The child with spinal injury

Muscles and ligaments supporting the vertebrae are more elastic in children than in adults (Atesok et al., 2018). This can allow vertebrae movement and spinal cord stretching without vertebral injury. The child has a larger head-to-body ratio predisposing greater flexion/extension movement. In small children the vertebral body endplate can break away, the intervertebral discs can longitudinally expand and there is greater structural provision for vertebral movement from facet joint and process variations (Brolin et al., 2015; Carroll et al., 2015).

Paediatric patients with spinal injuries do not always have detectable bony injury. This is referred to as spinal cord injury without radiographic abnormality (SCIWORA). Most commonly seen in children < 9 years old, it is almost entirely a paediatric presentation (Atesok et al., 2018; Carroll et al., 2015; Farrell et al., 2017; Martin et al., 2004; Shin et al., 2016). Out-of-hospital responders must maintain high suspicion for SCIWORA when managing any child with potential for spinal trauma but is without bony tenderness (Brown et al., 2001). Magnetic resonance imaging (MRI) may be useful in detecting SCIWORA (Boese et al., 2015).

Vertebrae have growth plates susceptible to compression injury, with near-full growth not achieved before 8 years of age. By then ligaments strengthen and bone calcification occurs. The younger the child, the more likely spinal injury will be higher cervical given the fulcrum effect of the relatively larger head and weaker neck (Carroll et al., 2015; Cirak et al., 2004; Leonard et al., 2014; Lustrin et al., 2003; Martin et al., 2004). Road trauma is a common cause of spinal injury in children. Though the cervical spine is most at risk, the thoracolumbar spine is also occasionally (Atesok et al., 2018), particularly when restrained only by a lap seatbelt.

> **PRACTICE TIP**
>
> Children should not be cleared of spinal injury in the out-of-hospital setting due to anatomical differences.

Usual adult car restraints do not necessarily offer adequate child protection from spinal injury with differing contact points over the abdomen or nearer the neck unless a booster seat is included or is rearward facing (Brolin et al., 2015; Eberhardt et al., 2016; Kroeker et al., 2015; Reilly, 2007). Air bag deployment is also associated with increased cervical injury risk. Children tend to have more forward movement due to their proportionally heavy head when using adult restraints and the air bag deploys more directly into the head (Lustrin et al., 2003) causing hyperextension of the cervical spine.

Children are commonly distressed and non-communicative after trauma. As with adult patients who cannot provide reliable examination, suspicion for spinal injury should be maintained with children. Smaller children tend to be provided with spinal immobilisation less frequently than larger children. Reasons for this are unclear but may include inadequate paediatric equipment, uncertainty and variations in presentation failing to raise adequate suspicion. It may be difficult to explain requirement for immobilisation to a small child, and they may resist application and increase agitation and movement. This is concerning as smaller children tend to have injuries higher up the cervical spine (C1–C4) than larger children with greater mortality risk (Shin et al., 2016; Skellet et al., 2002).

 CASE STUDY 1

Case 10464, 1522 hrs.

Dispatch details: A 17-year-old male thrown from a motorcycle. He is conscious, alert and oriented.

Initial presentation: The paramedics find the patient lying beside a creek where his friends have dragged him. He is in wet clothing including jacket, jeans and motorcycle boots. His helmet is still on.

 ASSESS

Patient history

The patient was riding his motorcycle along a dirt track beside a creek with friends. Hitting an unseen rock, he lost control and was thrown over the handlebars. He rolled from the track ending up partly in the creek. He was immediately communicative with those who ran to his aid. His helmet is damaged from striking the ground. He was unable to pull himself from the creek afterwards or to stand.

He complains of neck pain and tingling in his arms. He cannot feel his legs and is unable to move any limb. On close physical examination he has abrasions on his left thigh and appears to have a closed left lower leg fracture.

He is normally healthy and takes no medications.

In this case the major clue is the history. The traumatic mechanism can produce primary SCI. His helmet damage highlights vulnerability of his neck and neurological changes suggest spinal cord involvement.

Airway

Patients with spinal injuries have greater airway complication risk: associated head and facial trauma can cause obstruction; conscious state alterations can reduce airway reflexes and patients unable to move adequately may not be able to effectively clear blood or vomitus from the airway without assistance. In this case the patient's airway is adequate.

Breathing

Respiratory complications are the major cause of mortality and morbidity post-SCI (Berlowitz et al., 2016; Sirvent et al., 2017). Particular complications include aspiration, atelectasis, pulmonary embolism and pulmonary infections (Kumar et al., 2017). Respiratory muscles chiefly include the diaphragm and the intercostals. The diaphragm is controlled by the phrenic nerve arising from C3–C5. Each thoracic spinal cord segment controls a level of intercostal muscles. Injuries above C4 interrupt central nervous breathing control resulting in need for the patient to be placed on a ventilator. Injuries between C4 and T6 have diaphragmatic innervation and, depending on the level, some intercostal contribution retaining ability to breathe.

Cervical and higher thoracic spinal injuries cause reduced lung volumes and forced expiration, pulmonary secretion accumulation and reduced cough capacity (Berlowitz et al., 2016; Kumar et al., 2017). Breathing is relatively normal for T6–T12 injuries, with only some residual difficulty coughing. Respiratory function improvement is common post-SCI with most patients no longer requiring ventilation (Zimmer et al., 2007).

Paradoxical respiration observed with higher injury level is from failure of the chest to expand during inspiration due to flaccid intercostal muscles (Berlowitz et al., 2016). Abdominal protrusion on inspiration can be noted. When sitting, flaccid abdominal muscles allow abdominal content to spread in a wider abdominal girth. In turn, the diaphragm lowers resulting in lessened ability to expand the chest. Supine position allows the diaphragm to sit higher for greater ventilation (Berlowitz et al., 2016; Berly & Shem, 2007).

Cardiovascular

Sympathetic innervation is conducted via the spinal cord while parasympathetic innervation is predominantly via cranial nerves outside the spinal cord. Injury to the thoracic spine or above, especially cervical, can severely interrupt sympathetic outflow from the spinal cord nerves. These injuries reduce sympathetic innervation and allow parasympathetic system domination. The heart has both sympathetic and parasympathetic innervation; most peripheral blood vessels are only sympathetic. Following SCI, brief initial rise in blood pressure from noradrenaline release occurs. Soon afterwards, vagal tone from the intact cranial vagus nerve goes largely unopposed, with bradycardia the predominant effect. Bradycardia denotes injury above the level of innervation of the sympathetic chain. Typically, pulse and blood pressure in SCI patients is lowered following reduced sympathetic activity below the level of the lesion (Berlowitz et al., 2016; Furlan et al., 2016). As hypotension is a frequent finding, paramedics must differentiate between differing causes: neurogenic shock or hypovolaemia from another injury. Blood pressure of 80–100 mmHg systolic may be normal in the SCI patient.

This patient presents with borderline bradycardia and marginal blood pressure of 90/50 mmHg. This is suggestive of SCI and within the normal or expected parameters for a patient with such injury.

Suspicion or clearance

Spinal suspicion

Injury patterns with SCI potential should raise automatic suspicion including trauma patients with GCS < 13, significant head trauma or any neurological symptoms. Major traumatic mechanisms evoke SCI suspicion. Trauma involving lesser force in those more vulnerable including patients over 55 years of age or those with a history of bone disease (such as osteoporosis or osteoarthritis) or muscular weakness (such as muscular dystrophy) increases SCI risk. These people have weakened structural support of the vertebral column and spinal cord. Patient history, including witness descriptions, can assist the recognition of injury potential, particularly in children (Atesok et al., 2018).

Significant painful or gross injuries can be distracting for both patient and paramedic; concurrent spinal care should be provided.

This patient has clear injury mechanism making spinal injury suspicion easy. His injured lower leg should be painful, with absence further suggestive of SCI.

Spinal clearance

Much out-of-hospital focus is on cervical spine; however, lower parts can also be injured. Patient handling and immobilisation must consider the whole of the spine. That said, the cervical spine is more likely to be injured and more easily moved or aggravated without support. Spinal immobilisation of all trauma patients is simply not feasible and burdensome for patients, paramedics and hospitals. A number of spinal clearance algorithms have been developed to identify those patients who should receive immobilisation. Some, including the Canadian C-Spine Rule (see Fig 37.3) and the National Emergency X-Radiography Utilisation Study (NEXUS) Low Risk Criteria (NLC), are primarily designed to direct hospital patients towards radiographic investigations but are partly transferable to out-of-hospital practice. Other derivations guide paramedics away from unnecessary spinal immobilisation (see Fig 37.4). Only patients with genuine SCI potential warrant immobilisation and subsequent radiographic evaluation; wherever possible those with risk should not be cleared including those with: 1. midline posterior cervical pain or bony tenderness; 2. altered motor or sensation, even unilaterally; 3. unreliable history whether from drug and/or alcohol use, loss of consciousness during the event or preexisting confusion such as dementia; 4. increased vulnerability to injury including bony or neuromuscular disease or older aged; and 5. distracting injury (Connor et al., 2015; Stiell et al., 2003; Weber & Nance, 2016).

Depending on local guidelines, patients who meet defined criteria can be cleared of spinal injury and avoid spinal immobilisation (Larson et al., 2017). There are multiple differences between adults and children and adult clearance options should not be applied to children.

Neurological examination

The forehead provides a baseline for evaluation as its innervation arises from the trigeminal cranial nerve. Rub the patient's forehead to establish normal sensation. Moving anatomically down, in order rub the upper neck (C2), lower neck (C3), thumb (C6) and little finger (C8) to assess the cervical

> ### PRACTICE TIP
>
> Any evidence of neurological change should be managed as suspected SCI. Remembering that spinal nerves arise from spinal cord segments, the body surface they correspond to assists quick and accurate injury level assessment.

> ### Look for!
> - Hyperextension
> - Hyperflexion
> - Compression
> - Overstretching
> - Rotational force
> - Combinations

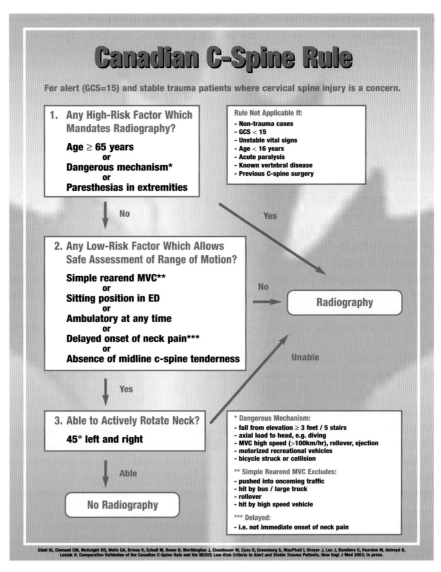

Figure 37.3
Canadian C-Spine Rule.
Source: Victorian Surgical Consultative Council, Department of Health Victoria.

spine. The upper chest (anterior and posterior) down to the waist corresponds in descending fashion to the thoracic segments (T2–T12). T4 is typically around the nipple line with T10 around the umbilicus. Finally, the upper leg corresponds to L1 and L2, while the lower leg corresponds to L4, L5 and S1 (see Fig 37.5). Gently rub, awaiting patient acknowledgment for each, to detect any dysfunction. Similarly, movement of the corresponding body surface, including the thumb, little finger and feet, assesses motor function at those levels.

Paramedics are not expected to specify precise injury level as this can be unreliable and evolve. Establishing baseline observation of neurological function allows appreciation of deficit progression.

A widely accepted method of classifying SCI is based on injury level and resultant motor and sensory dysfunction (Kirshblum et al., 2011).

- Tetraplegia replaces quadriplegia as the term for cervical-level injury resulting in neurological change in all four limbs. Depending on injury level, some tetraplegic injuries still allow some upper limb response.

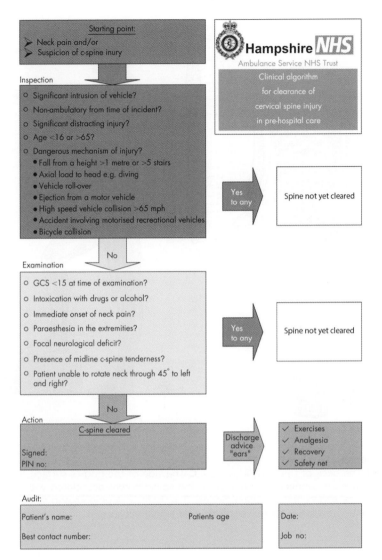

Starting point:
➤ Neck pain and/or
➤ Suspicion of c-spine inury

Inspection
○ Significant intrusion of vehicle?
○ Non-ambulatory from time of incident?
○ Significant distracting injury?
○ Age <16 or >65?
○ Dangerous mechanism of injury?
    • Fall from a height >1 metre or >5 stairs
    • Axial load to head e.g. diving
    • Vehicle roll-over
    • Ejection from a motor vehicle
    • High speed vehicle collision >65 mph
    • Accident involving motorised recreational vehicles
    • Bicycle collision

Yes to any → **Spine not yet cleared**

No

Hampshire NHS
Ambulance Service NHS Trust
Clinical algorithm for clearance of cervical spine injury in pre-hospital care

Examination
○ GCS <15 at time of examination?
○ Intoxication with drugs or alcohol?
○ Immediate onset of neck pain?
○ Paraesthesia in the extremities?
○ Focal neurological deficit?
○ Presence of midline c-spine tenderness?
○ Patient unable to rotate neck through 45° to left and right?

Yes to any → **Spine not yet cleared**

No

Action
C-spine cleared
Signed:
PIN no:

Discharge advice "ears" →
✓ Exercises
✓ Analgesia
✓ Recovery
✓ Safety net

Audit:
Patient's name: Patients age   Date:
Best contact number: Job no:

Figure 37.4
Hampshire Ambulance Service Spinal Clearance Guide.
Source: Armstrong et al. (2007).

- Paraplegia is the term for injury at thoracic, lumbar or sacral level and involves the lower limbs.

An SCI may be complete with no nerve impulse conduction past injury level. Incomplete injury varies with spinal tracts affected. A number of identifiable patterns have been described.

- **Central cord syndrome** is commonly associated with cervical injury and cord compression giving central cord ischaemia. Typically it occurs following a fall or head hyperextension, with the elderly more likely to be affected (see Box 37.1). It is characterised by greater upper limb weakness than lower due to cord centre injury where upper limb tracts are concentrated. Sometimes there is less spinal column injury, allowing good recovery prognosis (Todd et al., 2008).
- **Brown-Séquard syndrome** presents with dysfunction differing on either side of the patient. Injury to one side of the cord affects motor function on the same side of the injury but altered sensory and pain input on the opposite side (Medscape, 2014). Sensory fibres for fine touch running in

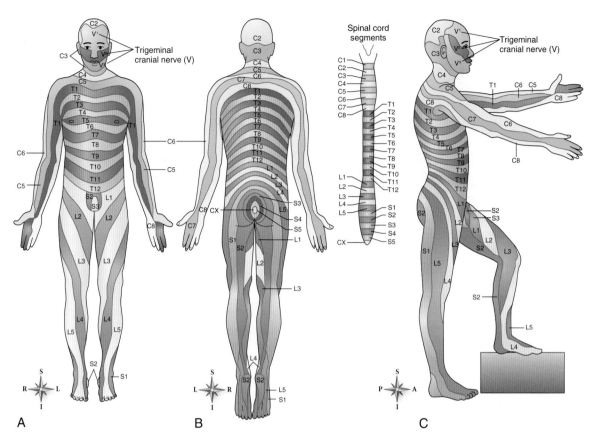

Figure 37.5
Dermatome distribution of spinal nerves.
A The front of the body's surface. **B** The back of the body's surface. **C** The side of the body's surface. The inset shows the segments of the spinal cord connected with each of the spinal nerves associated with the sensory dermatomes shown. C = cervical segments and spinal nerves; T = thoracic segments and spinal nerves; L = lumbar segments and spinal nerves; S = sacral segments and spinal nerves.
Source: Patton & Thibodeau (2012).

BOX 37.1 Common causes of falls in the elderly

- Medications such as:
  › antihypertensives
  › cardiac medications
  › hypoglycaemic agents
  › sedatives
  › anxiolytics or antidepressants
  › anticholinergic drugs
- Alcohol
- Acute illness
- Stroke/transient ischaemic attack
- Chronic illness
- Postural hypotension
- Visual disorders
- Confusion or cognitive disorders
- Gait disturbance due to arthritis
- Musculoskeletal disorders
- Balance disorders
- Weakness
- Environmental hazards: mats, slippery surfaces

the lateral spinal thalamic tract cross over at the level of entry to the cord, while those motor fibres running in the corticospinal tract cross over high above the cord itself.

- **Anterior cord syndrome** is commonly associated with anterior spinal column injury and subsequent interruption of the anterior spinal artery supply. It produces signs on both sides of the body as the tracts are affected equally. Motor function is usually more significantly altered with sensation frequently less affected given the lateral tracts used through the cord (Radiopaedia.org, 2014).
- **Conus medullaris syndrome** and **cauda equina syndrome** are injuries of the very distal end of the spinal cord. Conus medullaris syndrome affects both the lower and the upper motor neurons, usually presenting quickly and bilaterally. It is less severe than cauda equina syndrome which presents more slowly and unilaterally. Both syndromes most notably affect the bladder, bowel and lower limbs (Spector et al., 2008).

Other signs and symptoms
Spinal shock
'Spinal shock' does not refer to circulatory system collapse as do other shock forms. Rather it refers to loss of usual neurological activity at and below injury level including motor, sensory and autonomic function. This is when autonomic dysreflexia can occur (see long-term care). Loss of bladder and bowel control accompanies spinal shock.

Neurogenic shock
Hypotension results from both slowed heart rate and vasodilation. Vasodilation below the injury level reflects interruption to sympathetic supply. The skin is frequently warm and dry, without the usual sympathetic response redirecting peripheral blood. This classic presentation may be delayed or not occur at all with some injuries. Its absence should not be considered diagnostic (Guly et al., 2008).

Priapism
SCI with complete transection can cause priapism given unopposed parasympathetic stimulation. Without sympathetic vasculature tone, blood pools in the peripheries resulting in blood accumulation including in the penis. This occurs at injury time and usually resolves requiring no specific treatment (Todd, 2011).

Hypovolaemic shock
Neurogenic shock ensures normal body response to circulatory dysfunction cannot be mounted. The SCI patient is also a trauma patient, possibly severe multi-trauma. Hypotension cannot simply be assumed to be from SCI; consider blood loss from other injuries. Absence of clear SCI neurological deficit suggests hypotension is likely from some other cause. For patients with other injuries consistent with blood loss and hypovolaemia, managing hypotension is a priority. Conversely, unnecessary and excessive fluid resuscitation can cause acute pulmonary oedema in SCI patients (Berlowitz et al., 2016).

Temperature
Reduced thermoregulatory sensory input from and loss of sympathetically mediated vasoactive temperature control and sweat regulation make the SCI patient vulnerable to ambient temperature (Hagen, 2015). Hypothermia can quickly follow neurogenic shock. Vasomotor control is no longer under autonomic control below the injury level. Inability to redistribute blood from exposed periphery or generate heat through muscle activity creates dependence on ambient air temperature for body temperature.

Look for!
- Head injury
- Chest injury
- Abdominal injury
- Limb trauma

Consider!
Check the environment the patient is in and how long they have been there. SCI patients may be vasodilated and susceptible to heat loss, particularly if wet, lying on cold ground or exposed to the elements. Move them to a warm place, remove wet clothing and cover them as soon as possible without compromising spinal care.

The patient in this case is at risk of hypothermia being exposed, wet, immobile and vasodilated.

Other injuries

It is imperative to remember that any patient with potential spinal injury may have other injuries. Lack of proper sensation and motor function increase difficulty examining for physical injuries. Secondary examination should be undertaken concurrently with spinal examination. Rely more on visual clues rather than typical clues of pain and altered movement.

Initial assessment summary

Problem	Motorcycle accident, conscious but unable to move
Conscious state	GCS = 15
Position	Supine
Heart rate	60 bpm
Blood pressure	90/50 mmHg
Skin appearance	Pale, cool, dry (skin is wet from wet clothing)
Speech pattern	Normal
Respiratory rate	18 bpm
Respiratory rhythm	Even cycles
Chest auscultation	Good breath sounds bilaterally
Pulse oximetry	96%
Temperature	35.2°C
Motor/sensory function	Altered sensation in his arms and loss of sensation and motor function in his lower limbs
Pain	4/10 neck pain
History	As he went over the handlebars, he could have hit the ground face first (hyperextension), struck the back of his head (hyperflexion), hit his head directly on the ground (compression) or even suffered rotational trauma. He was then dragged by his friends, potentially causing further trauma to any injuries. He is also wet, with hypothermia developing.
Physical assessment	Neck pain, altered sensation in his arms and loss of sensation and motor function in his legs. Possible closed fracture of his left lower leg.

D: There are no dangers to patient or crew.

A: The patient is conscious with no current airway obstruction.

B: Respiratory function is currently normal.

C: Heart rate and blood pressure are both low.

The patient is hypotensive (with no obvious external haemorrhage) with a pulse at the lowest end of normal. This is not consistent with hypovolaemia but it is consistent with SCI. He has motor and sensory deficits. Given the mechanism, his whole spine is at risk.

② CONFIRM

The essential part of clinical reasoning is to confirm initial hypothesis with clinical signs. Challenge your diagnosis by exploring findings that do not fit your hypothesis: don't just ignore them.

Unlike medical cases where multiple possible causes need exclusion, trauma mechanism of injury is usually clearer. Obvious injuries are not always the most serious and visually dramatic and painful injuries can distract patient and paramedic from other possibilities.

DIFFERENTIAL DIAGNOSIS

Spinal injury
Or
- Stroke
- Stroke mimics
- Head injury
- Limb injury
- Preexisting injury
- Other cause of poor perfusion

What else could it be?

Medical illness

Perhaps the patient had a medical event precipitating the incident. History is an important discerning tool. Particularly consider neurological, cardiac or metabolic causes.

This patient's history does not suggest a medical cause for his presentation.

Head injury

Head injuries, particularly penetrating, may cause lower body neurological dysfunction similar to SCI. It is prudent for patients with significant head injury to be managed as if they have concurrent spinal injury.

Limb injury

Inability to move a limb does not mean there has been loss of central motor control. Localised injury may result in similar presentation to SCI.

Preexisting injury

New appearing presentation might in fact be preexisting injury. Search for history, vehicle disability stickers or a stored wheelchair.

③ TREAT

Emergency management

Injury above C4 may necessitate ongoing ventilation. Head trauma may alter consciousness. Airway management priorities depend on presentation. Secondary physical examination provides evidence of spinal and other presenting injuries enabling management prioritisation.

Box 37.2 outlines principles of management for spinal injury.

Helmet removal

One great first-aid conundrum is whether to remove an injured patient's helmet. Much available literature refers to sporting helmets; often of very different design to motorcycle helmets, removal need and principles not necessarily translatable. Potential complications for open-face helmet as opposed to full-faced variety may differ. In Australia, paramedics most frequently encounter helmets related to motorcycles or motor sport (excluding bicycle helmets). The helmet of a sports player or motorcyclist should be removed as soon as practicable by paramedics (as opposed to on-scene first-aiders) for reasons including:

- inability to assess and manage airway and breathing, including dealing with a soiled airway and performing intubation
- inability to place the head and neck in the neutral position—or worse, the head may be forced into undesirable flexion
- inability to apply a cervical collar or immobilise the spine

CLINICAL COMMENT

There is growing evidence routine application of rigid cervical collars to trauma patients is not routinely beneficial and can even cause harm. Judgement and consideration of potential complications has seen the 2015 report by the International Liaison Committee on Resuscitation (ILCOR) (Zideman et al., 2015) no longer support such application by first-aid organisations.

BOX 37.2 Principles of management

Spinal injury
- Safety of patient and rescuers
- Airway care
- Respiratory support
- Cervical care
- Antiemesis
- Spinal immobilisation
- Careful handling
- Temperature maintenance
- Perfusion support
- Management of other injuries

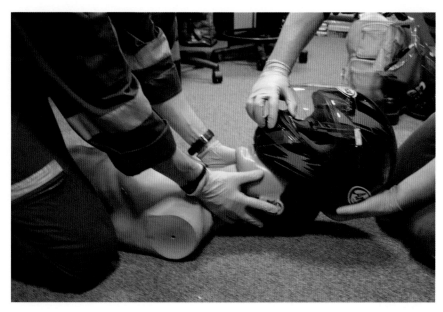

Figure 37.6
The helmet should be removed as soon as practicable.
Source: Jeff Kenneally.

- full-face helmets may cause rebreathing and CO_2 retention (Segan et al., 1993; Branfoot, 1994).

One method of helmet removal is to manage the patient (ideally supine) with one rescuer kneeling or lying above the patient's head holding the helmet stationary (see Fig 37.6). A second removes the patient's glasses (if worn) and undoes the helmet chin strap. This second rescuer takes responsibility for head stabilisation by holding the patient's jaw and under the patient's neck. They may need to take the weight of the patient's head and must be prepared to resist any movement from the first rescuer removing the helmet. The first rescuer should gently spread the helmet base and lift the chin-piece to the patient's nose. The helmet can then be carefully slid off, pulling the back of the helmet rotationally over the top towards the patient's face. Attempting to slide off backward over the face will snare the chin-piece on the patient's nose. Neutral position, with occipital padding, is then established with first rescuer continuing head and neck stabilisation.

The patient in this case is still wearing his helmet. It is a full-face helmet and requires two-person removal as soon as practicable.

Neutral position
No matter what position the patient is found in, the head should be returned to neutral unless that causes pain, resistance to movement is felt or the patient describes not being able to move the neck from the current position. In such a case, one rescuer must support the patient's head as found until immobilisation by a more secure method. Once a rescuer is tasked with cervical stabilisation, this remains continuous with that person unable to assist with any other function. Coordination of patient movement should occur via this person. Careful consideration should thus be given to the person allocated: they must be senior and assertive enough to perform the role yet remain expendable from other tasks.

The neutral position is relative and unique to each patient. When supine, the adult head falls back into a partially extended position in as many as 98% of people (Schriger et al., 1991). To maintain adult neutral position, padding is

> **PRACTICE TIP**
>
> Immobilisation should encompass a whole-of-spine approach: neither the head nor the body should be immobilised in isolation.

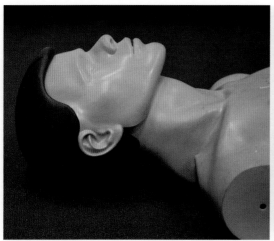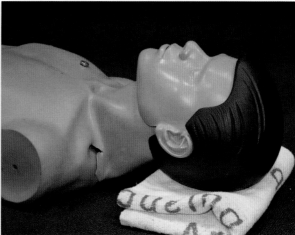

Figure 37.7
The neutral position.
Source: Jeff Kenneally.

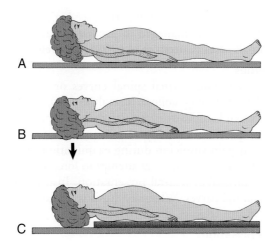

Figure 37.8
The neutral position in children varies with age and development.
Source: Roberts (2009).

placed beneath the occiput (Austin et al., 2014). The amount of padding varies targeting a range of no more than +/– 5° head flexion/extension (Boswell et al., 2001). Raising the occiput between 2 and 5 cm provides optimal positioning with the opening of the ear on the same plane as the mid-clavicle (De Lorenzo et al., 1995). Personalise position, avoiding flexion or extension (see Fig 37.7).

For patients with head injury and no spinal injury, the optimal position to balance intracranial pressure and cerebral perfusion pressure is 15–30° head-up posture flexed at the hips to facilitate cerebral venous drainage (Durward et al., 1983; Haddad & Arabi, 2012; Protheroe & Gwinnutt, 2011). However, the typical human head weighs 4–5 kg, providing significant downward force on any unstable cervical injury. Patients with potential spinal injury should be managed supine or lateral until clearance is provided or more substantial injury stabilisation occurs. For patients found in an upright position who cannot immediately be placed supine (such as in road trauma), the head should be returned to the position best approximating neutral and maintained there.

In children younger than 8 years, the relatively larger occiput may require either no padding or padding beneath the shoulders to raise the thorax and

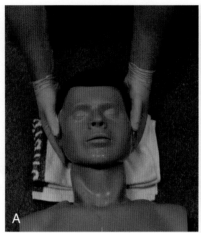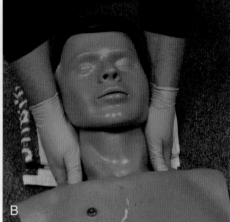

Figure 37.9
A Holding the head only. **B** Holding the head and clavicles.
Source: Jeff Kenneally.

prevent flexion of the head (Boswell et al., 2001; see Fig 37.8). Neutral position has been shown to be poorly managed in paediatric patients, with no single method reliable in all cases (Curran et al., 1995; Boswell et al., 2001).

Spinal abnormalities
Some conditions exaggerate normal spinal curves or produce curves when there should be none, including scoliosis (lateral curving), kyphosis (exaggerated upper spinal curve) and lordosis (exaggerated lower spine curve). Although history of previous spinal abnormality may be unknown to the paramedic, in many cases they may gain suspicion during examination, particularly if there are signs of disability. In any event, never attempt to force an unusually appearing spine back into a 'normal' or neutral presentation. Instead, support as found using padding to fill the curves. Where kyphosis is found, the neutral position must be tailored to suit (Rao et al., 2016).

Manual inline stabilisation
Manual inline stabilisation can be provided with the patient in any position, including seated, supine or lateral. The ideal method is with the rescuer's fingers spread across the greatest surface area of the patient's head to produce greatest stability (see Fig 37.9). Avoid contact with the patient's neck to avoid affecting venous return. By holding the head only, there is no direct support to the lower body allowing for uncoordinated movement between head and body, placing the cervical spine at risk. This is particularly so when the patient is being moved, such as during log rolling. Alternatively, the patient's head can be held between the rescuer's forearms with the fingers grasping the (uninjured) clavicles on either side. Where advanced airway techniques or ventilation support is required, the rescuer can use their own knees and thighs to provide some patient head stabilisation. Whichever method is used, traction is not applied as it may exacerbate any injury (Gerling et al., 2000).

Airway management
Airway management includes addressing current needs and considering ongoing needs including antiemetics, intubation and assisted ventilation. Usual oro-pharyngeal and nasopharyngeal airway devices may be necessary in the first instance, mindful of relative contraindications, including facial or skull fractures and avoidance of inducing gag reflex with head injury. Patients may be initially positioned laterally provided great care is taken to support the head in a neutral inline position (Hyldmo et al., 2015).

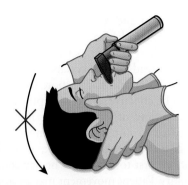

Figure 37.10
Head stabilisation during intubation.
Source: Adams (2008).

Intubation

Where necessary, intubation may be safely performed, provided parasympathetic response to airway manoeuvres has been blocked with atropine (avoiding dramatic unopposed parasympathetic-induced bradycardia). The usual positions for achieving the best view during intubation, such as occiput elevation, are best avoided, with the preference for the neutral position. Instead use supportive tools of direct laryngeal pressure and bougie use. A secondary assistant holding the patient's head and resisting any movement during the procedure is ideal (Nolan & Wilson, 1993) though this may conflict with laryngoscopy.

Cervical collar release for mouth opening is required during intubation with total reliance on manual axial inline stabilisation (see Fig 37.10). Such stabilisation reduces anteroposterior movement and may adversely impact view and delay intubation and ventilation (Austin et al., 2014; Manoach & Paladino, 2007). The Miller™ blade technique can reduce such movement (Gerling et al., 2000). Devices including video laryngoscopes may improve view without compromising cervical spine stabilisation (Akbar & Ooi, 2015; Suppan et al., 2016).

Movement during cricothyroidotomy is likely small and clinically insignificant (Crosby 2002; Malik et al., 2008). Rapid-sequence intubation remains safe and effective for securing the airway in a patient with cervical injuries (Criswell et al., 1994). Laryngeal mask airway devices are controversial given increased cervical spine displacement (Austin et al., 2014).

Cervical collar

The cervical collar is intended to minimise cervical spine movement. It does not provide complete neck immobilisation and provides no care for the rest of the spinal column (Kreinest et al., 2017). There are major questions as to whether it offers benefit in many patients, particularly those who are awake and alert (Phillips & Nutbeam, 2017). The collar is at best a component of a management package. A poorly fitted cervical collar may force the neck to remain in a position of poor alignment, which may affect the injury. Patients who are agitated or regain consciousness may attempt movement against the collar and further risk injury (Morris & McCoy, 2003). The cervical collar has been implicated in causing soft-tissue injury from prolonged application. More significantly, it can interfere with jugular venous return and potentially cause a rise in intracranial pressure with traumatic brain injury (Connor et al., 2015; Davies et al., 1996; Holly et al., 2002; Kreinest et al., 2017; Iida et al., 1999; Peck et al., 2018; Purvis et al., 2017; Raphael & Chotai, 1994).

Cervical collar application remains a short-term out-of-hospital option, used in conjunction with multiple other spinal care principles including gentle coordinated patient movement and manual head immobilisation. Even if the collar provides little benefit, its placement can highlight ongoing spinal care need to the patient and other medical personnel. A recent trend has been towards using soft collars instead of hard collars. These reduce movement even less but still serve as a reminder and flag to potential SCI.

For a cervical collar to be effective, it must be properly measured and fitted. Some collars come in a variety of sizes and are measured for each patient, while others can be adjusted to suit. The collar must be in close contact with the patient's skin across the chest, upper back, shoulders and jaw line, so clothing should be removed first to allow best fit. Jewellery should be removed to avoid discomfort or injury. Patient movement may prompt collar readjustment. The cervical collar can be applied with the patient in any position, only requiring the head in the neutral position first. Maintain manual stabilisation while the collar is fitted.

Patient extrication

Patient extrication methods evolved largely from the dogma of allowing no patient movement for fear of worsening SCI and the resulting litigation potential. Recent trends are moving away from this. For conscious patients able to move relatively freely, self-extrication from vehicles does not necessarily cause more movement or aggravate injury, with considerable self-protection demonstrated (Cowley et al., 2017). Patients with potential spinal injury may be found ambulating at the scene; this should not preclude appropriate spinal immobilisation. Consider supporting the head and upper body, such as by bringing the back of the bed upright and allowing the patient to lean into it, before lowering them supine. A patient lying themselves supine can cause the head weight to place strain on the unsupported cervical spine.

Where rescue is necessary, numerous methods can be used to immobilise the whole spine. Spineboards are common for extrication and sometimes carrying patients (see Fig 37.11).

There are purpose-built devices for extricating patients with spinal injuries while providing whole-of-spine care, such as the Kendrick Extrication Device®

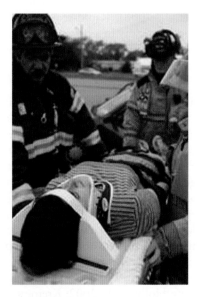

Figure 37.11
Spineboard immobilisation for extrication.
Source: Laerdal Medical (2011). https://www.laerdal.com/in/products/medical-devices/immobilisation/.

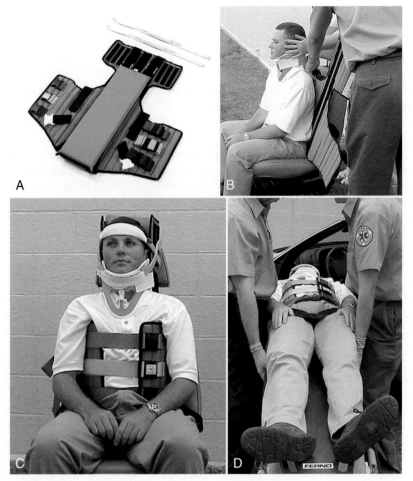

Figure 37.12
Kendrick Extrication Device®: for very small children the device can be inverted and used as a spineboard.
Source: Ferno-Washington Inc. (2011).

(see Fig 37.12). With such devices, a thoracic flexible frame is applied to the patient, which includes extension to the head and straps for harnessing the legs. The device can be applied to a patient in situ and has handles/straps to allow rescuers to lift and carry. Not all patients are found lying on the ground and the Kendrick Extrication Device® is useful for extricating patients found sitting. Some patients may be moved with a combination of spineboard and coordinated manual handling.

Patient extrication can be completed with coordinated lifting using a scoop stretcher, spineboard or flat lift. Scoop stretcher sides can be separated and placed under the patient. Although reducing the need to lift and roll the patient, it does not work on all surfaces and is not designed for immobilisation. Notwithstanding this, the scoop stretcher can be useful in spinal care (Krell et al., 2006; Moss et al., 2015).

Injury stabilisation

Out-of-hospital suspected spinal injury patient management includes careful handling to avoid worsening the injury and sometimes immobilisation. Spinal immobilisation has the same aim as other fracture management, to restrict movement and reduce pain and further injury. There are two key options:

- manual immobilisation
- immobilising devices.

Despite spinal immobilisation being common, it should not be considered lightly, being without supporting randomised controlled trials. Early prospective evidence pertaining to non-injured volunteers (Kwan et al., 2001) and retrospective evidence suggested immobilisation had little or no effect and may even increase neurological injury (Hauswald et al., 1998). For most patients, damage occurs at the time of injury and is not worsened by subsequent handling (Connor et al., 2015).

Complications can accompany spinal immobilisation. The most obvious is that it is uncomfortable and likely unwanted. Rigid cervical collars and hard backboards soon cause pressure areas (Connor et al., 2015; Ham et al., 2017; Ham et al., 2014). Movement restriction and chest strapping can adversely impact airway opening, breathing and lung ventilation and increases aspiration risk in supine patients (Ala et al., 2016; Bauer & Kowalski, 1988; Connor et al., 2015; Lieberman & Webb, 1994; Peck et al., 2018; Totten & Sugarman, 1999). The benefits must outweigh disadvantages. Many potential complications of spinal immobilisation result from prolonged immobilisation (in excess of 48 hours) and are of less out-of-hospital concern (Davis et al., 1995). Immobilisation methods are not indicated in penetrating neck trauma nor where there is other life-threatening complication such as severe haemorrhage (Connor et al., 2015; Kreinest et al., 2017).

Spineboards should be used for extrication only (Connor et al., 2015). They should no longer be used for immobilisation after extrication (Moss et al., 2015; White et al., 2014).

Whenever a patient is managed with spinal immobilisation, the head and body are never managed independently. Immobilising either independently allows movement or shearing between the parts exposing the neck to great risk.

A vacuum mattress can provide whole spine support conforming to the normal curves. These are usually more expensive and bulky to store than spineboards (see Fig 37.13) but have comfort, spine stability advantage (Luscombe & Williams, 2003; Moss et al., 2015; Rahmatalla et al., 2018) and superior thoracic spine immobilisation (Wampler et al., 2016; Johnson et al., 1996).

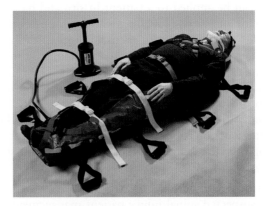

Figure 37.13
Vacuum mattress for spinal immobilisation.
Source: RAPP Australia Pty Ltd (2014). www.neann.com.au/neann-vim-vacuum-immobilisation-mattress-6-ft-157.

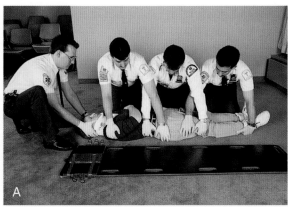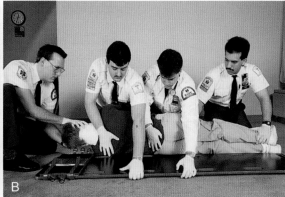

Figure 37.14
The team log roll.
Source: Swartz (2009).

For small children, immobilisation can be improvised using an inverted Kendrick Extraction Device® (see Fig 37.13) or standard adult vacuum mattress, paying attention to neutral position variations. Children are more likely to remain unsettled and immobilisation may require parental support. If too unsettling for the child, improvisation using a capsule or car seat may be possible.

There are two broad methods of moving any patient onto a bed or spineboard.

- *Log rolling* involves coordinated roll of the patient from supine to lateral and back (see Fig 37.14). It may initially involve the patient being turned from prone or similar. The head is returned to neutral before or during the rolling process. The rescuer providing head support is critical as they are the vital link between the patient's head and body. Cervical collar application may have to be delayed until after roll completion. Log rolling is not reliable for maintaining spinal alignment (Moss et al., 2015).
- *Team lifting* involves multiple rescuers lifting the patient while keeping them in a constant plane. This is potentially heavier for rescuers but could offer better head and body stability (Del Rossi et al., 2003).

Antiemesis
Since typically patients with spinal injuries are managed supine, nausea and vomiting risk is concerning. Patient movement to facilitate vomiting is problematic for spinal care. Cervical collars restrict mouth opening, increasing aspiration risk. Intubation should be considered for patients in an altered state of consciousness and unable to protect their own airway. For conscious patients where this is not appropriate, antiemetic prophylaxis can reduce the likelihood of vomiting. Ambulance transportation can produce motion sickness in supine patients, with an imbalance between vestibular system movement perception and the visual clues received.

General care
Pressure area formation is a lifelong risk for SCI patients. Body points contacting hard surfaces should be appropriately padded. Place limbs that cannot self-support into anatomically normal positions and do not allow them to hang dependently as further soft-tissue injury can occur or the limb can be injured during movement.

Fluid resuscitation/perfusion support
To compensate for vasodilation following spinal cord trauma, an initial fluid bolus is suitable for early resuscitation. For isolated SCI, up to 10 mL/kg maintains adequate mean arterial pressure and tissue perfusion. Fluid resuscitation must not become overzealous to avoid pulmonary oedema from fluid overload.

> ## PRACTICE TIP
>
> Depending on injury, body heat can be lost from vasodilation or conduction into cold surfaces (which they may not feel) or large fluid volume administration, or gain heat from a hot environment from which they cannot move. Spinal patients should have their temperature monitored and be managed carefully.

Where this does not correct blood pressure in isolated SCI assess for other injuries causing hypovolaemia and resuscitate accordingly. If adequate fluid resuscitation is ineffective, vasopressors may be required. Maintaining mean arterial blood pressure above 90 mmHg is associated with improved neurological outcome (Ahuja et al., 2016; Hawryluk et al., 2015).

Temperature management

Patients with spinal injury should be managed to maintain normal body temperature. Regular and ongoing temperature assessment is necessary. In this case, remove the wet clothing that is exacerbating heat loss, dry the patient and protect them from adverse ambient temperature.

④ EVALUATE
Hospital admission
Definitive spinal assessment

Radiological assessment is usually required for definitive exclusion of bony injury unless the patient can be confidently screened with preliminary assessment (Morris et al., 2004). Children may be screened using radiographs but where there is any uncertainty, computed tomography (CT) may be required (Slack & Clancy, 2004). Despite vertebral fractures being evident on most plain radiographs, some spinal column injuries are not easy to detect and MRI remains highly sensitive for evaluating ongoing concern (Ahuja et al., 2016). MRI is particularly effective in evaluating soft-tissue injuries such as ligament damage (Atesok et al., 2018; Hey et al., 2018; Maung et al., 2017; Morris & McCoy, 2004). Radiography and CT combinations can be reliable and effective in providing confident clearance, particularly where there is alteration in consciousness or intoxication (Badhiwala et al., 2015; Bush et al., 2016; Martin et al., 2017; Morris & McCoy, 2004; Tan et al., 2014).

Continued immobilisation

The spineboard has no role in transport, the ED or hospital admission (Vickery, 2001). Essential resuscitation should occur without interruption but remove the patient from the spineboard as soon as practicable once they are on the ambulance stretcher (Cooke, 1998; Moss et al., 2015; White et al., 2014; Yeung et al., 2006; Lubbert et al., 2005).

Respiratory care

Respiratory complications are a major acute SCI problem with most deaths occurring within days following injury. The more complete the injury, the more likely respiratory complications will occur (Berlowitz et al., 2016; Berly & Shem, 2007; Sirvent et al., 2017; van Silfhout et al., 2016) including respiratory failure from spinal or chest injury. Chest trauma, adult respiratory distress syndrome (ARDS) and overhydration for neurogenic shock can all cause pulmonary oedema (Berlowitz et al., 2016; Berly & Shem, 2007).

In-hospital management requires airway secretion removal and good hygiene. Monitoring of blood gases and clinical signs of respiratory failure is important. Mechanical ventilation is commonly employed to assist ventilation and avoid atelectasis. Postural drainage positioning and chest percussion assists effective ventilation.

Ongoing airway care may require tracheostomy. This offers increased patient comfort and easier care than an endotracheal tube and enables patient mobility where possible. An increase in the use of long-term ventilation has led to improved patient survival rates (Berlowitz et al., 2016).

Pharmacotherapy

Much of the secondary injury derives from inflammatory responses, with steroid therapy administered early (Ahuja et al., 2016; Atesok et al., 2018).

However, the inflammatory responses and the early administration of steroid therapy can increase sepsis and pneumonia rates so are not universally supported (Kreinest et al., 2017).

Spinal cord concussion

A few patients with initial SCI signs recover in a short period of time. Just as the brain can show temporary dysfunction signs when concussed, so too can the spinal cord. Spinal concussion occurs when a traumatic mechanism causes SCI deficits yet full recovery occurs within 48–72 hours (Asan 2018; Zwimpfer & Bernstein, 1990; Del Bigio & Johnson, 1989). The mechanism for this is not well understood. Long-term recovery is usually good. Absence of major structural injury is common.

Temperature

To combat greater influence of environmental temperature, body temperature is closely monitored and managed with temperature-controlled fluids, warmed environment and warming equipment such as Bair Hugger® therapy.

Bowel and bladder

SCI often causes loss of bladder and bowel control at the time of injury or afterwards. It may not be permanent. Changes vary with injury severity and location. Higher-level injuries may cause an increase in bladder tone, leading to frequency and incontinence. Lower-level injuries may cause loss of bladder tone, leading to urine retention and recurring infection risk (Sezer et al., 2015).

Bowel control loss presents similarly. Higher injuries can remove the ability to identify when a bowel motion is required. Bowel movements occur on a reflex basis with the anal sphincter retaining its tone; the patient stimulates this reflex at a suitable time. Lower injuries may remove anal sphincter tone and cause faecal retention. Depending on symptoms, a combination of manual stimulation techniques, diet management, medications, laxatives and enemas may become regular life (Sezer et al., 2015).

The first few days post-SCI are frequently accompanied by paralytic ileus. This usually self-resolves and requires only nasogastric tube insertion to facilitate drainage. Unopposed parasympathetic activity increases gastric ulcer prevalence.

Deep vein thrombosis

Limb stasis predisposes to deep vein thrombosis—another lifelong complication. Anticoagulation and compression stockings are common management.

Length of hospital stay

Hospital stay length varies with injury severity and other injuries. Typically, SCI patients have a median stay of 16 days in acute care followed by a median of 133 days in a rehabilitation unit. Duration of hospital stay for persisting SCI varies between 77 and 221 days. The overwhelming majority of patients are discharged home, with only a small percentage moving to a nursing home. In Australia, care costs approach $500 million annually (Norton, 2010). Given that the typical injury age is 25 years, the ongoing care cost is huge.

Long-term issues and care

Pressure areas

Pressure area care is required for life for all SCI patients (Hagen, 2015). Healing pressure ulcers is a major healthcare cost, with the best strategy avoiding the problem in the first place (Cobb et al., 2014).

Coronary heart disease

Coronary heart disease and its risk factors is more common and seen earlier in those with SCI. The reasons are unclear but may be related to adrenergic system dysfunction, lipids, cholesterol and insulin resistance changes (Chopra et al., 2016; Myers et al., 2007).

Respiratory muscle training

Various training techniques such as forced breathing against resistance of a blocked airway (Berlowitz et al., 2016; Liaw et al., 2000; Van Houtt et al., 2006) can increase strength and respiratory muscle use. Improvement in inspiratory muscle use can increase vital capacity and reduce atelectasis. Improvement in expiratory muscle effectiveness can increase cough ability and secretion clearing and reduce infections (Roth et al., 2010).

Phrenic and diaphragm nerve pacing

Intramuscular electrodes can be implanted into the diaphragm of a ventilator-dependent patient enabling increases in inspiratory effort and tidal volume and periods without ventilator support. Similarly, direct phrenic nerve stimulation can produce diaphragm activity (Berlowitz et al., 2016; DiMarco et al., 2002, 2005; Zimmer et al., 2007).

Abdominal muscle electrical stimulation can sometimes help overcome disadvantages of flaccidity on diaphragm position and chest expansion (McCaughey et al., 2016).

Autonomic dysreflexia

Although SCI is usually permanent, return of spinal cord reflexes below the injury site eventually occurs. Autonomic dysreflexia is an abnormal and excessive spinal reflex response involving alpha-adrenoreceptor hyperresponsiveness producing excessive pressor response (Partida et al., 2016; Sezer et al., 2015; Teasell et al., 2000). This is a true medical emergency. For SCI above T6 level a dangerous hypertensive crisis can result. Intact peripheral nerves return stimuli to the cord from sources including distended bladder, bowel motion, pain, illness or even mild discomfort such as sheets tucked in tightly. These sensory impulses, though blocked at the injury level, can set up a reflex arc response in the cord itself leading to an uncontrolled sympathetic response. Peripheral vasoconstriction and hypertension can ensue. The brain becomes aware of hypertension via baroreceptors linked to cranial nerves. Response to halt the crisis cannot pass the cord injury so proves largely ineffective. The other response is compensatory bradycardia.

Typically a patient with autonomic dysreflexia presents with headache, flushing and profuse upper body sweating from upper compensatory vasodilation. In contrast, the lower body may be pale and cold. Key to effective management is recognition and prompt response. Search for possible stimuli and manage accordingly, including catheter bag clearing and draining, clearing impacted bowel and loosening clothing or bedding. Analgesia may be required even if pain cannot be described by the patient. If these options fail, a vasodilator, particularly glyceryl trinitrate, in a regimen similar to treatment of cardiac chest pain is appropriate.

Life expectancy for SCI survivors

SCI survivor life expectancy is considerably reduced. Varying with injury severity, the most common causes of death include infection (septicaemia, pneumonia and urinary tract disease), heart disease, pulmonary embolism and, tragically, suicide (Chamberlain et al., 2015; Soden et al., 2000). Survival post-SCI has not changed substantially for decades (Shavelle et al., 2015).

Ⓒs CASE STUDY 2

Case 11054, 1530 hrs.

Dispatch details: A four-year-old boy has been struck by a motor vehicle in the street. He is conscious and crying and still lying in the road.

Initial presentation: There is a crowd of people around the child. A bystander is waving at oncoming cars to slow down as police are not yet in attendance. The ambulance is parked to block traffic from proceeding past the scene.

1 ASSESS

1538 hrs Primary survey: The child is conscious, talking and crying.

1539 hrs Chief complaint: The child has an obvious forehead abrasion and appears to be in considerable left mid-thigh pain.

1541 hrs Vital signs survey: Perfusion status: HR 120 bpm, strong and regular; BP 90/50 mmHg; skin cool and dry.

Respiratory status: RR 28 bpm; good, clear air entry bilaterally, no accessory muscle use.

Conscious state: GCS = 15.

1542 hrs Pertinent hx: The child was riding his bicycle when he was struck by the vehicle, which was travelling at approximately 40 km/h. He was thrown across the car bonnet before landing on the road a few metres away. He was wearing his bicycle helmet and did not get up afterwards. There is no apparent loss of consciousness.

1545 hrs Secondary survey: There are no visible injuries or pain to the chest or abdomen. His left mid-thigh is markedly swollen compared to the right and is painful. A small temple haematoma has minimal bleeding. There is no neck pain or tenderness. He can move all limbs except his left leg.

2 CONFIRM

What else could it be?

Head injury

Event history and the forehead abrasion indicate blunt head strike against either the car or the ground. Assess for loss of consciousness described by bystanders. The child's age and distressed state increase the difficulty of assessing neurological function.

Spinal injury

The injury pattern suggests possible spinal column or cord injury. The left thigh pain is a distracting injury. Opioid analgesia can relieve pain, but may also alter his conscious state adding to assessment difficulty.

Any child with a mechanism or pattern of injury suggesting spinal injury should be managed as such and only cleared after medical and/or radiological assessment.

Something else

The incident was traumatic. Injury extent is not known, apart from left mid-thigh pain suggestive of a fracture. Secondary survey is required to identify other injuries including chest, abdominal and pelvic injuries with this mechanism.

> **DIFFERENTIAL DIAGNOSIS**
>
> **Fractured left femur**
> Or
> - Head injury
> - Spinal injury
> - Something else

3 TREAT

Treat the patient as multi-trauma. Provide manual inline spinal immobilisation, reassurance and build rapport. Consider cervical collar application and immobilisation. Splint the suspected fractured femur; administer analgesia as per local guidelines.

1545 hrs: Paramedics request other resources as appropriate (e.g. intensive care or aeromedical retrieval) and administer intranasal fentanyl for pain.

1547 hrs: Inline manual spinal immobilisation is commenced. The left leg is immobilised with splinting.

1553 hrs: A cervical collar is applied but he tries to remove it and shakes his head around; they decide to remove it. Manual immobilisation continues.

1554 hrs: IV access is established with fluid TKVO (to keep vein open) and analgesia titrated to patient weight and response.

1557 hrs: Further analgesia settles the patient, allowing soft cervical collar and spinal immobilisation using a vacuum mattress.

 EVALUATE

Clinical intervention evaluation can provide clues to initial diagnosis accuracy and management effectiveness. New findings in patients who are difficult to assess may come with time.

In this case the patient would be expected to remain stable during transport with any deterioration triggering reassessment. Positional discomfort and over-sedation from analgesia are possible complications.

 CASE STUDY 3

Case 10983, 0830 hrs.

Dispatch details: An 80-year-old woman has been found lying on the floor at home. She is conscious and has a head laceration.

Initial presentation: The crew are led inside a private house by a carer who found the patient. She is lying on her back in the bedroom.

 ASSESS

0841 hrs Chief complaint: Pain at the back of her head and inability to get up.

0841 hrs Vital signs survey: Perfusion status: HR 96 bpm, weak and irregular; BP 95/50 mmHg; skin cool and dry; temperature 34.1°C.

Respiratory status: RR 14 bpm; good, clear air entry; L = R; normal work of breathing; no dyspnoea.

Conscious state: GCS = 14; confused to time, place and event.

0842 hrs Secondary survey: She is able to move all limbs.

0843 hrs Pertinent hx: She is normally unsteady with a history of falls. Despite this, she lives independently at home with limited daily help. She is in her pyjamas and cannot say how long ago she fell. She has been incontinent of urine. The bedside table has been knocked over, suggesting she struck it as she fell.

0845 hrs Secondary survey: There are no visible chest or abdomen injuries or pain. Similarly, all limbs appear free from pain or injury. There is dried blood on the back of her head with a small amount observable on the bedside table. She has neck pain and tenderness.

This patient has a visible head injury. She is confused: is this 'normal' for her or a result of the injury? If in any doubt, consider any change a result of or contributing to the fall. She is more susceptible to sustaining spinal injury from a low-level fall.

② CONFIRM

The essential part of the clinical reasoning process is to seek to confirm your initial hypothesis by finding clinical signs that should occur with your provisional diagnosis. You should also seek to challenge your diagnosis by exploring findings that do not fit your hypothesis: don't just ignore them because they don't fit.

What else could it be?

Cardiac event

Her falls have been attributed to unsteadiness. Although this may be the cause, it is prudent to consider whether an event may have precipitated it including a cardiac event such as arrhythmia. An ECG can be evaluated, but it may not show signs now. Explore for cardiac symptoms.

Stroke

A neurological event precipitating the fall is also possible. While not definitive, neurological assessment is prudent to determine stroke symptoms.

Metabolic cause

An assessment of past history and blood glucose allows hypo- or hyperglycaemia consideration.

Infection

While fever is one infection indicator, in the elderly it is unreliable given autonomic nervous system changes. Recent illness, including symptoms including cough, chest consolidation or urinary, give clues to infection.

③ TREAT

Regardless of the cause of the fall, her age and current presentation dictate the need for spinal care. Pad bony prominences and curves such as the occiput, lumbar region and iliac crests. The ideal tool is a vacuum mattress. Accommodate abnormal spinal curvature or deformity.

0855 hrs: One paramedic maintains manual inline cervical support with her head returned midline. The other considers a cervical collar but forgoes it given her kyphosis. Instead she provides padding behind the patient's neck and occiput. They remove her wet clothing, covering her in warm blankets and attending to her wounds.

0905 hrs: The patient is spinally immobilised using a vacuum mattress.

④ EVALUATE

In this case the patient would be expected to remain stable during transport. Her body temperature should rise slowly. If any discomfort presents, this can be modified for her comfort.

DIFFERENTIAL DIAGNOSIS

Fall
Or
- Cardiac event
- Stroke
- Metabolic cause
- Infection

PRACTICE TIP

Complications of lying on the floor for a prolonged period of time include:
- hypothermia
- dehydration
- crush syndrome.

Future research

During the inflammatory phase, significant demyelination can occur resulting in permanent nervous tissue injury. One promising research area is neuroregeneration and cell transplantation, including stem cells, early in the acute phase to enable either new cellular growth or remyelination of remaining cells. This includes ways to improve or enhance remaining demyelinated nerve actions. Research includes investigation of optimal time for such activities, with some promise of neuronal regrowth, albeit insufficient, in post-acute stages. Strategies revolve around directly enabling cellular regrowth and enhancing the environment for it to occur (Ahuja et al., 2016; Kanno et al., 2015; Rowland et al., 2008).

Scar tissue in CNS injury, known as glial scar, inhibits axonal tissue regrowth. Various models for cellular transplant and enhancing the environment

657

for scar inhibition, thus allowing regrowth, are being explored (Rowland et al., 2008; Silver & Miller, 2004).

Neuroprotection is a future focus with evaluation of means to preserve tissue and reduce secondary injury development. This principally revolves around therapeutic hypothermia—which is difficult to timely initiate, yet may have future out-of-hospital implications—and pharmacotherapy options (Ahuja et al., 2016; Siddiqui et al., 2015).

Rehabilitation methods continue to be explored to enhance recovery from SCI. In particular, electrical stimulation and activity therapy aim to maintain existing muscle structures to help maintain life skills including writing, eating and self-care (Ahuja et al., 2016).

Summary

Spinal column injury and spinal cord injury are different, with potentially different long-term care pathways. SCI often leads to multiple body responses, resulting in the need to consider all systems throughout recovery and rehabilitation. SCI must be a primary out-of-hospital consideration for all patients who have experienced even low trauma levels, particularly if they have greater vulnerability. Avoidance of further injury is a primary out-of-hospital goal.

References

Adams, J. G. (2008). *Emergency medicine*. Philadelphia: Saunders.

Ahuja, C. S., Martin, A. R., & Fehlings, M. (2016). Recent advances in managing a spinal cord injury secondary to trauma. *F1000Research, 5*.

AIHW: Tovell A. (2018). *Spinal cord injury, Australia, 2012–13*. Injury research and statistics series no. 99. Cat. no. INJCAT 175. Canberra: AIHW.

Akbar, S. H., & Ooi, J. S. (2015). Comparison between C-MAC video-laryngoscope and Macintosh direct laryngoscope during cervical spine immobilization. *Middle East Journal of Anaesthesiology, 23*(1), 43–50.

Ala, A., Shams-Vahdati, S., Taghizadieh, A., Miri, S. H., Kazemi, N., Hodjati, S. R., & Jalilzadeh-Binazar, M. (2016). Cervical collar effect on pulmonary volumes in patients with trauma. *European Journal of Trauma and Emergency Surgery, 42*(5), 657–660.

Anwar, M. A., Al Shehabi, T. S., & Eid, A. H. (2016). Inflammogenesis of secondary spinal cord injury. *Frontiers in Cellular Neuroscience, 10*, 98.

Armstrong, B. P., Simpson, H. K., & Deakin, C. D. (2007). Prehospital clearance of the cervical spine: does it need to be a pain in the neck? *Emergency Medicine Journal, 24*(7), 501–503.

Asan, Z. (2018). Spinal concussion in adults: transient neuropraxia of spinal cord exposed to vertical forces. *World Neurosurgery, 114*, e1284–e1289.

Atesok, K., Tanaka, N., O'Brien, A., Robinson, Y., Pang, D., Deinlein, D., Manoharan, S. R., Pittman, J., & Theiss, S. (2018). Posttraumatic spinal cord injury without radiographic abnormality. *Advances in Orthopedics, 2018*.

Austin, N., Krishnamoorthy, V., & Dagal, A. (2014). Airway management in cervical spine injury. *International journal of critical illness and injury science, 4*(1), 50.

Badhiwala, J. H., Lai, C. K., Alhazzani, W., Farrokhyar, F., Nassiri, F., Meade, M., Mansouri, A., Sne, N., Aref, M., Murty, N., & Witiw, C. (2015). Cervical spine clearance in obtunded patients after blunt traumatic injury: a systematic review. *Annals of Internal Medicine, 162*(6), 429–437.

Bauer, D., & Kowalski, R. (1988). Effect of spinal immobilisation function in the healthy, non-smoking man. *Annals of Emergency Medicine, 17*(9), 915–918.

Berlly, M., & Shem, K. (2007). Respiratory management during the first five days after spinal cord injury. *The Journal of Spinal Cord Medicine, 30*(4), 309–318.

Berlowitz, D. J., Wadsworth, B., & Ross, J. (2016). Respiratory problems and management in people with spinal cord injury. *Breathe, 12*(4), 328.

Boese, C. K., Oppermann, J., Siewe, J., Eysel, P., Scheyerer, M. J., & Lechler, P. (2015). Spinal cord injury without radiologic abnormality in children: a systematic review and meta-analysis. *The Journal of Trauma and Acute Care Surgery, 78*(4), 874–882.

Boswell, H. B., Dietrich, A., Shiels, W. E., King, D., Ginn-Pease, M., Bowman, M. J., & Cotton, W. H. (2001). Accuracy of visual determination of neutral position of the immobilized pediatric cervical spine. *Pediatric Emergency Care, 17*(1), 10–14.

Branfoot, T. (1994). Motorcyclists, full-face helmets and neck injuries: can you take the helmet off safely, and if so, how? *Journal of Accident & Emergency Medicine, 11*, 117–120.

Brolin, K., Stockman, I., Andersson, M., Bohman, K., Gras, L. L., & Jakobsson, L. (2015). Safety of children in cars: a review of biomechanical aspects and human body models. *IATSS research, 38*(2), 92–102.

Brown, R. L., Brunn, M. A., & Garcia, V. F. (2001). Cervical spine injuries in children: a review of 103 patients treated consecutively at a level 1 pediatric trauma center. *Journal of Pediatric Surgery, 36*(8), 1107–1114.

Bush, L., Brookshire, R., Roche, B., Johnson, A., Cole, F., Karmy-Jones, R., Long, W., & Martin, M. J. (2016).

Evaluation of cervical spine clearance by computed tomographic scan alone in intoxicated patients with blunt trauma. *JAMA Surgery, 151*(9), 807–813.

Carroll, T., Smith, C. D., Liu, X., Bonaventura, B., Mann, N., Liu, J., & Ebraheim, N. A. (2015). Spinal cord injuries without radiologic abnormality in children: a systematic review. *Spinal Cord, 53*(12), 842.

Chamberlain, J. D., Meier, S., Mader, L., Von Groote, P. M., & Brinkhof, M. W. (2015). Mortality and longevity after a spinal cord injury: systematic review and meta-analysis. *Neuroepidemiology, 44*(3), 182–198.

Chopra, A. S., Miyatani, M., & Craven, B. C. (2016). Cardiovascular disease risk in individuals with chronic spinal cord injury: prevalence of untreated risk factors and poor adherence to treatment guidelines. *The Journal of Spinal Cord Medicine, 41*(1), 2–9.

Cirak, B., Ziegfeld, S., Knight, V. M., Chang, D., Avellino, A. M., & Paidas, C. N. (2004). Spinal injuries in children. *Journal of Pediatric Surgery, 39*(4), 607–612.

Cobb, J. E., Bélanger, L. M. A., Park, S. E., et al. (2014). Evaluation of a pilot Pressure Ulcer Prevention Initiative (PUPI) for patients with traumatic spinal cord injury. *Journal of Wound Care, 23*, 211–226.

Connor, D., Greaves, I., Porter, K., & Bloch, M., Consensus Group, Faculty of Pre-Hospital Care. (2015). Prehospital spinal immobilisation: an initial consensus statement. *Trauma, 17*(2), 146–150.

Cooke, M. W. (1998). Use of the spinal board within the accident and emergency department. *Journal of Accident & Emergency Medicine, 15*, 108–113.

Cowley, A., Hague, A., & Durge, N. (2017). Cervical spine immobilization during extrication of the awake patient: a narrative review. *European Journal of Emergency Medicine, 24*(3), 158–161.

Criswell, J. C., Parr, M. J. A., & Nolan, J. P. (1994). Emergency airway management in patients with cervical spine injuries. *Anaesthesia, 49*(10), 900–903.

Crosby, E. (2002). Airway management after upper cervical spine injury: what have we learned? *Canadian Journal of Anaesthesia, 49*(7), 733–744.

Curran, C., Dietrich, A. M., Bowman, M. J., Ginn-Pease, M. E., King, D. R., & Kosnick, E. (1995). Pediatric cervical spine immobilisation: achieving neutral position. *The Journal of Trauma, 39*(4), 729–732.

Davies, G., Deakin, C., & Wilson, A. (1996). The effect of a rigid collar on intracranial pressure. *Injury, 27*(9), 647–649.

Davis, J. W., Parks, S. N., Detlefs, C. L., Williams, G. G., Williams, J. L., & Smith, R. W. (1995). Clearing the cervical spine in obtunded patients: the use of dynamic fluoroscopy. *The Journal of Trauma, 39*, 435–438.

De Lorenzo, R. A., Olson, J. E., Boska, M., Johnston, R., Hamilton, G. C., Augustine, J., & Barton, R. (1995). Optimal positioning for cervical immobilization. *Annals of Emergency Medicine, 28*(3), 301–308.

Del Bigio, M. R., & Johnson, G. E. (1989). Clinical presentation of spinal cord concussion. *Spine, 14*(1), 37–40.

Del Rossi, G., Horodyski, M., & Powers, M. E. (2003). A comparison of spine board transfer techniques and the effect of training on performance. *Journal of Athletic Training, 38*(3), 204–208.

DiMarco, A. F., Onders, R. P., Kowalski, K. E., Miller, M. E., Ferek, S., & Mortimer, J. T. (2002). Phrenic nerve pacing in a tetraplegic patient via intramuscular diaphragm electrodes. *American Journal of Respiratory and Critical Care Medicine, 166*(12), 1604–1606.

DiMarco, A. F., Onders, R. P., Ignagni, A., Kowalski, K. E., & Mortimer, J. T. (2005). Phrenic nerve pacing via intramuscular diaphragm electrodes in tetraplegic subjects. *Chest, 127*(2), 671–678.

Durward, Q. J., Amacher, A. L., Del Maestro, R. F., & Sibbald, W. J. (1983). Cerebral and cardiovascular responses to changes in head elevation in patients with intracranial hypertension. *Journal of Neurosurgery, 59*(6), 938–944.

Eberhardt, C. S., Zand, T., Ceroni, D., Wildhaber, B. E., & La Scala, G. (2016). The seatbelt syndrome—do we have a chance? A report of 3 cases with review of literature. *Pediatric Emergency Care, 32*(5), 318–322.

Farrell, C. A., Hannon, M., & Lee, L. K. (2017). Pediatric spinal cord injury without radiographic abnormality in the era of advanced imaging. *Current Opinion in Pediatrics, 29*(3), 286–290.

Fatima, G., Sharma, V. P., Das, S. K., & Mahdi, A. A. (2015). Oxidative stress and antioxidative parameters in patients with spinal cord injury: implications in the pathogenesis of disease. *Spinal Cord, 53*(1), 3.

Furlan, J. C., Verocai, F., Palmares, X., & Fehlings, M. G. (2016). Electrocardiographic abnormalities in the early stage following traumatic spinal cord injury. *Spinal Cord, 54*(10), 872.

Gerling, M. C., Davis, D. P., Hamilton, R. S., Morris, G. F., Vilke, G. M., Garfin, S. R., & Hayden, S. R. (2000). Effects of cervical spine immobilization technique and laryngoscope blade selection on an unstable cervical spine in a cadaver model of intubation. *Annals of Emergency Medicine, 36*(4), 293–300.

Guly, H. R., Bouamra, O., & Lecky, F. E. (2008). The incidence of neurogenic shock in patients with isolated spinal cord injury in the emergency department. *Resuscitation, 76*(1), 57–62.

Haddad, S. H., & Arabi, Y. M. (2012). Critical care management of severe traumatic brain injury in adults. *Scandinavian Journal of Trauma, Resuscitation and Emergency Medicine, 20*(1), 12.

Hagen, E. M. (2015). Acute complications of spinal cord injuries. *World Journal of Orthopedics, 6*(1), 17.

Ham, W., Schoonhoven, L., Schuurmans, M. J., & Leenen, L. P. (2014). Pressure ulcers from spinal immobilization in trauma patients: a systematic review.

The Journal of Trauma and Acute Care Surgery, 76(4), 1131–1141.

Ham, W. H., Schoonhoven, L., Schuurmans, M. J., & Leenen, L. P. (2017). Pressure ulcers in trauma patients with suspected spine injury: a prospective cohort study with emphasis on device-related pressure ulcers. *International Wound Journal, 14*(1), 104–111.

Hauswald, M., Ong, G., Tandberg, D., & Omar, Z. (1998). Out-of-hospital spinal immobilization: its effect on neurologic injury. *Academic Emergency Medicine: Official Journal of the Society for Academic Emergency Medicine, 5*(3), 214–219.

Hawryluk, G., Whetstone, W., Saigal, R., Ferguson, A., Talbott, J., Bresnahan, J., Dhall, S., Pan, J., Beattie, M., & Manley, G. (2015). Mean arterial blood pressure correlates with neurological recovery after human spinal cord injury: analysis of high frequency physiologic data. *Journal of Neurotrauma, 32*(24), 1958–1967.

Hey, H. W. D., Lau, B. P. H., & Tan, W. T. (2018). Answer to the Letter to the Editor of A. Malhotra concerning 'The utility of magnetic resonance imaging in addition to computed tomography scans in the evaluation of cervical spine injuries: a study of obtunded blunt trauma patients' by B. P. H. Lau, et al. (Eur Spine J [2017]; doi:10.1007/s00586-017-5317-y). *European Spine Journal, 27*(1), 249–250.

Holly, L. T., Kelly, D. F., Counelis, G. J., Blinman, T., McArthur, D. L., & Cryer, H. G. (2002). Cervical spine trauma associated with moderate and severe head injury: incidence risk factors and injury characteristics. *Journal of Neurosurgery, 96*, S285–S291.

Hyldmo, P. K., Vist, G. E., Feyling, A. C., Rognås, L., Magnusson, V., Sandberg, M., & Søreide, E. (2015). Does turning trauma patients with an unstable spinal injury from the supine to a lateral position increase the risk of neurological deterioration? A systematic review. *Scandinavian Journal of Trauma, Resuscitation and Emergency Medicine, 23*(1), 65.

Iida, H., Tachibana, S., Kitahara, T., Horiike, S., Ohwada, T., & Fujii, K. (1999). Association of head trauma with cervical spine injury, spinal cord injury or both. *The Journal of Trauma, 46*, 450–452.

Johnson, D. R., Hauswald, M., & Stockhoff, C. (1996). Comparison of a vacuum splint device to a rigid backboard for spinal immobilization. *The American Journal of Emergency Medicine, 14*(4), 369–372.

Kanno, H., Pearse, D. D., Ozawa, H., Itoi, E., & Bunge, M. B. (2015). Schwann cell transplantation for spinal cord injury repair: its significant therapeutic potential and prospectus. *Reviews in the Neurosciences, 26*(2), 121–128.

Kirshblum, S. C., Burns, S. P., Biering-Sorensen, F., Donovan, W., Graves, D. E., Jha, A., Johansen, M., Jones, L., Krassioukov, A., Mulcahey, M. J., & Schmidt-Read, M. (2011). International standards for neurological classification of spinal cord injury (revised 2011). *The Journal of Spinal Cord Medicine, 34*(6), 535–546.

Kreinest, M., Ludes, L., Türk, A., Grützner, P. A., Biglari, B., & Matschke, S. (2017). Analysis of prehospital care and emergency room treatment of patients with acute traumatic spinal cord injury: a retrospective cohort study on the implementation of current guidelines. *Spinal Cord, 55*(1), 16.

Krell, J. M., McCoy, M. S., Sparto, P. J., Fisher, G. L., Stoy, W. A., & Hostler, D. P. (2006). Comparison of the Ferno scoop stretcher with the long backboard for spinal immobilisation. *Prehospital Emergency Care, 10*, 46–51.

Kroeker, A. M., Teddy, A. J., & Macy, M. L. (2015). Car seat inspection among children older than three: using data to drive practice in child passenger safety. *The Journal of Trauma and Acute Care Surgery, 79*(3 Sup 1), S48–S54.

Kumar, N., Pieri-Davies, S., Chowdhury, J. R., Osman, A., & El Masri, W. (2017). Evidence-based respiratory management strategies required to prevent complications and improve outcome in acute spinal cord injury patients. *Trauma, 19*(1_suppl), 23–29.

Kwan, I., Bunn, F., & Roberts, I. G. (2001). Spinal immobilization for trauma patients. *The Cochrane Database of Systematic Reviews*, (2), CD002803.

Larson, S., Delnat, A. U., & Moore, J. (2017). The use of clinical cervical spine clearance in trauma patients: a literature review. *Journal of Emergency Nursing*.

Lee, B. B., Cripps, R. A., Fitzharris, M., & Wing, P. C. (2014). The global map for traumatic spinal cord injury epidemiology: update 2011, global incidence rate. *Spinal Cord, 52*(2), 110.

Leonard, J. R., Jaffe, D. M., Kuppermann, N., Olsen, C. S., & Leonard, J. C., Pediatric Emergency Care Applied Research Network and Cervical Spine Study Group. (2014). Cervical spine injury patterns in children. *Pediatrics*, e1179–e1188.

Liaw, M. Y., Lin, M. C., Cheng, P. T., Wong, M. K. A., & Tang, F. T. (2000). Resistive inspiratory muscle training: its effectiveness in patients with acute complete cervical cord injury. *Archives of Physical Medicine and Rehabilitation, 81*, 752–756.

Lieberman, I. H., & Webb, J. K. (1994). Cervical spine injuries in the elderly. *The Journal of Bone and Joint Surgery. British Volume, 76*(6), 877–881.

Lubbert, P. H. W., Schram, M. E., & Leenen, L. P. H. (2005). Is there a reason for spine board immobilization in the emergency department for patients with a potential spinal injury? *European Journal of Trauma and Emergency Surgery, 31*(4), 375–378.

Luscombe, M. D., & Williams, J. L. (2003). Comparison of a long spinal board and vacuum mattress for spinal immobilisation. *Emergency Medicine Journal, 20*(5), 476–478.

Lustrin, E. S., Karakas, S. P., Ortiz, O., Cinnamon, J., Castillo, M., Vaheesan, K., Brown, J., Diamond, A., Black, K., & Singh, S. (2003). Pediatric cervical spine:

normal anatomy, variants and trauma. *Radiographics: A Review Publication of the Radiological Society of North America, Inc, 23*, 539–580.

Malik, M. A., Maharaj, C. H., Harte, B. H., & Laffey, J. G. (2008). Comparison of Macintosh, Truview EVO2, Glidescope and Airwayscope laryngoscope use in patients with cervical spine immobilization. *British Journal of Anaesthesia, 101*(5), 723–730.

Manoach, S., & Paladino, L. (2007). Manual inline stabilization for acute airway management of suspected cervical spine injury: historical review and current questions. *Annals of Emergency Medicine, 50*(3), 236–245.

Martin, B. W., Dykes, E., & Lecky, F. E. (2004). Patterns and risks in spinal trauma. *Archives of Disease in Childhood, 89*(9), 860–865.

Martin, M. J., Bush, L. D., Inaba, K., Byerly, S., Schreiber, M., Peck, K. A., Barmparas, G., Menaker, J., Hazelton, J. P., Coimbra, R., & Zielinski, M. D. (2017). Cervical spine evaluation and clearance in the intoxicated patient: a prospective Western trauma association multi-institutional trial and survey. *The Journal of Trauma and Acute Care Surgery, 83*(6), 1032–1040.

Maung, A. A., Johnson, D. C., Barre, K., Peponis, T., Mesar, T., Velmahos, G. C., McGrail, D., Kasotakis, G., Gross, R. I., Rosenblatt, M. S., & Sihler, K. C. (2017). Cervical spine MRI in patients with negative CT: A prospective, multicenter study of the Research Consortium of New England Centers for Trauma (ReCONECT). *The Journal of Trauma and Acute Care Surgery, 82*(2), 263–269.

McCance, K., & Huether, S. (2014). *Pathophysiology: the biologic basis for disease in adults and children* (7th ed.). Philadelphia: Mosby.

McCaughey, E. J., Borotkanics, R. J., Gollee, H., Folz, R. J., & McLachlan, A. J. (2016). Abdominal functional electrical stimulation to improve respiratory function after spinal cord injury: a systematic review and meta-analysis. *Spinal Cord, 54*(9), 628.

Medscape. (2014). *Brown-Sequard Syndrome*. Retrieved from http://emedicine.medscape.com/article/321652-overview. (Accessed 28 October 2014).

Morris, C. G., McCoy, E. P., & Lavery, G. G. (2004). Spinal immobilization for unconscious patients with multiple injuries. *British Medical Journal, 329*, 495.

Morris, C. G. T., & McCoy, E. (2003). Cervical immobilization collars in ICU: friend or foe? *Anaesthesia, 58*(11), 1051–1053.

Morris, C. G. T., & McCoy, E. (2004). Clearing the cervical spine in unconscious polytrauma victims, balancing risks and effective screening. *Anaesthesia, 59*(5), 464–482.

Moss, R., Porter, K., & Greaves, I. (2015). Minimal patient handling: a Faculty of Pre-Hospital Care consensus statement. *Trauma, 17*(1), 70–72.

Myers, J., Lee, M., & Kiratli, J. (2007). Cardiovascular disease in spinal cord injury: an overview of prevalence, risk, evaluation and management. *American Journal of Physical Medicine and Rehabilitation, 86*(2), 142–152.

Nolan, J. P., & Wilson, M. E. (1993). Orotracheal intubation in patients with potential cervical spine injuries. *Anaesthesia, 48*(7), 630–633.

Norton, L. (2010). *Spinal Cord Injury, Australia 2007–08*. Injury Research and Statistics Series No. 52. Cat. no. INJCAT 128. Canberra: AIHW.

Partida, E., Mironets, E., Hou, S., & Tom, V. J. (2016). Cardiovascular dysfunction following spinal cord injury. *Neural regeneration research, 11*(2), 189–194.

Patton, K. T., & Thibodeau, G. A. (2012). *Anatomy and physiology* (7th ed.). St Louis: Mosby.

Peck, G. E., Shipway, D. J. H., Tsang, K., & Fertleman, M. (2018). Cervical spine immobilisation in the elderly: a literature review. *British Journal of Neurosurgery*, 1–5.

Phillips, R., & Nutbeam, T. (2017). Should cervical spinal immobilisation be applied to alert adult patients following blunt traumatic injury? *Trauma, 19*(3), 226–227.

Protheroe, R. T., & Gwinnutt, C. L. (2011). Early hospital care of severe traumatic brain injury. *Anaesthesia, 66*(11), 1035–1047.

Purvis, T. A., Carlin, B., & Driscoll, P. (2017). The definite risks and questionable benefits of liberal pre-hospital spinal immobilisation. *The American Journal of Emergency Medicine, 35*(6), 860–866.

Radiopaedia.org. (2014). Retrieved from http://radiopaedia.org/articles/anterior-cord-syndrome. (Accessed 28 October 2014).

Rahmatalla, S., DeShaw, J., Stilley, J., Denning, G., & Jennissen, C. (2018). Comparing the efficacy of methods for immobilizing the thoracic-lumbar spine. *Air Medical Journal, 37*(3), 178–185.

Rao, P. J., Phan, K., Mobbs, R. J., Wilson, D., & Ball, J. (2016). Cervical spine immobilization in the elderly population. *Journal of Spine Surgery, 2*(1), 41.

Raphael, J. H., & Chotai, M. B. (1994). Effects of the cervical collar on cerebrospinal fluid pressure. *Anaesthesia, 49*(5), 437–439.

Reilly, C. W. (2007). Pediatric spine trauma. *The Journal of Bone and Joint Surgery. American Volume, 89*(1), 98–107.

Roberts, D. (2009). *Clinical procedures in emergency medicine* (5th ed.). St Louis: Elsevier.

Roth, E. J., Stenson, K. W., Powley, S., Oken, J., Primack, S., Nussbaum, S. B., & Berkowitz, M. (2010). Expiratory muscle training in spinal cord injury: a randomized controlled trial. *Archives of Physical Medicine and Rehabilitation, 91*, 857–861.

Rowland, J. W., Hawryluk, G. W. J., Kwon, B., & Fehlings, M. G. (2008). Current status of acute spinal cord injury pathophysiology and emerging therapies: promise on the horizon. *Neurosurgical Focus, 25*(5), E2.

Schriger, D. L., Larmon, B., LeGassick, T., & Blinman, T. (1991). Spinal immobilization on a flat backboard: does it result in neutral position of the cervical spine? *Annals of Emergency Medicine, 20*(8), 878–881.

Segan, R. D., Cassidy, C., & Benkowski, J. (1993). A discussion of the issue of the football helmet removal in suspected cervical spine injuries. *Journal of Athletic Training, 28*(4), 294, 296, 298, 300, 302, 304–305.

Sezer, N., Akkuş, S., & Uğurlu, F. G. (2015). Chronic complications of spinal cord injury. *World Journal of Orthopedics, 6*(1), 24–33.

Shavelle, R. M., DeVivo, M. J., Brooks, J. C., Strauss, D. J., & Paculdo, D. R. (2015). Improvements in long-term survival after spinal cord injury? *Archives of Physical Medicine and Rehabilitation, 96*(4), 645–651.

Shin, J. I., Lee, N. J., & Cho, S. K. (2016). Pediatric cervical spine and spinal cord injury: a national database study. *Spine, 41*(4), 283–292.

Siddiqui, A. M., Khazaei, M., & Fehlings, M. G. (2015). Translating mechanisms of neuroprotection, regeneration, and repair to treatment of spinal cord injury. *Progress in Brain Research, 218*, 15–54.

Silver, J., & Miller, J. H. (2004). Regeneration beyond the glial scar. *Neuroscience, 5*, 146–156.

Sirvent, J. S., Castillo, M. P., Belmonte, M. A. R., Alarcón, D. C., Beltran, S. M., González, E. R., Obregon, P. L., Garrido, A. G., González-Viejo, M. Á., & Sancho, J. F. (2017). Respiratory complications in acute traumatic spinal cord injury. *European Respiratory Journal, 50*, PA4746. doi:10.1183/1393003.congress-2017.PA4746.

Skellet, S., Tibby, S. M., & Durward, A. (2002). Immobilisation of the cervical spine in children. *BMJ, 324*, 591.

Slack, S. E., & Clancy, M. J. (2004). Clearing the cervical spine of paediatric trauma patients. *Emergency Medicine Journal, 21*(2), 189–193.

Soden, R. J., Walsh, J., Middleton, J. W., Craven, M. L., Rutkowski, S. B., & Yeo, J. D. (2000). Causes of death after spinal cord injury. *Spinal Cord, 38*, 604–610.

Spector, L. R., Madigan, L., Rhyne, A., Darden, B., & Kim, D. (2008). Cauda equina syndrome. *The Journal of the American Academy of Orthopaedic Surgeons, 16*(8), 471–479.

Stiell, I. G., Clement, C. M., McKnight, R. D., Brison, R., Schull, M. J., Rowe, B. H., Worthington, J. R., Eisenhauer, M. A., Cass, D., Greenberg, G., & MacPhail, I. (2003). The Canadian C-spine rule versus the NEXUS low-risk criteria in patients with trauma. *The New England Journal of Medicine, 349*(26), 2510–2518.

Suppan, L., Tramèr, M. R., Niquille, M., Grosgurin, O., & Marti, C. (2016). Alternative intubation techniques vs Macintosh laryngoscopy in patients with cervical spine immobilization: systematic review and meta-analysis of randomized controlled trials. *British Journal of Anaesthesia, 116*(1), 27–36.

Swartz, M. (2009). *Textbook of physical diagnosis* (6th ed.). Philadelphia: Saunders.

Tan, L. A., Kasliwal, M. K., & Traynelis, V. C. (2014). Comparison of CT and MRI findings for cervical spine clearance in obtunded patients without high impact trauma. *Clinical Neurology and Neurosurgery, 120*, 23–26.

Teasell, R. W., Arnold, J. M. O., Krassioukov, A., & Delaney, G. A. (2000). Cardiovascular consequences of loss of supraspinal control of the sympathetic system after spinal cord injury. *Archives of Physical Medicine and Rehabilitation, 81*(4), 506–516.

Todd, A. J., Moe, L. R., & Joon, L. Y. (2008). *Cervical spine surgery challenges: diagnosis and management.* Thieme Medical Publishers.

Todd, N. V. (2011). Priapism in acute spinal cord injury. *Spinal Cord, 49*, 1033–1035.

Totten, V. Y., & Sugarman, D. B. (1999). Respiratory effects of spinal immobilization. *Prehospital Emergency Care, 3*(4), 347–352.

Van Houtt, S., Vanlandewijck, Y., & Gosselink, R. (2006). Respiratory muscle training in persons with spinal cord injury: a systematic review. *Respiratory Medicine, 100*(11), 1886–1895.

van Silfhout, L., Peters, A. E. J., Berlowitz, D. J., Schembri, R., Thijssen, D., & Graco, M. (2016). Long-term change in respiratory function following spinal cord injury. *Spinal Cord, 54*(9), 714.

Vickery, D. (2001). The use of the spinal board after the prehospital phase of trauma management. *Emergency Medicine Journal, 18*, 51–54.

Wampler, D. A., Pineda, C., Polk, J., Kidd, E., Leboeuf, D., Flores, M., Shown, M., Kharod, C., Stewart, R. M., & Cooley, C. (2016). The long spine board does not reduce lateral motion during transport—a randomized healthy volunteer crossover trial. *The American Journal of Emergency Medicine, 34*(4), 717–721.

Weber, A. D., & Nance, M. L. (2016). Clearing the pediatric cervical spine. *Current Trauma Reports, 2*(4), 210–215.

White, C. C., IV, Domeier, R. M., & Millin, M. G., Standards and Clinical Practice Committee, National Association of EMS Physicians. (2014). EMS spinal precautions and the use of the long backboard–resource document to the position statement of the National Association of EMS Physicians and the American College of Surgeons Committee on Trauma. *Prehospital Emergency Care, 18*(2), 306–314.

White, N. H., & Black, N. H., 2016. *Spinal cord injury (SCI) facts and figures at a glance. National spinal cord injury statistical center, facts and figures at a glance.*

Witiw, C. D., & Fehlings, M. G. (2015). Acute spinal cord injury. *Journal of Spinal Disorders & Techniques, 28*(6), 202–210.

Yeung, J. H. H., Cheung, N. K., & Graham, C. A. (2006). Reduced time on the spinal board: effects of guidelines and education for emergency department staff. *Injury*, *37*(1), 53–56.

Zideman, D. A., De Buck, E. D. J., Singletary, E. M., Cassan, P., Chalkias, A. F., Evans, T. R., Hafner, C. M., Handley, A. J., Meyran, D., Schunder-Tatzber, S., & Vandekerckhove, P. G. (2015). *European Resuscitation Council Guidelines for Resuscitation 2015 Section 9.*

First aid. European Resuscitation Council. October: 278–287.

Zimmer, M. B., Nantwi, K., & Goshgarian, H. G. (2007). Effect of spinal cord injury on the respiratory system: basic research and current clinical treatment options. *The Journal of Spinal Cord Medicine*, *30*(4), 319–330.

Zwimpfer, T. J., & Bernstein, M. (1990). Spinal cord concussion. *Journal of Neurosurgery*, *72*(6), 894–900.

CHAPTER 38

Burns

By Toby St Clair and Yvonne Singer

OVERVIEW

- Burn injuries encompass a wide range of mechanisms and severity.
- Patients at the greatest risk of a poor outcome after a burn injury are infants and the elderly.
- Patients at the highest risk of sustaining a burn injury are young children, the elderly and young males.

- Burn injuries present particular challenges in pain management, fluid administration and advanced airway management.
- Early and effective intervention can result in significant and lifelong improvement in functional and cosmetic outcomes.

Introduction

In Australia, approximately 10,000 people are hospitalised every year as a result of a burn-related injury (Harrison & Steel, 2006); fortunately, however, severe burns are uncommon. Approximately 80% of the 3500 people transferred to the 17 dedicated Australian and New Zealand burns units for specialist burn care each year have burn injuries involving less than 10% total body surface area (TBSA); 70% were adults and 70% were male (Burn Registry of Australia and New Zealand [BRANZ], 2018). The predominant cause of burn injury in younger adults are flame burn injuries, usually involving an accelerant such as petrol, whereas scald burns, generally caused by hot beverages, are the most common cause of burns in children. High-risk groups include children aged between 1 and 2 years, which represented 33% of all paediatric cases, and adult males aged between 20 and 29 years, which represented 25% of all adult cases. Other types of burn injuries are uncommon, with chemical burn accounting for 7% of adult burn presentations and less than 1% of paediatric presentations, and electrical burn injury accounting for less than 2% of all injuries (BRANZ, 2018) (see Tables 38.1 and 38.2).

Burns injuries can be confronting and challenging to manage in the out-of-hospital setting. Multiple early priorities exist for the paramedic. Once scene safety has been established, a rapid assessment of the extent of the patient's injuries is needed to accurately initiate effective treatment and expedite transfer to the most appropriate destination. Despite major advancements in in-hospital management of burn injury, out-of-hospital burns care remains poorly researched and its impact on patient outcomes unclear; however, expert sources agree that effective management in the immediate 24 hours after injury directly correlates to decreased morbidity and mortality (ISBI Practice Guidelines Committee, 2016; Pham et al., 2008). In Australia and New Zealand, 28% of adult cases and 16% of paediatric cases were transferred directly from the scene by paramedic services with over 50% of cases resulting in secondary transfer via another regional hospital (BRANZ, 2018). The median transfer time from time of injury to arrival at the burns unit was 19 hours for adults and 18 hours for children, with regional differences due to geographical size and population distribution. Clearly, the effectiveness and efficiency of care received by paramedics prior to arrival at a specialist burns unit contributes to the patient's long-term recovery, and further research into effective out-of-hospital care should be a priority for out-of-hospital and burn professional communities.

Anatomy of the skin

The skin is the largest organ of the body, consisting of two layers—the epidermis and the dermis—beneath which is a layer of subcutaneous fat (see Fig 38.1). The skin acts as a physical barrier to infection and fluid loss, regulates body temperature and acts as a sensory interface with the external environment. Any one of these functions may be compromised by burn injury and, if severe enough, the consequence of the burn injury can rapidly become life-threatening.

The outermost layer, the epidermis, forms the barrier to fluid loss and infection, contains no blood vessels or nerve endings, and is comprised largely of layers of slowly maturing epithelial cells that form at the junction between the dermis and the epidermis. These epithelial cells are 'pushed' towards the surface by growth of newer cells forming beneath and progressively lose their normal cellular contents, becoming flattened, infused with keratin and ultimately shed as they reach the skin surface (Herndon, 2007).

Table 38.1 Most common causes of burn injury in children

Cause	Subcause	N	%
Scald	Hot beverages	190	20
Scald	Water from saucepan/kettle/jug/billy/urn	130	13
Scald	Food (liquid/solid)	81	8
Contact	Coals/ashes	63	6
Scald	Water from tap/bath/shower	43	4
Scald	Fat/oil	42	4
Contact	Vehicle exhaust	42	4
Friction	Treadmill	36	4
Flame	Campfire/bonfire/burn-off	34	4
Scald	Other source	26	3
Contact	Iron	21	2
Contact	Hot metal	18	2
Contact	Wood heater	18	2
Flame	Lighter/matches	17	2
Scald	Water from hot-water bottle	15	2

Primary subcause of burn injury in paediatric cases (BRANZ, 2015–2016)

Source: BRANZ (2018).

Table 38.2 Most common causes of burn injury in adults

Cause	Subcause	N	%
Flame	Campfire/bonfire/burn-off	306	14
Scald	Fat/oil	150	7
Flame	Other	127	6
Scald	Water from saucepan/kettle/jug/billy/urn	125	6
Chemical	Alkali	113	5
Flame	Other source	91	4
Flame	Vehicle/engine parts	87	4
Flame	Gas/gas bottle	75	3
Contact	Coals/ashes	65	3
Contact	Contact hot/metal	63	3
Flame	Welder/grinder	63	3
Scald	Food liquid/solid	60	3
Scald	Hot beverages	60	3
Friction	Vehicle/motorbike	60	3
Contact	Vehicle exhaust	42	2

Primary subcause of burn injury in adult cases (BRANZ, 2015–2016)

Source: BRANZ (2018).

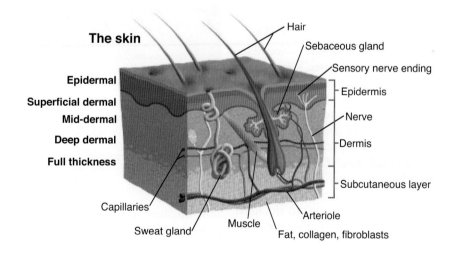

Figure 38.1
The skin and burn depth.
Source: Image re-produced with permission of the Victorian Adult Burn Service at The Alfred.

The dermis is a relatively thin layer directly underneath the epidermis, composed primarily of connective tissue rich in blood vessels, pain and pressure nerve receptors, sebaceous (sweat) glands and hair follicles. The dermis also provides the skin with its elasticity and strength, and its rich blood flow allows for control of thermoregulation and provides nutrients to the growing cells in the lower epidermis. The dermis is divided into two layers: the thin and superficial *papillary region* (so named because of its irregular surface) and the deeper and stronger *reticular region* where the hair follicles and glands reside. The dermis has variable depth across the body, with less than half a millimetre on parts of

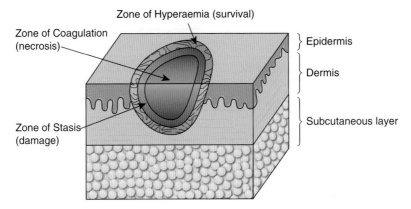

Figure 38.2
Jackson's thermal wound model demonstrates how the inflammatory response to burn injury needs to be managed in order to maximise the patient's chances of quick and scar-less recovery.

the face but up to 3 mm thick on the back (Scott & Fong, 2004; Herndon, 2007). The degree of damage to the dermis following burn injury determines the capacity of the dermis to spontaneously regenerate, or whether surgical intervention is required.

Below the dermis is a layer of fat sometimes referred to as the hypodermis. Although not considered part of the skin, this subcutaneous tissue is rich in fat cells and white blood cells and anchors the skin to underlying bone or connective tissue.

Pathophysiology of burn injury

Burn injury is sustained when tissues are subjected to excessive heat. As the temperature rises, human cells remain stable to a point, but denature rapidly once they exceed a temperature threshold. They become irreversibly damaged when cell temperature rises above 45°C, and the rate of cell death doubles with each degree above 45°C (Pham & Gibran, 2007).

The 'Jackson's thermal wound model' is used commonly to describe burn injury (Jackson, 1953; see Fig 38.2). The zone at the centre of the burn (the Zone of Coagulation) was closest to the heat source, where the damage is greatest. This zone has irreversible tissue necrosis due to exposure to heat, chemicals or electricity. The extent of this injury is dependent on the temperature (or concentration) and the duration of exposure. Immediately surrounding the Zone of Coagulation, both laterally and beneath, is the Zone of Stasis, an area where tissue is ischaemic and/or injured, but may survive if managed correctly. This zone has been shown to react positively to initial first aid but can progress to a deeper burn injury if not properly managed in the immediate stages following injury (Shupp et al., 2010). Finally, in the Zone of Hyperaemia cells are not damaged by the heat but are affected by the

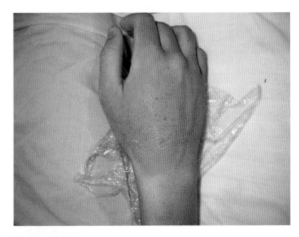

Figure 38.3
Epidermal burns.
Epidermal burns are red and painful to touch. The epidermis is damaged but not broken, so they do not form blisters. They usually heal within 7–10 days with no scarring.
Source: Image reproduced with permission of the Victorian Adult Burn Service at The Alfred.

inflammatory mediators (Gray & O'Reilly, 2009) causing an increased blood supply, which gives the skin surounding the burn a red colour (see Fig 38.3).

Burn injury severity

In clinical terms, burn injury severity is classified by depth and size.

Depth

The depth of burn injury is proportional to the duration of exposure, the energy involved and the conductivity of the tissues affected. Burn depth can involve all anatomical structures including the epidermis, dermis and subcutaneous tissue, as well as underlying muscle, bone and organs. Many factors can affect the appearance of the damaged tissue, making it difficult to assess wound depth: even experienced specialist clinicians struggle to correctly assess burn depth in more than 70% of cases (Johnson & Richard, 2003; Jaskille et al., 2010). In the out-of-hospital setting, the important distinction is between superficial and deeper burns, because deeper injuries will require specialist treatment.

Historically, burn depth was classified as first, second or third degree; however, the descriptors epidermal, dermal partial-thickness and full-thickness are now commonly used in Australia (Australian and New Zealand Burn Association [ANZBA], 2015) (see Table 38.3).

Epidermal burns involve only the epidermis, and do not penetrate or damage the dermis. They are red and painful to touch, and due to the intact underlying dermis, do not form blisters. Importantly, epidermal burns are not included in calculating % TBSA burn estimations. In the acute phase, epidermal burns often only require symptomatic treatment of pain and they spontaneously heal within 7 days without any cosmetic defect (Pham & Gibran, 2007). Contact injuries caused by household cooking, domestic appliances and sunburn generally fit into this category of epidermal injury (see Fig 38.4).

Full-thickness burns are their own category and dermal partial-thickness burns comprise of three subclassifications which are categorsied according to the depth that the injury extends into the dermis: superficial dermal, mid-dermal and deep dermal.

- **Superficial dermal partial-thickness burns** extend into the upper (papillary) region of the dermis. They are extremely painful to exposure and touch. The dermis will have a brisk capillary return to pressure (< 2 seconds), indicating good preservation of dermal circulation. If the epidermis remains intact this will result in blisters, but if the epidermis is broken or burnt away the exposed dermis will appear red and moist. Superficial partial-thickness burns generally heal in less than 14 days with minimal scarring (see Fig 38.4).

- **Mid-dermal partial-thickness burns** extend further into the dermis resulting in some damage to vasculature and nerve endings that manifests as slow capillary return and altered pain sensation on assessment. They take longer to heal, usually within 14–21 days, which increases the risk of scarring (see Fig 38.5).

- **Deep dermal partial-thickness burns** extend into the deeper reticular dermis and damage structures such as sweat glands and hair follicles. They exhibit absent or, at most, sluggish capillary refill to pressure (Pham & Gibran, 2007), and pain sensation is significantly reduced due to damaged nerve endings. The burn can appear pale or mottled (pink and pale white) in colour because of reduced blood flow, and at other times may have a cherry red appearance caused by the extravasation of red blood cells into the soft tissues. Deep dermal burns can take weeks to months to heal, resulting in significant scarring if left to heal spontaneously, and are usually managed similarly to full-thickness burns (see Fig 38.6).

Table 38.3 Depth assessment of burns

Classification	Description
Epidermal	Dry and red, blanches with pressure, no blisters. May be painful. Heals with no scarring.
Superficial dermal partial-thickness burns	Pale pink with fine blistering, blanches with pressure. Usually extremely painful. Can have colour-match defect. Low risk of hypertrophic scarring.
Mid-dermal partial-thickness burns	Dark pink with large blisters. Capillary refill sluggish. May be painful. Moderate risk of hypertrophic scarring.
Deep dermal partial-thickness burns	Blotchy red, may blister, no capillary refill. In child may be dark lobster red with mottling. High risk of hypertrophic scarring.
Full-thickness burns	White, waxy or charred. No blisters. No capillary refill. Will scar.

Source: Based on Craft et al. (2011).

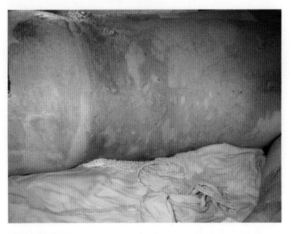

Figure 38.4
Superficial dermal partial-thickness burns.
These extend into the dermis and are extremely painful. They are moist, the epidermis can be detached or semidetached, and blisters are often present.
Source: Image reproduced with permission of the Victorian Adult Burn Service at The Alfred.

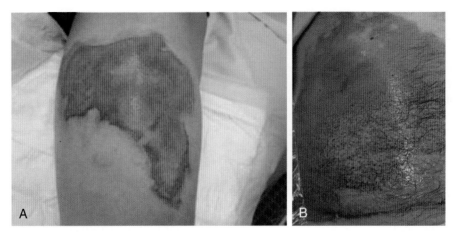

Figure 38.5
Mid-dermal partial-thickness burns.
Capillary return is present, but it is delayed and pain is present, albeit less severe than the pain of superficial burns. Blisters may be present and the underlying dermis is a variable colour (pale to dark pink).
Source: Image reproduced with permission of the Victorian Adult Burn Service at The Alfred.

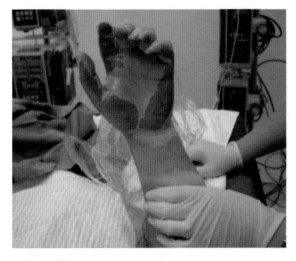

Figure 38.6
Deep dermal burns.
Deep dermal partial-thickness burns tend to be dry, with diminished fluid exudates compared with more superficial burns.
Source: Image reproduced with permission of the Victorian Adult Burn Service at The Alfred.

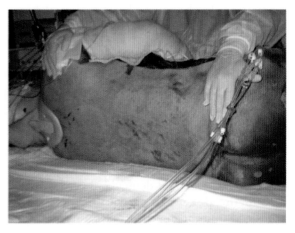

Figure 38.7
Full-thickness burns.
Full-thickness burns involve destruction of both layers of skin (epidermis and dermis) and may penetrate more deeply into underlying structures. These burns have a dense white, waxy or even charred appearance. The coagulated dead skin has a leathery appearance, called eschar.
Source: Image reproduced with permission of the Victorian Adult Burn Service at The Alfred.

• **Full-thickness burns** involve all skin layers, extending through the epidermis and dermis to the subcutaneous tissue (see Fig 38.7). Common characteristics include the absence of both capillary return and painful sensation, as all of the dermis has been destroyed. They can be charred or pale in colour depending on the applied heat source, and the burn eschar is 'leathery' in texture. After arrival to the burns unit, full-thickness burns, as well as deep dermal partial-thickness burns, are usually managed with early complete surgical excision (Ong et al., 2006) and wound closure by traditional skin grafting, or more modern skin substitution techniques, as soon as possible (Gacto-Sanchez, 2017). This important early surgical intervention that improves mortality, morbidity and length of stay outcomes relies on the quality care in the out-of-hospital environment to ensure the patient is stable and warm enough to immediately undergo the surgical procedure after leaving the ED (Ong et al., 2006).

Burn injuries, in particular thermal burns such as flame or scald injuries, rarely present as

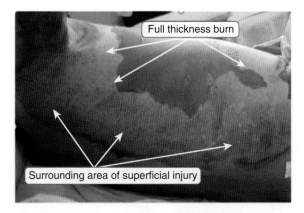

Figure 38.8
Mixed depth.
Mixed depth burn injury to torso.
Source: Image reproduced with permission of the Victorian Adult Burn Service at The Alfred.

a single depth of injury, and are usually heterogeneous (Hettiaratchy & Papini, 2004). Full-thickness thermal burns will almost certainly be surrounded by an area of more superficial burns and the pain associated with these 'lesser' areas is likely to be severe, even if the centre of the burn is desensitised due to nerve damage, and it is important to consider this in effective out-of-hospital pain management. As seen in Figure 38.8, the injury involves a central full-thickness burn area underneath the axilla, characterised by the white/yellow area which possibly extends underneath the damaged brown epidermis. There is also a surrounding area of partial and superficial burns, characterised by the red areas, away from the central area extending along the arm, towards the back and hip.

Surface area

The extent of injury is best described as % TBSA affected by the burn. In the out-of-hospital setting, the % TBSA of burns gives indications for fluid resuscitation requirements and transfer destination (see discussion below in the section Treat). There are several methods of assessing burn size. Regardless of the specific method used, it is essential that erythema is not included in the calculation (Connolly, 2011). The following are the three most commonly used tools to assess burn surface area in the emergency setting.

1. **Lund and Browder.** This is predominantly used to assess paediatric burn injury size. It assigns different percentages to body areas according to the child's age, allowing for adjustments in the surface area of the head and neck relative to the surface area of the limbs that are seen during the stages of normal childhood development (see Fig 38.9).

2. **Rule of Nines.** This is commonly used to assess adult burn injuries. It is similar to Lund and Browder but divides the body into **sections** that represent 9% of the body surface area, and does not accommodate the differences in paediatric stages of growth (see Fig 38.10).

3. **Palmar method.** Common in current clinical practice is the use of the surface area of the patient's hand (palm plus fingers adducted) to represent 0.8% TBSA and 0.5% TBSA if palm alone. This technique is useful for calculating scattered burns or estimated burns < 15% or very large burns > 85% where unburnt skin is counted; however, it can be inaccurate for medium-sized burns (Hettiaratchy & Papini 2004).

Several studies have compared the various methods of estimating burn surface. The Lund and Browder chart has been demonstrated to be more accurate than either the Rule of Nines or the palmar method in identifying % TBSA burns in children, whereas the Rule of Nines is faster and more convenient to use for adult burn patients in emergency situations. A number of studies have highlighted inaccuracies in TBSA assessment (Wachtel et al., 2000; Harish et al., 2015; Freiburg et al., 2007). Overestimation of burn size area can result in excessive fluid resuscitation with subsequent pulmonary complications, as well as a greater risk of compartment syndrome and need for escharotomy. Underestimation can lead to circulatory collapse and renal failure because of insufficient fluid resuscitation (Chan et al., 2012). Inaccurate % TBSA burn assessment can also lead to inappropriate transfers, which are costly and consume unnecessary healthcare resources.

The inflammatory response to burn injury

As described in detail in Chapter 4, the inflammatory response is the body's normal reaction to injury and is the start of the healing process. There are a range of triggers and substances that drive this response, but the net result of all these inflammatory mediators is to increase blood flow to the injured area while simultaneously increasing the permeability of the capillaries close to the injured tissue. These reactions facilitate the movement of white blood cells from the capillaries to the extracellular space to help fight infection and remove cellular detritus.

Local inflammatory effects

At the local tissue level, the changes to the microvascular blood flow and vessel permeability caused

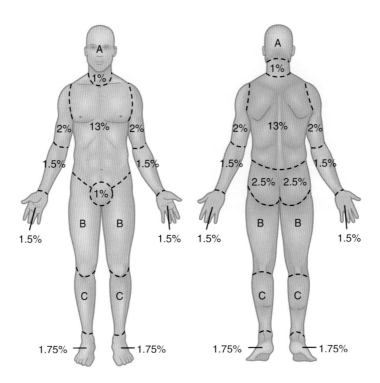

Relative percentages of areas affected by growth

Age	Half of head (A)	Half of one thigh (B)	Half of one leg (C)
Infant	9.5	2.75	2.5
1 yr	8.5	3.25	2.5
5 yr	6.5	4	2.75
10 yr	5.5	4.25	3
15 yr	4.5	4.25	3.25
Adult	3.5	4.75	3.5

Figure 38.9
Lund and Browder chart.
Source: Marx et al. (2014).

by burn injury result in a shift of fluid, electrolytes and protein from the intravascular space into the interstitial space (Latenser, 2009). Most of the oedema forms within minutes to hours of the injury and reaches its maximum by 24 hours post-injury (Demling, 2005; Tricklebank, 2009). While the inflammatory response is essential for healing, an overly aggressive response can direct so much blood to an area, causing so much oedema, that damaged but viable cells surrounding the injury (the Zones of Stasis and Hyperaemia) can become inadequately perfused and further compromised, increasing the likelihood of burn wound progression. Furthermore, if the inflammatory response extends beyond the burn site, as in cases of severe burn injury, it can lead to widespread vasodilation and oedema and progress to burns shock (see Figs 38.11 and 38.12).

Systemic inflammatory effects— burns shock

In larger burn injuries the consequences of the inflammatory response can extend far beyond the burn site, and cause systemic vasodilation and increased capillary permeability. This initial stage following burn injury, known as the 'hypodynamic phase', can cause substantial fluid shifts that can lead to hypovolaemia and tissue oedema. It is suspected that inflammatory mediators (histamine, prostaglandins, thromboxane and nitric oxide) released by local tissue damage are supported by additional inflammatory mediators such as interleukins to produce far-reaching, widespread systemic effects (Schwartz & Balakrishan, 2004). The involvement of these mediators occurs most frequently when the dermal partial-thickness burn area exceeds 20% of TBSA and some authors describe this

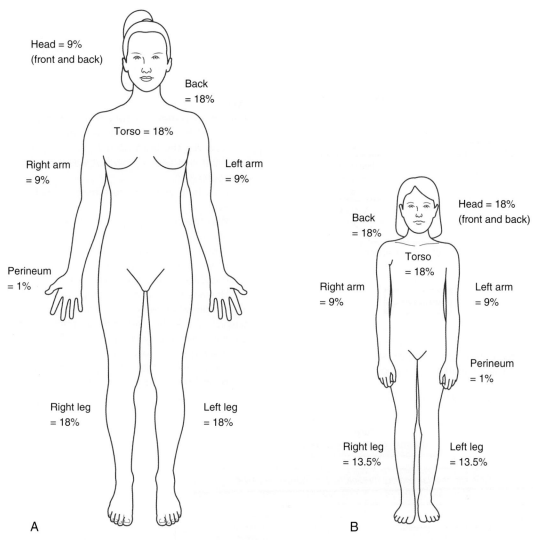

Figure 38.10
The Rule of Nines.
A Adult, **B** Child.
Source: Smith et al. (2010).

situation as the entire body becoming the Zone of Hyperaemia (Connolly, 2011) (see Fig 38.12). The inflammation and hypermetabolic response are thought to persist for long periods, years even, post-injury (Nielson et al., 2017).

It has reported that in the first few hours post burn in ≥ TBSA 40% and above, up to half of the total plasma water can be lost from the vascular compartment (Vaughn & Beckel, 2012). Compounded with the evaporative fluid loss from the burn site itself, this form of distributive shock can cause hypotension and organ hypoperfusion, which is often referred to as 'burns shock' (Schwartz & Balakrishan, 2004). The priority during this phase is intravascular volume resuscitation to maintain end-organ perfusion and function.

This resuscitation is not without consequence, however, leading to a decreased capillary oncotic pressure; worsening oedema ensures. Oedematous swelling, characteristic of the fluid shifts into the interstitial spaces, is called angio-oedema, and is often first noted in the feet, hands, face (lips and eyelids) and upper airway which may be observed as changes to the patient's voice (Shupp et al., 2010).

The second phase begins roughly 24 to 72 hours post injury and is known as the 'hypermetabolic flow phase'. This phase is characterised by a reduction in vascular permeability, increased heart rate and decreased peripheral vascular resistance. This is likely due to a redistribution of peripheral blood flow to the burn wound and the beginning of healing within the microvasculature (Bittner et al., 2015).

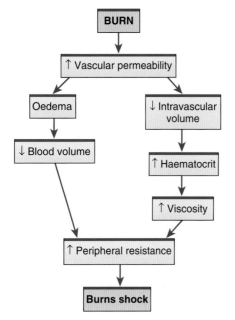

Figure 38.11
After surviving the initial insult, the greatest initial threat to a patient with a major burn is hypovolaemic shock as the inflammatory response spreads away from the burn site.
Source: Brown & Edwards (2012).

The cardiac output is reported to be more than 1.5 times and an elevation of basal metabolic rate threefold of that of a non-burned equivalent patient 3–4 days post burn injury (Nielson et al., 2017).

> **Ask!**
> **Important patient history to understand nature of burn and possible injuries**
> - How did the burn occur?
> - What was and/or how hot was the heat source?
> - How long was exposure time to heat source?
> - Was the burn exposure in an enclosed space?
> - When did the burn occur?
> - How old is the patient?
> - Past history and comorbidities
> - Has any first aid been completed already?
>
> This information aids in generating an 'index of suspicion' (i.e. the likely risk of immediate or evolving respiratory compromise). Burns incurred in an enclosed environment always produce a high index of suspicion for airway injury and respiratory compromise.

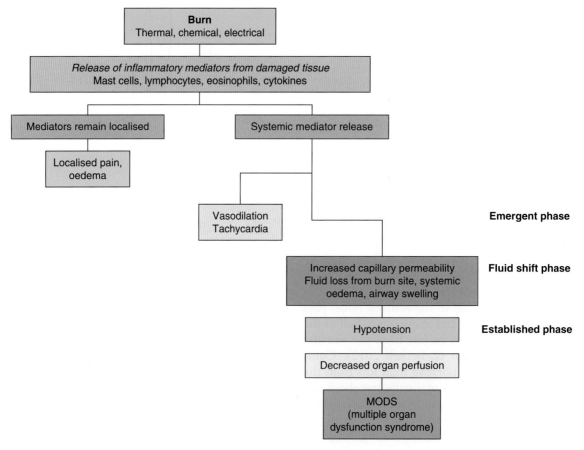

Figure 38.12
Phases of burns shock.

CASE STUDY 1

Case 54046, 1800 hrs.

Dispatch: A 30-year-old male has burns after a gas explosion.

Initial presentation: A 30-year-old male is seated indoors, with wet towels on his face and arms. He is conscious and in clear discomfort. He is shivering.

Pertinent Hx: The patient was working in the garage of his family home. Gas was leaking from the barbeque gas bottle that was not fully turned off after the family lunch. The gas was ignited by the pilot light on a hot-water service causing a flash 'explosion' and the flames briefly consumed him. He rolled to the ground, took off his t-shirt to smother his hair and then walked into his house. He stood in the shower for 10 minutes and now has wet towels over his face and arms.

ASSESS

Danger

As always, paramedics must first ensure that the scene is safe—in this setting, in conjunction with other emergency services. This may involve moving the patient to a safe location. Heat sufficient to cause tissue damage can remain in clothes and jewellery for a considerable period of time, particularly if the heat source is a liquid. In this case, the fire was extinguished and the patient's t-shirt was removed prior to the crew's arrival. Where spilled accelerants are involved, clothing may still be a potential fire hazard and should be removed, even from non-burned areas. It is important to note that accelerants and other flammable substances may irritate or produce burns to the skin if they are not removed and flushed away or diluted with water. Following confirmation of scene safety, a structured physical assessment must be prioritised (see Table 38.4).

1809 hrs Primary survey: The patient is conscious and responding.

1810 hrs Vital signs survey: RR 18 bpm, increased work of breathing, speaking in short sentences, shortness of breath.

No obvious haemorrhage. HR 106, sinus tachycardia, BP 110/85 mmHg, skin pale and cool, tympanic temperature is 35.2°C.

The patient has red, burnt, semidetached areas of skin to the face and bilateral arms.

Chief complaint: 'My face and arms hurt.'

Airway

Airway stability should be assessed as a matter of priority. Assessment of the airway commences by first looking for physical signs and symptoms suggestive of direct structural injury. These include burns to the face, neck and chest wall. Injuries to the face may involve the mouth, tongue, nasopharynx, oropharynx and larynx. Airway obstruction in the first 12 hours post injury is caused by direct thermal injury and/or chemical irritation of the upper airways (Mlcak et al., 2007). Assessment should include a visual inspection of the patient's oral

Table 38.4 Principles of emergency management: initial assessment of the burn patient

Airway	• Is the airway secure or at risk? • Look for signs of pending obstruction/inhalation injury: face, mouth or neck burns, carbonaceous sputum, flame burns in enclosed space, respiratory distress, stridor.
Breathing	• Assess respiratory rate, effort, breath sounds, dyspnoea, wheeze, hoarse voice, SpO$_2$. • Expose the chest to observe for equal bilateral chest expansion.
Circulation	• Observe for signs of haemorrhage. • Assess heart rate, blood pressure, colour, capillary refill, skin turgor.
Disability	• Assess conscious state using the Glasgow Coma Scale or AVPU. Consider differential diagnosis for altered states of consciousness. • Consider hypoglycaemia in diabetics.
Exposure	• Expose the patient and assess the extent of the burn injury. • Assess for any concomitant injuries. • Take the patient's temperature.
Pain	• Assess the severity, nature and location of pain.
Burn injury	• Estimate % TBSA burns; consider the extent of deep injury versus superficial.

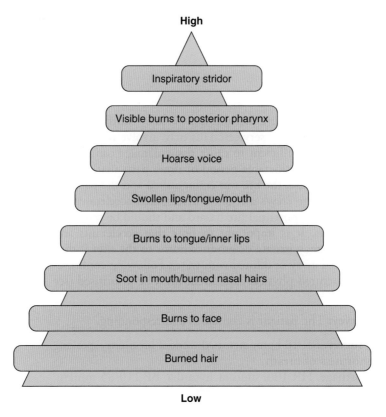

Figure 38.13
Risk stratification for development of airway obstruction from burn.
Source: Adapted from Sanders (2007).

and nasal cavities to assess for redness, swelling, and/or burnt lips, oral mucosa or tongue, as these can swell significantly if burnt. This airway inspection will help determine whether an immediate threat is present and provide clues to the extent of airway involvement.

Second, assessment should determine whether there are signs and symptoms suggestive of inhalation injury (see Fig 38.13). Hoarseness and/or stridor are late signs indicative of possible pending airway obstruction. Ask the patient if there are any changes to their voice, or whether they have difficulty swallowing or experience pain or discomfort when coughing or talking, as irritation of the airway and vocal cords from heat, chemical irritants and/or inflammatory response changes may alter speech. Signs and symptoms of inhalation injury include:

- carbonaceous sputum
- soot in the oral cavity
- singed nasal hairs and eyebrows
- intraoral burn
- stridor
- hoarseness with vocalisation
- wheezing
- persistent coughing.

The first four signs indicate that the face and oral cavity are affected; stridor and hoarseness indicate that the structural components of the pharyngeal and laryngeal regions are compromised; and wheezing and coughing indicate that the bronchial tree is affected. The presence of any of these signs aids in determining how much of the airway may have been compromised. If all signs are present, the whole airway is likely to have been involved. The final element of assessment examines any indications of systemic effects of airway burn injury. These include:

- asphyxia
- dyspnoea
- altered conscious state
- confusion
- cyanosis or skin flushing
- hypoventilation
- poor SpO_2 despite adequate ventilation.

Systemic complications arise when inhaled contaminants enter the central circulation. When this occurs susceptible organs can be damaged. Complications causing organ dysfunction can initiate a separate cascade of complications many hours, days or weeks after a burn event.

Breathing and ventilation

Once the airway is secure, the paramedic should then assess respiratory rate, effort, breath sounds and oxygen saturation. Breathing can be compromised following flame burn injury if people inhale smoke, especially in enclosed spaces, which can cause damage to the lungs and toxic poisoning from substances such as carbon monoxide or cyanide. Only small quantities of toxic irritants or super-heated gases are required to injure the delicate tissues of the small airways. This is likely to cause bronchospasm and subsequent wheezing, a common finding for paramedics during the assessment of a patient with burns (see Ch 17). Paramedics should remain vigilant for signs of worsening respiratory compromise such as wheezing, coughing, difficulty speaking or swallowing, copious sputum production or an increased work of breathing (Haberal et al., 2010).

Inhalation of smoke, especially from burning furniture and carpets, can also lead to systemic complications such as carbon monoxide poisoning, cyanide poisoning or other toxic contamination of the bloodstream, organs and tissues (Reade et al., 2012). A history of exposure to noxious gases in an enclosed environment should raise serious concerns. Oxygen saturation is an unreliable oxygenation assessment parameter in patients with carbon monoxide poisoning. The SpO_2 monitor interprets saturation of haemoglobin and cannot differentiate carbon monoxide from oxygen, giving a false-positive reading when the patient may actually be profoundly hypoxic. Therefore, routine

> **Ask!**
> **Key patient history questions related to suspected inhalation injury**
> - Do you feel breathless or anxious or are you finding it difficult to catch your breath?
> - Is your voice different?
> - If a flame or explosion burn: Did the injury occur in an enclosed environment?
> - What was the environment of the exposure?
> - What materials are you likely to have breathed in?
> - How long did you breathe them in for?

administration oxygen should be given regardless of the oxygen saturation when treating a patient at risk of exposure to harmful contaminates. Consider carbon monoxide poisoning in patients who sustain burns in an enclosed area. Carbon monoxide has a 280 times greater affinity for haemoglobin than oxygen does. A history of altered consciousness associated with the accident, the presence of neuropsychiatric or cardiac abnormalities and a cherry pink appearance to the skin indicate potential carbon monoxide or cyanide poisoning, and where available, carboxyhaemoglobin (COHb) blood levels should be taken in the secondary survey.

The patient's chest should be exposed to determine whether chest expansion is adequate and bilaterally equal. Deep circumferential burns of the chest or abdomen can have a tourniquet effect that can restrict chest expansion, limit respiratory excursion and subsequently compromise ventilation. These patients require urgent transfer in case an urgent escharotomy is required to facilitate adequacy of ventilation (see Figs 38.14 and 38.15 and Box 38.1).

Circulation

Inspect for any signs of haemorrhage and apply direct pressure to any external wounds. Haemorrhage is rare in isolated burn injuries, but consider the potential for internal bleeding and haemorrhagic shock in multi-trauma burn injury cases. Parameters including blood pressure, heart rate and unburnt skin colour provide important clues to circulatory status. Burns shock takes some time to evolve and is generally preceded by tachycardia, although tachycardia is considered normal in the context of increased catecholamine response following thermal injury which makes diagnosis difficult (American Burn Association, 2011). Furthermore, circulatory assessment can be problematic: measuring blood pressure, applying cardiac electrodes or palpating painful tissue may not be feasible; alternative sites may be required (e.g. apply a blood pressure cuff to the thigh or the calf, place ECG dots in alternative locations); and some assessments may need to be delayed until after analgesia is administered or avoided completely. Despite these potential difficulties, all vital signs should be obtained whenever possible.

Examination of the perfusion of all extremities should complete circulatory assessment and involve evaluation of skin colour, presence of pulses, capillary

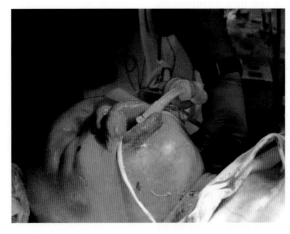

Figure 38.14
Airway obstruction in the first 12 hours post injury is often caused by direct thermal injury to the face, mouth and neck.
Source: Image reproduced with permission of the Victorian Adult Burn Service at The Alfred.

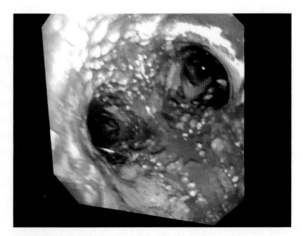

Figure 38.15
Emergency department bronchoscopy.
Patient fell asleep while smoking a cigarette in an enclosed room, causing a house fire.
Source: Image reproduced with permission of the Victorian Adult Burn Service at The Alfred.

BOX 38.1 Inhalation injury

Inhalation injury has a wide spectrum of clinical consequence and is associated with high mortality (Latenser, 2009). Burns can compromise the airways' supraglottic, tracheobronchial and parenchymal structures, manifesting in varying degrees of severity of upper and lower airway oedema, inflammation, epithelial sloughing, increased mucus production, atelectasis, respiratory failure, obstruction and carbon monoxide intoxication. In general terms, airway burn injury has one or more of three basic components.

1. **Structural component**: heat source causes direct physical injury to exposed structures (e.g. face/neck).
2. **Inhalational component**: inhalation of heated toxic gases and debris deposited into the airways.
3. **Systemic component**: carbon monoxide leading to hypoxaemia.

   These can occur in isolation or collectively. For example, a patient may receive facial burns resulting from a scald or flame without inhaling hot or toxic gases, while inhalational injury can occur from noxious gas or smoke without injury to external airway structures. Burn events may also involve all three, such as airway and facial burns and smoke inhalation from a house fire. The nature of the environment, the duration and level of exposure and the materials combusted during exposure are key elements in determining the likely degree and subsequent risk of respiratory compromise.

The variable presentation of inhalation injury and delayed onset of symptoms can lead to ambiguity in diagnosis and delayed management. There is no definitive evidence available yet to distinguish people with burn injury that require intubation from those who do not. Fibreoptic bronchoscopy is a simple and safe method used often after arrival at the ED to assist in the diagnosis of acute inhalation injury; however, it is not readily available in the out-of-hospital setting. The absence of high-quality scientific evidence regarding which patients should be intubated and the unavailability of out-of-hospital diagnosis aids make paramedic clinical decisions regarding who should be intubated difficult, and delaying the procedure will make it increasingly difficult to intubate later as symptoms and swelling progress. All cases with signs and symptoms of pending airway obstruction and/or obvious inhalation injury should be intubated, and consideration should also be given to protecting the airway in cases where symptoms and the progression of airway compromise remains unclear, as delaying the procedure makes it increasingly difficult later.

refill, warmth and pain. Particular attention should be paid to distal circulation beyond circumferentially burned extremities. Burnt skin loses its elasticity quickly in deep burns that can have a tourniquet effect if the injury is circumferential, when non-expandable eschar is combined with rapidly accumulating underlying burn oedema (see Fig 38.16 and Box 38.2).

Disability

Conscious state can be challenging to assess in patients with thermal injury, substance use, hypoxia or inhalation injury; preexisting illness or associated injury can affect the patient's mental state. The Glasgow Coma Scale (GCS) and the AVPU mnemonic are internationally recognised measures for rapid neurological assessment to establish a baseline mental status on trauma patients. Altered level of consciousness indicates the need for repeated evaluation of the patient's airway and ventilation in case the airway needs to be protected.

Exposure

The patient should be completely exposed to assess the extent of injuries. Examine the patient from head to toe, and log roll to check posterior surfaces, inspect for concomitant injuries as well as remove any contaminants that might prolong contact with heat sources and get the first estimation of burn % TBSA. Clothing including nappies, jewellery, contact lenses and other accessories should be removed early in the evaluation process as they may have a tourniquet effect as swelling progresses.

BOX 38.2 Circumferential burns and escharotomy

Circulation and/or breathing can be compromised in circumferential burn injuries due to increased pressure caused by the oedema and swelling in the tissue deep to the burn interfacing with the unyielding overlying burnt skin ('eschar'), which acts like a tourniquet. Patients with circumferential limb burns with compromised circulation exhibit:

- loss of distal circulation and pulses
- cool limbs
- numbness or pain
- reduced peripheral pulse oximetry.

The onset of circulatory compromise is slowly progressive, and escharotomy is not usually required within 6 hours of injury. Escharotomy may be indicated, and this is a high-risk procedure performed by surgeons or ED doctors in consultation with the appropriate burns unit to optimise outcomes and minimise risks. In the out-of-hospital setting, elevation of the affected limb can help minimise swelling and improve blood flow to buy time until arrival at the burns unit or regional ED where urgent interventions can be performed.

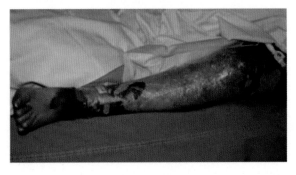

Figure 38.16

Circumferential burn example

Eschar from circumferential deep full-thickness burns of an extremity can have a tourniquet effect on distal circulation as vascular supply becomes compromised by worsening underlying oedema and the unyielding overlying eschar. Monitor neurovascular observations and elevate the affected area.

Source: Image reproduced with permission of the Victorian Adult Burn Service at The Alfred.

People with severe burn injuries lose their ability to thermoregulate and can lose heat quickly. Those at risk of hypothermia following burn injury include: patients with large surface area burns; children due to their large body surface area relative to size; the elderly, as the body's ability to regulate and sense temperature lessen with age; and intubated patients who are unable to shiver following the administration of deep sedation and paralysing agents. This patient's temperature is now 35.9°C.

Efforts should be made to minimise heat loss to avoid the detrimental effects of hypothermia. Complications of hypothermia in burns patients include coagulopathies and delay to definitive surgery in a burns theatre until normothermia is re-established. Stop burn wound cooling if the patient's core temperature is < 35°C, and during examination expose only those necessary areas of the body being inspected. Keep other areas covered to preserve warmth and cover again as soon as possible. Remove any wet dressings, sheets or clothing that can accelerate evaporative heat loss. A warmed environment and readily available clean blankets can prevent or limit heat loss during transfer. Heat loss minimisation measures should commence immediately from the time the crew arrive and should not be delayed while initiating other procedures.

Ambulance IV fluids are often stored at less than body temperature and, given the high volumes to be administered, this can increase the risk of hypothermia. Where fluid warmers are fitted in ambulances, paramedics should consider using warmed normothermic fluids.

Initial assessment summary

Problem	Burns to face, upper torso, neck, arms and hands
Conscious state	GCS = 15; increasingly restless and distressed
Heart rate	108 bpm
Blood pressure	135/75 mmHg
Inspection	Facial burns, carbonaceous sputum, singed facial hair
Speech pattern	Patient is yelling in pain, speaking in words
Respiratory assessment	RR = 34, increased work of breathing, tracheal tugging, expiratory stridor, reduced bilateral air entry, widespread expiratory wheeze, O_2 saturation 93%

D: The heat source has been removed and the scene made safe.
A: Currently patent, signs of inhalation injury and pending airway obstruction.
B: Respiratory function is compromised and requires frequent reassessment.
C: Heart rate is elevated but he has sufficient blood pressure.
I: The patient has a potential airway injury and 15% TBSA burns that are capable of producing a systemic inflammatory reaction that could cause cardiovascular collapse.

2 CONFIRM

Immediate consideration should focus on airway protection

This patient presents with ominous warning signs of potential airway injury. He has signs of both a possible structural upper airway injury and an inhalational injury. Facial burns, carbonaceous sputum and singed facial hair suggest at least superficial burns to the upper airway, and the presence of widespread expiratory wheeze indicates an inflammatory response in progress in the distal airways given he has no past history of restrictive airways disease (see Boxes 38.3 and 38.4).

In this scenario, the paramedics elect to conduct a drug-facilitated intubation according to local guidelines. The extra risks in this situation are significant and include mechanical obstruction due to oedema and eschar, the hyper-reactivity of the pharynx, the altered laryngeal appearance due to inflammation and oedema, and a significantly reduced tolerance to respiratory depression and/or apnoea from the induction medications. An urgent surgical airway should be considered as a genuine possibility and all equipment and practitioners prepared.

Important aspects of the secondary survey

Patient history

A comprehensive history from the patient or bystanders can provide important information regarding the extent and severity of the burn, the likelihood of inhalation injury or associated injuries, and any potential safety hazards. Paramedics should determine the mechanism of injury to help identify hazards as well as prioritise treatment options (e.g. cardiac management in electrical injury) and the likely pattern of injury and possible complications (e.g. fluid resuscitation for significant thermal burns). For flame or explosion-related injuries, ascertaining whether the burn occurred in an enclosed space will help with the early identification of the risk of airway compromise. Vapour combustion from ignited accelerants is a common source of burn injury, particularly in

BOX 38.3 Intubation

Direct thermal exposure to the face, neck, mouth and oral mucosa can cause upper airway injuries that can rapidly obstruct the airway and require early intubation to protect it. Patients requiring intubation should be identified early, as it becomes increasingly difficult with the onset of oedema, especially once fluid resuscitation has commenced. As discussed, there is no definitive evidence regarding which patients require intubation; furthermore, guidelines and protocols based on expert opinion are often imprecise, and variation in protocols and unnecessary intubation outcomes exist. While prophylactic intubation can be beneficial by immediately ensuring airway protection, it is not without risks of significant morbidity and mortality including increased rates of pneumonia, increased fluid volume requirements, hypothermia and unnecessary healthcare costs. An evidence base to determine exactly which signs or symptoms can be confidently used to determine who to intubate and when is required.

Expect any patient with symptoms of airway burns to require out-of-hospital intubation. Ensure scene times are kept to a minimum and pre-notify the receiving hospital to ensure that the trauma and resuscitation team are informed and therefore prepared for an urgent airway intervention. Depending on local protocols, paramedics capable of advanced airway intervention may be requested and a rendezvous en route arranged.

males, and ignition is typically very fast and can cause an instinctive inhalation reflex in the patient (Rainey et al., 2007).

The patient's age and medical history will help identify those at risk of poor outcomes. Age guides both how the case will be managed (e.g. paediatric pain relief guidelines are often different from adult guidelines), the likely outcome (increasing age is strongly associated with increased morbidity and mortality) and transfer destination.

Establishing the time of the burn injury is of particular importance given the onset of airway and cardiovascular complications and the potential for burn wound 'progression'. For patients suffering burns in remote areas, there can be long delays before definitive treatment is available. Establishing the time of injury will also determine whether cooling remains a worthwhile intervention if medical care or first aid has been delayed. Establishing these facts at the outset allows the creation of a patient injury profile, facilitating the treatment pathway most likely to provide maximum clinical benefit.

Concomitant trauma

Although the force of the explosion did not knock the patient over or cause loss of consciousness, the secondary survey should determine whether there are any eye or barotrauma injuries. In this case, the patient has normal vision and hearing.

Burn area and depth

Recall that large areas of erythema may be present immediately or soon after the injury. These superficial reddened and hot areas with brisk capillary refill, although painful, have relatively minor injury that will heal spontaneously. Erythema will gradually subside as the burn cools (or is cooled), the inflammatory response mediates and the skin heals. It may, however, complicate initial TBSA calculations.

This patient has burns to his face, neck, bilateral upper limbs extending from the hands to upper arms, and upper chest. The burns on the upper chest and face appear more severe: large patches of skin have been burnt, with some

BOX 38.4 To intubate or not?

Several studies have reported a high incidence of likely unnecessary out-of-hospital intubations, with high extubation rates (> 40–65%) within the first 48 hours. A 10-year retrospective observational study which reviewed 416 out-of-hospital intubations that arrived to one burns unit found that patients who had flame burn injuries are more likely to be intubated, and those cases which were extubated in < 48 hours were more likely to have been burnt outside in an unenclosed space. They proposed the following guidelines for the intubation of burn patients (from Romanowski et al., 2015).

1. Patient safety should not be compromised, and patient status is the ultimate determinant of intubation need.
2. Standard indications for intubation should be followed including but not limited to shortness of breath, wheezing, stridor, hoarseness, combativeness or decreased level of consciousness.
3. Contact should be made with the burn unit as soon as is safely feasible to discuss the events surrounding the burn and need for intubation.
4. If the patient is clinically stable with no signs or symptoms of a compromised airway, they have a low likelihood of requiring intubation. The following types of burns also have a lower need for intubation before transfer:
   › burns that occur from causes other than flame injury
   › burns that do not occur in enclosed spaces
   › burns less than 20% TBSA
   › burns with no third degree burns to the face
   › within a reasonable distance to a burn service (approximately 3 hours transfer time).

Another retrospective study compared the American Burn Association (ABA) criteria for intubation with traditional criteria for intubation. Of 218 reviewed cases, the specificity of the ABA criteria was 77% compared to 22.5% specificity of the traditional criteria (Badulak et al., 2018).

ABA indications for intubation	Traditional indications for intubation
Full-thickness facial burns	Suspected smoke inhalation
Stridor	Oropharynx soot
Upper airway trauma	Dysphagia
Haemodynamic instability	Hoarseness
Respiratory distress	Singed facial hair
Swelling on laryngoscopy	Oral oedema
Altered mentation	Oral burn
Hypoxia/hypercarbia	Non-full-thickness facial burn

Of the traditional criteria for intubation, suspected smoke inhalation and singed facial hair were associated with long-term intubation, so the authors proposed the Denver criteria when considering intubation. Any of the following signs or symptoms, either in isolation or combination, support the potential need for intubation:

- full-thickness facial burns
- suspected smoke inhalation
- stridor
- upper airway trauma
- singed facial hair
- haemodynamic instability
- respiratory distress
- swelling on laryngoscopy
- altered mentation
- hypoxia/hypercarbia.

blistering, and areas of epidermal detachment reveal red and moist tissue underneath. Assessment using the Rule of Nines gives an estimated burned TBSA of < 20% (see Fig 38.17).

TREAT AND EVALUATE

Emergency management

Table 38.5 outlines the principles of emergency management for thermal burns.

Ongoing airway vigilance

As discussed previously, oxygen should be administered to all patients with severe burn injury, especially so for burns received in enclosed spaces. This patient's airway is now secured via endotracheal tube, and his ventilatory status is relatively improved; the patient has been placed onto a mechanical

Table 38.5 Initial management of the burn patient

Airway	• Enact plan to secure the airway
Breathing	• Administer high-flow oxygen
Circulation	• Establish IV access • Commence IV fluids and titrate to estimated amount according to local fluid protocols

Pain	• Administer fast-acting analgesia according to local protocols. Estimates include:
	  › Children: 0.1 mg/kg IV morphine repeated every 5 minutes
	  › Young adults: 2–5 mg IV morphine repeated every 5 minutes
	  › Older people: 1–2 mg IV morphine repeated every 5 minutes
	• Reassess and readminister until pain control satisfactory

Cooling	• Cool the burn with 20 minutes of cool running water
	  › Stop cooling if patient is hypothermic (temperature < 35°C)
	  › Consider delaying transfer to complete first aid for non-severe burns
	  › Transfer should not be delayed to complete first aid for severe burns

Wound Care	• Cover the wound with cling wrap/film (longitudinally), or as per local guidelines • Sit the patient with facial burns up to minimise facial oedema • Elevate affected limbs in transit to minimise oedema
Warmth	• Minimise exposure time during care procedures to reduce heat loss • Cover the patient with blankets to minimise heat loss • Consider warming the ambulance and administer warm IV fluids where available

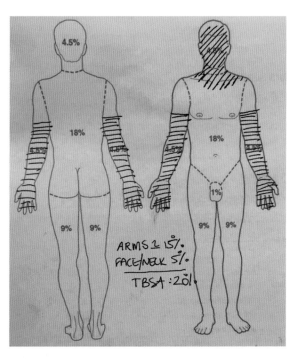

Figure 38.17
Lund and Browder chart: TBSA % calculation for Case study 1

ventilator and is ventilating without complication. His SpO$_2$ is 99%, EtCO$_2$ is 38 mmHg and GCS = 3 following ongoing sedation and analgesia infusions.

In cases where the airway is not secured, paramedics must remain vigilant during transport for early identification of worsening airway compromise. Consider whether early treatment with inhaled bronchodilators (salbutamol) and steroidal medications (where provided in local guidelines) is required.

BOX 38.5 Modified Parkland formula

This formula for estimating fluid resuscitation requirements determines the total fluid load as follows:

$$3\text{--}4 \text{ mL/body weight (kg)/\% TBSA burnt/24 hours}$$

with:
- 50% in the first 8 hours after injury
- 50% in the remaining 16 hours.

Controlling a deteriorating airway through endotracheal intubation is much more likely to be successful if attempted before swelling obstructs the airway.

Perfusion support

Mechanisms that control protein and fluid loss from the vascular space are severely compromised following severe burns. Changes in microvasculature caused by direct thermal injury and the systemic inflammatory response increases total body capillary permeability, creating a rapid equilibrium between intravascular and interstitial fluid compartments.

The overall aim of fluid resuscitation is to restore circulating intravascular volume, preserve vital organs and maintain tissue perfusion. Secondly, it is important that the right amount of fluid is given to try to avoid complications of both under- and over-resuscitation. During the first 8–12 hours following burn injury, the majority of IV fluid administered will largely end up as oedema. Trigger points for the commencement of fluid resuscitation vary between jurisdictions and no universal consensus exists. ANZBA recommends fluid resuscitation in patients with burn injuries ≥ 20% TBSA. The most widely used formula to estimate fluid resuscitation requirements is the Modified Parkland formula (see Box 38.5).

Any isotonic fluid is suitable, although several fluid types have been considered including colloids, albumins and crystalloids. At this time, definitive evidence on the best fluid alternative is lacking.

Early fluid replacement is one of the highest priorities for patients with severe burn injuries and is associated with improved morbidity and mortality outcomes. Delayed fluid resuscitation can result in inadequate perfusion potentially causing ischaemic injury to the kidneys and other organs, cardiovascular shock and/or eventual multisystem organ failure, and is associated with poor patient outcomes (Warden, 1992; Kramer et al., 2007; Diver, 2008). As a result, all of Australia's inclusive trauma systems now employ early fluid resuscitation in the field, typically commencing fluid resuscitation and then adjusting using a standardised formula such as the Modified Parkland formula.

Fluid resuscitation formulas were developed during the mid-20th century to prevent acute kidney injury (AKI). While a recent meta-analysis of AKI in burn injury reported incidence of AKI in burn patients as high as 43%, it is uncommon during the resuscitation phase in the 21st century (Wu et al., 2016). Serious complications of over-resuscitation are now more prevalent, with the term 'fluid creep' used to describe burn patients requiring and receiving much more resuscitation fluid than predicted by widely accepted formulas. Fluid creep has been reported in 30% to 90% of patients with major burns and increasing burn size is an associated risk factor. Importantly, excessive fluid given in the initial hours after injury predisposes to fluid creep (Chung et al.,

CALCULATING FLUID REQUIREMENTS FOR CASE 54046

- **Weight:** 80 kg
- **% TBSA burns:** 20%
- **Modified Parkland formula:**
  4 mL/80 kg/20% TBSA burns/24 hours = 6400 mL/24 hours
  - 3200 mL by 0200 hours
  - 3200 mL by 1800 hours

Note: 4 mL used to account for insensible loss from suspected inhalation injury.

2009). Characteristics of fluid creep usually emerge around 8–12 hours after injury following arrival at the trauma centre/burns unit in cases who have received substantially more fluid than required, when markers of perfusion indicate a need to increase fluid requirements well beyond formula predictions. This has downstream effects on the emergence of oedema-related complications. Complications of fluid creep are not insignificant and include massive swelling of the face and airway necessitating intubation, respiratory and cardiac failure, extremity compartment syndromes requiring escharotomy, and abdominal compartment syndrome that, while an uncommon outcome of extreme over-resuscitation, has an associated mortality of 75% (Dulhunty et al., 2008; Ivy et al., 2000; Strang et al., 2014).

Therefore, it is necessary to monitor markers of fluid and perfusion status, including blood pressure and heart rate and measure urine output (if a urinary catheter has been inserted during an inter-hospital transfer) so that fluids can be adjusted accordingly to avoid complications of over- and under-resuscitation. Problems arise when fluid resuscitation is NOT titrated to perfusion markers, especially in cases where the patient's weight and % TBSA burns calculations could be inaccurate, subsequently making fluid resuscitation calculations inaccurate. Maintaining an accurate fluid balance chart will assist in ongoing fluid resuscitation once the patient arrives at the burns unit.

Pain relief

Burns induce mechanical and thermal hyperalgesia in human skin. The experience of immediate pain following burn injury is caused by the stimulation of skin nociceptors responding to heat, mechanical distortion and inflammatory mediators, in particular histamine, serotonin, bradykinin and prostaglandins. The severity of burn pain during the immediate stage after injury can range widely, from none to severe, and pain is often the most frequent complaint. Pain assessment tools are essential for a standardised measure of burn pain and the effectiveness of treatment. In the adult burn patient population, the most common pain assessment tools are verbal self-report instruments that measure pain intensity, such as the '0 to 10' numeric rating scale. Particular attention should be given to the management of pain in cases complicated by acute alcohol or drug intoxication, which may have been a precipitant to injury, but can also adversely interact with analgesic and anxiolytic medications.

The patient in this scenario requires early administration of effective analgesia. IV administration of analgesia is the preferred route for delivery in this case because of potential problems with absorption of intranasal analgesia in the presence of inhalation injury, and the potential problems with enteral absorption related to decreased gut perfusion.

Doses of IV opioid, usually morphine or fentanyl in the Australian out-of-hospital setting, should be titrated according to pain level as per local guidelines, and consultation with senior clinicians should occur before guideline analgesic limits are reached. Pain from burns can be severe and the doses described in some paramedic guidelines may be insufficient to provide adequate pain relief.

Initial management with an inhaled opioid analgesic such as intranasal (IN) fentanyl is ideal in the out-of-hospital setting, providing rapid and effective pain relief while IV access is obtained in cases without inhalation injury. Ketamine is used in some out-of-hospital jurisdictions; there is in-hospital evidence of its efficacy for the management of burn pain and out-of-hospital evidence for its use in acute burn pain is emerging (Reid et al., 2011). Ketamine may be administered intranasally, adding to its usefulness in the management of burns. Methoxyflurane may be considered for small, painful burns on limbs, as it is

BOX 38.6 Intravenous access in burn patients

IV access needs to be established to commence fluid resuscitation where necessary and provide pain relief. Peripherally inserted venous catheters (PIV) can be inserted with relative ease to establish immediate short-term IV access rapidly in the out-of-hospital environment and are routinely used. Patients with severe burns require significant amounts of IV fluids for resuscitation and often require more than one PIV to meet resuscitation targets. Establishing peripheral venous access can be challenging for paramedics when patients are obese, or have stenosed or thrombotic veins from previous therapeutic or illicit use. To improve longevity and minimise mechanical failure risks, the forearm is the recommended site for insertion of PIVs (Gorski, 2017; Wallis et al., 2014); however, studies in hospital environments demonstrate that compliance is poor (Alexandrou et al., 2018).

In adult populations, 20-G PIV catheters are recommended (Marsh et al., 2018; Cicolini et al.,

2009) to minimise risks of thrombosis or dislodgement associated with large or smaller gauge PIVs (Wallis et al., 2014; Marsh et al., 2018). The PIV and insertion site should be covered with a sterile dressing (Moureau et al., 2012). Studies have demonstrated that PIVs inserted in emergency environments increases the risks of *Staphylococcus aureus* bacteraemia, and IV access devices are usually removed and re-established in controlled conditions on arrival to the burn unit.

Where possible select sites for vascular access devices that are away from burnt skin to reduce risks associated with infective complications. However, this is not possible in some circumstances where injury characteristics present no alternative access sites., and this necessary procedure will unfortunately increase the risk of blood stream infection (Ciofi Silva et al., 2014; Tao et al., 2015).

---

quick-acting and has no cardiovascular side effects. However, even small burns may need subsequent IN or IV opioid analgesics due to the short, variable duration and intensity of analgesia obtained with methoxyflurane (Wasiak et al., 2014). Given these limitations, IN/IV opioids are the preferred option. Inhaled analgesics are not suitable when lung function or mechanical ventilation has been compromised. Deep ventilation is likely to cause a significant increase in pain where chest wall injury is present, which will affect the availability and effectiveness of inhaled analgesic medication. Furthermore, the patient is unlikely to be able to effectively self-administer in this circumstance. Inhaled analgesics should never be used where the patient presents with respiratory distress and signs of inhalation injury, such as wheezing and coughing, stridor or changes to voice (see Box 38.6).

Burn first aid

Current evidence-based best practice guidelines recommend cooling the burn wound with cool running tap water for 20 minutes within 3 hours of injury. This is the recommendation of the Australian and New Zealand Burn Association and the Australian Resuscitation Council, as well as many Australian and international out-of-hospital services and burn care organisations. These recommendations are based on several animal model studies that examined the temperature and histological reaction of porcine skin to burns treated with cool running water for 5, 10, 20 and 30 minutes to determine the most effective cooling timing in reducing the impact of burn wound injury. Burns cooled for 20 minutes showed the most signs of re-epithelialisation on histological analysis at 9 or 14 days post injury. While its immediate application may reduce the actual burn severity by reducing the temperature of the tissue, there is increasing evidence that cool running water has beneficial effects even when there are delays between the burn injury and the period of cooling. In addition to providing effective pain relief, cooling suppresses the inflammatory response, limits the progression of the burn injury and reduces scarring (Yuan et al., 2007; Bartlett et al., 2008; Rajan et al., 2009). The mechanism by which cool running water suppresses the inflammatory response is not fully understood but it appears to be effective in preserving and reducing damage to the dermal collagen framework, facilitating the likelihood of re-epithelialisation of injured areas (Cuttle et al., 2009; Shupp et al., 2010).

Data from the Burn Registry of Australia and New Zealand (BRANZ) showed that 68% of patients had burn wound cooling provided before arrival to Australian and New Zealand burns units, with at least 46% receiving the recommended 20 minutes of cooling. Importantly, the data showed that first aid was associated with a reduction in burn injury severity, and hospital length of stay, as well as a statistically significant reduction in the probability for skin grafting and/or ICU admission (Wood et al., 2016). While there is no universal consensus on the best water temperature for cooling, between 15°C and 18°C is considered optimal, with a range between 8°C and 25°C (Cuttle et al., 2009). Iced water should not be used as it increases the risk of hypothermia and its vasoconstrictive effects may worsen the injury. BRANZ data shows that 60% of adult injuries and almost 80% of paediatric burn injuries occur in the home environment where access to cool running water should be readily available, suggesting that access to cool running water is not prohibitive in the Australian context, and patients or family can often attend to first-aid measures before the paramedics arrive (BRANZ, 2018).

This patient has been in a cool shower for 10 minutes before the paramedics arrived. Further cooling can be considered while the crew establishes IV access, implements other interventions and prepares the patient for transport. The 20-minute cooling time can have implications for scene management, as it is difficult to maintain cool running water in transport. Unless airway issues, secondary trauma or cardiac complications manifest, a full 20 minutes of cooling should be completed at the scene before transport to hospital. Modified approaches to cooling can be undertaken en route (e.g. using rotating wetted soaks or mist spraying), albeit they have been shown to be inadequate in wound cooling compared with cool running water (Yuan et al., 2007). However, transport should not be delayed at the scene for ongoing cooling of patients in high-risk groups, including those with severe burns such as this case. In this situation, the patient's baseline temperature of 35.9°C, coupled with the effects of intubation on further heat loss, and the severity of the overall injury, further burn wound cooling that would delay departure was not warranted.

Hydrogel dressings are used in some out-of-hospital settings as an alternative to water first aid, though fortunately this is decreasing in usage. These dressings are open-cell foam sheets impregnated with a gel containing a small quantity of melaleuca oil. Studies indicate that these dressings do not cool the burn as effectively as running water (Cuttle et al., 2009), and they have not been investigated in out-of-hospital trials, thus the clinical benefits of these dressings remain uncertain and in need of further research. They are contraindicated as a first-aid measure for chemical burns, which require copious irrigation to dilute chemical irritants. Duplication of cooling using both cool running water and hydrogel dressings may increase the risk of hypothermia (Allison, 2002). These dressings are portable, sterile and provide good short-term pain relief, so are useful for the treatment of minor burns where risk of hypothermia is negligible, or in austere situations where there may be no access to water. However, in most situations where it is available, use of cool running water should prevail as the gold standard first-aid measure because of its superior benefits of wound damage mitigation compared to hydrogel dressings.

Minimising heat loss

Minimising heat loss is a priority, especially in the early management of severe burns as hypothermia is associated with significantly increased morbidity and mortality (Singer et al., 2010). While mechanisms that contribute to hypothermia following burn injury are poorly understood, patients lose their ability to thermoregulate when dermal integrity is lost, and they lose heat due to continued exposure during paramedic tasks and treatments such as first aid. It is fundamental that paramedics ensure that efforts are made to minimise heat loss and that the patient is kept as warm and dry as possible while maintaining treatment. This includes covering non-affected areas during cooling procedures and using ambulance heaters during transport, irrespective of the ambient temperature. Warming of the patient should commence immediately from the time the crew arrive and should not be delayed while initiating other procedures. Ambulance IV fluids are often stored at less than body temperature and, given the high volumes to be administered, patients can easily become hypothermic. Where fluid warmers are fitted in ambulances, paramedics should consider using only normothermic fluids.

Wound care

Definitive burn wound care will be achieved after arrival at the appropriate burns unit. The goals of initial wound care at the scene, particularly following severe burn injury, is to keep it short and sweet, cool the wound, decontaminate if possible and cover the wound quickly to minimise heat loss. Initial wound care in cases with severe burns should be rapid, and transfer should not be delayed by performing meticulous dressings, which will be removed on arrival. Covering the burn wound often results in a marked reduction in pain, which suggests a contribution to pain of the exposure of the wound and nerve endings.

Cling wrap is often used in the out-of-hospital setting to provide temporary and quick burn wound coverage; it is clean and unlikely to complicate infection risk. It is also cheap, simple to use, non-adherent and transparent, making visualisation of the underlying wound easy. It may also slow evaporative fluid loss. Limbs must not be wrapped circumferentially with cling wrap, as this may limit limb expansion with ensuing progressive oedema and compartment syndrome may develop. Small overlapping or longitudinal layers should be applied to ensure that the limb is not tightly encircled.

There is little evidence that supports the efficacy of one type of dressing over any other (Wasiak et al., 2008). Burn dressings, including hydrogel and silver products, are available for use by transferring facilities; however, the benefits of applying expensive dressings prior to burns unit arrival is questionable given the absence of evidence regarding dressing efficacy and because they will undoubtedly be removed on arrival to the burns unit to facilitate comprehensive burn wound assessment. In circumstances where transfer is delayed more than a few hours, the use of burn dressings should be considered; however, this is likely to be a responsibility of the transferring hospital rather than the out-of-hospital services (see Fig 38.18).

Infection risk and antibiotic therapy

Infection is a leading cause of morbidity and mortality in patients with severe burns, and diagnosis is complicated by the reduced specificity of fever and elevation of systemic inflammatory markers, both driven by the injury itself. Prophylactic administration of antibiotics is not routine in either the hospital or the out-of-hospital environment, and there is a uniform consensus in the current literature that systemic antibiotic prophylaxis should not be given because of the potential induction of antibiotic resistance. A systematic review which pooled evidence from 17 randomised controlled trials showed a discrepancy

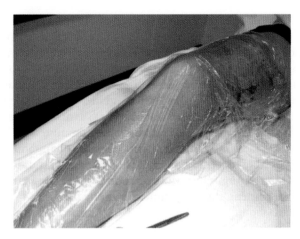

Figure 38.18
Cling Wrap placed longitudinal example.
Source: Image reproduced with permission of the Victorian Adult Burn Service at The Alfred.

between evidence and current guideline recommendations, demonstrating a 50% reduction in all-cause mortality when systemic antibiotic prophylaxis was implemented (Avni et al., 2010). Systemic perioperative prophylaxis was associated with a reduction in pneumonia and a reduced rate of burn wound infection, although there was an increase in resistance of bacteria to the antibiotic used for prophylaxis. However, there is a paucity of trials and poor methodological quality involving unclear and/or inadequate randomisation in available trials making the quality of evidence in the systematic review weak. As such, prophylaxis is currently only recommended perioperatively for patients with severe burns, with further randomised controlled trials required before any further recommendations regarding prophylactic antibiotic use can be made.

Burn wounds can be contaminated if cooled by water from a tank, bore, dam or other untreated source. Irrigation with clean water or sterile solutions (e.g. normal saline) at the earliest opportunity may reduce the level of contamination, although the effectiveness of this approach is yet to be confirmed in studies. Nonetheless, some cleansing of the wound may be achieved without risking complications; this may also remove loose or adhered material from the wound. It is important that burns unit handover include information regarding potential burn wound contamination so that subsequent mitigating strategies can be implemented to reduce the risks of infection, such as the use of antimicrobial dressings, rigorous daily assessment and early decontamination and/or debridement. If possible, providing a sample of the cooling water can assist in the planning of early targeted antibiotic treatment.

Transport

In Australia and New Zealand, burn care is regionalised and patients with severe or complex burn injuries are transported to one of the 17 specialised burns units across the two nations, which are staffed and equipped appropriately to manage burns (see Fig 38.19). Australian burns units operate within inclusive trauma systems with defined geographical regions that involve the coordination of out-of-hospital and acute medical services to match patient needs to the rapid definitive care required. It is likely that for patients who meet severe burn injury criteria and/or the ANZBA Referral Criteria, consultation with the burns unit will occur before arrival to ensure time-critical care is complete and appropriate transfer arrangements organised as necessary.

Hospitals with Designated Burns Units Across Australia and New Zealand

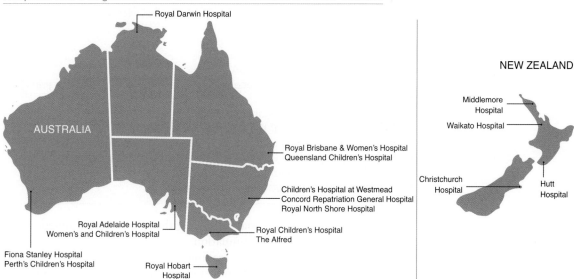

Figure 38.19
Australian and New Zealand Specialist burns centre locations.
Source: ANZBA Annual Report (2018-19).

Unless the patient's situation is immediately life-threatening, there is evidence that transport directly to a specialist burns unit improves patient outcomes (ACI, 2011). These guidelines should be used together with local protocols to determine the best destination for the patient. Aeromedical transfer should be considered for patients with severe burns, especially if the distance to the burns unit may delay definitive care. Aeromedical transportation is well tolerated by burn patients, but presents unique physiological stressors caused by the changes to altitude and barometric pressures, especially with concurrent traumatic injuries (Treat et al., 1980; Klein et al., 2007; Carreras-Gonzalez & Brio-Sanagustin, 2014; Warner et al., 2016). Fluctuations in blood pressure and core temperature and increased oxygen demands are caused by decreased oxygen partial pressure, temperature and humidity that occur at altitude, and barometric pressure changes can lead to volume gas expansion that is problematic for patients with pneumothorax. Acute barometric pressure fluctuations during ascent and descent can induce additional haemodynamic stressors that add significant risks to severe burn cases who may already have hypothermia and/or hypovolaemic shock.

Hospital admission (burns unit)

The choice of patient destination is a critical consideration for paramedics, particularly where large or deep burns are involved (Gabbe et al., 2011). Specific transfer criteria enable out-of-hospital clinicians to triage patients to the most appropriate facility. In Australia and New Zealand, most services use the ANZBA criteria listed in Box 38.7.

On admission to the burns ward/intensive care unit, the following procedures are standard care:

- continuous cardiorespiratory, haemodynamic, temperature and oxygen saturation monitoring
- carboxyhaemoglobin estimation
- intubation and ventilation; a tracheostomy may be performed if long-term ventilation is required

> ### PRACTICE TIP
>
> Sit the patient up in transit to help minimise swelling to the face and neck. Elevating burnt areas, including limbs in transit, should occur where possible to reduce oedema and its effects on tissue perfusion.

BOX 38.7 ANZBA criteria for transfer to a specialist burns unit

- Burns > 10% TBSA or > 5% in a child
- Full-thickness burns > 5% TBSA
- Burns of special areas (i.e. face, hands, feet, perineum and major joints)
- Electrical or chemical burns
- Burns with associated inhalation injury
- Circumferential burns of the limbs or chest
- Burns at the extremes of age (i.e. children and the elderly)
- Burn injury in patients with preexisting medical disorders that could complicate management, prolong recovery or affect mortality
- Any burn patient with associated trauma

- frequent arterial blood gas analysis during the acute stage of illness
- central venous and arterial cannulation
- nasogastric tube and nasogastric feeding
- IV fluid replacement; close monitoring of fluid volumes is essential, as excessive resuscitation is as problematic as inadequate resuscitation
- indwelling urinary catheter with hourly urine output measure
- regular monitoring of infection markers
- ± prophylactic therapy for gastric ulcers.

Prophylactic systemic antibiotic therapy is not recommended. Wound cleansing and debridement are often performed initially in the operating theatre. Oedema, increased blood viscosity and the poor perfusion that occur with burns can cause compartment syndrome. This is particularly problematic in circumferential burns and venous stasis and ischaemia distal to the burn may result. Escharotomy and/or fasciotomy may be required. Rehabilitation begins on admission to maximise functional recovery.

 CASE STUDY 2

Case 220702, 1015 hrs

Dispatch details: An older male has burns.

Initial presentation: The patient's wife directs the paramedics to their bathroom.

1029 hrs Primary survey: The patient is conscious and responding. GCS 15.

1029 hrs Chief complaint: 79-year-old male describes slipping in the shower this morning, and accidentally bumped the cold tap off. He was caught under the hot running tap for approximately 5 minutes before he could reach the tap to turn it off, and pressed his personal medical alarm. The patient was found shivering in the shower recess and has managed to cover himself with a towel which is now wet.

1030 hrs Vital signs survey:
Respiratory status: RR 28 bpm, good air entry, L = R, normal work of breathing, speaking in phrases.

Perfusion status: HR 125 bpm; sinus tachycardia; BP 90/45 mmHg; skin cold, pale and clammy.

Conscious state: GCS = 14.

Temperature: 33.1°C.

The scene is safe.

1 ASSESS

Burns cause significant physiological stress. Older or frail patients have reduced physiological reserves to cope with or adapt to the stress of burn injury, resulting in a decreased ability to physiologically compensate. His hypotension, tachycardia and pallor are evidence of cardiovascular compromise. He is also hypothermic. Older adults are at risk of hypothermia because a normal physiological response to cold may be diminished by chronic medical conditions, along with some medications (Soreide, 2014; Hostler et al., 2013; Singer et al., 2010).

Of particular concern is the precipitant for the incident: did he fall or collapse, and was there a loss consciousness? Falls and collapses are common in the elderly, so precipitating and consequent combinations of injury or illness must always be considered and managed. A broad assessment of potential causative factors is essential (see Key considerations).

Ageing is complex, involving structural and biochemical changes to the skin, immune system and many organs. These changes can have a significant negative impact on the normal trajectory of burn recovery. Older people have been consistently shown to have a disparate and higher morbidity and mortality following burn injury relative to younger age groups with equivalent burn injury (Manktelow et al., 1989). Age is one of several independent predictors of in-hospital mortality, which is reflected in various burn outcome prediction tools including the Baux score (Rani & Schwacha, 2011; Makrantonaki, 2012). Burn injuries in older people meet ANZBA referral criteria because of their complex nature, and the higher morbidity and mortality risks require specialist care to optimise patient outcomes (see Fig 38.20).

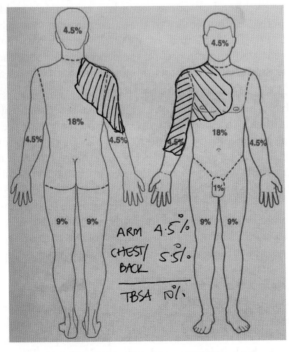

Figure 38.20
Rule of Nines chart: TBSA % calculation for Case Study 2

Key considerations

- What is the size and depth of the burn?
- What caused the fall? Was it a mechanical fall? Or was it loss of consciousness caused by syncope, cerebrovascular accident/transient ischaemic attack or diabetic hypoglycaemia? Do these possible events explain why the patient was unable to turn the tap off?
- Are there other injuries associated with the fall and the prolonged period of immobility?
- Will the patient's preexisting comorbidities affect out-of-hospital treatment?
- What effect will the comorbidities have on the clinical course of recovery and how they are managed?
- Did the burns result from deliberate abuse?

1035 hrs Secondary survey: The patient has burns over his left shoulder, partially down the left side of his back, right arm and upper chest. His right leg is externally rotated suggesting a fracture of the neck of the femur. On palpation he has acute localised bony tenderness at the proximal portion of his right thigh. He also has a red bump on his forehead.

1036 hrs Pertinent Hx: Lives at home alone, past history of hypertension, congestive cardiac failure, controlled atrial fibrillation, type 1 diabetes, chronic renal failure. Independent with activities of daily living and receives home care once per fortnight.

What else needs to be considered?

Comorbidities

Comorbidities in older people further reduce the functional reserve of integral organ systems, which can lead to earlier systemic deterioration or failure than seen in younger age groups. Sequelae of this patient's preexisting comorbidities may be contributing to the early presentation of both signs and symptoms of cardiovascular compromise. This patient has type 1 diabetes, and this should be considered as a cause of the collapse and altered conscious state; importantly, it also has long-term immunosuppressive effects on recovery (Mandell et al., 2013). As will be discussed, his cardiac and renal comorbidities will need to be managed with great care once burns treatment commences.

Secondary trauma

Secondary trauma should always be suspected and investigated where a fall is noted. Falls from a standing height are sufficient to cause fractures in elderly patients, as bony disease is common. This can lead to spinal trauma or limb/joint injury even where the impact was with a relatively soft surface (such as carpet). In particular, fractures of the pelvis and long bones can cause significant internal haemorrhage. This patient has a fractured right neck of femur. In conjunction with a major burn injury, secondary trauma can lead to profound cardiovascular complications and an inadequate perfusion state. It is important not to become so focused on the burn injury during the secondary survey as to overlook the likelihood of serious secondary trauma in an elderly patient. A prolonged period of immobility in the same position may also cause local tissue damage. Pressure sores and even muscle breakdown, rhabdomyolysis and compartment syndrome can occur if the patient is immobile for a protracted period. Skin tears and other wounds should be dressed as soon as possible.

Burn injury

The patient has a burn of 10% TBSA. The initial assessment of burn depth is frequently difficult in elderly patients. Due to changes to the skin caused by the normal ageing process, including the loss of dermis, injuries which cause superficial injuries in younger people are more likely to cause deeper burns in older people who also have a reduced potential to re-epithelialise and take longer to heal (Rani & Schwacha, 2011; Farage et al., 2013). Burns that initially appear superficial often convert to deeper injuries over the subsequent few days. Although the total area of the burn is 10%, this should nonetheless be considered a significant burn in the context of the patient's age, secondary traumatic injuries and existing comorbidities—collectively presenting a potentially lethal clinical situation.

Cause of fall

Although the patient reports that he fell in the shower, syncope, a transient ischaemic attack and a cerebrovascular accident are all possible differential diagnoses that should be considered. The patient's preexisting conditions predispose him to both ischaemic and arrhythmic events. This could include acute coronary syndrome, myocardial infarction or dysrhythmias. The patient

BOX 38.8 Burns injuries in older people

Reduced physical abilities and capacity to react quickly, as well as multiple comorbidities such as impaired vision, high risk of falls and short-term memory problems place older people at increased risk of burn injury. The Australian Institute of Health and Welfare (AIHW, 2018) reported in 2016 that 1 in 7 Australians was aged 65 or over. Populations in developed countries show increasing longevity, and by 2046 it is estimated that 35% of Australia's population will be between 75 and 84 years old, and 19% of people will be aged 85 and over. Older people are at increased risk of burn injury so therefore it is expected that the number of older Australians to suffer burn injuries will also increase. In 2019, people ≥ 65 years old accounted for 12.0% of adult patients recorded by BRANZ, and the incidence of burn injuries in older adults was reported as 7.4 per 100,000 people (Tracy et al., 2020). The predominant mechanism of injury for burns in 42% of older adult patients were scald burns, which is consistent with other reported incidences (Klein et al., 2011). In addition to greater risk for injury, the older adult burn patient has a longer hospital stay than middle-aged patients. Five per cent of older adults succumb to their injuries, dying during their hospital admission—a rate far higher than their middle-aged and younger adults comparators at 2% and 1% respectively (Tracy et al., 2020).

is inadequately perfused, which may have resulted from one or more of these pathologies. A 12-lead ECG and cardiac assessment should be performed to detect any abnormal cardiac ischaemia or dysthymias. A neurological examination looking for focal neurological signs is also indicated (see Ch 26). Neurological impairment (reduced cognitive function) or motor deficits may explain why the patient had difficulty getting up from the shower recess. Diabetics can experience overnight dips in blood glucose levels, particularly if long-acting oral anti-hyperglycaemics or subcutaneous insulin are used in the setting of reduced or absent dietary intake. A blood glucose assessment should be performed, especially if there are signs of neurological changes.

Hypothermia

Hypothermia is associated with greater incidence of morbidity and mortality in trauma patients, and the effects of hypothermia are profound in elderly burn victims (Ireland et al., 2011). Heat loss can occur from exposure, evaporation from the burn wound and immobility (no muscle thermogenesis). Hypothermia can also be exacerbated by, and complicates, hypovolaemia and poor perfusion states. Coagulopathies and acidosis, as well as complications caused by the burn injury, can combine to significantly impact morbidity and mortality. While he is alert and orientated, in some cases hypothermia may complicate neurological assessment, as it can affect cognitive function (see Box 38.8).

③ TREAT

Respiratory support and monitoring

Inhalation injury is uncommon following scald burn injury. This patient should be treated with supplemental oxygen. In the elderly, close monitoring of respiratory parameters is mandatory, particularly once fluid replacement commences in patients with preexisting cardiac or other comorbidities. Elderly patients have a lower threshold for ventilator support during treatment due to decrease in functional lung reserve and subsequent fatigue. Where clinically possible, sitting patients upright in transport will help to optimise respiratory capacity (Keck et al., 2009).

PRACTICE TIP

Patients with facial and neck burns should be sat upright in transit where clinically appropriate to minimise swelling and airway compromise. Similarly, elevation of burnt limbs can help reduce limb swelling and oedema.

Perfusion support

The patient requires IV fluid as he has well-established signs and symptoms of hypovolaemia. Fluid replacement or resuscitation of elderly burn patients with compromised cardiovascular, renal or pulmonary responses should be approached carefully. Age is associated with increased volume requirements in the acute stage following burn injury; however, in patients with preexisting organ dysfunction, rapid or excessive resuscitation may quickly result in fluid overload, elevation of central venous pressure or pulmonary oedema complications further aggravating decreased tissue perfusion (Hayek et al., 2011; Rani & Schwacha, 2011; Farage et al., 2013; Huang et al., 2008). Application of established guidelines may need to be adapted, as fluid requirements may differ to accommodate for the complexities of preexisting comorbidities and their effects on both under- and over-resuscitation. The close monitoring of effects of fluid resuscitation in elderly patients is vital—it cannot be understated.

Secondary trauma management

Fracture management, including splinting and immobilisation, will need to be undertaken for this patient in concert with other clinical care. While basic immobilisation of the fractured femur may be accomplished in the supine position, and is also appropriate for spinal care, this must be considered in the context of the burn wounds.

Warming and cooling

In this case, burn wound cooling is likely to contribute to further lowering the patient's body temperature and the ramifications of the complications present. The patient already presents with hypothermia, poor perfusion and secondary trauma. Furthermore, the injuries in context of a complex clinical background and scenario should be considered time-critical, and transport to hospital should not be delayed for extended cooling. Active re-warming measures should be implemented, including head-to-toe covering and heating once in the ambulance to prevent further heat loss and worsening hypothermia.

Pain relief

IN/IV opioids are the preferred method of pain relief. IN fentanyl provides a more sustained analgesic effect than inhaled anaesthetics such as methoxyflurane, and is quick and easy to deliver at the outset prior to further IV management. Due to the patient's age and comorbidities, IV/IN doses of powerful opioids like fentanyl and morphine should be given in small initial increments: 1–2 mg of morphine or 25 micrograms of fentanyl (subject to local guidelines), with ongoing monitoring of blood pressure, respirations and conscious state. Frequent doses are likely to be needed until substantial pain relief has been achieved. Caution is advised with dosage intervals: elderly patients may not metabolise drugs as quickly as younger adults and so peak effect times may be extended. Pain relief should continue until effective analgesia has been achieved or the onset of significant side effects. Maximum doses may be subject to local guidelines and high doses of opioid are often required in this patient group: consultation for ongoing opioid analgesics is recommended.

Wound management

Burn wounds need to be covered with cling wrap, taking care to wrap the right arm longitudinally to allow for any subsequent swelling and avoid dressing constriction. Cling wrap allows easy inspection of the burn without exposure. Simply covering the wound alone (with any dressing) will greatly assist in reducing pain. Never leave a burn wound uncovered as this exacerbates pain and evaporative fluid and heat loss, and leaves the wound unprotected at further risk of infective contamination. Avoid handling the wound and never be tempted to manipulate blisters or loose skin; this can be attended to on arrival at the hospital destination in much more controlled conditions. Hydrogels should *never* be used as a wound dressing when the patient has a large burn injury, has hypothermia, is at risk of hypothermia or when cooling has already been completed.

Transport

This patient needs assessment at a specialist burns unit and trauma service. The paramedics should consult with their local resources to activate this response immediately and follow prearranged trauma transport guidelines. In transit, important clinical parameters including respiratory, perfusion and neurological reassessment need to be closely monitored in case care is required to be adapted in response to the patient's potentially rapidly changing condition (see Boxes 38.9 and 38.10).

BOX 38.9 Elder abuse

Elder abuse is an unfortunate reality and is under-reported in comparison with child abuse. If patients are not living alone and their story contains inconsistencies, the paramedics should explore the details again when they are in a safe environment. Elderly victims often find themselves trapped and are reluctant to volunteer a story that might make the situation worse for them in the long term.

BOX 38.10 Frailty

Frailty may represent a more accurate predictor of adverse outcomes and mortality than chronological age. Several studies in the burn literature demonstrate the usefulness of Frailty scoring systems in predicting outcome following burn injury. Patients with lower frailty scores on admission were more likely to survive burn injury, and those with higher frailty scores had an increased risk of mortality, or survivors were more likely requiring supported nursing care facilities on discharge (Romanowski et al., 2015). Furthermore, even in the absence of a formal frailty diagnosis, a frail appearance has been demonstrated to influence clinical decision to have Goals of Care discussions with patients and/or relevant family members, and set treatment limitation parameters after severe thermal injury (Tarik et al., 2018).

 CASE STUDY 3

Case 50999, 1938 hrs.

Dispatch details: An 18-month-old girl has been burnt with hot tea.

Initial presentation: The patient is an 18-month-old child who has pulled a mug of boiling hot tea off a table, spilling it down her chest and abdomen. She is distressed and screaming. There is an obvious red mark where the tea has burned her skin.

PRACTICE TIP

Avoid overhandling the child, and maintain eye-level contact and speak quietly. Use distraction or comparison with items familiar to the child's age group, such as using a doll to show how a stethoscope is applied. However, if life-threating or serious physical compromise is imminent, the parent or other caregivers may need to restrain the child so that emergency treatment can be provided.

1 ASSESS

1950 hrs Primary survey: The patient is conscious and responding with a clear airway and normal breathing.

1951 hrs Vital signs survey: Perfusion status: HR 140 bpm, sinus tachycardia, BP not taken, skin warm and pink, capillary refill < 2 seconds on non-injured areas.

Respiratory status: RR 40 bpm, good air entry, L = R, normal work of breathing, screaming.

Conscious state: GCS = 15.

Temperature: 35.9°C.

1953 hrs Pertinent Hx: The patient pulled the mug of hot tea onto herself and immediately started crying. Her parents removed her clothing and nappy and quickly placed her under a cool shower.

1954 hrs Secondary survey: The child has blistered and reddened skin from the base of her neck, down her sternal area and in a narrow line down her abdomen. Below the umbilicus the reddened areas spread horizontally in a 1-cm wide line to her hips. This coincides with the top of her nappy, which has since been removed. Skin has peeled away in many of these areas, particularly on her chest, and is reddened with small blisters in other areas.

Paediatric assessment: general principles

Assessing a child with burns can be extremely difficult because pain and fear often mean the child is inconsolable, unapproachable and uncooperative. Many children will seek refuge in the arms of parents or family and they can be used as valuable allies in gaining the child's trust and cooperation. Furthermore, the child may not be able to describe events or symptoms or answer questions in a meaningful manner. Assessment tools such as the paediatric subjective pain score, the paediatric assessment tool and modified GCS assessment are useful to elicit clinical information. An assertive but sensitive approach may be required.

This patient is conscious and responding, with normal breathing. She has less than 10% superficial and partial-thickness burns. The paramedics find no other injuries on examination. The child is in severe pain and is shivering. The parents and child will need reassurance.

2 CONFIRM

In many cases paramedics are presented with a collection of signs and symptoms that do not appear to describe a particular condition. A critical step in determining a treatment plan in this situation is to consider what other conditions could explain the patient's presentation. In this case it is obvious that burns are the problem. The issues are what anatomical structures are involved and the severity of the burns.

What else needs to be considered?

Airway burns

Airway compromise should always be considered; however, in this case there is no evidence that the child inhaled hot steam or fluid. She is also screaming loudly in a normal voice, suggesting no laryngeal inflammation or airway compromise.

Burn area and depth

Most scald injuries are superficial or superficial partial-thickness injuries as most hot liquids cool rapidly when exposed to air (Hettiaratchy & Dziewulski, 2004). The heat in more viscous oils may persist longer. Unlike thermal burns caused by flames and contact with hot surfaces, burns caused by hot liquids can affect body regions away from the original burn site as the liquid spills or splashes.

Look for burns adjacent to undergarments and nappies in footwear and socks. Also examine posterior, non-adjacent or counterintuitive body surface locations.

Prolonged scalding from liquids soaked into clothing or undergarments may increase the extent and severity of injury. Scald injury is deepest in areas of thick clothing, in natural creases in the body and where clothing is compressed into those creases. The area of a child's skin covered by a nappy is a common location where this may occur, as disposable nappies contain hydrogels with high water absorbency. The groin is also a particularly sensitive and vulnerable area. Burns to the groin in children meet admission requirements for a specialist burns unit, as they may require specialist intervention. In scald injuries, it is therefore essential to remove nappies and other items of clothing to minimise the extent of the burn and to accurately assess burn size. It is also important to remember that children have thinner skin and this may affect burn depth estimations. An apparently superficial or partial-thickness injury may in fact be a deeper burn.

Non-accidental burns

Unfortunately, burns are sometimes associated with abuse, and a burn that does not seem to coincide with the stated mechanism of injury should raise suspicions in this area. Any suspicious burn should be reported and investigated by those with expertise in this field.

③ TREAT

Pain management

Particular care must be taken regarding pain management in paediatric burn victims, as chronic debilitating pain and stress disorders can ensue if pain is inadequately managed. Opioids remain the cornerstone of analgesic options, but administration must be carefully titrated to effect and the onset of side effects. The pharmacokinetics of opioids in burn patients are reported to be similar to the effects seen in patients without burns.

Although analgesia can be difficult to administer to young children, IN fentanyl is easy to administer, is highly effective and has a relatively rapid onset. The dose depends on the size of the child and should be directed by local guidelines. Repeat doses will probably be required but ensure the child is alert and breathing normally and reassess pain scores before subsequent administration. Supplemental oxygenation (where tolerated) is recommended with all opioid administration, particularly where frequent increments or large doses are required, as respiratory rate and tidal volume may decrease with the onset of opioid action.

Hospital staff should be given an accurate handover of analgesic doses and times of administration. Opioid analgesics have powerful and potentially long-lasting side effects and the patient will require careful monitoring after paramedic care is completed.

Avoiding hypothermia

Body mass and surface area differences between children and adults mean that children lose heat and fluid more readily, predisposing them to an increased risk of hypothermia. Furthermore, neonates have underdeveloped thermoregulatory mechanisms so more obvious signs of cooling such as shivering may not be apparent. Absence of shivering may not truly reflect the level of core body temperature loss—and it might lull the paramedic into a false sense of security in relation to hypothermia risk. It is also interesting to note that shivering in children can occur for many reasons unrelated to hypothermia. In addition, children are less able to adopt behaviours to mitigate burn risk or complications such as anticipating dangers, protecting themselves from a heat source, mitigating hypothermia effects through self-warming or applying first-aid measures to their own burns.

In this case, the patient is starting to shiver, exhibiting the first signs of hypothermia. A tympanic temperature reading must be taken as early as possible after drying the patient. Tympanic thermometers may be affected by cold water in the ear canals, so the ears must be dried before attempting a reading. Readings should be taken quickly, with a parent lightly restraining the child while the reading is taken. Monitoring trends in temperature changes enables assessment of the effectiveness of warming and aids in the avoidance of hypothermia.

Warming

The importance of effective warming in vulnerable high-risk groups cannot be overstated. Warming needs to be commenced expeditiously, as first aid before the paramedics arrived may have already lowered the patient's core body temperature. While cooling proceeds, aim to warm as much of the non-burned area as possible. Once cooling is completed, gently dry the patient; water remaining on the skin will evaporate rapidly, accelerating overall heat loss. Either a heat-reflective foil blanket or an ordinary blanket is effective, but a foil blanket is easier to use in a wet environment. Warming does not end at the scene, continuing throughout care. This includes heating the ambulance as much as is tolerable.

Cooling at the scene

Cooling should continue for the recommended 20 minutes wherever possible unless hypothermia is noted (< 35°C), the burn is large or deep, or airway compromise or poor perfusion is present. In such situations there is a need to expedite transport and manage treatment en route. The presence of burns in certain anatomical locations (such as groin, hands, feet and face) requires that the patient be transported to a specialist burns unit, but does not necessarily require that cooling be immediately ceased. Nonetheless, transport should never be unduly delayed, even for cooling: the aim is to use the available time efficiently.

Continued cooling at the scene for this patient will provide further pain relief and contribute to reducing burn progression, both important considerations. Where possible the burned area should be exposed to cool running water while the rest of the child is kept dry and warm and preparations are made for transport.

Cooling en route to hospital

If cooling has been accomplished at the scene for a full 20 minutes, applying wet dressings or further cooling en route to hospital will have only limited analgesic benefit. Management of hypothermic risk must not be compromised in belated attempts to reduce pain by cooling a burn, especially as this can be accomplished with appropriate IV analgesia. This is crucially important in paediatric and other high-risk patients. If rotated wet dressings are applied, these should be limited to short periods and reassessed for effect. The patient is often the best source of information to determine the effectiveness of treatments and subjective pain score analysis should be undertaken frequently.

Wound management

Specific burn dressings should be applied as per local guidelines. Cling wrap enables observation of the wound while also providing barrier protection and aiding in pain relief by preventing exposure to the ambient environment.

Transport

Since the criteria for a major burn is > 5% TBSA in children, this child should be referred to a burns unit. She should be transported with at least one parent, who will provide reassurance as well as feedback on the child's pain and wellbeing. Analgesic narcosis is likely to result from delivery of opioids once the source of stimulation has been reduced, so the child will be more settled during transport than at the scene. Children in this age group are often suspicious or frightened of strangers and this has ramifications for assessment, treatment and ongoing care.

(4) EVALUATE

Evaluating the effect of any clinical management intervention can provide clues to the accuracy of the initial diagnosis. Some conditions respond rapidly to treatment so patients should be expected to improve if the diagnosis and treatment were appropriate. In this case the primary aims are to continue cooling the burned area, avoid hypothermia and provide adequate pain relief. Titrating to this patient's pain will require more analgesia than most paramedics usually administer to children. An effective level of pain relief would be when the child is restful when there is no intervention or examination being conducted. Respiratory depression is rarely a complication of carefully administered opioids in these cases.

The child's vital signs may not improve during transport, even with adequate analgesia, and deteriorating signs of perfusion combined with a long transport time indicate the need for IV fluid support.

Other types of burns

Chemical burns

Chemicals continue to destroy tissue as long as they are in contact with the skin. Death from a chemical injury is rare, although they can occur in cases with extensive burns, or because of severe systemic toxicity of absorbed chemicals. During the secondary survey it is important to ascertain the extent of tissue damage by determining the following:

- type and amount of agent involved
- strength and concentration of the agent
- site of contact and whether it was swallowed or inhaled
- manner and duration of contact
- mechanism of action of the chemical.

Appropriate medical management includes decontamination of the burn injury with water irrigation for longer than 20 minutes.

High-risk industries usually have evidence-based protocols for management of common chemicals exposure. They often include the use of buffering or neutralising agents such as Diphoterine (Alexander et al., 2017). Paramedics who attend industry-related chemical burn cases where neutralising agents have been applied should reconsider applying further first aid, as dilution of the agents with water will reduce their effectiveness. There is some evidence that Diphoterine improves chemical burn wound outcomes, especially when applied immediately following injury.

Safety and first aid for chemical burns

- Personal protective equipment (PPE) such as protective overalls, gloves and glasses should be considered mandatory for healthcare providers who assist a person with a chemical burn injury.
- Prolonged irrigation with water flow is the mainstay of immediate treatment of most chemical burns. Irrigation should occur as soon as possible and continue while pain persists.
- Remove contaminated clothing from patient.
- Powdered agents should be brushed from the skin while protecting the paramedics.
- Avoid washing the chemical over unaffected skin.
- For burns to the eye, always ensure the unaffected eye is uppermost when irrigating, to avoid contamination.

High-voltage electrical burns (> 1000 volts)

Electrical burn severity is determined by the voltage, current, type of current, duration of contact and resistance at contact points. High-voltage electrical injuries (> 1000 volts) occur as a result of contact with overhead powerlines and other sources of high-voltage electrical currents. These burns are commonly associated with other traumatic injuries, and tend to be characterised by deep, extensive tissue damage with three general patterns of injury:

- 'true' electrical injury caused by current flow
- electrical arc injury caused by arc of current from source to object
- flame injury from ignition of clothes etc.

Safety, first aid and initial management of high-voltage electrical burns

- Turn off mains power at the source.
- Ensure your own safety.
- Apply cool running water to the affected area for 20 minutes.

- Spinal precautions are mandatory.
- Perform primary and secondary survey, and initial management.

Management considerations
Cardiac support
Electrical injuries may result in a variety of cardiac arrhythmias, including asystole and ventricular fibrillation which manifest very soon after injury.
- CPR should be initiated for those in cardiac arrest.
- Monitor cardiac rhythm.

Fluid resuscitation
Fluid resuscitation requirements following high-voltage electrical burn are usually more than that indicated by the extent of the cutaneous burn. Muscle damage that is not immediately evident can cause fluid loss which is not accounted for by the Modified Parkland formula. It is important to always titrate fluid resuscitation according to urine output goals.

Management of myoglobinuria
Muscle damage can result in myoglobinuria and haemoglobinuria. These pigments can exacerbate acute renal failure. Prompt diuresis will help to protect against pigment deposition in the renal tubules and kidney damage. If pigment is evident in the urine, IV fluids should be increased to create a urine output of 75–100 mL/hr to 'flush' the kidneys. Diuretics may be required as an adjunct.

Entry and exit points
Look for entry and exit points to determine the path of the current. Consider possible damage to tissue in any organs that the path of the current crosses.

Compartment syndrome
Patients with high-voltage electrical injuries are at risk of developing compartment syndrome. Damaged muscle swells and the high pressure within the investing fascia can obliterate blood flow and result in further muscle necrosis. Signs of compartment syndrome include:
- 'tight' muscle compartments in limbs
- pain at rest
- increased pain on passive extension of digits
- decreased distal sensation
- decreased distal perfusion.

Elevate affected areas to help to minimise swelling. If multi-compartment fasciotomy is required, transfer should be time critical; consult with the appropriate burn unit.

Future research
There are well established and internationally recognised clinical processes for the initial assessment and management of trauma and burn patients. These include the primary and secondary survey for rapid and systematic assessment, as well as initial treatments including oxygen therapy and establishing IV access to provide fluids and analgesia. Nevertheless, large evidence gaps remain in out-of-hospital burn care that offer potentially significant improvements to patient outcomes (Muehlberger et al., 2010).

Further research priorities for out-of-hospital burn care include identifying precision in guidelines on which patients benefit from early intubation, in a hope to reduce the number of unnecessary intubations, adding to clinical risk and costs to out-of-hospital and hospital systems. Furthermore, future studies on out-of-hospital interventions to ascertain their effect on long-term patient outcomes, the ever-increasing sophistication of out-of-hospital and hospital patient information systems as well as clinical quality registries will aid opportunities in this space.

In particular, future research into the volume and quality of out-of-hospital fluid resuscitation and its effects on oedema formation, organ ischaemia and/or fluid creep can help make out-of-hospital fluid resuscitation more precise to mitigate adverse effects. The type of fluid used in burn resuscitation is the subject of ongoing controversy. Crystalloids, colloids or albumin or a combination of these have all been proposed but have not been adequately researched in the out-of-hospital field. Research opportunities exist in the optimal analgesic for acute out-of-hospital burn pain. It has been suggested that excessive narcotic use or 'opioid creep' may further contribute to excessive IV volume resuscitation (Nielson et al., 2017); therefore, better evidence to help titrate out-of-hospital analgesia for burn injury can help to mitigate any potentially negative effects.

Further research should focus on enhancing communication between out-of-hospital and burn care providers. The variety of portable digital media available offers great potential to support paramedics to undertake accurate assessment and quality care of burn patients at the scene before transfer. In particular, it can help with the out-of-hospital estimate of burn size and depth. Furthermore, while cling wrap is recommended for burn wound coverage, this is based on consensus; expert opinion and future research could help to identify the ideal out-of-hospital burn wound coverage.

Summary
Patients with burns present the paramedic with a range of clinical and logistical challenges. The mantra of *'cool the burn and warm the patient'* is not always logistically simple, and is influenced significantly by the severity of burn injury and the age of the

patient. Understanding the pathophysiology of burn progression along with the importance of ongoing airway assessment for risk, titrated and targeted volume resuscitation and analgesia, and accurate TBSA and weight calculation will all aid paramedics in prioritising care. A low threshold for seeking intervention to secure an airway at risk must be at the forefront of the paramedic's mind when assessing and treating the burns patient, especially when the mechanism involves an enclosed-space burn. Analgesia is of the utmost importance in patients with superficial burns. However, some patients may present without pain, often indicating the burns involved are severe. Wherever possible and in accordance with local protocols, the patient with complicated burns, large % TBSA or preexisting significant comorbidities should be transported to a specialist burns centre in the first instance, recognising that subsequent transfer adds to delay in definitive burn care. Finally, burns can be confronting and traumatic for paramedics and recognition may have lasting effects; mental health and wellbeing should be considered and discussed in accordance with local support systems.

References

Agency for Clinical Innovation (NSW) (ACI). (2011). *Model of Care*. Chatswood: ACI Statewide Burn Injury Service, NSW Agency for Clinical Innovation.

Alexander, K. S., Wasiak, J., & Cleland, H. (2018). Chemical burns: diphoterine untangled. *Burns: Journal of the International Society for Burn Injuries, 44*(4), 752–766. doi:10.1016/j.burns.2017.09.017. Jun.

Alexandrou, E., Ray-Barruel, G., Carr, P., Frost, S. A., Inwood, S., Higgins, N., Lin, F., Alberto, L., Mermel, L., & Rickard, C. M. (2018). Use of short peripheral intravenous catheters: characteristics, management, and outcomes worldwide. *Journal of Hospital Medicine*, doi:10.12788/jhm.3039.

Allison, K. (2002). The UK pre-hospital management of burn patients: current practice and the need for a standard approach. *Burns: Journal of the International Society for Burn Injuries, 28*(2), 135–142.

American Burn Association (ABA). (2011). *Advanced Burn Life Support (ABLS) Provider Course Manual*. Retrieved from http://www.ameriburn.org/ABLS/ABLSCourseDescriptions.htm/ [accessed 22.09.15].

Australian and New Zealand Burn Association (ANZBA). (2016). *Annual Report*. 1st July 2015–30th June 2016. ANZBA, Brisbane.

Australian and New Zealand Burn Association (ANZBA) and Education Committee (2015). *Emergency management of severe burns (EMSB): Course Manual*. ANZBA, Brisbane.

Australian Institute of Health and Welfare. (2018). *Older Australia at a glance [Internet]. Canberra: Australian Institute of Health and Welfare*, [cited 2020 Jun. 4]. Retrieved from https://www.aihw.gov.au/reports/older-people/older-australia-at-a-glance.

Avni, T., Levcovich, A., Ad-El, D., Leibovici, L., & Paul, M. (2010). Prophylactic antibiotics for burns patients: systematic review and meta-analysis. *The British Medical Journal, 340*, c24.

Badulak, J., Schurr, M., Sauaia, A., Ivashchenko, A., & Peltz, E. (2018). Defining the criteria for intubation of the patient with thermal burns. *Burns: Journal of the International Society for Burn Injuries, 44*(3), 531–538.

Bartlett, N., Yuan, J., Holland, A. J. A., Harvey, J. G., Martin, H. C. O., La Hei, E. R., Arbuckle, S., & Godfrey, C. (2008). Optimal duration of cooling for an acute scald contact burn injury in a porcine model. *Journal of Burns Care & Research, 29*(5), 828–834.

Bittner, E. A., Shank, E., Woodson, L., & Martyn, J. A. (2015). Acute and perioperative care of the burn-injured patient. *Anesthesiology, 122*, 448–464.

Brown, D., & Edwards, H. (2012). *Lewis's Medical-surgical nursing* (2nd ed.). Sydney: Elsevier.

Burn Registry of Australia and New Zealand (BRANZ). (2018). *Annual Report*. 1st July 2016–30th June 2017. Retrieved from https://www.monash.edu/__data/assets/pdf_file/0005/1411349/BRANZ-8th-Annual-Report-Jul-16-Jun-17_0.pdf.

Carreras-Gonzalez, E., & Brio-Sanagustin, S. (2014). Prevention of complications in the air transport of the critically ill pediatric patient between hospitals. *Anales de Pediatria (Barc), 81*(4), 205–211.

Chan, Q. E., Barzi, F., Cheney, L., Harvey, J. G., & Holland, A. J. (2012). Burn size estimation in children: still a problem. *Emergency Medicine Australasia: EMA, 24*(2), 181–186.

Chung, K. K., Wolf, S. E., Cancio, L. C., Alvarado, R., Jones, J., McCorcle, J., King, B., Barillo, D., Renz, E., & Blackbourne, L. (2009). Resuscitation of severely burned military casualties: fluid begets more fluid. *The Journal of Trauma and Acute Care Surgery, 67*(2), 231–237.

Cicolini, G., Bonghi, A. P., Di Labio, L., & Di Mascio, R. (2009). Position of peripheral venous cannulae and the incidence of thrombophlebitis: an observational study. *Journal of Advanced Nursing, 65*(6), 1268–1273.

Ciofi Silva, C. L., Rossi, L. A., Canini, S. R., Gonçalves, N., & Furuya, R. K. (2014). Site of catheter insertion in burn patients and infection: a systematic review. *Burns: Journal of the International Society for Burn Injuries, 40*(3), 365–373.

Connolly, S. (2011). *Clinical Practice Guidelines: Summary of Evidence. Chatswood: ACI Statewide Burn Injury Service, NSW Agency for Clinical Innovation.*

Craft, J., Gordon, C., & Tiziani, A. (2011). *Understanding pathophysiology.* Sydney: Elsevier.

Cuttle, L., Pearn, J., McMillan, J. R., & Kimble, R. M. (2009). A review of first-aid treatments for burn injuries. *Burns: Journal of the International Society for Burn Injuries, 35*(6), 768–775.

Demling, R. H. (2005). The burn edema process: current concepts. *Journal of Burn Care & Rehabilitation, 26*(3), 207–227.

Diver, A. J. (2008). The evolution of burn fluid resuscitation. *International Journal of Surgery, 6*(4), 345–350.

Dulhunty, J. M., Boots, R. J., Rudd, M. J., Muller, M. J., & Lipman, J. (2008). Increased fluid resuscitation can lead to adverse outcomes in major-burn injured patients, but low mortality. *Burns: Journal of the International Society for Burn Injuries, 34*(8), 1090–1097.

Farage, M. A., Miller, K. W., Elsner, P., & Maibach, H. I. (2013). Characteristics of the aging skin. *Advances in Wound Care, 2*(1), 5–10.

Freiburg, C., Igneri, P., Sartorelli, K., & Rogers, F. (2007). Effects of differences in percent total body surface area estimation on fluid resuscitation of transferred burn patients. *Journal of Burn Care and Research, 28*(1), 42–48.

Gabbe, B., Cleland, H. J., & Cameron, P. A. (2011). Profile, transport and outcomes of severe burns patients within an inclusive, regionalized trauma system. *ANZ Journal of Surgery, 81*(10), 725–730.

Gacto-Sanchez, P. (2017). Surgical treatment and management of the severely burn patient: review and update. *Medicina Intensiva, 41*(6), 356–364.

Gorski, L. (2017). The 2016 infusion therapy standards of practice. *Home Healthcare Now, 35*(1), 10–18.

Gray, T., & O'Reilly, G. (2009). Burns. In P. Cameron, G. Jelinek, A. M. Kelly, L. Murray & A. F. T. Brown (Eds.), *Textbook of adult emergency medicine.* Churchill Livingstone.

Haberal, M., Abali, A. E. S., & Karakayali, H. (2010). Fluid management in major burn injuries. *Indian Journal of Plastic Surgery, 43*(3), 29–39.

Harish, V., Raymond, A. P., Issler, A. C., Lajevardi, S. S., Chang, L. Y., Maitz, P. K., & Kennedy, P. (2015). Accuracy of burn size estimation in patients transferred to adult Burn Units in Sydney, Australia: an audit of 698 patients. *Burns: Journal of the International Society for Burn Injuries, 41*(1), 91–99.

Harrison, J., & Steel, D. (2006). *Burns and scalds. Cat. no. INJ 92.* Canberra: AIHW.

Hayek, S., Ibrahim, A., Abu Sittah, G., & Atiyeh, B. (2011). Burn Resuscitation: is it straight forward or a challenge? *Annals of Burns and Fire Disasters, 24*(1), 17–21.

Herndon, D. N. (2007). Total burn care. *Elsevier Health Sciences, 12*(2), 110–111.

Hettiaratchy, S., & Dziewulski, P. (2004). Pathophysiology and types of burns. *British Medical Journal, 328*(7453), 1427–1429. Jun 12.

Hettiaratchy, S., & Papini, R. (2004). ABC of burns: Initial management of a major burn: II—assessment and resuscitation. *British Medical Journal, 329*(7457), 101–103.

Hostler, D., Weaver, M. D., & Ziembicki, J. A. (2013). Admission temperature and survival in patients admitted to burn centers. *Journal of Burn Care and Research, 34*(5), 498–506.

Huang, S. B., Chang, W. H., Huang, C. H., & Tsai, C. H. (2008). Management of elderly burn patients. *International Journal of Gerontology, 2*(3), 91–97.

Ireland, S., Endacott, R., Cameron, P., Fitzgerald, M., & Paul, E. (2011). The incidence and significance of accidental hypothermia in major trauma—a prospective observational study. *Resuscitation, 82*(3), 300–306.

ISBI Practice Guidelines Committee. (2016). ISBI practice guidelines for burn care. *Burns: Journal of the International Society for Burn Injuries, 42*(5), 953–1021.

ISBI Practice Guidelines Committee. (2018/2019). *ISBI Practice Guidelines for Burn Care.* (Ahead of Print).

Ivy, M. E., Atweh, N. A., Palmer, J., Possenti, P., Pineau, M., & D'Aiuto, M. (2000). Intra-abdominal hypertension and abdominal compartment syndrome in burn patients. *The Journal of Trauma and Acute Care Surgery, 49*(3), 387–391.

Jackson, D. (1953). The diagnosis of the depth of burning. *British Journal of Surgery, 40*(164), 588–596.

Jaskille, A. D., Ramella-Roman, J., Shupp, J., Jordan, M., & Jeng, J. (2010). Critical review of burn depth assessment techniques: part II. Review of laser Doppler technology. *Journal of Burn Care and Research, 31*(1), 151–157.

Johnson, R. M., & Richard, R. (2003). Partial-thickness burns: identification and management. *Advances in Skin and Wound Care, 16*(4), 178–187.

Keck, M., Lumenta, D. B., Andel, H., Kamolz, L. P., & Frey, M. (2009). Burn treatment in the elderly. *Burns: Journal of the International Society for Burn Injuries, 35*(8), 1070–1079.

Klein, M. B., Lezotte, D. C., Heltshe, S., Fauerbach, J., Holavanahalli, R. K., Rivara, F. P., & Engray, L. (2011). Functional and psychosocial outcomes of older adults after burn injury: results from a multicenter database of severe burn injury. *Journal of Burn Care and Research, 32*(1), 66–78.

Klein, M. B., Nathens, A. B., Emerson, D., Heimbach, D. M., & Gibran, N. S. (2007). An analysis of the long-distance transport of burn patients to a regional burn center. *Journal of Burn and Care Research, 28*(1), 49–55.

Kramer, G., Hoskins, S., Copper, N., Chen, J., Hazel, M., & Mitchell, C. (2007). Emerging advances in burn resuscitation. *Journal of Trauma-Injury Infection & Critical Care*, 62(6), S71–S72.

Latenser, B. A. (2009). Critical care of the burn patient: the first 48 hours. *Critical Care Medicine*, 37(10), 2819–2826.

Makrantonaki, E. (2012). Challenge and promise: human skin ageing. *Dermato Endocrinology*, 4(3), 225–226.

Mandell, S. P., Pham, T. B., & Klein, B. M. (2013). Repeat hospitalization and mortality in older adult burn patients. *Journal of Burn Care and Research*, 34(1), 36–41.

Manktelow, A., Meyer, A., Herzog, S., & Peterson, H. (1989). Analysis of life expectancy and living status of elderly patients surviving a burn injury. *The Journal of Trauma*, 29(2), 203–207.

Marsh, N., Webster, J., Larson, E., Cooke, M., Mihala, G., & Rickard, C. M. (2018). Observational study of peripheral intravenous catheter outcomes in adult hospitalized patients: a multivariable analysis of peripheral intravenous catheter failure. *Journal of Hospital Medicine*, 13, 83–89.

Marx, J. A., Hockberger, R. S., & Walls, R. M. (2014). *Rosen's emergency medicine*. Philadelphia: Elsevier Saunders.

Mlcak, R. P., Suman, O., & Herndon, D. (2007). Respiratory management of inhalation injury. *Burns: Journal of the International Society for Burn Injuries*, 33(1), 2–13.

Moureau, N. L., Trick, N., & Nifong, T. (2012). Vessel health and preservation (Part 1): a new evidence-based approach to vascular access selection and management. *The Journal of Vascular Access*, 13(3), 351–356.

Muehlberger, T., Ottomann, C., Toman, N., Daigeler, A., & Lehnhardt, M. (2010). Emergency pre-hospital care of burn patients. *The Surgeon: Journal of the Royal Colleges of Surgeons of Edinburgh and Ireland*, 8(2), 101–104.

Nielson, C., Duethman, N., Howard, J., Moncure, M., & Wood, J. (2017). Burns: pathophysiology of systemic complications and current management. *Journal of Burn Care and Research*, 38(1), 469–481.

Ong, Y. S., Samuel, M., & Song, C. (2006). Meta-analysis of early excision of burns. *Burns: Journal of the International Society for Burn Injuries*, 32(2), 145–150.

Pham, T., Cancio, L. C., & Gibran, N. S. (2008). American Burn Association practice guidelines burn shock resuscitation. *Journal of Burn Care Research*, 29(1), 257–266.

Pham, T. N., & Gibran, N. S. (2007). Thermal and electrical injuries. *Surgical Clinics of North America*, 87(1), 185–206.

Rainey, S., Cruse, C. W., Smith, J., Smith, K., Jones, D., & Cobb, S. (2007). The occurrence and seasonal variation of accelerant-related burn injuries in central Florida. *Journal of Burn Care and Research*, 28(5), 675–680.

Rajan, V., Bartlett, N., Harvey, J. G., Martin, H. C. O., La Hei, E. R., Arbuckle, S., Godfrey, C., & Holland, A. J. A. (2009). Delayed cooling of an acute scald contact burn injury in a porcine model: is it worthwhile? *Journal of Burn Care & Research*, 30(4), 729–734.

Rani, M., & Schwacha, G. (2011). Ageing and the pathogenic response to Burns. *Ageing and Disease*, 2(6), 171–180.

Reade, M. C., Davies, S. R., Morley, P. T., Dennett, J., & Jacobs, I. C. (2012). Australian Resuscitation Council review article: management of cyanide poisoning. *Emergency Medicine Australasia: EMA*, 24(3), 225–238.

Reid, C., Hatton, R., & Middleton, P. (2011). Case report: prehospital use of intranasal ketamine for paediatric burn injury. *Emergency Medicine Journal*, 28(4), 328–329.

Romanowski, K. S., Barsun, A., Pamlieri, T. L., Greenhalgh, D. G., & Sen, S. (2015). Frailty score on admission predicts outcomes in elderly burn injury. *Journal of Burn and Care Research*, 36(1), 1–6.

Scanlon, V. C., & Sanders, T. (2007). *Essentials of anatomy and physiology* (5th ed.). Philadelphia: F.A. Davis Co.

Schwartz, L. R., & Balakrishan, C. (2004). Thermal burns. In J. E. Tintinalli, et al. (Eds.), *Tintinalli's emergency medicine: a comprehensive study guide* (8th ed.). Boston: McGraw-Hill.

Scott, A. S., & Fong, E. (2004). *Body structures and function* (10th ed.). Canada: Thomson Delmar Learning.

Shupp, J. W., Nasabzadeh, T. J., Rosenthal, D., Jordan, M., Fidler, P., & Jeng, J. (2010). A review of the local pathophysiologic bases of burn wound progression. *Journal of Burn Care & Research*, 31(6), 849–873.

Singer, A. J., Taira, B. R., Thode, H. C., McCormack, J. E., Shapiro, M. D., Aydin, A., & Lee, M. D. (2010). The association between hypothermia, prehospital cooling, and mortality in burn victims. *Academic Emergency Medicine: Official Journal of the Society for Academic Emergency Medicine*, 17(4), 456–459.

Smith, J. A., Fox, J. G., Saunder, A. C., & Ming, K. Y. (2010). *Hunt & Marshall's clinical problems in surgery* (2nd ed.). Sydney: Churchill Livingstone.

Soreide, K. (2014). Clinical and translational aspects of hypothermia in major trauma patients: from pathophysiology to prevention, prognosis and potential preservation. *Injury*, 45(4), 647–654.

Strang, S. G., Van Lieshout, E. M., Breedervelt, R. S., & Van Waes, O. (2014). A systematic review of intra-abdominal pressure in severely burned patients. *Burns: Journal of the International Society for Burn Injuries*, 40(1), 9–16.

Stuart, R. L., Cameron, D. R., Scott, C., Kotsanas, D., Grayson, M. L., Korman, T. M., Gillespie, E. E., & Johnson, P. D. (2013). Peripheral intravenous catheter-associated Staphylococcus aureus bacteraemia: more than 5 years of prospective data from two tertiary health services. *The Medical Journal of Australia*, 198(10), 551–553.

Tao, L., Zhou, J., Gong, Y., Liu, W., Long, T., Huang, X., Luo, G., Peng, Y., & Wu, J. (2015). Risk factors for central line-associated bloodstream infection in patients with major burns and the efficacy of the topical application of mupirocin at the central venous catheter exit site. *Burns: Journal of the International Society for Burn Injuries*, *41*(8), 1831–1838.

Tarik, D., Madni, M. D., Nakonezny, P., Wolf, S., Joseph, B., Mohler, M., Imran, J., Clark, A., Arnoldo, B., & Phelan, H. (2018). The relationship between frailty and the subjective decision to conduct a goals of care discussion with burned elders. *Journal of Burn Care & Research*, *39*(1), 82–88.

Tracy, L. M., Rosenblum, S., & Gabbe, B. J. (2020). *Burns Registry of Australia and New Zealand (BRANZ) 2018/19 Annual Report*. Department of Epidemiology and Preventive Medicine, Monash University. Melbourne, Australia.

Treat, R. C., Sirinek, K. R., Levine, B. A., & Pruitt, B. A. (1980). Air evacuation of thermally injured patients: principles of treatment and results. *Journal of Trauma, 20*, 275–279.

Tricklebank, S. (2009). Modern trends in fluid therapy for burns. *Burns: Journal of the International Society for Burn Injuries*, *35*(6), 757–767.

Vaughn, L., & Beckel, N. (2012). Severe burn injury, burn shock, and smoke inhalation injury in small animals. Part 1: burn classification and pathophysiology. *Journal of Veterinary Emergency and Critical Care (San Antonio)*, *22*(2), 179–186.

Wachtel, T., Berry, C., Wachtel, E., & Frank, H. (2000). The inter-rater reliability of estimating the size of burns from various burn area chart drawings. *Burns: Journal of the International Society for Burn Injuries*, *26*(2), 156–170.

Wallis, M., McGrail, M., Webster, J., & Marsh, N. (2014). Risk factors for PIV catheter failure: a multivariate analysis from a randomized control trial. *Infection Control and Hospital Epidemiology*, *35*(1), 63–68.

Warden, G. D. (1992). Burn shock resuscitation. *World Journal of Surgery*, *16*(1), 16–23.

Warner, P., Bailey, J., Bowers, L., Hermann, R., James, L., & McCall, J. (2016). Aeromedical pediatric burn transportation: a six-year review. *Journal of Burn and Care Research*, *37*(1), 181–187.

Wasiak, J., Cleland, H., & Campbell, F. (2008). Dressings for superficial and partial thickness burns. *The Cochrane Database of Systematic Reviews*, (4), CD002106.

Wasiak, J., Mahar, P. D., Paul, E., Menezes, H., Spinks, A. B., & Cleland, H. (2014). Inhaled methoxyflurane for pain and anxiety relief during burn wound care procedures: an Australian case series. *International Wound Journal*, *11*(1), 74–78.

Wood, F. M., Phillips, M., Jovic, T., Cassidy, J. T., Cameron, P., & Edgar, D. W. (2016). Water first aid is beneficial in humans post-burn: evidence from a Bi-National Cohort Study. *PLoS ONE*, *11*(1), e0147259.

Wu, G., Xiao, Y., Wang, C., Hong, X., Sun, Y., Ma, B., Wang, G., & Xia, Z. (2017). Risk factors for acute kidney injury in patients with burn injury: a meta-analysis and systematic review. *Journal of Burn Care and Research*, *38*(5), 271–282. Sept/Oct.

Yuan, J., Wu, C., Holland, A. J. A., Harvey, J. G., Martin, H. C. O., La Hei, E. R., Arbuckle, S., & Godfrey, T. C. (2007). Assessment of cooling on an acute scald burn injury in a porcine model. *Journal of Burn Care & Research*, *28*(3), 514–520.

CHAPTER 39

Mass-Casualty Incidents

By Dr Erin Smith

OVERVIEW

- A mass-casualty incident (MCI) is an incident where the location, number, severity or type of casualties requires external assistance or resources.
- MCIs can take a variety of forms including natural disasters (e.g. earthquakes, bushfires, cyclones, floods), transportation incidents (e.g. road traffic, railway, aircraft), industrial incidents (e.g. chemical spills), building collapses and explosions. MCIs can also result from poisonings (e.g. from sources such as restaurants or water supplies) and outbreaks of disease.
- Safety during MCIs should focus on self (of the responders), scene and survivors.
- Communication is often reported as the most common failing at the scene of an MCI.
- The management of MCIs will involve some sort of initial assessment (triage) of the injured, basic treatment at the scene and transport of patients.

- A number of contemporary out-of-hospital MCI triage systems have been developed largely based on physiological parameters associated with clinical instability. These systems classify patients into one of four categories.
  - Priority 1: Patients who are critically injured and require immediate attention.
  - Priority 2: Patients who require urgent attention but can tolerate a delay.
  - Priority 3: Patients who do not require immediate attention.
  - Priority 4: Deceased patients or patients not expected to survive.
- MCIs can result in mass fatalities, which pose unique challenges for disaster management.

Introduction

Mass-casualty incidents (MCIs) are incidents where the location, number, severity or type of casualties requires external assistance or resources.

MCIs can be classified as either natural or man-made. A natural MCI is the result of a naturally occurring event, such as an earthquake, bushfire, cyclone, flood or infectious disease. Man-made MCIs can result from human-caused events like terrorist attacks and transport-related attacks. They can also result from technological events.

The 'all-hazard' response to MCIs

The 'all-hazard' approach to MCIs can be adopted by all responding emergency services. The approach is encapsulated in seven generic key principles.

1. Command and control

Command

Each emergency service involved with the response to an MCI will have a commander. Command is vertical within each service. There are three tiers of command at a major incident.

Bronze

The bronze area is the area of immediate hazard, and is where initial triage and treatment will take place. The boundary of the bronze area can be referred to as the inner cordon. Each emergency service may designate a bronze commander. Depending on the type of MCI, there may be more than one bronze area and set of bronze commanders within the MCI.

Silver

The silver area is the entire scene and the boundary is known as the outer cordon. Each emergency service will provide a silver commander. Unlike the bronze area, there is only one silver area for an MCI, except in an incident over a wide area (e.g. an earthquake, with multiple MCIs).

Gold

Gold represents the highest level of command for the incident. Gold command is remote from the scene and may be identified by a local authority or by a regional, county, state or national boundary (see Fig 39.1).

Control

At the scene of an MCI, overall responsibility will be taken by one service and this service is said to have control. Control is therefore horizontal across the services.

Each emergency service at the scene of the major incident will have a commander. These commanders are responsible for all single service

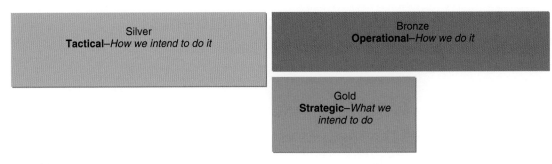

Figure 39.1
Command cordons for an MCI.

assets. One service will have overall responsibility, or scene control. Who has scene control will differ depending on the type of MCI that is taking place.

The commander of the emergency service that has overall responsibility at the scene of an MCI should clearly introduce himself or herself and establish who the key personnel are that are present at the briefing. The commander should provide a brief description of the type of incident, the time of the incident and subsequent response, the estimated total number of casualties and the estimated number of casualties remaining on the scene.

The commander should also be able to summarise the size of the medical response. This includes the number of ambulance personnel on scene, the number of immediate care doctors and the number of hospital teams on scene. They should also be able to describe the incident site including the boundaries of the bronze and silver areas, and any important features such as access routes, railways, pylons, obstacles and hazards (see Box 39.1).

2. Safety
The code of safety for MCIs is remembered as 'SSS': Self, Scene, Survivors.

Self
The first priority for paramedics at the scene of an MCI should be their own personal safety. Paramedics should ensure that they wear appropriate protective equipment. This may include a high-visibility jacket or tabard/vest, protective boots, hard hat, goggles or visor, ear protectors, gloves and appropriate airway protection. Responders should not approach the scene of an MCI when hazards are known to exist without permission from the most appropriate commander (see Box 39.2).

Scene safety
It is useful to remember the THREE Cs of immediate MCI scene safety: CONFIRM the nature of the incident and any hazards; CLEAR the area of bystanders and walking casualties; and CORDON the area to prevent further casualties.

Survivor safety
Occasionally it will be necessary to move casualties if there is an immediate threat to life at the scene of an MCI such as fire, secondary devices or toxic chemicals. This will usually be done without the usual precautions employed during controlled extrication (e.g. spinal immobilisation). Measures must also be taken to avoid additional casualties depending on the location and climate at the MCI scene. For example, measures may need to be taken to prevent hypothermia, exposure, heat illness, exhaustion and dehydration.

3. Communication
Communication will be integral to effective MCI response and must take place within emergency agencies (intra-agency communications) and across different agencies (inter-agency communications). Effective communication between the incident commanders must be established early and arrangements made for regular liaison.

Failures in communication can lead to very serious consequences, including injury and death. Indeed, the communication failures inherent with the response to the terrorist attacks in the United States on 11 September 2001 (9/11) potentially led to the deaths of hundreds of first responders (Fig 39.2 and Box 39.3).

4. Assessment
A rapid assessment of the scene of an MCI should be undertaken to estimate the number and severity of injured. The information gathered is used to determine the initial response to the scene and to estimate the number of casualties for receiving hospitals.

5. Triage
When an MCI occurs, rapid assessment and treatment of victims is a priority. This rapid assessment is referred to as 'triage'. Coming from the French word 'trier' (which means to 'sort'), triage will play an important role in this initial assessment, especially when resources are constrained.

BOX 39.1 Activity

You are the ambulance commander and in control of the following MCI.

Disaster-town is a small island town with an area of 95 square kilometres and a population of 42 371. Many of the inhabitants commute over one of two bridges that connect Disaster-town to mainland Crisisville. The Jameston Bridge is a combined road and railway bridge and was the only connection to the mainland until the Hollywood Crossing Bridge was built in 2006. The Hollywood Crossing Bridge runs alongside the Jamestown Bridge. It has four lanes with a 100-kilometre per hour speed limit and does not have a hard shoulder. It is unlit and has no warning signs. The bridge is 1270 metres long.

At 0715 hrs today, a road traffic accident occurred on the Hollywood Crossing Bridge. When the accident happened there was a very thick fog and visibility was reduced to about 20 metres. The initial call to 000 reported a car-versus-car crash. No mention was made of the low visibility. Subsequent calls started to come in from other cars involved in the accident.

It was difficult for 000 call-takers to determine how many individual cars had been involved in the accident, but it appeared initially to be at least five cars.

The first ambulance crew arrives on scene at 0726 hrs as the fog is lifting.

You are one of the paramedics on that ambulance and assume the role of ambulance commander. The first police crew arrives at 0727 hrs. The first fire crew arrives at 0734 hrs.

As ambulance commander, you have your first meeting with other emergency services at 0740 hrs.

As you begin to assess the scene, it quickly becomes evident that the pile-up involved cars extending across most of the bridge.

Despite heavy fog and low visibility, some drivers approached the bridge at speed and without lights. This culminated in a pile-up involving more than 120 cars. The bridge is now inaccessible. There are hundreds of people milling around on the bridge, which in addition to safety issues, makes it difficult to assess and triage casualties.

Between 0728 hrs and 0735 hrs three other ambulance crews arrive on the scene. You instruct them to establish a casualty clearing station (CCS). Your partner who arrived with you has been instructing the walking wounded (Priority 3/minimal patients) to move off the bridge and in the direction of where the CCS will be set up.

You assign one crew (of two paramedics) to triage the walking wounded once they arrive at the CCS while the other two ambulance crews on scene are sent to triage the casualties who remained on the bridge.

As the fog lifts, the temperature reaches 30°C and the prolonged period stranded outside begins to put those remaining on scene at risk from dehydration and exacerbation of preexisting illnesses.

First assessment: More than 200 people are assessed at the scene and 69 of these require hospital treatment.

There are four fatalities.

What is included in your initial briefing?

BOX 39.2 Personal protective equipment

Personal protective equipment (PPE) is a key aspect of ensuring responder safety during a major incident and disaster response. Proper selection of PPE for individual responders must be based on a careful assessment of two factors:

1. the hazards anticipated to be present, or are present, at the scene
2. the probable impact of the hazards based on the role of the individual.

Developed as a wartime necessity, the earliest use of triage was employed by the Chief Surgeon of Napoleon's army in the 1790s, who was credited not only with the concept of triage, but the organisational structure necessary to manage the growing number of casualties in modern warfare (Robertson-Steel, 2006).

During an MCI, triage can be used to ensure that medical resources are directed at achieving the greatest good for the greatest number of people. A number of contemporary out-of-hospital MCI triage systems have been developed largely based on physiological parameters associated with clinical instability. These triage systems can be broadly classified as either primary or secondary triage (Jenkins et al., 2008).

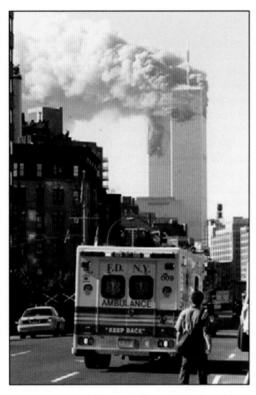

Figure 39.2
Terrorist attacks on the World Trade Centre in New York on 11 September 2001.
Source: Editorial, The Lancet (2011).

Primary triage systems are utilised at the scene of an MCI and include the Simple Treatment and Rapid Transport (START) method, the Sacco Triage Method (STM), the CareFlight Model, the Manchester Sieve and Sort model and the Sort/ Assess/Lifesaving Intervention/and Treatment/ Transport (SALT) model. Secondary triage is the re-evaluation of the victim's condition after initial medical care. It helps to establish the order in which patients receive care at the receiving hospital or, in the case of delayed transportation, at the scene of the MCI. Secondary triage systems include the Secondary Assessment of Victim Endpoint (SAVE) and Triage Sort models.

All of these out-of-hospital MCI triage systems, with the exception of the STM (which is based on a simple physiological score; e.g. respiratory rate, pulse, best motor response), are algorithms that classify patients into one of four categories (see Fig 39.3 and Box 39.4).

These different priorities are usually associated with a specific coloured tag that is attached to the patient.

Priority 1 patients
A Priority 1 patient requires immediate care for a good probability of survival. These patients will be classified as the highest priority to receive care.

BOX 39.3 Communication failures on 9/11

From the first moments of the response to the 9/11 terrorist attacks on New York City to the last, the efforts of the emergency first responders were plagued by failures of communication, command and control. When the firefighters needed to communicate, their radio system failed, just as it had in those same buildings 8 years earlier during the response to the 1993 World Trade Centre (WTC) bombing.

No other agency lost communications on 9/11 as broadly, or to such devastating effect, as the Fire Department of the City of New York (FDNY). The FDNY communication system failed frequently that morning and problems escalated once the vital communication infrastructure that was located on the roof of the South Tower of the WTC was destroyed when the tower fell. Even if the radio network had been reliable, it was not linked to the communication systems of other emergency response agencies.

This failure was further compounded by the lack of interagency communication. Minutes after the South Tower of the WTC collapsed, NYPD police helicopters above the remaining North Tower communicated to police officers on the ground that the building looked like it was ready to collapse.

Those clear warnings captured on police radio tapes were transmitted 21 minutes before the North Tower fell. The warning was relayed to police officers in the building, but unfortunately fire, police and emergency medical services (EMS) operated on different communication channels and were not routinely sharing information. While most police officers heard the order to evacuate and escaped the North Tower, most firefighters and EMS responders never heard those warnings.

Ultimately, this breakdown in communication contributed to the loss of 343 firefighters and 10 paramedics and emergency medical technicians (EMTs) that day.

Common injuries in this category include:
- airway obstruction
- sucking chest wounds
- tension pneumothorax
- unstable chest and abdominal wounds
- incomplete amputations
- exsanguinating haemorrhage
- second- or third-degree burns involving 40–60% of the total body surface area.

A patient's respiratory rate will also be important to assess. In general, anything less than 10 breaths

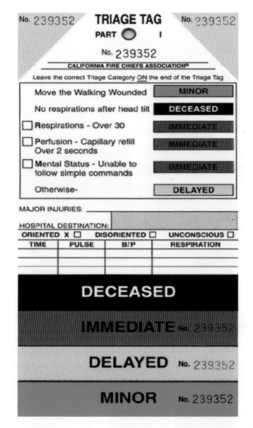

Figure 39.3
Example triage tag.
Source: Schultz & Koenig (2018).

BOX 39.4 Triage categories

Priority 1 (Immediate; red)
Patients who are critically injured and require immediate attention.
Priority 2 (Delayed; yellow)
Patients requiring urgent attention but can tolerate a delay.
Priority 3 (Minor/Minimal; green)
Patients where any necessary intervention can be delayed.
Priority 4 (Deceased/Expectant; black)
Patients who are deceased or expectant patients who are not expected to survive.

BOX 39.5 Examples of Priority 1 patients

1. A 45-year-old female with a large laceration to her right thigh that has uncontrolled bleeding.
2. A 75-year-old man who is breathing but has no palpable radial pulse.
3. A 4-year-old girl with acute respiratory distress.

BOX 39.6 Examples of Priority 2 patients

1. A 20-year-old male who is having acute abdominal pain but is alert with normal vital signs.
2. A 5-year-old boy with a laceration and deformity to his right forearm. He is able to move his arm and his vital signs are good.
3. A 35-year-old pregnant female with abdominal pain.

per minute, or greater than 30 breaths per minute, would place someone in the Priority 1 category (see Box 39.5).

Priority 2 patients
Priority 2 patients require care that can be safely delayed without affecting the probability of survival. The delayed category is used for casualties requiring medical intervention for survival, but who have a condition that is less time-sensitive to those classified as immediate.

Common injuries in this category include:
- stable abdominal wounds without haemodynamic instability
- traumatic crush injuries without crush syndrome
- traumatic amputation with controlled bleeding
- smoke inhalation without respiratory distress
- major orthopaedic injuries requiring manipulation, debridement or external fixation
- most eye and central nervous system injuries
- second- or third-degree burns involving 15–40% of total body surface area (see Box 39.6).

Priority 3 patients
The Priority 3 category is used for casualties who have minor injuries or illness and are expected to survive even if they do not receive medical attention. Common injuries in this category include:
- superficial wounds
- closed, uncomplicated fractures
- first- and second-degree burns involving < 15% of total body surface area (see Box 39.7).

Priority 4 patients
Priority 4 patients will either be deceased or expectant. An expectant patient is one who is not expected to survive.

No further time in the MCI setting should be spent with lifesaving procedures for these patients. If the patient is still alive once all Priority 1 and 2 patients have been assessed, these patients may be

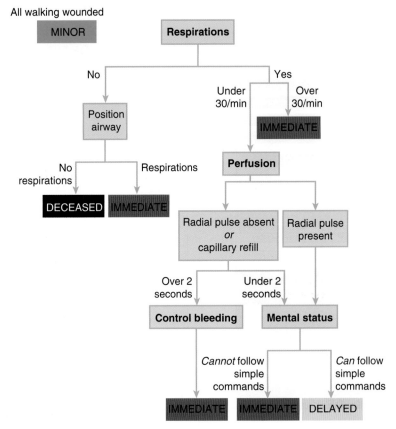

Figure 39.4
Example triage algorithm.
Source: Schultz & Koenig (2018).

BOX 39.7 Examples of Priority 3 patients

1. A 40-year old male with bruises, abrasions and non-bleeding lacerations.
2. A 14-year old female with left lower leg pain, but no deformity, a good pulse and normal vital signs.
3. A 75-year old male with a headache but no evidence of head trauma and normal vital signs.

BOX 39.8 Examples of Priority 4 patients

1. An 18-year-old female with third-degree, full-thickness burns to over 80% of her body.
2. A 26-year-old male with an obvious trauma to the head with brain matter exposed.
3. A 30-year-old female with nil respirations or pulse.

---

re-assessed and further treatment and transport options can then be considered.

Common injuries in this category include:

- agonal respirations
- unresponsive individuals with penetrating head injuries
- multiple explosive wounds involving multiple anatomic sites
- second- and third-degree burns involving > 60% of total body surface area (see Fig 39.4 and Box 39.8).

The evidence base for MCI triage

Surprisingly, there has been very little research validating or evaluating any of these existing triage systems. The lacking evidence base for MCI triage systems is largely due to the difficulties involved in prospectively studying MCIs.

Questions remain as to when and how triage algorithms are best used, and how the triage decision should be displayed or documented.

Additionally, it is unclear what training methods are most effective to ensure responders are well versed in the application of such algorithms.

The general principles of mass-casualty triage

Triage provides a method for organising casualties at the scene of an MCI and is based around three broad considerations:

1. the presence of a life-threatening condition
2. the immediately available lifesaving interventions that can be delivered
3. the availability of transportation assets.

Because triage balances patient condition with available resources, a casualty with a life-threatening injury will not always be assigned the highest triage category.

It is also important to note that triage is a dynamic concept. A patient that is initially triaged to one category may have their category changed if their condition changes or if there is a secondary triage process at the scene.

Triage in practice

The first action a paramedic will undertake as part of triage is to conduct an initial assessment. One useful way of initially sorting patients is as follows.

Step 1: Sorting to determine Priority 3 patients

Action

Paramedic: 'If you can hear my voice and you can move, please make your way over to [insert specific location].'

These patients will become the Priority 3s initially as they can hear and obey commands and walk.

Step 2: Sorting to determine Priority 2 patients

Action

Paramedic: 'If you can hear my voice but you can't walk, raise a limb in the air or wave if you can.'

These patients will initially become Priority 2s. They are alert as they can hear and obey commands, but they have injuries or are trapped and cannot walk.

Step 3: Sorting to determine Priority 4 patients

The patients remaining who are not moving or have obvious injuries need to be assessed first. Some of these will become Priority 1s and some will become Priority 4s.

Let's consider how a paramedic could conduct this assessment. Initially, the use of applicable lifesaving interventions should be used on these patients. These interventions include controlling major haemorrhage, opening the airway and chest decompressions.

Secondary assessment

After all immediately life-threatening injuries are identified and treated in the primary assessment,

Action 1

Assessment 1: Are they breathing?
  No: Priority 4 (deceased)
  Yes: Move on to Assessment 2.

Action 2

Assessment 2: Do they obey commands or make purposeful movements? Do they have a peripheral pulse? Are they in respiratory distress? Is major haemorrhage controlled?
  No to any of these:
    Likely to survive?
    No: Priority 4
    Yes: Priority 1
  Yes:
    Minor injuries only?
    No: Priority 2
    Yes: Priority 3

the secondary assessment can begin. A consistent and methodical approach to casualty history and physical examination should be used.

Triage of paediatric patients

Some MCIs, like school shootings, will involve paediatric victims. It is important to understand the unique challenges associated with triaging paediatric patients.

Difficulties in the out-of-hospital care of children in non-MCI situations have historically been well documented, including the lack of proper equipment, the relative lack of practice for technical skills and lack of paediatric-specific continuing education (Graham et al., 1993; Youngquist et al., 2008; Zaritsky et al., 1994). These paediatric-specific challenges in normal day-to-day out-of-hospital care are likely to be exacerbated in an MCI (Lyle et al., 2009).

The distinctive physiological, developmental and psychological attributes of children make them one of the most challenging populations to treat during major incidents. Because of their unique biological, social and ethical factors, it is crucial that paediatric needs are incorporated into major incident planning and training. Box 39.9 highlights some of the key vulnerabilities of children that can influence the management of mass casualties.

During an MCI, paediatric patients can be triaged using the Paediatric Triage Tape (PTT), an easy-to-use major incident primary triage tool based on a modification of the Triage Sieve. It is a vinyl waterproof tape derived from, and using exactly the same flow process as, the Triage Sieve. It has specific

BOX 39.9 Vulnerabilities in children

- Anatomically, children's solid organs are proportionately larger, closer together and not as well protected as adult organs.
- Children have respiratory and heart rates that are faster than adolescents and adults, increasing their susceptibility to airborne chemical and biological agents that will quickly spread throughout a young child's circulatory system.
- Children also have a different respiratory physiology that varies by age.
- Children metabolise drugs differently to adults, requiring varying dosages of medications and antidotes.
- Children are a particularly vulnerable group during chemical, biological, radiological, nuclear and explosive (CBRNE) events. Many chemical agents, including certain gases such as sarin and chlorine, have a high vapour density and are heavier than air, which means that they 'settle' close to the ground, in the airspace used by children.
- Children also have more permeable skin than adults, so they receive proportionally higher doses of agents that either contact or seep into the skin.
- Fluid and electrolyte balance may be difficult to maintain in young children.
- Children can become easily dehydrated and suffer circulatory collapse because they possess minimal fluid reserve.
- Developmentally, children are particularly vulnerable because of physical and mental limitations based on developmental milestones.
- Infants do not have the motor skills to escape from the site of a biological or chemical incident. Even if they can walk, infants, toddlers and young children lack the self-preservation and cognitive skills developmentally that enable them to know how to react.

Sources: Allen et al. (2007); Burke et al. (2010); Markenson & Reynolds (2006).

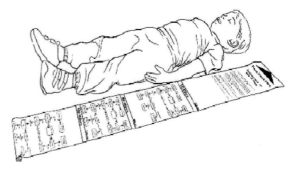

Figure 39.5
Paediatric Triage Tape.
Source: Wallis & Carley (2005).

BOX 39.10 Triage quiz

Try triaging the following patients to Priority 1, 2, 3 or 4. Once you have finished, check your answers at the end of the chapter.
1. A 16-year-old female walking around the scene with a broken arm.
2. A 68-year-old female who is unresponsive and has brain matter showing.
3. A responsive 44-year-old male with pale, moist skin and respirations of 32 breaths per minute.
4. A 23-year-old female with a traumatic amputation of the arm with controlled bleeding.
5. An unresponsive male patient who has snoring respirations. His breathing improves when you open his airway.
6. A 42-year-old female with a broken arm and a broken leg. She is alert with a respiratory rate of 20 breaths per minute.
7. A 14-year-old male who is ambulatory and says he is 'okay'.
8. A 32-year-old woman with no obvious injuries and without a carotid pulse.
9. An 8-year-old boy with full-thickness burns to 85% of his body and still breathing.
10. A 16-year-old female with a large laceration to her right arm and bruising to her left leg. She is crying.

triage blocks for children measuring < 50 cm, 50–80 cm, 80–100 cm, 100–140 cm, and > 140 cm (see Fig 39.5 and Box 39.10).

6. Treatment

The aim of treatment at an MCI is to 'do the most for the most'; that is, to identify and treat the salvageable. The actual treatment delivered will reflect the skills of the providers, the severity of the injuries and the time the patient spends on the scene.

7. Transport

During an MCI, emergency ambulance vehicles will move most casualties to hospital. Other forms of transport can be used and it is the responsibility of the health service commanders to ensure that patients are transported in an appropriate vehicle, with the necessary in-transit care.

Managing the scene at an MCI

The first ambulance on scene at an MCI will need to start a log and record their time of arrival. The paramedics should ensure they are wearing protective clothing, a helmet and high-visibility coat or tabard.

This crew will make the METHANE assessment and send the METHANE report. Used by the Major Incident Medical Management and Support (MIMMS) course and adopted widely by emergency services worldwide, METHANE is the mnemonic for remembering the key information that should be conveyed immediately as part of declaring a major incident (actual or 'standby').

METHANE

Emergency services widely use the METHANE acronym to build a report for alerting others about a major incident (see Box 39.11).

The first ambulance crew on scene should also consider where arriving ambulances should park and where the casualty clearing station should be placed. This should be a safe distance from the site of the incident and where possible using available shelter. Ideally this should be discussed with fire services on site. This crew should also be considering a suitable location for a helicopter landing site should this be needed. This may need to be discussed with police.

The first ambulance crew on scene also adopts the command and triage responsibilities ensuring pertinent information is received and relayed to ensure appropriate resources are available and utilised as required.

The scene commander and triage officer are to complete their tasks until relieved by a senior clinician or supervisor. The scene commander provides an initial windscreen sitrep and is the contact between the scene and the communication centre.

Determining incident complexity

A number of factors may influence the complexity of an MCI and should be taken into consideration during the initial and subsequent assessments.

1. Simple incident

A simple MCI can be managed using routine patient distribution models where casualties are managed within the usual hospital and health system capacities. No extraordinary measures are needed to cope with casualty numbers.

2. Complex incident

A complex MCI has the potential to overwhelm available hospitals and health systems, requiring significant multi-agency response for potential casualties (e.g. bushfire, earthquake, cyclone, epidemic or terrorist attack). The nature of the incident means there could be high media interest.

3. Restricted incident

The location of the incident may prevent access to necessary and specialist services. A restricted MCI has the potential to overload specialist services without coordination between networks or the request for national assistance (e.g. multiple serious burns).

A restricted incident may require specialist equipment or plans to be in place (e.g. chemical, biological, radiological, nuclear and explosive [CBRNE]/hazardous materials [HAZMAT]) and may compromise health services or facilities (e.g. loss of key acute and public healthcare infrastructure, long term power loss, disruption to water supply or loss of workforce).

MCIs that have a significant impact on the aged care sector should be considered restricted by nature of the demand for medical and health services, which can result from compromises to aged care facilities and services.

Determining major incident level

Level 1

A Level 1 major incident is one where the number of casualties and/or complexity/restriction requires a coordinated approach. This may result in a coordinated response for creation of capacity and distribution of casualties across more than one region. A Level 1 major incident may also require a coordinated response due to a disruption to normal business, which may include loss of facilities or services. This may therefore require coordination of resources across networks or regions, escalation of utility reconnection and assistance from other agencies through state arrangements. A Level 1 major incident may also require multiple/all networks to assess their capacity and report on capacity to accommodate a surge in the immediate future.

Level 2

A Level 2 major incident is where the number of casualties and/or complexity/restriction of the event is beyond the capacity and/or capability of the health system without adopting extraordinary measures.

Decontamination

In the setting of an MCI, first responders may have to manage a scene where there is potential

BOX 39.12 Special considerations

- Special consideration must be given to children as they are at higher risk of hypothermia.
- If possible, gender mixing should be avoided during decontamination due to potential cultural sensitivities.

contamination due to the release (accidental or intentional) of CBRNE agents. In some services and under some command structures, specially trained HAZMAT teams are dispatched to the scene to provide decontamination services.

On-scene decontamination

On-scene decontamination of patients, usually performed by the fire service, is preferred but not always possible. An all-hazards management plan for receiving and dealing with contaminated patients arriving at healthcare facilities should be in place, including prearranged decontamination areas. Overflow capacity should also be considered and security needs taken into account (see Box 39.12).

Five stages of decontamination

1. **Crowd control.** Patients should be moved through a corridor.
2. **Triage.** There is a need to identify the contaminant, degree of contamination and degree of patient distress. Toxidromes can be used to help determine the type of contaminant. Smell, sight and information from victims can help indicate contamination. Emergency resuscitation can be performed in the decontamination area but remember all equipment is then contaminated.
3. **Remove contaminated clothing.** This will remove 70–85% of the contaminant. Remember to keep the patient's clothes, as they may be required later as evidence by law enforcement personnel.
4. **Cleaning and washing.** The best method is using tepid water and mild soap. Where possible, self-decontamination is encouraged. For specific decontaminants there are particular substances available for decontamination. However, if unsure of the type of contamination, water is best.
5. **Management of contaminated materials.** This includes clothing, equipment and run-off.

Wet versus dry decontamination

In an MCI involving the release of a chemical agent, the majority of victims are going to have been exposed to a vaporised agent. The traditional approach of wet decontamination (washing patients down in showers) will not be effective. Even if a victim has been exposed to an agent requiring wet decontamination, simply removing the clothing and washing them down will remove approximately 80% of the contamination. Patients who have been exposed to a vaporised agent do not require decontamination beyond the removal of clothes.

Specific agent decontamination
Chemical agents
Chemical agents can spread rapidly and cause extensive damage. In the case of chemical contamination, external evidence of contamination is likely. People will probably present en masse.
Biological agents
Biological contamination may go undetected and patients may present later. Basic decontamination is all that is required (strip and shower) and simple infection control may be suitable. People are more likely to present as individuals or in small groups. Decontamination does not play a major role in the management of biological events.
Radiological agents
Victims exposed but not contaminated don't require decontamination. However, they may need significant medical management. Direct radiological contamination may be easy to recognise. As well as the radioisotope contamination, it is likely that victims will have been exposed to a dispersal device and therefore have subsequent evidence of blast injury.
Nerve agents
Nerve agents are extremely lethal. The majority of patients exposed to liquid nerve agents will die within minutes of exposure. Most patients with vapour exposure will require dry decontamination only.
Vesicants
Vesicants are highly reactive and may cause tissue damage immediately. However, symptoms may also be present for hours after exposure. Early wet decontamination is essential.
Choking agents
Choking agents dissolve poorly in water and pose an inhalational risk. Dry contamination is adequate.
Cyanide
Cyanide commonly presents as a vapour hazard and dry decontamination is adequate. However, if there is skin contamination due to liquid exposure, wet decontamination will also be indicated (see Box 39.13).

BOX 39.13 Tokyo subway sarin gas attack

On 20 March 1995, five makeshift chemical devices were placed on three subway lines in Tokyo between 8.09 am and 8.13 am. Two bombs released sarin gas at the government station; three others were discovered either before or after their trains had reached the target area. The poisonous vapours were intended for the government employees who worked in the Kasumigaseki area and the release was scheduled to affect the peak point of rush hour, just before the start of the 8.30 am workday.

Subway passengers reported seeing people leave packages or noticed unaccompanied packages spilling oily substances on the floor. Symptoms of those mildly to moderately affected varied from headaches and miosis to vomiting and convulsions. Firefighters were the first emergency crews to arrive on the scene. The firefighters were not only unauthorised to give antidotes, they were also completely unaware of what substance they were dealing with. While some attempts were made at triaging the patients on the scene, those less severely affected left the scene on foot and hailed passing cars and taxis for transportation to hospitals.

Upon arrival at the hospitals the extent of decontamination of the casualties varied from hospital to hospital, and even within a single hospital. Sarin caused secondary contamination among medical staff through patients' clothing.

Ambulances transported 688 patients and nearly 5000 people reached hospitals by other means. Hospitals saw almost 6000 patients, 17 of whom were deemed critical, 37 severe and 984 moderately ill. The attack killed 12 people.

Source: Smithson & Levy (2000).

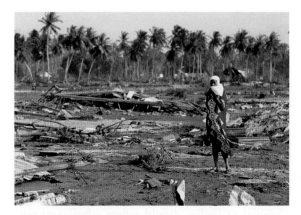

Figure 39.6
Indian Ocean tsunami.
Source: McCall (2014).

While local arrangements may be able to manage small numbers, they are rarely able to cope with the hundreds or thousands of fatalities that may occur following an MCI. When the number of bodies exceeds normal local mortuary arrangements, mass fatality management plans may be activated to provide the additional capacities.

Typically the events that result in the highest numbers of fatalities are located in regions with increased risk and vulnerable populations; this is often compounded by limited infrastructure and integration of the health system into disaster preparedness, response and recovery.

As in all cases of unnatural death, there are legal implications for mass fatalities concerning the identity of the deceased, the cause of death and determining who is responsible for the disaster. All of these factors can make the management of mass fatality incidents overwhelming for any local jurisdiction, and often requires a coordinated effort at the local, state and national level.

Three phases of mass fatality management
The overall response to a mass fatality incident can be divided into three phases.
Phase 1
Begins when the first responders arrive at the scene and incident command structure is set up. Emergency services commence their roles.
Phase 2
Begins when the relevant disaster plans are activated and the predetermined responders and officials take on their designated roles. Emergency services continue their role. Support services are established to assist rescue workers and survivors. A public information officer coordinates with the media. Additional resources and assistance are obtained as needed.

Managing mass fatalities
A mass fatality incident is a situation resulting in a loss of life that exceeds the death investigation resources of the local community. Natural disasters, man-made disasters and large-scale accidents have the potential to produce a devastating number of fatalities. The bombing of the Alfred P. Murrah Federal Building in Oklahoma City in 1995 claimed 168 lives, and the attacks on the World Trade Centre buildings in New York in 2001 killed nearly 3000 people. The Indian Ocean Tsunami killed over 225,000 people and the 2010 earthquake in Haiti recorded estimates of over 200,000 deaths (see Fig 39.6).

Phase 3

The resolution phase, which involves the removal and transport of any human remains, coordination of morgue services and continued family support.

Challenges associated with mass fatalities

One of the main challenges associated with the management of mass fatalities is inadequate capacity to deal with dead bodies, which may result in distress to families and the community.

Inappropriate practices may also cause distress among the bereaved if they are unable to perform funeral rites in accordance with local customs. Disposal of bodies should reflect ethnic and religious sensitivities where possible and appropriate. Where able, access to support mechanisms should be provided for survivors, relatives and those dealing with fatalities.

It is important for the psychosocial wellbeing of the living, including responders, survivors, relatives and the wider community, that the dead are managed with dignity and respect.

Health risks

The health risk to responders of dead bodies arising from a natural disaster is negligible. There may be health risks through secondary contamination from fatalities as a result of exposure to chemical or radiological agents.

There are no reports of infection arising from contact with a dead body following natural disasters, although long-term follow-up of disaster responders is yet to be undertaken.

The majority of health effects following a natural disaster include injury/strain from lifting bodies, and injury from debris during body recovery.

Risk assessments need to be made where fatalities arise following epidemics of infectious disease or exposure to chemical or radiological agents to prevent infection and/or secondary contamination. It is important in all cases that universal precautions are adhered to when handling dead bodies, including wearing gloves and washing hands.

Additional personal protective equipment may be needed when handling fatalities occurring as a result of chemical, biological and radiological incidents and specialist advice should be sought.

The challenge of mass fatalities during pandemics

A severe pandemic has the ability to overwhelm healthcare systems with predicted surge in demand. Outbreaks of Severe Acute Respiratory Syndrome (SARS) in 2003, H1N1 (Swine) influenza in 2009 and Ebola Virus Disease (EVD) in 2014 served as a warning that this scenario is not only possible, but probable (Naylor et al., 2004; Kruk et al., 2015).

During the 2020 COVID-19 coronavirus pandemic, this anticipated surge in patients was witnessed in some countries like Italy and the United States, but attendance at accident and emergency departments in the United Kingdom was reported to have decreased following the introduction of national lockdown, with anecdotal reports suggesting that heart attacks and strokes had 'vanished from hospitals' and that such patients 'delay seeking help' (Bernstein, 2020; Spinney, 2020).

This reported decrease in accident and emergency department presentations was not reflected by a reduction in ambulance callouts for these two conditions associated with lockdown (Lumley Holmes et al., 2020). Ambulance callouts in some Australian cities were reported to have dropped by as much as 25% since the introduction of COVID-19 restrictions. In three states and territories, ambulance staff reported attending fewer car crashes (Roberts, 2020).

The impact on health systems will not only come from patient surge during a pandemic, but also from the effect it has on paramedics. During SARS, around half of Toronto's out-of-hospital workforce was exposed to the disease within days of the outbreak (Bielajs et al., 2008). Of the more than 850 paramedics exposed to SARS from patients, 436 were placed in 10-day home quarantine and four were hospitalised with probable SARS (Gershon et al., 2009).

During the COVID-19 pandemic, more than 3300 healthcare workers had been infected by early March 2020 and, according to local media, by the end of February at least 22 had died. In Italy, around 20% of responding healthcare workers were infected. Reports from medical staff describe physical and mental exhaustion, the torment of difficult triage decisions and the pain of losing patients and colleagues, all in addition to the infection risk (Editorial, 2020). In China, transmission from healthcare workers to family members was reported, with asymptomatic individuals transmitting the disease to multiple family members (Bai et al., 2020). Preliminary Australian data suggested that community acquisition of COVID-19 was more likely to occur in healthcare workers than work-related acquisition (Muhi, 2020).

During a pandemic, local authorities will have to be prepared to manage additional deaths over and above the number of fatalities from all causes routinely expected during the interpandemic period. Within any locality, the total number of fatalities (including those resulting from influenza and all other causes) occurring during a 6–8-week pandemic wave is estimated to be similar to that which typically occurs over 6 months in the interpandemic period.

BOX 39.14 Triage quiz answers

1. Priority 3
2. Priority 4
3. Priority 1
4. Priority 2
5. Priority 1
6. Priority 2
7. Priority 3
8. Priority 4
9. Priority 4
10. Priority 2

Summary

MCIs are incidents or events where the location, number, severity or type of casualties requires external assistance or extraordinary resources. They can pose unique challenges for first responders in terms of safety, decontamination and the management of mass fatalities (see Box 39.15).

References

Allen, G. M., Parrillo, S. J., Will, J., & Mohr, A. (2007). Principles of disaster planning for the pediatric population. *Prehospital and Disaster Medicine, 22*(06), 537–540.

Bai, Y., Yao, L., Wei, T., Tian, F., Jin, D.-Y., Chen, L., & Wang, M. (2020). Presumed asymptomatic carrier transmission of COVID-19. *JAMA*, doi:10.1001/jama.2020.2565.

Bernstein, L., & Stead Sellers, F. (2020). Patients with heart attacks, strokes and even appendicitis vanish from hospitals. *Washington Post.* 20 April. Retrieved from https://www.washingtonpost.com/health/patients-with-heart-attacks-strokes-and-even-appendicitis-vanish-from-hospitals/2020/04/19/9ca3ef24-7eb4-11ea-9040-68981f488eed_story.html.

Bielajs, I., Burkle, F. M., Jr, Archer, F. L., & Smith, E. (2008). Development of prehospital, population-based triage-management protocols for pandemics. *Prehospital and Disaster Medicine, 23*(5), 420–430.

Burke, R. V., Iverson, E., Goodhue, C., Neches, R., & Upperman, J. S. (2010). Disaster and mass-casualty events in the pediatric population. *Seminars in Pediatric Surgery, 19*(4), 265–270.

Editorial. (2011). 9/11: ten years on. *The Lancet, 378*(9794), 849.

Editorial. (2020). COVID-19: protecting health-care workers. *The Lancet, 395*(10228), P922.

Gershon, R. R. M., Vandelinde, N., Magda, L. A., Pearson, J. M., Werner, A., & Prezant, D. (2009). Evaluation of a pandemic preparedness training intervention of emergency medical services personnel. *Prehospital and Disaster Medicine, 24*(6), 508–511.

Graham, C. J., Stuemky, J., & Lera, T. A. (1993). Emergency medical services preparedness for pediatric emergencies. *Pediatric Emergency Care, 9,* 329–331.

Jenkins, J. L., McCarthy, M. L., Sauer, L. M., Green, G. B., Stuart, S., Thomas, T. L., & Hsu, E. B. (2008). Mass-casualty triage: time for an evidence-based approach. *Prehospital and Disaster Medicine, 23*(1), 3–8.

Kruk, M. E., Myers, M., Varpilah, S. T., & Dahn, B. T. (2015). What is a resilient health system? Lessons from Ebola. *The Lancet, 385*(9980), 1910–1912.

Lumley Holmes, J., Brake, S., Docherty, M., Lilford, R., & Watson, S. (2020). Emergency ambulance services for heart attack and stroke during UK's COVID-19 lockdown. *The Lancet, 355*(10237), e93–e94. doi:10.1016/S0140-6736(20)31031-X.

Lyle, K., Thompson, T., & Graham, J. (2009). Pediatric mass casualty: triage and planning for the prehospital provider. *Clinical Pediatric Emergency Medicine, 10*(3), 173–185.

Markenson, D., & Reynolds, S. (2006). The pediatrician and disaster preparedness. *Pediatrics, 117*(2), e340–e362.

McCall, C. (2014). Remembering the Indian Ocean tsunami. *The Lancet, 384*(9960), 2095–2098.

Muhi, S., Irving, L. B., & Buising, K. (2020). COVID-19 in Australian healthcare workers: early experience of the Royal Melbourne Hospital emphasises the importance of community acquisition. *The Medical Journal of Australia.* Published online 23 April 2020.

Naylor, C. D., Chantler, C., & Griffiths, S. (2004). Learning from SARS in Hong Kong and Toronto. *JAMA, 291*(20), 2483–2487.

Roberts, L., & Heaney, C. (2020). Coronavirus has changed the workload of paramedics across Australia. *ABC News.* 17 April. Retrieved from: https://www.abc.net.au/news/2020-04-17/coronavirus-changes-ambulance-callouts-across-australia/12149090.

Robertson-Steel, I. (2006). Evolution of triage systems. *Emergency Medicine Journal, 23,* 154–155.

Schultz, C. H., & Koenig, K. L. (2018). Disaster preparedness. In R. M. Walls, R. S. Hockberger & M. Gausche-Hill (Eds.), *Rosen's emergency medicine: concepts and clinical practice* (9th ed., pp. 2406–2417). Philadelphia: Elsevier.

Smithson, A. E., & Levy, L. A. (2000). *Chapter 3 – Rethinking the lessons of Tokyo,* in: Ataxia: The Chemical and Biological Terrorism Threat and the US Response

(Report). Henry L. Stimson Centre. Report No. 35. pp. 91–100.

Spinney, L. (2020). Concern as heart attack and stroke patients delay seeking help. *The Guardian (Australia edition)*. 16 April. Retrieved from: https://www.theguardian.com/world/2020/apr/16/coronavirus-concern-heart-attack-stroke-patients-delay-seeking-help.

Wallis, L. A., & Carley, S. D. (2005). Validation of the paediatric triage tape. *Emergency Medicine Journal, 23*(1), 47–50.

Youngquist, S. T., Henderson, D. P., Gausche-Hill, M., Goodrich, S. M., Poore, P. D., & Lewis, R. J. (2008). Paramedic self-efficacy and skill retention in pediatric airway. Management. *Academic Emergency Medicine: Official Journal of the Society for Academic Emergency Medicine, 15*, 1295–1303.

Zaritsky, A., French, J. P., Schafermeyer, R., & Morton, D. (1994). A statewide evaluation of pediatric prehospital and hospital emergency services. *Archives of Pediatrics & Adolescent Medicine, 148*, 76–81.

SECTION 13:
The Paramedic Approach to the Patient With an Environmental Condition

In this section:

A 50-year-old male scuba diver on his first deep dive suddenly surfaces and is struggling to talk. Has he suffered a decompression injury due to his rapid ascent, or did he ascend rapidly because he suffered a cerebrovascular accident while diving? Similarly, did the elderly woman found semiconscious in her backyard one cold night fall because she had a cardiac arrhythmia, or is the arrhythmia a result of her hypothermia? Injuries caused by exposure to extreme temperatures, pressures and toxic substances are particularly challenging to assess and manage as they tend to affect entire body systems and can mimic other disease presentations. In all the cases presented in this section the impact of the environment must be incorporated into patient assessment and management.

CHAPTER 40

Hypothermia and Hyperthermia

By Brian Haskins

OVERVIEW

- Core body temperature of 37°C is one of the most tightly regulated parameters of human physiology (Kurz, 2008). When the core temperature drops to 20°C or exceeds 41°C, the threat to life is extreme.
- The hypothalamus is the dominant thermoregulatory structure in mammals but temperature is also moderated by the skin, deep abdominal and thoracic tissues, the spinal cord and other portions of the brain.
- Although the mechanisms remain unclear, core temperature is also thought to be moderated by noradrenaline, dopamine, 5-hydroxytryptamine, acetylcholine, prostaglandin E_1 and neuropeptides (Sanders, 2012).
- Under normal conditions, body temperature fluctuates by around 0.5°C daily with circadian rhythm and hormonal activity such as menstruation.
- The cerebral metabolic rate decreases 5–7% for each degree Celsius drop in body temperature (Kurz, 2008).
- The mechanisms that decrease heat production include a reduction in muscle tone and voluntary activity, decreased hormone secretion and decreased appetite (Sanders, 2012).

- Hypothermia can have metabolic, neurological, traumatic or infectious causes but it is most often a result of exposure to cold environments.
- Many neural processes are temperature dependent (Kiyatkin, 2011).
- Shivering and cutaneous vasoconstriction are the body's major autonomic defences against cold.
- Rapid recognition and treatment of hypothermia is critical to maximising patient survival and post-survival function.
- Therapeutic hypothermia following a cardiac arrest is understood to be neuroprotective.
- Exposure, extreme exercise, anaesthetics, surgery, injury, infection, food intake, hypo- and hyperthyroidism and drugs (including alcohol, nicotine, sedatives, as well as illicit drugs such as ecstasy) can disrupt the thermoregulatory system.
- All patients presenting with a core temperature in excess of 39°C require rapid assessment, cooling and transport to hospital.
- Uncorrected severe hyperthermia is a potentially life-threatening condition that can result in multiple organ failure and death.

Introduction

Thermoregulation refers to the body's sophisticated, multisystem regulation of core body temperature (Kurz, 2008). This hierarchical system extends from highly thermosensitive neurons in the pre-optic region of the brain proximate to the rostral hypothalamus, down to the brainstem and spinal cord. Coupled with receptors in the skin and the spine, central and peripheral information on body temperature is integrated to inform and activate the homeostatic mechanisms that maintain our core temperature at 37°C (Boulant, 2000).

Body heat is lost through the skin, via respiration and excretions. The skin is perhaps the most important organ in regulating heat loss. The control of temperature needs to be precise as a number of essential metabolic functions operate only within a narrow range of temperatures. Outside of this range the processes can fail or produce toxic side effects. This leads to physical and cognitive changes, but a detailed history and physical examination can usually identify the cause and direct treatment.

The normal adult core temperature ranges from 36–38°C and may increase to as much as 40°C during exercise. Heat transfer facilitated by flowing blood is thought to be one of the most important heat-exchange pathways in the body (Gonzalez-Alonso, 2012). Measurements of core temperature (e.g. rectal, oesophageal, bladder or intravascular) are typically around 0.5°C higher than measurements of oral or tympanic temperature and fluctuate with circadian rhythm (Connolly & Worthy, 2000).

Thermoregulation around the 37°C set-point is usually managed by two key temperature-regulating centres in the hypothalamus: 1. the posterior hypothalamic heat maintenance centre, which is stimulated by the sensation of cold; and 2. the anterior hypothalamic heat maintenance centre, which is stimulated by an increase in circulating blood temperature. These regulation centres activate mechanisms that increase heat loss and decrease heat production (Kurz, 2008).

Hypothermia

Hypothermia is defined as a core body temperature less than 35°C (Brown et al., 2012). As with hyperthermia, hypothermia is assessed on a graduating scale of three key stages: mild, core temperature 32–35°C; moderate, core temperature 28–32°C; and severe, core temperature < 28°C (Brown et al., 2012). Hypothermia can be the main presenting problem or it can complicate an underlying injury or illness. Hypothermia may be accidental or induced for clinical benefit (i.e. therapeutic hypothermia). Temperatures capable of causing hypothermia do not need to be extreme and can occur even in low-level temperate areas across Australia and New Zealand. Although external environmental conditions are the most common cause of accidental hypothermia, they are not the only cause. Other causes include metabolic imbalance, trauma, neurological and infectious disease and exposure to toxins such as organophosphates. Organophosphate poisoning can have a significant effect on thermoregulation causing initial hypothermia followed by a rebound fever (Moffatt et al., 2010).

In some circumstances, hypothermia may be induced to protect neurological functioning as a result of the associated decrease in cerebral metabolism and energy consumption. This is known as **therapeutic hypothermia**. Mild hypothermia has been used as an effective treatment confirmed clinically for improving the neurological outcomes of a comatose patient following cardiac arrest (Donnino et al., 2015).

Accidental hypothermia

There are three progressive stages of accidental hypothermia. Each has specific clinical features indicative of the stage of challenge to the body's thermoregulation systems.

In **mild hypothermia** (32–35°C) the reduction in temperature produces dermal vasoconstriction, tachycardia, increased cardiac output, increases in plasma catecholamine levels, diuresis and hyperglycaemia. In most cases, pituitary, adrenal and thyroid function remain within normal limits (Elliot & Kiran, 2006).

When exposed to cold, the body's immediate response is to conserve heat through peripheral vasoconstriction and increase in central nervous system (CNS) metabolism. Heart rate, respiratory rate and blood pressure increase dramatically. Other mechanisms of heat production include shivering, increased muscular activity and increased secretion of adrenaline and noradrenaline. To protect against heat loss, vasoconstriction and piloerection also occur.

All of these actions act in concert with some form of behaviour modification in the affected individual, such as putting on extra clothes or seeking an external source of warmth like a fire or warmer environment. Shivering is a sign that the body is attempting to generate heat. In normal individuals, shivering usually occurs when the core temperature is reduced by 0.7°C and it increases the metabolic rate by as much as fivefold (Elliot & Kiran, 2006; Mallett, 2002). At 35°C, shivering is uncontrollable. Studies have shown that even mild systemic hypothermia (32–35°C) influences platelet adhesion, aggregation and coagulation reactions (Che et al., 2011).

Moderate hypothermia (28–32°C) is characterised by the cessation of shivering as a result of the depletion of glucose stores and the consequent loss of insulin available for glucose transfer (Flouris, 2011). Once these energy stores are depleted, shivering stops and the body rapidly loses heat. At this point, all major organ systems are at extreme risk. Muscles and joints become stiff and the individual begins to feel lethargic and drowsy and often falls asleep. Pulse rate, blood pressure and respiratory rate are all depressed at this point.

In **severe hypothermia** (< 28°C) the body has lost its ability to spontaneously return to normal temperature due to the failure of the body's thermoregulatory mechanisms (Kiyatkin, 2011). If an external heat source is not found and/or internal heat production is not restored, there is a further decline in respiratory rate, heart rate and blood pressure; blood pH drops; and electrolyte imbalances emerge. Hypovolaemia occurs as a consequence of the movement of fluid out of the vascular space and the excretion of fluid via diuresis. Cold diuresis is thought to be a response to pronounced vasoconstriction, which raises preload, increasing cardiac output, the glomerular filtration rate and the secretion of atrial natraemic factor. Bradycardia develops and progresses as the body continues to cool. Prolonged PR, QRS and QT intervals are present on ECG readings; P waves may be absent or obscure. Osborn waves (see Fig 40.1), or J waves, are waves seen occurring at the J point and are associated with hypothermia, as are U waves, which occur after the T wave. Osborn waves are positive

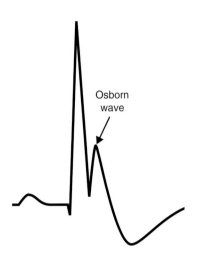

Figure 40.1
Osborn waves of hypothermia.

deflections that occur at the conclusion of the QRS complex. To the inexperienced clinician they can mimic ST elevation but the narrow nature of the wave is distinct and is not typical of myocardial infarction. Death is the result of respiratory and cardiac arrest.

At temperatures below 28°C we can expect the individual to be unconscious and areflexic, pupils will be fixed and dilated and signs of life may be difficult to detect. Both bradycardia and atrial fibrillation occur at temperatures below 30°C and ventricular fibrillation may occur at temperatures below 28°C. The respiration rate will be slow and may be reduced to as little as 1–2 breaths per minute.

The physiological and physical effects of accidental, uncontrolled hypothermia can be understood in terms of three progressive stages of reduction in core temperature and their associated clinical signs, but it is important to understand that the clinical picture does not always correlate well with the degree of hypothermia experienced. Accidental deaths from hypothermia are relatively rare events but individuals who are elderly, socially disadvantaged and/or isolated are at greatest risk. Most deaths from an accidental hypothermic episode are in fact caused by associated arrhythmias and sepsis.

Therapeutic hypothermia

It is now well-accepted that hypothermia provides neuroprotection against the oxidative reactions that occur in tissues that have been deprived of oxygen and can protect patients from the brain injury that typically follows a cardiac arrest. Mild hypothermia is known to cause a 50-fold reduction in H_2O_2 (hydrogen peroxide) production, which allows neurons to retain their normal cell morphology and viability (Zitta et al., 2010). Therapeutic hypothermia provides neuroprotection by preventing the development of hyperthermia resulting from the secondary causes of neurotoxicity such as ischaemia, disrupted blood flow, lipid peroxidation, oxidative stress, acidification and inflammation (Kuffler, 2012). It is a highly controlled and monitored intervention during which the patient is cooled to around 33–36°C and maintained at this temperature for between 12 and 48 hours following a prolonged cardiac arrest (Soar et al., 2010).

Cold water drowning

When a drowning occurs in cold water less than 6°C, the cold-water-induced hypothermia may provide some protection against anoxia (Suominen et al., 1997). Many EMS systems now use mechanical CPR devices to safely transport hypothemic patients to hospitals with extracorporeal rewarming capabilities. If this is not possible, resuscitation attempts should continue on scene until a core temperature of > 35°C is achieved (Callaway et al., 2015). However, survival is extremely unlikely if the victim is submerged for longer than 90 minutes in cold water (< 6°C) and 30 minutes in warm water (> 6°C) (Tipton & Golden, 2011).

CS CASE STUDY 1

Case 10464, 0630 hrs.

Dispatch details: A 19-year-old male who has been missing in mountainous terrain for about 15 hours has been located.

Initial presentation: The patient has been found by his motorbike. He is conscious and breathing but is aphasic.

1 ASSESS

Patient history

The patient was trying to access a back-country area to meet with friends on a camping trip but his motorbike ran out of fuel on the fire trail at about 3 pm yesterday. The alarm was raised at 9 pm when he tried contacting police by mobile phone, but due to an unseasonal blizzard search parties were unable to commence searching until daybreak this morning. Overnight temperatures in the area dropped to −12°C with sleet and the patient was not equipped for an overnight stay.

Initial assessment summary

Problem	Hypothermia and altered conscious state in an otherwise fit and healthy male
Conscious state	GSC = 8 (E 2, V 1, M 5)
Position	Supine
Heart rate	38 bpm
Blood pressure	Unrecordable
Skin appearance	Exposed extremities are cold, mottled
Speech pattern	Unable to determine
Respiratory rate	8 bpm
Respiratory rhythm	Even cycles
Chest auscultation	Clear chest sounds bilaterally
Pulse oximetry	Does not sense
Temperature	32°C
BGL	'Low'
ECG	Evidence of atrial fibrillation; QRS and QT intervals with prominent J or Osborn waves in leads II and V3–V6
History	The 19-year-old male has been missing in high mountainous terrain for about 15 hours, where overnight temperatures dropped to −12°C with snow and sleet; he has no previous significant medical history
Physical assessment	No obvious external signs of injury

D: The ongoing low temperatures present a danger to the crew and the patient.
A: The patient is conscious with no airway obstruction.
B: Respiratory function is poor but consistent with hypothermia. There are no adventitious sounds. Tidal volume is decreased.
C: Heart rate is very slow and blood pressure is not recordable.

The patient is presenting with poor perfusion and an altered conscious state. He is bradycardic and hypotensive and the crew cannot get recordings for SpO$_2$ and BGL. Given the history, environmental setting and the patient's presentation, it is evident that he is suffering from moderate hypothermia.

2 CONFIRM

Hypothermia disrupts a number of physiological processes and even in the absence of any other injuries it will cause abnormal vital signs. For the paramedic dealing with a trauma patient who is hypothermic, it can be difficult to distinguish between vital signs that have been altered by temperature or by other injuries or illnesses. Before concluding that the patient is just hypothermic, it is important to check whether he may be hypothermic with other injuries.

What else needs to be considered?

Hypoglycaemia

With no history of diabetes, it is unlikely that hypoglycaemia is the underlying problem in an otherwise fit young male. The most likely cause of the low BGL reading is stagnant blood flow in the extremities from which the sample was taken. Retesting the blood from a more central source reveals a level of 5.9 mmol/L so the crew are able to discard this diagnosis.

Arrhythmia

While it is possible that a poorly perfusing arrhythmia led to the patient becoming lost and collapsing, it is not consistent with the medical or immediate history. Arrhythmias that cause such poor perfusion do not typically persist for hours without resolving or deteriorating further. The bradycardia is most likely a result of the hypothermia but will need to be carefully managed.

CVA

Although the patient is aphasic there is no unilateral dysfunction with his face or limbs, and although weak, his motor response is equal left and right.

Spinal injury/trauma

Spinal injuries can cause immobility, bradycardia and hypotension. One of the complicating factors of hypothermia is that it can obscure underlying injuries, and the fact that the patient was riding a motorcycle increases the chance he may have had an accident prior to becoming immobile. The history doesn't seem consistent with a traumatic injury but a thorough secondary survey should be completed as soon as it is practicable to expose the patient without causing further temperature loss.

Thermal injury (frost bite)

It is difficult to assess the extent and depth of cold tissue damage in exposed and unprotected parts of the body in the first instance. However, as a general rule of thumb, if the tissue springs back after being depressed, the injury is likely to be superficial (see Box 40.1).

③ TREAT

Emergency management

Safety

Moving the patient to a safe, warm environment and removing all of his wet clothing is a priority. The paramedics need to cut his clothes and gently remove them, as they are yet to confirm he has no traumatic injuries and because too much activity can return cold and stagnant blood to the central circulation.

Passive rewarming

Rewarming is critical for this patient and in the out-of-hospital setting it can be facilitated by covering his head and body with space blankets and warmed blankets. This form of treatment is termed *passive rewarming* (or endogenous

BOX 40.1 Frost bite

Frostbite is a cold-induced injury that has been classified by degree of damage, but it is more useful to use the terms *superficial* and *deep*. Superficial frostbite affects the skin and subcutaneous tissues, while deep frostbite also affects the bones, joints and tendons. Management comprises rewarming and then waiting to see which parts retain viability and which need to be amputated. With superficial frostbite rewarmed skin has clear blisters, whereas with deep frostbite rewarmed skin has haemorrhagic blisters (see Fig 40.2; Biem et al., 2003).

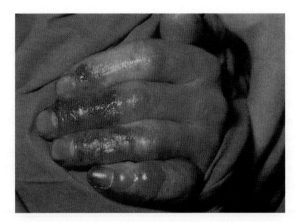

Figure 40.2
Frostbite of the hand of a mountaineer. On rewarming, the hand became painful, red and oedematous, with signs of probable gangrene in the fifth finger.
Source: Forbes & Jackson (2003).

warming) and for most patients with mild hypothermia this is sufficient to resolve the condition. It should also be used in more serious cases but will need to be combined with close monitoring and other strategies.

In the out-of-hospital care of frostbite, non-adherent wet clothing should be removed and local rewarming should begin only if refreezing will not occur in transit. Rubbing affected areas worsens tissue damage (Biem et al., 2003).

Active rewarming

Moderate hypothermia generally requires some form of *active rewarming* techniques such as forced air or warm humidified oxygen. Active warming should be conducted slowly, so it usually occurs during transport. Warm water bottles and external radiant heat sources can be applied if available but only once IV access has been achieved. Warm fluids may be considered according to local guidelines and if available. However, warm fluids should be given cautiously as there is a chance of after-drop cooling. After-drop cooling happens when the increased vascular volume leads to increased perfusion of the cold extremities, thus returning cold blood to the core.

Oxygen

The low SpO_2 reading is most likely due to poor perfusion but supplemental oxygen is not contraindicated in hypothermia and should be used until a definitive reading is collected.

ECG monitoring

The patient may have suffered a degree of pressure injury from inactivity and rewarming could trigger a number of arrhythmias. Continuous monitoring is advisable even if management of any arrhythmia that might develop will be conservative.

4 EVALUATE

Hypothermic patients who undergo rewarming should be considered dynamic and need frequent evaluation. The process of rewarming can cause complications or reveal previously hidden conditions. In particular, be aware of dehydration and hyperglycaemia.

Dehydration

A 'cold diuresis' will have occurred. Cold diuresis is believed to be due to a response to pronounced vasoconstriction that raises preload, increasing cardiac

> **PRACTICE TIP**
>
> The role of a space blanket is to prevent the transfer of heat by acting as a heat reflector; it is therefore applied outside the layer of warm blankets. A further layer of blankets may be placed over the top to anchor the space blanket.

output, the glomerular filtration rate and secretion of atrial natraemic factor. Another explanation that has been suggested is that cold diuresis is due to a defect in distal tubular sodium and water reabsorption, cold-induced glycosuria or inhibition of antidiuretic hormone (Biem et al., 2003). Fluid sequestration in damaged tissues may also add to volume depletion.

Hyperglycaemia

Insulin is known to be inactive at less than 30°C. Hyperglycaemia on rewarming occurs in part due to loss of insulin activity and in part due to a decreased metabolic demand. While hyperglycaemia is common in hypothermic patients it should be managed conservatively until sufficient rewarming has occurred to restore endogenous insulin activity and metabolic activity.

Ongoing management

Hospital management of moderately hypothermic patients continues on from out-of-hospital care. Active peripheral rewarming may effectively increase the vascular volume in a patient who has not got enough volume to fill this expanded space. If IV access is not achieved, a slow and conservative approach to rewarming is logical, allowing time for gradual adaptation to the increasing vascular space.

Rewarming will continue slowly (1°C per hour) in hospital and may be facilitated by warmed IV fluids or invasive techniques such as active core rewarming via extracorporeal circulation or cardio-pulmonary bypass (Paal et al., 2016).

Active rewarming using an external energy supply (e.g. heated blankets, heaters or a warm bath) or more aggressive core rewarming through infusion of warmed fluids, warm lavage of body cavities, cardiopulmonary bypass or corporeal shunt rewarming, obviously provides faster results but needs detailed monitoring of electrolytes, blood gases and haemodynamic parameters. As a general rule, unless in a resuscitation setting rapid rewarming is less desirable than a steady controlled rewarming at about 1°C per hour.

Hypothermia summary

Effective management of the patient with accidental hypothermia requires paramedics to be alert to the potential for the development of arrhythmias as rewarming progresses. Where rehydration is required but only cold fluids are available, core temperature management takes precedence over the need for rehydration, especially in the early stages. The use of cold fluids in an already hypothermic patient will clearly exacerbate the patient's condition. Where tissue damage is evident it requires careful assessment and management. Careful removal of frozen or wet clothing to prevent unnecessary skin tearing is important, particularly in the context of the increased risk of sepsis in these patients. Most of the physiological changes associated with hypothermia are reversible with rewarming, but some of the pathological effects are related more to this corrective process than to the hypothermia itself (Mallett, 2002).

Hyperthermia

The term **hyperthermia** or heat illness is defined as a core body temperature greater than 40°C for more than 60 minutes. At higher-than-normal temperatures the body's ability to regain normothermia can fail. There are several stages of heat stress that represent points along a continuum of heat-related illness from relatively mild and easily corrected physiological distress to a life-threatening condition that may result in long-term disability or death. Symptoms of hyperthermia include headache, nausea and weakness, dizziness and fainting, confusion and loss of coordination, muscle cramps, seizures and, ultimately, coma and cardiac arrest.

> **DIFFERENTIAL DIAGNOSIS**
>
> **Hypothermia**
> And/or
> - CVA
> - Arrhythmia
> - Spinal injury/trauma

Pathophysiology

Hyperthermia occurs when there is an imbalance between the metabolic and external heat accumulated in the body and an inability to dissipate heat (Epstein et al., 2004). It should be considered as a spectrum of illness that ranges from mild and reversible to severe and life-threatening (see Fig 40.3). Even at rest the body generates heat that needs to be dissipated.

Heat stress
1. Moist, clammy skin
2. Normal or subnormal temperature

Heat stroke
1. Dry, hot skin
2. Very high body temperature

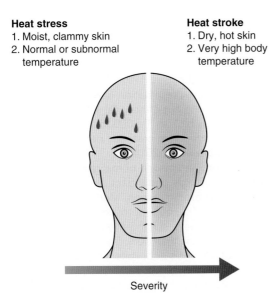

Severity

Figure 40.3
Hyperthermia should be considered a continuum of illness that starts with the mild symptoms of heat stress such as cramps and progresses through to heat stroke. At its most severe it can lead to multi-organ failure and should be considered a medical emergency.

> ## BOX 40.2 Causes of increased heat production
>
> - Overexertion
> - Thyroid storm
> - Malignant hyperthermia
> - Neuroleptic malignant syndrome
> - Phaeochromocytoma
> - Delirium
> - Brainstem infarct (hypothalamic haemorrhage)
> - Poisoning (sympathomimetics, anticholinergics, ecstasy)

The body normally loses heat by a combination of conduction, convection, radiation and evaporation, with peripheral vasodilation and sweating the most effective mechanisms. Increased ambient heat and/or increased humidity can limit the effectiveness of these measures and, combined with increased heat production (see Box 40.2), the body's core temperature can rise to dangerous levels.

As core temperature rises, CNS dysfunction is one of the early signs and the altered mental function that results can reduce the individual's ability to seek strategies to cool down. As the temperature rises further the dysfunction can extend to all the organ systems including renal, cardiovascular, musculoskeletal and hepatic functions. If the high temperature persists, skeletal muscle can start to break down, leading to rhabdomyolysis. Apart from the long-term loss of muscle tissue, in the acute state the breakdown leads to hyperkalaemia (which can cause cardiac arrhythmias) and myoglobinuria (causes renal failure).

Most chronic environmentally induced heat illnesses occur after 3–4 days of exposure to higher-than-normal ambient temperatures and relative humidity (Nitschke et al., 2011; Tomlinson et al., 2011; Mastrangelo et al., 2007). The body's ability to acclimatise is relatively robust but that ability is compromised by chronic illness and the inability to effectively reduce body temperature by changes in behaviour. In these conditions, exercise, illness and age may predispose some individuals to higher-than-usual risk of hyperthermia.

Individuals exercising or working in hot and humid environments are obviously at increased risk of heat illness, but the situation in which they are found often makes the diagnosis self-evident. The elderly, however, can develop heat stress at much lower ambient temperatures and without significant exertion, making the diagnosis and suitable treatment more difficult. Medications, limited mobility, poverty and mental illness can all contribute to heat illness in the elderly (Hausfater et al., 2010). Antihypertensives such as beta-blockers can limit the ability of the cardiovascular system to dissipate heat while suppressing sweat gland activity. Diuretics can also make it difficult to remain hydrated, while a lack of air-conditioning and inappropriate clothing can limit heat loss. Other medications can also inhibit sweat production or increase heat production, and these are commonly prescribed for the elderly. Anticholinergics for chronic obstructive pulmonary disease (COPD) or Parkinson's, lithium and antidepressants for mental illness and alpha-blockers for urinary dysfunction can all affect thermoregulation and predispose users to heat stress. In younger patients, alcohol, ecstasy and amphetamines can increase the risk of heat illnesses by either increasing heat production or promoting dehydration (or both).

Hyperthermia in the cool setting
There are a number of conditions where heat illness can arise without the individual being in a hot environment. For example, hyperthyroidism, phaeochromocytoma or acute stroke can produce

BOX 40.3 Malignant hyperthermia

Malignant hyperthermia is a rare response to a range of agents used in anaesthesia. The pharmacogenetic disorder of skeletal muscle is triggered when a susceptible individual receives a depolarising muscle relaxant such as suxamethonium or one of the volatile anaesthetic agents such as halothane, enflurane or isoflurane (Epstein et al., 2004). The pathophysiology of malignant hyperthermia relates to the inappropriate rise in skeletal muscle myoplasmic calcium ion concentration and results in a hypermetabolic state. This hypermetabolism is characterised by accelerated cellular processes that lead to increased oxygen consumption and the production of CO_2 and heat. Adenosine triphosphate stores are consequently depleted and lactic acid is produced. Acidosis hyperthermia and adenosine triphosphate depletion cause the destruction of sarcolemma, causing a marked release of potassium, myoglobin and creatine kinase into the extracellular fluid (Epstein, 1997). Relatively little is known about the presentation of malignant hyperthermia in the out-of-hospital setting, although rates as high as 1:5000 to 1:10,000 have been reported in anaesthetic patients (Schneiderbanger et al., 2014).

Survival from an episode of malignant hyperthermia is highly dependent on early recognition and prompt action. Mortality was once as high as 70%, but improved drugs and early recognition have significantly reduced the mortality rate to less than 10%. Dantrolene is used to treat this crisis in hospital and has been described as the cornerstone of management of this condition. It inhibits intracellular calcium release from the sarcoplasmic reticulum to facilitate muscle relaxation, although not to the point of paralysis (Glahn et al., 2010; Kugler & Russell, 2011).

excessive heat that may exceed the body's ability to dissipate it.

Malignant hyperthermia is 'an inherited subclinical myopathy characterised by a hypermetabolic reaction during anaesthesia. The reaction is related to skeletal muscle calcium dysregulation triggered by volatile inhaled anaesthetics and/or succinylcholine' (Capacchione & Muldoon, 2009; see Box 40.3). Presentation includes skeletal muscle rigidity, mixed metabolic and respiratory acidosis, tachycardia, hyperpyrexia, rhabdomyolysis, hyperkalaemia, elevated serum creatine kinase, multi-organ failure, disseminated intravascular coagulation and death (Nelson, 2002). This is a rare but serious side effect of some of the drugs used by paramedics and should be treated as per other heat-related illnesses.

Finally, profound dehydration can also produce heat stress in a temperate setting because it restricts the amount of sweat produced. Patients with poor fluid intake or high outputs due to diarrhoea or diuretic use are particularly at risk.

Exertional hyperthermia

Exercise increases heat generation and, particularly in conditions of high humidity and high temperature, can lead to a state of hyperthermia. **Exertional hyperthermia** causes a complex cascade of cellular damage. Some of this occurs as a direct effect of heat on the cells but many of the changes that contribute to mortality are multi-factorial and share pathways with sepsis, poisoning and systemic inflammation. The effects are so widespread that they produce neurological, metabolic, circulatory and renal injury. Of particular concern is the progression to multi-organ failure and most patients require admission to ICU for close monitoring and support of major organ systems. In contrast to environmental hyperthermia, the metabolic presentation of exertional hyperthermia is complex and challenging to manage (see Table 40.1).

Table 40.1: Electrolyte and enzyme responses to hyperthermia

Environmental hyperthermia	Exertional hyperthermia
Mixed respiratory alkalosis	Severe metabolic acidosis
Normal potassium	Hyperkalaemia
Normal calcium	Hypocalcaemia
Normal phosphate	Hyperphosphataemia
Hyperglycaemia	Hypoglycaemia
Moderately raised creatine kinase	Markedly raised creatine kinase
Markedly raised hepatic enzymes	Moderately raised hepatic enzymes

CASE STUDY 2

Case 11134, 1030 hrs.

Dispatch details: An 83-year-old female has been found by her home and community care nurse. The patient is confused and agitated.

Initial presentation: When the paramedics arrive they find the patient conscious and sitting in her recliner chair.

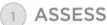

① ASSESS

Patient history

The patient lives alone and suffers from severe osteoarthritis. She has been sleeping in her recliner chair under the fan for the past 4 days due to a heatwave. She is unable to provide a reliable report of how much she has had to eat or drink in the last 24 hours. Under normal circumstances, she is reported to be in full command of her cognitive faculties. The nurse reports that when she arrived this morning the house was extremely hot. The patient managed to open the front door for her but other doors and windows were closed. The patient was sitting in the front room with the ceiling fan on but no other means of circulating air. The nurse placed a damp face washer on the patient's forehead and opened doors and windows to try to 'catch the breezes'. The patient is wearing a dress over a singlet.

Airway

Unless heat stress has caused a significant alteration of mental state, airway patency is rarely compromised in heat stress, but dry and cracked lips and thick white sputum are signs of dehydration and decreased fluid intake.

Breathing

Patients with heat stroke present with a mixed respiratory and metabolic acid–base disturbance. The predominant findings on admission are those of metabolic acidosis followed by respiratory alkalosis. An increased respiratory rate is the body's response to the acidotic state: blowing off CO_2 (Hashim, 2010) is a typical early sign of the body reacting to the metabolic acidosis.

Circulation

As a patient begins to heat up, the heart rate increases to maintain sufficient cardiac output to support perfusion of the internal organs in the context of redistribution of blood to the skin for thermoregulatory purposes (reducing peripheral vascular resistance). Despite the increased heart rate associated with hyperthermia, in severe hyperthermia cardiac output is not adequate to maintain blood pressure as stroke volume falls. This lowering of stroke volume is a combined effect of a reduction in cardiac filling pressure due to reduced central venous pressure (CVP) and a shorter diastolic filling time that reduces both left and right ventricular end-diastolic volumes (Nybo, 2007). Heat transfer from the body core to the skin depends on the perfusion of the skin and the core-to-skin temperature difference. In hot conditions, the temperature gradient between the body core and the skin narrows and thermoregulation mechanisms increase skin blood flow, increasing the transfer of heat to the skin. In late stages, however, the loss of circulating volume will lead to poor peripheral perfusion.

Skin

Adequate sweat production is essential for heat dissipation through evaporation, but dehydration will eventually reduce the amount of sweat produced and hot dry skin is the hallmark of heatstroke.

Conscious state

Cerebral perfusion is reduced due to the reduced perfusion pressure as blood volume falls as a result of dehydration, while the increased metabolic demand further reduces the oxygen supply/demand ratio. The increase in brain temperature implies that the global cerebral metabolic rate increases due to the effect of temperature on metabolism rates affecting cerebral tissue energy turnover (Cameron et al., 2009). When oxygen uptake increases and cerebral blood flow decreases, cerebral and motor function are affected (Nybo, 2007). Hyperventilation results in a lowered arterial CO_2 tension and consequently cerebral vasoconstriction that reduces cerebral blood flow by as much as 20–25% (Nybo, 2007). At a late stage, cerebral oedema raises the intracranial pressure further thus reducing cerebral perfusion, as cerebral perfusion pressure is a function of mean arterial pressure minus intracranial pressure.

Renal function

Renal function can be impaired by both fluid loss (and thus a decrease in glomerular filtration pressures) and the influx of myoglobin generated by muscle damage. This creates a pathological accumulation of myoglobin in the kidney tubules. This results in damage to the glomerular membrane and red/brown urine stained with myoglobin may be seen. The early stages of acute renal failure or acute kidney injury may be asymptomatic and reversible, but patients found to have developed oliguria or anuria tend to have more severe kidney impairment than those without oliguria.

Initial assessment summary

Problem	Dizzy, confused and feeling unwell
Conscious state	GCS = 14, confused
Position	Sitting in a recliner chair
Heart rate	120 bpm
Blood pressure	100/70 mmHg sitting, 90/60 mmHg standing
Skin appearance	Dry and flushed
Speech pattern	Normal
Respiratory rate	20 bpm
Respiratory rhythm	Even cycles
Chest auscultation	Clear breath sounds bilaterally
Pulse oximetry	98% on room air
Temperature	38.2°C
BGL	5.4 mmol/L
Physical assessment	The patient has tenting of the skin on her forearm and evidence of pitting oedema in both ankles. She states that she hasn't been to the toilet recently but is not complaining of pain or irritation. There is no obvious smell of a urinary tract infection (UTI).

D: There are no dangers.
A: The patient is conscious with no current airway obstruction.
B: Respiratory function is currently normal. The respiratory rate is elevated but ventilation is normal.
C: Heart rate is elevated but there is a sufficient blood pressure.

The environmental conditions and patient's temperature indicate that she is likely to be suffering from heat stress. In these circumstances excessive sweating and the associated dehydration, electrolyte imbalance, low blood pressure and inadequate cerebral and peripheral perfusion could explain her unusual confusion and peripheral oedema.

② CONFIRM

The essential part of the clinical reasoning process is to seek to confirm your initial hypothesis by finding clinical signs that should occur with your provisional diagnosis. You should also seek to challenge your diagnosis by exploring findings that do not fit your hypothesis: don't just ignore them because they don't fit.

What else could it be?

Infection
The patient may have an infection that has resulted in her increased temperature. The sources of infection in the elderly are usually respiratory or urinary tract and neither appears involved in this case. Nonetheless, infection cannot be entirely discarded until the patient is placed in a cool environment and her temperature is allowed to resolve. If she remains hyperthermic in this setting, an infection is the most likely cause.

Stroke
A CVA should always be a differential diagnosis in elderly patients presenting with confusion and an altered conscious state. In this case the lack of any one-sided deficit assists in ruling this diagnosis out. It is also far more likely that the temperature has caused an altered mental state than a stroke causing the temperature.

Hypoglycaemia
Hypoglycaemia usually presents with cool and clammy skin and is ruled out by the patient's normal BGL reading.

③ TREAT

Emergency management

Evaporative cooling
Cooling and rehydration are important first steps in the treatment of this patient. The community nurse has begun the process by opening up the house, attempting to draw cooler air into the property and placing a damp face washer on the patient's forehead. In addition to this, damp towels should be placed around the patient's neck and in her axilla and groin if possible, and additional fanning should be established. Evaporative cooling is the fastest and most efficient non-invasive technique for cooling and can reduce core body temperature by approximately 0.3°C per minute. Any tight, restrictive or excessive clothing should be loosened or removed while maintaining the patient's dignity as much as possible.

Rehydration
Some degree of dehydration will occur in all patients suffering heat illness. In mild hyperthermia, oral fluids should be encouraged for both rehydration and internal cooling, but given the severity of this patient's symptoms and clear evidence of dehydration, intravenous (IV) fluid replacement is recommended provided there is no evidence of pulmonary oedema. IV administration of a balanced sodium chloride solution, cooled if possible, should be titrated to her perfusion status and not her temperature: attempting to reach a target temperature with cooled fluid risks fluid overload. The fluid should be commenced slowly in the field and continued in a controlled fashion in hospital. This patient has taken some time to get this dry and she should be rehydrated

---

PRACTICE TIP

Increased temperature associated with infection and fever should not be confused with hyperthermia. In fever, the effect on the hypothalamus is caused by endogenous pyrogens released by phagocytic leucocytes. Antipyretics can reverse fever but have little role in hyperthermia.

DIFFERENTIAL DIAGNOSIS

Heat exhaustion
Or
- Infection
- Stroke
- Hypoglycaemia

---

slowly to allow time to balance out osmolality and electrolytes. She is not deteriorating rapidly so there is no urgent need to provide large quantities of fluid in a hurry.

Topical cooling

Some local guidelines recommend applying cooling directly to the head. Research has demonstrated that cognitive impairment is one of the effects of heat stress. In particular, impairment in working and short-term memory has been noted (Hunter et al., 2006). These studies also note that head cooling restores efficiency to frontal lobe functions but is less efficient with other brain functions.

 ## EVALUATE

Evaluating the effect of any clinical management intervention can provide clues to the accuracy of the initial diagnosis. Some conditions respond rapidly to treatment so patients should be expected to improve if the diagnosis and treatment were appropriate. A failure to improve in this situation should trigger the clinician to reconsider the diagnosis.

Improvements in mental status can occur quickly but the combined effects of dehydration and hyperthermia can also take hours to resolve. A rapid improvement should not be expected in this patient.

Ongoing management

The patient's temperature should be monitored every 5 minutes and recorded. Cardiovascular monitoring including ECG is indicated, with attention to blood pressure monitoring en route to hospital. The use of antipyretic agents, steroids and prophylactic antibiotics has not been shown to be effective.

Hospital admission

More aggressive cooling measures such as ice packs and gastric lavage are unlikely to be required in this patient. Given her age and concurrent health issues, this patient would be admitted to hospital for fluid replacement and monitoring and, barring complications, would expect to remain an inpatient for at least 24 hours until all her observations have become normalised.

Investigations

The electrolyte imbalances that occur secondary to heat stress will prompt the hospital staff to measure serum electrolytes and possible arterial blood gases. Urine output and composition will be closely monitored to measure hydration and renal function, while blood tests for liver enzymes, creatine kinase and other proteins will try to identify impending organ failure.

Follow-up and long-term impact

This patient could be expected to recover and return home with support in the short term. Advice about prevention of heat stress should be provided and regular contact with a community support agency established. The outcome for this patient is largely dependent on the ability to correct metabolic function and on the degree of long-term damage to major organs that may have been done. Recovery from heat stroke can take between days and months and long-term impacts are not uncommon. These can include impaired renal function and, in extreme cases, brain damage.

Hyperthermia across the lifespan

Exertional heat stroke and heat stress are more common in young, physically active adults than in other age groups. However, heat-related illnesses affect all age groups and several subpopulations are known to be at particular risk. Elderly people and those with chronic health conditions are at higher risk of heat-related illness, especially those with diabetes. Chronic illnesses such as diabetes impair the body's ability to institute initial temperature-modifying actions such as sweating.

Central temperature regulation systems are intact in infants but careful attention to the maintenance of normal temperature range during extreme heat events is important. Maintaining adequate fluids in the context of increased perspiration and choosing appropriate clothing and external environments should be sufficient to prevent heat stress in normal, healthy infants.

CASE STUDY 3

Case 11054, 1230 hrs.

Dispatch details: A 23-year-old male jogger has been found unconscious on a popular running track in the inner city in the middle of a hot summer day.

Initial presentation: The paramedics find the patient red in the face and with hot, dry skin, although there is evidence of extreme sweating on his clothes. His water bottle is empty. Bystanders have loosened his clothing but have had access to only a little water, which they have splashed on his face. He has not regained consciousness.

1 ASSESS

1250 hrs Primary survey: The patient is unconscious but is breathing regularly.

1251 hrs Vital signs survey: Perfusion status: HR 145 bpm, sinus tachycardia, BP 110/70 mmHg.
   Respiratory status: RR 30 bpm, good tidal volume, regular and even rhythm.
   Conscious state: GCS = 6, weak withdrawal to sensory challenge, moaning.
   Temperature: 40.9°C.
   BGL: 5.4 mmol/L.

1254 hrs Pertinent hx: Temperatures have been in the high 30s for the last 3 days and humidity is around 60%. The patient is not carrying any identification and the paramedics are unable to establish any medical history.

1255 hrs Secondary survey: There are no obvious external signs of injury.
   This patient is unconscious but is ventilating adequately and his blood pressure is sufficient: neither explains his altered conscious state. His blood sugar is within normal limits. However, he is hyperthermic and the presentation is consistent with the environment.

2 CONFIRM

In many cases paramedics are presented with a collection of signs and symptoms that do not appear to describe a particular condition. A critical step in determining a treatment plan in this situation is to consider what other conditions could explain the patient's presentation.

What else could it be?
Syncopal episode
A brief episode of either a bradycardic or a tachycardic arrhythmia could have temporarily reduced the patient's blood pressure and caused him to collapse. However, his blood pressure and ECG are now normal; while it is not possible to rule out syncope as the initial cause of his collapse, there are no signs of external injury, so it makes it unlikely.

DIFFERENTIAL DIAGNOSIS

Hyperthermia
Or
- Syncopal episode
- Acute myocardial infarction (AMI)
- CVA
- Head trauma

Ask!
If informed bystanders are present, ask about the patient's known chronic health conditions such as diabetes, epilepsy, heart problems or allergies.

Look for!
- Any medications the patient might be carrying or a medical alert bracelet/pendant
- Rapid respiratory rate: tachypnoea (RR persistently exceeding 20 bpm) or hyperpnoea (slower, deeper breaths than seen in tachypnoea)
- Tachycardia and hypotension (hypotension and decreased cardiac output in a patient with suspected heat stroke are prognostic of a poor outcome)

AMI

AMI could lead to either an arrhythmia or decreased cardiac output sufficient to lead to a collapse, but alterations in the ECG or a return of consciousness once his blood pressure resumed a normal value would be expected.

CVA

The patient does not appear to be in a high-risk category for CVA and for an injury large enough to render him unconscious it would be expected that his motor responses would not be equal. CVA cannot be ruled out at present but hyperthermia is more consistent with his presentation.

Head trauma

It is possible that the patient tripped while running and suffered a head strike sufficient to cause prolonged unconsciousness. While there is no clear evidence of a head strike it cannot be ruled out. Importantly, hyperthermia increases the risk of secondary head injury (see Ch 34) and is a reversible cause of unconsciousness: it needs to be corrected while managing the potential for a traumatic head injury; the patient should be transported to a trauma-capable hospital if possible as a precaution.

③ TREAT

This patient's severe hyperthermia is consistent with his presentation and should be considered a medical emergency.

Airway

With such a poor level of consciousness some local guidelines will recommend intubation, possibly with the use of depolarising neuromuscular blocking agents and pharmacological paralysis. This management has been shown to be safe and effective for severe isolated traumatic brain injury but due to the metabolic derangement associated with hyperthermia it needs to be considered on a case-by-case basis.

This patient is currently maintaining a patent airway, shows no signs of vomiting and is ventilating spontaneously and adequately. Attempting to secure his airway with any adjunct that causes a gag reflex could raise his intracranial pressure leading to a reduction in cerebral blood flow (see Ch 34). Given these facts and the metabolic challenges that RSI drugs may present, a conservative airway management strategy would be recommended.

Breathing

This patient is ventilating adequately but additional oxygen via a non-rebreather mask is recommended. The increased basal metabolic rate (BMR) can raise oxygen consumption by a factor of four.

Circulation

Cooled IV fluids can help correct both dehydration and temperature. Fluids containing potassium, such as Hartmann's solution, should be avoided if rhabdomyolysis is suspected (Khan, 2009). In most patients, blood pressure should rise to normal during the cooling process; this is the consequence of large volumes of blood returning from the peripheral to the central circulation.

Cooling

In addition to cooling with IV fluids, external cooling using wet sheets is effective. Preparing the vehicle for the patient by leaving it idling with the air-conditioning running will help. If the scene time is likely to be prolonged, provide shade over the patient and loosen or remove restrictive clothing while maintaining the patient's dignity. Towels soaked in tepid water can be effective, especially if a fan can create a breeze to enhance evaporative cooling. Given the severity of this patient's condition, additional cooling from ice wrapped

DEFINITION

Rhabdomyolysis: skeletal muscle damage from heat releases proteins from the muscle cells. These myoglobin molecules damage the filtration and reabsorption membranes in the kidneys and result in acute renal failure. An early sign is darkly stained urine.

in wet towels and applied to the axilla, groin and neck arteries should be used. Towels should be re-soaked and replaced at regular intervals.

It is important to avoid rebound hypothermia. In the out-of-hospital setting this is best done by ceasing cooling methods when the temperature reaches 39°C and allowing further cooling to be undertaken in hospital under controlled conditions.

(4) EVALUATE

Vigilant and continuous reassessment of patients with suspected heat stroke is essential.

- Continue cooling to 39°C but be vigilant for hypothermic rebound.
- Continue to take tympanic temperature regularly to monitor clinical progress.
- Avoid fluid overload and be vigilant for early signs of pulmonary oedema.
- Seizures are associated with CNS deterioration; be prepared to manage these according to local guidelines (often midazolam).
- Monitor the patient for cardiac arrhythmias due to electrolyte imbalance.
- Note any urine output and keep if possible.
- Constantly monitor the airway and ventilation.
- Ensure the receiving hospital is notified.

Paramedics should understand the progression of symptoms to ensure effective preparation for the more serious complications, should they arise.

Hyperthermia summary

Rapid identification of and response to a heat-related illness are critical to the patient's immediate and long-term outcome. Hyperthermia is considered a medical emergency and cooling and restoration of the body's homeostasis are critical.

Research has demonstrated that trauma patients admitted to hospital with a core temperature less than 36°C or more than 38°C experienced poor outcomes (Wade et al., 2011). This provides further indication of the importance of establishing and maintaining normal body temperature in the out-of-hospital emergency setting.

Paramedics themselves are not, of course, immune to the effects of heat: careful monitoring of fluid intake and working conditions during heatwaves is important for organisational efficiency and personal performance.

References

Biem, J., Niels, K., Classen, D., & Dosman, J. (2003). Out of the cold: management of hypothermia and frostbite. *CMAJ: Canadian Medical Association Journal = Journal de l'Association Medicale Canadienne, 168*(3), 305–311.

Boulant, J. A. (2000). Role of preoptic-anterior hypothalamus in thermoregulation and fever. *Clinical Infectious Diseases, 31*, S157–S161.

Brown, D. J. A., Brugger, H., Boyd, J., & Paal, P. (2012). Accidental hypothermia. *The New England Journal of Medicine, 367*, 1930–1938. Retrieved from https://www.nejm.org/doi/full/10.1056/NEJMra1114208.

Callaway, C. W., Donnino, M. W., Fink, E. L., Geocadin, R. G., Golan, E., Kern, K. B., Leary, M., Meurer, W. J., Peberdy, M. A., Thompson, T. M., & Zimmerman, J. L. (2015). Part 8: post–cardiac arrest care: 2015 American Heart Association guidelines update for cardiopulmonary resuscitation and emergency cardiovascular care. *Circulation, 132*(18_suppl_2), S465–S482.

Cameron, P., (Ed.). (2009). *Textbook of adult emergency medicine* (3rd ed.). Sydney: Elsevier.

Capacchione, J. F., & Muldoon, S. M. (2009). The relationship between exertional heat illness, exertional rhabdomyolysis and malignant hyperthermia. *Anesthesia and Analgesia, 109*(4), 1065–1069.

Che, D., Li, L., Kopil, C. M., Lui, Z., Guo, W., & Neumar, R. W. (2011). Impact of therapeutic hypothermia onset and duration on survival, neurologic function and neurodegeneration after cardiac arrest. *Critical Care Medicine, 39*(6), 1423–1430.

Connolly, E., & Worthy, I. G. (2000). Induced and accidental hypothermia. *Critical Care and Resuscitation, 2*, 22–29.

Donnino, M. W., Andersen, L. W., Berg, K.M., Reynolds, J. C., Nolan, J. P., Morley, P. T., Lang, E., Cocchi, M. N., Xanthos, T., Callaway, C. W., Soar, J., ILCOR ALS Task Force. (2015). Temperature management after cardiac arrest: an advisory statement by the advanced life support task force of the International Liaison Committee on Resuscitation and the American Heart Association Emergency Cardiovascular Care Committee and the Council on Cardiopulmonary, Critical Care, Perioperative and Resuscitation. *Circulation*, 132, 2448–2456.

Elliot, E., & Kiran, A. (2006). Accidental hypothermia. *British Medical Journal*, 332(7543), 706–709.

Epstein, Y. (1997). Predominance of type 2 fibres in exertional heat stroke. *The Lancet*, 350, 83–84.

Epstein, Y., Hadad, E., & Shapiro, Y. (2004). Pathological factors underlying hyperthermia. *Journal of Thermal Biology*, 29, 487–494.

Flouris, A. (2011). Functional architecture of behavioural thermoregulation. *European Journal of Applied Physiology*, 111, 1–8.

Forbes, C. D., & Jackson, W. F. (2003). *Color atlas and text of clinical medicine* (3rd ed.). London: Mosby.

Glahn, K., et al. (2010). Recognizing and managing a malignant hyperthermia crisis: guidelines from the European Malignant Hyperthermia Group. *British Journal of Anaesthesia*, 105(4), 417–420.

Gonzalez-Alonso, J. (2012). Human thermoregulation and the cardiovascular system. *Experimental Physiology*, 97(3), 340–346.

Hashim, A. (2010). Clinical biochemistry of hyperthermia. *Annals of Clinical Biochemistry*, 47, 516–523.

Hausfater, P., Megarbane, B., Dautheville, S., Patzak, A., Andronikof, M., Santin, A., André, S., Korchia, L., Terbaoui, N., Kierzek, G., Doumenc, B., Leroy, C., & Riou, B. (2010). Prognostic factors in non-exertional heatstroke. *Intensive Care Medicine*, 36, 272–280.

Hunter, J., Gregg, K., & Damani, Z. (2006). Rhabdomyolysis. *Continuing Education in Anaesthesia, Critical Care & Pain*, 6(4), 141–143.

Kämäräinen, A., Hoppu, S., Silfvast, T., & Virkkunen, I. (2009). Prehospital therapeutic hypothermia after cardiac arrest—from current concepts to a future standard. *Scandinavian Journal of Trauma, Resuscitation and Emergency Medicine*, 17, 53. doi: doi.org/10.1186/1757-7241-17-53.

Khan, F. Y. (2009). Rhabdomyolysis: a review of the literature. *The Netherlands Journal of Medicine*, 67(9), 272–283.

Kiyatkin, E. A. (2011). Brain temperature homeostasis: physiological fluctuations and pathological shifts. *Frontiers in Bioscience (Landmark Edition)*, 15, 73–92.

Kuffler, D. P. (2012). Maximising neuroprotection: where do we stand? *Therapeutics and Clinical Risk Management*, 8, 185–194.

Kugler, Y., & Russell, W. J. (2011). Speeding dantrolene preparation for treating malignant hyperthermia. *Anaesthesia and Intensive Care*, 39(1), 84–88.

Kurz, A. (2008). Physiology of thermoregulation. *Best Practice & Research. Clinical Anaesthesiology*, 22(4), 627–644.

Mallett, M. L. (2002). Pathophysiology of accidental hypothermia. *Journal of Medicine*, 95, 775–785.

Mastrangelo, G., Fedeli, U., Visentin, C., Milan, G., Fadda, E., & Spolaore, P. (2007). Pattern and determinates of hospitalisation during heat waves: an ecologic study. *BMC Public Health*, 7, 200–208.

Moffatt, A., Mohanned, F., Eddleston, M., Azher, S., Eyer, P., & Buckley, N. A. (2010). Hypothermia and fever after organophosphate poisoning in humans: a prospective case series. *Journal of Medical Toxicology: Official Journal of the American College of Medical Toxicology*, 6, 379–385.

Nelson, T. E. (2002). Malignant hyperthermia: a pharmacogenetic disease of Ca++ regulating proteins. *Current Molecular Medicine*, 2, 347–369.

Nitschke, M., Tucker, G. R., Hansen, A. L., Williams, S., Zhang, Y., & Peng, B. (2011). Impact of two recent extreme heat episodes on morbidity and mortality in Adelaide, South Australia: a case-series analysis. *Environmental Health: A Global Access Science Source*, 10, 42–51.

Nybo, L. (2007). Hyperthermia and fatigue. *Journal of Applied Physiology*, 104, 871–878.

Paal, P., Gordon, L., Strapazzon, G., Maeder, M. B., Putzer, G., Walpoth, B., Wanscher, M., Brown, D.,Holzer, M., Broessner, G., & Brugger, H. (2016). Accidental hypothermia–an update. *Scandinavian Journal of Trauma, Resuscitation and Emergency Medicine*, 24(1), 111.

Sanders, M. J. (Ed.), (2012). *Mosby's paramedic textbook* (4th ed.). St Louis: Elsevier.

Schneiderbanger, D., Johannsen, S., Roewer, N., & Schuster, F. (2014). Management of malignant hyperthermia: diagnosis and treatment. *Therapeutics and Clinical Risk Management*, 10, 355–362. https://doi.org/10.2147/TCRM.S47632.

Soar, J., Perkins, G. D., Abbas, G., Alfonzo, A., Barelli, A., Bierens, J. J., Brugger, H., Deakin, C. D., Dunning, J., Georgiou, M., Handley, A. J., Lockey, D. J., Paal, P., Sandroni, C., Thies, K. C., Zideman, D. A., & Nolan, J. P. (2010). European Resuscitation Council Guidelines for Resuscitation 2010 Section 8. Cardiac arrest in special circumstances: electrolyte abnormalities, poisoning, drowning, accidental hypothermia, hyperthermia, asthma, anaphylaxis, cardiac surgery, trauma, pregnancy, electrocution. *Resuscitation*, 81(10), 1400–1433.

Suominen, P. K., Korpela, R. E., Silfvast, T. G., & Olkkola, K. T. (1997). Does water temperature affect outcome of nearly drowned children? *Resuscitation*, 35(2), 111–115.

Tipton, M. J., & Golden, F. S. C. (2011). A proposed decision-making guide for the search, rescue and resuscitation of submersion (head under) victims based on expert opinion. *Resuscitation, 82*(7), 819–824.

Tomlinson, C. J., Chapman, L., Thornes, J. E., & Baker, C. J. (2011). Including the urban heat island in spatial health risk assessment strategies: a case study in Birmingham, UK. *International Journal of Health Geographics, 10*, 42–56.

Wade, C. E., Eastbridge, B. J., McManua, J. G., & Holcomb, J. B. (2011). Admission hypo- and hyperthermia and survival after trauma in military and civilian environments. *International Journal of Emergency Medicine, 4*, 35–41.

Zitta, K., Meybohm, P., & Bein, B. (2010). Hypoxia-induced cell damage is reduced by mild hypothermia and post-conditioning with catalase in-vitro: application of an enzyme-based oxygen deficiency system. *European Journal of Pharmacology, 628*(1–3), 11–18.

CHAPTER 41

Decompression Injuries

By Andrew Bishop

OVERVIEW

- The changes in pressure that occur during diving can cause symptoms ranging from minor ear pain to sudden death.
- Diagnosis of decompression injuries is by clinical presentation and response to treatment, but some symptoms overlap with non-pressure-induced medical conditions and these can present challenges in clinical reasoning.

- All patients with health complaints emerging after diving should seek some form of medical advice. Some may need to be reviewed at a specialist hyperbaric unit.
- While the pathology that generates symptoms may vary, the initial management is consistent.

Introduction

The term **decompression illness (DCI)** describes both decompression sickness and arterial gas embolus (Gorman, 1991) and is commonly used in the field as it can be impossible to differentiate between these conditions (they may coexist) and their emergency management is the same. In most cases it affects divers who ascend too quickly. While the history of a dive provides strong diagnostic clues of a patient's condition, the physical stresses of diving (temperature, exertion, dehydration, hunger) can also contribute to the development of other medical conditions and these need to be excluded or treated if the patient is to have the best chances of recovery (see Fig 41.1).

Although pressure-related injuries typically afflict underwater divers after a poorly managed ascent from depth, aviators flying in inadequately pressurised aircraft are also at risk.

Pathophysiology

Decompression sickness (DCS) refers to the symptoms that occur when metabolically inert gas (typically nitrogen) dissolved in body tissues under pressure is allowed to precipitate out of solution and form bubbles. **Arterial gas embolism (AGE)** occurs when blood flow is blocked distal to gas bubbles (gas embolus). These bubbles can develop within the blood from inert gas as a result of decompression or they can be forced into the bloodstream as a result of trauma to the lungs. Rupturing of lung tissue will force air from the lungs into the blood vessels and is referred to as barotrauma. Tissue damage from the rapid expansion of air can also occur outside the lungs and, although less serious, this form of barotrauma can be extremely painful.

Barotrauma

Barotrauma refers to physical damage to tissues caused by changes in the volume of gas-filled spaces as a consequence of changes in pressure. It arises as a consequence of Boyle's law, which states that at a constant temperature, the volume of a gas is directly proportional to the pressure of that gas. This means that if the pressure of a gas doubles, its volume will halve, and vice versa. The pressure at sea level is about 100 kilopascals or one atmosphere absolute (ATA). Pressure increases by one atmosphere for every 10 m a diver descends in seawater (see Table 41.1).

Barotrauma can occur as the diver is descending or ascending. *Descent barotrauma* is caused by gas-filled spaces becoming smaller as the surrounding (i.e. ambient) pressure increases and the trapped gas is unable to escape. This results in damage to the tissues surrounding the space and filling of the space by blood and oedema. Descent barotrauma typically occurs in the ears and sinuses. *Ascent barotrauma* is caused by gas-filled spaces becoming bigger as ambient pressure decreases, resulting in traumatic disruption of the tissues. The lungs and eyes are most commonly affected by ascent barotrauma but any gas-filled space in the body can be affected.

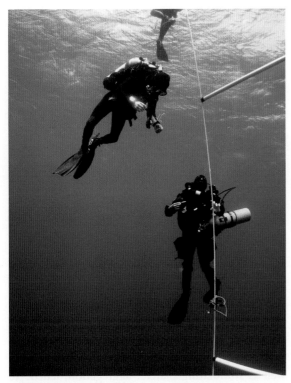

Figure 41.1
The changes in pressure that occur during diving can either cause or exacerbate existing conditions. The challenges in managing these patients are significant and require an understanding of the potential causes and presentations.
Source: Shutterstock/LauraD.

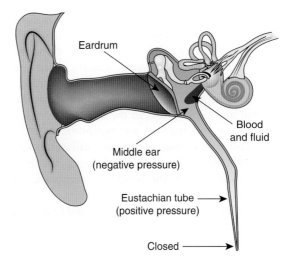

Figure 41.2
During descent, the eustachian tube collapses due to external pressure and air in the middle ear cannot escape to the nasopharynx. The pressure generated by the trapped air causes pain and tissue damage.

Table 41.1 Pressure changes during seawater descent

Depth (m)	Pressure (ATA)	Gas volume (%)	Gas density
Surface	1	100	1
10	2	50	2
20	3	33	3
30	4	25	4
60	7	16	7

Barosinusitis

Sinus barotrauma (barosinusitis) usually occurs on descent. As the pressure surrounding the diver rises, the volume of gas in the sinuses tends to decrease unless it is replaced by air drawn in through the sinus connections to the nasopharynx. If those connections are blocked, the pressure in the sinuses decreases in relation to the rising environmental pressure and the tissues lining the sinuses swell to replace the volume lost. Unless the pressure difference is relieved by unblocking, or an ascent towards the surface, the sinus spaces will fill with blood and mucus to equalise the pressure. Symptomatically the diver will often experience pain in the sinuses, which is relieved when the pressure equalises. On ascent the volume of gas in the sinuses will increase again and the mucus and blood may be expelled through the nose. Sinus barotrauma is usually self-limiting and does not cause serious morbidity. However, subsequent infection can occur and requires treatment; also, rarely, the delicate bony walls of the sinuses may rupture, resulting in more serious infection.

Ears

Ear barotrauma occurs most commonly on descent but may occur on ascent as well. The middle ear is like a cube, surrounded by bone on four sides, plus the inner ear and tympanic membrane. A passage from the middle ear to the pharynx, called the eustachian tube, allows air to move in and out of the middle ear space. On descent, the volume of gas in the middle ear decreases unless more gas is added from the pharynx via the eustachian tube (middle ear equalisation). As the volume of gas decreases, the tympanic membrane is pushed inwards, usually causing pain (see Fig 41.2). If descent continues, there will be bleeding into the tympanic membrane and the middle ear fills with oedema and blood. At worst, the tympanic membrane can rupture, which immediately relieves the pain but may cause severe vertigo as cold water enters the middle ear.

On ascent, *middle ear barotrauma* can occur if the eustachian tube becomes blocked during the dive, but it is rare. This results in the tympanic membrane moving outwards, causing pain and possibly rupture. A patient suffering from middle ear barotrauma will complain of varying degrees of ear pain and hearing loss in the affected side. It is self-limiting and requires just symptomatic treatment and prohibition of diving until symptoms have resolved—ranging from 1 week for mild disease to 6 weeks if the tympanic membrane has ruptured.

The tympanic membrane is connected to the oval window of the inner ear via a chain of three tiny bones called the ossicles. Sudden large movements of the tympanic membrane may cause a pressure wave in the inner ear between the oval and round windows that may result in the rupture of either window. This results in a leak of perilymph from the inner ear into the middle ear, leading to sensorineural hearing loss and vertigo, both of which may be severe. *Inner ear barotrauma* often requires surgery to repair the damage, and hearing loss may be permanent. Persistent hearing loss, tinnitus, vertigo and/or nausea after a dive indicate the possibility of inner ear barotrauma. Expert diving medical advice should be sought.

Lungs

Pulmonary barotrauma most often occurs during a rapid and uncontrolled ascent from a compressed-gas dive. The pressure differential required to cause rupture of an alveolus is as little as 1 m of water near the surface (Neuman, 2004). Theoretically, this means that if a diver takes a full breath from a compressed-gas source just 1 m below the surface and ascends without exhaling, alveolar rupture may occur. Although humans are much more likely to hold their breath while immersed (Neuman, 2004), the natural reflex is to exhale as they ascend. Pulmonary barotrauma is commonly seen in breath-hold ascents due to panic among novice divers, but it can also occur if the airway is obstructed (e.g. by bronchospasm). If pulmonary barotrauma does occur it may manifest as either direct damage to lung tissue or arterial gas embolus (Neuman, 2004).

The gas from an alveolus ruptured by overpressure may move into the pulmonary interstitium and then into the pleural cavity (causing a pneumothorax), the mediastinum (causing pneumomediastinum and pneumopericardium) and the subcutaneous tissues (causing subcutaneous emphysema). There may also be damage to the pulmonary parenchyma causing alveolar haemorrhage and haemoptysis. The most common presentation of pulmonary barotrauma is cough, haemoptysis and substernal chest pain (Elliott et al., 1978). The presentation and management of pulmonary barotrauma–induced pneumothorax is identical to non-diving-related pneumothorax, although the patient needs to be monitored for neurological manifestations of arterial gas embolus and, if present, recompression treatment needs to be sought.

Arterial gas embolus

Arterial gas embolus occurs secondary to pulmonary barotrauma when gas is forced into the pulmonary vasculature. When gas from alveolar rupture enters the pulmonary capillaries, it travels via the pulmonary veins and left side of the heart to the arterial blood. Arterial bubbles move through the arterial circulation where they may be trapped at a vessel bifurcation, with larger bubbles blocking larger vessels. These bubbles cause problems in two ways: 1. they physically obstruct the circulation, causing ischaemia distal to the blocked vessel as well as stimulating platelet aggregation, leucocyte activation and aggregation and fibrin deposition; and 2. they damage the vessel endothelium, activating the complement and clotting cascades (Pollock & Buteau, 2017).

Most tissues tolerate arterial bubbles reasonably well, with the exception of the brain (cerebral arterial gas embolus [CAGE]) and the heart (coronary arterial gas embolus). CAGE causes neurological problems occurring within seconds to minutes of the diver surfacing (Neuman, 2004) that may range in severity from mild sensory changes to seizures to coma or sudden death. There appears to be an inverse relationship between the severity of symptoms and the time of onset. Approximately 4% of victims suffer from the classic and most severe form of AGE, which presents catastrophically with collapse, loss of consciousness, apnoea and cardiac arrest (Neuman, 2002). Symptoms of AGE typically present rapidly, often within 10 minutes of surfacing. In contrast, symptoms of DCS normally appear within 6 hours after surfacing but they may not become apparent for more than 24 hours (Pollock & Buteau, 2017). By blocking the coronary circulation, coronary arterial gas embolus may cause myocardial ischaemia, but this is a rare occurrence (Neuman, 2004).

Decompression sickness

Decompression sickness is an acute condition that occurs following a reduction in ambient pressure. It is caused by bubbles that form when the partial pressure of a gas dissolved in blood or tissue exceeds the ambient pressure. DCS was first described in tunnel workers who used compressed air in the 19th century (caisson disease) and was subsequently observed in divers, high-altitude pilots and astronauts. Bubbles can form in the venous blood in any tissue and are usually harmless unless they are transmitted to the arterial circulation or are so voluminous as to overwhelm the heart ('the chokes'). If bubbles arise in the tissues, they may cause symptoms via direct mechanical effects and by causing damage at the cellular and tissue level. Bubbles can cause endothelial disruption, complement activation, platelet activation, nitric oxide production and leucocyte activation. Commonly affected tissues are detailed in Table 41.2.

Table 41.2 Areas commonly affected by DCI

Tissue/organ affected	Effects
Joints/bones	Local pain (may be severe) Bone necrosis if repeated
Spinal cord	Neurological symptoms
Veins	Spinal cord venous stasis and infarction Cardiopulmonary collapse with massive bubble load blocking the pulmonary venous circulation Arterial bubbles if there is a right to left shunt present
Brain	Any conceivable neurological symptom or sign
Inner ear	Vertigo and hearing loss
Skin	Rash and bruising

Source: Francis & Mitchell (2004).

 CASE STUDY 1

Case 10780, 1530 hrs.

Dispatch details: A 24-year-old female is in an altered conscious state following a diving accident.

Initial presentation: The paramedics find the patient dressed in a wetsuit. She is lying on the pier receiving high-flow oxygen via a facemask. They are near the southern Queensland border, 20 minutes from the nearest tertiary hospital and 75 minutes by road from the nearest hyperbaric chamber.

 ASSESS

Patient history

The patient was involved in a shallow-water training dive just offshore when she panicked and rapidly ascended to the surface. She cried out on surfacing and appeared very anxious. She was helped onto a low pier next to where the training dive was being conducted. Initially she appeared confused and distressed. She was complaining of chest pain but over the next 5 minutes her speech gradually became slurred and she was unable to support herself in a seated position.

For any patient presenting soon after a dive the length and depth of the dive are important factors, along with the number of dives in the past 24 hours and the ascent of the most recent dive. Modern dive watches can record these details and should always accompany the patient to hospital. It is important to remember that the patient's symptoms may not be related to the dive, so a past medical history is also important.

HISTORY

Ask!

- What are the details of the dive (depth, duration, first dive of the day, ascent details)?
- Are your symptoms improving or getting worse over time?
- Has oxygen been administered? If so, for how long, and did it appear to help?
- What is your past medical history?

Airway

The patient is sufficiently conscious to maintain her own airway but she may deteriorate. If the crew are not skilled in advanced airway management (i.e. endotracheal tube) they should consider requesting the help of a crew who can perform these skills, as this patient is likely to deteriorate. Checking the patient's sputum for any traces of blood is a strong indicator of pulmonary barotrauma. There is no evidence of angio-oedema or swelling.

Breathing

The patient is ventilating normally and although she does not appear to be in respiratory distress this should also be considered dynamic and prone to deterioration if barotrauma has occurred. Wheezes and crackles are commonly auscultated in the area of injury.

Circulation

The patient is normotensive but slightly tachycardic. At this point there is no significant issue with her perfusion but there remains the potential for a pneumothorax to develop and extend into a tension pneumothorax. Establishing a set of baseline observations will assist in early detection if this occurs.

Skin

Underneath her wetsuit the patient is warm to touch and does not appear to have any rash or erythema.

Neurological status

The patient appears dazed and confused; she is dysphasic with significant slurring. She appears to have difficulty finding her words. Her right arm has no response to painful stimuli but her right leg appears to have normal sensation and movement.

Initial assessment summary

Problem	Decompression illness
Conscious state	GCS = 13; confused and agitated
Position	Left lateral
Heart rate	105 bpm
Blood pressure	135/85 mmHg
Skin appearance	Pink, damp, warm
Speech pattern	Slurring, difficulty finding her words
Respiratory rate	18 bpm
Respiratory rhythm	Even
Chest auscultation	Sounds clear but the patient is agitated and auscultation is difficult
Pulse oximetry	97% on oxygen
Temperature	36.4°C
Motor/sensory function	She has a dense right hemiparesis
Pain	Unable to ascertain
History	The patient was training on a 10-m dive for 10 minutes when she panicked and ascended rapidly; upon reaching the surface she cried out and became agitated
Physical assessment	No injuries noted

D: There are no immediate dangers to the patient or the crew.

A: The patient is conscious with no current airway obstruction but needs frequent reassessment.

RESPIRATORY STATUS

Look/listen for!
- Airway swelling
- Wheezes/crackles
- Localised decreased breath sounds

PERFUSION STATUS

Look for!
- Tachycardia
- Hypotension: late sign
- Altered conscious state
- Erythema
- Pruritus
- Hives

B: Respiratory function is currently normal but needs frequent reassessment. The respiratory rate is elevated but ventilation is normal.

C: Heart rate is elevated but there is a sufficient blood pressure.

The patient presents in an altered conscious state but with normal perfusion. The neurological deficits are unilateral and consistent with a cerebral emboli or haemorrhage. Given the patient's age and recent diving history this is likely to be due to a rapid decompression injury.

② CONFIRM

The essential part of the clinical reasoning process is to seek to confirm your initial hypothesis by finding clinical signs that should occur with your provisional diagnosis. You should also seek to challenge your diagnosis by exploring findings that do not fit your hypothesis: don't just ignore them because they don't fit.

What else could it be?
Anaphylaxis/envenomation
Diving exposes participants not only to changes in temperature, pressure and inhaled gases but also to an environment filled with toxins and antigens. A past history of anaphylaxis can identify atopy but the absence of any allergic history doesn't rule out anaphylaxis (see Ch 28). The lack of bronchospasm, gastro-intestinal complaints and skin changes is strongly suggestive that anaphylaxis is not the cause.

A number of marine animals are capable of injecting neurotoxins (see Ch 44) but their effects are systemic and do not produce the unilateral weakness seen in this case. It is always possible that the patient was stung or bitten by a harmless animal or plant and this caused her panicked ascent: trying to identify what the patient was doing immediately prior to the ascent can be helpful.

Hypoxia/hypercapnia
Hypoxia, hypercapnia, hypotension, hypoglycaemia and hypothermia should be remembered as the 'reversible causes' of an altered conscious state. With divers there is a slim chance that the compressed gas they were breathing was contaminated, so hypoxia and hypercapnia should be considered. In this case the patient is ventilating normally, so both should be self-correcting once the patient was removed from the circuit. Although the neurological symptoms may be attributed to a generalised hypoxic state, the focal nature and rapid onset make this cause unlikely. Carbon monoxide (CO) is a potential contaminant, so SpO_2 readings should be considered in the context of the entire clinical picture as CO will falsely elevate SpO_2 readings.

Hypothermia
Water disperses heat very efficiently and even in warmer regions divers can become hypothermic. Neurological changes (especially slurring) are among the early signs of hypothermia but unilateral weakness is not typical. Measuring the tympanic temperature will help eliminate this differential entirely.

Hypoglycaemia
This patient does not have a history of diabetes, but nevertheless her blood sugar level should be measured, as it should be for all patients with an altered level of consciousness, no matter what the apparent cause. Neurological changes are among the early signs of hypoglycaemia, but unilateral weakness is not typical. Measuring the BGL will help eliminate this differential.

Subarachnoid haemorrhage/CVA
A CVA could well give focal signs and this patient's presentation could be consistent with a subarachnoid haemorrhage or an embolic CVA, both of which would give a sudden onset of neurological symptoms. While it is likely

> ## DIFFERENTIAL DIAGNOSIS
>
> **Cerebral arterial gas embolus**
> Or
> - Anaphylaxis/envenomation
> - Hypoxia/hypercapnia
> - Hypothermia
> - Hypoglycaemia
> - Subarachnoid haemorrhage/cerebrovascular accident (CVA)
> - Pneumothorax

that the diving environment contributed to the event, it is possible that the patient has suffered a spontaneous cerebral bleed. Given her age this is likely to be a subarachnoid haemorrhage. Although it does not alter the immediate management, the potential that blood rather than air has caused her symptoms might direct the choice of receiving hospital.

Pneumothorax

Barotrauma can tear the lung wall and allow air to escape into the pleural space (see Ch 20). Although a large pneumothorax can cause hypoxaemia and hypotension and lead to an altered conscious state, this is not apparent in this case. The potential for a pneumothorax to develop remains, however, and it should be considered if there is an increase in respiratory distress with a concurrent decrease in blood pressure.

 TREAT

Emergency management

The principles of management for decompression illness are outlined in Box 41.1.

Positioning

Air emboli tend to 'float' so positioning the patient with their head raised may allow more emboli to travel to the brain. Because of this, it is important that patients with possible CAGE are kept supine. This can sometimes be difficult if there is coexisting pulmonary barotrauma causing significant respiratory distress. In this event, the patient may need to be managed in a position of comfort and monitored carefully.

If bubbles travel to whichever part of the body is highest, it would seem to make sense to transport patients feet up. The problem is that it is often difficult to differentiate between AGE and DCS in the early stages. Patients with DCS almost always have bubbles in their venous circulation. As many as 30% of the population have a potential communication between their right and left atria across the patent foramen ovale (PFO), which is a flap valve between the atria that is important in fetal circulation (Hagen et al., 1984). Normally, the PFO is held closed because left atrial pressure is higher than the right. Elevation of a patient's legs causes an increase in right atrial pressure, which may open the PFO and allow shunting of blood from the right atrium to the left. Normally this doesn't matter but if there are bubbles in the venous blood this shunting will convert benign, right-sided bubbles that are filtered out of the circulation in the lungs into left-sided bubbles, which can cause AGE. In addition, raising the patient's legs can exacerbate breathing difficulties, if present.

Oxygen

Oxygen is currently indicated for all patients with significant diving-related illness regardless of their SpO_2. Bubbles that form in the blood as a result of rapid decompression are composed mainly of nitrogen and by reducing the

---

BOX 41.1 Principles of management

Decompression illness
- Positioning: Keep the patient supine at all times if possible.
- Oxygen: Administer 100% oxygen concentration.
- Fluids: Administer to maintain perfusion.
- Transport: Transport to a recompression facility.
- Supportive: Manage pain and nausea as required.

BOX 41.2 The Diver's Alert Network

The Diver's Alert Network (DAN) is the diving industry's largest association dedicated to scuba diving safety. DAN provides emergency assistance, medical information resources, educational opportunities and more. By phoning the hotline number paramedics can access a hyperbaric specialist for diagnostic and treatment advice as well as liaison with local hyperbaric facilities.
- 1800 088 200 (toll free within Australia)
- +61-8-8212 9242 (from outside Australia)
- https://www.danap.org/emergency/hotline_numbers.php

amount of inhaled nitrogen these bubbles will dissolve more quickly due to a higher partial pressure gradient. With an AGE from barotrauma the bubbles are likely to be composed of more oxygen (the gas has been forced into the vessels from the lungs) but oxygen should not be denied as the increased dissolved oxygen in the plasma may offset the embolic insult to the micro-vasculature and surrounding tissues.

Transport

Definitive management of AGE is recompression in a hyperbaric oxygen facility and the patient should be transported to a hospital with a hyperbaric facility. Unless procedures such as endotracheal intubation and resuscitation are immediately required, transport should not be delayed. Notification of the receiving hospital with the patient's details (including the details of the dive) is important to assist in preparing the hospital. Contacting the Diver's Alert Network (see Box 41.2) or the local hyperbaric centre can help paramedics with expert advice.

4 EVALUATE

Evaluating the effect of any clinical management intervention can provide clues to the accuracy of the initial diagnosis. Some conditions respond rapidly to treatment so patients should be expected to improve if the diagnosis and treatment were appropriate. A failure to improve in this situation should trigger the clinician to reconsider the diagnosis.

While some patients with CAGE will improve quickly, others will show no change or will deteriorate. There is no guide to the effectiveness of treatment but any deterioration should trigger a re-evaluation of the differential diagnoses to check if the change has made a diagnosis more probable.

Is the patient:
- Protecting their airway and ventilating adequately?
- Adequately perfused?

Ongoing management

Definitive treatment for decompression illness is obviously not usually available in the out-of-hospital setting so management of conscious patients should be supportive of symptoms and all efforts should be focused on delivering the patient to definitive care.

Fluids

Divers are often dehydrated after diving due to immersion diuresis and from breathing dry gas. Administration of fluids to support perfusion should be commenced according to local guidelines. Consultation with the receiving hospital is recommended

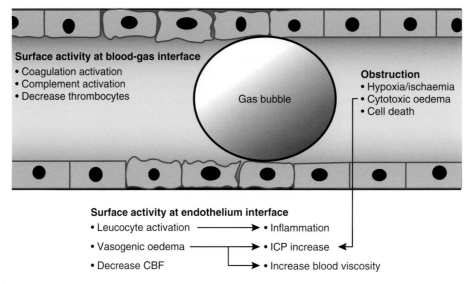

Figure 41.3
In addition to occluding blood supply to the tissues distal to the gas emboli, the bubbles also trigger a number of inflammatory changes in the endothelium that promote localised oedema and further compromise of local tissue perfusion.
Source: Papadakos et al. (2008).

and transport must not be delayed in order to gain IV access.

Endothelial damage caused by bubbles causes vasodilation and increased capillary permeability, loss of circulating blood volume and swelling in the tissues around the obstruction. The subsequent cerebral oedema is consistent with that which occurs following a stroke or head trauma (see Fig 41.3). While paramedics should not aim for blood pressure greater than normal, avoiding hypotension can assist in maintaining cerebral perfusion pressure.

Pain relief
Opioid pain relief should be considered according to local guidelines for patient comfort but with careful consideration of side effects.

Steroids
Steroids have been used in the past in an attempt to reduce inflammation and damage to brain tissue but there is no evidence to support the practice.

Airway
The ability to deliver 100% FiO_2 to intubated patients suggests that patients with CAGE should be considered for intubation. However, there are significant risks and complications associated with elective intubation, with the drugs used to facilitate intubation impacting on blood pressure and cerebral perfusion. Intubation may also restrict access to some hyperbaric chambers and if positive pressure ventilation is required it may create new gas emboli. In this circumstance endotracheal intubation should be reserved for comatose patients where maintaining adequate oxygenation and ventilation is not otherwise possible.

Hospital admission
Hyperbaric oxygen therapy (HBOT) is supported by a long series of case reports and although there are no randomised controlled trials demonstrating a positive effect, HBOT remains the preferred treatment. The combination of high oxygen concentration and high pressure promotes resorption of nitrogen from the bubbles and a reduction in bubble size. With the pressures commonly used (2.8 ATA, which is the equivalent of 18 m of seawater) bubble size can be reduced by nearly half, allowing the bubbles to pass through the smaller vessels and resolve the occlusion. Hyperbaric oxygen also has a number of beneficial physiological effects, including reduction in platelet activity, changes in neutrophil marginalisation and changes in nitric oxide levels. All Australian and New Zealand hospital hyperbaric facilities can offer full intensive care treatment and monitoring of patients in the hyperbaric chamber.

Long-term impact
Most patients with DCI will recover fully if they are treated relatively promptly in a hyperbaric

chamber and early treatment is associated with better outcomes. Patients with more severe neurological problems may be left with permanent sequelae. Less serious DCS (e.g. pain only, isolated skin involvement, very minor neurological symptoms) will often completely resolve even without recompression, especially if adequate high-concentration oxygen administration (usually in excess of 4 hours) has been provided.

 CASE STUDY 2

Case 10489, 1115 hrs.

Dispatch details: A 40-year-old male has surfaced after a 90-m dive and developed vertigo and vomiting shortly afterwards.

Initial presentation: The paramedics are met at a paddock gate by a group of divers and escorted to the patient, who is lying on the ground wearing a drysuit. They are told that the diver became unwell shortly after climbing 15 m up a rope ladder following a 2-hour, 90-m decompression dive using a closed-circuit rebreather, breathing trimix (a mixture of helium, oxygen and air). The other divers are adamant that the patient cannot be suffering from DCI because they dived strictly according to the profiles provided by their computers. It is at least 4 hours by road to the nearest hyperbaric facilities. The local hospital has an emergency department with 24-hour staffing and a high-dependency unit.

1 ASSESS

1150 hrs Primary survey: The patient is lying supine; he is conscious, but very distressed. He says that the world is spinning around and he is very nauseous, retching frequently.

1151 hrs Vital signs survey: Perfusion status: HR 115 bpm, sinus rhythm, BP difficult to assess due to clothing, skin cold and clammy.
   Respiratory status: RR 24 bpm, SpO_2 96% (air).
   Conscious state: GCS = 15.

1153 hrs Pertinent hx: The patient denies any significant past medical history or allergies. He had a small amount of trouble clearing his ears at the start of the dive, which was otherwise uneventful. He felt well until just after he finished climbing the ladder.

1154 hrs Secondary survey: Profound nystagmus with rapid phase to the left. No other abnormalities found.
   BGL: 6.1 mmol/L.
   Temperature: 36.2°C.

> HISTORY
>
> **Ask!**
> - What is your past medical history?
> - Have you taken any illicit drugs or alcohol?

2 CONFIRM

In many cases paramedics are presented with a collection of signs and symptoms that do not appear to describe a particular condition. A critical step in

DIFFERENTIAL DIAGNOSIS

Vestibular decompression sickness
Or
- Inner ear barotrauma
- Labyrinthitis
- Stroke/subarachnoid haemorrhage (SAH)

determining a treatment plan in this situation is to consider what other conditions could explain the patient's presentation.

This patient has experienced a very deep dive and now has symptoms that could be consistent with vestibular decompression sickness. While the dive has been controlled, followed the dive computers and used a helium oxygen mixture, it is still possible that the patient could be suffering from vestibular decompression sickness. The picture is initially far from clear, with inner ear barotrauma also a possibility.

What else could it be?

Inner ear barotrauma

The patient's symptoms are entirely consistent with inner ear barotrauma. The history of some difficulty with his ears at the start of the dive supports this diagnosis.

Labyrinthitis

The symptoms are consistent with labyrinthitis as a diagnosis but it would be highly coincidental to develop the symptoms immediately after a dive. Inner ear barotrauma is far more likely.

Stroke/subarachnoid haemorrhage

Stroke and SAH are possible but much less likely. However, they cannot be completely excluded.

This case has the potential to challenge the paramedic who is unfamiliar with the intricacies of mixed-gas, closed-circuit decompression diving. The diagnostic uncertainty in this case is a major issue, in that recompression is mandatory to prevent significant disability if the patient does have DCI, but it will possibly do more harm if the diagnosis is inner ear barotrauma. The main issue is to involve people with the expertise to resolve this uncertainty as soon as possible, and this expertise may well not exist in a regional hospital.

③ TREAT

1201 hrs: The paramedics administer oxygen at 15 L/min via bag-valve-mask with reservoir or non-rebreather mask.

1202 hrs: The paramedics gain IV access and commence antiemetic administration.

1205 hrs: The paramedics administer crystalloid fluids to 20 mL/kg.
A fixed-wing aircraft pressurised to sea level can evacuate the patient.

④ EVALUATE

Evaluating the effect of any clinical management intervention can provide clues to the accuracy of the initial diagnosis. Some conditions respond rapidly to treatment so patients should be expected to improve if the diagnosis and treatment were appropriate. A failure to improve in these cases should trigger the clinician to reconsider the diagnosis.

In this case it is unlikely that the patient will either improve or deteriorate significantly if the diagnosis of inner ear barotrauma is correct. The extension of symptoms to the limbs would suggest DCI but the two conditions can coexist. With the limited resources available in the out-of-hospital setting, paramedic treatment should focus on providing relief and transporting the patient to an appropriate facility that is aware of his condition.

Summary

The mechanism of injury provides a strong clue for the diagnosis of divers who arrive at the surface complaining of illness, but the physical stresses of diving (temperature, exertion, dehydration, hunger) can trigger a range of conditions unrelated to pressure injury that paramedics will need to exclude (where possible). There is also the possibility that divers can suffer both pressure- and non-pressure related injuries simultaneously and an understanding of the pathology of the injuries is essential if treatment is to be safely prioritised. While paramedics working in coastal areas are often familiar with local hyperbaric resources, it is important to note that diving and pressure-related injuries can occur far from the coast: divers may develop symptoms on commercial flights taken too soon after diving, and deep-diving caves exist in inland areas.

References

Elliott, D. H., Harrison, J. A. B., & Barnard, E. E. P. (1978). Clinical and radiological features of eighty-eight cases of decompression barotrauma. *Paper presented at the Proceedings of the Vth Symposium on Underwater Physiology, Bethesda, MD.*

Francis, T. J. R., & Mitchell, S. J. (2004). Manifestation of decompression disorders. In A. O. Brubakk & T. S. Neuman (Eds.), *Bennett and Elliott's physiology and medicine of diving*. Philadelphia: Saunders.

Gorman, D. F. (1991). A proposed classification of dysbarism. In T. J. R. Francis & D. H. Smith (Eds.), *Describing dysbarism*. Bethesda, MD: Undersea and Hyperbaric Medicine Society.

Hagen, P. T., Scholz, D. G., & Edwards, W. D. (1984). Incidence and size of patent foramen ovale during the first 10 decades of life: an autopsy study of 965 normal hearts. *Mayo Clinic Proceedings, 59*(1), 17–20.

Neuman, T. S. (2002). Arterial gas embolism and decompression sickness. *News in Physiological Sciences, 17,* 77–81.

Neuman, T. S. (2004). Arterial gas embolism and pulmonary barotrauma. In A. O. Brubakk & T. S. Neuman (Eds.), *Bennett and Elliott's physiology and medicine of diving*. Philadelphia: Saunders.

Papadakos, P. J., Lachmann, B., & Visser-Isles, L. (2008). *Mechanical ventilation: clinical applications and pathophysiology*. Philadelphia: Elsevier Saunders.

Pollock, N. W., & Buteau, D. (2017). Updates in decompression illness. *Emergency Medicine Clinics of North America, 35*(2), 301–319.

CHAPTER 42

Snakebite Envenoming

By Julian White

OVERVIEW

- Australia has some of the most venomous snakes in the world.
- Most snake bites do not result in significant envenoming and do not require antivenom.
- All patients with a history of a possible snake bite should be assessed, managed and transported to hospital.
- Fatalities are now rare due to the availability of antivenom; most fatalities are a consequence of medical events occurring within a few hours of the snake bite.
- Basic first aid such as appropriate pressure bandaging and immobilisation (PBI) appears to be effective and may have been a factor in the reduced death rate from snake bite in recent decades.

- Antivenom is indicated for all patients who present with clinical and laboratory evidence of envenoming.
- Antivenom should be given early. This horse-derived antibody is associated with producing allergic reactions in approximately 25% of patients and anaphylaxis in 5%.
- Using the clinical presentation and geographical location it is often possible to determine which antivenom to administer: while killing the offending snake should be discouraged, if it has been killed and is available, it should be brought with the patient as it is a valuable resource for absolutely identifying the culprit species, but care should be exercised in handling the dead snake, to avoid contact with the head area.

Introduction

Envenoming is the injection of venom into the body (Harris et al., 2010). Australia has the dubious and arguably undeserved reputation of being potentially one of the most dangerous locations in which to go for a walk or a swim. In fact, lethal envenoming is rare in Australia (snake bite in Australia has a fatality rate of about 0.01/100,000 per year compared to a global figure of about 1.32). Approximately 500–1000 people per year suffer snake bites in Australia (see Fig 42.1), with an average death rate in recent years of 2.2 deaths per year. Most of these deaths follow an out-of-hospital cardiac arrest, with few deaths among patients who reach hospital without having suffered a major medical event such as cardiac or respiratory arrest. This may reflect the ready availability of both antivenom and high-quality medical care. However, the majority of snake bites do not cause envenoming (Ireland et al., 2010). Climate change and the creep of the suburbs into wilderness areas may speculatively lead to more interactions between people and venomous snakes in the future. A number of dangerously venomous snakes have adapted to urban environments and snake bites do occur in major urban areas, including inside homes; therefore, city-based paramedics need to be aware of the challenges in diagnosis and management.

Pathophysiology

Snake venoms are complex mixtures of substances, particularly toxins, that have evolved to target prey species that are often physiologically different from, and much smaller than, humans. The venom of any particular snake species will contain many toxins, so when injected into a human it can produce a range of symptoms and presentations. While these can be unpredictable and challenging to the paramedic, for most snake species there is usually a distinctive pattern of envenoming effects characteristic for that species. Some of the symptoms will be nonspecific and not immediately recognisable as life-threatening (nausea, vomiting, headache, abdominal pain, lethargy), but the most serious effects occur when the toxins target entire systems. These systemic effects can be divided as follows:

- neurotoxicity, either paralytic or neuroexcitatory (disruption of the nervous system)
- haemostasis disorders (disruption of blood clotting)
- cardiovascular dysfunction
- rhabdomyolysis (damage to muscles)
- renal dysfunction (acute kidney injury [AKI])
- intravascular haemolysis
- local bite/sting site tissue injury/necrosis.

Disruption of the nervous system

Paralysis is a classic symptom of snake bite and is mostly caused by toxins in the venom blocking the presynaptic or postsynaptic transmission of nerve impulses at the neuromuscular junction (NMJ), resulting in flaccid paralysis of voluntary and respiratory muscles. Nerve impulses reaching the synaptic cleft trigger the release of acetylcholine (ACh). ACh diffuses across the NMJ,

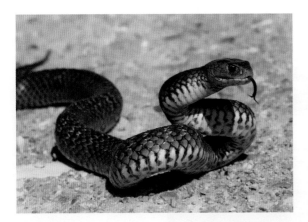

Figure 42.1
The Eastern Brown (*Pseudonaja textilis*) is considered the second most venomous snake in the world and this genus is responsible for the majority of fatal bites in Australia. Its widespread distribution, daytime activity and nervous nature when cornered most likely contribute to its bite rate. The snake's colour can range from deep brown to silvery grey, sometimes with a dark head, or broad dark bands on the body, or dark speckles. Some other dangerous Australian snakes may also be coloured brown, causing confusion with non-expert identification.
Source: Shutterstock/Kristian Bell.

binds to receptor proteins on the muscle end plate and causes the muscle cell membrane to depolarise and the muscle to contract (see Fig 42.2). In order to allow the muscle to relax and be ready for further contractions, an enzyme (acetylcholinesterase) breaks down the ACh, removing the stimulus from the muscle. Toxins that block the release of ACh from the nerve ending (terminal axon) are known as presynaptic neurotoxins (the nerves cannot trigger muscle activity; see Fig 42.3). Presynaptic neurotoxicity is present in most dangerous Australian snake venoms, but clinically is characteristic of bites by tiger snakes, rough-scaled snakes and taipans. Presynaptic neurotoxicity can take days to weeks to resolve, because the internally damaged nerve cells at the NMJ must regrow. Once such paralysis is established, antivenom cannot reverse it because antivenom can neither reach the inside of cells, nor repair damaged cells. It follows that detecting envenoming early, before major nerve damage has occurred, and giving adequate doses of antivenom at that time is more likely to prevent onset of full paralysis unresponsive to antivenom.

Postsynaptic neurotoxins bind with the ACh receptor proteins on the muscle cell membrane in the end plate region, blocking the normal binding of ACh and thereby block the receptor from activation, resulting in failure to initiate muscle contraction. Because the binding of the neurotoxin is extracellular it is potentially accessible to antivenom, which can sometimes fully reverse postsynaptic paralysis. All dangerous Australian snakes have postsynaptic neurotoxins in their venom and for some species, such as death adders and copperheads, postsynaptic paralysis may be a dominant clinical feature in envenomed humans. However, the presence of neurotoxins in venom does not always mean paralysis will be a significant feature in envenomed humans. Members of the black snake genus rarely cause significant paralysis in humans, despite the presence of neurotoxins in their venom, but cats and dogs bitten by these snakes often develop paralysis.

Clinically in humans the effects of snake neurotoxins, whether presynaptic or postsynaptic, are first evident in the cranial nerves. Bilateral ptosis is the classic first sign, followed by diplopia and partial then complete ophthalmoplegia and fixed dilated pupils, drooling and loss of upper airway protection. The effects then 'descend' to involve limb weakness and progressive respiratory muscle involvement. Without treatment in severe envenoming, death may occur secondary to respiratory paralysis.

> ## NEUROLOGICAL ASSESSMENT
> ### Look for!
> - Ptosis
> - Diplopia
> - Partial or complete ophthalmoplegia
> - Facial palsy
> - Drooling
> - Limb weakness
> - Decreased or absent deep tendon reflexes
> - Weak respirations

Haemostasis disorders

Most of Australia's dangerous venomous snakes contain toxins that interfere with the blood's ability to coagulate, in some cases dramatically. Brown snakes, tiger snakes, the rough-scaled snake, the broad-headed snake group (*Hoplocephalus* spp.) and taipans all have potent prothrombin activators in their venom that cause a complex cascade of effects on blood clotting resulting in either complete or partial defibrination coagulopathy (also referred to by some authors as 'venom-induced consumptive coagulopathy'). In this process there is an initial activation of circulating prothrombin to thrombin which then converts fibrinogen to fibrin and promotes some cross-linkage of fibrin strands, so minor thrombi may briefly exist, prior to consumption of fibrin by the simultaneously activated fibrinolytic system. The whole process can progress in a matter of minutes to consume all circulating fibrinogen, at which point the patient is no longer able to make blood clots. Other clotting factors are also consumed in this process. Therefore, although these toxins are powerful clot-promoting substances, their effect in humans is to render the

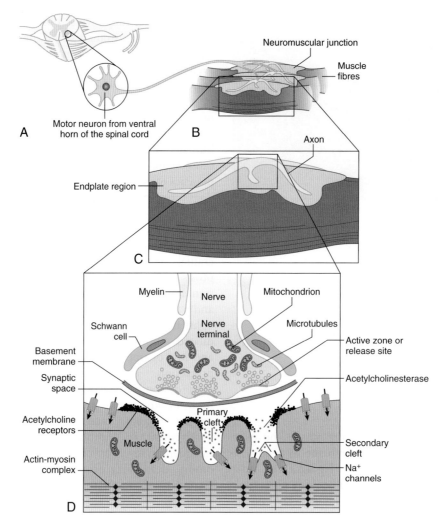

Figure 42.2
Structure of the adult neuromuscular junction showing the three cells that constitute the synapse: motor neuron (i.e. nerve terminal), muscle fibre and Schwann cell.
A The motor nerve originates in the ventral horn of the spinal cord or brainstem. **B** As the nerve approaches its muscle fibres and before attaching itself to the surface of the muscle fibre, the nerve divides into branches that innervate many individual muscle fibres. **C** Each muscle receives only one synapse. The motor nerve loses its myelin and further subdivides into many presynaptic boutons to terminate on the surface of the muscle fibre. **D** The nerve terminal, covered by a Schwann cell, has vesicles clustered about the membrane thickenings, which are the active zones towards its synaptic side and mitochondria and microtubules towards its other side. A synaptic gutter or cleft made up of a primary and many secondary clefts separates the nerve from the muscle. The muscle surface is corrugated, and dense areas on the shoulders of each fold contain acetylcholine receptors. Presynaptic toxicity is a characteristic of tiger snake, rough-scaled snake and taipan venom, while death adder venom acts at the postsynaptic site in most cases.
Source: Miller et al. (2009).

blood incoagulable, so clinically it appears to be profound anticoagulation with increased tendency to bleed, particularly from any vascular breach such as insertion of intravenous (IV) lines or intramuscular (IM) injections, or blunt trauma. Coagulation function will return to normal only once all the venom procoagulants have either been neutralised (by antivenom) or have naturally broken down, and then normal homeostasis has progressively replaced depleted clotting factors (especially fibrinogen), a

process that may take more than 6 hours, during which time the patient remains at risk of increased bleeding. Mulga and black snake venom contain a true anticoagulant toxin which inhibits clotting factors, but does not cause consumption of factors, so is quickly reversible using antivenom to neutralise the toxins.

The increased tendency to bleed is an important factor in patients who suffer traumatic injuries (particularly head injuries) subsequent to envenoming.

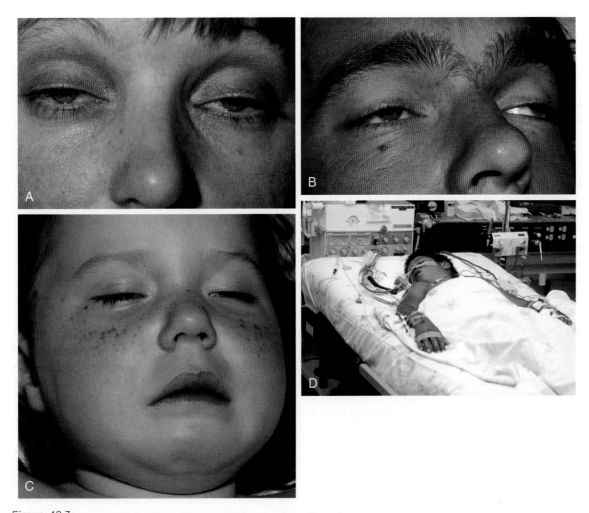

Figure 42.3
Effects of Australian snake neurotoxins which cause a progressive descending flaccid paralysis.
A Mild bilateral ptosis as the early sign of developing neurotoxicity. **B** Mild bilateral ptosis and divergent squint on being asked to look laterally, due to neurotoxic paralysis of the muscles moving the eye medially. **C** flat facies indicative of developing neurotoxicity in a young child (tiger snake bite). **D** Patient intubated and ventilated in ICU because of neurotoxic paralysis of all voluntary and respiratory muscles; this patient required ventilation in ICU for 4 weeks (tiger snake bite).
Source: All photos copyright © Julian White.

BLEEDING

Look for!
- Bleeding from: 1. intravenous (IV) sites and wounds; 2. gums; 3. bite site; 4. any other wounds
- Extensive bruising
- Collapse/loss of consciousness

CARDIOVASCULAR

Look for!
- Collapse/loss of consciousness
- ECG changes

RENAL

Look for!
- Oliguria/anuria
- Dark urine

LOCALISED SYMPTOMS

Look for!
- Swelling at bite site
- Local erythema
- Persistent blood ooze from bite
- Local bruising

Cardiovascular dysfunction

Hypotension is a known complication of envenoming but its mechanism is probably multifactorial; although in many patients, envenoming is associated with hypertension, at least in the hospital setting. Loss of consciousness and collapse shortly after untreated snake bite, particularly by brown snakes (*Pseudonaja* spp.) is common, but the causation remains uncertain, is likely to be multifactorial and may not always be associated with sudden hypotension. The possible role of early procoagulant coagulopathy remains speculative in humans, as does the role of these toxins in early out-of-hospital cardiac collapse and cardiac arrest, which is most often seen with brown snake bites and is currently the leading factor associated with snake-bite fatalities in Australia.

Rhabdomyolysis

Many snake venoms contain toxins based on a phospholipase A_2 (PLA_2) molecule, with a multitude of possible targets and effects, but for Australian snake bite evolved PLA_2 toxins which target muscle, particularly skeletal muscle, are clinically important. For some snakes these PLA_2 toxins are both presynaptic neurotoxins and myolysins which damage muscle (e.g. tiger snakes, rough-scaled snake, taipans), while for others the PLA_2 toxin just targets muscle (mulga and black snake genus, *Pseudechis* spp.). For all these snakes the extent of muscle damage is highly variable from case to case but can be very severe, extensively damaging skeletal muscles throughout the body and manifesting clinically as muscle pain, decreased strength, grossly elevated blood CK and myoglobinuria, with potential secondary effects including secondary AKI, hyperkalaemia and cardiac toxicity. However, it should be noted that even severe myoglobinuria following snake bite is not routinely associated with AKI, unlike some other causes of rhabdomyolysis. While other snakes may also contain such PLA_2 toxins targeting muscle, clinically in humans muscle damage is either absent or minor (e.g. death adders, possibly copperheads), or never reported clinically (brown snakes, *Pseudonaja* spp.; broad-headed snake group, *Hoplocephalus* spp.).

Renal dysfunction

Kidney damage (AKI) can occur following Australian snake bite, uncommonly, usually secondary to other envenoming-related problems such as coagulopathy, rhabdomyolysis (uncommonly) or a period of hypotension. In most cases the AKI results in short-term kidney dysfunction, which may range from just a rise in creatinine/urea levels through to full anuric renal failure requiring a period of dialysis. Full renal recovery is expected for most patients. No specific kidney-toxic toxins have been reported from Australian snake venoms.

Intravascular haemolysis

Many snake venoms contain toxins that can, in laboratory testing, cause destruction of red blood cells (haemolysis), but intravascular haemolysis after Australian snake bite is uncommon and usually associated with a syndrome that is similar in some ways to haemolytic uraemic syndrome (HUS) and thrombotic thrombocytopenic purpura (TTP). This haemolytic syndrome following snake bite, often called 'microangiopathic haemolytic anaemia' (MAHA) and incompletely understood, is thought to be associated with coagulopathy and fibrin strand deposition in small blood vessels, the key features being thrombocytopenia, intravascular haemolysis, anaemia and secondary AKI. Most cases are self-limited, with ultimate recovery.

Local bite/sting site tissue injury/necrosis

Symptoms that occur at the site of the bite vary widely and may reflect the high number of dry bites (the snake bites but does not inject venom) inflicted by some Australian snakes. Australian snake venom does not contain the tissue-damaging factors that cause the local tissue necrosis associated with bites from some exotic snakes such as the Malayan pit viper (*Calloselasma rhodostoma*). Mulga/black snakes and, to a lesser extent, tiger snake bites are associated with significant local reactions such as pain and swelling, but rarely extend to local necrosis. Brown snake bites are often associated with minimal local effects, with the small fang size sometimes making it difficult to identify bite marks, yet such apparently trivial local effects can still be associated with life-threatening systemic envenoming. Patients may sometimes be unaware of having been bitten because of the lack of local effects, which can complicate diagnosis. Bites from some whip snakes (*Demansia* spp.) sometimes cause significant local pain and swelling, but without major systemic envenoming.

CASE STUDY 1

Case 10694, 1530 hrs.

Dispatch details: A 38-year-old male has suffered a snake bite. The property is 1 hour's drive from nearest city or major country hospital.

Initial presentation: The crew find the patient sitting down. His skin is warm and dry, and he is conscious but very anxious. He is holding his left wrist tightly with his right hand.

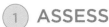 **ASSESS**

Patient history

Determining the underlying cause of the patient's presentation is not difficult as he saw the snake strike. The key to effective clinical reasoning in this case is therefore not in determining what is wrong with the patient now but what is likely to develop and how it can best be managed. After being bitten by the snake the patient attempted to slow the progression of the venom by applying a tourniquet of sorts with his other hand. He then ran back to the house. He is normally fit and well. Always ask if the snake was killed, or photographed with a mobile phone (it wasn't in this case).

Airway

Given the potential for paralysis with some venoms, the patient's airway should always be monitored but it is unlikely to become a problem unless the patient loses consciousness.

Breathing

The patient is currently in respiratory distress, but this could possibly be attributed to anxiety at this early stage. Given the potential for paralysis, his respiratory function must be monitored to ensure adequate tidal volume and adequate protection of the upper airway.

Cardiovascular

Hypotension may occur in snake-bite victims, but some envenomed patients become hypertensive. At this stage, the patient is adequately perfused.

CNS

Snake venom can significantly affect neurological function. Patients must be monitored closely for symptoms of neurological dysfunction. Earliest signs of developing neurotoxic flaccid paralysis appear in cranial nerves, with bilateral ptosis the classic first sign, which must always be checked for in snake-bite patients regularly, just as pulse and BP are checked. This patient is holding his left wrist tightly in an attempt to contain the venom to the site of the bite on his left hand. He has some altered sensation in his fingers on this hand, but this could be due to limited perfusion as a result of the pressure he is applying. Seizure activity is also a possibility but it is a late sign and if seizures commence, he should be managed according to local guidelines.

The bite site

There is a single puncture wound on the back of the patient's hand and a reddened 5-mm scratch about 1 cm from the puncture wound. Always ensure

HISTORY

Ask!

- What did the snake look like, including how long?
- What was the geographic location?
- How many times were you bitten?
- Did the snake hang on when biting or was it a very brief glancing strike?
- When were you bitten?
- What type of first aid did you apply and how long after the bite?
- Were you physically active before or after applying first aid?
- Are the symptoms better or worse now?
- Do you have any difficulty seeing, speaking, swallowing, breathing or moving your limbs?
- Are you on any medications?
- Do you have any preexisting medical conditions?

that there is not more than one bite site. Multiple bites are associated with more severe envenoming.

Initial assessment summary

Problem	Snake bite
Conscious state	GCS = 15
Position	Sitting
Heart rate	105 bpm
Blood pressure	120/80 mmHg
Skin appearance	Pink, warm, dry
Speech pattern	Normal
Respiratory rate	32 bpm
Respiratory rhythm	Even cycles
Chest auscultation	Good breath sounds bilaterally
Pulse oximetry	98%
Temperature	37.2°C
Motor/sensory function	No ptosis or other cranial nerve defect detected; altered sensation in left fingers, possibly due to the tight grip the patient has around his left wrist
Pain	8/10
History	The patient was collecting wood from behind a shed when he saw a short, fat, black snake lying coiled in the pile. He instinctively struck at it with the piece of wood in his hand but missed and the snake bit him on the back of his hand. The snake was not killed or photographed. He encircled his wrist with his other hand and ran 20 m back to the house where he sat while his wife called the ambulance.
Physical assessment	He is complaining of severe burning pain at the bite site and mild nausea. There is a single puncture wound on the back of his hand and a reddened 5-mm scratch about 1 cm from the puncture wound.

D: The patient has moved away from the snake.

A: The patient is conscious with no current airway obstruction but needs frequent reassessment.

B: Respiratory function is currently normal but needs frequent reassessment. The respiratory rate is elevated but ventilation is normal.

C: Heart rate is elevated but there is a sufficient blood pressure.

The patient has suffered a single snake bite and is displaying localised symptoms but no systemic effects at this stage.

DIFFERENTIAL DIAGNOSIS

Snake envenoming
Or
- Anxiety
- Anaphylaxis

---

② CONFIRM

The essential part of the clinical reasoning process is to seek to confirm your initial hypothesis by finding clinical signs that should occur with your provisional diagnosis. You should also seek to challenge your diagnosis by exploring findings that do not fit your hypothesis: don't just ignore them because they don't fit.

What else could it be?

Anxiety

The most common mimic associated with snake bite is anxiety and it is not uncommon for victims to develop persistent symptoms despite subsequent tests showing no envenoming. In this case it is reasonable for the patient to be anxious and without testing for venom the crew will need to assume that the patient has been envenomed.

Anaphylaxis

Anaphylactic reactions to snake bite are known but usually occur in snake handlers who have experienced multiple envenomings and in persons working with snake venom. In cases where the patient presents with poor perfusion, diarrhoea and abdominal pain it is extremely difficult to exclude this pathology but outside of snake handlers envenoming is the more likely cause.

 TREAT

Emergency management

The principles of management for envenoming are outlined in Box 42.1.

Safety

The patient did not attempt to capture or kill the snake. Identifying the species can assist in selecting the antivenom, but the description of the snake and the area where it was living may provide sufficient detail to isolate a species. If the snake has been killed, it should be brought with the patient if possible; if photographed on a mobile phone, this image should be made available to the treating doctors once at a hospital. At this point the paramedics have to assume that the patient may have been envenomed and may require antivenom. Remember, the size of the bite does not correlate with the degree of envenoming. The primary focus is to apply a **pressure bandage and immobilisation (PBI)** and transport the patient to a facility that has antivenom, while supplying supportive management until that point.

Pressure bandage and immobilisation/splinting

Many components of snake venom are proteins too large to pass through capillary walls; therefore, applying pressure to the entire affected limb to stop the venom travelling through the lymph system remains the primary emergency management, despite it lacking high-level evidence. A wide (15 cm) elastic bandage should be applied over the bite site, then the whole limb using the same pressure that would be used to wrap a sprained ankle. Once wrapped, a mouldable or board splint should be used to further immobilise the limb and reduce the chances of muscle activity 'pumping' venom (see Fig 42.4). If the limb is already bandaged but the coverage is inadequate, bandage *over* the original dressing: do not remove it. However, beware applying multiple instances of PBI over the top of previous applications, which may result in excessive pressure to the underlying limb and can then act as a tourniquet, with increased pain in the limb and the risk of hypoxic and direct limb damage.

The concept of immobilisation should be extended to the entire patient: do not allow the patient to walk and try to minimise any physical exertion (Australian Resuscitation Council, 2011). If the site of the bite is marked on the outside of the bandage, identification swabs of the bite site can be taken through a small hole without disturbing the pressure bandage.

PRACTICE TIP

Do not wash the bite site or discard any dressings that have been applied over the site: they can be swabbed to assist in identifying the species of snake.

BOX 42.1 Principles of management

Envenoming
- Immobilise: Place a pressure bandage and immobilisation/splint (PBI) on the affected limb.
- Minimise: Restrict patient movement.
- Adrenaline: Administer IM adrenaline if anaphylaxis is suspected.
- Supportive: Manage the patient's pain, nausea and hypotension as required.
- Transport: Convey the patient to a facility to receive antivenom if required. PBI to remain in place until antivenom is ready to be administered.

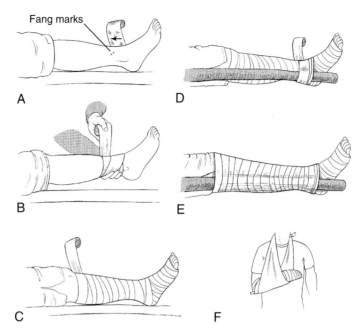

Fang marks

A

B

C

D

E

F

Figure 42.4
Pressure immobilisation.
Venom contains toxins of varying sizes, some quite large, and research indicates that at least some key toxins in snakebite principally reach the general circulation via the lymphatic system. This is the basis for the 'pressure bandage and immobilisation (PBI)' first aid method for Australian snakebite. However, the original technique has been modified by various groups, so that consensus on correct application is arguably absent. The following is based on ARC recommendations, but with some modifications. **A-C** Pressure bandage: If the bite location permits, consider applying a cloth or gauze pad (6–8 cm x 6–8 cm x 2 cm thick) directly over the area and hold it firmly in place with a circumferential bandage 15–18 cm wide applied at lymphatic-venous occlusive pressure (not ARC policy). The circumferential bandage may be used alone (ARC policy), particularly if a cloth or gauze pad is not available. Extend the bandage over the rest of the bitten limb, over the top of clothing where appropriate. Take care not to occlude the arterial circulation, as determined by the detection of arterial pulsations and proper capillary refill. Fingers/toes should be immobilised, but with nail beds visible to assess circulation. **D-F** Immobilising the limb: Splint the limb, keeping the limb and patient as immobile as possible and do not release the bandage until after the patient has been transported to definitive medical care, or as advised by a medical expert. Take care to check frequently that swelling beneath the bandage has not compromised the arterial circulation; seek expert medical advice if in doubt about viability of circulation.
Source: Auerbach (2013).

Transport

Definitive management of snake envenoming is antivenom and transport should not be delayed. Effective PBI can delay the onset of symptoms for several hours in patients who have been envenomed and local medical providers who do not have access to antivenom should be bypassed in order to deliver the patient to definitive care, unless procedures such as endotracheal intubation and resuscitation are required immediately and are beyond the skills of the crew in attendance. Providing notification to the receiving hospital with patient details (including past history of snake bites, allergies, renal disease and uses of drugs such as aspirin, warfarin and non-steroidal anti-inflammatory drugs) and a description of the snake can assist in preparing the hospital. Some smaller hospitals may hold sufficient antivenom only for an initial dose and can use the time to arrange for supplemental deliveries or transfer to a larger hospital once initial treatment is complete.

4 EVALUATE

Evaluating the effect of any clinical management intervention can provide clues to the accuracy of the initial diagnosis. Some conditions respond rapidly to treatment so patients should be expected to improve if the diagnosis and treatment were appropriate. A failure to improve in this situation should trigger the clinician to reconsider the diagnosis. In the setting of snake bite, out-of-hospital treatment is aimed at managing symptoms rather than providing definitive care.

Continuous reassessment of suspected snake-bite victims is essential as the progression of symptoms allows paramedics to plan and prepare for more serious complications. Look for the early signs of paralysis, such as ptosis, that may progress to respiratory failure and require airway and ventilatory support. A transient loss of consciousness shortly after envenoming is regularly reported and although the mechanism is unclear it is suspected that this occurs at about the time of onset of the various coagulopathies. This needs to be anticipated and the patient protected from falls or other injuries.

Seizures are regularly associated with worsening symptoms and paramedics should be prepared to manage these according to local guidelines (usually with the administration of midazolam). Any urine production should be noted and kept if possible.

Ongoing management

Paramedics do not have immediate access to antivenom, so management of conscious patients should be supportive of symptoms and all efforts should be focused on delivering the patient to definitive care.

Breathing

Respiratory failure due to developing neurotoxic paralysis, either loss of upper airway protection or respiratory paralysis (usually takes many hours to develop), is the most immediate concern. The paramedics should monitor the patient carefully for signs of neurotoxicity and be prepared to provide respiratory support.

Fluids

Some snake venoms may cause vasodilation and increased capillary permeability leading to inadequate perfusion. Administration of fluids to support perfusion should be commenced according to local guidelines. Consultation with the receiving hospital is recommended and transport must not be delayed in order to gain IV access. Coagulopathy will develop in some patients if antivenom is not provided, so IM injections and multiple IV attempts should be avoided. Avoid IV insertion in sites where controlling bleeding may prove difficult (femoral, jugular, subclavian veins). Once coagulopathy develops, expect bleeding from around IV sites and haematoma formation at IM sites. An initial IV load of fluid is recommended before administering antivenom, but paramedics should consult local guidelines and experts. To minimise secondary kidney injury, fluid resuscitation should be titrated to maintain a urine output of 1–2 mL/kg/hr.

Antiemetics

Symptomatic relief of nausea with IV antiemetics should be administered according to local guidelines. Some antiemetics such as metoclopramide can produce extrapyramidal side effects that may be mistaken for the ptosis and ophthalmoplegia that are early signs of neurotoxicity: consultation with a senior ambulance clinician or the receiving hospital is recommended before administration.

Pain relief

Opioid pain relief for patient comfort should be considered according to local guidelines, but with careful consideration of side effects. Since severe pain is not a feature of most Australian snake bites, a patient complaint of severe pain in the bitten and bandaged limb is a reason to check on the tightness of the PBI and vascular function in limb extremities (fingers or toes). If it is clear that the PBI is too tight and causing vascular compromise, immediately seek expert advice on whether to loosen or remove the PBI.

Hospital management

Antivenom

The symptoms of envenoming are often not obvious when clinicians first assess patients who have had appropriate first aid (Isbister et al., 2013). Antivenom carries some risk (anaphylaxis) and administration should be stratified according to the patient's presentation. Antivenom is not routinely given to all victims of snake bite: it is reserved for those showing systemic features of envenoming as determined by

Table 42.1: Indications for antivenom

Absolute indication	Relative indication	No indication
Out of hospital		
Ptosis, paralysis	Vomiting, diarrhoea, abdominal pain	Bite marks with no neurological or haematological symptoms (persistent bleeding from bite site or IV site)
Seizure	Headache	Positive result on snake venom detection kit but no symptoms
Collapse or cardiac arrest		No symptoms within 12 hours of bite after PBI removed
Active major bleeding secondary to coagulopathy	Evidence of active coagulopathy	
In hospital		
Evidence of defibrination coagulopathy (gross elevation of D-dimer, decreased fibrinogen, elevated/prolonged INR/aPTT)	Leucocytosis	
Evidence of anticoagulant coagulopathy (prolonged aPTT, normal fibrinogen, D-dimer)	Lymphopenia	
Evidence of active bleeding secondary to suspected coagulopathy		
Evidence of developing neurotoxicity	Minor neurotoxic signs (ptosis, partial ophthalmoplegia) without evidence of progression over more than 6 hours	
Evidence of developing rhabdomyolysis	Creatine kinase > 1000 U/L	
Evidence of acute kidney injury		
History of post-bite cardiac collapse or convulsions		

their clinical presentation or laboratory testing (see Table 42.1). Clinical evidence of envenoming is generally classified as:

- paralysis of any degree (ptosis, ophthalmoplegia, limb weakness and respiratory muscle failure)
- loss of consciousness
- seizure activity
- anuria, oliguria, myoglobinuria
- bleeding disorders (abnormal bleeding from IV sites, bite site, gums, nose or wounds or haematoma formation at IM sites).

This means that patients presenting with isolated general symptoms such as vomiting, abdominal pain and headache do not normally qualify for antivenom, but a combination of these symptoms should be considered with a strong suspicion.

Swabbing the bite site is the most accurate method of venom detection but in patients already displaying signs of systemic envenoming urine may be used, although this is unreliable for some snake species including brown snakes. Blood testing is also

unreliable. A positive swab for snake venom does *not* confirm envenoming and antivenom should only be administered in patients displaying evidence of systemic envenoming. Venom detection should never be used as a screening test for snake bite. If there is clinical evidence of envenoming (or laboratory testing confirms it) and antivenom is required, then the choices are to use a polyvalent antivenom (higher risk and cost), a combination of two different monovalent antivenoms (but you must know which snakes may be involved, based on geographic location) or (ideally) give a monovalent antivenom specifically targeting the snake involved. To follow the latter, ideal course implies that the identity of the snake is reasonably assured. This is straightforward if the snake has been killed and then expertly identified or if the snake was a captive specimen of known identity; however, in most cases the snake identity will not be known. In this latter, common setting the most reliable course is to use a two-factor system, combining results from a diagnostic algorithm for snake bite (available since 1994) and separate venom detection (Snake Venom Detection Kit [SVDK]). If both give a similar answer, choosing an appropriate antivenom is straightforward; however, if they give quite different answers then it will be necessary to give polyvalent antivenom or, sometimes, a mixture of two monovalent antivenoms.

If the patient does not display evidence of systemic envenoming, the antivenom and other drugs should be prepared for administration but not given unless necessary and the PBI should be released. Antivenom should never be drawn up unless it is definitely going to be used. Leaving the PBI in place simply delays absorption and does not deactivate the venom, so once all preparations are in place it can be removed and the patient closely monitored for symptoms. If the patient is displaying systemic effects, the PBI should not be removed until the initial antivenom therapy has been completed.

Dosages and intervals of antivenom administration vary according to the degree of symptoms and the type of antivenom available, but it is usually diluted 1:10 with crystalloid fluids and given over 30 minutes. Clinicians should be guided by expert consultation regarding the exact dose, dilution and rate of infusion. Given in an effective dose, antivenom will stop the progression of presynaptic neurotoxicity but will not reverse the already established paralysis. However, postsynaptic neurotoxicity is sometimes rapidly reversed, as are the effects of anticoagulant toxins. Antivenom will also stop the progression of procoagulant toxins but it can take up to 48 hours for the recovery of a normal coagulation pattern, although return to detectable clotting parameters (INR, aPTT, fibrinogen) should occur within 6–8 hrs of giving a sufficient dose of the appropriate antivenom.

Fresh frozen plasma and whole blood

Appropriate doses of antivenom prevent the progression of coagulopathies but in the case of defibrination coagulopathy it can take several hours for the body to regenerate sufficient clotting factors to protect the patient from serious haemorrhage. Administration of fresh frozen plasma (FFP) and/or cryoprecipitate to assist in regeneration of a normal clotting profile is not recommended as a routine procedure, but may be beneficial in patients with active major and life-threatening bleeding who have already received an appropriate dose of antivenom. Administration of whole blood is rarely required.

Adrenaline

Allergic responses to antivenom occur in about 5% of cases and snake handlers who have previously had antivenom are more susceptible. Premedication prior to giving antivenom has not been a recommended procedure in Australia for many years. Steroids and antihistamines have no proven benefit in prophylaxis of acute adverse reactions to antivenom, but subcutaneous adrenaline (0.1–0.3 mg in adults) 5 minutes before commencing the antivenom infusion may have benefit in specific situations, such as patients with known allergy to antivenom. If an anaphylactic reaction does occur, the antivenom infusion should be suspended until the reaction is controlled. Reactions can be related to the rate of infusion and a slower rate once symptoms have resolved can be effective.

Steroids

Serum sickness can occur 4–14 days following antivenom administration and some centres recommend a prophylactic course of oral corticosteroids.

Investigations

In-hospital investigations of patients include generic full blood examinations, extended coagulation studies, electrolytes, creatine kinase, renal function and urine output. The patient's motor and sensory function, as well as their wound, should be monitored for changes (see Table 42.2).

Hospital admission

While there are no universally accepted guidelines for the length of time an asymptomatic patient should be observed before being cleared of envenoming, in Australia 12 hours is the generally recommended minimum time for observation, or longer if the discharge time occurs during the night. These times can be extended for snakes that have longer-acting venoms, such as death adders.

Infections at the bite site are rare and any local swelling usually resolves without treatment. As such, antibiotics are not routinely prescribed but prophylactic treatment for tetanus is recommended, although this should only be administered after any coagulopathy has resolved.

Long-term impact

Recovery from severe envenoming can take months if paralysis, rhabdomyolysis, AKI or other severe complications occur. Changes in smell, taste and other cranial nerve functions can also persist for months and in some cases may be permanent.

Snake bites across the lifespan

Detecting snake bites in children can be difficult if the attack was not witnessed: bite marks can easily

Table 42.2: Clinical and laboratory profiles following snake bites

Laboratory profile	Clinical profile	Snake
Defibrination coagulopathy	No paralysis or myolysis Bite site has minimal pain No significant bruising or redness Slight ooze of blood	Brown snake Broad-headed snake (Stephens' banded snake and pale-headed snake)
Defibrination coagulopathy + paralysis, no myolysis	Variable paralysis Bite site has usually minimal pain No significant swelling Oozing of blood from bite site	Brown snake (rare presentation; nearly all brown snake bites do not develop features of paralysis)
Defibrination coagulopathy + paralysis ± mild myolysis	Bite site is variable Slight ooze of blood	Taipan and inland taipan
Defibrination coagulopathy + paralysis + moderate to severe myolysis	Bite site is usually painful Mild swelling Bruising, redness Ooze of blood evident	Tiger snake Rough-scaled snake
Moderate to marked myolysis + anticoagulant coagulopathy	No paralysis (beware major myolysis mimicking paralysis) Bite site is painful Marked swelling and bruising Persistent blood ooze not common	Mulga snake Collett's snake Spotted black snake Red-bellied black snake
Moderate to marked myolysis	No paralysis (beware major myolysis mimicking paralysis) No coagulopathy Bite site is usually painful Marked swelling and bruising	Mulga snake Collett's snake Spotted black snake Red-bellied black snake Eastern small-eyed snake
Paralysis (usually postsynaptic which may reverse with antivenom) ± (rarely) mild anticoagulant coagulopathy	No myolysis and renal damage unlikely Bite site often painful Little swelling, redness or bruising Persistent blood ooze unlikely	Death adder Copperhead
No paralysis or coagulopathy No or mild myolysis	General symptoms of envenoming (headache, nausea, vomiting, diarrhoea, abdominal pain, dizziness, collapse)	Red-bellied black snake Spotted black snake Collett's snake Yellow-faced whip snake Other large whip snakes

be confused with everyday scratches and marks. The early signs can also be difficult to detect. Children are at greater risk of developing systemic effects as their reduced body weight effectively increases the venom dose. The pattern of envenoming and management for snake bite in children is similar to that in adults, although children are more likely to develop an early episode of collapse and sometimes convulsions. There may be significant difficulties in obtaining an accurate history from children because they are too young to verbalise a meaningful history, or the child may not recognise a snake, may not have seen the snake, or was bitten and did not realise the importance of snake envenoming. As a clinician it is important to recognise any potential bite as a snake bite/envenoming through accurate history taking and all clinical investigations should be carried out, including transport to hospital for

confirmation of negative envenoming. Children require the same dose of antivenom as adults.

The presence of preexisting medical conditions may adversely influence the outcomes in elderly people who have been envenomed by a snake. The prevalence of preexisting conditions increases significantly with age and certainly for those elderly patients envenomed by snakes such as the tiger snake, defibrination coagulopathy can be a rapid feature that may lead to cerebral haemorrhage. This is especially true for those patients on drugs like anticoagulants ('blood thinners') that will enhance this process.

In addition to seeking immediate medical assistance, the public and health professionals can contact their nearest Poisons Information Centre for further advice about the presenting symptoms (see Box 42.2).

BOX 42.2 Sources of expert advice

Clinical toxinology service

For health professionals there is a specialised clinical toxinology service available through the Women's & Children's Hospital, Adelaide; 08-81617000; ask for the duty clinical toxinologist.

Poisons information centres

There are four Poisons Information Centres operating in Queensland, New South Wales, Western Australia and Victoria. Each centre has trained staff who provide telephone consultations 24 hours per day to medical professionals and the general public in cases of acute and chronic poisonings. They provide toxicological advice on the management of exposure to prescription and non-prescription pharmaceuticals, household and industrial chemicals, plants, animal envenomings, pesticides and other agricultural products.

To contact the nearest Poisons Information Centre, telephone 13 11 26 or check these websites:

- Queensland Poisons Information Centre: www health.qld.gov.au/poisonsinformationcentre
- Victorian Poisons Information Centre: www. austin.org.au/poisons
- Western Australia Poisons Information Centre: www.scgh.health.wa.gov.au/Clinicians/ Services/PoisonInformationCentre.html
- New South Wales Poisons Information Centre: www.chw.edu.au/poisons

CASE STUDY 2

Case 19433, 1220 hrs.

Dispatch details: A 59-year-old male has been found unconscious by the dam on his property. He is breathing. The crew will be met at the farmhouse and directed to the patient.

Initial presentation: The crew are met at the house by the patient's son and follow him 500 m to the dam. The patient is lying on his right side near the top of the dam wall.

1 ASSESS

1230 hrs Primary survey: The patient is unconscious. GCS = 6 (E1, V2, M3).

1231 hrs Vital signs survey: Perfusion status: HR 135 bpm; sinus tachycardia; BP 80/50 mmHg; skin cool, pale and clammy.

Respiratory status: RR 10 bpm, shallow respirations, no adventitious sounds, normal pattern, air entry L = R. SpO$_2$ not sensing.

Conscious state: GCS = 6.

1232 hrs Pertinent hx: The patient's wife left home at 9.30 am. The patient said he was going to check the dam pump after slashing the paddock. She arrived back at 12.15 pm and saw his tractor parked at the dam. When she couldn't find him she went down to the dam and discovered him. He was prone when found and was rolled onto his right side.

1233 hrs secondary survey: The patient has a small graze on his forehead, which is oozing blood. His pupils are dilated and sluggish. He has an abrasion and swelling to the left hand and wrist area. There may be a small puncture wound under the abrasion but it is difficult to confirm.

1234 hrs Past hx: The patient is normally well and takes no medications.

The clinical presentation is consistent with snake bite and the hand wound may be a bite. The persistent bleeding from the head wound is also consistent (coagulopathy). Snake-bite envenoming is a likely explanation for the patient's presentation, but in the absence of any clear corroborating history or findings the potential diagnosis is still wide open.

② CONFIRM

In many cases paramedics are presented with a collection of signs and symptoms that do not appear to describe a particular condition. A critical step in determining a treatment plan in this situation is to consider what other conditions could explain the patient's presentation.

What else could it be?

Cardiovascular

While the patient is poorly perfused, this is not so dramatic as to be the underlying cause of his altered conscious state. The ECG is normal. This requires further investigation.

Stroke

A cerebral bleed would explain the altered conscious state but is inconsistent with the poor perfusion.

Hypoglycaemia

The symptoms are consistent with hypoglycaemia: altered conscious state, poor perfusion and diaphoresis. The lack of history cannot be used to rule this out, so a BGL should be taken.

Infection/sepsis

The lack of a fever cannot be used to exclude sepsis, especially in a patient who has been outside for a period of time, but the deterioration from when he was last seen well to becoming unconscious would be very atypical.

Trauma

The tractor is parked 10 m away. The minor head injury does not explain the lack of perfusion but the possibility of cervical injury needs to be considered. A cervical spine collar should be applied before transport.

Near-drowning

There are no tracks leading from the water. The patient is damp but not drenched and his chest sounds are clear. This possibility is unlikely.

Poisoning

The farm does not use organophosphates and there is no spraying equipment on the tractor.

Anaphylaxis

The poor perfusion is typical of anaphylaxis and given the number of allergens in the surrounding area this cannot be confidently excluded. The lack of erythema or urticaria does not preclude anaphylaxis. This cannot be excluded at this stage.

This is a case where it is impossible to definitely make a diagnosis in the field and the paramedics must manage the patient symptomatically and resolve the basic issues of airway, breathing and circulation before reassessing to see whether the underlying cause has become clearer.

③ TREAT

1240 hrs: The paramedics initiate oxygen at 8 L/min via a bag-valve-mask and his breathing is supplemented to 12–16 bpm at 8–10 mL/kg. They

---

> ### DIFFERENTIAL DIAGNOSIS ②
>
> **Snake envenoming**
> Or
> - Cardiovascular
> - Stroke
> - Hypoglycaemia
> - Infection/sepsis
> - Trauma
> - Near-drowning
> - Poisoning
> - Anaphylaxis

administer 0.3 mg of adrenaline IM to his left lateral thigh, as anaphylaxis is impossible to rule out and the IM route is safe and quick. They apply a PBI and splint to his left arm, then establish IV access and fluid load initially at 10–20 mL/kg. Finally, they apply a cervical collar.

1250 hrs: Perfusion status: HR 124 bpm, sinus tachycardia, BP 90/50 mmHg, skin cool and clammy.

Respiratory status: RR 12 bpm, air entry L = R, normal work of breathing.
Conscious state: GCS = 6.

The patient's symptoms are unresolved despite a slight improvement in perfusion.

1252 hrs: The paramedics repeat 0.3 mg of adrenaline IM in his left lateral thigh. (They consider IV infusion, referring to local guidelines.) They continue IV fluid.

1257 hrs: Perfusion status: HR 124 bpm, sinus tachycardia, BP 90/50 mmHg, skin cool and clammy.

Respiratory status: RR 12 bpm, air entry L = R, normal work of breathing.
Conscious state: GCS = 6.

④ EVALUATE

Evaluating the effect of any clinical management intervention can provide clues to the accuracy of the initial diagnosis. Some conditions respond rapidly to treatment so patients should be expected to improve if the diagnosis and treatment were appropriate. A failure to improve in this situation should trigger the clinician to reconsider the diagnosis.

In this case the treatment for anaphylaxis should have generated an improvement in the patient's condition. The patient's failure to improve, in combination with his poor respiratory effort, suggests that envenoming is the primary cause.

The paramedics focus on supporting the patient's ventilations and if this cannot be achieved effectively with non-invasive techniques, they will consider endotracheal intubation according to local guidelines. They also notify the receiving hospital of the suspected envenoming and expedite transport. It is unlikely that the patient will improve significantly during transport and progressive respiratory failure due to paralysis should be expected.

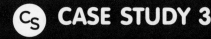

CASE STUDY 3

Case 16563, 1115 hrs.

Dispatch details: A 19-year-old male is complaining of numbness. He has no traumatic injuries. He is being carried to a riverside carpark.

Initial presentation: The crew are met at the carpark where a bushwalking group have carried their companion for approximately 1 km.

HISTORY

Ask!
- Have you had any falls recently?
- Have there been any changes to your medications recently?
- What is your medical history?
- Do you have a history of depression?
- Have you taken any illicit drugs or alcohol?

DIFFERENTIAL DIAGNOSIS

Snake envenoming
Or
- Cardiovascular problem
- Anaphylaxis
- Stroke

PRACTICE TIP

Seizure activity is sometimes associated with envenoming, particularly in young children.

ASSESS

1150 hrs Primary survey: The patient is lying supine and is semiconscious. He moans to painful stimuli but moves his limbs weakly. There is no obvious injury.

1151 hrs Vital signs survey: Perfusion status: HR 115 bpm, sinus rhythm, BP 70/P; skin warm, pink, clammy.

Respiratory status: RR 6 bpm, air entry L = R, no adventitious sounds, shallow regular breaths, SpO_2 = 92% on room air.

Conscious state: GCS = 10 (E = 4, M = 4, V = 2); weak withdrawal, moaning quietly.

1153 hrs Pertinent hx: The group have spent the last 3 days bushwalking and were almost back at the carpark when one member complained of 'numbness' in his right leg. The group leader examined his leg but found no abnormalities. Over the next 10 minutes the patient developed a facial paralysis that started to spread down his chest. He described the sensation to the group as if his face was 'falling off'. The group called for help using a mobile phone and started to carry him along the trail to the carpark. The patient's partner states that he has no significant medical history, was not complaining of anything prior to the paralysis and did not suffer any falls during the walk.

1154 hrs Secondary survey: Pupils dilated and sluggish, ptosis. Multiple scratches to both legs. The patient is wearing shorts and high-top boots.

BGL: 6.1 mmol/L.

Temperature: 36.2°C.

The pressure to reach a diagnosis can often delay management which the patient needs immediately.

CONFIRM

In many cases paramedics are presented with a collection of signs and symptoms that do not appear to describe a particular condition. A critical step in determining a treatment plan in this situation is to consider what other conditions could explain the patient's presentation.

Envenoming is a possibility in this case and a lack of a clear history of a bite does not mean it can be excluded. It is not uncommon for patients to have been bitten but not to have noticed it when walking or working in rough bushland, particularly for brown snakes.

What else could it be?
Cardiovascular problem
While the patient is poorly perfused, this does not offer an explanation for the underlying cause of his altered conscious state. The ECG is normal. This requires further investigation.

Anaphylaxis
The poor perfusion is typical of anaphylaxis but the paraesthesia and paralysis are not consistent.

Stroke
A cerebral bleed would explain the altered conscious state, but is inconsistent with the poor perfusion and is unusual for the patient's age.

TREAT

The patient suddenly moans and experiences a tonic–clonic seizure. Regardless of the provisional diagnosis, generalised seizure activity needs to be managed immediately.

1155 hrs: The paramedics administer midazolam 0.1 mg/kg IM.

1158 hrs: The patient's seizure activity ceases.

1158 hrs: Perfusion status: HR 125 bpm; sinus rhythm; BP 70/50 mmHg; skin cool, pale and clammy.

Respiratory status: RR 6 bpm, air entry L = R, no adventitious sounds, shallow regular breaths, SpO_2 = 90% on 100% oxygen.

Conscious state: GCS = 3.

1201 hrs: The paramedics administer crystalloid fluids at 20 mL/kg.

1202 hrs: The paramedics apply a PBI to the patient's right leg as this was the first point where symptoms were noted.

 4 EVALUATE

Evaluating the effect of any clinical management intervention can provide clues to the accuracy of the initial diagnosis. Some conditions respond rapidly to treatment so patients should be expected to improve if the diagnosis and treatment were appropriate. In this case it is unlikely that the patient will improve significantly if the diagnosis of envenoming is correct.

With the limited resources available in the out-of-hospital setting, paramedic treatment should focus on providing symptomatic support and transporting the patient to an appropriate facility that is aware of his condition. The paramedics notify the receiving hospital of the suspected envenoming and expedite transport. Progressive respiratory failure due to paralysis should be expected.

Future research

The discovery of the effect of the Brazilian jararaca (*Bothrops jararaca*) venom on the inflammatory mediator bradykinin eventually led to the development of the antihypertensive group of drugs known as angiotensin converting enzyme (ACE) inhibitors. The complex effects and mechanisms of snake venom hold the promise of new drugs and treatments for a variety of conditions.

Summary

Envenoming from snake bite is a life-threatening emergency that can present with a variety of symptoms, and is often complicated by delayed access and prolonged transport. Paramedics are regularly the first healthcare professionals to assess these patients and astute assessment, management and planning can reduce fatalities and complications. Seeking in-field consultations from experts is strongly recommended. A specialised clinical toxicology service is available for healthcare professionals through the Women's and Children's Hospital, Adelaide on 08 8161 7000; ask for the duty clinical toxinologist.

References

Auerbach, P. S. (2013). *Field guide to wilderness medicine* (4th ed.). St Louis: Mosby.

Australian Resuscitation Council. (2011). *Guideline 9.4. Envenoming: Australian Snake Bite.* Retrieved from: www.resus.org.au/policy/guidelines/index.asp. (Accessed 15 December 2011).

Harris, P., Nagy, S., & Vardaxis, N. (2010). *Mosby's dictionary of medicine, nursing & health professions* (2nd ed.). Sydney: Elsevier.

Ireland, G., Brown, S. G., Buckley, N. A., Stormer, J., Currie, B. J., White, J., Spain, D., Isbister, G. K.,

Australian Snakebite Project Investigators. (2010). Changes in serial laboratory test results in snake-bite patients: when can we safely exclude envenoming? *The Medical Journal of Australia, 193*, 285–290.

Isbister, G. K., Brown, S., Page, C. B., McCoubrie, D., Greene, S. L., & Buckley, N. A. (2013). Snake bite in Australia: a practical approach to diagnosis and treatment. *The Medical Journal of Australia, 199*, 11.

Miller, R. D., Eriksson, L., Fleisher, L., Wiener-Kronish, J., & Young, W. (2009). *Miller's anesthesia* (7th ed.). Philadelphia: Elsevier.

CHAPTER 43

Spider Bites

By Julian White

OVERVIEW

- In Australia most spider bites occur during the warmer months between December and April.
- Almost three-quarters of spider-bite cases involve bites to the patient's upper or lower extremities.
- Any bite from a large > 2 cm dark-coloured spider in Sydney, the Blue Mountains, the Central, Northern and Southern Highlands, the South Coast of New South Wales and Southeast Queensland should be considered as a potentially dangerous bite (Australian Resuscitation Council [ARC], 2014).

- Basic first aid such as an icepack or a cold compress is an effective management regimen for some spider bites and may reduce pain.
- The redback spider bite is the most common envenoming requiring antivenom in Australia. Antivenom may be indicated for patients who present with clinical evidence of envenoming by a redback spider, but symptoms may be more severe in the young and the elderly.

Introduction

In Australia, envenoming by several species of spider requires treatment. These species include:

- redback spider
- funnel-web spiders (numerous species)
- mouse spider (several species).

Bites by other species require either no treatment, or only minor first aid and pain management. These species include:

- trap-door spiders
- garden orb-weaving spiders
- Saint Andrew's Cross spider
- huntsman spiders
- wolf spiders
- white-tailed spiders
- black house spiders.

Pathophysiology

Redback spider

Only the female redback spider is considered dangerous. It can grow to approximately 10 mm in abdomen size, and has a round black body, usually with a distinct red, orange or brown stripe on the back, with a smaller cephalothorax (front part of body) (see Fig 43.1). The spider generally does not bite unless provoked by direct contact, handling or squeezing. The venom may take several hours to act in some cases, causing significant regional or systemic envenoming, the latter delayed up to about 24 hours in some cases. However, not all bites cause envenoming and only a minority develop systemic envenoming. The venom is rarely life-threatening in adults. Prior to the introduction of

redback antivenom in 1956, 13 deaths from redback bites were reported in Australia. There have been no reported deaths since the introduction of the antivenom.

The cardinal symptoms of redback spider envenoming include pain at the site of the bite with or without erythema and local sweating, developing within minutes to an hour of the bite, which may then progress over hours to involve the entire limb and draining lymph nodes in the axilla or groin. The area around the bite can be quite pale and sweaty, with surrounding erythema. In more severe cases the pain may spread to other parts of the body, potentially causing severe chest pain mimicking myocardial ischaemia, or abdominal pain mimicking acute abdomen. The pain is often accompanied by localised, regionalised or generalised profuse sweating and sometimes hypertension and nausea, less commonly vomiting. In patients with delayed presentation irrespective of the site of the bite, symptoms may gravitate to both legs, with burning pain in the feet, and pain and profuse sweating below the knees. In infants envenoming may present as a very irritable crying child with widespread erythema.

Patients presenting even many hours after the bite will usually respond to antivenom, even if given 24 hours later. The pain relief from administration of antivenom is rapid and dramatic, becoming established within minutes to an hour or so of administration. However, a 2014 clinical study (RAVE-II; Isbister et al., 2014) claimed to show that antivenom was ineffective, in conflict with over 50 years' clinical experience in Australia. Unless this study is replicated independently, it seems unwise

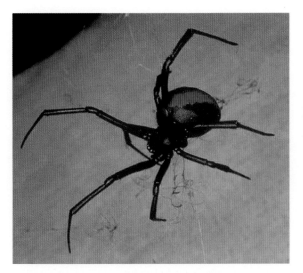

Figure 43.1
Redback spider (*Latrodectus hasselti*).
Females have a pea-shaped abdomen with a
distinctive red marking and long slender legs.
Females are larger than males, which tend to brown
rather than black and lack the red stripe (they may
have a white stripe). The spider lives in tight, dark
spaces (e.g. under logs, hard rubbish).
Photo copyright © Julian White.

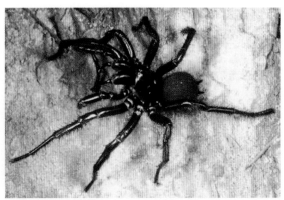

Figure 43.2
Funnel-web spider (*Atrax robustus*).
The Sydney funnel-web is found within 100 km of
Sydney and ranges from 1 to 5 cm in body length.
The male is smaller but both sexes are glossy and
hairless and range from blue-black to black or brown
in colour.
Photo copyright © Julian White.

to mandate a change in clinical practice, especially
given that the alternative 'treatment' has not proven
effective when in particular compared with historical
and overseas experience with antivenom. There is
no evidence-based effective first aid for redback
spider envenoming and pressure bandaging and
immobilisation (PBI) should not be used as it may
increase severity of local pain.

Funnel-web spiders

Funnel-web spiders are arguably the most dangerous
spiders in the world. There are about 35 species in
the *Hexathelidae* family with three genera (*Atrax,
Hadronyche, Illawarra*). Although there are numerous big black spiders throughout Australia, clinical
reasoning is based around the geography of where the
patient was bitten as many spiders look similar to the
funnel-web but are not dangerous. The distribution
of the funnel-web is roughly coastal New South Wales
(see Fig 43.2), Southeast Queensland and some parts
of Victoria and South Australia (although they may be
found further afield when unintentionally transported
with agricultural goods). The toxicity of the spider's
venom is considered due to potent neuro-excitatory
delta-atracotoxins: the amino acid structure differs
between different species of funnel-web spiders, possibly based on their geographical location (Graudins
et al., 2002). Once bitten, delta-atracotoxins bind to

the outer surface of tetrodotoxin-sensitive sodium
channels and induce excitability, resulting in a major
outpouring of autonomic nervous system activity.
A sympathetic storm comprised of acetylcholine,
noradrenaline and adrenaline is responsible for the
clinical findings of funnel-web envenoming (Graudins
et al., 2002). The introduction of a specific funnel-
web spider antivenom in about 1981 dramatically
changed the outlook for envenoming by these spiders,
with most cases rapidly responding to antivenom
and no reported fatalities. The rapidity of onset of
systemic envenoming mandates urgent PBI first aid
and transport to a hospital where the antivenom
can be given.

Mouse spiders

Mouse spiders are medium-to-large size spiders with
a length of up to 35 mm and are Mygalomorph
spiders related to funnel-
web spiders. In one species
the males have a distinctive
red anterior cephalothorax
('head'). These spiders may
potentially be dangerous
to humans, particularly
to the young, although
most recorded bites have
been minor, with only one
case with major systemic
envenoming, in a child.
The fangs are large and
firm and can cause a
painful bite. Their venom
has similarities to funnel-
web spider venom.

> ## SPIDER BITES
> **Look for!**
> - Immediate pain at the site that may progress over 5–10 minutes
> - Hot, red, swollen bite site
> - Localised sweating around the bite site
> - Nausea, vomiting and abdominal cramps
> - Swollen, tender glands in the groin or armpit of the envenomed limb

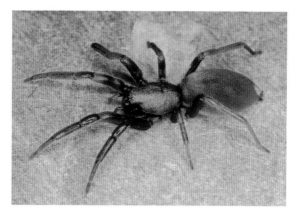

Figure 43.3
White-tailed spider (*Lampona cylindrata*).
The white-tailed spider is a nocturnal hunter of other spiders. It has a dark-grey body with legs tending to reddish brown and the front two pairs are angled forwards. The abdomen may have a dull-white spot at the tip.
Photo copyright © Julian White.

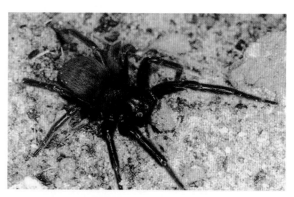

Figure 43.4
Black house spider.
This spider is commonly found behind a lacy funnel-like web in small cracks on buildings and trees. It is fearsome looking but usually timid.
Photo copyright © Julian White.

White-tailed spider

Although the white-tailed spider (see Fig 43.3) may cause pain and mild inflammation at the site of envenoming, there have been no reported cases of local tissue destruction as once thought (ARC, 2014). Despite significant studies into the spider's venom, no reported toxicity has been identified (ARC, 2014) and this spider should not be considered as medically significant.

Black house spider

This brown-black spider measures about 15 mm in length (see Fig 43.4). Its bite is not considered dangerous to humans. Symptoms include localised pain, and uncommonly, sweating, dizziness, headache and vomiting.

Wolf spider

The common wolf spider is grey to brown in colour, although there are many species, with varying colours. It ranges in size from 15 to 30 mm. Like the black house spider, it is not considered dangerous.

Huntsman spider

These are common both outside and inside houses. There are numerous species, many large and able to deliver initially painful bites that may draw blood, but significant envenoming is not expected.

Orb-weaving spider

There are numerous species of orb-weaving spider, which has a diverse appearance and is able to deliver a bite that often causes only minor localised pain, without systemic effects. Classically, this spider may be found in washing left on the line overnight and a bite occurs when someone puts on one of these items of clothing.

 CASE STUDY 1

Case 10107, 1115 hrs.

Dispatch details: A 3-year-old girl has been bitten by a spider. She is distressed.

Initial presentation: The crew find the patient sitting on her mother's lap—she is crying inconsolably. There is an icepack on the bite site but the child keeps pushing it away.

① ASSESS

Patient history

Determining the underlying cause of the child's presentation in this case is not difficult. The child's parents state that she was playing in her father's shed when she suddenly screamed out in pain. Her father ran to the shed where he saw a spider with a distinct red stripe and approximately 10 mm in length sitting on the child's hand. He instinctively swiped at it with his hand and then stood on the spider, killing it. The child was taken inside and consoled by her mother while an icepack was applied to the bite site. Approximately 2 hours post-bite the child started to become progressively more distressed and complained of abdominal pain.

The key to effective clinical reasoning in this case is not being complacent that this is just a redback spider bite and the child will recover: this child has progressively deteriorated and is likely to need antivenom. The primary focus is to provide further pain relief if necessary and commence transporting the patient to a facility that has antivenom. An initial set of vital signs will act as a baseline against which to measure any changes.

Airway

The patient does not have any airway involvement. The airway should always be assessed, as some venoms do produce an anaphylactic-type response that can involve the airway. Respiratory distress is not a likely problem in redback spider envenoming.

Breathing

This child has no trouble with breathing, but again, this must be thoroughly assessed.

Cardiovascular

This child is still crying, so she has a moderate level of perfusion. Ongoing assessment should be carried out to determine trends in her presentation. Is her blood pressure measurable (difficult in a distressed 3 year old) and, if measurable and elevated, is this due to distress and crying, or an underlying envenoming effect?

Gastrointestinal

The child is complaining of abdominal pain.

The bite site

At the bite site there is localised sweating around a small puncture wound. The father says the area where the spider was sitting when he found his daughter became hot and red immediately.

Initial assessment summary

Problem	Redback spider envenoming
Conscious state	GCS = 15
Position	Sitting on her mother's lap
Heart rate	120 bpm
Blood pressure	Unable to measure due to patient distress, but capillary refill < 2 seconds
Skin appearance	Pink, warm, dry
Speech pattern	Crying inconsolably
Respiratory rate	30 bpm
Respiratory rhythm	Appears even, child crying
Chest auscultation	Difficult to assess, but appears clear, normal work of breathing

HISTORY

Ask!
- What did the spider look like? What markings did it have?
- When were you bitten? What were the circumstances of the bite?
- Are the symptoms getting better or worse now?
- What treatment, if any, have you initiated?
- Were any symptoms evident prior to the bite?

Pulse oximetry	Unable to apply probe to child
Temperature	37.2°C
Motor/sensory function	Appears normal
Pain	Appears severe: she is crying inconsolably and guarding her abdomen and the site of the bite
History	Bitten by a redback spider approximately 2 hours ago
Physical assessment	Localised redness and swelling around the puncture site

D: The patient has moved away from any dangers.

A: The patient is conscious with no current airway obstruction but needs frequent reassessment.

B: Respiratory function is currently normal but needs frequent reassessment. The respiratory rate is elevated but ventilation is normal.

C: Heart rate is elevated but perfusion appears adequate.

There is no evidence of the cutaneous, respiratory or cardiovascular symptoms of an anaphylactic reaction.

② CONFIRM

The essential part of the clinical reasoning process is to seek to confirm your initial hypothesis by finding clinical signs that should occur with your provisional diagnosis. You should also seek to challenge your diagnosis by exploring findings that do not fit your hypothesis: don't just ignore them because they don't fit.

The clinical reasoning in this case revolves around whether or not the patient's current symptoms are associated with a redback spider bite or could be caused by some other pathology and the redback spider is a coincidental element in the scenario.

What else could it be?

Acute abdominal issue

The abdominal pain may be consistent with a patient suffering appendicitis or another acute abdominal complaint. However, it seems to have developed too rapidly for this to be considered a likely diagnosis.

Anxiety

The most common issue surrounding children receiving painful animal bites is anxiety and it is not uncommon for children to develop persistent symptoms such as inconsolable crying due to the bite. In this case it is reasonable for the patient to be anxious and the paramedics need to assume she is suffering from envenoming until proven otherwise.

Allergic reaction

In cases where the patient presents with poor perfusion, diarrhoea and abdominal pain, it is extremely difficult to exclude this pathology. If there is a history of sensitisation and the signs are consistent with a generalised anaphylaxis, the paramedics should treat with adrenaline as for any anaphylaxis. Treatment with adrenaline will not have an adverse effect on the management of spider-bite envenoming.

③ TREAT

Emergency management

Safety

The child's father was instrumental in removing and killing the spider, as well as identifying the species.

Pressure immobilisation and splinting

The pressure immobilisation technique is not used in patients who have been envenomed by a redback spider as the venom acts slowly and any attempt to restrict the movement of the venom increases the local pain.

DIFFERENTIAL DIAGNOSIS ②

Spider envenoming
Or
- Acute abdominal issue
- Anxiety
- Allergic reaction
- Drug reaction
- Analgesia-seeking behaviour

Ice and/or analgesia

There is no clear evidence that an icepack application, in an attempt to reduce the pain, is effective. Oral and/or parenteral analgesia may be considered according to local guidelines.

Antiemetics

Symptomatic relief of significant nausea with intravenous/intramuscular (IV/IM) antiemetics should be administered according to local guidelines, though this is not commonly required in redback spider envenoming; however, administration in paediatric patients may be contraindicated. In addition, some antiemetics such as metoclopramide can produce drowsiness: if a patient deteriorates and becomes drowsy, paramedics should remember to consider their interventions as a possible cause.

④ EVALUATE

Evaluating the effect of any clinical management intervention can provide clues to the accuracy of the initial diagnosis. Some conditions respond rapidly to treatment so patients should be expected to improve if the diagnosis and treatment were appropriate. A failure to improve in this situation should trigger the clinician to reconsider the diagnosis. In the setting of spider bites, treatment is generally aimed at managing symptoms rather than providing definitive care, but there are exceptions to this. In particular, for bites by funnel-web spiders, causing medically significant systemic envenoming, neutralisation of circulating venom using specific antivenom is both definitive and lifesaving. Since this antivenom was introduced in the 1980s there have been no confirmed deaths following funnel-web spider bite, compared to at least 13 deaths prior to availability of antivenom.

Continuous reassessment of suspected redback spider victims is essential as the progression of symptoms allows paramedics to plan and prepare for more serious complications. Sometimes the progression can be slow and if, in the paramedic's clinical judgment, the patient does not need to be transported to hospital, clear and concise advice should be left with the patient's carer explaining the potential delay in symptoms and what to look out for. However, deciding this may be beyond the scope of paramedics who should always consider seeking expert advice in such situations.

Is the patient:
- Still suffering significant pain?
  › Consider oral and/or parenteral pain relief.
- Deteriorating?
  › Fully reassess the patient to rule out other potential underlying causes.
- Showing clinical signs of significant regional or systemic envenoming?
  › Ensure that the receiving hospital is notified.

Ongoing hospital management

Unless the patient is showing signs of significant envenoming not adequately responding to analgesia, antivenom administration should be reserved until at least major regional or systemic signs are showing, which may be 1–3 hours post-bite and in some cases up to 24 hours. The antivenom consists of a small volume (~0.5–1.5 mL) of an antibody that is derived from horse serum. There is a low incidence of allergic reaction. Administration has historically been given IM, as recommended in the product information, but there is an increasing trend to use it IV as this provides more rapid significant circulating levels. Certainly if envenoming is severe IV administration should be considered by medical staff. The commonly recommended initial dose is 2 vials (not 1 vial as stated in the PI). Because redback spider bite is most unlikely to cause rapid life-threatening envenoming, it is usually inappropriate to consider antivenom administration in an out-of-hospital setting; therefore, it is unlikely a paramedic will be justified in giving antivenom out of hospital.

Hospital admission

There are no universally accepted guidelines for the length of time an asymptomatic patient should be observed before being cleared of envenoming. Infections at the bite site are rare and any local swelling usually resolves without treatment. As such, antibiotics are not routinely prescribed. For uncomplicated minor redback spider bites not requiring antivenom, discharge after 6 hours would be routine.

Long-term impact

Patients who have received antivenom may develop serum sickness (an immune complex-mediated hypersensitivity reaction) 4–14 days post-injection. They should be advised of the symptoms, which can include fever, rash, arthritis and joint pain. Paramedics should also be aware of the symptoms

in case they are called to a patient suffering these signs and symptoms and the patient history shows that they have been administered antivenom.

Spider bites across the lifespan

Bites are equally common in children and adults, but as is the case with envenoming of any aetiology, children who are envenomed may suffer more severe signs and symptoms because of the greater venom toxicity per kilogram of body weight. Death is now an unheard-of outcome from redback spider bite, even in children, and the reasons for fatalities in the pre-antivenom era are unclear. The dose of redback antivenom should not be reduced for children.

The presence of preexisting conditions may adversely influence the outcome in elderly patients who have been envenomed by a redback spider. The prevalence of preexisting conditions increases significantly with age.

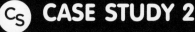

CASE STUDY 2

Case 10515, 1720 hrs.

Dispatch details: A 29-year-old pregnant female has been found unconscious by her husband in the family home near Gosford, New South Wales.

Initial presentation: The paramedics are met at the house and follow the patient's husband to a bedroom located at the rear of the property. The patient is lying in a supine position with obvious frothy sputum around her mouth.

 ASSESS

1723 hrs Primary survey: The patient is unconscious: GCS = 3 (E1, V1, M1).

1724 hrs Vital signs survey: Perfusion status: HR 135 bpm; sinus tachycardia; BP 180/90 mmHg; skin cool, pale and sweating. SpO_2 = 88%.

Respiratory status: RR 32 bpm, shallow respirations with bilateral coarse crackles consistent with pulmonary oedema.

Conscious state: GCS = 3.

1726 hrs Pertinent hx: The patient's husband received a phone call from her 20 minutes ago. She was very agitated and stated that she felt unwell and was bitten by a large black spider that hung on and had to be shaken off. He rushed home and found his wife in the bedroom, unresponsive. When he couldn't wake her he called the ambulance.

1727 hrs Secondary survey: Abrasion and two bite marks to the patient's left hand. No other abnormalities found.

1727 hrs Past hx: The patient is normally well and takes no medications. She is 24 weeks' gestation with no reported complications with the pregnancy. This is her first pregnancy.

The patient is unconscious with pulmonary oedema, tachycardia and tachypnoea. The potential causes of this presentation are many and without a specific indication implicating spider envenoming other causes must be considered. The marks on her left hand are apparently two puncture marks with no significant local reaction.

② CONFIRM

In many cases paramedics are presented with a collection of signs and symptoms that do not appear to describe a particular condition. A critical step in determining a treatment plan in this situation is to consider what other conditions could explain the patient's presentation.

In this situation the clinical reasoning component is about acknowledging that while envenoming by a funnel-web spider is a likely diagnosis, other possible causes of collapse should also be considered in the differential diagnosis.

What else could it be?
Cardiovascular issue
While the patient is suffering from tachycardia, hypertension, pulmonary oedema and unconsciousness, such sudden deterioration in a patient with no medical history or comorbidities does not offer an explanation leading towards a cardiovascular issue. The ECG is also normal.

Severe allergic reaction
The tachycardia and hypertension may be a result of a severe allergic reaction without cardiovascular collapse, but poor perfusion, being pale, cold and sweaty and the pulmonary oedema are atypical of a severe allergic reaction. The lack of erythema does not preclude severe allergic reaction but it is a very unlikely presentation.

Drug overdose
Although the symptoms are also consistent with an adrenergic stimulant drug overdose such as amphetamines, the socioeconomic environment and the patient's lack of unusual behaviour make this less likely, particularly given the history.

Subarachnoid haemorrhage
The raised intracranial pressure than can result from a subarachnoid haemorrhage (SAH) can trigger the Cushing reflex but this is usually characterised by hypertension and bradycardia. When the patient phoned her husband prior to her collapse she made no mention of the classic headache caused by a SAH.

Pregnancy-induced hypertension/eclampsia
The typical signs of tachycardia, hypertension and pulmonary oedema are significant signs of pregnancy-induced hypertension with the possibility of eclampsia occurring. There is a high index of suspicion that this is pregnancy-induced hypertension, although the lack of history of pregnancy-induced hypertension throughout her pregnancy are not consistent with this diagnosis. The paramedics should contact the local obstetrician to discuss the possibility of pregnancy-induced hypertension or risk factors that may cause sudden clinical deterioration.

Infection/sepsis
The lack of a fever cannot be used to exclude severe infection. The sudden deterioration from when the patient was last seen well to being unconscious

---

DIFFERENTIAL DIAGNOSIS

Unconsciousness and pulmonary oedema
Associated with:
- Cardiovascular issue
- Severe allergic reaction
- Drug overdose
- Subarachnoid haemorrhage (SAH)
- Pregnancy-induced hypertension/eclampsia
- Infection/sepsis
- Poisoning
- Envenoming

is atypical of infection, as is the lack of an increasing state of being unwell. Infection is unlikely, but possible.

Poisoning

The house does not contain obvious poisons and there are no other chemicals around that would explain the patient's clinical condition. The tachycardia is not typical of organophosphates.

Envenoming

The clinical presentation is consistent with a funnel-web spider bite and her hand wound may be a spider bite. The unconsciousness, non-cardiogenic pulmonary oedema and autonomic nervous system signs are consistent with this type of envenoming and given the clear history of a spider bite typical of a funnel-web spider, this is a probable diagnosis.

This is a case where it is possible to make a provisional diagnosis in the field, even though the patient is now unable to give a history, because of the early history provided to the partner, with the patient identifying that she was bitten by a spider. In the absence of a definitive diagnosis, treating symptomatically provides a strong treatment pathway. The incidence of funnel-web spiders in the patient's community and the patient's history, signs and symptoms provide a high index of suspicion that this is funnel-web spider envenoming; as such, treating symptomatically as well as applying a PBI would be recommended.

③ TREAT

1730 hrs: The paramedics manage the patient's airway by positioning her laterally to allow postural drainage and suction as required. They then administer oxygen at 15 L/min via a bag-valve mask and undertake intermittent positive pressure breathing to improve tidal volume.

1733 hrs: The paramedics apply a PBI and splint to the patient's left arm, then gain IV access.

④ EVALUATE

Evaluating the effect of any clinical management intervention can provide clues to the accuracy of the initial diagnosis. Some conditions respond rapidly to treatment so patients should be expected to improve if the diagnosis and treatment were appropriate. A failure to improve in this situation should trigger the clinician to reconsider the diagnosis.

1735 hrs: Perfusion status: HR 124 bpm, sinus tachycardia, BP 90/50 mmHg, skin cool and clammy.

Respiratory status: RR 32 bpm, air entry L = R, full field crackles.

Conscious state: GCS = 3.

The patient has progressed from being hypertensive to hypotensive. This is consistent with envenoming, anaphylaxis or cardiogenic shock. The absence of any ECG changes does not rule out cardiogenic shock but it is unlikely in a patient of this age and history.

With no antivenom to hand, rapid transport and maintaining the patient's perfusion and respiratory status are the fundamentals of management. Intravenous fluids are usually contraindicated for patients with acute pulmonary oedema so an inotrope infusion may be necessary to support the patient's blood pressure. Now that the patient has developed hypotension, anaphylaxis should be reconsidered as a cause and an IM dose of adrenaline would then be indicated, even if acute pulmonary oedema is not a common sign of anaphylaxis. However, in this case the evolving clinical picture is consistent with severe systemic envenoming by a funnel-web spider, which can evolve rapidly. The most urgent need is to administer specific antivenom, so rapid transport to a hospital with funnel-web spider antivenom is a top priority.

If the patient remains unresponsive to perfusion management and the paramedics are not able to adequately ventilate her using non-invasive means, they should consider endotracheal intubation according to local guidelines. The receiving hospital needs to be advised that the patient is pregnant.

 CASE STUDY 3

Case 16543, 1115 hrs.

Dispatch details: A 55-year-old male is complaining that his hand is going to 'fall off' as a result of a spider bite.

Initial presentation: The paramedics are met at a local residence and once inside are confronted by the patient who states that he has been bitten by a white-tailed spider and believes his hand is going to 'fall off'. He tells them that he looked up the spider species on the internet and found that it causes flesh to come off as a result of a bite.

---

1 ASSESS

1150 hrs Primary survey: The patient is standing in his lounge room fully conscious. There is a red mark on the webbing between his thumb and forefinger on his right hand. He is complaining of mild persistent pain.

1151 hrs Vital signs survey: Perfusion status: HR 85 bpm; sinus rhythm; BP 145/85 mmHg; skin warm, pink, dry.

Respiratory status: RR 16 bpm, air entry L = R, no adventitious sounds, normal regular breaths, SpO_2 = 97% on room air.

Conscious state: GCS = 15.

1153 hrs Pertinent hx: The patient states he has no significant medical history and that he was looking for some socks in the bottom of his cupboard when he felt a sting on his right hand. He saw the spider, which he killed, and then proceeded to look it up on the internet.

1154 hrs Secondary survey: There is a red mark on the patient's right hand and a constant mild pain described by the patient. There are no other abnormalities.

> ## HISTORY
>
> **Ask!**
> - What is your past medical history?
> - What other symptoms do you have (e.g. nausea, vomiting, cramps)?
> - What medications do you take?
> - When did you last eat?
> - Can you describe the pain?

2 CONFIRM

In many cases paramedics are presented with a collection of signs and symptoms that do not appear to describe a particular condition. A critical step in determining a treatment plan in this situation is to consider what other conditions could explain the patient's presentation.

The patient has given a good description of the spider and it does not fit the description of either a redback or a funnel-web. He lives in a region that is outside the normal distribution for funnel-web spiders. He does not have extreme pain or any sign of physiological compromise.

(3) TREAT

Treatment comprises reassurance, paracetamol for pain analgesia in line with local guidelines and advice from his general practitioner.

(4) EVALUATE

From a purely clinical standpoint there is no reason to transport this patient to an emergency department. With the passage of time and the absence of developing symptoms he will be more confident and ready to accept reassurance. Unfortunately, if he is still concerned about a delayed effect sometime in the future he may require reassurance from someone other than the paramedics, such as his general practitioner. Taking the time to arrange for him to discuss his concerns with his general practitioner is part of the paramedic role. Hopefully this extra reassurance will prevent him from unnecessarily attending the emergency department at a later time.

Summary

Spider envenoming is not generally a life-threatening emergency, the exception being some funnel-web spider bites. It can present with a variety of symptoms but, depending on the species of spider, may be complicated by a delayed response to the envenoming. Paramedics are regularly the first healthcare professionals to assess patients and perceptive assessment, management and planning can reduce patient suffering regarding unnecessary pain and complications from severe envenoming, especially in children. Paramedics' awareness of serum sickness is valuable in the field when attending patients who have recently been administered antivenom.

References

Australian Resuscitation Council (ARC). (2014). *Guideline 9.4.2. Spider Bite. July*. Retrieved from: https://resus.org.au/guidelines/.

Graudins, A., Wilson, D., Alewood, P. F., Broady, K. W., & Nicholson, G. M. (2002). Cross-reactivity of Sydney funnel-web spider antivenom: neutralization of the in vitro toxicity of other Australian funnel-web (Atrax and Hadronyche) spider venoms. *Toxicon, 40*(3), 259–266.

Isbister, G. K., Page, C. B., Buckley, N. A., Fatovich, D. M., Pascu, O., MacDonald, S. P. J., Calver, L. A., & Brown, S. G. A., on behalf of the RAVE Investigators. (2014). Randomized controlled trial of intravenous antivenom versus placebo for latrodectism: the second redback antivenom evaluation (RAVE-II) study. *Annals of Emergency Medicine*, https://doi.org/10.1016/j.annemergmed.2014.06.006.

CHAPTER 44

Marine Envenoming

By Julian White

OVERVIEW

- Australian and New Zealand coastal waters contain a number of venomous animals.
- Envenoming by marine animals is rarely fatal but can produce immense pain. Reactions range from mild and localised to systemic and life-threatening.
- Box jellyfish (*Chironex fleckeri*) envenoming is considered the most deadly marine envenoming worldwide and is capable of killing a human in under 5 minutes.
- Irukandji syndrome refers to a spectrum of signs and symptoms that can occur post irukandji envenoming.

- Marine envenoming can mimic or exacerbate medical conditions and envenoming needs to be considered when treating people at or near ocean beaches.
- Antivenom is available for a number of marine species but there is lack of evidence to support immediate and emergency treatment and conflicting advice is not uncommon.

Introduction

There is a threat of marine envenoming in almost all Australian and New Zealand waters, although the risks are greater in tropical and subtropical waters. Stonefish, blue-ringed octopuses, sea snakes, jellyfish, corals, anemones, stingrays and cone snails contribute to more than 40,000 cases of envenoming a year, with jellyfish making up around one-quarter of these (Winkel & Nimorakiotakis, 2003). Although mortality is rare, morbidity can be significant. The overall mortality may be underestimated, however, as some drownings may occur secondary to envenoming.

Pathophysiology

A diverse array of marine animals can cause envenoming. Some cause envenoming through substantial penetration of the skin, either through biting (e.g. sea snakes, blue ring octopus), or through stinging with some form of spine or similar (e.g. stinging fish such as the stonefish, stingrays, sea urchins, cone snails). Others cause envenoming through micro-penetration of the skin, mostly using nematocysts (specialised stinging organelles; found in jellyfish, corals and so on). The local appearance at the bite/sting site can assist in diagnosis. For most marine venomous animals, envenoming effects are principally or wholly local, but for some systemic envenoming can occur and it is these which are more likely to prove life-threatening (e.g. sea snakes, certain jellyfish, blue-ringed octopus, cone snails). However, those causing local envenoming effects can only threaten life when the skin penetration is extensive, deep or involves the chest or abdomen (e.g. stingrays). In this latter situation it is often the mechanical trauma which is of paramount importance, rather than envenoming. The mechanism and subsequent management of the injury and envenoming varies significantly between the species involved and depends on the type of toxin and type of wound involved (see Box 44.1 and Fig 44.1).

Penetrating wounds
Sea snake
Australian waters host more than half the world's diversity of sea snakes and although they possess some of the most potent venoms of all snakes, bites are rare and fatalities have very rarely been reported in Australia (Winkel & Nimorakiotakis, 2003). Outside of Australian waters, sea snakes have, at least in the past, been a significant cause of bites and fatalities among traditional fisherman in the Indo-Pacific, although modern fishing techniques have reduced that risk. Sea snakes (see Fig 44.2) are generally timid and most of the recorded bites have occurred when the snakes have been handled. The bite is usually painless and, like terrestrial snakes, envenoming is not common even when the snake strikes. Fisherman sorting fish from commercial nets are probably most at risk, though most sea snakes caught in modern nets will have drowned by the time they are hauled aboard ship.

BOX 44.1 Toxins: mechanisms of action

Envenoming must be distinguished from the symptoms caused by anxiety. Some people who believe that they have been stung by a jellyfish (even if this is not the case) will hyperventilate, resulting in perioral or diffuse paraesthesia or rigidity and tetany of the hands from a decrease in the free plasma Ca^{++} concentration due to respiratory alkalosis. Others experience dizziness or syncopal tendencies, even vasovagal syncope. A few people will become agitated and may list a series of bizarre symptoms they think are related to the event. Having a clear understanding of the types of toxins and the sequence of the symptoms they cause can assist in eliminating the emotional elements from the presentation. Toxins are generally divided into categories according to the area they affect (Tibballs et al., 2001):

- *Tetrodotoxins* affect the axon, inhibiting the passage of depolarisation from reaching the motor end plate. These toxins act rapidly and their effect may last for hours with no actual damage to the nerve fibre. This can occur with blue-ringed octopus envenoming, which

induces respiratory paralysis. If the patient's respirations are maintained through mechanical ventilation, the nerve function is gradually restored as the toxin is metabolised or excreted.
- *Neurotoxins* target the neuromuscular junction (see Fig 44.1), blocking the initiation of muscle depolarisation. Cone shells affect this area with their toxins.
- *Haemolytic toxins* cause rupture of erythrocytes and therefore haemoglobin is released into the bloodstream. *Chironex fleckeri* envenoming and stonefish stings can release haemolytic toxins.

Dermonecrotic effects may occur as a direct or indirect effect of toxin activity. Box jellyfish stings sometimes result in necrosis along tentacle contact tracks, which can be extensive. The role of antivenom in reducing necrosis remains uncertain. Other marine animals associated with a necrotic reaction include stingrays, sea urchins and, uncommonly, stonefish.

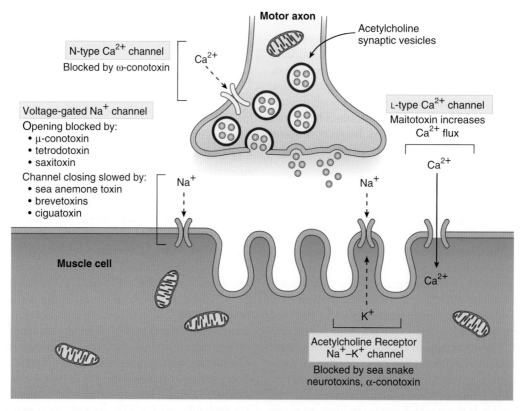

Figure 44.1
Schematic representation of a motor axon synapse and the sites of action of various marine neurotoxins.
Source: Goldman & Schafer (2012).

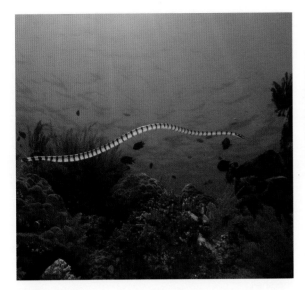

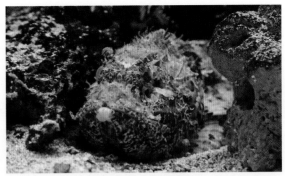

Figure 44.3
Exquisitely camouflaged, the stonefish has a row of sharp and tough dorsal spines that can penetrate shoes. The spines inject a painful but rarely lethal venom.
Source: iStock/Thinkstock/tane-mahuta.

Figure 44.2
Sea-snake venom is extremely toxic but sea snakes rarely bite unless handled and often don't envenomate.
Source: iStock\Thinkstock\Divelvanov.

The clinically relevant toxins in sea-snake venom are a combination of postsynaptic neurotoxins and myotoxins. The neurotoxins cause descending flaccid paralysis by competitively binding to postsynaptic nicotinic acetylcholine receptors at the neuromuscular junction (see Fig 44.1). Ptosis is usually the first sign to develop, with vision impairment, eye muscle paralysis (ophthalmoplegia) and mydriasis all developing subsequently, followed by limb weakness in more severe cases. Respiratory muscle paralysis can develop in severe cases. The potent myotoxins can cause significant rhabdomyolysis (with associated pain). Unlike its land counterparts, sea-snake venoms do not affect blood coagulation.

Pressure bandaging and immobilisation (see Ch 42) is recommended and tiger snake antivenom may be effective if sea-snake antivenom is not available.

Scorpionfish and stonefish
In New Zealand the scorpionfish family is represented by the widely distributed *Scorpaena cardinalis* (scorpionfish, Grandfather Hāpuku). Two species of stonefish are found in Australian waters (*Synanceia trachynis* and *S. verrucosa*) and they are considered to be the most dangerous stinging fish in the world (Winkel & Nimorakiotakis, 2003). These fish reside in shallow water near coral reefs, are superbly camouflaged and have a row of sharp dorsal spines, enveloped by venom glands, along their back (see Fig 44.3). The venom is purely for defence and is injected when the spine is pressed. Fatalities have

been recorded in the Pacific region, though details are not sufficient to determine actual cause, but not in Australia or New Zealand (Fenner, 1998) and it is unclear if these fish should even be considered as potentially lethal.

The venom is a mixture of myotoxins, neurotoxins, cytotoxins and cardiotoxins (Winkel & Nimorakiotakis, 2003), but clinical effects in humans do not reflect this venom diversity, as it is the local effects that dominate envenoming. The symptoms are immediate onset of severe pain from the site of injection, which may extend up the extremity (usually a leg). Swelling may occur and there are apparently rare cases of local necrosis around the bite site.

Antivenom is available and is considered effective (Gomes et al., 2011; White, 2013); immersing the leg in hot water (45°C) may also provide some relief. The area immediately surrounding the puncture can appear bluish or discoloured, but this is not a sign of developing necrosis. Severe inflammation of the site is probably indicative of infection; spines may break and become lodged acting as a nidus for infection, but this may be uncommon to rare.

Blue-ringed octopus
Growing up to 20 cm in diameter, these small octopuses (there are at least six species) can inflict a usually painless bite with its bony beak and inject venom from its salivary glands, the most important component of which is tetrodotoxin (see Fig 44.4). Found in shallow waters from India to New Zealand, there have been only a handful of recorded fatalities as a result of paralysis from the toxin, which blocks nerve conduction and leads to rapid flaccid paralysis and respiratory arrest. Paraesthesia, weakness, numbness, chest tightness and difficulty breathing indicate

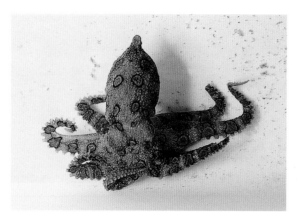

Figure 44.4
Blue-ringed octopus.
This small octopus is found in shallow rock pools and can painlessly inject a toxin that causes a flaccid respiratory paralysis. Envenoming is usually associated with handling of the octopus.
Source: Tyring et al. (2006).

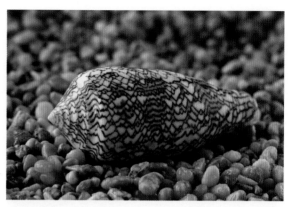

Figure 44.5
Usually found on coral reefs and sandy bottoms of tropical, subtropical and temperate waters, the cone shell can inject a painful but rarely lethal poison from a harpoon-like barb that extends from the apex of the shell.
Source: Dreamstime.com/John Anderson.

envenoming and usually occur within 15 minutes. The effects depend on the amount of venom and symptoms can resolve in as little as 10 minutes or persist for hours. There is no antivenom but giving the victim mouth-to-mouth or mechanical ventilation prior to cerebral hypoxia can provide an effective outcome. The pressure bandaging and immobilisation (PBI) technique may slow the spread of venom and should be applied (RCHM, 2013). Nearly all envenomings have occurred when the octopus has been handled out of the water (White, 2013).

Cone snail

These predatory snails live in shallow tropical, subtropical and temperate waters and can inject a complex venom via small tethered harpoon-like radula 'teeth' fired from the proboscis that extends from the apex of the shell (see Fig 44.5). Injection occurs only when the snail is handled or molested, so most stings are on the hands, or on parts of the body adjacent to clothing pockets, if the cone snail has been picked up and placed in a pocket. The sting may cause immediate pain, or be virtually painless, and the subsequent local effects vary from minimal to local swelling and numbness. Life-threatening cases develop generalised weakness, confusion and disturbances of coordination, speech and vision. Several deaths have been recorded across the Pacific region, with respiratory arrest from paralysis the most likely cause. There is no antivenom and PBI is generally recommended, but there is no evidence to either support or refute its effectiveness. Survival depends on active support of compromised vital functions, especially maintenance of effective

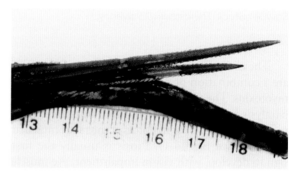

Figure 44.6
The serrated edges of stingray barbs can inflict severe lacerations, while puncture wounds can extend up to 30 cm.
Source: Tyring et al. (2006).

respiration, either by mouth-to-mouth expired air or by more formal ventilation.

Stingray

Stingrays inhabit all Australian and New Zealand waterways and many, but not all, species carry a cartilaginous barb on their tails. The barbs can be up to 30 cm in length: they can resemble a serrated knife blade, but are covered in a mucus sheath that contains a venom gland producing a venom which, at least for some species, contains a necrotic toxin (see Fig 44.6). Most injuries occur to the lower limbs when the ray responds to being stepped on. The ray whips the tail and attached barb up, around and forwards and can leave a deep, ragged laceration contaminated by toxins and barb debris (see Fig 44.7). Occasionally, the barb may puncture the chest, abdomen or groin and transect a major vessel

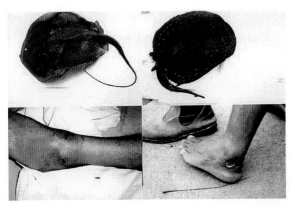

Figure 44.7
The cartilaginous barb located on the tail of the stingray can produce a severe laceration or puncture wound. The necrotoxin in the mucus sheath that surrounds the barb produces severe pain but also impedes healing and the wounds often ulcerate.
Source: Tyring et al. (2006)

to create an uncontrollable bleed, or penetrate an internal organ.

While the laceration can be severe, the venom also causes intense local pain. There is no antivenom and hot-water immersion (45°C; see Box 44.2) is widely recommended for pain relief. Opioids and nerve blocks may be required to reduce the pain. While systemic signs such as weakness, nausea, vertigo, headache, hypotension and arrhythmias have been reported occasionally, mostly from outside Australia, current evidence does not indicate that stingray injuries cause primary systemic effects, though secondary systemic effects are possible (for instance, shock from exsanguinating injuries to major vessels). The combination of toxins and remnants of the mucus sheath may predispose stingray lacerations to infection. It is important not to prematurely surgically close the wound, instead allowing healing by secondary intention. The use of prophylactic antibiotics and packing the wound with alginate-based dressing before allowing it to heal by secondary intention could be considered. PBI is not recommended.

Non-penetrating (surface) wounds

Cnidaria (includes jellyfish, anemones and some corals) use specialised stinging organelles, nematocysts, to envenom their prey. A *nematocyst* is a venom-filled organelle found in specialised cells on the surface of the cnidarian (e.g. tentacles and sometimes the bell on jellyfish) (see Fig 44.8). Nematocysts contain a coiled, hollow, threadlike tube that can extend explosively and act like a tiny hypodermic needle to inject venom. The trigger for nematocysts to fire can be mechanical, electrical

BOX 44.2 Hot-water immersion for pain relief

Immersing body parts affected by jellyfish or fish-spine stings in hot water is widely recommended but there isn't a large body of evidence to support the practice (Atkinson et al., 2006). One theory is that the proteins in the venom can be deactivated at temperatures greater than 43°C. However, this temperature is just a few degrees less than the temperature at which human skin is damaged and patients have reported pain relief at significantly lower temperatures (Briars & Gordon, 1992). Another theory is that hot-water immersion alters the pain receptors and leads to a reduced interpretation of pain from the nociceptors (Muirhead, 2002).

Regardless of the mechanism, there is no evidence against the practice and hot-water immersion should be used for fish-spine stings and may be useful in some jellyfish stings provided the tentacles are removed prior to immersion. Immersion in water as warm as the patient can stand for up to 30 minutes appears to be both safe and effective.

or chemical stimulation. In each case the stimulus causes the nematocyst to propel the shaft or tubule into its victim and this can penetrate below the skin surface, in some cases into underlying capillaries, which can result in rapid and potentially severe systemic envenoming, as is the case with major box jellyfish stings (Bailey et al., 2003).

In most cases people unknowingly come into contact with jellyfish tentacles and are envenomed instantly. The severity of envenoming depends on:

- the size of the area stung and the size of the patient
- nematocyst contact with the skin
- the length of time between actual envenoming and treatment.

Critically, tentacles can be attached to the skin with nematocysts that have not yet fired but may be triggered when the patient or responders try to remove the tentacles. In the case of a standard jellyfish envenoming, millions of nematocysts will discharge into the patient. The venom is deposited along the entire length of the discharged nematocyst tubule. Over such a large surface area it is reasonable to suspect that some tubules will pierce the microvasculature of the dermis while the rest of the toxin pools in the tissues, but the exact mechanism for venom transport around the body is still uncertain.

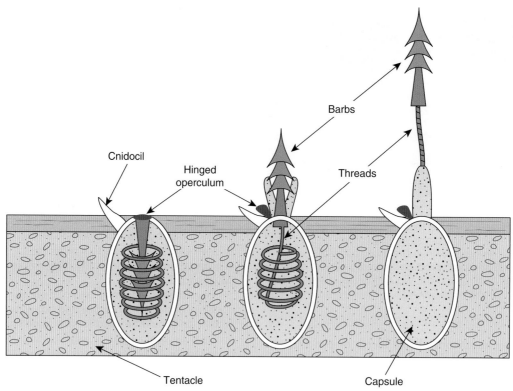

Figure 44.8
When the nematocyst is triggered by chemical or mechanical contact, the 'lid' covering the top of the capsule flips open: the barb hinges outwards and the thread expands explosively with a twisting motion. The barbs consequently 'drill' into the skin of the victim and release the venom.
Source: Adapted from Spaully, http://en.wikipedia.org/wiki/File:Nematocyst_discharge.png, licensed under a CC BY SA 1.0.

Box jellyfish

The box jellyfish *Chironex fleckeri* is the most dangerous jellyfish in the world and in Australia it has killed 67 people since reporting began (CDC, 2012). The last 10 deaths in the Northern Territory have all been children in remote coastal communities (CDC, 2012). Stings are more common from September to May but can occur year round and the distribution of the jellyfish (see Fig 44.9) may spread with climate change. The box jellyfish is a large creature (the bell can grow up to 30 cm in diameter) and its 10–15 tentacles can extend up to 3 m but its lack of colour makes it difficult to see in the water. In total one jellyfish has up to 180 m of tentacles: as little as 5 m of tentacles can cause fatal envenoming (Winkel & Nimorakiotakis, 2003).

Box jellyfish venom is complex and its action is incompletely understood but it certainly contains potent cardiotoxins and dermonecrotic components

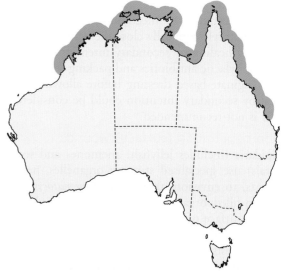

Figure 44.9
Box jellyfish distribution.

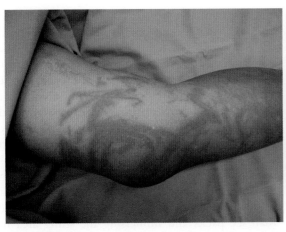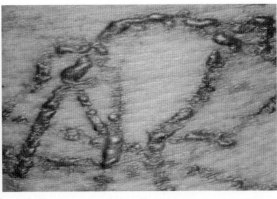

Figure 44.10
Widespread welts are typical of a severe *Chironex fleckeri* sting and can involve an entire limb.
Source: Courtesy Bart Currie.

that cause immediate intense pain and can lead to severe scarring (see Fig 44.10). Most stings are minor, although extremely painful, but some victims have been known to sustain cardiac arrest irrespective of respiratory function and it is likely there is a cardiotoxic nature to the venom that possibly blocks conduction in the heart (Tibballs et al., 2001; Winkel & Nimorakiotakis, 2003). This direct cardiotoxic action of the venom is seen in animal models. A neurotoxic component of the venom has been previously postulated, leading to weakness and respiratory paralysis, but more recent studies indicate it is pore-forming toxins that damage and can kill cells, especially in the heart, that are the main cause of observed pathology, not any neurotoxic effect. The first signs are pain and erythematous lines that develop as the nematocysts discharge their venom. The extent of welts can indicate the severity of envenoming. Stings involving an area equivalent to half of a lower limb are considered potentially lethal. The pain generally increases for the first 15–20 minutes by which time signs of cardiovascular compromise may have developed, although in severe stings cardiac collapse can occur within 5 minutes of a sting.

Although there is no rigorous evidence to support the practice, and some recent evidence indicating vinegar may actually accentuate envenoming, it still remains widely recommended that the immediate treatment is to inactivate the nematocysts with liberal amounts of vinegar before attempting to remove the tentacles that this jellyfish tends to leave on the skin. An antivenom is available.

Irukandji syndrome
Irukandji envenoming is a syndrome, not limited to envenoming by a single jellyfish species; however, it is particularly associated with a jellyfish often referred to as the irukandji. In contrast to *Chironex fleckeri* and its mass of tentacles, the irukandji (*Carukia barnesi*) is a relatively small box jellyfish, measuring just 25 mm across the bell with a single tentacle on each corner extending up to 1 m. The irukandji is found north of the Tropic of Capricorn. An irukandji sting starts with mild pain and sometimes just a pinkish stain to the area where the tentacle has made contact with the skin, or sting contact marks may be difficult to locate. The irukandji doesn't typically leave tentacles on the skin. Within 20 minutes, the venom appears to cause a hypercatecholaminergic state and the effects are known as *irukandji syndrome* (Macrokanis et al., 2004). The exact mechanism of the venom remains incompletely understood, but the syndrome is characterised by severe muscle, joint, back and abdominal pain, distress and a sense of impending doom. The effects of increased catecholamine secretion are displayed as hypertension, flushing of the face, sweating, tachycardia and chest pain. The potentially extreme hypertension can cause a cerebrovascular accident (CVA) in susceptible patients and is also associated with acute pulmonary oedema, which can be rapid in onset and severe. There are only two known possible fatalities from irukandji syndrome, both associated with preexisting major pathology that are likely to have co-contributed to the outcome. However, even in healthy young adults, a major sting, though trivial in local appearance, may cause severe and life-threatening envenoming with extreme pain, severe hypertension and severe pulmonary oedema. While the envenoming can cause marked hypertension, this is likely to be exacerbated by secondary hypertension in response to the extreme pain.

In the early stages the condition is easy to confuse with decompression illness if a diver has recently surfaced. Treatment is the same as for the box jellyfish (copious vinegar) but there is no antivenom. There are a number of trials underway involving the use of glycerol trinitrate (GTN) or magnesium to manage hypertension, but the results are not yet conclusive. The use of magnesium is controversial, with evidence both favouring and deprecating its use.

Bluebottle jellyfish

Possibly the most common source of jellyfish sting is the bluebottle jellyfish (*Physalia utriculus*). Found across wide areas of Australia and New Zealand this small jellyfish can have tentacles up to 8 m in length and they are especially adhesive to skin. The tentacles can produce a painful sting but have not been associated with any severe systemic events or fatalities. The nematocysts contain a venom that has neurotoxic and myotoxic properties (Tibballs, 2006) that cause localised erythematous welts and pain, but are not reported as neurotoxic or myotoxic in envenomed humans. The tentacles do not seem as responsive to vinegar, so removing the tentacles from the skin needs to be done gently (Adams, 2007). There has been controversy about first aid and pain relief, with both ice and heat recommended, but more recent studies indicate heat is more likely to be effective than ice packs and immersing the stung area in hot water, to about 45°C, is currently considered the most appropriate first aid by most authorities. A hot shower is often effective. Applying alcohol directly will increase the activity of the nematocysts and should be avoided. Topical pain relief is usually sufficient and antihistamines and oral paracetamol can reduce ongoing discomfort. Allergic reactions, both local and occasionally systemic, are reported for a number of jellyfish species, but appear particularly likely for bluebottle stings, though still representing only a small fraction of all stung patients.

CASE STUDY 1

Case 20806, 0900 hrs.

Dispatch details: A 32-year-old male is in severe pain after swimming in the ocean north of Cairns.

Initial presentation: The paramedics find the male lying near the shoreline screaming in pain. A bystander is putting dry, fine beach sand onto the patient's legs and palms. There are no obvious injuries.

 ASSESS

Patient history

Determining where the patient was when envenomed can assist in diagnosis and developing a treatment plan: was the patient walking in shallow water, swimming or handling an item from the sea for example? The time period between when the patient first noticed the pain and how quickly it progressed can also help identify the species involved. Likewise, a description of the patient's appearance in the water may be suggestive: the literature suggests that patients may be jerked backwards due to the extent of box jellyfish envenoming, either as a sudden response to the severe immediate pain or possibly due to contraction of a large mass of tentacles if a large jellyfish.

An associated medical history (such as asthma or hypertension) might suggest risk factors if the envenoming continues to develop, but it is often hard to obtain and should not delay treatment. In this case, the patient was seen swimming before calling out for help. As he left the water, red welts were obvious on his legs.

The patient is a member of the local rugby league community and is known to be quite fit.

Airway

Anaphylaxis is a potential outcome of any envenoming and there are rare cases where the sting or bite occurs on the face. The patient's airway needs to be assessed for any obstruction as a result of angio-oedema. In this case, there is none.

Breathing

Envenoming with neurotoxins has the potential to paralyse the muscles of respiration, while anaphylaxis can produce severe bronchospasm. However, while box jellyfish venom is reported to contain neurotoxic activity, it is unclear whether true neurotoxic paralysis occurs with envenoming by this species or any other jellyfish. Assessing breathing and chest sounds will differentiate between these two abnormalities. Pain and anxiety may act as a confounder in the assessment of breathing, as both of these presentations are often quite marked in patients who have been envenomed. In this case, the patient appears to have some respiratory distress.

Circulation

Circulatory compromise is a real possibility in any patient who has been envenomed either directly through cardiac toxins or secondary to profound and prolonged hypoxia. Hypertension is indicative of irukandji syndrome, while hypotension suggests anaphylaxis. For major box jellyfish stings, massive rapid envenoming with consequent acute cardiac toxicity is the major threat to life and cardiac arrest can occur within 5 minutes of a major sting.

Initial assessment summary

Problem	Severe pain after swimming in the ocean; query marine envenoming
Conscious state	GCS = 15
Position	Lying on the sand
Heart rate	140 bpm
Blood pressure	135/90 mmHg
Skin appearance	Cool, diaphoretic
Speech pattern	Speaking in phrases between screams of pain
Respiratory rate	30 bpm
Respiratory rhythm	Even cycles
Chest auscultation	Clear breath sounds
Pulse oximetry	99%
Temperature	37.2°C
Motor/sensory function	Appears normal, but difficult to assess given the patient's level of agitation
Pain	10/10
History	The patient was swimming in the ocean and was seen to yell out and start thrashing around in the water.

AIRWAY

Look for!
- Swelling of the lips or tongue

Listen for!
- Stridor
- Hoarseness

BREATHING

Look for!
- Increased/decreased work of breathing
- Respiratory rate
- Decreased tidal volume

Listen for!
- Wheezes

| Physical assessment | The patient has red erythematous whip-like marks across his lower legs. |

D: There is an ongoing danger of further envenoming for the patient as well as for the paramedics if this is a box jellyfish sting with still active tentacles in situ. The paramedics should don gloves before applying copious amounts of vinegar to help remove the tentacles (note: the role of vinegar, long the recommended standard of care, is currently being re-evaluated and while it is still recommended first aid at time of writing, this may change in the future).

A: His airway appears clear.

B: There are no abnormal lung sounds. The oxygen saturation is normal but his respiratory rate is elevated, which may be a reaction to the pain.

C: The patient is tachycardic (possibly due to the pain) and his skin is cool, but his blood pressure is normal.

The patient is in severe pain, has an elevated respiratory rate and is tachycardic. In the absence of obvious injuries it is highly likely he has suffered some type of marine envenoming. From the location, he is at risk of box jellyfish or irukandji envenoming, but the latter is unlikely because of the severity of immediate pain..

② CONFIRM

The essential part of the clinical reasoning process is to seek to confirm your initial hypothesis by finding clinical signs that should occur with your provisional diagnosis. You should also seek to challenge your diagnosis by exploring findings that do not fit your hypothesis: don't just ignore them because they don't fit.

What else could it be?

Anaphylaxis

The lack of respiratory and gastrointestinal symptoms is not consistent with anaphylaxis. The erythematous welts are also confined to his legs. Anaphylaxis may yet develop but it is not consistent with the presentation at the moment.

Irukandji syndrome

There are irukandji in the region but the welts and sudden onset of pain are not typical: they are more likely from a box jellyfish.

Stonefish envenoming

Severe sudden pain is typical of stonefish envenoming, but the pain radiates from the source and generally spreads slowly; the puncture wound is often made while walking. The welts are not consistent with stonefish envenoming.

Stingray envenoming

Stingray venom is painful but is usually associated with lacerations from the barb and occurs while walking. The history, welts and physical examination are not consistent with stingray attack.

Non-lethal jellyfish sting

Given the severity of the pain, the welts and the geographical region it is far safer to manage the patient as suffering from box jellyfish envenoming than to suggest a severe episode from a less lethal species.

It is usually difficult to recognise which species of jellyfish has caused a sting unless it has left a significant marking, such as the 'ladder-like' sting pattern left by the box jellyfish. Management should be based on the risk of the most serious sting known in the geographical region. Determining treatment lies with the possible physiological effects on the cardiovascular and respiratory system that may be predicted. The paramedics must treat for the worst, anticipating a significant deterioration. They will therefore treat the patient for box jellyfish envenoming. If available, taking a nematocyst sample using

DIFFERENTIAL DIAGNOSIS

Box jellyfish envenoming
Or
- Anaphylaxis
- Irukandji syndrome
- Stonefish envenoming
- Stingray envenoming
- Non-lethal jellyfish sting

a piece of sticky tape placed over a stung area of skin may be useful, as it may sometimes assist a marine biologist in later identifying the most likely jellyfish species involved, but this is a low priority compared to acute care.

 TREAT

Emergency management

Safety

If tentacles are still adhered to the patient, any undischarged nematocysts will fire off when an attempt is made to remove them, causing further envenoming to the patient and possible injury to the paramedic. Examination gloves may protect the paramedic from envenoming.

Application of vinegar is recommended and early application is essential to stop the sting getting worse (see earlier note). It has been reported that 4–7% acetic acid causes permanent chemical sealing of the nematocysts. A minimum of 8 L of vinegar is recommended to irrigate the area, or more if required.

Circulation

Maintaining adequate circulation is a priority. If the patient is in cardiac arrest then immediate cardiopulmonary resuscitation is paramount and should be continued with some optimism, if necessary for a prolonged period of at least 20 minutes, probably an hour, to allow time for the stunned heart to recover from the acute envenoming shock. For patients in cardiac arrest, in addition to resuscitation, consider also giving specific box jellyfish antivenom, either intravenous (IV) or, if that is not possible, intramuscular (IM antivenom is much less likely to be effective, even in a patient with non-compromised circulation, but especially if in cardiac arrest). If antivenom is given in this setting, up to 6 vials may be required. Note that the effectiveness of antivenom in reversing established major venom-induced cardiac toxicity is controversial, although antivenom remains a recommended treatment for cardiac arrest following box jellyfish stings. The role of magnesium infusion in management of box jellyfish stings also remains controversial, but in cases unresponsive to antivenom it is considered reasonable adjunctive treatment.

Airway and breathing

Airway management should be considered as appropriate for the patient's level of consciousness. Oxygenation may be required to maintain the SpO_2 above 94%. Manual ventilation may be required if paralysis/respiratory arrest occurs.

Pain management

Due to the significant pain that occurs with box jellyfish envenoming, an inhaled analgesic should be considered initially until IV access is obtained and narcotic analgesia administered.

Antivenom

If the patient has unrelieved pain, envenoming to at least half of one limb and abnormal vital signs, box jellyfish antivenom should be considered. Box jellyfish antivenom is only registered as effective for stings by this jellyfish and is not indicated for irukandji syndrome or other jellyfish stings. The antivenom is available through emergency responders in some areas but is usually administered in hospital; however, see earlier notes about management of cardiac arrest.

 EVALUATE

Evaluating the effect of any clinical management intervention can provide clues to the accuracy of the initial diagnosis. Some conditions respond rapidly to treatment so patients should be expected to improve if the diagnosis and treatment were appropriate, while other conditions are characterised by a lack of improvement even when treated correctly.

> **PRACTICE TIP**
>
> Vinegar causes nematocyst discharge for some jellyfish stings, including the bluebottle, and is therefore only recommended for tropical areas where box jellyfish and irukandji stings occur.

Patients suffering box jellyfish envenoming are unlikely to improve significantly in the short term and stabilising the patient's pain should be considered an effective response. Cardiorespiratory arrest is the major risk and although uncommon and restricted to extensive stings, should always be considered, so continuous reassessment of patients with suspected box jellyfish envenoming is essential. Look for the early signs of severe envenoming that may progress to respiratory and cardiac failure and require airway, ventilatory and particularly cardiac support. The following symptoms are associated with rapid progression into cardiac arrest:

- decreased level of consciousness
- cardiac and/or respiratory failure
- total surface area affected by the sting is greater than half the surface area of one limb
- intractable pain.

Hospital management

Box jellyfish antivenom is preferably given IV but may be given IM. The recommended dose is 20,000 units (1 vial) by slow IV injection or 60,000 units (3 vials) by IM injection. For a patient suffering cardiac arrest as a result of box jellyfish envenoming, the recommended dose is 60,000 units IV (3 vials), but up to 6 vials may be used. Premedication is not recommended.

After stabilising the patient, general and supportive management in the ICU is continued for up to 48 hours. The sting site is typically treated as a burn. A delayed hypersensitivity rash may develop 1–2 weeks after the sting and usually responds to corticosteroid cream.

Long-term impact

Recovery from severe envenoming can take months to years and the patient may be left with scarring.

Envenoming across the lifespan

There is no change in management for box jellyfish envenoming depending on the patient's age. The dose of antivenom for box jellyfish is the same for both children and adults, including the elderly. Children are more likely to suffer severe envenoming because of their surface-to-body-area ratio. The 2002 deaths of two tourists in north Queensland from irukandji syndrome identified that adults may be more at risk due to comorbidities. Both tourists were deemed to have died from intracerebral haemorrhage from the hypertension caused by irukandji syndrome, but in association with other risk factors.

 CASE STUDY 2

Case 10484, 1020 hrs.

Dispatch details: An 18-year-old female in a local hotel is complaining of feeling unwell. Her friends state she is getting worse, with agitation, restlessness and severe pain.

Initial presentation: The paramedics find the patient lying on the bed in her hotel room, clearly uncomfortable with pain.

1 ASSESS

1024 hrs Primary survey: The patient is conscious. GCS = 15 (E4, V5, M6). She is agitated, restless and in severe pain.

1026 hrs Vital signs survey: Perfusion status: HR 140 bpm strong and regular, BP 180/90 mmHg, skin cool and diaphoretic.

Respiratory status: RR 32 bpm, good air entry bilaterally, slightly increased effort, SpO_2 98% on a non-rebreather mask at 10 L/min.

Conscious state: GCS = 15.

1028 hrs Pertinent hx: The patient says she was swimming at the local beach approximately 30 minutes ago. She came back to the hotel and felt unwell after having a shower.

1033 hrs Secondary survey: Localised sweating. Erythema is obvious on her left lower leg. Generalised severe pain, nausea and vomiting with abdominal cramps. BGL 5.7 mmol/L.

1034 hrs Past hx: The patient is normally well and takes no medications.

The patient was swimming and appears to have a local response on her left lower leg associated with tachycardia, hypertension, diaphoresis and tachypnoea. She is in severe pain. Envenoming from a marine sting seems the most likely initial diagnosis.

2 CONFIRM

In many cases paramedics are presented with a collection of signs and symptoms that do not appear to describe a particular condition. A critical step in determining a treatment plan in this situation is to consider what other conditions could explain the patient's presentation.

In this case the presence of erythema on the patient's leg confirms that she has been stung; the question is whether the rest of her symptoms are attributable to the envenoming or to another cause.

What else needs to be considered?

Food poisoning
Food poisoning could cause nausea and diffuse abdominal pain and be associated with tachycardia, sweating and tachypnoea. The onset of abdominal symptoms from food poisoning can be very rapid and therefore this differential diagnosis should be explored. A dietary history/illness history of the whole group of friends would be helpful.

Acute abdomen
An intraabdominal acute event such as appendicitis, cholecystitis, pancreatitis or gastritis could give diffuse abdominal pain and nausea and might be associated with tachycardia and the autonomic response. It would be very unusual, however, for the intra-abdominal pathology to have appeared so quickly, so this is less likely.

Drugs or drug withdrawal
Many drugs act on the sympathetic system to produce tachycardia and relative hypertension. Withdrawal of drugs, particularly opiates, can produce symptoms of tachycardia, sweating and abdominal cramping. The patient reports a very sudden onset after swimming and does not appear to be regularly using drugs, so this is an unlikely diagnosis, but not impossible.

Heat exhaustion/heat illness
The symptoms of heat exhaustion and heat illness can include nausea and abdominal cramps. However, the patient has just been swimming, which is ideal for cooling down, so this seems unlikely.

DIFFERENTIAL DIAGNOSIS

Irukandji envenoming
Or
- Food poisoning
- Acute abdomen
- Drugs or drug withdrawal
- Heat exhaustion/heat illness

This is a case where it is impossible to make a definitive diagnosis based on the clinical signs alone and requires adequate history taking combined with paramedic clinical knowledge for the diagnosis to become clearer.

 TREAT

1040 hrs: The crew administer oxygen at 10 L/min via a non-rebreather mask.

1041 hrs: The crew apply copious amounts of vinegar over the affected site for 1 minute. Although not proven to inhibit nematocyst discharge of all jellyfish causing irukandji syndrome, the application of vinegar is considered good first-aid practice (Australian Resuscitation Council, 2010).

1044 hrs: The crew administer 5 mg of IV morphine and repeat the dose 1 minute later. This would usually be considered an excessive loading dose for most types of pain, but in a study on irukandji syndrome incidents in the Northern Territory 70% of patients required narcotic analgesia with a dose range from 2 to 82.5 mg (Currie & Jacups, 2005).

Patients are often hypertensive, likely due to pain and a catecholamine-like effect of envenoming. Glyceryl trinitrate is a first-line agent for hypertension in some local protocols. The use of GTN to counter an acute hypertensive reaction in this situation is reasonable, given that the two known fatalities following irukandji stings were associated with extreme hypertension and intracranial bleeds, and is completely different from considering GTN for potentially chronic hypertension when rapid lowering of the blood pressure would be considered dangerous and likely to risk cerebral hypoperfusion.

4 EVALUATE

Evaluating the effect of any clinical management intervention can provide clues to the accuracy of the initial diagnosis. Some conditions respond rapidly to treatment so patients should be expected to improve if the diagnosis and treatment were appropriate.

In this case significant doses of pain relief are likely to be needed. Even if adequate pain relief is supplied, the effects of the toxin may see the hypertension persist.

This patient requires careful ongoing evaluation of her cardiovascular and respiratory status looking for trends and changes. If irukandji syndrome is suspected then it is essential to monitor for development of acute pulmonary oedema, a potentially life-threatening complication of envenoming. The effectiveness of the analgesic strategies also requires frequent evaluation and the dose of opiates used may need to exceed local guidelines to be effective: early consultation with the receiving hospital is likely to be required.

Hospital management

These patients require ongoing monitoring and assessment. They will also need analgesia for some time. There is no antivenom available for irukandji syndrome, therefore treatment is always supportive. Modest doses of benzodiazepines such as diazepam may facilitate anxiolysis.

Magnesium sulphate may be considered. Magnesium decreases both catecholamine release and sympathetic terminal receptivity to catecholamines via multiple sites of action, including most calcium channel subtypes (both at the cell membrane and intracellularly), as well as modifying other cation fluxes. It reduces catecholamine-induced myocardial necrosis in phaeochromocytoma (Fawcett et al., 1999). The only randomised controlled trial into the use and efficacy of magnesium found no benefit (McCullagh et al., 2012), but some lower levels of evidence suggest that magnesium sulphate improves analgesia and lowers blood pressure (Nickson et al., 2009). Its use has been incorporated as a second-line agent in some management guidelines (Barnett et al., 2004). It is administered IV as a loading dose followed by a constant infusion, which is progressively withdrawn as the illness settles.

The use of antihistamines as an adjunct to analgesia is unclear. The addition of a medication with a significant risk of side effects needs to be balanced against the risk of opiate toxicity.

The control of severe hypertension is a priority. Many patients' hypertension will settle with analgesia and/or magnesium sulphate. If this is not the case, antihypertensive agents should be initiated. Some authorities advocate the use of GTN spray while awaiting infusions to be prepared. IV GTN by infusion is commonly used as it is familiar to many practitioners and readily available. Use of catecholamine antagonists such as alpha-blockers (e.g. phentolamine) has been described as effective and associated with improved analgesia in some cases. Patients requiring this level of intervention need to be discussed with the local area clinician or referral centre if this has not already happened.

CASE STUDY 3

Case 10249, 1015 hrs.

Dispatch details: A 7-year-old female has suddenly collapsed at a beach on the Capricorn Coast in Central Queensland. She was walking through some rock pools 5 minutes prior to the collapse.

Initial presentation: The paramedics are met at a beachside carpark and taken to the patient by a family friend. The 7 year old is unconscious and looks to be cyanosed.

① ASSESS

1020 hrs Primary survey: The patient is lying supine and is unconscious. Her respiratory effort is depressed. There is no obvious injury.

1021 hrs Vital signs survey: Perfusion status: HR 130 bpm; sinus rhythm; BP 70/P; skin warm, pink, clammy.

Respiratory status: RR 2 bpm, shallow and uneven, absent lung sounds; SpO_2 not reading.

Conscious state: GCS = 3 (E1, M1, V1).

1022 hrs Pertinent hx: The parents tell the paramedics that their daughter was in the rock pools looking for some crabs. When she returned she told them that she had seen some crabs and some small fish. Over the next 5 minutes she developed a facial paralysis that rapidly deteriorated until she became unconscious. Her mother states she has no significant medical history and that she did not scream out or complain of anything before she collapsed.

1024 hrs Secondary survey: Pupils dilated and sluggish.

BGL: 5.2 mmol/L.

Temperature: 36.2°C.

The patient has deteriorated very suddenly from a normal state to respiratory failure and unconsciousness. She didn't complain of pain, but rapidly developed paralysis. The most likely diagnosis is envenoming by a blue-ringed octopus.

HISTORY

Ask!

- What is the patient's medical history?
- Did the patient suffer a fall or any trauma prior to losing consciousness?
- Was there any indication that the patient interacted with marine creatures?
- Could the patient have consumed any medications or drugs?
- Has this occurred to the patient before? Does the family have any history of sudden paralysis?

DIFFERENTIAL DIAGNOSIS

Blue-ringed octopus envenoming
Or
- Accidental drug poisoning
- Stonefish envenoming
- Cone-shell envenoming
- Sea-snake envenoming

② CONFIRM

In many cases paramedics are presented with a collection of signs and symptoms that do not appear to describe a particular condition. A critical step in determining a treatment plan in this situation is to consider what other conditions could explain the patient's presentation.

What else could it be?
Accidental drug poisoning
While the parents state that there are no medications lying around, the scene would have to be investigated for any prescribed medications or illicit drugs that the child may have found. However, a rapid onset within 5 minutes is not consistent with oral ingestion of a toxicant.

Stonefish envenoming
Despite the presence of myotoxic, neurotoxic and cardiotoxic components of the venom, stonefish envenoming is characterised by immediate extremely painful sting with pain extending rapidly up the limb and associated rapid local swelling, without neurotoxic effects: this is not consistent with the history.

Cone-shell envenoming
Although the patient is unconscious with paralysis, the cone-shell sting may cause a sharp pain, with the stung area potentially becoming swollen and pale: none of these signs is evident on the child. Cone snails are also arguably far less likely to be found in coastal rock pools, so the location makes this an unlikely differential diagnosis.

Sea-snake envenoming
A sea-snake bite is usually relatively painless. The clinical features are paralysis and/or myolysis but they are not expected to occur in such a short period of time (the timeframe is quoted as within 4 hours in most cases: White, 2013). A rock pool is also an unlikely setting for exposure to a sea snake.

This case reflects the uncertainty often involved in out-of-hospital emergency care and that a diagnosis is not always achievable. Managing the patient's airway, breathing and circulation is the primary concern. The presentation is consistent with envenoming, with a pertinent part of the history describing what marine life caused the envenoming.

③ TREAT

1025 hrs: The paramedics prepare a laryngeal mask (or endotracheal tube insertion with intermittent positive-pressure ventilation [IPPV] as per local guidelines) as this patient requires artificial ventilation until the effects of the venom wears off (usually 24–48 hours).

1026 hrs: The paramedics apply a PBI even though no envenoming site is noted (see Fig 44.11) as the PBI technique is recommended (Australian Resuscitation Council [ARC], 2010).

1029 hrs: The patient is rapidly transported to the nearest appropriate facility to maintain artificial ventilation and close observation until the venom wears off.

④ EVALUATE

Evaluating the effect of any clinical management intervention can provide clues to the accuracy of the initial diagnosis. Some conditions respond rapidly to treatment so patients should be expected to improve if the diagnosis and treatment were appropriate.

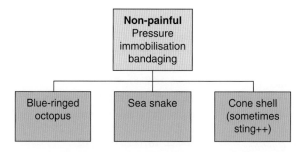

Figure 44.11
A PBI is not recommended for all marine envenomations but given that it is often difficult to identify the source, a useful criterion is pain. Painless envenomation is most likely to be due to sea snake or blue-ringed octopus and these patients should receive a PBI. Patients with cone-shell envenomation should also receive a PBI, but may occasionally present with pain.

In this case there is no way to reverse the effects of the toxin and they will need hours to abate. In the meantime, the patient's perfusion and oxygen saturations should return to normal values provided the patient is adequately ventilated. Importantly, if this occurs the patient may regain consciousness 'underneath' the paralysis but not be able to communicate with the paramedics. Providing pain relief to reduce any discomfort is advisable and communicating with the patient about the events and treatment is essential.

Future research

Research is currently being undertaken into techniques to slow or reduce envenoming in patients who have been stung by all varieties of jellyfish (Nickson et al., 2009). The distribution of the box jellyfish appears to be changing, with specimens now being found further south, though still in tropical waters. This has particular relevance for those living in the previously clear areas further south and may be a result of climate change. Ongoing mapping studies may expand the current risk area.

Further research is required to determine the optimal management of patients with irukandji syndrome. The mainstays of medical treatment are provision of analgesia, control of severe hypertension and support if severe complications occur. In most patients the acute phase does not require any complex intervention and settles over 6–24 hours. Despite adverse publicity, the rates of severe complications are low and fatalities are exceedingly rare.

Summary

Australian and New Zealand coastal waters contain a number of venomous animals. Marine envenoming can result in intense and difficult-to-relieve pain but episodes are rarely fatal. Depending on the species and degree of envenoming, the reaction can range from mild and localised to systemic and life-threatening.

Envenoming from the box jellyfish is considered to be the most likely to cause fatal injuries, but irukandji syndrome may also be the cause of several unreported deaths. South of the tropical areas where these jellyfish occur, stingrays and non-lethal jellyfish may inflict painful but rarely fatal stings. Treatment of marine envenoming varies widely according to the species, and some treatments can worsen the condition if applied to the wrong type of envenoming. Paramedics should be aware of the classic signs of injury and the recommended treatment for each species. Marine envenoming can also mimic or exacerbate preexisting medical conditions and envenoming needs to be considered when treating patients at or near ocean beaches.

Antivenom is available for a number of marine species but there is lack of evidence to support immediate and emergency treatments and conflicting advice is not uncommon.

References

Adams, S. (2007). Bites and stings. Marine stings. *Journal of the Accident and Medical Practitioners Association, 4*(1), 1–10.

Atkinson, P. R. T., Boyle, A., Hartin, D., & McAuley, D. (2006). Is hot water immersion an effective treatment for marine envenoming? *Emergency Medicine Journal, 23*, 503–508.

Australian Resuscitation Council (ARC). (2010). *Guideline 9.4.5. Jellyfish Stings.* Retrieved from www.resus.org.au/policy/guidelines/index.asp.

Bailey, P. M., Little, M., Jelinek, G. A., & Wilce, J. A. (2003). Jellyfish envenoming syndromes: unknown toxic mechanisms and unproven therapies. *The Medical Journal of Australia, 178*, 34–37.

Barnett, F. I., Durrheim, D. M., Speare, R., & Muller, R. (2004). Management of irukandji syndrome in Northern Australia. *Remote and Rural Health, 5*(369), 1–10.

Briars, G. L., & Gordon, G. S. (1992). Envenoming by the lesser weever fish. *The British Journal of General Practice, 42*, 213.

Centre for Disease Control (CDC). (2012). Chironex fleckeri *(box jellyfish).* Accessed 20 November 2013. Retrieved from https://digitallibrary.health.nt.gov.au/prodjspui/bitstream/10137/1209/1/Box%20Jellyfish%20Sept%202015.pdf.

Currie, B. J., & Jacups, S. P. (2005). Prospective study of *Chironex fleckeri* and other box jellyfish stings in the 'top end' of Australia's Northern Territory. *The Medical Journal of Australia, 183*, 631–636.

Fawcett, W. J., Haxby, E. J., & Male, D. A. (1999). Magnesium: physiology and pharmacology. *British Journal of Anaesthesia, 83*, 302–320.

Fenner, P. J. (1998). Dangers in the ocean: the traveler and marine envenoming II. Marine vertebrates. *Journal of Travel Medicine, 5*(4), 213–216.

Goldman, L., & Schafer, A. (2012). *Goldman's Cecil medicine* (24th ed.). Saunders.

Gomes, H. L., Menezes, T. N., Carnielli, J. B., Andrich, F., Evangelista, K. S., Chávez-Olórtegui, C., Vassallo, D. V., & Figueiredo, S. G. (2011). Stonefish antivenom neutralises the inflammatory and cardiovascular effects induced by scorpionfish *Scorpaena plumieri* venom. *Toxicon, 57*(7–8), 992–999.

Macrokanis, C. J., Hall, N. L., & Mein, J. K. (2004). Irukandji syndrome in northern Western Australia: an emerging health problem. *The Medical Journal of Australia, 181*(11), 699–702.

McCullagh, N., Pereira, P., Mulcahy, R., Little, M., Gray, S., & Seymour, J. (2012). Randomised trial of magnesium in the treatment of Irukandji syndrome. *Emergency Medicine Australasia: EMA, 24*(5), 560–565.

Muirhead, D. (2002). Applying pain theory in fish spine envenoming. *South Pacific Underwater Medicine Society Journal, 32*, 150–153.

Nickson, C. P., Waugh, E. B., Jacups, S. P., & Currie, B. J. (2009). Irukandji syndrome case series from Australia's Tropical Northern Territory. *Annuals of Emergency Medicine, 54*(3), 395–403.

Royal Children's Hospital Melbourne (RCHM) (2013). *Clinical Practice Guidelines.* Accessed December 2013. Retrieved from www.rch.org.au/clinicalguide/guideline_index/Envenoming_and_Bites/#marine.

Tibballs, J. (2006). Australian venomous jellyfish envenoming syndromes, toxins and therapy. *Toxicon, 48*, 830–859.

Tibballs, J., Hawden, G., & Winkel, K. (2001). Mechanisms of cardiac failure in irukandji syndrome and first aid therapy for stings [letter]. *Anaesthesia and Intensive Care, 29*, 552.

Tyring, S., Lupi, O., & Hengge, U. (2006). *Tropical dermatology.* Philadelphia: Elsevier.

White, J. (2013). *CSL clinicians guide to Australian venomous bites & stings.* Melbourne: bioCSL.

Winkel, K. D., & Nimorakiotakis, B. (2003). Marine envenomings: part 1 and part 2. *Australian Family Physician, 32*(12).

Tropical Medicine

By Peter A Leggat

OVERVIEW

- Paramedics are key members of an increasingly mobile global workforce, which are encountering tropical diseases in their practice.
- Tropical medicine is the specialty area addressing the burgeoning load of tropical disease globally. It is increasingly becoming a required part of training in paramedicine.
- A range of tropical diseases, in particular malaria, human immunodeficiency virus and tuberculosis, stand out as major concerns for international operations and deployments, but other common problems, such as arboviral diseases and diarrhoeal disease, also need to be addressed in both a local and an international setting.
- Various national and international groups contribute substantially to tropical disease research and the development of guidelines and policies for delivery of effective countermeasures to infectious and tropical diseases associated with a mobile workforce.

Introduction

With the professionalisation of paramedics as healthcare providers and recognition by health practitioner registration agencies, paramedics are key members of the workforce who, in many cases, are the sole primary healthcare provider in remote areas, and more particularly for offshore mining, petroleum and other facilities and operations. Paramedics are also playing a role at major events, such as the Olympics and Paralympics, as well as having an increasing presence on humanitarian missions. Many of the remote areas in Australia and more particularly abroad carry significantly increased risks of disease outbreaks and exposure to a variety of tropical diseases. It is important to be able to recognise the more common infectious diseases, including important tropical diseases that can be life-threatening.

General approach

While a paramedic working in most Western countries is unlikely to encounter many of the more exotic tropical diseases, there are situations where they can also encounter these conditions among increasingly mobile patients, including the increasing influx of travellers from tropical disease endemic areas. Some of the tropical diseases that might be encountered by paramedics might include malaria, human immunodeficiency virus (HIV)/acquired immunodeficiency syndrome (AIDS) and tuberculosis, as well as a number of other vector-borne and vaccine-preventable diseases. More recently, the emerging infectious disease COVID-19 (a coronavirus, SARS-CoV-2) was also spread through travel and the community required sustained infection control and prevention measures, including wearing of masks (Cheng & Williamson, 2020). One of the most important questions to ask is regarding the patient's travel history, including their itinerary, to gain an understanding of potential exposures to tropical diseases, as well as a history concerning any immunisations or prophylaxis taken. This may open a different range of diagnoses. As always, up-to-date medical reference material and local clinical guidelines should be followed in all cases where immunisations and medical treatment are delivered. When working overseas or in areas with high rates of tropical disease, patient education is a great way to reduce or prevent the acquisition or spread of many diseases. Knowing how a disease is contracted and how it is spread is useful information that can be passed on to the local population.

Guidelines

Comprehensive guidelines in tropical medicine have not been published in a consolidated form; however, various key government, international, non-governmental and commercial organisations have produced a range of relevant publications; these provide guidelines and advice for tropical medicine practice (see Box 45.1). There are also online resources that provide valuable information on disease distribution and prevention (see Box 45.2). *International Travel and Health* (World Health Organization, 2012), produced by the World Health

BOX 45.1 Key guidelines and related resources used in tropical medicine

Guidelines	Scope of coverage
Therapeutic Guidelines: Antibiotic (Antibiotic Expert Group, 2019)	Chemoprophylaxis and treatment guidelines for malaria, travellers' diarrhoea and other tropical diseases
Australian Immunisation Handbook (National Health and Medical Research Council, 2018)	National guidelines on vaccine-preventable diseases, including travellers' vaccinations
Pharmacopoeia, such as *The MIMS Annual* (MIMS Australia, 2018) and similar drug references	Pharmaceutical items for clinical practice and their use
International Travel and Health (WHO, 2012)	Yellow fever areas; general reference on travel-related conditions

BOX 45.2 Major online resources for tropical medicine practice

Name of resource	Internet address
Australian Immunisation Handbook (Australian Technical Advisory Group on Immunisation [ATAGI], 2018)	https://immunisationhandbook.health.gov.au/
International Travel and Health (WHO, 2012)	http://www.who.int/ith
Health Information for International Travel (Yellow Book) (Centers for Disease Control and Prevention, 2020a)	https://wwwnc.cdc.gov/travel/page/yellowbook-home
Communicable Diseases Intelligence (Australian Government Department of Health, 2020)	http://www.health.gov.au/cdi
Weekly Epidemiological Record (WHO, 2020g)	http://www.who.int/wer
Morbidity and Mortality Weekly Report (Centers for Disease Control and Prevention, 2020b)	http://www.cdc.gov/mmwr

Organization (WHO), is designed to assist in determining destinations that might require yellow fever vaccination, in addition to providing broader travel health advice. The WHO provides updates to this publication from time to time (WHO, 2012).

The Centers for Disease Control and Prevention (CDC) also produces a publication, *Health Information for the International Traveler*, which provides similar advice and has some useful maps on yellow fever endemic areas (CDC, 2020a).

 CASE STUDY 1

Case 180416, 1025 hrs.

Dispatch details: A 38-year-old female presents as a walk-in patient with a skin rash.

Initial presentation: On arrival, the paramedics find the female well, but she presents with curious itchy skin lesions on both feet.

1 ASSESS

History

The patient has returned from a holiday in Koh Samui, Thailand about 10 days previously. The symptoms started a few days after she returned and have worsened. She now presents with what she describes as itchy skin lesions on both feet. She indicates that she had spent most of her time at the beach and around the resort where she was staying.

Closer inspection of the skin lesions on each foot show they are both linear and serpiginous (having a wavy margin). They appeared as tracks on the dorsum of the skin and are quite erythematous. The patient describes the margins as seeming to move around. It looks like worm tracks under the skin.

She is otherwise well with normal observations.

This is typically a spot diagnosis and the condition is called cutaneous larva migrans (CLM) or creeping eruption.

2 CONFIRM

CLM or creeping eruption results from infection with larval stages of animal (dog and cat) or zoonotic hookworms (usually *Ancylostoma* spp.). The history of exposure on a beach where dogs and cats roam free, such as Koh Samui, was important.

Diagnosis of CLM or creeping eruption is generally made on the basis of the typical serpiginous, erythematous tracks that appear in the skin and is associated with intense itchiness and mild swelling. The tracks may spread up to a few centimetres daily. It usually appears 1 to 5 days after skin penetration, but the incubation period may be 1 month or more.

Usual locations are the feet and buttocks, although any skin surface coming into contact with contaminated soil or sand can be affected (the latter in this case). The history of possible exposure is important and in this case it was the beach. There are a lot of stray dogs that inhabit the area around the beaches of Koh Samui and they tend to be heavily infected with hookworms.

What else could it be?

Very rarely, other organisms could cause something similar, such as erythema migrans of Lyme borreliosis, impetigo, scabies, tinea pedis and larva currens. The location on the feet is not typical of larva currens from autoinfection of larval worms of strongyloidiasis. This latter condition is more often seen around the buttocks.

This case study reveals a typical instance of CLM or creeping eruption. As a parasitic worm causes the condition, it is worth understanding the lifecycle of the animal hookworms. The life cycle is given in Figure 45.1 and shows the developing larva penetrating the skin of their animal host. However, in humans the immature larva in animal hookworms tend to not develop any further after penetration of the skin and infect only the skin with subsequent migration of the larvae through the skin, leading to the skin reaction of CLM.

3 TREAT

CLM is not infectious to others, as the immature worms are under the skin and they may or may not be viable. The routine use of gloves by paramedics is sufficient protection. CLM is usually self-limiting, but treatment can alleviate symptoms. Therapeutic options include deworming tablets. These might be either ivermectin (adult and child 15 kg or more) 200 microgram/kg orally with fatty food as a single dose, or albendazole 400 mg (child 10 kg or less: 200 mg) orally with fatty food once daily for 3 days (Antibiotic Expert Group, 2019). The patient can also be reassured that they have been given deworming

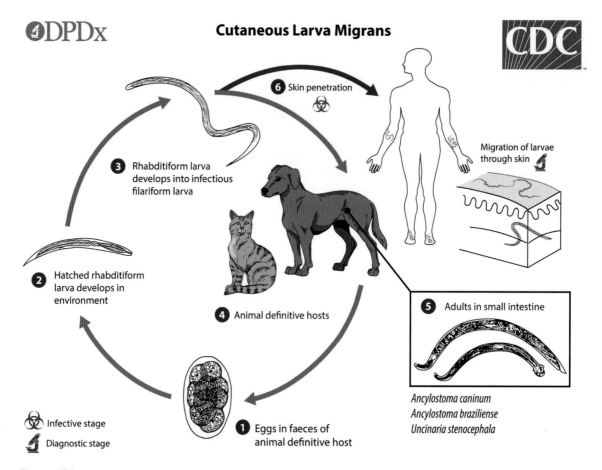

ODPDx

Cutaneous Larva Migrans

CDC

6 Skin penetration

3 Rhabditiform larva develops into infectious filariform larva

Migration of larvae through skin

2 Hatched rhabditiform larva develops in environment

4 Animal definitive hosts

5 Adults in small intestine

Ancylostoma caninum
Ancylostoma braziliense
Uncinaria stenocephala

Infective stage

Diagnostic stage

1 Eggs in faeces of animal definitive host

Figure 45.1
Life cycle of cutaneous larva migrans.
Source: Centres for Disease Control and Prevention. https://www.cdc.gov/dpdx/zoonotichookworm/index.html (accessed 19 June 2020).

tablets but that they should return or contact paramedics if symptoms worsen or they get generalised symptoms, such as those that might result from an allergy to the deworming tablet given.

It is important to also look out for secondary bacterial infections, which can result from excessive scratching. Sometimes when the itchiness is intense the patient might need an antihistamine, antipruritic agent, topical anaesthetic or even a sedative. In the case of sedating medications, they may need time off work or restricted duties.

4 EVALUATE

It is important to evaluate the effectiveness of treatment. In this case, the patient should be advised to return in 1–2 weeks. When this patient returns, her condition has cleared almost completely in about 2 weeks, which is typical of CLM. It is important to check for any side effects concerning the medications given. Generally, there are none with the deworming tablets mentioned, but the patient should be advised to return if they are getting drowsy using antihistamines, as they should not operate motor vehicles or machinery if they are affected.

As mentioned previously, it is important to check for evidence of secondary bacterial infections, which can result from the patient's excessive scratching.

Malaria and other vector-borne diseases

Vector-borne diseases remain among the greatest problems for overseas operations in the tropics. Some vector-borne diseases also represent a potential public health problem when personnel return home. Malaria (see Box 45.3) remains the single most important vector-borne disease problem for overseas deployments; however, arboviral diseases such as dengue and Japanese encephalitis (see Box 45.4) are becoming important health problems during deployment. Some vector-borne diseases are important for operations within Australia as well as international deployments (e.g. scrub typhus, which affected personnel in northern Australia and the South-East Asian region; McBride et al., 1999). Other vector-borne diseases, such as lymphatic filariasis (see Box 45.5), pose some concerns for operations in the Asia–Pacific region, where the disease is endemic.

Many infectious diseases of travellers can be prevented by immunisation. There are few mandatory vaccines for which certification is necessary; these include yellow fever and meningococcal meningitis, which is prescribed by the WHO (2012), when travelling to/from certain countries. In addition to routine and national schedule vaccinations, specific vaccinations may be required for particular destinations. It seems prudent to vaccinate against diseases that might be acquired through food and water, such as hepatitis A, typhoid and polio

---

BOX 45.3 Malaria

The WHO estimates that there are more than 216 million cases of malaria and 445,000 deaths due to malaria worldwide each year (WHO, 2020c). Most serious cases and deaths are due to infection with *Plasmodium falciparum*; however, *P. vivax* infection remains important, especially as dormant liver stages can cause relapses for months. Other species include the much less common *P. ovale* (can also cause relapses), *P. malariae* and *P. knowlesi* (a potentially deadly 'monkey malaria' emerging in South-East Asia) (WHO, 2020c). Malaria is transmitted by *Anopheles* sp. mosquitoes, which generally bite at night.

Malaria countermeasures include chemoprophylaxis, personal protective measures against mosquito bites (PPMs), environmental health measures against disease vectors and eradication treatment for parasite liver stages on return to Australia. Current recommended chemoprophylaxis includes doxycycline, mefloquine and Malarone (atovaquone plus proguanil) (Antibiotic Expert Group, 2019). Current eradication treatment for malaria is primaquine, although tafenoquine (a longer half-life primaquine analogue) has recently been approved in Australia and other jurisdictions (Therapeutic Goods Administration, 2018).

Because of the possible associated incidence of neuropsychiatric effects, such as anxiety and nightmares, patients should be screened for conditions that might preclude the use of mefloquine (Antibiotic Expert Group, 2019). Trial doses should be considered, possibly commencing as early as 2–3 weeks before departure (Ingram & Ellis-Pegler, 1997). It is also advisable that patients be given trial doses of other antimalarial agents that they are taking for the first time, such as doxycycline and Malarone (atovaquone/proguanil). This allows time to consider alternative drugs if necessary (Antibiotic Expert Group, 2019).

Opinions vary on how long antimalarial agents should be continued after leaving a malaria area. For drugs that have no pre-erythrocytic effects on the liver stages of the parasite, such as doxycycline and mefloquine, drugs should be continued for up to 4 weeks. This relates to the time it takes for residual parasites to develop in the liver and infect the bloodstream. Malarone, which has some effects on the hepatic stages of *P. falciparum*, may be given for shorter periods (1 week) after return (Antibiotic Expert Group, 2019).

For more remote areas, standby treatment may be useful. This consists of a course of drugs that travellers to malaria endemic areas can use for self-treatment if they cannot obtain medical advice within 24 hours of becoming unwell (Antibiotic Expert Group, 2019). A medical kit may be supplied with a thermometer, possibly an immunochromatographic test (ICT) malaria diagnostic kit and written instructions, an appropriate malaria treatment course and written instructions. Medical advice should be sought as soon as possible. Drugs that may be useful for standby treatment include Malarone and Riamet (20 mg artemether and 120 mg lumefantrine) (Antibiotic Expert Group, 2019). Malarone should not be used for standby treatment, if also used for chemoprophylaxis. Treatment of malaria is detailed elsewhere (Antibiotic Expert Group, 2019; WHO, 2015).

BOX 45.4 Arboviral diseases

Many arboviral diseases may be encountered in Australia and the region. Two of the most important arboviruses in the region are dengue and Japanese encephalitis, as they are prevalent in South-East Asia. Both diseases are transmitted by various species of mosquitoes, some of which exist in Australia, especially in north Queensland. Others of recent concern include Zika and chikungunya.

Dengue

The WHO estimates that there are more than 96 million clinical cases of dengue per year (WHO, 2020a). It is a viral illness, and infection may range from subclinical to fever, arthralgia and rash, or be complicated by haemorrhagic diatheses or shock syndromes (severe dengue). Severe dengue may be more common in those becoming infected with a subsequent infection with a different serotype of dengue (there are four serotypes, 1–4) (WHO, 2020a). It is spread throughout the tropical regions of the world, especially in urban areas. The vector is mosquito, generally *Aedes aegypti* or *Aedes albopictus* (WHO, 2020a). Treatment is supportive, and management of the problem is directed towards preventing transmission upon return to Australia. Outbreaks of dengue in north Queensland have been attributed to travellers returning with the disease. A study of soldiers returning from East Timor during the incubation period of the disease showed that a collaborative effort by military and civilian public health authorities to contain and prevent the transmission of the disease is vital (Kitchener et al., 2002). Although a dengue vaccine is available, it provides limited protection for workers and travellers abroad and prevention still depends on personal protective measures (PPMs) and environmental health measures against disease vectors (WHO, 2020a). The vaccine has been registered in a number of countries to assist in the public health control of dengue.

Japanese encephalitis

Japanese encephalitis (JE) is a flavivirus (same group as dengue and yellow fever) and is the leading cause of viral encephalitis in Asia. The WHO estimates that there are more than 68,000 cases annually in South-East Asia (WHO, 2019b). Up to a third of patients with clinical disease die and about half have permanent residual neurological sequelae (WHO, 2019b). Several effective vaccinations are available (WHO, 2019b).

Zika

Zika is a flavivirus (same group as dengue and yellow fever) that is transmitted by the *Aedes aegypti* mosquito (WHO, 2018). Symptoms are generally mild and include fever, rash, conjunctivitis, muscle and joint pain, malaise or headache. Symptoms typically last for 2–7 days. This arbovirus came to prominence through a finding of increased microencephaly in South American outbreaks. The WHO has now determined that there is a causative link between Zika and microcephaly and also Guillain-Barré syndrome (WHO, 2018). The WHO has provided advice for those women who are pregnant and intending to become pregnant (WHO, 2018). There is no vaccine. PPMs remain the first line of defence in endemic areas.

Chikungunya

Chikungunya is an alphaviral disease (same group as Ross River Virus) transmitted to humans by infected mosquitoes. It causes fever and severe joint pain. Other symptoms include muscle pain, headache, nausea, fatigue and rash (WHO, 2017). Joint pain is often debilitating and can vary in duration. Mosquitoes involved in transmission include *Aedes aegypti* and *Aedes albopictus*. The disease shares some clinical signs with dengue and Zika, and can be misdiagnosed in areas where they are common (WHO, 2017). There is no vaccine. PPMs remain the first line of defence in endemic areas.

(Australian Technical Advisory Group on Immunisation [ATAGI], 2018), as well as using other measures to combat these diseases. The most common vaccine-preventable disease is hepatitis A (ATAGI, 2018); typhoid vaccination should also be considered for travel to many developing countries. Polio vaccination is rarely required these days, but may be required in situations where polio outbreaks have been reported (ATAGI, 2018).

Other infectious diseases, such as hepatitis B, Japanese encephalitis and rabies, are also vaccine preventable. The development of combination vaccines, such as hepatitis A plus typhoid and hepatitis A plus B, has greatly reduced the number of injections required (ATAGI, 2018). The development of rapid schedules for those departing at short notice has been useful in providing protection within 4 weeks (ATAGI, 2018).

Other tropical diseases, such as leptospirosis and rickettsial diseases, are not vaccine preventable and may affect workers and travellers in rural areas of Australia and overseas. Prevention of diseases may

BOX 45.5 Lymphatic filariasis

Lymphatic filariasis is the second most common vector-borne disease, after malaria. It is caused by three species of nematode parasites, which can be spread by a wide range of mosquito species. The WHO estimated the global burden of infection to be 120 million, with nearly 900 million people at risk of infection (WHO, 2020b). Lymphatic filariasis is also the second most common cause of long-term disability with about 40 million disfigured or incapacitated from the disease (WHO, 2020b). It has a widespread geographic distribution, mainly in tropical regions, including most of Australia's neighbouring countries in the tropics. Given its widespread distribution and the increase in mining and other operations in filarial-endemic areas, steps should be taken to prevent transmission of lymphatic filariasis among personnel, which mainly relate to PPMs. There is no vaccine. Treatment is described elsewhere (WHO, 2020b).

require the use of personal protective measures by personnel and in some cases chemoprophylaxis with doxycycline (Antibiotic Expert Group, 2019).

Tuberculosis

Tuberculosis (TB) is caused by a bacterial infection with *Mycobacterium tuberculosis* and a number of non-human mycobacterial species. There are about 10 million people who fall ill each year from TB and about 1.6 million people who die (WHO, 2020f). It can lie dormant in people for many years. Spread is through aerosols and the main presentation is pulmonary TB, but it can present as an extra-pulmonary infection (WHO, 2020f). At-risk groups for infection include those who have had close contact with an infected person, immigrants from places with high rates of TB, various other groups of people with increased transmission rates and people who work closely with groups of people that have an increased transmission rate (e.g. healthcare workers).

Common signs and symptoms of pulmonary TB include a cough persisting for over 3 weeks, which may be productive (blood or sputum), and may be associated with chest pain, weakness, fatigue and weight loss (often due to loss of appetite). Often, the patient will have a fever, accompanied by chills and night sweats. Extra-pulmonary TB symptoms depend on the organs or system affected. Screening

tests are available. For healthcare workers, the use of personal protective equipment (PPE) or respiratory devices is recommended such as a properly fitting N95 mask. TB screening should be considered before deployment abroad and upon return. Treatment regimens are prescribed by the WHO and by Australian guidelines. Although TB vaccination exists, it is not useful in adult population (WHO, 2020f).

Human immunodeficiency virus

Human immunodeficiency virus (HIV) is a retrovirus that attacks the patient's immune system, specifically CD4 T-cells, weakening the body's ability to respond to infections and some cancer. As the infection continues to destroy and impair immune function, individuals become immunodeficient (WHO, 2019a). If HIV is left untreated, it leads to the development of acquired immunodeficiency syndrome (AIDS), the most advanced stage of HIV infection, defined by the development of infections and some cancers. Once infected with HIV, individuals carry it for life.

The WHO estimates that there are 36.9 million people living with HIV and there are around 1.8 million new cases annually. There are nearly 1 million HIV deaths annually. There is no cure for HIV infection and there is no vaccine. However, effective antiretroviral (ARV) drugs can control the virus and help prevent transmission so that people with HIV, and those at substantial risk, can enjoy healthy, long and productive lives (WHO, 2019a). Post-exposure prophylaxis is also available.

Other tropical and emerging diseases

Many other tropical diseases exist in different countries. Many of these are considered neglected tropical diseases (NTDs) (see Box 45.6). For many of these NTDs, there tends to be need for better treatments, such as Leishmaniasis and Trypanosomiasis (WHO, 2020d).

Future research

Despite the significant scientific advances in tropical medicine in the 20th and early part of the 21st century, much needs to be done to combat traditional and emerging communicable diseases as well as the emerging non-communicable disease burden in developing countries. In addition to the longstanding excellence of work coordinated by international agencies, such as the WHO's Special Program for Research and Training (WHO, 2020e), governments, commercial interests (such as pharmaceutical companies), and non-government organisations (such as the Gates

BOX 45.6 Neglected tropical diseases

- Buruli ulcer
- Chagas disease
- Dengue and Chikungunya
- Dracunculiasis (guinea-worm disease)
- Echinococcosis
- Foodborne trematodiases
- Human African trypanosomiasis (sleeping sickness)
- Leishmaniasis
- Leprosy (Hansen's disease)
- Lymphatic filariasis
- Mycetoma, chromoblastomycosis and other deep mycoses
- Onchocerciasis (river blindness)
- Rabies
- Scabies and other ectoparasites
- Schistosomiasis
- Soil-transmitted helminthiases
- Snake-bite envenoming
- Taeniasis/cysticercosis
- Trachoma
- Yaws (endemic treponematoses)

Source: WHO (2020d)

Foundation) have joined the fight against health problems in the tropics. Countries in the region, including Australia, remain in the forefront of tropical disease research. This augurs well for development of tropical medicine in Australasia and the potential elimination of some tropical diseases in the 21st century.

Summary

Tropical diseases may be encountered in paramedicine, particularly through overseas deployment. They may be encountered by workers and travellers abroad to countries with endemic tropical diseases and may present in workers, travellers and migrants entering Australia. Australia has a relatively long tradition of academic courses in tropical medicine, with programs continuing today in tropical medicine and its applications such as travel medicine and international public health. A professional organisation in tropical medicine, the Australasian College of Tropical Medicine (ACTM), has been established for Australasia with similar bodies in other countries. The ACTM maintains a body of knowledge in tropical medicine relevant for the region. With enhanced prospects for academic training, professional recognition and development, as well as research, perhaps we are entering a new golden age in tropical medicine.

References

Antibiotic Expert Group. (2019). *Therapeutic guidelines: antibiotic*. Version 16. North Melbourne: Therapeutic Guidelines Limited.

Australian Government Department of Health. (2020). *Communicable Diseases Intelligence*. Retrieved from http://www.health.gov.au/cdi. (Accessed 19 June 2020).

Australian Technical Advisory Group on Immunisation (ATAGI). (2018). *Australian Immunisation Handbook*. Canberra: Australian Government Department of Health. Retrieved from https://immunisationhandbook.health.gov.au. (Accessed 20 July 2020).

Centers for Disease Control and Prevention. (2020a). *Health Information for International Travel*. Retrieved from. https://wwwnc.cdc.gov/travel/yellowbook/2020/table-of-contents. (Accessed 19 June 2020).

Centers for Disease Control and Prevention. (2020b). *Morbidity and Mortality Weekly Report*. Retrieved from. http://www.cdc.gov/mmwr. (Accessed 19 June 2020).

Cheng, A. C., & Williamson, D. A. (2020). An outbreak of COVID-19 caused by a new coronavirus: what we know so far. *The Medical Journal of Australia, 212*(9), 393–394, e1. https://doi.org/10.5694/mja2.50530.

Ingram, R. J., & Ellis-Pegler, R. B. (1997). Mefloquine and the mind. *The New Zealand Medical Journal, 110*, 137–138.

Kitchener, S., Leggat, P. A., Brennan, L., & McCall, B. (2002). The importation of dengue by soldiers returning from East Timor to north Queensland, Australia. *Journal of Travel Medicine, 9*, 180–183.

McBride, W. J. H., Taylor, C. T., Pryor, J. A., & Simpson, J. D. (1999). Scrub typhus in north Queensland. *The Medical Journal of Australia, 170*, 318–320.

MIMS Australia. (2018). *The MIMS Annual 2018*. Sydney: MIMS Australia.

Therapeutic Goods Administration. (2018). *1.19. Tafenoquine succinate*. Retrieved from https://www.tga.gov.au/book-page/119-tafenoquine-succinate. (Accessed 5 October 2018).

World Health Organization. (2012). *International travel and health*. Geneva: WHO. Retrieved from http://www.who.int/ith. (Accessed 19 June 2020).

World Health Organization. (2015). *Guidelines for the treatment of malaria* (3rd ed.). Geneva: WHO. Retrieved from http://www.who.int/malaria/publications/atoz/9789241549127/en/. (Accessed 19 June 2020).

World Health Organization. (2017). *Chikungunya. Factsheet*. Updated 12 April 2017. Retrieved from http://www.who.int/news-room/fact-sheets/detail/chikungunya. (Accessed 19 June 2020).

World Health Organization. (2018). *Zika Factsheet.* Updated 20 July 2018. Retrieved from http://www.who.int/news -room/fact-sheets/detail/zika-virus. (Accessed 19 June 2020).

World Health Organization. (2019a). *HIV/AIDS. Factsheet 1.* Updated 15 November 2019. Retrieved from http:// www.who.int/news-room/fact-sheets/detail/hiv-aids. (Accessed 19 June 2020).

World Health Organization. (2019b). *Japanese Encephalitis. Fact Sheet.* Updated 9 May 2019. Retrieved from http:// www.who.int/news-room/fact-sheets/detail/ japanese-encephalitis. (Accessed 19 June 2020).

World Health Organization. (2020a). *Dengue and dengue haemorrhagic fever. Fact Sheet No. 117.* Updated 2 March 2020. Retrieved from http://www.who.int/news-room/ fact-sheets/detail/dengue-and-severe-dengue. (Accessed 19 June 2020).

World Health Organization. (2020b). *Lymphatic filariasis. Factsheet.* Updated 2 March 2020. Retrieved from http:// www.who.int/news-room/fact-sheets/detail/ lymphatic-filariasis. (Accessed 19 June 2020).

World Health Organization. (2020c). *Malaria. Fact Sheet 94.* Updated 14 January 2020. Retrieved from http:// www.who.int/news-room/fact-sheets/detail/malaria. (Accessed 19 June 2020).

World Health Organization. (2020d). *Factsheets: Neglected Tropical Diseases.* Retrieved from http://www.who.int/ topics/tropical_diseases/factsheets/neglected/en/. (Accessed 19 June 2020).

World Health Organization. (2020e). *Special program for research and training.* Retrieved from. http://www.who.int/ tdr. (Accessed 19 June 2020).

World Health Organization. (2020f). *Tuberculosis.* Updated 24 March 2020. Retrieved from http://www.who.int/ news-room/fact-sheets/detail/tuberculosis. (Accessed 19 June 2020).

World Health Organization. (2020g). *Weekly Epidemiological Record.* Retrieved from http://www.who.int/wer. (Accessed 19 July 2020).

SECTION 14:
The Paramedic Approach to Complex Cases: Specific Challenges to Paramedic Reasoning and Management

In this section:

While a standardised approach to patient assessment and clinical reasoning underpins every patient encounter, paramedics will regularly need to adapt their tendency to view their work from a purely clinical focus. The opportunity to respond to patients in their own homes adds a unique aspect to paramedic practice and often presents challenges not encountered by clinicians who operate in specialist medical facilities. The chapters in this section focus on patients whose environment, ethnicity or social situation renders their assessment and management even more complex than usual. In many cases it can be quickly determined that there is no need for immediate medical intervention, but that does not mean there is no role for the paramedic.

Identifying patients who have become socially isolated and are struggling to manage their health is a unique aspect of paramedic practice, but one that is largely ignored in clinical practice guidelines. Similarly, being called on when the family members of a terminally ill patient are confronted by a sudden deterioration in their loved one's condition requires a much broader understanding of the paramedic role than determining the underlying pathophysiology of the condition. In this case, the confidence to withhold clinical care requires an especially strong approach to clinical reasoning.

Finally, it is well recognised that ethnicity has significant influences on health. It is also clear that there are genetic aspects that influence the frequency and severity of certain diseases. We now have a better understanding of how social and cultural influences alter patients' views of their illness and how they engage with the healthcare system. Paramedics are often the interface between these patients and the greater healthcare system. We look at the unique aspects of two Indigenous groups—Indigenous Australians and Māori—and examine how their cultural beliefs need to be incorporated into the clinical reasoning process.

This section reinforces that while paramedics maintain a clear clinical focus, they must be able to incorporate non-clinical factors into their assessment and management. Managing these patients in their complex environments and situations is an excellent illustration of the value of the reasoning professional paramedic over a procedure- or protocol-driven technician.

CHAPTER 46

The Socially Isolated Patient

By Jessica Lacey

OVERVIEW

- Humans are social beings and the absence of contact with others can lead to feelings of loneliness, low self-esteem and depression.
- Social isolation is associated with negative health outcomes and an increased rate of mortality.
- Disease and illness can impair mobility, decrease the ability to communicate and/or create a sense of shame. These can all contribute to social isolation.

- Specific groups within society are at a greater risk of social isolation. These include older people, people with mental health issues, the unemployed and refugees.
- Working in the community setting, paramedics will be exposed to socially isolated patients and need to both adapt their treatment to the conditions and use the opportunity to engage patients in the wider healthcare system where appropriate.

Introduction

The definition of **social isolation** has evolved from simply meaning a loss of social attachments and community ties to a broader description that incorporates an individual's feelings of being socially cut-off, combined with an actual lack of engagement with others—social contacts are few in number and superficial or non-supportive (Nicholson, 2008). It differs from loneliness, which is entirely subjective, and varies between people according to their need for companionship and attachment through relationships. It is also distinct from social exclusion, where an individual's non-participation is beyond their control.

Disease and illness can affect mobility, decrease the ability to communicate and/or create a sense of shame. Similarly, an inability to interact with society can directly affect an individual's health by excluding them from visiting their doctor or pharmacist. Isolation from friends and family also removes the ability of these groups to monitor the health of the patient. Paramedics need to be aware of the propensity for some patients to be socially isolated and adapt their treatment plans accordingly, as well as taking the opportunity to engage these people in the wider healthcare system where appropriate.

Background

Much of the research on social isolation has been undertaken among the older population. This group is exposed to many of the causes of isolation and is at a higher risk of becoming isolated. Addressing issues that impact on the health and wellbeing of older adults is becoming more important because the number of older people living in Australia and New Zealand is growing rapidly. The number of centenarians living in Australia increased between 2000 and 2016 from 2000 to 3500 people (Australian Bureau of Statistics [ABS], 2016b). In addition, the current age-structure transition, as the Baby-Boomer generation ages, is increasing the proportion of older people within the total population (ABS, 2016a).

The health consequences of social isolation

Humans need and desire contact and relationships with others. Social connectedness and integration are associated with a wide range of positive health outcomes including an improvement in life expectancy, comparable with the benefits of smoking cessation (Holt-Lunstad et al., 2010). People with strong social relationships also report higher levels of health than those with weaker social connections (Cornwell & Waite, 2009; Hawton et al., 2010). In contrast, social isolation has been linked to a range of negative health outcomes such as poor nutrition (Locher et al., 2005), heavy alcohol consumption, greater chance of rehospitalisation (Mistry et al., 2001), depression, cognitive decline (Cacioppo et al., 2006) and increased susceptibility to dementia (Fratiglioni et al., 2000).

Factors associated with the development of social isolation

The identification of social isolation in an individual typically includes some, or all, of the following features:

- an extremely low number of social contacts
- a failure to initiate contact with others, contact with others that does not add to wellbeing or is even abusive
- a feeling of not belonging

- a lack of fulfilment in present relationships (Nicholson, 2008).

The main precursors of social isolation are a lack of relationships with a partner, family, friends and/or colleagues (de Jong Gierveld & Havens, 2004). For older adults, the combination of losing a life-partner and close contacts through death, adult children relocating, pursuing a career or raising their own family and not participating in the workforce can all lead to a drastic decrease in the number and quality of social contacts. For recently arrived refugees, the loss of a partner and family members (often in traumatic circumstances), difficulties entering the workforce and joining social organisations in their adopted country, and the absence of their extended family and the wider community from their country of origin can lead to a nexus of isolation.

As well as an absence of relationships, physical, psychological, environmental and economic factors contribute to a lack of social connection (Nicholson, 2008). Poor health, disability and declining mobility can act as physical barriers to sharing in social events and activities. Psychological conditions such as depression or dementia and increasing frailty combined with the fear of falling can lead to withdrawal. Where the individual lives and their distance from social contacts also limits participation; vulnerable groups typically do not have access to private transport and public transport may be infrequent, impractical or dangerous. In addition, housing design, typified by blocks of flats with poor access, can contribute to isolation. Finally, poverty can act as an economic barrier to participation in society.

Implications of social isolation for paramedic practice

The proportion of people living alone in Australia increased from 12% of the population in 2009 to 24.4% in 2016. In addition, living alone becomes increasingly common with age; in 2016 those aged over 85 years were more likely to be living alone than any other age group (ABS, 2016a). As social isolation is prevalent in the elderly population, it is anticipated that the increase in older people living alone in the community will lead to a rising number of cases of social isolation. The elderly are more likely to have chronic health conditions and may be frequent users of ambulance services. When paramedics attend older patients they should use it as an opportunity to make a holistic assessment of the person's wellbeing and to determine whether they are sufficiently supported within the community. In some cases, the only contact with any health services may be through the ambulance service and

the paramedics attending in their own home (Ross et al., 2017). Unlike many other health services, paramedics can assess patients within their own home, so they need to be able to identify people at risk of social isolation and to be aware of the associated negative health outcomes. They should also be familiar with, and know how to access, services that support elderly people living in the community by providing social contact. Unfortunately, systems that paramedics can use to refer at-risk patients for multidisciplinary assessment and intervention are not widely established (Snooks et al., 2006). Telephone befriending services are one means of re-engaging older people in society that has been demonstrated to increase participants' feelings of wellbeing and self-esteem (Cattan et al., 2011). This intervention has an affinity with the wider role of ambulance service providers and some organisations provide this service as part of their community programs.

Social isolation and falls in the older patient

Falls are common among the elderly and can have serious consequences, including injury and death. In the United States, the prevalence of having a fall in a year, for people living in the community and who are over the age of 65, is 1 in 3, while for those over the age of 80, this increases to 1 in 2 (Chang et al., 2004). In addition, the most common location for a fall to occur is within or outside the home, accounting for 70% of falls involving people over 65 (Australian Institute of Health and Welfare [AIHW], 2018). After falling, the patient typically suffers a reduction in quality of life and physical activity and this can trigger a negative cycle of decreasing functionality and increasing social isolation, ultimately leading to dependency, institutionalisation and death (Snooks et al., 2006). Even when the fall does not result in injury, patients may restrict their activities out of a fear of falling again and may withdraw from contact (Davison & Marrinan, 2007; see Fig 46.1).

Falls and related injuries frequently require medical attention and the ambulance service is often the first point of contact for patients. They are a significant component of the ambulance service workload, accounting for approximately 5% of all emergency ambulance responses in Australia. Of these falls, almost 75% required transport to an emergency department (ED) with 46% of these falls resulting in an injury. The injuries that are most commonly seen after a fall are hip fractures, traumatic brain injuries and soft tissue and upper limb injuries (Simpson et al., 2013).

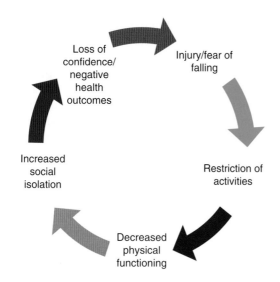

Figure 46.1
Potential negative cycle resulting from falls.
Falls in older people are not uncommon as mobility, eyesight and balance are affected by age. Even if a patient does not suffer an acute injury after a fall, fear and loss of confidence as a result of the fall can lead to a restriction of activities and increased social isolation. Visiting patients in their homes, paramedics have a unique opportunity to assess both the patient and the home for the risk of falls.

Falls incur high financial costs for the health system: in the United Kingdom (UK), falls account for approximately 3% of the total health budget (Snooks et al., 2006). By 2051 it is estimated that the cost of falls to the Australian healthcare system will be $1375 million per annum and that an additional 2500 hospital beds will be required to manage falls alone (Moller, 2003). In Australia in 2014–2015, more than 111,200 people aged over 65 were hospitalised as a result of a fall. The majority were women and the rate of subsequent hospitalisation as a result of the fall was also higher for women than men (AIHW, 2018). Although more women suffer falls than men, the rate of fatal falls is higher among men than women of the same age. The World Health Organization (WHO) reports that fall-related deaths is the second leading cause of unintentional injury death in the world with death rates highest for those over the age of 60 (WHO, 2018a). Rates of falls also increase with age: in Australia, of all the cases of hospitalised people over the age of 65 as a result of a fall, 63% of them were 80 years and over (AIHW, 2018).

Refugees

The experience of living as a refugee is different for each individual but typically refugees suffer ongoing physical, psychological and social consequences due to the events they have endured. Many have witnessed or suffered severe brutality, including abuse and torture. Having survived a dangerous journey, they must then live in overcrowded refugee camps, which frequently have limited provision of the necessities of life such as food, sanitation and medical care, and are unsafe due to attacks from both other inhabitants and external agents. Female refugees are particularly vulnerable to violence and exploitation. They are often the head of their family unit and are entirely responsible for the welfare of their dependants. Low levels of literacy and education, a consequence of sexual discrimination in their homeland, contribute to their position of powerlessness. In many cases they have been subjected to frequent and extreme levels of sexual violence (DeSouza, 2012).

Refugees arriving under quota or humanitarian programs participate in a coordinated resettlement program. The Australian government provides a 5-day Australian Cultural Orientation Program prior to arrival and the Humanitarian Settlement Program delivers an individualised case management approach to settling refugees (Department of Social Services, 2018). Further resources are administered at state level. In New Zealand, newly arrived refugees attend a 6-week residential orientation program, which includes general orientation, medical screening and treatment, some English lessons and assistance with accommodation and employment (Ministry of Health, 2012). However, the early stage of resettlement is often a confusing and overwhelming time and information is not always retained. Asylum seekers do not have an organised program of support and are not always aware of their entitlements.

Determinants of social isolation among refugees

Refugees have a high risk of becoming profoundly socially isolated. Many refugees have lost partners and close family members to violence or while fleeing from their country. Establishing social contacts and new relationships within their adopted country is difficult due to a lack of fluency in English. Acquiring new friendships outside of their own culture is difficult if they are not involved in an organised activity such as study or work. Feelings of being different are reinforced by different clothing, speaking with a different accent, differences in religious beliefs and cultural customs, and racism (DeSouza, 2012). For women especially, the impact of the changed family structure (where they may be the sole adult in the household) and the reduction in family size with a resultant lack of family support can be profound. In addition, neighbours may be less likely to be involved in their lives than in their previous community. Community organisations for refugees are thus an important source of social contact as well as support and information.

As well as a lack of relationships, refugees experience physical barriers to social activity as a result of injuries, disability and sickness. The profound grief for family members they left behind and at being exiled from their homeland forms psychological barriers to participation. While humanitarian programs provide assistance to find housing, it is not always close to where refugees from the same country have settled. New arrivals may become isolated from the established refugee community if they need to travel long distances to socialise. This geographical barrier to maintaining contact, compounded by the physical difficulties of travelling on public transport with young children and the financial barrier of transport costs if they have difficulty entering the workforce, increase the likelihood of social isolation. Even when refugees are housed near others from their country of origin, social isolation can occur if deep-seated group differences, such as religious beliefs or clan membership, are retained in the new country (Ministry of Health, 2012).

 CASE STUDY 1

Case 10489, 1530 hrs.

Dispatch details: A personal alarm belonging to a 73-year-old female has been activated and she hasn't replied to a telephone call from the emergency key holder, a neighbour. The patient lives alone and has a history of falls.

Initial presentation: The paramedics arrive and find the patient sitting on her kitchen floor; she is visibly upset. She states that she has fallen and cannot get up.

---

1 **ASSESS**

The paramedics' questions should be clear and concise and they should weigh all facets of the patient's past and present medical history against the four risk categories for falls: biological, behavioural, environmental and socioeconomic. The cause of the patient's fall may range from a complex interaction of medical conditions to simple mechanics. It is important not to underestimate the significance of what may appear to be a simple fall but is actually indicative of a more serious underlying problem. This patient does not appear to have any injuries but she is unable to get up unassisted. She refuses transport to a medical facility. People aged 60–90 years are characteristically stoical by nature and often reject medical attention or fuss. There is a great deal of fear among the elderly that their independence will be lost and apprehension about what the future will bring if they are moved from their home.

The clinical reasoning behind a decision to leave an 'at-risk' person at home alone must be weighed against the risk of a subsequent fall and therefore the increased risk of morbidity or mortality. A patient who suffers recurrent falls is at higher risk of suffering a fall-related fracture (Tromp et al., 2001). A closer investigation of the patient's living conditions—including the state of the bedding, the bathroom facilities and what food and fluids are in the fridge and cupboards—can reveal a more detailed picture of the potentially isolated client.

LOOK!

- Is the house clean?
- Is there any fresh food in the fridge?
- Is the garden neglected?
- Are there any trip hazards?
- Does the patient have a medical alert bracelet/ pendant?

Initial assessment summary

Problem	Fall
Conscious state	GCS = 15
Position	Sitting
Heart rate	65 bpm
Blood pressure	165/95 mmHg
Skin appearance	Warm and dry
Speech pattern	Normal
Respiratory rate	14 bpm
Respiratory rhythm	Even cycles
Chest auscultation	Good breath sounds bilaterally
Pulse oximetry	96%
Temperature	36.2°C
Motor/sensory function	Normal sensation
Pain	The patient denies any pain.
History	The patient has fallen in the kitchen. She claims she just needs assistance to get up and doesn't want to go to hospital.
Physical assessment	No abnormalities detected.

D: There are no dangers to the patient or the crew.
A: The patient is fully conscious and protecting her own airway.
B: The patient is breathing normally.
C: Her perfusion is within normal limits.
At the moment, this patient appears simply in need of help to get up from the floor and, provided she receives appropriate follow-up/support, many would consider that she doesn't need to be transported to a medical facility.

 ## CONFIRM

The essential part of the clinical reasoning process is to seek to confirm your initial hypothesis by finding clinical signs that should occur with your provisional diagnosis. You should also seek to challenge your diagnosis by exploring findings that do not fit your hypothesis: don't just ignore them because they don't fit.

What else could it be?
A fall with an underlying medical cause
There are a large number of possible factors that could have caused this patient to fall.

- Biological causes should be investigated by reviewing body systems, with particular emphasis on:
  › the cardiovascular system, including myocardial ischaemia and infarction, cardiac arrhythmias, orthostatic hypotension, syncopal attack, stroke and transient ischaemic attack
  › the gastrointestinal system, particularly low food and fluid intake, which can cause hypoglycaemia and hypotension, respectively
  › the musculoskeletal system and its impact on stability and gait
  › the genitourinary system, as urinary tract infections are commonplace among the elderly and can cause gait imbalance
  › the central nervous system, including changes in vision.
- Behavioural causes for the fall should be explored and include:
  › Has the patient inadvertently overdosed or underdosed on her prescribed medications?
  › Is alcohol a factor?

DIFFERENTIAL DIAGNOSIS

A simple fall with no underlying medical condition and no traumatic injury
Or
- A fall with an underlying medical cause, resulting in syncope, loss of balance or loss of motor power
- A fall that has resulted in an occult traumatic injury (e.g. a fractured pubic ramus)

Finally, the environment should be examined for possible contributory factors to a mechanical fall, such as:

> loose mats
> slippery surfaces
> obstacles.

This patient is not suffering any arrhythmia and did not complain of symptoms typical of poor perfusion prior to making the call. Her blood sugar, temperature and behaviour are normal and do not suggest any underlying medical cause.

A fall that has resulted in an occult traumatic injury

The patient denies any pain and has normal movement, strength and sensation of all limbs.

A thorough investigation and an open mind are essential to avoid errors in clinical judgment caused by cognitive biases such as anchoring, confirmation bias, overconfidence bias and premature closure (Croskerry, 2002).

③ TREAT

Initial management

Safety

Older people living alone are at a particular risk of falls as most falls occur in the home. Being able to quickly and competently assess a patient's ability to perform their activities of daily living is a complex task. The need for training within paramedicine programs on both physical assessment of the elderly and assessment of their homes is becoming more apparent. Paramedics have the opportunity to refer patients to a social services team: if patients are referred early enough, the potential for a subsequent fall with a worse outcome may be averted. Factors that reduce the chance of referral include a lack of well-established local care pathways, paramedics being unaware of these care pathways or referral being outside the paramedic's scope of practice. Most ambulance services, however, are actively engaging in falls management programs and with the expansion of registration within paramedic fields around the world and paramedic practitioners becoming more common, these services and programs within the community are becoming increasingly available.

Pain management

If the patient has signs of pain or is complaining of pain, their underlying injuries need to be assessed and managed. It is not unusual for older patients to minimise their complaints to the point where there is a risk that significant injuries may be overlooked. This behaviour may simply be an attempt to avoid causing a fuss but it may also be an attempt to avoid transport for further treatment. Assessing the patient thoroughly after assisting them to stand is important in order to detect hidden injuries. Providing the patient with oral pain relief should be done with caution and only after more serious injuries have been excluded. Non-steroidal anti-inflammatory drugs (NSAIDs) are often contra-indicated in the elderly so consultation with the patient's GP is advisable.

Transport

The decision to transport an elderly patient from their home environment should be balanced and well-considered. Anxiety and apprehension often place increased stressors on the frail and already vulnerable, and overcrowding in hospital EDs and the paramedic's unwillingness to expose a patient to a long wait in hospital can add to the pressure not to transport the patient. Leaving a patient with no apparent injuries at home would be considered the correct course of action, because keeping people independent is vital for patient wellbeing and reducing healthcare costs. However, research from the UK has shown that 49% of patients who were not transported to hospital after a fall had a second healthcare attendance within 2 weeks and an increased risk of death and hospitalisation compared with their peers (Snooks et al., 2006). Emerging evidence within out-of-hospital research suggests that leaving a patient at home with advanced out-of-hospital support through the use of extended care paramedics and appropriate social and medical follow-up may lead to a reduction in secondary admissions (Thompson et al., 2014). Improvements in health integration, in linking relationships between paramedics and GPs and in the assessment skills of extended care paramedics will enable more sound clinical decisions regarding which patients to transport and which to leave at home.

The process of safely arranging the support strategies to leave someone at home and documenting this thoroughly takes a lot longer than simply transporting the patient, although in the long run it may be a much better option. Across various ambulance services, the minimum criteria for leaving a patient at home may include the following.

- A medical cause for the fall has been excluded.
- Traumatic injury has been excluded.
- A clinical review program has been implemented.
- The person has immediate social support (not living alone).
- The person has food and is capable of preparing it.
- The person is capable of attending to their own daily living needs.
- The above has been well documented, along with a series of vital sign observations proving stability.
- A call-back plan has been established, including triggers and actions to follow if problems occur.

4 EVALUATE

Even for patients who are left at the scene, a period of time should be allocated to evaluate the patient again after they have been assisted from the floor. A fall in blood pressure, uneven gait and confusion can all indicate an underlying medical cause that may have been missed in the first assessment. Spending a few minutes evaluating the patient can also reveal risk factors for future falls such as a loss of balance or vision problems; in many cases the patient may not have noticed the slow deterioration in these abilities.

> **PRACTICE TIP**
>
> Home alarm devices are popular among the elderly, their families, carers and GPs. Knowing that help can easily be summoned increases the older person's confidence to continue living at home but it also increases ambulance attendance for non-medical–related calls. This is further reinforced as some elderly people may not want to bother family members with medical-related issues, further increasing the likelihood of ambulance attendance. In addition, these alarms can be seen as a further tool that socially isolates the elderly: family members may believe their loved one is fine and will simply 'push the button' if something is wrong.

Ongoing management

Pain relief

Polypharmacy is rife within the older population and adherence to prescription treatment regimens is variable. Simple oral analgesics such as paracetamol and ibuprofen may well suffice for the majority of falls victims and classic soft-tissues injuries and muscular strains can be well-managed with these relatively simple, cost-effective and low-risk medications. Stronger medications like codeine may have negative dissociative effects and a more prolonged anaesthetic effect than is required. Inhaled medications like methoxyflurane may have varied results due to compliance and reduced capacity to inhale effectively, but can be very effective for one-off movements such as standing or rolling, alignment of fractured limbs and difficulty with vascular access. Opioid-based products (synthetic and natural) and benzodiazepines have a high potency and are typically rapid-acting in the IV form. Titrating small aliquots of these medications may lead to very effective results in a short period of time. Care should always be taken when using pharmaceutical management for fall-related injuries in the elderly, as they have a decreased ability to metabolise and eliminate medications (Mangoni & Jackson, 2003).

Social isolation

Family and friends are a vital part of the network required by older people to feel socially accepted and part of a community. Social isolation is associated with an increased risk of mortality and a fall exponentially increases the risk of morbidity and mortality (Dickens et al., 2011). Offering social activity and support within a group format and interventions in which older people are active participants appears to be an effective means of reducing social isolation within the elderly.

Falls prevention

Falls prevention programs aim to reduce the number of people who have a fall. Outcomes of fall prevention programs in the UK saw emergency call-outs for falls decrease by 75% between 2006 and 2011, leading to increased capacity for emergency services to deal with higher-acuity calls (NHS Confederation, Ambulance Service Network and Community Health Services Forum, 2012). Several falls prevention models exist within Australian and New Zealand governmental agencies promoting strategies on how best to reduce falls. Multifaceted programs including environmental modifications (occupational therapists), physical exercise, review of medications (general practitioner) and review of visual acuity or aids are among some of the methods that have been shown to reduce fall numbers. Behavioural changes to adopt a healthy lifestyle, including reducing alcohol intake, smoking cessation, maintaining weight within normal parameters and self-health initiatives such as walking, are fundamental to healthy ageing. Emergency medical service providers have a role to play in health promotion and many already include falls prevention in their community programs.

Hospital admission

Following any medical intervention in hospital, the patient will often be assessed in terms of their safety and independence. Questions to be considered include:

- Is this patient safe at home?
- Did any underlying pathology cause this fall?
- Is there an alternative care pathway or support service available to the patient?
- Is the patient able to perform activities of daily living?
- Is the patient socially integrated with family and/or community, with systems in place to cope with a change in circumstance?

CS CASE STUDY 2

Case 10980, 1453 hrs.

Dispatch details: A 28-year-old woman is complaining of feeling unwell with abdominal pain.

Initial presentation: The paramedics are met by a volunteer refugee support visitor, who is visiting the patient for the first time and called the ambulance. She explains that the patient is a Somali refugee who arrived within the last 2 months with two of her children.

---

(1) ASSESS

Assessing a patient who is a refugee can be a challenging experience for paramedics for a number of reasons, including language-based communication difficulties and the patient's possible lack of understanding of the healthcare system, previous experiences of abuse and/or feelings of shame about their health problems. Patients who speak some English may find it difficult to communicate in such a stressful situation or may agree with what is said out of confusion or politeness. Some paramedics may use family members or friends as informal interpreters but this has the potential to create miscommunication.

Some cultures have strong beliefs about the appropriateness of contact between males and females and mixed crews should offer a same-sex paramedic where the patient clearly prefers this (Kansu in Burnett & Peel, 2001; see Box

BOX 46.1 Strategies for interacting with patients who are refugees

- Be flexible and if possible offer the choice of a same-sex paramedic.
- Speak slowly and clearly.
- Use simple words; do not use slang or jargon.
- Be specific and offer the patient clear choices.
- Avoid making assumptions and generalisations based on your cultural biases.
- Consider family participation, especially as a translator.
- Avoid asking closed (yes/no) questions.
- Encourage the patient to ask you questions in order to confirm they have understood.

Source: Burnett & Peel (2001).

46.1). If the patient has suffered abuse or torture they may be suspicious or fearful of physical examination, or they may react aggressively towards people wearing uniforms who are assumed to be authority figures. Out-of-hospital emergency care is not an appropriate setting to address or explore these issues and doing so may cause the patient anguish or psychological harm.

In addition, there are some extra potential issues to consider clinically. The patient may not have received routine childhood immunisations and they may demonstrate disease specific to the region they came from—for example, tuberculosis is still prevalent in Asia and the Indian subcontinent, malaria is a definite concern in Southeast Asia and for patients with an African background sickle-cell anaemia is worth considering.

Effective communication is a critical paramedic skill. Establishing rapport with this patient and gaining her trust sufficiently to be able to assess her, to some degree, is vital. If it is not possible to gain her permission to carry out an assessment, or if undertaking the assessment is causing her great distress, the paramedics' aim should be to rule out the worst-case scenario. They should treat the patient with respect and not probe with questions that are more to satisfy their curiosity than to treat the patient.

In this case the patient appears seated upright but has a very flat affect, speaks very quietly and refuses to make eye contact but does not appear discomforted. She moves freely and is holding her youngest child. She is more animated when addressing the child. She is complaining of abdominal pain but the paramedics' ability to use history and examination to clarify the situation will be impaired in this case. They need to enlist the assistance of interpreters and support strategies to ensure that the patient's pain is appropriately investigated and managed. It is likely that this cannot be achieved effectively in the out-of-hospital environment.

DIFFERENTIAL DIAGNOSIS · 2

Undifferentiated abdominal pain
Or
- An unrelated medical condition described as abdominal pain
- An expression of distress described as abdominal pain

CONFIRM

In many cases paramedics are presented with a collection of signs and symptoms that do not appear to describe a particular condition. A critical step in determining a treatment plan in this situation is to consider what other conditions could explain the patient's presentation.

What else could it be?
An unrelated medical condition
Refugees can have multiple, complex or unusual health conditions that are not commonly seen, or are not seen at all, in the general population. For this patient, in addition to the usual differential diagnoses, the paramedics need

to consider whether a common presentation is complicated in some way or an unfamiliar condition is present.

Abdominal pain in a woman of child-bearing age always requires consideration of ectopic pregnancy or a complication of pregnancy. Female genital mutilation (FGM) is a traditional but harmful body modification prevalent in the Horn of Africa and is estimated to affect 97.9% of women in Somalia (Ministry of Health, 2012). It is defined by the WHO as 'partial or total removal of the external genitalia or other injury to the female genital organs whether for cultural or other non-therapeutic reasons' (WHO, 2018b). Paramedics should be aware of the complications caused by FGM in obstetric and gynaecological conditions such as spontaneous abortion or imminent childbirth.

Abdominal pain can be caused by infectious and parasitic diseases. For example, infection with *Helicobacter pylori* is high among the general refugee population and is associated with peptic ulcers and persistent abdominal discomfort. Parasitic worms are common in underdeveloped countries, entering the human host through contaminated food or drinking water. Infections of some parasitic worms, such as schistosomiasis, can be asymptomatic for years before causing serious disease, with symptoms including abdominal pain (Abdul Rahim et al., 2017).

A sickle-cell crisis is identified by severe pain that can occur in a number of sites including the abdomen. Sickle-cell disease is a genetically inherited blood disorder found in Africa and parts of the Middle East and causes significant morbidity and mortality. People with sickle-cell disease suffer from a crisis in response to hypoxia, which causes the haemoglobin to clump, changing the shape of the red blood cells. The abnormally shaped red blood cells block capillaries, causing ischaemia and infarction of the distal tissue (El-Hazmi et al., 2011).

An expression of distress

Abdominal pain can be a symptom of psychological disorders such as depression, anxiety or an eating disorder. Refugees are especially prone to feelings of intense guilt, loss and homesickness, which place them at a higher risk of developing psychological disorders. Abdominal pain could also arise from the ongoing physical effects of prolonged malnutrition, physical abuse, sexual abuse or sexually transmitted infection.

③ TREAT

This patient does not appear to be in any form of physiological distress or to have any overt symptoms that suggest a particular disease process. The likely progression of her abdominal pain is difficult to predict, however, and any suspicion that her presentation is primarily a response to social stress cannot override the possibility that she may also have a physical complaint. Her normal vital signs and lack of overt symptoms suggest that the paramedics have some time to make their decision regarding treatment and that immediate transport to hospital may not be the best management path for her. Ultimately, although she needs further medical assessment to exclude any serious pathology, alternatives such as being assessed by a local doctor or having a refugee support service arrange a medical examination may be better than delivering her to a crowded ED with limited resources to support her needs. Assessment and planning may take a lot longer than usual, allowing for time to gain the patient's confidence, sort out interpreters and provide support for the family.

④ EVALUATE

Evaluating the effect of any clinical management intervention can provide clues to the accuracy of the initial diagnosis. Some conditions respond rapidly to treatment so patients should be expected to improve if the diagnosis and treatment were appropriate. A failure to improve in this situation should trigger the clinician to reconsider the diagnosis.

In this case the recent onset of symptoms, combined with the lack of any physiological signs, suggests that the patient is unlikely to deteriorate during transport. Given the possible social factors involved in this case, an improvement in the patient's anxiety and discomfort once she has been transported from the site may provide some clues to the cause of her symptoms but a physical cause should not be completely ruled out.

Summary

Socially isolated patients are disconnected from society and lack relationships with a partner, family or friends. Physical, psychological, environmental and economic barriers may act to limit the individual's ability to engage with others. Social isolation is strongly associated with morbidity and mortality. Paramedics are in the unique position of attending to patients in their own homes. This gives them the ability to make a holistic assessment of the person's living situation and to refer isolated patients to appropriate services.

References

Abdul Rahim, N. R., Benson, J., Grocke, K., Vather, D., Zimmerman, J., Moody, T., & Mwanri, L. (2017). Prevalence of *Helicobacter pylori* infection in newly arrived refugees attending the migrant health service, South Australia. *Helicobacter, 22*(2), doi:10.1111/hel.12360.

Australian Bureau of Statistics. (2016a). *Census of population and housing: reflecting Australia.* Canberra, ACT: ABS.

Australian Bureau of Statistics. (2016b). *The Way we live now.* Canberra, ACT: ABS.

Australian Institute of Health and Welfare (AIHW). (2018). *Trends in hospitalised injury due to falls in older people 2002-03 to 2014-15.* Canberra, ACT: AIHW.

Burnett, A., & Peel, M. (2001). Health needs of asylum seekers and refugees. *British Medical Journal, 322,* 544–547.

Cacioppo, J. T., Hughes, M. E., Waite, L. J., Hawkley, L. C., & Thisted, R. A. (2006). Loneliness as a specific risk factor for depressive symptoms: cross-sectional and longitudinal analyses. *Psychology and Aging, 21*(1), 140–151. doi:10.1037/0882-7974.21.1.140.

Cattan, M., Kime, N., & Bagnall, A. (2011). The use of telephone befriending in low level support for socially isolated older people: an evaluation. *Health and Social Care in the Community, 19,* 198–206.

Chang, J. T., Morton, S. C., Rubenstein, L. Z., Mojica, W. A., Maglione, M., Suttorp, M. J., Roth, E. A., & Shekelle, P. G. (2004). Interventions for the prevention of falls in older adults: systematic review and meta-analysis of randomised clinical trials. *British Medical Journal, 328*(7441), 680. doi:10.1136/bmj.328.7441.680.

Cornwell, E. Y., & Waite, L. J. (2009). Social disconnectedness, perceived isolation, and health among older adults. *Journal of Health and Social Behavior, 50,* 31–48.

Croskerry, P. (2002). Achieving quality in clinical decision making: cognitive strategies and detection of bias. *Quality in Clinical Decision Making, 9,* 1184–1204.

Davison, J., & Marrinan, S. (2007). Falls. *Reviews in Clinical Gerontology, 17,* 93–107. doi:10.1017/S0959259808002426.

de Jong Gierveld, J., & Havens, B. (2004). Cross-national comparisons of social isolation and loneliness: introduction and overview. *Canadian Journal on Aging, 23*(2), 119–123.

Department of Social Services (DSS). (2018). *Humanitarian settlement services.* Canberra, ACT: Australian Government.

DeSouza, R. (2012). *Doing it for ourselves and our children: refugee women on their own in New Zealand.* Auckland: Centre for Asian and Migrant Health, AUT University.

Dickens, A. P., Richards, S. H., Greaves, C. J., & Campbell, J. L. (2011). Interventions targeting social isolation in older people: a systematic review. *BMC Public Health, 11,* 647–669. doi:10.1186/1471-2458-11-647.

El-Hazmi, M. A. F., AlHazmi, A. M., & Warsy, A. S. (2011). Sickle cell disease in Middle East Arab countries. *The Indian Journal of Medical Research, 134*(5), 597–610. doi:10.4103/0971-5916.90984.

Fratiglioni, L., Wang, H., Ericsson, K., Maytan, M., & Winblad, B. (2000). Influence of social network on occurrence of dementia: a community-based longitudinal study. *The Lancet. Neurology, 355,* 1315–1319.

Hawton, A., Green, C., Dickens, A. P., Richards, S. H., Taylor, R. S., Edwards, R., Greaves, C. J., & Campbell,

J. L. (2010). The impact of social isolation on the health status and health-related quality of life of older people. *Quality of Life Research, 20,* 57–67.

Holt-Lunstad, J., Smith, T. B., & Layton, J. B. (2010). Social relationships and mortality risk: a meta-analytic review. *PLoS Medicine, 7,* 1–20.

Locher, J., Ritchie, C., Roth, D., Baker, P., Bodner, E., & Allman, R. (2005). Social isolation, support, and capital and nutritional risk in an older sample: ethnic and gender differences. *Social Science & Medicine, 60,* 747–761.

Mangoni, A. A., & Jackson, S. H. D. (2003). Age-related changes in pharmacokinetics and pharmacodynamics: basic principles and practical applications. *British Journal of Clinical Pharmacology, 57*(1), 6–14. doi:10.1046/j1365-2125.2003.02007.x.

Ministry of Health. (2012). *Refugee health care: a handbook for health professionals.* Wellington: Ministry of Health.

Mistry, R., Rosansky, J., McGuire, J., McDermott, C., & Jarvik, L. (2001). Social isolation predicts re-hospitalization in a group of older American veterans enrolled in the UPBEAT program. *International Journal of Geriatric Psychiatry, 16,* 950–959.

Moller, J. (2003). *Projected cost of falls-related injury to older persons as a result of demographic change in Australia.* Canberra: Commonwealth Department of Health and Ageing.

NHS Confederation, Ambulance Service Network and Community Health Services Forum. (2012). *Falls Prevention. New Approaches to Integrated Falls Prevention Services.* Retrieved from www.nhsconfed.org/Publications/Documents/Falls_prevention_briefing_final_for_website_30_April.pdf.

Nicholson, N. R. (2008). Social isolation in older adults: an evolutionary concept analysis. *Journal of Advanced Nursing, 65*(6), 1342–1352.

Ross, L., Jennings, P. A., Smith, K., & Williams, B. (2017). Paramedic attendance to older patients in Australia, and the prevalence and implications of psychosocial issues. *Prehospital Emergency Care, 21*(1), 32–38. doi:10.1080/10903127.2016.1204037.

Simpson, P. M., Bendall, B. C., Patterson, J., Tiedemann, A., Middleton, P. M., & Close, J. C. (2013). Epidemiology of ambulance responses to older people who have fallen in New South Wales, Australia. *Australasian Journal on Ageing, 32*(3), 171–176. doi:10.1111/j.1741-6612.2012.00621.x.

Snooks, H. A., Halter, M., Close, J. C. T., Cheung, W., Moore, F., & Roberts, S. E. (2006). Emergency care of older people who fall: a missed opportunity. *Quality and Safety in Health Care, 15,* 390–392.

Thompson, C., Williams, K., Morris, D., Lago, L., Kobel, C., Quinsey, K., Eckermann, S., Andersen, P., & Masso, M. (2014). *HWA Expanded Scopes of Practice Program Evaluation: Extending the Role of Paramedics Sub-Project Final Report.* NSW: Centre for Health Service Development, Australian Health Services Research Institute, University of Wollongong.

Tromp, A. M., Pluijm, S. M., Smit, J. H., Deeg, D. J., Bouter, L. M., & Lips, P. (2001). Fall-risk screening test: a prospective study on predictors for falls in community-dwelling elderly. *Journal of Clinical Epidemiology, 54,* 837–844.

World Health Organization (WHO). (2018a). *Falls.* Geneva: WHO.

World Health Organization (WHO). (2018b). *Female genital mutilation.* Geneva: WHO.

Further resources

- Learn more about telephone befriending services at www.stjohn.org.nz/What-we-do/Community-programmes/Caring-Caller.
- Understand more about female genital mutilation with information and resources for health professionals at www.fgm.co.nz/contact.

CHAPTER 47

The Dying Patient

By Auston Rotheram and Peter Lucas

OVERVIEW

- Patients who are expected to die of an established disease often engage with ambulance services during episodes of sudden deterioration.
- Differentiation of reversible and inevitable deterioration requires decisions about active treatment versus active comfort measures.
- The physiological changes associated with dying include a gradual shutdown of organ function that may have no obvious effect for periods but then causes episodes of sudden change.

- Immunological compromise, immobility and pain-relieving medications can all lead to an acute change in the patient's condition. These changes are not caused directly by the underlying terminal condition and are often treatable.
- The psychological aspects of care of both the patient and their family are part of the holistic management of the dying patient.

Introduction

Paramedics, as with many other health professionals, are regularly faced with patients suffering from terminal conditions for which treatment is futile. Paramedic training, however, is heavily focused on responses to acute events where the goal is to restore the patient to health. As one of the few healthcare providers able to respond to patients in the community setting, paramedics are often faced with the difficult situation of an acute exacerbation of a terminal condition for which their clinical guidelines are inappropriate or ineffective. This chapter provides an overview of the clinical decision-making process pertaining to the challenging circumstances surrounding end-of-life care.

Caring for a person during the last few weeks and days of life can be stressful and demanding. Many different feelings and emotions may surface at this time (Palliative Care Australia, 2018). In many cases advance care planning will determine what the person's goals are regarding their end-of-life care. This planning process may result in an advance care plan or directive that sets out the person's values and preferences for end-of-life care often involving the appointment of an advocate or proxy decision-maker (palliAGED, 2017). Death from terminal conditions is rarely linear and many patients will have some episodes of sickness, decline and hospitalisation when dealing with a health crisis. Patients receiving end-of-life care may experience a range of conditions including increased and noisy respirations or alterations in conscious state that can be distressing to family members. This may trigger a call for emergency assistance. For paramedics the decision-making process must consider the advance care plan as well as whether the presenting acute condition is treatable or part of the dying process, all while considering the patient's and family's emotional wellbeing.

Palliative care aims to 'improve the life of those who have a life-limiting illness, their families and carers. The care provided does not endeavour to shorten or extend the life of patients, rather it helps give those with a life-limiting illness a better quality of life through care and support' (Department of Health and Ageing, 2011). End-of-life care is typically provided by an interdisciplinary team of specialist palliative care professionals and takes place in a variety of settings including the patient's home as well as hospitals, aged care facilities, specialist palliative care inpatient settings or hospices (Wiese et al., 2009).

The paramedic's role includes calm explanations to allay the patient's and family's fear and anxiety and liaison with the treating palliative care team or GP to arrange hospital admission. Research shows, however, that many paramedics feel poorly prepared to manage such situations (Stone et al., 2009).

Death and dying across the lifespan

In recent years Australia's death rate has stabilised at 5.4 deaths per 1000 population, down from 6.1 in 2006 and 12.7 in 1971 (ABS, 2016b). These rates have fallen due to a range of factors including advances in medicine, public health strategies and public awareness. Deaths from ischaemic heart disease declined from 99.1 per 100,000 in 2007 to 62.4 per 100,000 in 2016. In the same period deaths from dementia and Alzheimer's disease increased from 5.3% of all deaths in 2007 to 8.3% in 2016 (ABS, 2016a). Men continue to die at a younger age compared with women, but the gap is shrinking (ABS, 2016a). Malignant neoplasms and circulatory diseases take over as the main causes of death for those aged over 45; respiratory disease is notable from age 65 and falls become a feature for those aged over 75 (ABS, 2016a).

Pathophysiology

Identifying when a terminally ill patient is suffering a reversible condition that may be related to their treatment, rather than being part of a dying trajectory, is a challenging aspect of end-of-life care. Differences in the trajectories of certain other conditions further complicates this. For example, in some patients a terminal cancer trajectory can have periods of exacerbation and remission with a return to relative health before an ultimately sharp decline at the end of life. Compared to chronic diseases such as chronic obstructive pulmonary disease (COPD), the trajectory of remission and exacerbation rarely sees the patient returning to former health: their decline is more linear and can take much longer from the time of diagnosis to death (Downey & Engelberg, 2010).

People who are imminently dying have noticeable physiological changes in the way their body functions. These changes may occur over a period of hours or days prior to death and this course is both unpredictable and inevitable. There will likely be variations between individuals who have different diagnoses, such as the presence or absence of particular symptoms like nausea and vomiting or haemorrhaging. Where a gradual decline is experienced before death, the following physical changes may be observed.

Central nervous system

As death approaches alterations in a patient's conscious state often lead to the person becoming more introspective and socially isolated, sleeping more and spending less time interacting with those around them. Common symptoms in the dying patient included dysphagia, drowsiness, headache, seizures, agitation and delirium and death rattle. In some instances a terminally ill patient's conscious state progresses steadily to coma as the person approaches death (Gofton et al., 2012). A broad range of symptoms are common in patients with terminal illness; however, with appropriate assessment and diagnosis these can often be relieved (Ferris et al., 2002).

Physiologically, these changes may be a result of accumulating toxins from tissue destruction caused, for example, by a tumour or hypoxia. Almost 90% of individuals suffering a terminal disease will experience some form of delirium in the last weeks of life (Moyer, 2011). Hypoactive delirium is relatively common and occurs in almost 30% of cases (Moyer, 2011). Typically represented by moaning and groaning, delirium can take a hyperactive form with hallucinations, florid speech, paranoia, restlessness and confusion, or myoclonic seizures (Keeley, 2009). These signs can be particularly distressing for relatives. Peripheral reflexes decrease as circulation to the periphery decreases. This also results in reduced peripheral sensation, so touch perception may be reduced, although pressure sensation may still be present, in addition to pain (Bush et al., 2014).

Circulation

As cellular function deteriorates approaching death, cardiac rate and rhythm may be altered and arrhythmias such as tachycardia and bradycardia are common. As cardiac output diminishes, pulse pressure decreases, peripheral pulses are less palpable and heart sounds fainter. With less peripheral circulation, skin may become pale and waxen. In cases where hypoxia contributes to cell death, there may be increased peripheral or central cyanosis. As peripheral circulation diminishes, core temperature may increase, while the periphery cools and sweating in order to cool the body occurs.

Cardiac failure, both right- and left-sided, is a feature of end-stage cardiac decline. The drop in cardiac output results in poor perfusion, which in turn generates inflammatory mediators. This may cause fluid to enter the interstitial spaces, leading to peripheral or (more often) pulmonary oedema.

Respiratory system

In people with cancer, the elderly and those with terminal illnesses pneumonia can be common (Wee & Hillier, 2008). Infection can lead to consolidation of fluids resulting in reduced air entry which, in turn, contributes to poor gas exchange at the alveoli, resulting in dyspnoea. Excess bronchial exudates may also contribute to increased cough; however, the cough reflex diminishes as the dying trajectory extends. Air hunger, as a result of lung failure at the end of life, can cause severe distress and restlessness and rapid grunting respirations.

There are other common significant changes to respirations as a person is dying. One is Cheyne-Stokes breathing, which refers to alternating periods of apnoea and hyperpnoea with a crescendo–decrescendo pattern (Hui et al., 2014). This sign appears in the comatose patient, indicating interruption of the respiratory drive mechanisms in the brainstem. The normal drive to breathe is driven by CO_2 levels, but as death approaches the respiratory centre's response to varying CO_2 levels can become erratic. The presence of this clinical sign in a person with terminal illness indicates biochemical changes associated with either hypoxaemia or chemical mediators associated with tissue breakdown.

The second change, terminal respiratory secretions, occurs later in the dying trajectory and is often referred to as the death rattle (Eastern Metropolitan Region Palliative Care Consortium [EMRPCC], 2016). This respiratory noise may develop as a result of both upper and lower airway changes (Wilson & Giddens, 2016). The coarse crackles associated with this phase can develop as a result of left ventricular failure causing pulmonary oedema or because secretions pool in the upper airways. At this stage the patient is often unable to clear these secretions and the noise becomes louder, which can be particularly distressing for family members and carers. As terminal secretions are low in the airway, suctioning may be of limited use and may in fact contribute to the distress of the patient, family and carers. Repositioning rather than suctioning is often more effective in reducing upper airway noises (Wee & Hillier, 2008).

Gastrointestinal system

Gastrointestinal motility and absorption diminish as circulation to the gut decreases which often results in weight loss and constipation. Often, family members and carers may be concerned about lack of eating and attempt to 'force feed' the person, which only results in nausea and vomiting. Dysphagia, or difficulty swallowing, may make taking oral medications difficult and this should be anticipated, as most drugs necessary at the end of life can be administered by the subcutaneous route. Thirst due to dehydration is not a common problem at the end of life, despite a reduction in fluid intake. Reduced hydration may assist in reducing other more noxious symptoms such as fluid accumulation in the lungs, vomiting and incontinence. Drying of the tongue and lips is not uncommon but may not be directly related to hydration levels; rather, it may be the result of an increased respiratory rate, the side effects of medications or oral candidiasis (Dalal & Bruera, 2004).

Renal system

Urine output decreases with a reduction in hydration and circulation. This is unlikely to cause symptoms, but incontinence or retention caused by loss of sensation to the bladder may contribute to agitation. Urinary concentration and stasis may contribute to the development of urinary tract infection, resulting in increasing pain, which can contribute to agitation.

Hepatic system

With the failing perfusion status comes a reduction in liver function and, therefore, a reduction in the body's ability to clear drugs (Sun et al., 2006). It is not uncommon to see a reduced need for opiates in the last stages due to the reduction in drug clearance that occurs. Drug administration should be guided by symptoms and acknowledgment that there may be a reduction in drug clearance (Abel, 2013).

Other changes

Haemorrhage occurs in up to 20% of patients with palliative care needs (NHS Scotland, 2014), particularly those with haematological malignancies (McGrath & Leahy, 2009). It may, however, be associated with liver failure, comorbid haematological disorders, chemotherapy, medications, radiotherapy, surgery and the underlying disease progression, such as damage of blood vessels by tumour (Hulme & Wilcox, 2008). Bleeding may be episodic, a low-volume oozing or catastrophic depending on the underlying cause (McGrath & Leahy, 2009). Bleeding may present as bruising, melaena, haemoptysis, haematuria, haematemesis, epistaxis or vaginal or rectal bleeding. The site of the bleeding may give some indication of the cause and provide direction for management.

Patients at risk of catastrophic bleeding should have advance care plans in place and standing orders for sedation and pain management available if they are being cared for in their own home. Paramedics should contact the patient's GP and community-based palliative care providers before starting aggressive resuscitation for bleeding. In addition, simple measures such as using dark-coloured towels to disguise the colour and amount of bleeding can reduce the family's distress (McGrath & Leahy, 2009). The patient's family and carers often require reassurance that the patient is in an altered conscious state and that any pain is being managed (McGrath & Leahy, 2009). Administration of sedation during a catastrophic bleed is standard palliative care practice but sits outside the normal guidelines used by paramedics: consultation with the patient's care team is strongly recommended in this situation.

Spinal cord compression may be caused by a primary tumour and have an insidious onset or commonly by metastases from lung, breast, prostate or renal primary malignancies. Displacement of the spinal cord is caused by the metastatic lesion affecting function and leading to irreversible paralysis if not treated (Quraishi & Esler, 2011). The signs and symptoms may include back pain, limb weakness or sensory changes and bladder dysfunction, followed by ataxia and paralysis if it progresses (Quraishi & Esler, 2011). The skeleton is the third most common site for metastases after the lungs and liver (Patchell et al., 2005). Bony metastases most commonly occur in the vertebrae (Selvaggi & Abrahm, 2006). Spinal cord compression occurs in 5–14% of patients with a cancer diagnosis and is considered a palliative care emergency that requires immediate hospitalisation (Patchell et al., 2005).

CASE STUDY 1

Case 14058, 0435 hrs.

Dispatch details: An unconscious 67-year-old man with a history of lung cancer is in respiratory distress and an altered conscious state.

Initial presentation: The paramedics are taken to the bedroom by the patient's distressed partner. The patient is lying supine in bed on three pillows. He appears cachexic, pale and diaphoretic, and his breathing is stertorous. Peripheral cyanosis is also noted.

---

1 ASSESS

Patient history

Determining the underlying cause of a patient's deterioration is important. In particular, identifying whether the patient's condition is due to a reversible side effect of medical treatment or an end-of-life trajectory is key to determining the paramedic's next step. Patients with advanced cancer are likely to have recently had medical advice about their condition and treatment options. Asking the patient's partner or carer about medical discussions in relation to their illness and treatment is important. Asking questions about the cultural and religious backgrounds of the patient and their family is an important assessment step to ground the context of ongoing psychosocial care.

A more thorough physical assessment is sometimes appropriate. The paramedic should check the patient's temperature and ask about their recent cancer treatment. Some cancer treatments such as chemotherapy can increase the risk of infection by causing neutropenia. This risk will be at its maximum within approximately two weeks of chemotherapy. Possible sites of infection such as lungs or urine should also be checked.

The paramedic should also ask what medications the patient is taking and any recent changes to these medications. Patients with cancer pain can be on significantly large doses of opioid analgesics but this is unlikely to be the cause of this patient's condition if they have been on a slowly increasing dose over time. The introduction of new opioids or large dose changes, however, should be investigated. The patient's central nervous system response should be checked by repeating the assessment of consciousness (Glasgow Coma Scale [GCS]) and pupil size and response to light.

Asking the patient's partner or carer about the patient's condition over the last few days, particularly relating to sleep–wake cycles and food and fluid intake, may indicate a pattern of deterioration. The paramedic should not conclude a dying trajectory, however, until they have determined that changes

PRACTICE TIP

Cancer Institute of NSW (2011) identifies cancer patients with multiple febrile events as possible medical emergencies. A temperature of at least 38.3°C (or at least 38°C on two occasions) should be viewed as a time-critical event.

in medications such as increases in opioids are not contributing to this decreased conscious state. Additionally, they should check peripheral circulation and reflexes; lack of plantar and radial pulses, peripheral cyanosis and coolness and sluggish plantar reflexes may be a result of reduced cardiovascular function in a dying patient.

Initial assessment summary

Problem	Altered conscious state
Conscious state	GCS = 6; no eye opening, no verbal response, minimal attempt at withdrawal to pain
Position	Semi-recumbent in bed
Heart rate	70 bpm, irregular, shallow
Blood pressure	100 on palpation
Skin appearance	Pale, diaphoretic, peripherally cyanosed
Speech pattern	No speech
Respiratory rate	15 bpm
Respiratory rhythm	Shallow, irregular with periods of apnoea
Chest auscultation	Widespread coarse crackles bilaterally
Pulse oximetry	Not sensing
Temperature	36.1°C
History	Recent decline in health; partner was woken by patient's noisy breathing and was unable to rouse them
Physical assessment	Patient cachexic (characterised by weight loss, muscle atrophy and weakness in someone who is not actively attempting to lose weight)

This patient appears to be in the terminal phase of his illness.

(2) CONFIRM

The essential part of the clinical reasoning process is to seek to confirm your initial hypothesis by finding clinical signs that should occur with your provisional diagnosis. You should also seek to challenge your diagnosis by exploring findings that do not fit your hypothesis: don't just ignore them because they don't fit.

There are a number of possible reasons for this patient's deterioration. The patient's cancer may be progressing and they may in fact be near death. Alternatively, they may be septic as a result of cancer treatment suppressing their immunity or they may have experienced an overdose of medications.

What else could it be?

Sepsis

If sepsis is assessed as the primary problem, the patient may have an increased body temperature; however, patients who have suppressed immunity may not exhibit the same response to infection as people with normal immunity (refer to Ch 32; Cancer Institute of NSW, 2011). The lack of tachycardia normally associated with sepsis may be a result of the patient's terminal state and cannot be used to definitively exclude sepsis. The risk of infection is increased by both the patient's bed-ridden state and their underlying disease, but infection may not be the cause of such sudden deterioration.

Medication change

In opioid overdose, patients often have a decreased level of consciousness, bradycardia and hypoventilation, as does this patient. A brief assessment of the patient's conscious level using the GCS to assess psychomotor response and pupil size will assist in differentiating between drug overdose and disease progression. Constricted pupils are often present in patients who have been on narcotics for a long period of time. In this case the patient's pupils are

---

LOOK FOR!

- Grunting respirations and use of accessory muscles to breathe
- Malodourous urine
- Lower abdominal pain on palpation

ASK ABOUT!

- Medication history
- Medication chart or record
- Palliative care record or referral
- Mental state over past 24 hours
- Patterns of eating and drinking
- Last medical discussions

DIFFERENTIAL DIAGNOSIS

Terminal stage of cancer (dying)
Or
- A reversible condition associated with sepsis
- A reversible condition associated with a change in medication

normal. Understanding the patient's recent medication history is likely to assist in the exclusion of drug overdose. Consulting with the patient's GP, district nurse or palliative care provider may clarify questions about medication usage, medical management plan and goals of care.

③ TREAT

Emergency management

The challenge for paramedics faced with this situation is not necessarily to initiate the emergency care that a patient displaying these vital signs would normally require. The primary concern in managing a terminally ill patient in the community is to slow decision-making down as much as possible to ensure that the patient's wishes are respected, family members are supported and the patient is kept comfortable. Using a palliative approach to care is necessary in order to ensure the comfort and safety of the patient and their family (Baillie et al., 2018).

If the patient is imminently dying as a result of their progressive cancer, there is nothing that can be done to prevent death. Determining the patient's wishes in the circumstances, however, is important. Some patients may have indicated their wishes in terms of the place of their death and their desire not to experience medical interventions such as trips to hospital or resuscitation by discussing this with family members, documenting a refusal of treatment, appointing a proxy decision-maker in an enduring power of attorney or preparing an advance care plan. A careful and sensitive discussion with the patient's carer may determine the patient's wishes and guide the treatment plan (Detering et al., 2010).

There are numerous reasons family members may call an emergency paramedic instead of the community nurse, palliative care provider, GP or other family members, even contrary to instructions or plans. Human mortality has been found to increase outside of regular working hours (Zhou et al., 2016), when other support services are often unavailable. Other conditions such as terminal restlessness can be distressing for families (Brajtman, 2003) and gentle assistance to recall the agreed plan of care in these circumstances may be helpful. Even when families have discussed death and options such as the patient's desire to remain at home or to refuse further medical interventions, family members may not be sure if these decisions apply to the particular situation they find themselves in. Sometimes they need reassurance that their loved one is dying in order to acknowledge that they can put an agreed plan into action.

Sometimes, the use of oxygen via a mask or nasal cannula will improve oxygenation and enable the patient to participate in these discussions. Gentle and appropriate oropharyngeal suction may also be used to reduce the secretions causing stertorous breathing (EMRPCC, 2016). The procedure may irritate an otherwise peaceful patient and is not always effective as the fluid is often low in the airway and re-accumulates. Patients with stertorous breathing are normally unconscious and dyspnoea is not apparent, but the noise is often distressing for family members.

If the following documents have been completed by the patient, they may assist in determining appropriate treatment in the event of imminent death by identifying either the patient's wishes or a proxy who has an understanding of the patient's wishes:

- Medical Goals of Care
- Refusal of Treatment
- Enduring Medical Power of Attorney (MPOA)
- Advance Care Plan.

A community palliative care service plan of care for end of life may include standing orders of helpful medications for symptoms such as pain, nausea, vomiting, agitation and noisy breathing. Phoning the palliative care service,

> ## BOX 47.1 Ethical issue: double effect
>
> The principle of double effect was identified by St Thomas Aquinas to describe circumstances in which an action may have good and bad effects but still be morally acceptable (Boyle, 2004; Jolly & Cornock, 2003). A good example of this is that the means of managing intractable symptoms may inadvertently shorten a patient's life. The intent of the treatment is to palliate the symptoms and death is a foreseen but unintended consequence of that treatment (Boyle, 2004). The principle of double effect does not simply allow bad outcomes because they are not intended, however: the requirement of a 'proportionally grave reason' for harmful side effects must give appropriate weight and consideration to the moral justification for the action (Boyle, 2004). Some palliative care legislation is enlightened enough to specifically mention and support the situation where management improves quality of life but may shorten it.

GP or nurse involved in the patient's care may assist the paramedic in clarifying the patient's condition and plan of care.

In some situations, the decision will be made to transport the patient to hospital for end-of-life care, based on clarification of the patient's wish not to die at home or consideration that the family is unable to provide care at home. Moving a patient who has very poor cardiac output into a sitting position in order to transfer them to a stretcher can reduce venous return sufficiently to completely compromise cardiac output and cause a sudden deterioration. This should be considered when making the decision to move the patient (Ingleton et al., 2009).

If an opioid overdose is suspected, extreme care, and preferably advice from the patient's medical practitioner, should be taken in attempting to reverse the overdose with a narcotic antagonist (see Box 47.1). A lack of careful titration is likely to cause severe rebound pain in the terminally ill person, either necessitating emergency hospital admission for some days to re-establish pain control or leading to an excruciatingly painful death if death is imminent. Supportive care is preferable with oxygen/ventilation support until the serum concentration of the narcotic has reduced and the patient's conscious state has improved, although this may take some time. Often CO_2 retention is a significant factor in opiate-induced respiratory failure causing a decreased conscious level: this will reverse with a few full breaths using a bag/mask. When all other options have been exhausted or if imminent death as a result of overdose is suspected, an opioid reversal protocol (not more than 100 micrograms intravenous [IV] per dose titrated to effect) devised for palliative care may be used.

Depending on the patient's wishes it may be appropriate to either aggressively manage sepsis or actively not manage it. If sepsis as a result of neutropenia is suspected and active management is selected, time to first treatment with antibiotics is a significant factor in survival: 1 hour is recommended. The septic shock is managed with oxygen and IV fluids to maintain blood volume during immediate transport to hospital (Cancer Institute of NSW, 2011).

Verification of death

In some jurisdictions approved paramedics are permitted to verify death by undertaking clinical assessment of a body and establishing that death has occurred although legislation differs across individual jurisdictions (see Box 47.2).

4 EVALUATE

Continuous reassessment of the patient's condition and interventions is important. Liaison with palliative care services or the patient's GP should also occur in conjunction with the patient's family.

> ## BOX 47.2 Criteria for the verification of death
>
> - No palpable pulse and
> - No heart sounds heard for 2 minutes and
> - No breath sounds heard for 2 minutes and
> - Fixed (non-responsive to light) pupils and
> - No response to centralised painful stimulus and
> - No motor response to peripheral painful stimulus
>
> *Source: Department of Health (2010).*

Ongoing management

While disease trajectories are unique to the individual they are also driven by pathophysiology, shaped by strategies used by patients, families and health professionals and affected by other issues such as access to treatment options and services. In the healthcare setting, clinical care pathways have been used to streamline care management and resource allocation. Clinical care pathways are structured multidisciplinary plans of care designed to support the implementation of clinical guidelines, clinical and non-clinical resource management, clinical audits and financial management. They provide detailed guidance for each stage in the management of a patient for a specific condition over a given time period and include progress and outcome details (Kinsman et al., 2010). Care pathways usually have four components:

1. a timeline
2. categories of care and interventions
3. intermediate and long-term outcome criteria
4. a record of deviations from the pathway and how they are managed.

They can be viewed as algorithms in that they offer a flow chart for stepwise decision-making for a particular patient group or condition.

In Australia, the majority of expected deaths of the elderly and those with non-palliative care conditions occur in hospitals or extended-care facilities (Jackson et al., 2009). The Liverpool Care Pathway has been adapted for use with patients in acute and extended-care facilities all over the world so as to best reflect local practices, needs and resource availability (Jackson et al., 2009). The end-of-life care pathway is patient- and family-focused, evidence-based and addresses the four key domains of physical, psychological, social and spiritual needs. Such pathways serve to guide generalist staff through basic palliative care principles and practices (Jackson et al., 2009).

A key to successful implementation of such pathways is helpful for identifying impending death early enough to facilitate a 'good death' for the patient and provide support for their family (Jackson et al., 2009). Using the pathway, medications, treatments and other interventions are reviewed and their value, in terms of how they support palliative care goals, is evaluated. Interventions and medications deemed unnecessary are discontinued. Recommended standing orders for medications to manage a range of potentially distressing symptoms that may accompany end of life are also included in the pathway. The most common symptoms are pain, terminal restlessness and agitation, excessive upper respiratory secretions, dyspnoea, and nausea and vomiting. Medications are balanced to provide the most effective level of symptom management possible. For non-specialist palliative care staff, the types of drugs used, the combinations and the dosage ranges may be unfamiliar and confronting. The recommended medication guidelines have been developed based on evidence-based palliative care practice (Jackson et al., 2009).

Hospital admission

Managing a 'good death' in a home setting is the goal of many palliative care plans but, failing this, admission to hospital or, less commonly, direct hospice admission are alternatives. The emergency department (ED) is the main portal of entry to hospital and, as such, has increasingly been accessed by those with end-of-life needs. The problem is that EDs, like paramedics, typically prioritise resuscitation and prolonging life over providing quality end-of-life care (Bailey et al., 2011). The focus on diagnosis, stabilisation and complying with performance measures such as waiting times and length of stay does not equip EDs with resources and pathways for palliation and explains why end-of-life care in this setting may be less than optimal

(Rosenberg & Rosenberg, 2013). In the ED there is little space or privacy for patients and families to prepare for impending death or for staff to be able to offer the quality of end-of-life care and family support that are hallmarks of quality palliative care (Quest et al., 2013).

A West Australian study reviewed hospital and ED use by people who were not living in residential aged care facilities but had a terminal illness and were expected to die. Over a one-year period, 61.5% of patients died in hospital and 4% had been seen in an ED on the day of their death (Bailey et al., 2011; Rosenwax et al., 2011). Rosenwax and colleagues (2011) suggest that such heavy reliance on the acute health system indicates gaps in palliative care service delivery to vulnerable people in the final stages of their life.

The likelihood of death while being transported to hospital by ambulance is another factor that needs to be considered. Discuss with family how the patient and family may be supported at home, particularly if the patient is close to death. Liaison with the patient's GP and community-based palliative care service provider is important for a plan of care to be complete. In some jurisdictions extended care paramedics have proved very competent in this area of care, working in conjunction with the patient's GP and palliative care teams. The patient may have been an inpatient in a specialist palliative care unit in the past and be known to the medical and nursing staff. If so, the GP or community palliative care service may be able to assist with admitting the patient directly into the palliative care unit, rather than an ED.

 CASE STUDY 2

Case 10045, 1600 hrs.

Dispatch details: A 78-year-old woman with a 5-year history of breast cancer has been found drowsy and disorientated by her daughter.

Initial presentation: The paramedics arrive at a private house and follow the daughter to the bathroom where they find the patient sitting against the vanity unit.

 ASSESS

1610 hrs Primary survey: The patient is disorientated to place and time.

1611 hrs Chief complaint: Drowsy and disorientated.

1612 hrs Vital signs survey: Perfusion status: HR 100 bpm strong and regular, BP 110/65 mmHg, skin pale and clammy.
  Respiratory status: RR 22 bpm, good clear air entry bilaterally.
  Conscious state: GCS = 12.

1615 hrs Pertinent hx: The daughter (the patient's carer) called her mother this morning at 11 and found that she had been vomiting; this was unrelieved by antiemetic. She arrived home from work at 4 to find her mother drowsy and disorientated. The patient has not had anything to eat or drink for 48 hours and has recently undergone chemotherapy. She is on cycle three and was reviewed by her GP a week ago, when her medications were reviewed. Initially the patient was diagnosed with ductal carcinoma of the breast with axillary lymph node involvement and had a right mastectomy and axillary clearance with radiotherapy. Two months ago she had liver metastases diagnosed following routine follow-up scans. She has had two cycles of chemotherapy with a limited response. She was referred to a palliative care consultant and community palliative care services in the local area.

1618 hrs Secondary survey: Alopecia related to chemotherapy; dry mouth, coated tongue; pupils equal and reacting; right mastectomy scarring well-healed; tense abdomen; bowel sounds present and normal; diffuse pain on palpation; nil rebound tenderness. The patient has been incontinent of urine and has a fine tremor in her hands.

The patient has a history of decline over the last 2 days and presents confused with a raised respiratory rate and signs of dehydration. The problem appears to be dehydration secondary to nausea and vomiting, but it is unclear what caused the nausea and vomiting in the first place. It is possible that this could be due to the drugs used in her chemotherapy.

② CONFIRM

In many cases paramedics are presented with a collection of signs and symptoms that do not appear to describe a particular condition. A critical step in determining a treatment plan in this situation is to consider what other conditions could explain the patient's presentation.

What could it be?

Side effect of medication

Nausea and vomiting are unfortunately a well-known side effect of many chemotherapy drugs and they can be difficult to manage effectively. Once a patient has started to vomit, administering oral antiemetics becomes difficult. The patient may respond to systemic administration of an appropriate antiemetic and consultation with the patient's care team is encouraged.

Cardiovascular stroke

A stroke could cause a decrease in the patient's conscious level. Patients with cancer can have an increase in coagulation factors and are at a higher risk of an embolic stroke. This would usually present with some unilateral signs, which do not appear to be present in this patient.

Sepsis

Infection is a possibility, with a relative lack of response to the infection being due to the immunosuppression associated with chemotherapy. If this cannot be confidently ruled out, empirical treatment as if this is sepsis is usually recommended.

Drug overdose of opiates

Opiates cause nausea and a decreased conscious state so could be responsible for this patient's presentation. Look for changes in drug use, noting that the patient may not have been following the prescribed recommendations exactly.

Bowel obstruction

The patient could have a bowel obstruction. Unfortunately, it is difficult to assess the patient's abdomen in this situation as diffuse tenderness is not diagnostic of a bowel obstruction. She wouldn't be expected to have passed much per rectum as she hasn't been eating, so this won't help the assessment. At the moment, this diagnosis remains a possibility.

Cerebral metastases

Cerebral metastases can present with nausea and vomiting and are quite likely in this setting. Lack of focal signs is reassuring but does not exclude the diagnosis. This diagnosis still remains a possibility.

Establishing the cause of the patient's nausea and vomiting becomes a process of elimination, which may well rely on in-hospital tests and investigations, as well as the patient's response to medication.

> **DIFFERENTIAL DIAGNOSIS**
>
> **Terminal stage of cancer**
> Or
> - Side effect of medication
> - Cardiovascular stroke
> - Sepsis
> - Drug overdose of opiates
> - Bowel obstruction
> - Cerebral metastases

TREAT

The patient's first need is for volume replacement and control of her nausea and vomiting. IV fluids and an IV antiemetic are an appropriate first measure. Her condition is complex and identifying the cause of the nausea and vomiting will lead to long-term management strategies. As health professionals, working within the greater healthcare team, this is the time for the paramedics to share the problem with the clinicians who know the patient's history well. A joint management plan between the paramedics and the treating palliative care team will probably involve an early review and investigations, either in hospital or as an outpatient.

4 EVALUATE

Evaluating the effect of any clinical management intervention can provide clues to the accuracy of the initial diagnosis. Some conditions respond rapidly to treatment so patients should be expected to improve if the diagnosis and treatment were appropriate. A failure to improve in this situation should trigger the clinician to reconsider the diagnosis.

In this case, the paramedics will evaluate whether they have relieved the patient's symptoms and returned her to a functional state. An improvement in her conscious level, a decrease in the nausea and vomiting and a decrease in her respiratory rate would all be indicative of an initial improvement. In conjunction with her treating team they will evaluate whether it is safe and appropriate to treat her at home or whether she needs hospital investigation for stabilisation and assessment.

Summary

Management of the dying patient in a palliative care situation is very different from the normal paramedic approach of treat and resuscitate. However, paramedics are in a position to be able to significantly improve quality of life for the remainder of the patient's life and to support their family and carers at the time of their death. Managing patients in this situation is very much a multidisciplinary team activity and the professional paramedic has an important role to play.

References

Abel, J. (2013). Withdrawing life-extending drugs at the end of life. *Prescriber, 24*(13–16), 17–20.

Australian Bureau of Statistics (ABS). (2016a). *Causes of Death, Australia, Cat. no 3303.0*. Retrieved from http://www.abs.gov.au/ausstats/abs@.nsf/Lookup/by%20Subject/3303.0~2016~Main%20Features~Summary%20of%20findings~1.

Australian Bureau of Statistics (ABS). (2016b). *Deaths, Australia. Cat. no. 3302.0*. Retrieved from http://www.abs.gov.au/ausstats/abs@.nsf/mf/3302.0.

Bailey, C., Murphy, R., & Porock, D. (2011). Trajectories of end-of-life care in the emergency department. *Annals of Emergency Medicine, 57*(4), 362–369.

Baillie, J., Anagnostou, D., Sivell, S., Van Godwin, J., Byrne, A., & Nelson, A. (2018). Symptom management, nutrition and hydration at end-of-life: a qualitative exploration of patients', carers' and health professionals' experiences and further research questions. *BMC Palliative Care, 17*(1), 60. doi:10.1186/s12904-018-0314-4.

Boyle, J. (2004). Medical ethics and double effect: the case of terminal sedation. *Theoretical Medicine and Bioethics, 25*(1), 51–60.

Brajtman, S. (2003). The impact on the family of terminal restlessness and its management. *Palliative Medicine, 17*(5), 454–460. doi:10.1191/0960327103pm779oa.

Bush, S. H., Leonard, M. M., Agar, M., Spiller, J. A., Hosie, A., Wright, D. K., & Lawlor, P. G. (2014). End-of-life delirium: issues regarding recognition, optimal management, and the role of sedation in the dying phase. *Journal of Pain and Symptom Management, 48*(2), 215–230.

Cancer Institute of NSW. (2011). *Immediate management of neutropenic fever*. Retrieved from https://www.eviq.org.au/clinical-resources/oncological-emergencies/123-immediate-management-of-neutropenic-fever.

Dalal, S., & Bruera, E. (2004). Dehydration in cancer patients: to treat or not to treat. *The Journal of Supportive Oncology, 2*(6), 467–479.

Department of Health. (2010). Guidance note for the 'Verification of Death'. Retrieved from http://www.health.vic.gov.au/__data/assets/pdf_file/0006/356667/Guidance-Note-for-the-Verification-of-Death-Feb-2010.pdf.

Department of Health and Ageing. (2011). *Guidelines for a Palliative Approach for Aged Care in the Community Setting*. Canberra: Australian Government Department of Health and Ageing.

Detering, K. M., Hancock, A. D., Reade, M. C., & Silvester, W. (2010). The impact of advance care planning on end of life care in elderly patients: randomised controlled trial. *British Medical Journal, 340*, c1345.

Downey, L., & Engelberg, R. A. (2010). Quality-of-life trajectories at the end of life: assessments over time by patients with and without cancer. *Journal of the American Geriatrics Society, 58*(3), 472–479.

Eastern Metropolitan Region Palliative Care Consortium (EMRPCC). (2016). *Management of respiratory secretions in the terminal phase*. Melbourne: EMRPCC.

Ferris, F. D., von Gunten, C. F., & Emanuel, L. L. (2002). Ensuring competency in end-of-life care: controlling symptoms. *BMC Palliative Care, 1*, 5. doi:10.1186/1472-684X-1-5.

Gofton, T. E., Graber, J., & Carver, A. (2012). Identifying the palliative care needs of patients living with cerebral tumors and metastases: a retrospective analysis. *Journal of Neuro-Oncology, 108*(3), 527–534. doi:10.1007/s11060-012-0855-y.

Hui, D., dos Santos, R., Chisholm, G., Bansal, S., Silva, T. B., Kilgore, K., & Perez-Cruz, P. E. (2014). Clinical signs of impending death in cancer patients. *The Oncologist, 19*(6), 681–687.

Hulme, B., & Wilcox, S. (2008). *Guidelines on the management of bleeding for palliative care patients with cancer*. Yorkshire Palliative Medicine Clinical Guidelines Group. Retrieved from http://www.Palliativedrugs.com.

Ingleton, C., Payne, S., Sargeant, A., & Seymour, J. (2009). Barriers to achieving care at home at the end of life: transferring patients between care settings using patient transport services. *Palliative Medicine, 23*(8), 723–730.

Jackson, K., Mooney, C., & Campbell, D. (2009). The development and implementation of the pathway for improving the care of the dying in general medical wards. *Internal Medicine Journal, 39*(10), 695–699.

Jolly, M., & Cornock, M. (2003). Application of the doctrine of double effect in end stage disease. *International Journal of Palliative Nursing, 9*(6), 240–244.

Keeley, P. W. (2009). Delirium at the end of life. *BMJ Clinical Evidence, 2009*, 2405.

Kinsman, L., Rotter, T., James, E., Snow, P., & Willis, J. (2010). What is a clinical pathway? Development of a definition to inform the debate. *BMC Medicine, 8*, 31. doi:10.1186/1741-7015-8-31.

McGrath, P., & Leahy, M. (2009). Catastrophic bleeds during end-of-life care in haematology: controversies from Australian research. *Supportive Care in Cancer, 17*(5), 527–537.

Moyer, D. D. (2011). Terminal delirium in geriatric patients with cancer at end of life. *American Journal of Hospice and Palliative Medicine®, 28*(1), 44–51.

NHS Scotland. (2014). *Scottish Palliative Care Guidelines*. Retrieved from http://www.palliativecareguidelines.scot.nhs.uk/guidelines/palliative-emergencies/.

palliAGED. (2017). *Advanced Care Planning*. Retrieved from https://www.palliaged.com.au/tabid/4389/Default.aspx.

Palliative Care Australia. (2018). *The Dying Process*. Retrieved from http://palliativecare.org.au/resources/the-dying-process.

Patchell, R. A., Tibbs, P. A., Regine, W. F., Payne, R., Saris, S., Kryscio, R. J., & Young, B. (2005). Direct decompressive surgical resection in the treatment of spinal cord compression caused by metastatic cancer: a randomised trial. *The Lancet, 366*(9486), 643–648.

Quest, T., Herr, S., Lamba, S., & Weissman, D. (2013). Demonstrations of clinical initiatives to improve palliative care in the emergency department: a report from the IPAL-EM initiative. *Annals of Emergency Medicine, 61*(6), 661–667. doi:10.1016/j.annemergmed.2013.01.019.

Quraishi, N. A., & Esler, C. (2011). Metastatic spinal cord compression. BMJ. *British Medical Journal, 342*.

Rosenberg, M., & Rosenberg, L. (2013). Integrated model of palliative care in the emergency department. *Western Journal of Emergency Medicine, 14*(6), 633–636. doi:10.5811/westjem.2013.5.14674.

Rosenwax, L. K., McNamara, B. A., Murray, K., McCabe, R. J., Aoun, S. M., & Currow, D. C. (2011). Hospital and emergency department use in the last year of life: a baseline for future modifications to end-of-life care. *The Medical Journal of Australia, 194*(11), 570–573.

Selvaggi, K., & Abrahm, J. (2006). Metastatic spinal cord compression: the hidden danger. *Nature Reviews. Clinical Oncology, 3*(8), 458.

Stone, S. C., Abbott, J., McClung, C. D., Colwell, C. B., Eckstein, M., & Lowenstein, S. R. (2009). Paramedic knowledge, attitudes, and training in end-of-life care. *Prehospital and Disaster Medicine, 24*(6), 529–534.

Sun, H., Frassetto, L., & Benet, L. Z. (2006). Effects of renal failure on drug transport and metabolism. *Pharmacology & Therapeutics, 109*(1), 1–11, doi. https://doi.org/10.1016/j.pharmthera.2005.05.010.

Wee, B., & Hillier, R. (2008). Interventions for noisy breathing in patients near to death. *The Cochrane Library*: CD005177.

Wiese, C. H., Bartels, U. E., Marczynska, K., Ruppert, D., Graf, B. M., & Hanekop, G. G. (2009). Quality of out-of-hospital palliative emergency care depends on the expertise of the emergency medical team—a prospective multi-centre analysis. *Supportive Care in Cancer, 17*(12), 1499–1506.

Wilson, S. F., & Giddens, J. F. (2016). *Health assessment for nursing practice* (6th ed.). Mosby.

Zhou, Y., Li, W., Herath, C., Xia, J., Hu, B., Song, F., Cao, S., & Lu, Z. (2016). Off-hour admission and mortality risk for 28 specific diseases: a systematic review and meta-analysis of 251 cohorts. *Journal of the American Heart Association, 5*(3), https://doi.org/10.1161/JAHA.115.003102. 9 March.

CHAPTER 48

Older Patients

By Judy Lowthian and Rosamond Dwyer

OVERVIEW

- The Australian population is ageing and older people are an increasing proportion of ambulance services call-outs.
- Underlying factors include population ageing, changes in social support, accessibility and pricing, and increasing community health awareness.
- Ageing is characterised by progressive decline of organ function and physiological reserve, albeit at

different rates that vary from individual to individual.
- Seemingly uncomplicated signs can mask serious underlying pathology.
- Management of older people with acute illness or injury requires a holistic approach including consideration of physical and mental state and social circumstances.

Introduction

Population ageing

Older people make up an increasing proportion of the world's population. A consequence of the significant improvement in life expectancy is the 'ageing' of the population, with the median age of the Australian population rising steadily from 32.1 to 35.2 to 37.2 years in 1990, 2000 and 2016, respectively (Australian Bureau of Statistics [ABS], 2017).

Between 1995 and 2015, the proportion of Australia's population aged 65 years and over increased from 11.9% to 15.0% including the proportion of people aged 85 years and over rising from 1.1% in 1995 to 2% in 2015 (ABS, 2015). If current trends continue, by 2033 the proportion of Australians aged 65 years and over will increase to 19%, with 3% of the population aged 85 years or more. Fast forward another 30 years to 2063, and the proportion of people aged 65 years and over would be 23%, including the proportion of people aged 85 years or more at 5% (ABS, 2014).

Increasing demand for emergency medical services by older people

Older people use more healthcare services per capita than younger age groups. People aged 70 years or older use emergency medical services (EMS) and emergency departments (ED) at higher rates and require more resources upon arrival in the ED. They are also more likely to experience adverse health outcomes after an acute health episode (Lowthian et al., 2015).

A study of emergency ambulance usage across Melbourne quantified the rise in demand, with an average annual growth rate of 4.8% over 14 years.

The transportation rate rose from 31.8 per 1000 people in 1994–95 to 57.6 per 1000 people of all ages. An acceleration in use by older cohorts was also identified as summarised in Table 48.1, with the highest increase apparent in people aged 85 years and over (Lowthian et al., 2011).

Epidemiological profile

Older people seek emergency care with medical problems related to chronic disease, multiple comorbidities, frailty and polypharmacy. Principal medical issues relate to cardiovascular, respiratory, neurological, musculoskeletal and abdominal conditions, to adverse drug reactions and to injury. In addition, there are usually numerous other intermingling contributing factors (Lowthian, 2016; Ross et al., 2017).

Medical factors

Studies from the United States, the United Kingdom and Australia concur that this is likely to be due to an increase in the prevalence of chronic medical conditions and the incidence of age-related acute illnesses alongside cognitive and physical dysfunction (Lowthian et al., 2011). Over 50% of Australians aged 65 or more report a disability, with one in five reporting profound limitations (ABS, 2003a, 2003b).

Certain comorbidities may increase the risk of requiring emergency care and ambulance call out. These include having a diagnosis of chronic obstructive pulmonary disease, congestive cardiac failure or diabetes or having a permanent indwelling device such as a urinary catheter or gastrostomy tube. Other signs of poor physical health such as low body mass index (BMI), pressure ulcers and functional dependence may also increase the risk of requiring acute medical intervention (Dwyer et al., 2015).

Table 48.1 Emergency ambulance transportation rates by age group, metropolitan Melbourne, 1994–95 to 2014–15

Emergency ambulance transportation rates		Rate per 1000 population		
		1994–95 (observed)	2007–08 (observed)	2014–15 (linear modelling forecasts)
All ages		31.8	57.6	77.9
45–69 years		33.6	53.4	64.6
70–84 years		147.0	211.2	255.5
≥ 85 years		247.6	474.0	651.0

Source: Lowthian et al., 2011.

In association with this is the growing concern of polypharmacy. Many older patients are prescribed large numbers of medications, increasing the risk of drug-related adverse effects, drug errors or potentially harmful drug interactions (Alder et al., 2017). Some drugs such as hypnotic or anxiolytic agents are particularly associated with increased frequency of requiring acute medical care (Alder et al., 2017). In addition, those who have recently commenced a new medication are increasingly likely to require an emergency hospital transfer (Dwyer et al., 2015).

Psychosocial factors

Changes in social structures and cultural norms in recent times have also been cited as underlying factors. The number of older people living alone has increased over the past 30 years (ABS, 2003a, 2003b). Concurrently, the increase in middle-aged women in the workforce, together with erosion of the extended family, has led to reduced capacity to care for parents and older relatives (Evans & Kelley, 2004). Furthermore, government policies encourage older people to remain living in their homes, with the majority of people aged 65 years or more doing so. Of those living in private dwellings, 62% live alone (ABS, 2003a, 2003b).

These changes in social support mechanisms, alongside reduced access to general practice (Australian Medical Association, 2004), leave the older person few alternatives for timely access to alternative transport or alternative healthcare, particularly after business hours.

Other factors

Increased health awareness from public health campaigns and changing community expectations regarding accessibility to healthcare may also contribute to increasing demand. Pricing and availability are also thought to play a role, with higher rates of use associated with cohorts entitled to free or low-cost transport (Ting & Chang, 2006).

Subgroups of older patients

As outlined in the next section, depending on varying social, psychological, genetic and pathological factors, different people may experience ageing in vastly different ways. One distinct group of older patients consists of those who have developed physical or cognitive impairments to such a degree that they require routine care, often leading to admission to residential aged care (RAC) homes. It has been demonstrated that this group of patients may vary significantly from those living in the community with rates of ambulance use up to four times higher than the community group.

Older people living in RAC and requiring emergency medical treatment frequently have high rates of chronic illness, frailty and cognitive impairment. These factors may complicate both the assessment and the treatment of acute injury and illness. This added complexity may also mean that there are times when an ambulance is called for non-urgent complaints in order to facilitate investigations or procedures that are difficult to perform in RAC (Dwyer et al., 2014; Dwyer et al., 2015).

Pathophysiology

The physiological changes of ageing alter the body's normal haemostatic mechanisms as well as response to illness and injury, making these important considerations for the paramedic in the evaluation and management of older adults. The ageing process is associated with an increase in prevalence of both acute and chronic conditions, deterioration of organ function and alteration in normal physiological processes. Of note is the fact that everyone experiences some decline with increasing age, but not everyone changes at the same rate (Health and Places Initiative, 2014).

Age-related change impacts almost every system. As outlined below, clinically significant physiological changes associated with ageing can occur across multiple organs including cardiovascular, respiratory, renal and neurological systems (Navaratnarajah & Jackson, 2017). In addition to impairing the ability of the body to respond to acute illness or injury, it is important to note that these physiological changes may lead to alterations in many baseline characteristics including 'vital signs' such as heart rate, oxygen saturation and blood pressure causing them to differ from values commonly found in younger populations and further complicating patient assessment.

Physiological changes

A number of predictable physiological changes occur with normal ageing.

Skin and connective tissue

With age skin atrophies, loses elasticity and thus becomes more prone to injury and infection. This may be exacerbated by reduced vascular supply and impaired skin repair. Wounds may then take longer to heal, develop chronic infection and the normal barrier and thermal insulation functions of skin are diminished (Marx et al., 2014).

Thermoregulation

Changes in hypothalamic function and end-organ responses lead to a reduced ability to regulate core body temperature; thus the patient may become more vulnerable to hypothermia or hyperthermia (Marx et al., 2014; Navaratnarajah & Jackson, 2017).

Musculoskeletal

Bone loss and reduction in density occurs with age, which increases the risk of fractures. Muscle mass and strength is also reduced which can lead to weakness and unsteadiness. In addition, degenerative changes in bones and joints lead to arthritis, pain, stiffness and joint instability (Marx et al., 2014; Navaratnarajah & Jackson, 2017).

Cardiovascular system

Reduced cardiac contractility and inotropic response can lead to impaired cardiac function and diminished capacity to increased cardiac output in response to stress or exertion. Additionally, hypertrophy and calcification of cardiovascular tissue may increase the risk of arrhythmias and conduction disorders. Increased peripheral vascular resistance may also lead to higher baseline blood pressure (Aalami et al., 2003; Navaratnarajah & Jackson, 2017).

Respiratory system

Tissue changes, including loss of elasticity, lead to a reduction in lung compliance and diffusion capacity and may contribute to ventilation–perfusion mismatch and impaired gas exchange. Additionally, response to hypoxia and hypercapnia via chemoreceptors may be blunted leading to overall impairment of the ability to compensate to increased respiratory demands whether due to illness or exertion (Aalami et al., 2003; Navaratnarajah & Jackson, 2017).

Immune system

Impaired cell-mediated and humoral responses lead to increased susceptibility to new infection as well as reactivation of latent infections such as tuberculosis (Aalami et al., 2003; Navaratnarajah & Jackson, 2017).

Liver and kidney function

A reduction in organ cellular mass and perfusion, and alteration in enzyme activity, may lead to impaired hepatic and renal function (Aalami et al., 2003; Navaratnarajah & Jackson, 2017).

Neurological system

Decreased neural density, slowing neural transmission and alterations in concentrations of some neurotransmitters can lead to slowing of some processes. Symptoms relating to these changes may be exacerbated by age- and disease-related hearing and visual impairment. Altered autonomic functioning may lead to less regulated haemodynamic responses and reduced ability to adequately compensate for changes in heart rate and blood pressure. Importantly, memory loss and dementia are not normal changes associated with ageing. However, the increase in prevalence of dementia necessitates consideration of cognitive problems including depression, delirium and dementia (Aalami et al., 2003; Navaratnarajah & Jackson, 2017).

Pharmacological considerations

Older patients are frequently prescribed multiple medications, so in addition to drug interactions it is important to recognise that many of these physiological changes will also have important pharmacological implications. The reduction in hepatic and gastrointestinal perfusion may influence both absorption and bioavailability of certain medications (Alder et al., 2017). Alterations in body mass including muscle atrophy, relative increase in adipose tissue and changes in total body water will impact drug distribution and may lead to increased serum levels and prolonged half-life of many agents (Alder et al., 2017). In addition, changes in enzyme activity and reductions in hepatic and renal perfusion may lead to reduced rates of clearance (Alder et al., 2017).

Frailty

Frailty is a distinct clinical syndrome that occurs in some older people and indicates a state of vulnerability to poor health outcomes. It encompasses a range of pathophysiological changes that are distinct from the normal ageing process and may be related

BOX 48.1 Considerations when managing older patients

1. Communication: hearing, visual and cognitive impairment; adapt communication as appropriate, ensure any hearing aids and glasses are kept with patient
2. General appearance: level of consciousness, mobility, social interaction, hygiene, discomfort
3. Frailty
4. Cognitive impairment: cognitive function, delirium, dementia
5. Attention to comprehensive assessment and management of pain
6. Mental health; for example, depression is an increasingly recognised problem in older adults and associated with more frequent interaction with emergency care services
7. Atypical signs and symptoms of disease
8. Potential for significant injury following low-impact mechanism of injury
9. Medications: polypharmacy, potential drug interactions, drug toxicity
   › Compare prescribed medication with what a person actually takes
   › Locate prescription bottles/boxes and take all meds to the ED
   › Note both high-risk medications such as anticoagulants, insulin and those that may alter physiological response to acute illness or injury (e.g. beta-blocker)
10. Elder abuse/neglect
    › Unexplained injuries
    › Poor living conditions, signs of neglect such as empty fridge, weight loss
11. Psychosocial circumstances
    › Living status: alone, social support networks
12. Caregiver needs and potential stressors
13. Presence of advance care directives

to physiological impairment, chronic immunological changes and multiple co-morbidities. There are a number of screening and measurement tools that aim to diagnose and quantify frailty in an individual, which may be used in varying clinical contexts. In general, the presence of frailty has been associated with increased risk of adverse health outcomes, progressive disability and increasing care needs. In particular, there is a strong association between frailty and falling, which may be both an indicator and an outcome of worsening physical health (Xue, 2011; Conroy & Elliott, 2017).

Approach to assessment

Acute medical problems in older adults share similarities with those of younger people; however, presentation can be atypical or can be masked by co-existing issues—making diagnosis a challenge. In addition, the older adult population may present with a wide variation in health status. Therefore, a holistic approach to assessment is recommended, encompassing evaluation of physical and mental state and social circumstances.

In general, patient assessment should follow the same format of history and examination, but with some important adaptations and considerations for this cohort. In particular, after seeking the patient's permission, and where possible, it may be helpful to obtain additional history from family members, carers or their general practitioner. With an increasing frequency of physical and cognitive disability, it is important to ensure efforts are made to maintain

and respect a patient's privacy, autonomy and dignity. Things to consider when assessing and treating older patients can be found in Box 48.1.

History

Obtaining a history may require more time than with a younger patient. Wherever possible, efforts should be made to optimise communication, including:

- correcting any hearing and visual deficit (e.g. ensuring the patient is wearing their hearing aids and glasses)
- minimising background noise and interruptions
- speaking clearly and with adequate volume, and
- ensuring adequate time and repeating questions as needed.

Be mindful of preexisting cognitive deficits and the potential for confusion and delirium to complicate acute illness. If the patient is known to have a cognitive or memory impairment, try to obtain an understanding of the baseline level of deficit compared with the presence of new deficits. Older patients more commonly have multiple chronic medical conditions, so it is important to explore those that may be either causing or contributing to the current presentation or those with the potential to complicate assessment and treatment.

Examination

The clinician should be aware of preexisting physical limitations that may limit some aspects of physical examination, and attention may have to be given to positioning the patient differently to how you might examine a younger person. As mentioned above, the clinician should be mindful that even when well, due to physiological changes of ageing, the presence of co-morbidity and prescribed medications, the vital signs of an older person may differ from those commonly given as 'normal values' and may not respond in a predictable way to stress and illness. For example:

- in an older person with long-standing hypertension a 'normal' systolic blood pressure of 110 mmHg may represent hypotension and indicate acute cardiovascular compromise
- an older person on a moderate dose of a beta-blocker may be unable to develop significant tachycardia and retain a 'normal' HR of 60 to 100 bpm despite the presence of pain, injury or acute illness.

Additionally, older people may not always demonstrate the same signs of illness commonly found in younger populations. For example:

- in acute abdominal conditions, age-related muscular atrophy and denervation may mean an older person will not demonstrate 'guarding' or 'rigidity', and may not be able to localise pain as specifically as younger patients
- older people may be less likely to produce a fever and, in some cases, may become hypothermic in response to acute infection
- acute confusional states and delirium may complicate a range of illness and injury and can lead to difficulty in detecting specific neurological deficits.

Specific considerations
Atypical presentations and pain
As outlined above, due to the presence of multiple medications, pathophysiological changes of ageing and presence of multiple comorbidities, older people with acute injury or illness may frequently present with minimal or atypical symptoms. For example:

- acute infection may present solely with delirium, without fever and with minimal localising symptoms
- acute abdominal infection such as appendicitis or cholecystitis may present with vague pain and without tachycardia, fever or guarding and palpable abdominal signs
- an acute myocardial infarct may present without pain ('silent infarct') and instead a patient may report more vague symptoms of dyspnoea, fatigue and general lethargy.

Additionally, many acute, severe conditions may occur more commonly in older patients such as myocardial infarct, bacterial infection and sepsis and an acute abdomen (Marx et al., 2014). It is

therefore important to entertain wide differential and to not exclude key diagnoses on symptomatology alone. This is also important for trauma presentations. Older patients may be more susceptible to significant injury from minor traumatic mechanisms and may also be less able to compensate physiologically and functionally for those injuries. Injuries may also be complicated by the presence of certain medications, in particular anticoagulant and antiplatelet agents that may increase the risk of life-threatening or life-altering haemorrhage. Pain is a key symptom of a multitude of conditions and can occur in both acute and chronic contexts.

- A number of studies have indicated that pain in older patients may be both under treated and under recognised. As mentioned above, many of the physiological indicators of pain such as tachycardia may not occur as commonly in older people and conditions affecting assessment and communication such as those due to hearing impairment, dementia or acute confusion may make it difficult to detect and quantify a patient's perception of pain (Horgas, 2017; White & Katz, 2012).
- In general, pain should be approached as in other age groups, with consideration given to treating the underlying condition causing the pain, attention to non-pharmacological modes of pain relief such as splinting and elevating injured limbs and then careful titration of multimodal analgesic agents (Galicia-Castillo & Weiner, 2017; Horgas, 2017).
- In older people on multiple medications or with chronic renal impairment, it may be necessary to avoid some agents such as NSAIDs and start with lower doses of more potent analgesic agents with careful titration to effect (Galicia-Castillo & Weiner, 2017).

Polypharmacy
Older people may frequently find themselves prescribed multiple medications. These leave a patient vulnerable to drug interactions, drug side effects and accidental drug omissions or overdoses, particularly in the setting of cognitive impairment or acute confusion. The presence of polypharmacy, as well as starting a new medication, may both be associated with increased risk of emergency transfer to hospital. In addition, there are particular types of drugs that may predispose to acute health deterioration, for example:

- anticoagulant agents may increase the risk of significant haemorrhage after minor trauma such as subdural haemorrhage after a low fall (Alder et al., 2017)

- drugs with sedative properties (e.g. benzodiazepines, opiates and antipsychotics) may increase the risk of falls and delirium (Alder et al., 2017)
- certain combinations of drugs may contribute to end-organ damage (e.g. the combination of diuretics with NSAIDs and certain anti-hypertensives, especially in the setting of an acute illness) (Alder et al., 2017)
- beta-blockers and calcium channel blockers may exacerbate conduction disease and lead to arrhythmias particularly in the presence of acute illness (Alder et al., 2017).

It is important to take a full medication history when assessing a patient and where possible observe how medication is stored and administered to gain an idea of potential errors or omissions.

Mental health

Current evidence suggests that common mental health disorders such as anxiety and depression may be prevalent and under reported among older adults with up to 16% of older adults experiencing clinically significant symptoms of depression and up to 20% experiencing symptoms of anxiety (Taylor, 2014; Hohls et al., 2018). Presence of mental illness is associated with chronic illness, cognitive impairment and social isolation and may lead to significantly higher risk of requiring both outpatient and inpatient medical care (Hohls et al., 2018). Pharmacological treatment of mental illness may contribute to polypharmacy and risk of drug-related adverse effects.

Social and functional history

As has been described above, some older people may develop significant functional limitations related to both acute and chronic health conditions. These limitations may compromise an individual's ability to safely and effectively care for themselves or others. Most adults are used to living independently and therefore it may be difficult for individuals to concede when they may no longer be able to perform tasks they once could. It is therefore important to build empathetic rapport with the patient and be mindful of the often sensitive nature of this aspect of history taking. As part of a comprehensive social history, it is important to gain an understanding of how the patient performs their normal daily tasks including dressing, cleaning and sourcing and preparing food, and whether or not these can be performed independently or require the assistance of a third party.

Paramedics who attend a patient in their home are also uniquely positioned to observe a person's domestic situation and will often gain valuable insight into aspects of their personal and social arrangements including mobility around their home and an individual's ability to maintain an adequate state of cleanliness and order. In addition to the individual patient, it is important to explore the role of informal caregivers in the individual's daily life. The role of assisting or caring for a debilitated older person often falls to a spouse or family member who themselves may not be adequately equipped or resourced to take on their role. The responsibility of caring for a loved one can be intensely demanding and so it is important for clinicians to be mindful of the health and wellbeing and support needs of carers when developing their management plan (Carmeli, 2014).

Elder abuse and neglect

As a person develops physical, cognitive or psychological vulnerabilities, they may also be at an increased risk of abuse. It has been estimated that up to 15% of older adults may experience some form of mistreatment (Yon et al., 2017). Elder abuse may occur in a number of ways including the following.

- Physical: where a patient is directly, physically harmed by another individual; for example, hitting and pushing. This type of abuse may also include sexual abuse, over-medication and physical restraint (Kurrle, 2003).
- Psychological: includes emotional and cognitive manipulation of the patient; for example intimidation, humiliation, isolation and shaming (Kurrle, 2003).
- Financial: where a patient's property, money or other belonging are inappropriately appropriated and include the manipulation of wills (Kurrle, 2003).
- Neglect: where a person responsible fails to provide an appropriate standard of basic care including food, shelter, clothing, bathing and attendance at medical appointments. Some patients may develop a degree of self-neglect if they are unwilling to accept necessary additional support services (Kurrle, 2003).

Elder abuse may not always be intentional and in some cases may be a symptom of insufficient caregiving, from a carer who may require additional support, education or resources (Teresi et al., 2016). In addition to the above it is important to recognise that older people may be equally vulnerable to other forms of abuse and violence, including domestic violence and drug- and alcohol-related harm.

Advance care directives (ACD)

For some older patients who have multiple significant comorbidities, cognitive impairment or notable disability, it may not be appropriate to perform invasive and potentially painful or uncomfortable resuscitative procedures. For these patients the goals of treatment may be directed more towards palliative aims of comfort and relief of potentially distressing symptoms such as pain, anxiety and dyspnoea. In addition, many people have their own thoughts and wishes with regard to resuscitation and may not wish to receive certain treatments. For these patients advance care directives (ACD) provide a written, legal document which healthcare providers can use to guide their treatment decisions, particularly when they are unable to communicate properly with the patient due to the acute illness or injury, cognitive impairment or profound disability. ACDs may also be known as do not resuscitate (DNR) and do not hospitalise (DNH) orders, advance directives (AD) and living wills (Dwyer et al., 2015). Unfortunately, prevalence and completeness of these documents may be quite variable among older people and may not always be present on scene.

CASE STUDY 1

Case 13971, 1000 hrs.

Dispatch details: An 86-year-old female with worsening confusion and agitation. Call from a staff member at an RAC home.

Initial presentation: On scene at 1200 hrs; ground floor of a large RAC home.

On arrival paramedics are escorted to the patient's room where the patient is lying in bed. The home appears well maintained. The nurse in charge is present at the patient's bedside and provides paramedics with a two-page summary containing a list of the patient's medications, medical diagnoses and contact details for the next of kin. The room is clean, the patient is in a fresh nightdress and her breakfast is on a tray next to the bed.

 1 ASSESS

Patient history

Paramedics engage the patient but she appears not to understand the questions asked and gives inappropriate answers, appearing to just name people from her past. The nurse in charge then provides further details. She reports that for the last 24 hours the patient has been noted to become more confused, did not eat dinner yesterday or breakfast this morning and has had periods of becoming agitated but over the last hour has become progressively drowsy. There have been no reports of a fall. The patient had her usual medications yesterday but has refused to take anything orally this morning. The nurse reports that she has not met this resident before and so is unsure of her baseline cognitive function.

The patient has a past medical history of dementia, ischaemic heart disease, osteoarthritis, chronic back pain and depression. She is taking a list of medications prescribed from her doctor including aspirin, metoprolol, paracetamol, frusemide and a fentanyl patch. The patient has lived in this care home for the last 5 years and is unable to mobilise independently from bed to a wheelchair. She requires assistance with bathing and dressing but is able to feed herself.

The patient has a son living interstate and a daughter nearby who is listed as the next-of-kin contact. The nurse was able to contact the daughter by phone, who reports she saw her mother 2 days ago and she appeared well, but she has noticed a general decline over the last 12 months. The daughter reports her mother can usually respond to yes/no questions appropriately but will not usually be oriented to person, place, time or date. The daughter reports she thinks her mother had previously indicated she wanted to die at home, but she never had a formal discussion with her about her wishes. No end-of-life care plan is present.

Initial assessment summary

Problem	Confusion and agitation
Conscious state	GCS = 12 (E3, V4, M5)
Position	Lying supine in bed
Heart rate	96 bpm, regular
Blood pressure	70/40 mmHg
Skin appearance	Pale, warm and dry
Respiratory rate	20 bpm
Chest auscultation	Difficult to hear, patient breathing softly, appears clear
Blood glucose level	5
Pulse oximetry	94% on room air
Temperature	35°C
Motor/sensory function	No facial droop, moving all four limbs equally
Secondary survey	No signs of trauma

(2) CONFIRM

Compared with older people living in the community, those living in RAC homes may be more likely to present to emergency care with severe acute illness, abnormal vital signs and multisystem disease (Dwyer et al., 2014). On initial assessment this patient appears acutely unwell. Key concerns from the initial history and examination includes new confusion and altered conscious state, tachypnoea, hypotension and low temperature. In addition, from preliminary assessment this patient appears to have a frailty syndrome and is therefore vulnerable to acute deterioration with high associated morbidity and mortality.

Differential diagnoses to consider include the following.

- Sepsis/infection. As mentioned above, older people may not mount a fever and may have variable cardiovascular parameters in response to infection. Potential sources include a urinary tract infection, respiratory infection and intra-abdominal source. Older people living in RAC are at higher risk of new infection and have increased rates of drug-resistant organisms.
- Stroke. It is always important to consider an intracranial cause of new neurological symptoms. On initial examination there were no obvious focal neurological deficits but it is often difficult to perform a comprehensive neurological assessment on an acutely agitated and confused patient.
- Acute myocardial infarct. Older patients who are also female have increased rates of atypical presentations for a number of conditions including acute coronary syndrome. Patients such as this may present with a sudden deterioration but without a report of chest pain, dyspnoea or other common cardiac symptoms.
- Dehydration and acute renal impairment. This patient is heavily reliant on others for food and drink. At times the behavioural and cognitive deficits associated with dementia render a person at risk of inadequate nutritional intake and hydration. This may be exacerbated by some medications such as diuretics.

- Pharmacological. This patient is on a number of medications that are at risk of causing confusion and delirium in older people, including opiate analgesics (fentanyl), antipsychotics (risperidone), anti-depressants (sertraline) and benzodiazepines (temazepam). Dose changes or changes in the patient's underlying physiology such as those affecting absorption and excretion of these drugs may precipitate acute medical deterioration and confusion. In addition, it is worth noting this patient is on a diuretic and anti-hypertensive which may be contributing to her haemodynamic instability.

Delirium

In addition to the underlying acute illness, it appears this patient has developed a delirium. In people with preexisting neurocognitive impairment it may be difficult to distinguish delirium from their underlying condition. Some key features of delirium include:

- development over hours to days
- fluctuation in symptoms
- disturbance in attention, awareness or conscious state
- findings from clinical assessment that suggest an acute illness or cause.

In this population of older patients delirium has a wide range of causes including infection, drug ingestion or withdrawal, trauma, neurovascular emergency and metabolic and nutritional disturbances (Yew & Maher, 2012; Francis, 2014; Hshieh et al., 2018).

TREAT

These patients may be highly complex to manage. This patient appears acutely unwell with signs of haemodynamic compromise, yet also has profound preexisting cognitive and physical disability and an associated high mortality risk; therefore, intensive and invasive resuscitation may not be appropriate. When present, ACDs can assist in appropriately guiding treatment. Even when providing resuscitative treatment, it is important to recognise a patient such as this may be nearing the end of their life and so it is also vital to provide concurrent care aimed at symptom relief, comfort and ensuring that next of kin, family and loved ones are informed and present where possible.

Some key aspects of management for this patient would include the following.

Appropriate resuscitation

Hypotension may be addressed with small fluid boluses titrated to response, and tachypnoea may be improved with supplemental oxygen.

Symptom control and delirium management

Pain can be an important contributor to the development of delirium and may be difficult to detect in a patient who is agitated and confused. It should be considered and then treated if appropriate while being mindful of conscious state and hypotension.

In addition to treating the underlying cause, there are a number of non-pharmacological and pharmacological treatments that may improve symptoms of delirium. Some to consider in the out-of-hospital setting, where possible, include:

- avoiding background noise and maintaining a calm, quiet environment
- maintaining adequate light
- ensuring the patient has their hearing aids and glasses, if used
- orientating the patient and having familiar family members or friends accompany them
- providing reassurance.

Identify and treat underlying cause and contributors

This includes a review of medications and withholding any that may be contributing to hypotension or delirium. It is important to search the patient for transdermal medications such as a fentanyl patch that might otherwise be missed.

Disposition

In the absence of an advance care plan it is likely that this patient will need to be taken to hospital. Many RAC homes are underequipped to treat patients undergoing acute medical illness, especially if end-of-life care plans have not been previously prepared.

However, if possible it is useful to check with the patient's GP, senior RAC staff and hospital outreach programs to see if acute medical care could be provided in the RAC home.

Hospital handover

This patient is highly dependent and unable to adequately communicate the extent of their personal and medical needs. It is therefore vital that a comprehensive handover occurs with detailed notes outlining out-of-hospital assessment and care. It is also important that family or next of kin are kept informed and encouraged to attend with the patient.

4 EVALUATE

This patient will need ongoing review and evaluation throughout their treatment and transport to hospital. This includes monitoring of response to medical interventions as well as further alterations in conscious state.

CS CASE STUDY 2

Case 17579, 2200 hrs.

Dispatch details: A 75-year-old male who fell from standing. Family member on scene.

Initial presentation: On scene at 2230 hrs. Private residence, two-storey house. Patient is lying on the floor of the upstairs bedroom.

Access to the front door is hindered by an overgrown garden. Backdoor leads through the kitchen to the stairs. Passing through the kitchen, it is noted that there are several bags of rubbish lying next to the door and plates and glasses are stacked on the table instead of in the cupboards above the sink. The narrow staircase leads to a small landing off which is the main bedroom.

1 ASSESS

Patient history

Patient reports he had gone to bed at approximately 2130 hrs, but then woke needing to go to the bathroom. He stood from the bed then reports waking on the floor. Patient is unable to describe how he fell; he thinks he may have tripped on the edge of the carpet but cannot remember falling. Patient reports discomfort to his left hip and is unable to move into a sitting position or to stand unaided. He currently denies headache or neck pain, or any other injury. The patient's wife was asleep and woke when he started calling out to her.

Past medical history

The patient has a past medical history of atrial fibrillation, hypertension, congestive cardiac failure and osteoarthritis and had a total knee replacement. He is on a list of medications prescribed from his doctor including atenolol, perindopril, frusemide and paracetamol.

Social history

The patient is a retired plumber who lives with his wife. He has two adult children who live 30 minutes away. The patient mentions that his wife has recently been diagnosed with dementia and he is concerned as she has wandered off and become lost on two occasional recently. He reports that he feels exhausted and is finding it difficult to manage household chores alongside providing extra care for his wife. He also reports his mobility is below average, and since his knee replacement he has used a walking stick. He drinks very little and gave up smoking 10 years ago.

Initial assessment summary

Problem	Fall
Conscious state	Alert and oriented; GCS = 15
Position	Lying supine on the floor
Heart rate	48 bpm, irregular
Blood pressure	145/92 mmHg
Skin appearance	Pink, warm and dry
Respiratory rate	12 bpm
Chest auscultation	Scattered crackles both bases
Pulse oximetry	94% on room air
Temperature	36.5°C
Motor/sensory function & secondary survey	No facial droop; moving right leg freely with normal power, movement of left leg is restricted by pain on flexing the hip, leg appears shortened and externally rotated; small abrasion to left temple—nil active bleeding

CONFIRM

There are a number of aspects of this presentation that need separate attention.

Cause of fall

It is sometimes difficult to distinguish a fall from a syncopal event and so both need to be considered.

Falls

Falls in older people are rarely simple and often have multiple contributory factors; some to be considered in this case include the following.

- Patient factors
  - › Arthritis causing joint instability and pain
  - › Poor balance potentially relating to previous knee replacement, underlying arthritis, age-related muscle wasting and decline in proprioception
  - › Visual impairment—patient appears to normally wear glasses
- Environmental factors
  - › Irregular carpet on the floor
  - › Nil use of walking stick—stick was not present at bedside

> Night—poor light contributing to poor visibility
> Slippers—if slippery or poorly fitting may contribute to instability

Syncope

Structural cardiac disease and cardiac arrhythmias can lead to syncope. The patient is known to have atrial fibrillation and congestive cardiac failure; he is also on multiple medications that affect cardiac conduction including a beta-blocker, calcium channel blocker and digoxin.

Postural hypotension

In addition to age-related diminution of the autonomic nervous system, this patient has known cardiac disease and is on multiple medications that may cause hypotension, bradycardia and inhibit the normal baroceptor response when moving from lying to standing.

Injuries sustained

As well as the cause of the fall, it is important to do a thorough assessment of potential injury. As mentioned above, older people may sustain significant injury from relatively low-impact mechanisms.

- Left hip injury. The hip appears shortened and is being held in external rotation. These may be signs of a hip fracture.
- Head injury: There is a new abrasion over the scalp which may indicate that the patient hit his head. In addition to this it is noted that the patient is taking an anticoagulant medication (rivaroxaban) and so is at increased risk of intracranial injury following a fall.

Social history

This patient's social circumstances and responsibilities will require dedicated attention in the management plan. The patient has already stated that he is finding it difficult to cope with caring for his wife and properly performing all the usual household chores, and that this may be exacerbated by his medical problems including arthritis and poor mobility.

On initial observation of the property it appears that there are some aspects of cleaning and maintenance that are not being attended to and support these concerns. These remarks also suggest this patient may be experiencing a significant degree of stress and fatigue from these responsibilities. Additional elements of history to consider are a systems review, review of past medical history and a review of medications.

On further questioning the patient denies chest pain, shortness of breath or palpitations but reports he has had two similar episodes in the last 6 months of becoming lightheaded upon standing. The patient denies any notable blood loss or change in bowel habit or stool. He reports he has felt more fatigued over the last couple of months and feels he is unable to walk further than 10 metres without stopping to rest.

The patient reports that he has been on most of his medications for at least 2 years but that recently his dose of atenolol was increased due to his blood pressure being too high.

③ TREAT

In this patient, ongoing evaluation and treatment should proceed side by side. Elements of management should include the following.

- Analgesia
  > This patient has a suspected fractured hip and so is likely to require additional analgesia during extrication and transport.
  > Simple measures such as supporting the hip and knee and avoiding unnecessary movement are important.

> This patient is already prescribed sustained release paracetamol and so paramedics should check that he has had an evening dose, or if there is room for additional dosing.
> It is likely this person will require a form of opiate analgesia. He is at risk of having impaired renal function and significant underlying cardiac disease and so may have an exaggerated cardiovascular response to medications. However, he also has a significant injury that is likely to cause moderate to severe pain. It would therefore be appropriate to consider starting with a lower dose intravenous agent and slowly titrating to effect.

- Disposition
  > There are a number of concerns that indicate this patient should be transported to hospital.
    - First, the cause of the fall is unknown and additional investigations will be beneficial in examining this further.
    - Second, this patient has a likely fractured hip which will require operative management.
    - Third, this patient has had a head injury while taking anticoagulant medication and so will likely need imaging of the head with a period of observation.
  > The second person to consider in disposition is the patient's wife. With underlying cognitive impairment, it may not be safe to leave her at home alone and it is likely she will require additional support while her husband is in hospital. Some options include transporting her with the patient to hospital or telephoning one of her adult children to look after her.
- Extrication and packaging for transport
  > This may be difficult given the upstairs location and current immobility of the patient.
  > Lying flat may be difficult for this patient given signs of mild cardiac failure and osteoarthritis.
  > Attention should be given to supporting the hip and leg during transport.
  > Early thought should be given to requesting additional crews and equipment.
- Further evaluation
  > Additional management that will be useful during treatment and transport include:
    - monitoring vital signs while titrating analgesia
    - observing the injured leg and regular checks of neurovascular status
    - ECG monitoring and a 12-lead ECG to examine for potential cardiac arrhythmia.
- Hospital handover
  > During a structured handover it is important that the different elements of the differential diagnosis are covered including the suspected cause of the fall and injuries.
  > It is also important to highlight the social concerns regarding ongoing care for this patient.
  > The patient is the sole carer for his wife who has a diagnosis of dementia.
  > Comprehensive assessment is required to determine the need for extra home help services, engagement with community supports including the GP and more detailed discussion with extended family about the changing care needs of the patient and his wife with a view to future planning.

(4) EVALUATE

Paramedics should attend to continuous reassessment and evaluation of both clinical state and analgesia requirements. With further history from the patient and his family it is likely the differential diagnoses will narrow and the management plan may need to be adapted.

Summary

Although not restricted to older adults, some important clinical features are far more common in this population and impact significantly on patient assessment, treatment and disposition. These include frailty syndromes, delirium, cognitive impairment, atypical presentations of disease, polypharmacy and multiple co-morbidity. Paramedics should be mindful of the added complexity these bring to patient management.

Older adults represent a significant and growing proportion of paramedic work and these patients require a thoughtful and holistic approach encompassing medical, psychological, functional and social aspects of care.

References

Aalami, O., Fang, T., Song, H., & Nacamuli, R. (2003). Physiological features of ageing persons. *Archive of Surgery, 138*, 1069–1076.

Alder, S., Caslake, R., & Mangoni, A. A. (2017). Practical advice for prescribing in old age. *Medicine, 45*(1), 11–14.

Australian Bureau of Statistics (2003a). *4102.0—Australian Social Trends—Housing Stock: Changes in Australian housing.* ABS.

Australian Bureau of Statistics (2003b). *4430.0—Disability, Ageing and Carers, Australia: Summary of Findings, 2003* ABS. Canberra.

Australian Bureau of Statistics (2014). *Does size matter? Population projections 20 and 50 years from 2013. 4102.0—Australian Social Trends, 2014* ABS. Canberra.

Australian Bureau of Statistics (2015). *Population by age and sex, Australia, States and Territories. 3101.0—Australian Demographic Statistics, Jun 2015* ABS. Canberra.

Australian Bureau of Statistics (2017). *3235.0—Population by Age and Sex, Regions of Australia, 2016* ABS. Canberra.

Australian Medical Association (2004). *Out-Of-Hours Primary Medical Care.* AMA.

Carmeli, E. (2014). The invisibles: unpaid caregivers of the elderly. *Frontiers in Public Health, 2*, 91.

Conroy, S., & Elliott, A. (2017). The frailty syndrome. *Medicine, 45*(1), 15–18.

Dwyer, R., Gabbe, B., Stoelwinder, J. U., & Lowthian, J. (2014). A systematic review of outcomes following emergency transfer to hospital for residents of aged care facilities. *Age and Ageing, 43*(6), 759–766.

Dwyer, R., Stoelwinder, J., Gabbe, B., & Lowthian, J. (2015). Unplanned transfer to emergency departments for frail elderly residents of aged care facilities: a review of patient and organizational factors. *Journal of the American Medical Directors Association, 16*(7), 551–562. 1 July 2015.

Evans, M. D. R., & Kelley, J. (2004). *Trends in Women's Labour Force Participation in Australia: 1984–2002.* Melbourne Institute of Applied Economic and Social Research, Melbourne University.

Francis, J. (2014). *Delirium and acute confusional States. UpToDate.* Wolters Kluwer. Retrieved from https://www .uptodate.com/contents/delirium-and-acute-confusional -states-prevention-treatment-and-prognosis?search =delirium&usage_type=default&source=search_result &selectedTitle=2-150&display_rank=2-H354892619. (Accessed 11th April 2018.)

Galicia-Castillo, M., & Weiner, D. (2017). *Treatment of persistent pain in older adults. UpToDate.* Wolters Kluwer. Retrieved from https://www.uptodate.com/contents/ treatment-of-persistent-pain-in-older-adults/print ?search=pharmacologygeriatric&source=search_result &selectedTitle=1-150&usage_type=default&display _rank=1. (Accessed 11th April 2017.)

Health and Places Initiative (2014). *Physiology and Psychology of Aging, Health, and Place—A Research Brief. H. College.* Harvard, United States. Version 1.0.

Hohls, J. K., Konig, H. H., Raynik, Y. I., & Hajek, A. (2018). A systematic review of the association of anxiety with health care utilization and costs in people aged 65 years and older. *Journal of Affective Disorders, 232*, 163–176.

Horgas, A. L. (2017). Pain management in older adults. *The Nursing Clinics of North America, 52*(4), e1–e7.

Hshieh, T., Inouye, S., & Oh, E. (2018). Delirium in the elderly. *Psychiatric Clinics of North America, 41*(1), 1–17.

Kurrle, S. (2003). *Elder Abuse—Revision of original paper, Australian and New Zealand Society for Geriatric Medicine.*

Lowthian, J. A. (2016). *Older adults in the emergency health care setting. Encyclopaedia of Geropsychology. Pachana NA* (p. 1). Singapore: Springer Science.

Lowthian, J. A., Cameron, P. A., Stoelwinder, J. U., Curtis, A., Currell, A., Cooke, M. W., & McNeil, J. J. (2011). Increasing utilisation of emergency ambulances. *Australian Health Review, 35*(1), 63–69.

Lowthian, J. A., McGinnes, R. A., Brand, C. A., Barker, A. L., & Cameron, P. A. (2015). Discharging older patients from the emergency department effectively: a systematic review and meta-analysis. *Age and Ageing, 44*(5), 761–770.

Marx, J., Hockberger, R., Walls, R., Biros, M., Danzl, D., Gausche-Hill, M., Jagoda, A., Ling, L., Newton, E., & Zink, B. (Eds.), (2014). *Rosen's emergency medicine: concepts and clinical practice*. Philadelphia: Elsevier Saunders.

Navaratnarajah, A., & Jackson, S. H. D. (2017). The physiology of ageing. *Medicine, 45*(1), 6–10.

Ross, L., Jennings, P. A., Smith, K., & Williams, B. (2017). Paramedic attendance to older patients in Australia, and the prevalence and implications of psychosocial issues. *Prehospital Emergency Care, 21*(1), 32–38.

Taylor, W. D. (2014). Clinical practice. Depression in the elderly. *The New England Journal of Medicine, 371*(13), 1228–1236.

Teresi, J. A., Burnes, D., Skowron, E. A., Dutton, M. A., Mosqueda, L., Lachs, M. S., & Pillemer, K. (2016). State of the science on prevention of elder abuse and lessons learned from child abuse and domestic violence prevention: toward a conceptual framework for research. *Journal of Elder Abuse and Neglect, 28*(4–5), 263–300.

Ting, J. Y. S., & Chang, A. M. Z. (2006). Path analysis modeling indicates free transport increases ambulance use for minor indications. *Prehospital Emergency Care, 10*(4), 476–481.

White, C., & Katz, B. (2012). *Australian and New Zealand. Society for Geriatric Medicine Position statement no. 21: Pain in older people, ANZSGM, Sydney.*

Xue, Q. L. (2011). The frailty syndrome: definition and natural history. *Clinics in Geriatric Medicine, 27*(1), 1–15.

Yew, T., & Maher, S. (2012). *Delirium in Older People, Australian and New Zealand Society for Geriatric Medicine.*

Yon, Y., Mikton, C. R., Gassoumis, Z. D., & Wilber, K. H. (2017). Elder abuse prevalence in community settings: a systematic review and meta-analysis. *The Lancet Global Health, 5*(2), e147–e156.

CHAPTER 49

Indigenous Australian Patients

By Abigail Trewin

OVERVIEW

- Australia's Indigenous peoples are culturally diverse with many languages and cultural practices.
- Interacting with patients from different cultural backgrounds requires a review of your own cultural expectations.
- The cultural beliefs of contemporary Indigenous Australians can be located on a continuum, spanning those who have had a traditional upbringing to those who may know they are Indigenous but have lost connections with their heritage and cultural traditions.

- Compared with other Australians, Indigenous Australians experience significant inequities in life expectancy, health status, health outcomes (morbidity and mortality) and access to a range of health services.
- The ability of paramedics to conduct a detailed health assessment and make sound clinical decisions when dealing with Indigenous patients may require an understanding of their culture and beliefs and how these shape their engagement with health providers.

Introduction

Both health professionals and the patients they attend are shaped by their experiences and cultural beliefs. These beliefs also shape how each group views disease and how they express disease to others. Most clinicians embrace the biomedical (or scientific) view of disease and often fail to accept that their patients do not always share this view. This can limit the clinician's ability to gain an accurate history, but also fails to engage the patient in the choice of treatment and ensure their adherence to therapy. This discrepancy between the clinician's view of disease and treatment and the patient's view can be exacerbated when the two are from significantly different cultures.

Culturally appropriate care extends the biomedical model to respect the patient's worldview, cultural values, beliefs and practices. Each person's concept of health, wellbeing and illness is developed within their sociocultural context. Identifying a person's concept of health, wellbeing or illness ensures that healthcare is both relevant to understanding why they have sought medical help and effective in addressing their health concerns (Wilson, 2008). Many Indigenous patients suffer a higher rate of socioeconomic disadvantage and chronic disease (AusMAT, 2011), with a higher number on treatment for preexisting conditions such as renal disease, diabetes, cardiac conditions (including rheumatic heart disease) and hypertension.

Indigenous Australians (Aboriginal and Torres Strait Islander peoples) comprise 2.5% of the country's total population. Almost 26% of people in the Northern Territory are estimated to be of Indigenous origin (ABS, 2017a), while in the other states and territories Indigenous Australians make up 2.8% of the total population (ABS, 2017b).

This chapter considers cultural aspects of traditional Indigenous Australian life. It is necessary that these matters are discussed in very broad and general terms and while the term 'Indigenous Australians' is used the authors acknowledge that it covers many different groups with different traditions, values and ways of life.

Kinship

Kinship can be defined as the relationship between members of the same family, or a feeling of being close or similar to other people or things (Bourke & Edwards, 2004). It is significant to every part of Indigenous Australian society and understanding the role that kinship plays will assist clinicians in managing Indigenous patients in a culturally safe way. Kinship dictates social organisation, but this will differ between regions and groups. Kinship describes whom an Indigenous person can speak to, how they are addressed and whom they are allowed to confide in. Kinship also describes 'avoidance' relationships, prohibiting individuals from approaching or speaking to another member of the group.

Within the kinship system everyone knows exactly how to behave towards everyone else. The basic principle is that people born of the same sex belong to the same sibling line and are viewed as essentially the same (Bourke & Edwards, 2004).

So in a community two brothers are considered equal: their children are referred to as brothers and sisters, not cousins, and they will view their father's brother not as their uncle but as another father. The same is true of sisters who have children: the children will refer to each sister as their mother, not their aunt. Their mother's brother, who is of the same sibling line but the other sex, is referred to as Uncle, and their father's sister is Auntie. It is therefore not uncommon to have many mothers and many fathers and many brothers and many sisters (Bourke & Edwards, 2004). In addition, many regions classify their community through 'skin names'. This is the name given at birth that describes the section/subsection that a person belongs to. The name relates to the child's parents' 'skin name' and divides the community further into relevant relationships.

When Indigenous Australians refer to someone to whom they are related they usually use the appropriate relationship term for that person, such as auntie; if they are unrelated, they are referred to as so and so's son or mother. Personal names are used with discretion as they are seen as essentially part of that person. When Indigenous Australians accept an outsider into their group, they name that person in relation to themselves in order for that person to fit into their society. This is because they need to know the kinship relationship of that person to themselves, and that person must have a defined social position. The value of the kinship system is that it structures people's relationships, obligations and behaviour towards each other, and this in turn affects matters such as who will look after children if a parent dies, who can marry whom, who is responsible for another person's debts or misdeeds and who will care for the sick and old.

Indigenous people raised in cities and towns may or may not follow kinship systems but they will still usually have close family networks in the area and socialise with other Indigenous people. Many maintain their links with family in remote or regional areas.

Culture

Australia is a culturally diverse country: 49% of the population were either born overseas or have a parent who was born overseas (ABS, 2017b). Migrants have enriched many aspects of Australian life, creating new influences while blending into a country of established traditions. The country's original inhabitants, Indigenous Australians, are the custodians of one of the world's oldest continuing cultural traditions.

Knowing how to behave to avoid offending patients and to demonstrate cultural sensitivity when managing patients is not simply learned through reading or attending a cultural awareness course. It involves continual learning through interaction, participation, reflection and engagement. A person's behaviour is influenced by a complex mix of human response to a crisis, personality differences and most importantly the culture the person brings to the situation (AusMAT, 2011). Many dimensions influence culture, such as gender equality in a society or the value of individualism, and these can lead to stereotyping of a particular race or group. While culture influences how people may behave, each person remains an individual. Stereotyping often leads to friction when behaviour doesn't match our expectations, but it is very difficult for people not to stereotype. Paramedics can adjust how they interact with patients by being aware of their own stereotypes and cultural biases, treating people as individuals and describing behaviour rather than judging it.

Given that paramedic encounters with younger patients (of all ethnicities) are strongly associated with drugs and alcohol (and sometimes traumatic injuries), dealing with cultural differences adds another dimension to conducting safe and accurate patient assessments.

Specific aspects of Indigenous culture
Indigenous representation in the cities
It is extremely simplistic to assume that Indigenous Australians who live in major cities or towns are not engaged with many of their traditional ceremonies, customs and beliefs. Culture is not static and, as a way of describing how people express themselves and structure their lives and relationships, it stretches across locations. Many Indigenous Australians maintain a strong connection to the land and describe themselves as coming from places that may not be as familiar to many as other Australian place names.

Despite local variations many Indigenous Australians share a similar history in terms of relationships with governments and healthcare systems. As a group they also share an experience of colonisation, albeit at different times and in different ways across the country. Being removed from their land, removing children from families and other discriminatory

> **PRACTICE TIP**
>
> You are encouraged to find out who the local Indigenous people are for the area in which you are working or studying (e.g. the Larakia, the Wurundjeri or the Jagera). Do they have particular customs? What you learn is likely to be far more precise than the generic cultural principles explained in this chapter.

practices by governments and government agencies stretch across this community to some degree and impact on how they interact with healthcare workers.

Payback

'Payback' is a term used in customary law, which is part of the kinship system. Kinship relationships determine the processes used to resolve disputes (Northern Territory Law Reform Committee, 2003). Payback is enacted when a wrongdoing has been committed. Public wrongs include breaches of sacred law, incest, sacrilege and murder by magic, while private wrongs include homicide, wounding and adultery. The essential difference lies in the manner in which the dispute is resolved. Elders are actively involved in public wrongs, whereas for private wrongs the person who has been harmed (and their relevant kin) generally determines the appropriate response (Williams, 1987). Therefore, under traditional law, families of the offender and the person who was harmed negotiate the outcome and kin relationships determine who inflicts the punishment (Trees, 2004). Families are involved in deciding the punishment because Indigenous Australian law demands satisfaction between families when a wrong has been committed (Law Reform Committee Western Australia, 2004).

Paramedics may sometimes be asked for a bandage for a perceived injury where none is detected. The wearing of a bandage often delays payback.

Underlying the emphasis on revenge is a general aim to restore balance and order. If punishment is inflicted properly, the matter is usually at an end; however, if the punishment goes too far as a result of an overemphasis on revenge, further conflict may result (Cousins, 2004). Unfortunately, payback is not always exacted in a traditional way, resulting in life-threatening injuries.

Indigenous legal systems including payback revolve around group rights and group control, whereas the Australian legal system has developed out of a more individualistic tradition, with greater emphasis on personal rights and freedoms.

Gender issues

Gender issues are important, with 'women's business' and 'men's business' being defined and held separate. This can prevent a practitioner from examining a person of the opposite sex (see Fig 49.1). It may be more appropriate to talk to or instruct family members or friends present to talk on behalf of the patient or to undertake basic treatment only (AusMAT, 2011).

Sorry business

Bereavement, known as sorry business, is a very important part of Indigenous Australian culture.

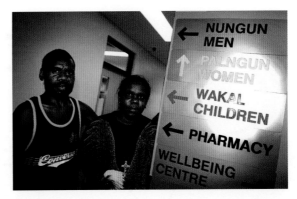

Figure 49.1
'Women's business' and 'men's business' are defined and held separate. Clinicians may find resistance from community members when they attempt to examine an Indigenous person of the opposite sex.
Source: AAP/Clive Hyde, Northern Territory Government.

When a person dies, sorrow is often expressed through wailing. Funerals can involve entire communities and the expression of grief may occasionally include self-injury. The relatives may cut off their hair or wear white pigment on their faces. The community will refrain from using the name of the deceased, but can refer to them by the name *Kwementyaye*; people with the same name as the deceased should also be called *Kwementyaye*. Photographs or videos of the deceased have to be destroyed (Sheldon, 2001).

Shame

Encroaching on any area that involves taboos or causes a person to feel judged may result in shame. When shame occurs it can impede treatment: a patient may get angry about being judged or feel very uncomfortable. This may result in ongoing silence and/or refusal of treatment/transport.

Communication

Introductory protocols are important: be prepared to spend more time than usual sharing personal information about yourself and the purpose of your visit. Remember that the patient may not have called for medical assistance: someone with greater authority within the community may have made the decision that the patient required an ambulance. While the patient may comply with this authority, they may be confused if they do not see their level of injury/illness as significant. Reluctance to engage may relate to not understanding why the community has decided that treatment is necessary.

The patient's story needs to be told, but who tells it is related to kinship. The patient may not engage in the story telling but expect an appropriate member of community to tell the story on their behalf. The use of silence should not be misunderstood. In many Indigenous communities it may be

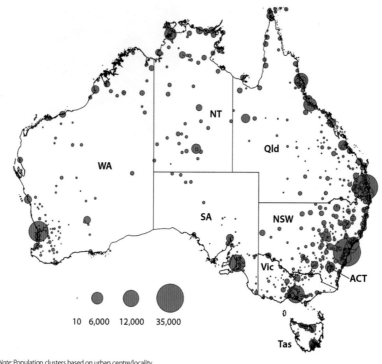

Note: Population clusters based on urban centre/locality.

Figure 49.2
Indigenous population clusters.
City-based paramedics need to be aware of the cultural and communication issues that can arise when dealing with the Indigenous community.
Source: AIHW (2011).

considered impolite to answer questions immediately and these pause intervals are a normal conversation style. Silence may also mean that the person does not want to express an opinion at that point in time or that they are listening and reflecting about what has been said (AusMAT, 2011). Rapid-fire direct questioning can cause confusion and does not allow the patient time to follow the question process, resulting in questions being ignored or not fully answered. Where possible explain why you have to ask so many questions, wait for the pause interval after each question and don't try to fill it.

Prolonged eye contact during conversations can make Indigenous people feel uncomfortable. Take your cues from the person: some will be very used to interacting with non-Indigenous people and have no issue with this, while others will refuse to look at you but are still listening—don't confuse this with dismissal.

Distribution

A high proportion of Indigenous Australians are considered socially and economically disadvantaged—and the socially and economically disadvantaged, no matter what their ethnicity, make up a large proportion of those needing emergency healthcare. This can be a challenge for young paramedics, who often have little experience with this section of the community. Many students may feel that they are unlikely to meet Indigenous patients in the major cities but in fact most Indigenous Australians live in major cities or towns: about one-third live in major cities, with only a quarter living in remote or very remote areas (ABS, 2017a; see Fig 49.2). However, no matter where Indigenous Australians live, their health status is remarkably similar and it is well-known that this is lower than for non-Indigenous Australians. The challenge is to ensure that clinicians are aware of the antecedents that may impact their clinical decision-making and care for Indigenous Australians so that the mistakes of the past are not repeated and the gap between Indigenous and non-Indigenous health is closed (see Fig 49.3).

Epidemiological profile
Morbidity
Rates of disease are much higher in the Indigenous population. Indigenous Australians also have a much higher rate of comorbidities, which, in turn, causes a greater burden of disease. Some diseases found in the Indigenous population are virtually unseen in the non-Indigenous population. These include trachoma and rheumatic heart disease (Australian

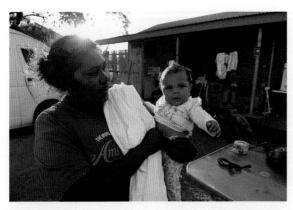

Figure 49.3
One of the factors in closing the gap between Indigenous and non-Indigenous health outcomes is providing a health service that recognises and responds to cultural factors. Encouraging early engagement with health services is a critical step in eliminating reduced life expectancy among the Indigenous population.
Source: AAP/Dan Peled.

Institute of Health and Welfare [AIHW], 2009). Paramedics working in areas with a large Indigenous population should try to develop their own knowledge of these conditions, as they are not often covered sufficiently in modern university courses.

Mortality

According to the Australian Bureau of Statistics (ABS, 2017c), the five leading causes of mortality for both Indigenous and non-Indigenous Australians are:

- ischaemic heart disease
- dementia
- cerebrovascular disease
- cancer
- chronic obstructive pulmonary disease.

For all but respiratory diseases, the mortality rate is far higher in the Indigenous population and almost always extends across a wider age range. According to the Australian Bureau of Statistics (2017c) the five main causes of death among the Indigenous population in 2017 were:

- ischaemic heart disease
- diabetes
- chronic lower respiratory disease
- malignant neoplasm of trachea, bronchus and lung
- intentional self-harm.

Medical information and treatment

Historically, health education and health-related information have not been delivered with reference to cultural views. As a result, information about organ functions, disease processes and so on is often delivered in a biomedical Western way, which is frequently not well understood or accepted. In addition, many people still consult traditional healers

(AusMAT, 2011) before seeking Western medicine. Seeking contemporary treatment may be delayed for a variety of other reasons including kinship responsibilities, finances, access to medical care and a lack of recognition of the urgency related to the illness. The resulting frustration for paramedics is often a deteriorating patient with a prolonged medical illness who has received minimal to no treatment prior to the ambulance being called.

Transport to hospital

Indigenous people with little experience of the healthcare system may assume that a trip to hospital means they won't return home alive as this may have happened to relatives in the past. They may be frighted of the 'unknown' and consequently reluctant to leave. Providing clear, simple explanations why transport is necessary and what the hospital will do for the patient is important to provide reassurance and reasoning for the patient and their family.

Alternatively, their reluctance to go to hospital may be related to the practicalities of being able to return home after they are discharged. If the patient has no money and no way of getting home, they may refuse to go to hospital. Convincing a patient to attend may be dependent on the paramedic being able to assist in the negotiation of guaranteed return travel through relatives or government travel schemes, such as taxi vouchers.

Be aware also that social issues may dictate why a patient is reluctant to be transported. If the patient's association with their community is likely to be adversely affected by their absence, they may simply refuse to go and it will be very difficult to convince them otherwise. Be sensitive to signals that alert you to this situation; for example, a patient refusing to be transported but giving no explanation and kin members refusing to accompany the patient.

When transporting an Indigenous patient to hospital take a relative too, where possible. A patient's reluctance to go to hospital can often be overcome when a suitable relative agrees to accompany them. In fact, kinship may require that a member of the family travel with the patient to provide emotional and social support.

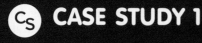

CASE STUDY 1

Case 14588, 2200 hrs.

Dispatch details: A 47-year-old male described as 'sick' by the caller for the past week is keeping the residents of his house awake with his coughing.

Initial presentation: The paramedics are waved down as they approach the address by a female who states that she is the patient's wife. She leads them to the patient, who is lying on the floor on a mattress covered in blankets. There is a tin cup next to the bed with what looks like green sputum in it. His wife tries to pull the blankets off her husband, but he grumpily argues with her and pulls them back over his head. The paramedics approach him and seek permission to examine him. He doesn't answer them, choosing to turn over and face the opposite direction. He appears short of breath. His wife chastises him. She explains that he has been sick for a week coughing 'that green stuff' and demands that the paramedics take him to hospital as she is too tired to continue watching him. The paramedics again ask the patient if they can examine him, explaining that they are here to help and that his wife is worried about him. He reluctantly pulls the blankets from his head and rolls onto his back. He looks flushed and unwell.

 ASSESS

Patient history

The patient is refusing to discuss his illness; only his wife can confirm his condition and the accuracy of her information is unknown. It is very easy for the paramedics to miss the importance of his wife relaying the information and instead demand that the patient talk to them directly. While this may be necessary in some situations, observing appropriate protocols when working with Indigenous people is critical to establishing positive and respectful relationships. Is the husband refusing to engage with the paramedics because he doesn't want to speak, because he wants a significant family member to disclose his story or because he doesn't want assistance? The clues lie in the fact that he has allowed the paramedics to examine him. He hasn't refused assessment and hasn't provided contradictory information over the story his wife has relayed in his presence.

Further confirmation can be sought by evaluating how other members of the house are behaving towards the patient and his wife. Are they supportive of her story or are they supporting the husband and stating he is okay? Support towards her will generally indicate that she has the right to relay his story. The patient participating in the examination also confirms that he is interested in the assistance offered. The community supporting the patient may indicate that the caller (his wife in this instance) may be involved in other social issues that may have prompted a request for removal of the patient, which may or may not be appropriate.

Once the patient's story has been relayed by his significant kin, there may be an opportunity to separate the wife from her husband, leaving the patient on his own to answer questions. Without significant kin present it is more likely that he will engage in questioning. Respect for her can still be shown by seeking information from her while she is away from him.

Initial assessment summary

Problem	Generally unwell
Conscious state	Alert
Position	Supine
Heart rate	115 bpm, regular
Blood pressure	100/80 mmHg
Skin appearance	Hot and dry
Speech pattern	Speaks in sentences
Respiratory rate	32 bpm, shallow
Respiratory rhythm	Even cycles
Chest auscultation	Widespread areas of coarse crackles that resolve/move with cough. Bronchial sounds are present in the lower right lobe.
Temperature	38.5°C
Pulse oximetry	94% on room air
History	The patient is complaining of dyspnoea. He continues to refuse to answer the crew's questions or make eye contact with them. His wife has answered all the questions to date and the patient's history is still quite sketchy. His wife is demanding that he be taken to hospital so she can get some sleep. The patient does not appear very happy with this option, but is clearly unwell.

D: There are no dangers.
A: The patient is conscious with no current airway obstruction.
B: Respiratory function indicates a chest infection. The respiratory rate is elevated and the volume is slightly reduced. The SpO$_2$ is at the lower range of normal.
C: Heart rate is elevated and blood pressure is on the lower limit, but the patient is not pale or clammy.

The patient is displaying respiratory distress consistent with pneumonia in the right lung.

 CONFIRM

The essential part of the clinical reasoning process is to seek to confirm your initial hypothesis by finding clinical signs that should occur with your provisional diagnosis. You should also seek to challenge your diagnosis by exploring findings that do not fit your hypothesis: don't just ignore them because they don't fit.

What else could it be?

Asthma
The patient's work of breathing is normal and there are no wheezes, so this diagnosis is not supported.

Acute pulmonary oedema
While crackles are present they are coarse, localised and resolve or move with a cough. The patient is also supine, which is atypical for acute pulmonary oedema, as sitting upright reduces the dyspnoea. This diagnosis is not supported.

Pulmonary embolism
The patient does not appear to have significant risk factors but this condition is difficult to exclude in the out-of-hospital setting. The lower blood pressure is a concern as it could indicate a significant obstruction to pulmonary blood flow.

> **DIFFERENTIAL DIAGNOSIS**
>
> **Pneumonia**
> Or
> - Asthma
> - Acute pulmonary oedema
> - Pulmonary embolism
> - Pleural effusion
> - Pneumothorax
> - Sepsis

Pleural effusion

This diagnosis is difficult to exclude in the out-of-hospital setting and is probably present to some degree if pneumonia is present.

Pneumothorax

Equal breath sounds and a lack of localised resonance help to exclude this diagnosis. The presence of bronchial sounds in the lower right lobe suggests consolidation of lung tissue (the 'solid' nature of the lung tissue is transmitting sounds more than air) and assists in excluding this diagnosis.

Sepsis

While the patient almost certainly has a lung infection, this does not preclude the infection from becoming systemic. Only a blood culture will confirm this finding, but given his vital signs, if he is not currently septic he is likely to progress to this state if left untreated.

The patient is indeed unwell and should be transported to hospital. In order to achieve this outcome some significant cultural considerations need to be evaluated.

 TREAT

Emergency management

Management of respiratory distress and sepsis is covered in Section 11 and Chapter 32, respectively, and so the issue here is the impact of the patient's Indigenous background in engaging with treatment. While the patient has the right to autonomy and to withhold consent, this can be defended only if he has been given and is capable of understanding the consequences of his decision. In this case the impediments to the patient agreeing to transport may go beyond those normally encountered by paramedics and they need to be addressed when considering the patient's wish to remain at the scene. For instance, if the patient was left untreated and succumbed to his illness, his significant kin could be punished by the community for not obtaining help for him. The paramedics should consider the following questions.

- Are his significant kin refusing to accompany him?
- Does the patient have the finances to return home?
- Is he likely to be disadvantaged by leaving his community or home?
- Is he afraid of what might happen when he goes to hospital?

They should then address each of these questions and again provide an opportunity for the patient to accompany them.

If the wife refuses to accompany her husband to hospital and there are no community members present to apply pressure to her to do so, the paramedics should ask for another person to accompany the patient. However, the person assigned to this role may not be the right person to advise in decision-making or have the right to tell the patient's story. As a result, they can provide support and company for the patient but won't be able to answer questions regarding treatment. If it is not possible to get another community member to accompany the patient, the paramedics should explain the seriousness of the situation to the patient's wife and encourage her to play her role in accessing help for the patient. In traditional Indigenous culture, if a significant kin member refuses to assist a person they are obligated to help and that person dies, there will be serious ramifications.

If return from hospital is an issue, the paramedics may be able to advise what services are available in the area to provide return transportation. This is particularly relevant where it is unlikely that the patient will be admitted to hospital. Alternatively, understanding what government schemes have been arranged may assist in persuading him to go to hospital. However, any arrangements must be communicated to the receiving hospital: one negative experience will not be forgotten and promises will mean little when the next paramedic makes one.

Belongings and finances are often shared within the kinship system. As a result, one member of the community may provide support for others and the patient may display a reluctance to leave their home or community if this support is likely to be interrupted. Allowing time for the patient to make alternative arrangements may be critical before they will agree to be transported.

The patient may not be familiar with the processes of care in the hospital setting and may be afraid of going to hospital. He may also be concerned about his rights being respected and whether his family will be allowed to be with him. Any such issues should be identified and addressed to put the patient's mind at ease.

4 EVALUATE

The response to the management of respiratory distress and sepsis is covered in Section 11 and Chapter 32, respectively.

CS CASE STUDY 2

Case 14590, 1630 hrs.

Dispatch details: Police request an ambulance at an alleged assault.

Initial presentation: The paramedics arrive and find a 49-year-old male arguing in the middle of a group of people. The police are in attendance and quickly resolve the situation and remove the patient from the group. The man, an Indigenous Australian male, was arguing with his wife when the quarrel became violent. An onlooker witnessed the violence and rang for the police when she saw blood.

---

1 ASSESS

Members of the group surround the police officers, insisting that the man deserved to be stabbed as he had been seen with a woman other than his wife. The patient is agitated, loudly declaring his innocence. He appears unaware of any injury and won't stay still long enough for a proper assessment.

1643 hrs Chief complaint: The paramedics notice a small tear in the upper leg of the patient's jeans and the crutch area and right leg of his jeans are soaked with blood down as far as the knee.

The police escort the patient to the rear of the ambulance and sit him down on the back steps. The paramedics then attempt an assessment.

1645 hrs Vital signs survey: Perfusion status: HR 120 bpm, BP 90/60 mmHg, skin cool and dry.

Respiratory status: RR 32 bpm, SpO$_2$ 94%.

Conscious state: GCS = 15.

1650 hrs Secondary survey: There is no obvious wound but a large amount of congealed blood around his upper right leg. On exposure a stab wound is located in the anterior right upper thigh, which pulsates bright-red blood when disturbed. Female members of the group start to wail loudly when they see his blood. No-one will confirm who the perpetrator is and his wife is insisting that she travel with him to hospital.

The clinical situation is relatively clear: a penetrating wound to the groin, combined with abnormal vital signs, requires immediate transport to hospital. Expediting transport and ruling out any other injuries will be difficult at this highly emotional scene.

2 CONFIRM

Determining the underlying cause of the patient's presentation is not difficult. Several witnesses saw him stabbed with a knife, the blood loss is obvious and the treatment is straightforward—immediate transport to definitive care. Assessing his vital signs confirms that he is most likely hypovolaemic and may have an internal bleed that cannot be controlled without surgery. He must be transported to hospital without delay, but there are significant cultural considerations that need to be addressed to enable this. The key to effective engagement in this case involves being culturally sensitive, describing behaviour without judging it and keeping calm. Impatience or assertive behaviour may further agitate the scene.

Marital problems aired publicly are likely to produce feelings of shame. Ideally, the treating paramedic should be the same gender as the patient when these issues are discussed, but even then permission needs to be sought from the patient before proceeding. It may be more appropriate for another member of the community to speak about these problems rather than the patient. It is important the patient does not feel judged as this will exacerbate the feeling of shame and make further management more difficult. The paramedics should preface any questions likely to induce these feelings with 'I'm not trying to shame you, but I need to know …' This is likely to facilitate more truthful conversations as the paramedics are describing why they should be included in the person's embarrassment. Acknowledgment of the shame builds rapport and allows the patient to understand that he is not being judged.

Wailing, mainly by females, demonstrates their sorrow at what has occurred. It is a mark of respect for the person and may occur even when the injury or illness is not life-threatening. As such, trying to explain the exact nature of an injury to them (if it is minor) may not resolve the reaction. In addition, understanding the meaning behind this reaction should enable paramedics to realise that attempting to console those who are wailing may not be necessary.

This patient is agitated and difficult to engage. The paramedics need to establish whether this is due to hypoxia, a sense of shame, the noise and stimulation at the scene or the fact that he is proclaiming his innocence but has received payback regardless. Confirmation can be sought by assessing how other members of the group are behaving towards the patient and his wife. Are they supportive of him or are they angry towards him? Support towards him will normally indicate that he has received payback and is forgiven and his agitation should diminish. Anger towards him could mean he has not taken the payback as he should and this could invoke shame and contribute to his agitated state.

The recruitment of an Indigenous male Elder may assist in getting the patient stationary long enough to take his vital signs. This person should be considered as an appropriate travel companion to keep the patient calm and approachable.

Amid the heightened emotions, the patient's wife asks to go with him to hospital but it is still not clear whether she is the alleged perpetrator. Consulting the patient is appropriate: if he agrees, the paramedics should ensure that his wife understands her role in the ambulance and will assist them and follow their directions. Due to the nature of the scene, giving the wife clear boundaries on what will and won't be acceptable behaviour, with consequences if she chooses not to follow the instructions, may be necessary to ensure the safety of both the patient and the crew.

3 TREAT

Safety

Depending on the circumstances, the patient may be at continued risk from the alleged perpetrator and other family members—as may be the paramedics. Consideration must be given to paramedic safety where violence is present. However, the aggression in this case is predominantly focused inwards and not towards the professionals trying to assist (see Fig 49.4 and Box 49.1).

The notion of privacy in Indigenous culture is different from traditional Anglo-Saxon Australia. Straightforward, loud conversations or arguments between individuals in a public forum are still considered private. Other community members who are not invited or of relevant kin should not join in, even though the argument can be heard publicly.

4 EVALUATE

Evaluating the effect of any clinical management intervention can provide clues to the accuracy of the initial diagnosis. Some conditions respond rapidly to treatment so patients should be expected to improve if the diagnosis and treatment were appropriate, whereas other conditions are unlikely to respond in the timeframes normally associated with ambulance transport times. In

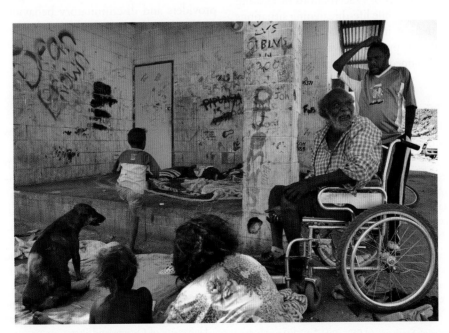

Figure 49.4
Violence rates among Indigenous Australians are regarded as high, but assaults occur more frequently in lower socioeconomic communities regardless of their cultural background.
Source: Corbis/Marianna Massey.

> ## BOX 49.1 Violence rates among Indigenous Australians
>
> Assault is among the five leading causes of death for Indigenous Australians, both males and females. Over the period 2001–2005, the Indigenous male age-specific death rates for 10-year age groups from 25 to 54 were between 11 and 17 times the corresponding age-specific rates for non-Indigenous males, while for females the rates ranged between 9 and 23 times the equivalent age-specific rates for non-Indigenous females (AIHW, 2009).

such cases, a failure to improve should not be considered an indication of a misdiagnosis.

In this case, haemorrhage control, IV fluid and pain relief should be effective in maintaining the patient's vital signs. Small reductions in his heart rate should be the first sign of a positive response to treatment. Improvements in blood pressure should occur once his heart rate starts to decrease.

Summary

Indigenous Australians live with significant health inequities that are compounded by not having access to the necessary determinants of care that optimise health outcomes and to quality health services. It is not unusual for some Indigenous Australians never to have seen a primary healthcare professional and paramedics may be the first health professionals to respond to their acute health conditions or exacerbations of existing chronic conditions. While life-threatening situations demand prioritisation, it is important to consider key cultural factors and appropriate ways to engage with these patients. Paramedics are in a unique position to facilitate patients' access to health services to have their health needs assessed and treated. To effectively engage and interact with Indigenous Australians, paramedics need to be aware of the stereotypes and prejudices they may hold that can adversely impact on their interactions with patients and their communities. This doesn't simply mean treating all patients the same: paramedics need to be aware that Indigenous Australians may have encountered negative healthcare providers and discriminatory behaviours; they also need to be genuine, respectful and non-judgemental, and aware of key cultural needs that should be respected.

References

AusMAT. (2011). *AusMAT Training, Version 3*. NCCTRC. Retrieved from www.nationaltraumacentre.nt.gov.au. (Accessed 2 October 2012).

Australian Bureau of Statistics (ABS). (2017a). *2016. Census Quick Stats, Northern Territory*. Retrieved from www.quickstats.censusdata.abs.gov.au/census_services/getproduct/census/2016/quickstat/7?opendocument.. (Accessed 6 November 2018).

Australian Bureau of Statistics (ABS). (2017b). *2016. Census Quick Stats, Australia*. Retrieved from www.quickstats.censusdata.abs.gov.au/census_services/getproduct/census/2016/quickstat/036?opendocument. (Accessed 6 November 2018).

Australian Bureau of Statistics (ABS). (2017c). *2016. Causes of Death, Australia 2017*. Retrieved from www.abs.gov.au/ausstats/abs@.nsf/Lookup/by%20Subject/3303.0~2017~Main%20Features~Australia's%20leading%20causes%20of%20death,%202017~2. (Accessed 6 November 2018).

Australian Institute of Health and Welfare (AIHW). (2009). *National Mortality Database: Recorded Crime: Victims*. Cat. no. 4510.0. Canberra: AIHW.

Australian Institute of Health and Welfare (AIHW). (2011). *The Health and Welfare of Australia's Aboriginal and Torres Strait Islander People, An Overview*. Retrieved from www.aihw.gov.au/WorkArea/DownloadAsset.aspx?id=10737418955. (Accessed 6 November 2014).

Bourke, C., & Edwards, B. (2004). Family and kinship. In *Aboriginal Australia* (2nd ed.). St Lucia, Queensland: University of Queensland Press.

Cousins, M. (2004). *Aboriginal justice: a Haudenosaunee approach*. Justice as Healing: a newsletter on Aboriginal concepts of justice (Native Law Centre), 1.

Law Reform Committee Western Australia. (2004). *Thematic Summaries of Consultations: Midland, 16 December 2002*. Perth: Law Reform Commission of Western Australia.

Northern Territory Law Reform Committee. (2003). *Aboriginal Communities and Aboriginal Law in the Northern Territory*. Background Paper No. 1 (21).

Sheldon, M. (2001). Psychiatric assessment in remote Aboriginal communities. *The Australian and New Zealand Journal of Psychiatry, 35*(4), 435–442.

Trees, K. (2004). *Contemporary Issues Facing Customary Law and the General Legal System. Roebourne: A Case Study*. LRCWA Project 94. Background Paper no. 6 (20).

Williams, N. (1987). *Two laws: managing disputes in a contemporary Aboriginal community*. Canberra: Australian Institute Studies Press.

Wilson, D. (2008). The significance of a culturally appropriate health service for indigenous Māori women. *Contemporary Nurse, 28*, 173–188.

CHAPTER 50

Māori Patients

By Haydn Drake and Denise Wilson

OVERVIEW

- Māori are the Indigenous people of Aotearoa (New Zealand) and they comprise 16% of the population.
- Contemporary Māori are not a homogenous group of people, but are diverse in terms of *iwi* (tribes) and experiences.
- The cultural beliefs of contemporary Māori are diverse and can be located on a continuum that spans those who have had a traditional upbringing to those who may know they are Māori but have lost connections with their heritage and cultural traditions.
- Compared to other New Zealanders, Māori experience significant inequities in life expectancy, health status, health outcomes (morbidity and mortality), quality of healthcare and access to a range of health services.
- The ability of paramedics to conduct a detailed health assessment and make sound clinical decisions may require an understanding of Māori culture and beliefs and how it shapes their engagement with health providers.
- Traditional Māori cultural worldviews are holistic and eco-spiritual in nature. This is evident in the collective (or group) orientation of Māori in contrast to the individual orientation of the dominant culture.

Introduction

Economic and social deprivations adversely affect health, and Indigenous groups generally have poorer outcomes and poorer survival chances (Whitehead, 1991). In New Zealand, the poor respiratory health experienced by many Māori can be linked to houses that lack insulation, and are cold and damp (Howden-Chapman et al., 2005). Research shows Māori (and Pacific) peoples have a high prevalence of multiple morbidity and polypharmacy (Stokes et al., 2018). Research also indicates that the extent and quality of care differs between non-Indigenous New Zealanders and Māori. For example, Māori are more likely to experience an adverse event while in hospital (Davis et al., 2006; Rumball-Smith et al., 2013), to postpone paying for a prescription medication (Jatrana et al., 2011), to notice differences in the quality of care they receive (Wilson & Barton, 2012) and to experience discrimination and racism within health services (Harris et al., 2012).

Despite their overrepresentation in avoidable mortality and morbidity statistics, Māori are less likely to access primary healthcare services (Ministry of Health, 2015). This may be because they do not have the opportunity due to remoteness, or because they do not consider the service appropriate to their needs. As a result, when the opportunity to engage with Māori patients does arise in the primary healthcare setting, the ability to engage effectively with their cultural beliefs as well as their illness may have a disproportionately positive and long-term effect.

Engaging with culturally distinct groups requires health professionals to undertake a process of reflection on their personal cultural background, professional values and beliefs, and the power they hold in their position. They then need to examine how these might impact on their professional practice when working with others from another culture, like patients and their *whānau* (extended family) (Wilson & Hickey, 2015).

Box 50.1 provides a glossary of Māori terms.

Specific aspects of healthcare for Māori

Quality of healthcare

Māori adults and children are most likely to report an unmet need for primary healthcare, and twice as likely not to have filled a prescription due to cost compared to other groups of people in New Zealand (Ministry of Health, 2016). A determinant of quality care and use of primary healthcare is having a continued relationship with a general practitioner (GP) and other health professionals; compromised access is a barrier for Māori receiving care quality without discrimination (Reid et al., 2016). Research with GPs confirms concerns about the quality of care that Māori may receive when they do access primary healthcare services (Crengle, 2007). GPs

BOX 50.1 Glossary

Aroha	Love, compassion
Hapū	A subtribe forming a basic political unit within Māori society
Hui	Gathering
Kia ora	Greeting, hello
Kuia	Older woman
Kupu	Māori words
Manaakitanga	Caring for others
Marae	Open courtyard in front of wharenui where formal gatherings are held
Mauri	Life force
Noa	Common, opposite to tapu
Rūnanga	Council or committee
Tane	Men
Tangihanga	Period of mourning
Tapu	Sacred, restricted, prohibited
Tēnā koe	Hello, thank you
Te whare tangata	Refers to women as bearers of children; the house of humankind
Te reo Māori	Māori language
Tikanga	Correct procedures, protocols
Tuku wairua	A verbal ritual said over those who are dying to ease the passage of the spirit into the afterlife
Wairua	Spirit, soul of a person
Wahine/wāhine	Woman/women
Whānau	Extended family
Whakamā	Shame, embarrassment
Whakapapa	Genealogy
Wharekai	Eating house
Wharenui	Meeting house
Whare tupuna	Ancestral meeting house

report that Māori are likely to have visits of shorter duration, have urgent presentations, are slightly less likely to have tests and investigations and are slightly more likely to have a prescription. Importantly, GPs report that their rapport with Māori patients is lower than that which they have with their other patients (Crengle, 2007). With this in mind and because Māori are an at-risk population, paramedics need to be mindful about screening for health conditions (e.g. rheumatic heart disease) and utilise local referral pathways.

Institutional racism

Māori, along with Pacific and Asian ethnic groups, have a higher prevalence of racial discrimination and multiple forms of other discrimination (such as family and marital status, sexual orientation, age,

and disability or health status) that is associated with poorer health and greater life dissatisfaction. These multiple forms of oppression intersect with compounding effects and are maintained by systems of privilege (Cormack et al., 2018). A system of privilege is evident where institutional racism exists that creates barriers to accessing health and social services for those living with high levels of deprivation, as many Māori do. Consequences include being unable to exercise choice and to access health services in the same way as people with less deprivation (see Fig 50.1). We should be mindful that the high rates of morbidity that Māori experience are caused by a complex set of factors, including not having the necessary resources (such as transport or money) to access healthcare services. Although publicly funded health systems are set up to give everyone

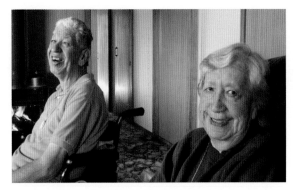

Figure 50.1
Eighty-three-year-old Rapaki Māori elder Rima Subritzky has helped raise 37 children from her *whānau* and continues to care for her son Charlie, who has disabilities. It is important that healthcare systems promote a cultural understanding of Māori communities to ensure that the specific needs of their people are met.
Source: Fletcher EQR (2013).

equal access (Morgan & Simmons, 2009), those living with high levels of social deprivation are not getting the healthcare they need.

Epidemiological profile

Ischaemic heart disease

Ischaemic heart disease (IHD) is the leading cause of premature death in New Zealand for Māori men and the second leading cause of death for Māori women (Ministry of Health, 2015). IHD death rates vary between ethnic groups within the population but are significantly higher for Māori than non-Māori. For Māori men and women, the age-standardised death rate from IHD is more than twice that of non-Māori men and women, with Māori women twice as likely to be hospitalised for IHD compared to non-Māori women (Ministry of Health, 2015). These figures take into account that Māori are a youthful population in comparison with the non-Māori population (only 5.4% of Māori live beyond the age of 65 years compared with 14.3% of non-Māori) and the actual difference in premature mortality rates is greater than these figures suggest (Statistics New Zealand, 2014).

Smoking

The health risks of smoking are well known, including the link between smoking and heart disease. Māori are almost three times more likely to smoke than other adults living in New Zealand: 40% of Māori women smoke (Ministry of Health, 2016). The health consequences of smoking extend beyond IHD to many other diseases such as lung cancer, which is the leading cause of death for Māori women.

Diabetes

The age-standardised rates of the diabetes-related complications of renal disease and lower limb amputation are more than five and three times higher, respectively, for Māori than non-Māori (Ministry of Health, 2016). Māori are also seven times more likely to die of complications related to diabetes than non-Māori (Harwood & Tipene-Leach, 2007). The ethnic disparities related to diabetes are complex and involve the interaction of various risk factors such as genetics, environment, social determinants of health (e.g. education, qualifications, income, employment, housing, access to transport) and interpersonal and institutional racism (Harwood & Tipene-Leach, 2007; Reid & Robson, 2007). The ethnic inequities related to diabetes (and other morbidities often experienced by Māori) are associated with reduced access to, and quality of, healthcare (Harwood & Tipene-Leach, 2007). In other words, absence or delay in the diagnosis and treatment of diabetes has detrimental effects on the health and lives of Māori and their *whānau* (Curtis et al., 2007).

Rheumatic heart disease

New Zealand has one of the highest prevalence rates of rheumatic heart disease (RHD) globally, with most cases occurring among Māori and Pacific peoples. Acute rheumatic fever (ARF) is a preventable autoimmune disease that may occur after pharyngitis caused by group A *streptococcus* (GAS) bacteria, with RHD being a severe consequence. ARF in childhood is associated with geographical region, ethnicity, social determinants of health such as poverty and overcrowding, high rates of streptococcal upper respiratory infections and a lack of access and use of health services (Wilson, 2010). ARF in childhood leads to chronic RHD for Māori. The highest rates of ARF in New Zealand are in Māori and Pacific children between the ages of 5 and 14 years (Webb & Wilson, 2013).

Primary prevention of ARF through antibiotic treatment of GAS pharyngitis is an essential part of ARF disease prevention, but not all *whānau* are able to access medical care for their children when needed. Barriers to access include geographical distance, access to transport, cost of petrol, difficulty getting appointments and not being able to get time off work (Anderson et al., 2017). There is an opportunity for paramedics to identify Māori patients presenting with sore throats who are at high risk for rheumatic fever, and refer them on to primary healthcare services for throat swabs and antibiotic treatment. Māori are greater than five times more likely to die because of RHD, with

Māori women more affected (Ministry of Health, 2015). The management of chronic RHD is compromised by factors such as geographical location, mobility, access to specialist care, lack of early diagnosis, comorbidities and cultural barriers (White et al., 2010). Paramedics need to be aware that Māori presenting with IHD might have underlying chronic RHD.

Driveway accidents

Accidents are a leading cause of death for Māori children aged between 1 and 4 years, with transport-related accidents accounting for 36% more deaths for Māori children compared with non-Māori children (Robson & Purdie, 2007). Of all the deaths caused by low-speed cars reversing, 48% were Māori children (Child and Youth Mortality Review Committee, 2011), despite Māori comprising only 15% of the New Zealand population. Māori children are also more likely to be killed in pedestrian accidents at home than non-Māori children: between 2002 and 2008 the rate was close to 15 per 100,000 among Māori children compared with 3 per 100,000 for non-Māori children (Child and Youth Mortality Review Committee, 2011). In the same period, the rate among the Pacific population was 20.5 per 100,000. This inequity in transport-related mortality rates continues throughout the lifespan, with the age-standardised mortality rate among Māori from motor vehicle accidents 18.4 per 100,000—more than twice that of the non-Māori population.

Family violence

I saw no quarrelling while I was there. They were kind to their women and children. I never observed either a mark of violence upon them, nor did I see a child struck.

Samuel Marsden in Elder *(1932).*

The above quote typifies observations documented by settlers and those sent to colonise New Zealand, and indicates that pre-colonisation violence did not exist in Māori *whānau*. Yet, similar to other colonised Indigenous peoples, Māori are overrepresented in child abuse and neglect, intimate partner and intrafamilial violence and deaths caused by a member within their *whānau*. Compared to non-Māori living in New Zealand, Māori are:

- 3 times more likely to be the deceased or offender of intimate partner violence deaths
- 4 times more likely to be killed as a child aged between 0 to 4 year of age
- 4 times more likely to be the deceased as a result of intrafamilial violence, and
- 5 times more likely to be the offender of an intrafamilial violence death (FVDRC, 2017).

While some argue that women and men are equally violent (Johnson et al., 2014), in New Zealand Māori women and children are at most risk of serious harm or death as a result of violence that occurs within their home.

It is important to understand that violence in *whānau* was not part of traditional Māori society (Kruger et al., 2004) and is a relatively recent development. In traditional Māori communities, women and children are held in high esteem and importance, especially their role in maintaining the *whakapapa* of a *whānau/hapū*; that is, women's role as bearers of, and children being, the future generations. Traditional values and practices provided *whānau* and *hapū* with mechanisms to keep women, children and men safe: however, colonisation and systems of patriarchy, capitalism, legislation, Christianity and assimilation (aided by urbanisation and policies of education) eroded the protective mechanisms inherent in the cultural traditions and support provided within *whānau* and *hapū*. Colonisation brought about marked depopulation of Māori, dispossession of their land and language, cultural and social disenfranchisement that destroyed important traditional mechanisms to keep women and children safe (Pihama et al., 2003).

The contemporary context of *whānau* violence is complex and requires an understanding of multiple intersecting and compounding effects on many Māori *whānau*: colonisation of Aotearoa and its ongoing impacts, historical trauma, contemporary socioeconomic deprivation and social marginalisation (including racism and discrimination). While displaying strengths and resilience (Evans-Campbell, 2008), ongoing intergenerational effects impacting the holistic wellbeing of many *whānau* (Pihama et al., 2016) requires an Indigenous *kaupapa* Māori approach (FVDRC, 2017).

New Zealand's Family Violence Death Review Committee (2016) stresses the need for those working with *whānau* to think differently about the violence occurring among their members; basically, they have complex lives and simple solutions lead to ineffective safety responses for those seeking help (see Box 50.2). Therefore, paramedics need to know and understand local

> **PRACTICE POINT**
>
> The safety of children is paramount.

> **PRACTICE POINT**
>
> Always consider the entangled form of child abuse, neglect and intimate partner violence; if a child is being abused, it is likely their mother is also being abused and vice versa.

BOX 50.2 Changing how we think about violence in *whānau*

Violence in *whānau* …	It is not …
Is a pattern of cumulative harm that occurs over time	An isolated or one-off event or 'just a domestic'
Requires knowing who is the primary victim and the predominant aggressor in a relationship	Mutual acts of violence involving both partners
Entraps victims in relationships with violent partners' who use coercive control and manipulation (e.g. threats against their children)	Possible for victims to simply leave a violent partner
Leads to victims using acts of resistance to keep themselves safe and to protect their children	Women being just as violent as men
Requires collective action for the safety of adult and child victims—this means paramedics need to work with other agencies to respond to keep them safe	Mothers negligently staying and not protecting their children from a violent partner
Involves the entanglement of the abuse and violence of victims and their children	Violence against women, and child abuse and neglect are separate issues
Is a form of cumulative and compounding trauma affecting adult and child victims' spiritual, psychological, social and physical wellbeing	Caused by alcohol or mental health problems

Source: NZ Family Violence Death Review Committee (2016)

agencies (government, non-government and community organisations) who work with *whānau* affected by violence.

Mental health

Māori understandings of mental illness are often at odds with Western biomedical understandings that inform mental health service delivery. First, Māori worldviews are holistic and based on the interrelationships between the spiritual, human and natural worlds: people's wellbeing is contingent on everything being in balance. *Te whare tapa whā*, the four-sided whare (house), symbolically shows the dimensions of Māori health and wellbeing: *taha wairua* (spiritual dimension), *taha whānau* (extended family dimension), *taha hinengaro* (the mental or psychological dimension) and *taha tinana* (the physical dimension). When an imbalance in one or more sides of a person's whare (house) occurs, the person's (and *whānau*) health and wellbeing is at risk (Durie, 1998). Second, there is a reluctance by some Māori to accept mental illness diagnoses, such as schizophrenia or psychosis, because it overlooks cultural and spiritual explanations that relate to imbalances, cultural disconnection or breaches of *tapu* (restrictions and sacredness) resulting in *mate Māori* (Māori illness). Colonisation has replaced this traditional knowledge and associated healing practices with Western biomedical explanations and treatments, including the belief that Māori

are predisposed to mental illness. This has been complicated by mainstream understandings of trauma, drug abuse, historical trauma and chemical brain imbalances (Taitimu et al., 2018).

It is important for paramedics working in primary healthcare settings to be aware of mental health issues affecting Māori health and wellbeing, and the need for culturally appropriate sociocultural and clinical assessments (Mulder, 2017). For Māori, mental health is situated within complex and varied contexts that include colonisation and its ongoing effects that contribute to significant life stressors (e.g. poverty, unemployment, poor or no housing), historical trauma, family violence, substance misuse and unmet health needs. Māori also report greater hazardous alcohol drinking and psychological distress than non-Māori (Ministry of Health, 2016). Such life contexts can cause or aggravate mental health leading to symptoms of depression, anxiety and posttraumatic disorders. Māori are 1.5 times more likely than non-Māori to have an anxiety or depressive disorder, with Māori men being twice as likely to have anxiety or depression compared to non-Māori men (Ministry of Health, 2015). Furthermore, research with pregnant women shows Māori women have a greater likelihood of depressive and anxiety symptoms, significant life stress and poor mood during their current pregnancy (Signal et al., 2017).

Paramedics should be mindful of the potential for substance use and cognitive impairments with Māori presenting with behaviours suggestive of mental illness. Māori are twice as likely (42%) to be acutely admitted to a mental health facility for serious mental illness (schizophrenia, bipolar disorder and schizo-affective disorder) and tend to be younger than non-Māori. Serious mental illness is also associated with smoking tobacco, misusing alcohol and substances (such as cannabis) (Dharmawardene et al., 2015) and higher prescribed dosages of antipsychotic medications that can lead to verbal memory, verbal learning and visual memory impairments (Kake et al., 2016).

Māori suicide rates are twice that of non-Māori, with Māori males—particularly 15–24 year olds—having significantly higher rates (Ministry of Health, 2015). The Suicide Mortality Review Committee (SUMRC, 2016) reported more than half of *rangatahi* Māori (15–24 year olds) suicide were those aged 15–19 years of age, with two-thirds being male. Their histories included prior self-harm and suicide attempts, sexual abuse (14%), family violence (22%), contact with child protective services (40%) and intimate relationship conflict or break-up. Importantly, in addition to *whānau* actively seeking help, almost half had previous contact with mental health services, with a third of young Māori having contact within 12 months before their death (SUMRC, 2016). Suicide is also the leading cause of maternal death in New Zealand; pregnant Māori women comprise over half (56%) of these deaths (Perinatal and Maternal Mortality Review Committee [PMMRC], 2017), highlighting the need for Māori women's antenatal and postnatal mental wellbeing to be considered and assessed (Signal et al., 2017).

Delayed access to healthcare

Health conditions and diseases can be prevented or treated at the community level through population-based health strategies, and at the individual level through timely access to primary healthcare. It is well-established that Māori are less likely to access primary healthcare and more likely to be admitted to hospital or to die from health conditions and injuries that could have been prevented or managed in the community (Ministry of Health, 2015). Paramedics are familiar with encountering patients who are seriously ill because they delayed seeking medical help due to the costs or difficulties in seeing a doctor. In addition to factors associated with socioeconomic deprivation, many Māori who live in rural or semi-rural areas face the added challenges of accessing distant health services. Delayed access to healthcare results in late diagnoses and deferments in receiving potentially life-saving treatments. Thus, the paramedic's role in gathering a patient's history

and undertaking observations and procedures, such as a 12-lead ECG, is crucial for identification of any problems and referral or transport to appropriate care.

Death among Māori populations

Māori, like other people, react in diverse ways to the news that someone they love has died. Some may express profound sadness, others may express anger. Some Māori women express their grief very emotionally by unreservedly crying or wailing loudly, while Māori men tend to grieve quietly: 'crying silently' (Salmond, 1976). Many, but not all, Māori hold traditional beliefs about death and dying and believe that following death a person's *wairua* (spirit) leaves the *tūpāpaku* (body) and lingers over it for several days prior to embarking on a journey to another dimension of life. A *tuku wairua* is performed (a verbal ritual said over those who are dying to ease the passage of the spirit into the afterlife), although it should be noted that different *iwi* have different beliefs about the nature of the journey that the *wairua* takes. The last breath of life signifies both the death of the *mauri* (life force), which then disappears, and the transition of the person to being a *tūpāpaku*. At this time the *tūpāpaku* is extremely *tapu* (sacred) and the person's *wairua* is released (Moko Mead, 2003). It is a commonly held belief by many Māori that the *tūpāpaku* should not be left alone, meaning close *whānau* will want to stay with the body.

The *whānau* may want to gather and have a *kaumātua* or church minister to say a *karakia* (as a form of last rites) over the *tūpāpaku*, especially as an illness or injuries that have led to the death are believed to weaken the *wairuai* (Moko Mead, 2003). It is vitally important to the *whānau* that the correct processes and protocols are carried out, such as saying the appropriate *karakia* and the *whānau* staying with the *tūpāpaku*. This enables the *tuku wairua* of their loved to be released and 'go in peace to the next world' (Barlow, 1994). It is believed that the *tuku wairua* watches the events and what people are doing: if things are not carried out correctly, they will not be at peace and will cause difficulties for the *whānau*. For this reason, it is important that the *whānau* are consulted about the correct spiritual and cultural protocols to be followed for the peace of mind of the *whānau* and for the *tuku wairua* to begin its journey peacefully (Moko Mead, 2003).

> ## PRACTICE POINT
> It is important not to assume that all Māori have traditional beliefs about death: ask and be guided by the *whānau* what their needs are.

CASE STUDY 1

Case 30635, 1123 hrs.

Dispatch details: A 46-year-old woman has collapsed. She is attending a *hui* (gathering) on a *marae* (open courtyard where formal gatherings are held) in a rural location, 45 minutes from the nearest tertiary hospital.

Initial presentation: The paramedics arrive and are led to the patient, who is sitting down in the *wharekai* (eating house) where she has been helping to prepare lunch. She is pale, sweaty and complaining of feeling dizzy.

 ASSESS

Patient history

As the patient is on a *marae* it is important for the paramedics to be respectful of and observe *tikanga*. A sound approach is to follow whoever greets them and observe any protocols such as removing their shoes prior to entering the *whare tupuna* (ancestral meeting house) or *wharenui* (meeting house). If time is critical, you can ask to enter the building without removing your footwear. In most circumstances paramedics will not be required to remove their footwear to enter the *wharekai*. If in doubt, ask. If the situation demands urgent action and involves breaching *tikanga*, quickly explain what you are doing and why. Research has shown that having a support person to assist Māori women to interpret and answer questions can reduce their stress (Wilson, 2008). If this is the case, allow time for the support person to interpret the questions and answers if language or hearing difficulties are involved.

This patient states that she was rushing to attend the *hui* and hasn't eaten beforehand. Once she arrived she was talking to friends when they said she briefly appeared confused before turning pale and stating she was dizzy. The friends helped her to sit on the ground and she says that made her feel better. Her friends noted that she was sweaty to touch after she nearly fainted. She denies any shortness of breath, chest pain or palpitations prior to this. She was not incontinent or unconscious at any time. She denies central chest pain but reports that she can feel a 'lump' in her throat. On further questioning you discover that she has no known medical history. She is overweight, but not obese.

Physical examination

Areas on a *marae* and in the homes of Māori living by traditional cultural values and *tikanga* are governed by the cultural concepts of *tapu* (sacred, restricted, prohibited) and *noa* (common, opposite to *tapu*). It is good practice to seek guidance about where to undertake observations and examinations and where to place equipment. For example, the *wharekai* is a place of *noa*.

In relation to people, body parts like the head, genitalia and heart are *tapu* at different times and in various situations. *Noa* is a state of safety without the impositions, protection and restrictions evident in *tapu* states (Durie, 1998). For example, while it is always good practice to avoid stepping over any patient, to Māori this would be particularly offensive. *Tapu* is particularly important when someone dies, as the *tūpāpaku* is very *tapu*. In these situations it is important to seek guidance from *whānau* about what is acceptable practice when someone dies.

Practically, trying to negotiate *tikanga* and making sure conditions of *tapu* and *noa* are observed is difficult when you are attending a call-out. Getting to know local *iwi* and/or the *rūnanga* (council or committee) in the area can assist clinicians who are unsure of appropriate behaviour. Guidelines for attending emergencies can then be established with the support of the community.

Initial assessment summary

Problem	The patient is complaining of atypical chest pain
Conscious state	Alert and orientated; GCS = 15
Position	Sitting upright in a chair
Heart rate	115 bpm, regular
Blood pressure	120/90 mmHg
Skin appearance	Pale, cool, clammy
Speech pattern	Speaking freely
Respiratory rate	24 bpm
Respiratory rhythm	Regular even cycles
Respiratory effort	No use of accessory muscles
Chest auscultation	Clear breath sounds, good bilateral air entry apices to bases
Pulse oximetry	97% on room air
Temperature	36.9°C
BGL	14.5 mmol/L
12-lead ECG	Sinus tachycardia, no ST abnormalities, intervals normal
Motor/sensory function	Normal
History	None known

D: There is no danger to the patient or the crew.
A: The patient is conscious with no airway compromise. Auscultation of the area around the 'lump' sensation reveals no stridor or abnormal sounds.
B: Respiratory function is currently normal.
C: Heart rate is increased and while her blood pressure is within normal limits the patient appears poorly perfused.

Following a near-fainting episode, the patient is displaying poor perfusion and complaining of throat discomfort. She has not eaten prior to this episode.

2 CONFIRM

The differential diagnoses following a near-fainting episode followed by chest pain was outlined in Chapter 35. While these differential diagnoses need to be considered, the patient's Māori heritage should be also taken into account. The types of issues the paramedics need to consider include:
- differences in terms of health and risk factors for Māori patients
- the fact that 46 years old is comparatively more aged for the Māori population than for the Caucasian population
- cultural differences in terms of the patient's willingness to access or enter into the healthcare system.

3 TREAT

Emergency management
Management of acute coronary syndrome is discussed in the chest pain chapter. This patient's increased risk of cardiac disease makes it likely that she is suffering an ischaemic event and needs to be treated accordingly.

COMMENT

When Māori come together, they usually engage in a process called *whakawhanaungatanga*. This involves introducing where you are from geographically, what you do and what your name is.

(4) EVALUATE

This patient's Māori background should have no impact on her response to treatment, but taking her cultural values into account may reduce her anxiety and have a positive effect on her ischaemia.

 CASE STUDY 2

Case 10234, 0725 hrs.

Dispatch details: A 16-month-old toddler has been struck at low speed by a car reversing out of the driveway. She is unresponsive.

Initial presentation: When the paramedics arrive they find the toddler lying motionless in the driveway surrounded by her parents and two other young children. There are several adults nearby who may be extended family or neighbours.

(1) ASSESS

0739 hrs Primary survey: The patient has an obvious severe head injury and no apparent respirations and the paramedics are unable to locate a carotid pulse.

(2) CONFIRM

The patient's failure to progress through the primary survey indicates that a differential diagnosis is not required.

(3) TREAT

0739 hrs: The paramedics commence CPR immediately. They attach the defibrillator and the first rhythm check reveals that the patient is in asystole. They also observe fixed dilated pupils. They continue CPR but after 20 minutes assess that there are no signs of life and terminate the resuscitation attempt.

When there has been a death at an accident scene, paramedics may arrive before the police and it can be helpful to notify the police that Māori *whānau* is involved, so that they can activate their cultural policies and involve their *iwi* liaison personnel (if available) to ensure that the spiritual and cultural needs of the *tūpāpaku* and *whānau* are addressed in the appropriate manner.

CASE STUDY 3

Case 11923, 1546 hrs.

Dispatch details: A 26-year-old woman has been assaulted. The call has come from police, who are in attendance.

Initial presentation: The paramedics arrive and find the woman outside her house talking to a police officer; there are two young children with her. She is standing but her left eye is bruised and slightly swollen. She refuses to be examined but talks to the paramedics.

1 ASSESS

1601 hrs Assessment: The patient reports that she tripped on the front doorstep and fell, knocking her head. She denies having any other injuries. Old bruising is visible on her forearms and one of her front teeth is missing but this does not appear to be a recent injury.

2 CONFIRM

The patient refuses close assessment but presents as orientated and alert. The paramedics explain the potential consequences of her injuries, and the patient appears to have sufficient capacity to refuse assessment and treatment (see Ch 13). Although this is never a comfortable position for an ambulance crew, patients have the right to autonomy provided they are supplied with sufficient information and their decision is not subject to coercion.

3 TREAT

In many cases paramedics (and other clinicians) view patients solely through a lens of clinical need; that is, do they require immediate medical intervention? In this case the patient does not appear to need immediate medical intervention and the crew do not have the right to enforce further assessment, but having been called out it does provide the paramedics with the opportunity to initiate treatments other than medical ones. The patient's preexisting injuries, combined with the complexities of cultural and personal factors (the perpetrator and the victim share custody of their child), suggests family violence. Providing her with the opportunity to be removed from the premises under the guise of medical treatment can offer her the chance to engage in support services. Away from the scene she may have the opportunity to reflect on her position and options and seek advice. In most jurisdictions the pathway in which paramedics are forced to operate (transport to an ED) is not particularly suited to this engagement, but it may be better than nothing. Providing the opportunity to the patient privately (away from police and family) can often allow them to engage in this pathway.

4 EVALUATE

The mild extent of injuries suggests that the patient's physiological condition is unlikely to change.

CASE STUDY 4

Case 30492, 1615 hrs.

Dispatch details: The *whānau* of a 64-year-old male with end-stage heart failure has called the ambulance. He has shortness of breath and has been deteriorating throughout the day. He lives at home under the care of his *whānau*, with home visits from a palliative care nurse.

Initial presentation: The paramedics arrive to find the patient lying in bed. He is pale with shortness of breath and chest pain.

 ASSESS

Patient history

The patient has a history of diabetes mellitus, RHD and hypertension. He is under palliative care for his end-stage heart failure and has become dependent on his *whānau* for assistance with his activities of daily living, including his medications. He has been well medicated up to this point for management of his symptoms with diuretics, ACE inhibitors, beta-blockers, spironolactone, digoxin and oral morphine. He has been deteriorating throughout the day with increasing dyspnoea and chest pain. He has mild confusion, which is an acute deterioration of his normal mental status.

Physical examination

The patient appears pale, has dyspnoea with mild wet lung sounds with oxygen saturations of 86%, and mild tachycardia. He has peripheral oedema, but this is not worse than has been normal for him.

2 CONFIRM

The patient has an established history of end-stage heart failure, and dyspnoea, pain and oedema are common features of this.

3 TREAT

The aim of end-of-life care should be to prevent and alleviate suffering by providing pain management as well as physical, psychosocial and spiritual support to the patient. This is usually managed by an interdisciplinary team and it is useful for paramedics to contact the hospice nurse or other member of the patient's palliative care team to discuss the best way to manage the patient's symptoms (Cobo-Cuenca & Martín-Espinosa, 2013).

4 EVALUATE

Providing care to a *whānau* member at the end of life is an important contribution *whānau* make to each other, as *whānau* wellbeing and that of the individual members are mutually inter-dependent. Moeke-Maxwell (2014) discussed the key concepts for *whānau* of *rangatiratanga* (autonomy and self-determination); *whānau kotahitanga* (unity through consensus); *aroha* and *manaakitanga* (hospitality, kindness, generosity); making meaning from illness and death; *tangihanga* (funerary customs); and *wairuatanga* (spiritual domain). Māori patients with life-limiting illness usually maintain their own *rangatiratanga* until their illness progresses and prevents them from doing so. The ill person then relies on the *rangatiratanga* of the *whānau* to make good end-of-life care decisions on their behalf. Through *whānau kotahitanga*, *whānau* come together to support each other and share the burden of care for the ill person, for the benefit of the ill person and the primary carer. Māori usually discuss *tangihanga* and their wishes after death with their *whānau* ahead of time, so the *whānau* will often have a clear idea of what process should happen. Māori place great importance on spiritual life and it is central to *whānau*-centred care. *Karakia* assists *whānau* at challenging times, and considered to help with healing and to ease suffering as an illness progresses. Paramedics need to be aware of the special relationship and role of *whānau* in caring for the ill person and their involvement in making decisions on their behalf. Paramedics should also be prepared to accommodate their spiritual and religious beliefs, and rituals such as *karakia* that *whānau* may want to perform.

CASE STUDY 5

Case 30709, 1040 hrs.

Dispatch details: A 7-year-old child has a sore throat. The call has come from the child's mother who is at home with two other children below school age.

Initial presentation: When the paramedics arrive they find the child lying on the couch, lethargic but responding normally.

1 ASSESS

Patient history

The child has had a sore throat and been away from school for the past three days. They are lethargic, but otherwise appears well and still able to take small amounts of oral fluids. The mother does not have transport to get to the GP.

Physical examination

The child is responding normally, and has clear lung sounds on auscultation with no increased work of breathing. The child appears flushed, and is febrile at 38°C. The child has had a reduced appetite but still tolerates oral fluids and there are no signs of dehydration.

2 CONFIRM

Pharyngitis is very common and usually get better on its own within about 4 days. ARF is a preventable inflammatory disease that can develop after pharyngitis caused by GAS bacteria that is not treated with antibiotics in at-risk children and young people. People at high risk of rheumatic fever are those with a personal, family or household history of ARF, or two or more of the following:

- Māori and Pacific people
- aged 3–35 years old
- living in crowded circumstances or lower socioeconomic areas of the North Island.

(3) **TREAT**

The child can be symptomatically treated by paramedics initially, for what is typically a low-acuity complaint. Being Māori between the age of 3–35 years, the child is in an at-risk group of ARF and needs referral to a primary health care centre for consideration of a throat swab and treatment with antibiotics.

(4) **EVALUATE**

Although assessment of pharyngitis and preventative management of ARF can be done through primary health care, not all Māori are able to access medical care for their children when needed. Common barriers to access include geographical distance, appointment costs, difficulty accessing transport, costs of transport and difficulty for *whānau* getting time off work (Webb & Wilson, 2013). Sole mothers are further disadvantaged in poorer health and suboptimal healthcare access, and may be separated by geographical distance from *whānau* support (Lee & North, 2013). Paramedics have the opportunity to ensure that parents are aware of the potential complications that may arise from sore throats, and provide advice, support and even transport for them to access the appropriate healthcare for further assessment and management.

Summary

Māori, like other Indigenous peoples, live with significant health inequities that are compounded by the fact that they have a higher level of socio-economic disadvantage and less access to quality health services, as well as cultural practices that mean they attempt to access healthcare less readily. When managing Māori patients, it is important to consider key cultural factors and appropriate ways to engage them in addition to the usual clinical considerations. Paramedics need to be aware of the stereotypes and prejudices they may hold and the cultural practices that can impact on the management of Māori patients and their *whānau*. Paramedics must remember that they are often the first point of contact for these patients on entering the healthcare system and they need to ensure that the shift into this system is met with as little resistance as possible.

References

Anderson, A., Mills, C., & Eggleton, K. (2017). Whānau perceptions and experiences of acute rheumatic fever diagnosis for Māori in Northland, New Zealand. *The New Zealand Medical Journal, 130*(1465), 80–88.

Barlow, C. (1994). *Tikanga whakaaro: key concepts in Māori culture.* Auckland: Oxford University Press.

Child and Youth Mortality Review Committee/Te Rōpū Arotake Auau Mate o te Hunga Tamariki Taiohi. (2011). *Low Speed Run Over Mortality. Wellington: Child and Youth Mortality Review Committee.* Retrieved from www.hqsc.govt.nz/assets/CYMRC/Publications/low-speed-report.pdf.

Cobo-Cuenca, A. I., & Martín-Espinosa, N. (2013). End of life in stage heart failure in elderly individuals. *Journal of Palliative Care and Medicine, 3*(4), doi:10.4172/2165-7386.1000157.

Cormack, D., Stanley, J., & Harris, R. (2018). Multiple forms of discrimination and relationships with health and wellbeing: findings from national cross-sectional surveys in Aotearoa/New Zealand. *International Journal for Equity in Health, 17*, 26.

Crengle, S. (2007). Primary care and Māori: findings from the national primary medical care survey. In B. Robson & R. Harris (Eds.), *Hauora: Māori health standards IV: a study of the years 2000–2005.* Wellington: Te Rōpū Rangahau.

Curtis, E., Harwood, M., & Riddell, T. (2007). Cardiovascular disease. In B. Robson & R. Harris (Eds.), *Hauora: Māori health standards IV: a study of the years 2000–2005.* Wellington: Te Rōpū Rangahau.

Dharmawardene, V., & Menkes, D. B. (2015). Substance use disorders in New Zealand adults with severe mental illness: descriptive study of an acute inpatient population. *Australasian Psychology, 23*(3), 236–240. https://doi.org/10.1177/1039856215586147.

Davis, P., Lay-Yee, R., Dyall, L., Briant, R., Sporle, A., Brunt, D., & Scott, A. (2006). Quality of hospital care for Māori patients in New Zealand: retrospective cross-sectional assessment. *The Lancet, 367*(9526), 1920–1925. doi:10.1016/s0140–6736(06)68847–8.

Durie, M. (1998). *Whaiora: Māori health development* (2nd ed.). Auckland: Oxford University Press.

Elder, J. R. (Ed.), (1932). *The letters and journals of Samuel Marsden*. Dunedin: Coulls, Somerville, Wilkie/A. H. Reed for the Otago University Council.

Evans-Campbell, T. (2008). Historical trauma in American Indian/Native Alaska communities. *Journal of Interpersonal Violence, 23,* 316–338.

Family Violence Death Review Committee 2016. *Fifth report: January 2014 to December 2015.* Wellington, New Zealand: Health Quality and Safety Commission.

Family Violence Death Review Committee 2017. *Fifth data report: January 2009 to December 2015.* Wellington, New Zealand: Health Quality and Safety Commission.

Fletcher, E. Q. R. (2013). *'I cried – it was so beautiful!' Rapaki homeowner overwhelmed by repair.* Accessed 6 November 2014. Retrieved from http://eqr.co.nz/news/i-cried-it-was-so-beautiful-rapaki-homeowner-overwhelmed-by-repair.

Harris, R., Cormack, D., Tobias, M. O., Yeh, L.-C., Talamaivao, N., Minster, J., & Timutimu, R. (2012). Self-Reported experience of racial discrimination and health care use in New Zealand: results from the 2006/07 New Zealand health survey. *American Journal of Public Health, 102,* 1012–1019.

Harwood, M., & Tipene-Leach. (2007). Diabetes. In B. Robson & R. Harris (Eds.), *Hauora: Māaori health standards IV: a study of the years 2000–2005.* Wellington: Te Rōpū Rangahau.

Howden-Chapman, P., Crane, J., Matheson, A., Viggers, H., Cunningham, M., Blakely, T., O'Dea, D., Cunningham, C., Woodward, A., Saville-Smith, K., Baker, M., & Waipara, N. (2005). Retrofitting houses with insulation to reduce health inequalities: aims and methods of a clustered, randomised community-based trial. *Social Science & Medicine, 61*(12), 2600–2610. doi:10.1016/j.socscimed.2005.04.049.

Jatrana, S., Crampton, P., & Norris, P. (2011). Ethnic differences in access to prescription medication because of cost in New Zealand. *Journal of Epidemiology and Community Health, 65,* 454–460. doi:10.1136/jech.2009.099101.

Johnson, M. P., Leone, J. M., & Xu, Y. (2014). Intimate terrorism and situational couple violence in general surveys: Ex-spouses required. *Violence Against Women, 20,* 186–207.

Kake, T. R., Garrett, N., & Te Aonui, M. (2016). Cognitive neuropsychological functioning in New Zealand Māori diagnosed with schizophrenia. *Australian & New Zealand Journal of Psychiatry, 50,* 566–576.

Kruger, T., Pitman, M., Grennell, D., McDonald, T., Mariu, D., & Pomare, A. (2004). *Transforming whānau violence: a conceptual framework. An updated version of the report from the former second Māori Taskforce on whānau violence* (2nd ed.). Wellington: Te Puni Kokiri.

Lee, R., & North, N. (2013). Barriers to Māori sole mothers' primary health care access. *Journal of Primary Health Care, 5*(4), 315–321.

Ministry of Health. (2015). *Tatau Kahukura Māori health chart book 2015.* Wellington, New Zealand: Ministry of Health.

Ministry of Health. (2016). *Annual update of key results 2015/16: New Zealand health survey.* Wellington, New Zealand: Ministry of Health.

Moeke-Maxwell, T. (2014). What whanau need at the end of life. *Nursing New Zealand, 20*(4), 12–14.

Moko Mead, H. (2003). *Tikanga Māori: living by Māori values.* Wellington: Huia.

Morgan, G., & Simmons, G. (2009). *Health Cheque: the truth we should all know about New Zealand's public health system.* Auckland: PIP.

Mulder, R. (2017). The heart of the matter: social and cultural factors impacting mental health. *Australian & New Zealand Journal of Psychiatry, 51,* 113–114.

Pihama, L., Jenkins, K., & Middleton, A. (2003). *Te Rito Action Area 13 Literature Review: Family Violence Prevention for Māori.* Retrieved from www.nzfvc.org.nz/PublicationDetails.aspx?publication=13532.

Pihama, L., Te Nana, R., Cameron, N., Smith, C., Reid, J., & Southey, K. (2016). Māori cultural definitions of sexual violence. *Sexual Abuse in Australia & New Zealand, 7,* 43–51.

Perinatal and Maternal Mortality Review Committee (PMMRC). (2017). *Eleventh annual report of the perinatal and maternal mortality review committee: reporting mortality 2015.* Wellington: Health Quality & Safety Commission.

Reid, P., & Robson, B. (2007). Understanding health inequities. In B. Robson & R. Harris (Eds.), *Hauora: Māori health standards IV: a study of the years 2000–2005.* Wellington: Te Rōpū Rangahau.

Reid, J., Cormack, D., & Crowe, M. (2016). The significance of relational continuity of care for Māori patient engagement with predominantly non-Māori doctors: findings from a qualitative study. *Australian & New Zealand Journal of Public Health, 40,* 120–125.

Robson, B., & Purdie, G. (2007). Mortality. In B. Robson & R. Harris (Eds.), *Hauora: Māori health standards IV: a study of the years 2000–2005.* Wellington: Te Rōpū Rangahau.

Rumball-Smith, J., Sarfati, D., Hider, P., & Blakely, T. (2013). Ethnic disparities in the quality of hospital care in New Zealand, as measured by 30-day rate of unplanned readmission/death. *International Journal of Quality in Health Care, 25,* 248–254.

Salmond, A. (1976). *Hui: a study of Māori ceremonial gathering* (2nd ed.). Retrieved from http://books.google.co.nz/books?id=TIEOAAAAQAAJ&printsec=frontcover#v=onepage&q&f=false.

Signal, T. L., Paine, S.-J., Sweeney, B., Muller, D., Priston, M., Lee, K., Gander, P., & Huthwaite, M. (2017). The prevalence of symptoms of depression and anxiety, and

873

the level of life stress and worry in New Zealand Māori and non-Māori women in late pregnancy. *The Australian and New Zealand Journal of Psychiatry*, *51*, 168–176.

Statistics New Zealand. 2014. *Quick stats: About culture and identity*. Retrieved from http://www.stats.govt.nz/Census/2013-census/profile-and-summary-reports/quickstats-culture-identity.aspx.

Stokes, T., Azam, M., & Noble, F. D. (2018). Multimorbidity in Māori and Pacific patients: cross-sectional study in a Dunedin general practice. *Journal of Primary Health Care*, *10*, 39–43.

Suicide Mortality Review Committee. (2016). *Nga rahui hau kura: suicide mortality review committee feasibility study 2014–15*. Wellington, New Zealand: Suicide Mortality Review Committee.

Taitimu, M., Read, J., & McIntosh, T. (2018). Ngā Whakāwhitinga (standing at the crossroads): how Māori understand what Western psychiatry calls 'schizophrenia'. *Transcultural Psychiatry*, *55*, 153–177.

Webb, R., & Wilson, N. (2013). Rheumatic fever in New Zealand. *Journal of Paediatrics and Child Health*, *49*(3), 179–184. doi:10.1111/j.1440-1754.2011.02218.x.

White, H., Walsh, W., Brown, A., Riddell, T., Tonkin, A., Jeremy, R., Brieger, D., Zeitz, C., & Kritharides, L. (2010). Rheumatic heart disease in Indigenous populations. *Heart, Lung and Circulation*, *19*(5), 273–281. doi:10.1016/j.hlc.2010.02.019.

Whitehead, M. (1991). The concepts and principles of equity and health. *Health Promotion International*, *6*(3), 217–228. doi:10.1093/heapro/6.3.217.

Wilson, D. (2008). The significance of a culturally appropriate health service for indigenous Māori women. *Contemporary Nurse*, *28*, 173–188.

Wilson, N. (2010). Rheumatic heart disease in Indigenous populations: New Zealand experience. *Heart, Lung and Circulation*, *19*(5), 282–288. doi:10.1016/j.hlc.2010.02.021.

Wilson, D., & Barton, P. (2012). Indigenous hospital experiences: a New Zealand case study. *Journal of Clinical Nursing*, *21*, 2316–2326.

Wilson, D., & Hickey, H. (2015). Māori health: Māori- and whānau-centred practice. In D. Wepa (Ed.), *Cultural safety in Aotearoa New Zealand*. Melbourne, Australia: Cambridge University Press.

CHAPTER 51

Family Violence

By Simon Sawyer

The legal response to family violence varies with each state and territory of Australia and New Zealand. The information presented in this chapter is intended as general advice. It is possible that some statements or recommendations may have been superseded by new or changing laws, and it is possible that individual states have their own laws and regulations with which paramedics must comply. Paramedics should ensure they are compliant with local legislation and policies.

OVERVIEW

- Family violence refers to all forms of physical violence, psychological or emotional abuse, and neglect occurring within a family.
- Family violence is complex and there is no single factor which leads to the occurrence of violence.

- Paramedics are frequently called to attend the victims of violence, and the management may extend to more than physical injuries.
- Paramedics will need to be able to recognise the signs of violence first, and then connect patients with referral services.

Introduction

Family violence is a common and highly damaging form of interpersonal violence. Family violence refers to all forms of physical violence, psychological or emotional abuse, and neglect occurring within a family, which can include children, siblings, parents, grandparents and extended family (Krug et al., 2002). As distinct from violence and abuse perpetrated by a stranger, family violence is unique in that the victim often lives with or maintains a close relationship with their abuser, often feeling trapped in a cycle of continuing and potentially escalating harm.

Types of family violence and abuse vary, and it can be difficult to clearly define which behaviours would be considered violent or abusive in which contexts. For example, most couples argue from time to time, and arguments might contain a level of physical contact or emotionally charged exchanges, but they wouldn't always be considered family violence. In most cases of family violence there is a power imbalance in the relationship, where one party is able to exert control over the other through coercive means, such as physical or psychological abuse or intimidation. Alternatively, neglect can occur where one party is dependent on the other for care, such as with young children, elderly, disabled or infirm patients. An abuser may neglect to provide proper care or may even use the victim's vulnerabilities to control them.

It is important to note that family violence or neglect, however it is perpetrated, is never the fault of the patient. A central tenet of responding to violence is the understanding and belief that *no one has the right to use violence or abuse against another person,* and excepting some situations of self-defence *it is never the fault of the victim that violence is used against them.* Understanding this is essential to ensuring an appropriate response as healthcare practitioners.

Paramedics are frequently called to attend the victims of violence, and while the management of physical injuries is important, there are additional factors which must be considered and managed in the context of family violence patients. For example, the isolated treatment of traumatic injuries often does not help prevent further violence, and patients experiencing family violence are likely to experience ongoing violence and abuse. Therefore, the response of paramedics has the potential to influence whether or not the violence, abuse or neglect continues.

While family violence patients may seek support from primary care providers such as general practitioners (GPs) (Hegarty & Bush, 2002) or self-present to emergency departments (EDs) (Wu et al., 2010) or other allied health practitioners (World Health Organization [WHO], 2014) it is believed that paramedics may also encounter these patients frequently in their practice (Sawyer et al., 2017b; Sawyer et al., 2015; Sawyer et al., 2014). Furthermore, as paramedics commonly assess patients in the home environment, they may be in a unique position to witness signs of violence, abuse or neglect which other healthcare workers do not see. The response of paramedics is largely to facilitate referrals for family violence patients to care, support and advocacy, which can help disrupt the cycle of violence (WHO, 2013b).

BOX 51.1 Key definitions

- **Family violence**: Violence, abuse or neglect occurring within a family. This can be any combination of patient and perpetrator including children, siblings, parents, grandparents and extended family such as uncles, aunts or cousins (Krug et al., 2002).
- **Child abuse**: Any type of physical violence, emotional ill-treatment, sexual abuse, neglect, negligence or exploitation of a child (ages vary across jurisdictions, generally less than 16 or 18 years old), which results in actual or potential harm to the child's health, survival, development or dignity in the context of a relationship of responsibility, trust or power (Renner & Slack, 2006). In addition, child abuse includes allowing a child to be exposed to family violence, due to the long-term damage caused to children who experience or witness parental intimate partner abuse (Butchart et al., 2006).
- **Intimate partner violence**: Violence and abuse transpiring between people who are, or

were formally, in an intimate relationship. This may include physical, sexual, psychological or other behaviours used to control or otherwise harm a partner (Krug et al., 2002).
- **Elder abuse**: Any type of abuse (physical, emotional, sexual, economic) or neglect of a person 65 years of age or over in a residential aged care facility, private care or living independently. It can be a single or repeated act, or lack of appropriate action, occurring within any relationship where there is an expectation of trust, which causes harm or distress to an older person (WHO, 2008).
- **Sexual violence**: Any sexual act, attempt to obtain a sexual act or other act directed against a person's sexuality using coercion, by any person regardless of their relationship to the victim, in any setting. This includes rape, which is defined as the physically forced or otherwise coerced penetration of the mouth, vulva or anus with a penis, other body part or object (World Health Organization, 2013b).

Four manifestations of family violence relevant to paramedics will be discussed in this chapter: *child abuse, intimate partner violence (IPV), sexual violence* and *elder abuse* (see key definitions in Box 51.1). This chapter will discuss the background to and prevalence of each of these family violence presentations; examine the expected response of paramedics to family violence; and discuss practical clinical skills and actions that paramedics can undertake in the out-of-hospital environment to help care and provide support for these patients.

Background to family violence
Defining family violence
Family violence (which includes abuse and neglect) can manifest itself in several forms and is not restricted to just physical injury. As previously discussed it is difficult to attempt to define violence or abuse through *behaviours*, as it is often the presence of a power imbalance which leads to the harm or neglect. Different behaviours that *might* constitute family violence are presented and discussed in Table 51.1.

Why does family violence happen?
The root causes of family violence are complex, variable and not entirely understood. One major theory used to explain the occurrence is the *ecological model*, which describes the known factors which make the presence of family violence more or less

likely, such as endorsement of gendered roles and male entitlement, unemployment and low socio-economic status, lack of adequate support services and experiencing or witnessing abuse as a child (Krug et al., 2002). It is important to understand that there is no single factor which leads to the occurrence of violence, and also that *everyone* in society can influence the success of strategies to end violence.

To further examine the root causes of family violence it is useful to examine the statistic: *the primary victims of family violence are female, and the primary perpetrators are male* (Krug et al., 2002). This does not imply that females can't perpetrate violence or that men can't be the victim, but the evidence shows that the majority of the most damaging violence is perpetrated by males against women (Krug et al., 2002; Victoria Police, 2009). One important factor that is known to influence the use of violence are our attitudes (Ellsberg et al., 2015). In this case the attitudes of males towards females and relationships appear to influence if they use violence in their relationships. For example, beliefs such as 'males have a right to sex' or 'women should obey their partner' are attitudes that are supportive of violence against women. While family violence is undoubtedly a gendered issue, it is important to note that *not all males are violent, and not all women experience violence*; in fact, most males aren't violent in their relationships and most women don't

Table 51.1: Defining family violence

Physical violence and abuse	Behaviours which actually, or could potentially, inflict pain or injury (e.g. pushing, slapping, hitting, kicking, beating and, in extreme cases, behaviours such as strangulation or attempts to murder or cause serious harm). This also includes the use of threats or weapons to intimidate, as well as destruction of property or the killing or harming of pets.
Emotional or psychological abuse	Causing psychological or emotional harm (e.g. verbal intimidation, constant belittling or humiliating, as well as threats of suicide from the perpetrator). This may be subtle or overt but is usually designed to scare or terrorise the victim, who may lose their confidence, self-esteem or self-determination.
Sexual assault or abuse	Adult sexual assault involves any type of sexual activity to which there is no consent. This might include physical contact, exposing the victim or perpetrator or penetration of the victim. It is important to note that certain individuals may be unable to consent, such as mentally disabled patients or patients with dementia. Child sexual assault may include forcing or enticing a child to take part in sexual activities, regardless of whether the child is aware of what is happening, as well as non-contact activities such as involving children in looking at, or in the production of, pornographic material, watching sexual activities or encouraging children to behave in sexually inappropriate ways. This also includes technology-facilitated sexual abuse such as 'revenge porn' or 'sexting'.
Controlling behaviours	Preventing freedom of movement, access or expression (e.g. isolating partners from their family and friends or from social, cultural or religious association, monitoring their movements or harassing them, or restricting their access to information, assistance, money or resources).
Neglect	The persistent failure to meet the basic needs of a person in your care (particularly a child or elderly dependant), including physical, emotional, medical and educational needs; failure to provide adequate food and nutrition, housing and clothing; with regards to children this includes a failure to protect them from violence or harm, or exposing them to intimate partner violence.

Source: Krug et al. (2002), The Royal Australian College of General Practitioners (2014).

experience violence in theirs (Krug et al., 2002; WHO, 2013a). There are some key populations that are at risk of experiencing violence, which are discussed in Box 51.2.

There also exists some common misunderstandings about why violence occurs in families and relationships, such as that alcohol abuse or experiencing abuse as a child are what cause violence. While alcohol abuse or experiencing violence as a child may increase the *likelihood* that a person uses violence, neither actually *cause* violence (Krug et al., 2002). Whenever someone consciously uses violence against another person, they are making a choice to do so. Certainly, there are some individuals who have endured significant trauma in their own past and have difficulty coping or understanding the impact of their behaviour; however, this does not justify the use of violence in their relationships. While there is no universal solution, or cure, to violence, a good start would be to change cultures that excuse violence or blame the victim, and embrace cultures that support individuals to change their attitudes and behaviours which are known to lead to violence. Paramedics can play a role in this, by modelling appropriate behaviours and attitudes.

Prevalence and impacts
Child abuse

Child abuse is a common occurrence for children and is usually perpetrated by someone known to the child, particularly their family (Hanson et al., 2003). Child abuse, which includes neglect, often leads to both immediate and long-term health and behavioural problems which can continue into adulthood. Not all cases of child abuse are wilful acts intended to cause harm; for example, neglect can often be the result of caregivers who are not adequately educated or supported. However, there are cases of wilful neglect and abuse, particularly emotional abuse from parents, as well as sexual abuse. In the majority of children physical injuries generally do less harm than the long-term impacts of violence and abuse on behavioural and emotional development (Norman et al., 2012). As the patient in these cases is not yet of legal age, there are special considerations which must be taken into account, particularly with regards to mandatory reporting obligations.

An Australian report for child abuse in 2016 found there were 162,175 children (aged < 18 years) receiving child protection services, and 45,714 children who were the subject of a substantiated

BOX 51.2 Key populations at risk

While family violence can occur to any person in any society, there are some groups that are particularly vulnerable.

- Aboriginal and Torres Strait Islander (ATSI) women are 35 times more likely to experience family violence, and are around 11 times more likely to be killed as a result of violent assault (Australian Productivity Commission, 2014). ATSI children are seven times more likely to receive child protection services than non-Indigenous children (AIHW, 2017). Family violence is not part of ATSI culture; however, the disadvantage that members of this population face, particularly with respect to intergenerational trauma, discrimination, poverty, homelessness and lower levels of literacy and numeracy, can lead to a higher risk of family violence occurring (Al-Yaman et al., 2006).
- Māori women have reported higher rates of both IPV victimisation and perpetration than non-Māori, as well as higher rates of injury related to IPV (Marie et al., 2008). Likewise, Māori adults are commonly overrepresented as victims in studies of interpersonal violence. Māori children are six times more likely to die from abuse or neglect (Kōkiri, 2017). Again, family violence is not part of Māori culture; however, they have similar disadvantages to ATSI populations which make its occurrence more likely.
- Culturally and linguistically diverse (CALD) and migrant peoples have been poorly studied; however, data indicates that both Australia and New Zealand have high migrant populations, and that while the evidence is unclear if CALD populations have a higher or lower risk of family violence, they do have high barriers to disclosing violence (Ghafournia, 2011). Barriers to disclosure for CALD communities include language

difficulties, accessing culturally specific services and knowledge of their rights in Australia and New Zealand (Vaughan et al., 2016). Patients from different backgrounds may hold different attitudes and beliefs about issues surrounding family violence, and paramedics should be open minded and non-judgmental. The patient is often a good source of information about their experiences and needs.

- The lesbian, gay, bisexual, transgender and intersex (LGBTI) communities are another understudied group. It appears they generally show similar rates of family violence to heterosexual couples (Blosnich & Bossarte, 2009); however, incidence may be more underreported, and victims may be less likely to seek support in this community (Irwin, 2008). Data does show that in Australia 63% of lesbian and bisexual women have reported experiencing violence in their lifetime (all violence not just family violence) compared with 37% of heterosexual women (McNair et al., 2005), and therefore it may be the case that these women are particularly vulnerable.
- Disabled patients commonly report higher rates of interpersonal violence (Hughes et al., 2011), particularly from family members or carers, and are especially vulnerable due to their social disadvantage and higher dependence. In particular these patients report other forms of abuse such as withdrawal of accessibility devices (such as walking frames, hearing or communication devices), or withholding of medication, medical care or socialisation, as well as the threat of institutionalisation. When a disabled patient is reliant on their abuser for care, or where their disability prevents or impacts communication, they can have little opportunity to access help and support.

report of child abuse and neglect (AIHW, 2017). Very young children (< 1 year old) had the highest rates of substantiated reporting, and children aged 15–17 years had the lowest. The most common form of abuse was emotional (45%), followed by neglect (25%), physical (18%) and sexual (12%). The most common co-occurrence was emotional abuse and neglect. Girls were more likely to experience sexual abuse than boys, and boys more likely to experience physical violence and neglect. Children living in families where there is parental substance

abuse, mental illness or family violence are at a higher risk of experiencing child abuse (Dawe et al., 2008).

Within New Zealand, research has shown that 14% of children were physically harmed by an adult at home in the last year, and that 20% of girls and 9% of boys have experienced unwanted sexual touching or other forced sexual acts (Rossen et al., 2009). There were 16,394 substantiated findings of child abuse or neglect in New Zealand (Ministry of Social Development, 2016).

The impact of child abuse can be significant, broad and long lasting. Children experiencing abuse report a higher incidence of mental health disorders (particular depression, anxiety and eating disorders), behavioural disorders, suicide attempts, drug use and risky sexual behaviours (Norman et al., 2012). Additionally, there is some limited evidence that conditions such as allergies, malnutrition, asthma, headaches, type 2 diabetes and obesity can be related to experiencing child abuse (Norman et al., 2012). In extreme cases child abuse can lead to death, with an estimated 25 children dying from abuse each year in Australia (AIHW, 2017). Research has shown that up to a third of children who died from child abuse were previously assessed by healthcare practitioners for injuries that were not recognised as stemming from abuse (King et al., 2006).

Intimate partner violence

As the name implies IPV (also called partner abuse) refers to violence and abuse occurring between intimate partners, which includes married and de facto relationships, dating couples or other informal relationships, and includes both heterosexual and same-sex couples (Krug et al., 2002). Due to IPV occurring largely within the home, and the difficulty that victims have in disclosing the violence, IPV is often a hidden problem. However, paramedics regularly assess patients in the home environment and are able to witness interactions between patients and perpetrators and observe scenes that are often unseen by other healthcare practitioners (Sawyer et al., 2015). This is why it is important that paramedics understand what IPV is, how to recognise the signs and how to help these patients.

As previously discussed, there is generally a power imbalance between the perpetrator of family violence and the victim. IPV goes beyond an isolated argument or heated exchange and arises when one partner begins to use violence or abuse as a means of coercion and control. As there is such disparity in what individuals accept from their partner in terms of physical, verbal and nonverbal interaction, what would constitute violence or abuse in one relationship may be acceptable in another. Therefore, it is difficult to define exactly what would constitute a violent or abusive act; it is largely up to the individual circumstances and characteristics of the relationship and the people involved.

Most relationships do not begin as violent or abusive, and many women who have left violent relationships state that the violence only began after a precipitating event (such as pregnancy). Once violence or abuse does begin, it can often continue in a *cycle*, where the perpetrator becomes violent or abusive and then later states they are remorseful, only to resume their behaviour once the victim has forgiven them (Walker, 1980). It is this cycle of violence that often makes the victim feel unsure about the nature of their relationship, sometimes not recognising that they are in a violent or abusive relationship.

Just because someone is in a violent relationship does not always mean that they want to leave their partner or that they no longer love them; often they just want the violence or abuse to end. Patients who are experiencing abuse want healthcare practitioners to talk to them about IPV, but this must be done in a supportive, non-judgmental and empathetic way (Feder et al., 2006). It is important that paramedics understand that their role is not to judge an IPV patient for their choices, or for what has happened to them, or even to offer advice, but to listen to their needs and help connect them with the right services.

IPV occurs across all cultures and communities; it is not limited to certain groups such as low socioeconomic status or CALD communities. IPV is one of the most common forms of violence against women in Australia and New Zealand (Australian Bureau of Statistics, 2013; Fanslow & Robinson, 2011). Australian statistics show that 17% of women over the age of 18 have experienced IPV at some point since the age of 15 (5.3% for men) and 1.5% had experienced it in the past 12 months (0.6% for men) (Australian Bureau of Statistics, 2013). The same dataset showed that around 25% had experienced emotional abuse from a current or past partner (14% for men).

Within New Zealand 35% of ever-partnered women reported experiencing physical and/or sexual violence at some point in their lifetime, which rises to 55% when psychological and/or emotional abuse are included (Fanslow & Robinson, 2011). For men 5% reported experiencing physical or sexual IPV in the last 12 months, which rose to 18% when psychological and/or emotional abuse were included.

IPV is the leading preventable contributor to death, disability and illness in young Australian women, and accounts for 8% of the burden of disease in Victoria, Australia (VicHealth, 2004), which is more than double any other risk factor. Common injuries as a result of IPV which require hospital attendance are injuries to the eyes, ears, head and neck as well as the breasts and abdomen (Campbell, 2002), and in extreme cases traumatic brain injury and strangulation (Black, 2011). On average one woman is killed each week in Australia by a current or past male partner for 'domestic motives', and homicides involving intimate partners account for 66% of domestic homicides (Dearden & Jones, 2008). There is also evidence that IPV is associated with an increased risk of a wide variety of conditions, including asthma, irritable bowel syndrome, diabetes, headaches, chronic pain, sleeping difficulties and poor general physical health (Black et al., 2011).

Women experiencing IPV have been shown to have a higher risk for several mental health outcomes including depression, anxiety, posttraumatic stress disorder and other mood and sleep disorders (Black, 2011). An Australian study found that women reporting IPV were nine times more likely to report having harmed themselves or having recent thoughts of doing so than women who had never experienced violence (Roberts et al., 1997). A study conducted by the WHO found that up to 50% of IPV patients developed substance abuse problems and that this was most prevalent among depressed patients (Astbury, 2000). It is important to note that the impacts of psychological or emotional IPV can be just as harmful as physical IPV (Coker et al., 2000), and women often report that the lasting psychological injuries are far greater and more damaging than any physical injury (Campbell, 2002).

Children are often present during acts of IPV, with one Australian study estimating that 25% of children and young people have witnessed IPV (Office of Women's Policy, 2002). Research has shown that childhood exposure to IPV increases their risk of behavioural and learning difficulties in the short term, and of developing mental health problems later in life (Edleson, 1999).

Elder abuse

Elder abuse refers to violence and abuse directed at elderly persons (WHO, 2008) (generally 65 years of age or over). The abuse itself can be a single or repeated act causing harm or distress, or the lack of appropriate action (such as neglect), occurring within any relationship. Elder abuse as a form of family violence is somewhat unique as it can occur both within the family home by members of the family and also within aged care facilities by nursing staff or volunteers, or even other elderly residents. As with other forms of abuse, there is an expectation of trust or care, particularly where the elder is dependent on the other person. Where the elder is reliant on another they can sometimes permanently exist in a state of power imbalance, and may have little or no recourse, particularly when frailty or dementia is present.

Elder abuse can be perpetrated in a number of different ways. For example, the adult children of elders may use violence or abuse to coerce their parents to provide money, housing or support. Alternatively, the abuse can come from an elderly partner, especially when there is a history of IPV. Another common pattern is when caregiver roles are reversed and the 'child' becomes the primary carer for the parent. The child can take up the role of the carer, sometimes reluctantly and without adequate support, and built-up frustration can lead to abusive behaviour (WHO, 2011). When an elderly patient becomes dependent on their children, family members or nursing home staff they may feel trapped or unable to seek help due to isolation or infirmity, and they may fear retribution from their carers if they do disclose the abuse (WHO, 2008).

The prevalence of elder abuse is poorly understood due to a lack of research focusing on elder abuse specifically. The WHO estimate prevalence rates of elder abuse in high- or middle-income countries ranges between 2% and 14%, though there was no Australian data included in this study (WHO, 2008). Australian literature has found between 2.3% and 5.4%, though further research is required (Kurrle et al., 1997; Livermore et al., 2001). It appears that financial abuse is most common, followed by physical, psychological and neglect, and then sexual abuse being relatively rare (Yon et al., 2017). It is expected that incidence of elder abuse will increase as the average age of the population is increasing around the world (WHO, 2011).

The presence of elder abuse is linked to several negative health outcomes, including trauma from injuries, higher risk of mental health conditions (particularly depression and anxiety) and even premature death (WHO, 2011). The consequences of abuse for the elderly can sometimes be disproportionately high, due to the inability of their ageing bodies to cope with even minor injuries (WHO, 2011).

Sexual assault

Sexual assault, also called sexual abuse, refers to unwanted or non-consensual sexual acts that can make a person feel intimidated, threatened or frightened (WHO, 2013b). Every person aged 16 years and over is able to choose freely about participation in sexual activity, but must be given the opportunity to freely consent. Both men and women who report sexual assault are more likely to have been sexually assaulted by someone they knew, usually a friend or family member, rather than a stranger. Research shows that half of victims are assaulted by a known person, including a family member in about a third of cases (Australian Institute of Criminology, 2013). Again, there are many myths which still pervade about sexual assault, such as rape being caused by how a person dresses or acts.

As with all forms of violence and abuse, sexual assault is never the fault of the victim.

In 2011, there were 17,238 reports of sexual assault in Australia (Australian Institute of Criminology, 2013). The same study found that 1 in 5 women and 1 in 20 men reported experiencing an act of sexual assault; however, many do not report the assault or seek help for the psychological and physiological impacts. Sexual assault is most common in children aged 10–14 years, and then declines as age increases; however, sexual assault against women is higher in all age groups compared with males (Australian Institute of Criminology, 2013).

In New Zealand research has found that 1 in 3 girls have been subject to an unwanted sexual experience by the age of 16 years (Fanslow et al., 2007), and 1 in 5 women have experienced sexual assault as an adult (Fanslow & Robinson, 2004). Rates for New Zealand males are unclear; however, estimates are that up to 1 in 7 young males will experience sexual violence (Rape Prevention Education New Zealand, 2011). As in Australia, young New Zealanders (16–24 years old) are at the highest risk of sexual violence (Rossen et al., 2009), and up to 90% of assaults are committed by a known person, often a family member (Morris et al., 2003).

Sexual assault can be a significantly traumatising experience and those who report sexual assault also report high rates of several adverse healthcare outcomes, including mental health conditions such as depression, anxiety and PTSD (Jozkowski & Sanders, 2012; Tjaden & Thoennes, 2000). In fact, there is evidence that almost a third of rape victims will develop PTSD, and are three times more likely to experience major depressive disorder (Green, 1993). Other health-related impacts include the presence of self-harm or suicidality, substance abuse, chronic gastrointestinal problems and unexplained pain, particularly in the pelvic or genital region (Tjaden & Thoennes, 2000; Jozkowski & Sanders, 2012).

Services offered for sexual assault patients, such as counselling and forensic medical assessments, are highly specialised and require specific training. While paramedics may be called on to assess and treat victims of sexual assault, it must be understood that the goal of care is to facilitate access to the right services to ensure clinicians with the appropriate training are able to provide the best possible outcomes for the patient.

The role of paramedics and ambulance services

Research on the links between family violence and paramedics is emerging, and at present it is unclear

exactly how or why family violence patients utilise the ambulance services. For example, it is unknown if patients call due to specific acts of violence, such as assault, or if they call for exacerbations of chronic conditions which are associated with their experiences of family violence. Young children and the elderly may be less likely to call an ambulance themselves, and it is likewise unclear which conditions or symptoms would provoke a caregiver to request an ambulance. As for victims of sexual assault, it appears unlikely they would request an ambulance unless there were traumatic injuries involved. It is possible that a high percentage of the family violence cases that paramedics see, particularly those involving sexual assault and child abuse, will be related to mental health presentations, such as self-harm, substance abuse and suicide attempts (WHO, 2014).

Despite not knowing exactly how or why a person experiencing family violence would utilise the ambulance service, it is believed that paramedics do encounter these patients regularly (Sawyer et al., 2017a; Sawyer et al., 2014; Weiss, Garza et al., 2000; Weiss, Ernst et al., 2000; Datner et al., 1999). Furthermore, there is a clear role that paramedics and ambulance services can play in the recognition and referral of family violence patients to care and support (Sawyer et al., 2015). The primary prevention of family violence (i.e. preventing violence before it occurs) requires a coordinated response from all members and communities in society, particularly healthcare groups. Ambulance services should ensure that their policies are appropriate and that their staff are well educated and demonstrate appropriate attitudes and behaviours.

Paramedics will be called to respond to family violence only after it happens. At this stage it is too late to prevent the violence, but the manner with which the paramedic responds may impact on the likelihood of further violence. The ability to recognise the signs of violence is the first step, followed by the ability to talk to patients and connect them with referral services that can provide the right care and support. The response of paramedics can be described in a four-step process: recognise, respond, refer and record.

Recognise

As discussed previously, it is not known exactly how a patient experiencing family violence would present to ambulance services, which makes recognition difficult but not impossible. There are common injuries and other family violence presentations which are known to result in presentation to other health services, including EDs and GP clinics, which

Table 51.2: Potential indicators of family violence

Feelings	• The patient appears depressed/withdrawn or anxious/distressed without an apparent reason • The patient or the patient's children/dependants appear fearful, particularly of a controlling person
Behaviours	• Suicidality or self-harm • Alcohol or other drug abuse • Repeated/suspicious callouts with no clear diagnosis • Inconsistent or implausible explanations for injuries/symptoms • Scene findings or behaviours of those on scene which indicate an unsafe environment (physically or psychologically), particularly for children, elderly or people with a disability
Medical signs	• Unexplained chronic symptoms (e.g. pain; gastrointestinal or genitourinary symptoms) • Pregnancy-related complications or trauma, or delays in care • Evidence of malnutrition or medical neglect, particularly in children, elderly or disabled patients
Controlling people	• The presence of intrusive or controlling people in the consultation (especially a partner or ex-partner) • The patient (or their children/dependants) are unwilling to respond without approval from controlling person • The presence of a controlling person who states things like the patient is 'crazy', 'mad', 'unstable' or other similar terms. • The presence of a potential abuser who attempts to minimise, distract or explain away injuries, or who states the patient is not to be believed (particularly with children, elderly or disabled patients) • The presence of withholding communication/mobility devices, access to funds/resources/services, over/under medication (especially for elderly or disabled patients)
Trauma	• A presentation related to an assault or suspicion of assault (e.g. there is the presence of weapons, or signs of violence) • The patient has suspicious bruises or injuries, especially to the neck, face, breasts or genitals. Note that toddlers are likely to have bruises, and therefore this may be a poor predictor in this group. • The patient states or indicates someone has threatened to kill or harm them, their children/dependants or their pets. • Evidence of sexual assault (actual or attempted)

can guide the suspicion of paramedics. The signs in Table 51.2 do not constitute an exhaustive list, but rather the signs that would be relevant and likely presentations which paramedics might witness.

In addition to the above listed indicators of potential family violence, there are several risk factors which are relevant to paramedics and are known to be associated with a higher likelihood of experiencing family violence. The presence of these risk factors does not indicate violence in themselves; however, an awareness of them may increase an individual paramedic's index of suspicion. Risk factors include young age, alcohol or other drug abuse (particularly in caregivers to children or other dependants), low socioeconomic status, separated or divorced marital status and pregnancy.

When a paramedic sees signs of family violence it is important that they don't ignore them or attempt to explain away what they saw. Patients living with violence can be helped and there are several things that paramedics can do to support them, which are discussed in the next section.

Respond

It is difficult to know when family violence is occurring based solely on indicators, which is why paramedics need to have a high index of suspicion and keep an open mind for the potential for family violence. When signs of family violence, abuse or neglect are noted, paramedics should respond appropriately based on the context of the scene, the patient and their presentation. Guidance for different patient classifications is given below.

For children or patients under the age of 18

In cases of suspected child abuse (including sexual abuse) **it is important that paramedics don't directly question children or others at the scene.** This is a difficult task that specialised, expert services perform. It may be appropriate to discuss some forms of abuse with older children (e.g. > 15 years); however, this should be done with extreme caution. Ideally paramedics should be conscious of the potential for child abuse and should respond by contacting the appropriate services (discussed below) for advice. Usually this involves the paramedic describing their scene findings, which allows the referral service to follow up as appropriate.

In some situations, such as neglect, it may be appropriate to discuss your concerns with the primary carer if they are on scene. For example, if you have encountered a child who appears neglected due to insufficient parental support and you believe the carer is genuinely concerned about their child, you might consider asking if they are getting enough support. This conversation must be done sensitively, and without judging the carer. Some carers either don't have the right education or aren't getting adequately supported, and in these situations you can help them access support, such as by referring them to their local GP or child and maternal health centre (see below).

If you do discuss this with a carer you should still document your scene findings and make any necessary reports to other services. You are not obliged to tell the carer you are going to do this, and you can arrange for them to be informed after you have left the scene.

Sexual assault

The response to sexual assault is complex, and except for the provision of comfort and any specific care needed there is little that paramedics can do to treat these patients. Informing the patient of the availability of specialised services is important, remembering that referrals must be done in consultation with the patient and with respect to their wishes (excepting situations involving mandatory reporting, discussed below).

Forensic evidence collection is another specialised medical service. Paramedics should ensure the patient is transported to an appropriately equipped and staffed hospital and ensure the patient's clothing is taken in a clean bag. The patient may wish to wash or shower; however, this may impact on the ability to collect further evidence. Patients should be informed of this but not prevented from making their own decisions.

For paramedics it is best that they consult with local experts. Most major cities in Australia and New Zealand have a sexual assault consultation line (see below).

In cases of sexual assault involving children, you are required by law to contact police regardless of the wishes of the patient or anyone else at the scene. If it is safe to remain on scene this is advised, but if there is a risk to paramedic safety you can await police from a safe location. Specifics regarding ages and definitions of sexual assault can vary with state and country legislation; paramedics are advised to seek clarification from their individual organisation.

IPV or elder abuse, and other forms of family violence against competent adults

For competent patients of legal age who you suspect are experiencing family violence, the correct response is to let them know that you are concerned for their safety and that you want to support them. Research shows that women experiencing family violence want to be asked by healthcare professionals, provided it is in a sensitive, empathetic and non-judgmental way (Feder et al., 2006).

Before asking them any questions first make sure that you are in a private environment. Never let anyone else know that you suspect family violence, and never ask a patient about family violence in front of anyone else. If it is safe to ask them at the scene you can do so there, but if you can't get the patient alone consider moving them to the ambulance or having your partner distract or move others on the scene.

Patients experiencing family violence often feel fear about disclosing, and letting them know that you will keep what they say confidential, and that they are in a safe place and won't be overheard can help them to feel comfortable disclosing. Remember that many patients will deny experiencing violence or abuse if they do not feel safe, so you should take your time to prepare the patient and the scene, build rapport and make them feel comfortable.

There is no one right way to ask a patient about abuse. It is recommended that *fear and safety* questions are used, which means questions that focus on how the patient feels about the events leading to the ambulance being called (WHO, 2014). This conversation should be natural and while memorising a screening question may be of use, it's best to adapt a simple questioning framework to the individual case. A sample conversation is provided in Box 51.3.

There are also many things that you shouldn't ask or say. Questions or comments that imply the patient was at fault or that excuse the violence, such as 'What did you do to make them angry?' or 'I'm sure they love you, this is just the way they show it', can be very damaging and can actually prevent the patient disclosing the violence or seeking help in the future (Feder et al., 2006). When in doubt it is best that paramedics just listen and respond with empathetic statements. If asked a question and you aren't sure what to say you can always say something like 'I'm not really sure I know the answer to that. Would it be okay if I referred you to an expert who can give you the right advice and support?' or similar.

When talking to patients consider that it is common for a patient to self-blame or make excuses for injuries; this does not mean they don't want

BOX 51.3

The following is a sample conversation with a patient experiencing family violence ('Sawyer et al., 2018).

- To broach the subject first assure the patient's confidentiality; for example, you might say: 'I'd like to ask a question but before I do I just want you to you know that your answers will be confidential and we won't be overheard'.
- Fear and safety questions are a good way to begin a conversation. Asking direct questions like 'Are you the victim of family violence?' is not generally encouraged. Example questions might be the following (you can use your own words if you wish): 'I'm wondering if what you're experiencing today might be related to feeling unsafe because someone is doing something to hurt or frighten you (or your children)' or 'I'm wondering if your injuries were caused by someone who wanted to hurt or frighten you'.
- You can leave a short pause allowing the patient to talk if they wish to. If they don't talk show them that you are concerned for them; for example, you might say: 'I'm concerned for your wellbeing and safety' or 'I want to make sure you are feeling safe'.
- Or you could offer support: 'If you'd like I can assist you to speak to someone who can offer confidential support or advice about this, would you like to do that?'
- If the patient discloses abuse or states they would like you to assist them, validate and reassure them before providing a referral. It's important that they feel that you believe them and you are supportive and non-judgmental. For example, you might say: 'Thank you for telling me this; it must have been difficult' and/or 'Everyone has the right to feel safe and I will do what I can to support you'.

you to ask about IPV and you should still offer care and support. It is also okay to ask the same patient about family violence again if you see them in subsequent consultations, even if they always decline help. It is likely that the more a patient is offered help and support the more likely they will be to seek help in the future. Your approach to questioning and your reaction to any disclosure can have a significant effect on the patient, and may impact their decision to follow up referral options or even if they will disclose the violence or abuse again in the future. Appropriate reactions are listening, believing and informing the patient without passing judgment.

If you feel you need to report the scene findings to specialist services, or if the patient accepts a referral, consider the local options as per the following section.

Refer

The needs of a person experiencing family violence can be very broad, and there is no one right referral option. It is important that, where possible, paramedics consult with patients and attempt to find a service that will meet their needs. Options will vary based on availability in the local area, and most ambulance services should maintain a list of local preferred referral options; however, as a guide you might consider national referral options in Australia and New Zealand (see Table 51.3).

Referrals can be made by providing details to patient's so that they can contact services in their own time. It is not advised that paramedics contact services on the patient's behalf or without their consent, unless in cases of mandatory reporting. It is also advised that ambulance services make printed referral materials available upon request, and additionally that materials are displayed in ambulances (WHO, 2013b).

Record

Recording encounters with family violence is important and must be done in an appropriate way. Of primary importance is the confidentiality of medical records. Individual ambulance services should have their own policies on medical records and these must be adequate to ensure confidentiality. Paramedics should make sure that any printed records are passed directly to whoever the patient is handed over to, and paramedics should consider and make sure any security risks are highlighted; for example, if the suspected perpetrator has joined the patient in the hospital the records must be kept secure. If draft copies are produced ensure secure destruction (such as shredding); never leave patient care records unattended where other people or the perpetrator may be able to access them.

Documentation of encounters should include the following.

- A description of the observed indicators, including a description of any injuries, indicative symptoms or behaviours, and any evidence or statements about who inflicted them. It can be useful to write direct quotes where appropriate.
- Note if there were any children or other witnesses present and if they were involved at all.
- If you discussed family violence with the patient or provided a referral include a note of which referral option was provided.

Table 51.3: National referral options for Australia and New Zealand

Patient category/needs	Australian national referral options	New Zealand national referral options
Information, counselling and support Advice and advocacy Safety planning Referrals to local/specialist support Safe house and refuge accommodation	**safe steps:** 1800 015 188, www.safesteps.org.au **1800RESPECT:** 1800 737 732, www.1800respect.org.au (referrals provided to local services)	**It's Not Okay:** 008 456 450, www.areyouok.org.nz (referrals provided to local services) **Shine:** 0508 744 633, www.2shine.org.nz
Protection from violence/abuse	**Police**	**Police**
Sexual assault (including children)	**1800RESPECT:** 1800 737 732, www.1800respect.org.au (referrals provided to local services) **Police**	**Rape Prevention Education:** https://rpe.co.nz/ (provides links to local services) **Police**
Medical care	**Emergency department** **Local GP services**	**Emergency department** **Local GP services**
Specialist patient services	**Aboriginal Family Domestic Violence Hotline:** 1800 019 123 **National Disability Abuse and Neglect Hotline:** 1800 880 052 **inTouch (Multicultural Centre Against Family Violence):** Ph. 1800 755 988, www.intouch.org.au	**Areyouok:** www.areyouok.org.nz/ (referrals provided to local services)
Legal Help	**1800RESPECT:** 1800 737 732 www.1800respect.org.au (referrals provided to local services)	**Community law centres:** http://communitylaw.org.nz/ (provides referrals to local services)
Child abuse and neglect	**Child Protection Services:** (contact local services) **Kids Helpline:** 1800 551 800 kidshelpline.com.au	**Child Protection Services:** (contact local services) **0800 What's Up:** 0800 942 8787, www.whatsup.co.nz
Elder abuse	**1800RESPECT:** 1800 737 732 www.1800respect.org.au (referrals provided to local services)	**Age Concern:** 0800 652 105, www.ageconcern.org.nz
Referral services for men who use violence and want help	**Men's Referral Service (No to Violence):** 1300 766 491, www.ntv.org.au	**It's Not Okay:** 008 456 450, www.areyouok.org.nz (referrals provided to local services)
Services for male victims of family violence	**MensLine Australia:** 1300 789 978, https://mensline.org.au	**It's Not Okay:** 008 456 450, www.areyouok.org.nz (referrals provided to local services)

- Any other relevant findings or statements made by the patient or potential perpetrators.
- It is also recommended that paramedics flag if police attended the scene. Paramedics and police are believed to frequently co-respond to family violence scenes and the ability to match patient records across services may benefit patients and researchers.

CASE STUDY 1

Case 21005, 2300 hrs.

Dispatch details: You are called to a 33-year-old female who has self-harmed via an intentional overdose of unknown medications. Patient is conscious and breathing.

Initial presentation: On arrival you are met by the patient's husband, who states his wife (Sharon) has attempted to overdose on medications. You enter the house which appears clean and tidy. There are no children present, though you notice assorted toys in a box in the corner and see children's drawings on the fridge. The patient is sitting on the couch and is clearly conscious and breathing, but she does not respond when you enter. You speak with the patient while your partner takes the husband into an adjoining room to talk with him.

 ASSESS

You approach the patient and say 'hello'. She looks up at you but doesn't speak. Sharon has red puffy eyes and it appears she has been crying. You ask if she knew you were coming and she nods but continues to look down. You introduce yourself and ask if you can sit next to her on the couch; she nods.

You say, 'Sharon, your husband has told us that you have taken an overdose of your medications. Is that right?' Again, she nods but does not look at you. You ask, 'Sharon, did you take the medications on purpose?' She nods. You ask, 'Sharon, did you do this to hurt yourself?' and she nods. You ask, 'Sharon, is it okay if I try and help you?' She doesn't move or respond.

At this stage your partner walks in and hands you 12 empty Panadol blister packs, and a note signed 'Sharon' that says goodbye to her daughter. He also hands you a note stating Sharon's full name and date of birth, and that she is currently taking Endep for depression, has no allergies and has a 3-year-old daughter with her husband.

You ask Sharon if she took all the Panadol and she nods. You ask when but she doesn't reply.

You say to Sharon, 'I can see you're upset and I want to help you. I want to take you into hospital so that you can see a doctor. You've taken a dangerous amount of Panadol and you need emergency care. Is that okay?' Sharon nods. You say, 'Before we go, is it okay for me to take a few observations like your pulse and blood pressure?' Sharon doesn't say anything but holds out her arm. Sharon has a BP of 120/80, a HR of 80, SpO$_2$ of 99%, a blood sugar level (BSL) of 5.3, Glasgow Coma Scale (GCS) of 15, and her pupils are equal and reactive to light (PEARL). You do not note any other unusual scene findings.

After you finish taking your observations, Sharon walks with you to the ambulance. On the way her husband tries to hug her but she pushes him away and walks ahead out the door. He looks at you and says, 'We've been fighting recently; she's never like this. I don't know what's happened'. The husband walks with you to the door and you ask if he will drive to the hospital. He states that he wants to come with you. You tell him that you think its best that he drives behind so he has transport back from the ED. The husband again states he wants to travel with you and that last time he travelled in the ambulance with his wife and it was fine. You explain that in this instance you aren't able to take him in the ambulance and that if he follows you to the ED and goes through reception he will be able to see his wife again; he agrees reluctantly.

During this conversation you begin to suspect that there may be more to this case than was immediately apparent, but you decide not to make your suspicions known to the husband.

② CONFIRM

In the back of the ambulance you place Sharon on the bed and ask if she is comfortable, she nods. You ask if it's okay to talk to her, she looks at you and nods. You ask her if there was something that happened today that made her take the medications, and she looks down and says, 'No, not really'. You ask if she has been having trouble at home and she doesn't reply. You wait a minute and Sharon says, 'I guess I'm pretty stressed'. You ask her if she knows why she is stressed and she says she's not sure. You ask if it is work that is stressing her, or if there is something else she is worried about and she says no. You say, 'Sharon, I'm wondering if there is someone who might be saying or doing something to hurt or frighten you, or maybe your children?' Sharon doesn't answer. You wait about 10 seconds and then add, 'Sharon, we believe that everyone has the right to feel safe in their home. If someone is hurting or frightening you, I can help connect you with people that can help you'. You wait for a response; you can see Sharon is thinking so you don't interrupt her. Eventually she says, 'It's not his fault. He's always so stressed with work and sometimes when he drinks he just goes too far. He's not a bad person, he just goes too far … he needs help'.

You place a hand on Sharon's shoulder and say, 'I understand, Sharon. Thank you for telling me that; it must have been hard'. Sharon starts crying again and says, 'I don't want him to get into trouble; I don't want you to do anything'. You say, 'Sharon, I understand and I'm not going to do anything that you don't want me too. If you like we can talk about some of the referral services that I can help you get in contact with. There are lots of services that you can access to get help and support and you can be in control of the process'. Sharon nods.

③ TREAT

You ask Sharon about what has been happening and she states that she has been having problems with her husband ever since she was pregnant with their first child. She states he has been 'different' ever since then; he calls her names and tells her she is stupid, and she thinks he might be monitoring her phone. You ask if he has ever been violent and she states he's never really hit her, but she is afraid sometimes when he is drinking that he will lose control. You ask if he acts this way with their daughter and she says no, they never fight in front of her. You ask her about her daughter, if she is happy and healthy, and she says she is doing really well.

You ask if she feels safe at home and she states that she doesn't think her husband would really hurt her; he can be rough and has hit her and pushed her in the past, but never really hard. She says it's more about their relationship failing; she feels trapped and doesn't know how to help him.

You explain to her there are several referral options available to her; some can help with information or advice, there is counselling or she can access legal advice. She asks you, 'I don't know, what do you think I should do?' You say to her that you know a little bit about family violence, but while you're not an expert, you think that if she needs advice she should contact the helpline, and that she can use the free-call number, or go online. They will be the best service to help answer any questions she has. Sharon agrees and you write the number down for her.

4 EVALUATE

After the conversation you ask Sharon if there is anything else you can help her with, she thanks you but says no. You ask her if it will be safe for her to contact the referral service and she says she can call from work one day. You remind her that if she ever feels unsafe she can always call 000 and ask for police, or she can call the ambulance back if she needs medical help. She thanks you again.

As you arrive at hospital you explain to Sharon that you need to explain what happened today to the nurse and doctor. You ask her if it is okay for you to tell them what happened and what you discussed in the ambulance. She asks you, 'What will they do? Will they call the police, or take my daughter away?' You reply that they won't call the police without your consent but they will probably want to ask her about her relationship with her husband and will want to help her. You tell her that you don't think they will try and take her children away from her. Sharon consents for you to explain what happened.

You complete your case notes, describing what happened on the job, what kinds of questions you asked and the patient's responses, and noted that you referred her to the helpline. You also note that there were no children present and police did not attend. When handing Sharon over to the nurse you quietly explain the nature of the case, stating that the patient disclosed family violence and that she is worried about what will happen to her husband and child. The nurse states that she will page the hospital's family violence unit worker to come and speak with her.

You say goodbye to Sharon and wish her luck in the future. She thanks you and you leave. As you get back in the ambulance you ask your partner what they thought of that job, they say it was pretty intense but they are okay with it. They ask you the same question and you say it was a very sad job and that it reminded you of some things that happened in your childhood. The two of you debrief while driving back to branch. At the end of the shift you partner reminds you that you can always call them if you want to talk more, and they offer to ask Peer-Support to call you. You say thanks but you're okay, and that you will seek support with Peer-Support or your local psychologist if you need to debrief further.

 CASE STUDY 2

Case 14762, 1450 hrs.

Dispatch details: You are dispatched code 1 to a 63-year-old male complaining of central chest pain.

Initial presentation: You arrive to find the patient's son (John) waiting for you. He states that his father (Sam) has been complaining of chest pain which has been getting worse so he called the ambulance. You enter the house which appears messy but mostly clean. John explains that Sam moved in 3 months ago after he could no longer care for himself at home due to the early stages of dementia.

1 ASSESS

You enter a small, messy bedroom. When you enter, Sam is lying in bed. You smell a strong odour of stale urine and there are dirty dishes around the room, some of which appear to have been there a while.

You assess Sam and find he has been experiencing intermittent chest pain for the past few weeks. He has been telling his son but John only called today due to Sam complaining it was hurting more. You do a full assessment and decide Sam is experiencing acute coronary syndrome and so decide to treat him as per your protocols.

You ask John about Sam's living arrangements. He says that his father had to move in with him as he could no longer care for himself at home and he can't afford to send him to a nursing home. John is a factory shift worker and is gone most days, leaving Sam to care for himself.

2 CONFIRM

You begin to wonder if John is able to provide adequate care for Sam. You ask him if he gets any help with his father and he says his brother lives interstate and can't really help so it's just him. You have a brief conversation and you feel it's clear that John wants to help his father, but also that he is struggling to care for him.

You ask John how often he checks on his father and he says he tries to check in on him most days, but it's not always possible due to him working long hours. He does his best to make sure his father is washed and fed regularly, but he admits it's difficult, and he often has to rely on his father caring for himself.

3 TREAT

In addition to providing treatment for Sam's chest pain, you discuss with John the possibility of arranging respite care or nursing care for Sam. You recommend that John goes to see Sam's GP and explain that he is having trouble providing adequate care for Sam, and he says that he will.

You state to John that you will also bring this up at ED and ask the staff to try and assist him access support to help him care for his father. John thanks you and says he's feeling like he's let his father down. You empathise with him saying that it's not easy caring for a parent and it's often helpful to recruit as much support as possible so that he can care for his father without stressing himself too much.

4 EVALUATE

You take Sam into the ED and hand over to the nurse, explaining what's been going on and that his son might need some help caring for him. The nurse replied that she will arrange the hospital's social worker to come and assess him.

In your case notes you make sure to document, in addition to your treatment for his chest pain, what you saw and discussed with John, and that you referred him to the GP and requested that the nursing staff at the ED review Sam's care needs.

Summary

Family violence is a common and highly damaging form of interpersonal violence which paramedics are likely to encounter in their practice. It is important that paramedics have a good knowledge of the definitions and background to the different manifestations of family violence, so that they are able to recognise the indications and respond appropriately. Victims of family violence can benefit from referrals to the right agencies, and paramedics can play a pivotal role in providing these referrals. Paramedics who have the right knowledge, attitudes and skills can be an effective resource for these patients to access care and support and end the violence.

References

Al-Yaman, F., Van Doeland, M., & Wallis, M. (2006). *Family violence among Aboriginal and Torres Strait Islander peoples*. Australia: Australian Institute of Health and Welfare Canberra.

Astbury, J. C. M. (2000). *Women's mental health: an evidence based review*. Geneva: World Health Organization.

Australian Bureau of Statistics. (2013). *2012 Personal Safety Survey, ABS Cat. No. 4906.0*. Canberra: ABS.

Australian Institute of Criminology. (2013). *Australian Crimes: Facts and figures*. Canberra: Australian Institute of Criminology.

Australian Institute of Health and Welfare (AIHW). (2017). *Child protection Australia 2015–16*. Child Welfare series no. 66. Cat. no. CWS 60. Canberra: AIHW.

Australian Productivity Commission. (2014). *Overcoming Indigenous Disadvantage—Key Indicators 2014*. Canberra: Australian Productivity Commission.

Black, M. C. (2011). Intimate partner violence and adverse health consequences implications for clinicians. *American Journal of Lifestyle Medicine, 5*, 428–439.

Black, M. C., Basile, K. C., Breiding, M. J., Smith, S. G., Walters, M. L., Merrick, M. T., Chen, J., & November, M. R. S. (2011). *National intimate partner and sexual violence survey*. Atlanta, GA: Centers for Disease Control and Prevention.

Blosnich, J. R., & Bossarte, R. M. (2009). Comparisons of intimate partner violence among partners in same-sex and opposite-sex relationships in the United States. *American Journal of Public Health, 99*, 2182–2184.

Butchart, A., Phinney Harvey, A., Mian, M., Furniss, T., & Kahane, T., World Health Organization. (2006). *Preventing child maltreatment: a guide to taking action and generating evidence*. Geneva: World Health Organization and International Society for Prevention of Child Abuse and Neglect.

Campbell, J. C. (2002). Health consequences of intimate partner violence. *The Lancet, 359*, 1331–1336.

Ministry of Social Development. (2016). *Oranga Tamariki— Ministry for Children—Key statistics and information for media*. https://www.msd.govt.nz/about-msd-and-our-work/publications-resources/statistics/cyf/.

Coker, A. L., Smith, P. H., Bethea, L., King, M. R., & McKeown, R. E. (2000). Physical health consequences of physical and psychological intimate partner violence. *Archives of Family Medicine, 9*, 451–457.

Datner, E. M., Shofer, F. S., Parmele, K., Stahmer, S. A., & Mechem, C. C. (1999). Utilization of the 911 system as an identifier of domestic violence. *The American Journal of Emergency Medicine, 17*, 560–565.

Dawe, S., Harnett, P. H., & Frye, S. (2008). *Improving outcomes for children living in families with parental substance misuse: what do we know and what should we do*. Australian Institute of Family Studies.

Dearden, J., & Jones, W. (2008). *Homicide in Australia: 2006-07 national homicide monitoring program annual report*. Australian Institute of Criminology.

Edleson, J. (1999). Children's witnessing of adult domestic violence. *Journal of Interpersonal Violence, 14*, 839–870.

Ellsberg, M., Arango, D. J., Morton, M., Gennari, F., Kiplesund, S., Contreras, M., & Watts, C. (2015). Prevention of violence against women and girls: what does the evidence say? *The Lancet, 385*, 1555–1566.

Fanslow, J. L., & Robinson, E. (2004). Violence against women in New Zealand: prevalence and health consequences. *The New Zealand Medical Journal, 117*(1206), U1173.

Fanslow, J. L., & Robinson, E. M. (2011). Sticks, stones, or words? Counting the prevalence of different types of intimate partner violence reported by New Zealand women. *Journal of Aggression, Maltreatment & Trauma, 20*, 741–759.

Fanslow, J. L., Robinson, E. M., Crengle, S., & Perese, L. (2007). Prevalence of child sexual abuse reported by a cross-sectional sample of New Zealand women. *Child Abuse & Neglect, 31*, 935–945.

Feder, G. S., Hutson, M., Ramsay, J., & Taket, A. R. (2006). Women exposed to intimate partner violence: expectations and experiences when they encounter health care professionals: a meta-analysis of qualitative studies. *Archives of Internal Medicine, 166*, 22–37.

Ghafournia, N. (2011). Battered at home, played down in policy: migrant women and domestic violence in Australia. *Aggression and Violent Behavior, 16*, 207–213.

Green, A. H. (1993). Child sexual abuse: immediate and long-term effects and intervention. *Journal of the American Academy of Child and Adolescent Psychiatry, 32*, 890–902.

Hanson, R. F., Kievit, L. W., Saunders, B. E., Smith, D. W., Kilpatrick, D. G., Resnick, H. S., & Ruggiero, K. J. (2003). Correlates of adolescent reports of sexual assault: findings from the National Survey of Adolescents. *Child Maltreatment, 8*, 261–272.

Hegarty, K. L., & Bush, R. (2002). Prevalence and associations of partner abuse in women attending general practice: a cross-sectional survey. *Australian and New Zealand Journal of Public Health, 26,* 437–442.

Hughes, R. B., Lund, E. M., Gabrielli, J., Powers, L. E., & Curry, M. A. (2011). Prevalence of interpersonal violence against community-living adults with disabilities: a literature review. *Rehabilitation Psychology, 56,* 302.

Irwin, J. (2008). (Dis) counted stories: domestic violence and lesbians. *Qualitative Social Work, 7,* 199–215.

Jozkowski, K. N., & Sanders, S. A. (2012). Health and sexual outcomes of women who have experienced forced or coercive sex. *Women and Health, 52,* 101–118.

King, W. K., Kiesel, E. L., & Simon, H. K. (2006). Child abuse fatalities: are we missing opportunities for intervention? *Pediatric Emergency Care, 22,* 211–214.

Kōkiri, T. P. (2017). *Māori Family Violence Infographic.*

Krug, E., Dahlberg, J., Mercy, J., Zwi, A., & Lozano, R. (2002). *World report on violence and health.* Geneva: World Health Organization.

Kurrle, S. E., Sadler, P. M., Lockwood, K., & Cameron, I. D. (1997). Elder abuse: prevalence, intervention and outcomes in patients referred to four Aged Care Assessment Teams. *The Medical Journal of Australia, 166,* 119–122.

Livermore, P., Bunt, R., & Biscan, K. (2001). Elder abuse among clients and carers referred to the Central Coast ACAT: a descriptive analysis. *Australasian Journal on Ageing, 20,* 41–47.

Marie, D., Fergusson, D. M., & Boden, J. M. (2008). Ethnic identity and intimate partner violence in a New Zealand birth cohort. *Social Policy Journal of New Zealand, 33,* 126.

McNair, R., Kavanagh, A., Agius, P., & Tong, B. (2005). The mental health status of young adult and mid-life non-heterosexual Australian women. *Australian and New Zealand Journal of Public Health, 29,* 265–271.

Morris, A., Reilly, J., Berry, S., & Ransom, R. (2003). *New Zealand national survey of crime victims 2001.* Ministry of Justice Wellington.

Norman, R. E., Byambaa, M., De, R., Butchart, A., Scott, J., & Vos, T. (2012). The long-term health consequences of child physical abuse, emotional abuse, and neglect: a systematic review and meta-analysis. *PLoS Medicine, 9,* e1001349.

Office of Women's Policy. (2002). *A policy framework: a co-ordinated approach to reducing violence against women, women's safety strategy.* Melbourne, Victoria: Office of Women's Policy.

Rape Prevention Education New Zealand. 2011. *Sexual violence against males* [Online]. Retrieved from http://rpe.co.nz/information/sexual-violence-against-males/. (Accessed 24 April 2018).

Renner, L. M., & Slack, K. S. (2006). Intimate partner violence and child maltreatment: understanding intra- and intergenerational connections. *Child Abuse & Neglect, 30,* 599–617.

Roberts, G. L., Lawrence, J. M., O'Toole, B. I., & Raphael, B. (1997). Domestic violence in the emergency department: I: two case-control studies of victims. *General Hospital Psychiatry, 19,* 5–11.

Rossen, F., Lucassen, M., Denny, S., & Robinson, E. (2009). *The Health and Wellbeing of secondary school students in New Zealand: results for young people attracted to the same or both sexes.* Aukland: Auckland University. researchspace.auckland.ac.nz.

Sawyer, S., Coles, J., Williams, A., Peter, L., & Williams, B. (2017a). Paramedic students' knowledge, attitudes, and preparedness to manage intimate partner violence patients. *Prehospital Emergency Care, 21,* 750–760.

Sawyer, S., Coles, J., Williams, A., Rotheram, A., & Williams, B. (2017b). The knowledge, attitudes and preparedness to manage intimate partner violence patients of Australian paramedics – A pilot study. *Prehospital Emergency Care,* 750–760. Published online: 22 Aug.

Sawyer, S., Coles, J., Williams, A., & Williams, B. (2015). Preventing and reducing the impacts of intimate partner violence: opportunities for Australian ambulance services. *Emergency Medicine Australasia: EMA, 27,* 307–311.

Sawyer, S., Coles, J., Williams, A., & Williams, B. (2018). Paramedics as a new resource for women experiencing intimate partner violence. *Journal of Interpersonal Violence,* doi: 10.1177/0886260518769363.

Sawyer, S., Parekh, V., Williams, A., & Williams, B. (2014). Are Australian paramedics adequately trained and prepared for intimate partner violence? A pilot study. *Journal of Forensic and Legal Medicine, 28,* 32–35.

The Royal Australian College of General Practitioners. (2014). *Abuse and violence: working with our patients in general practice* (4th ed.). Melbourne: The Royal Australian College of General Practitioners.

Tjaden, P., & Thoennes, N. (2000). *Full report of the prevalence, incidence, and consequences of violence against women (NCJ 183781).* National Institute of Justice, Office of Justice Programs, Washington, DC.

Vaughan, C., Davis, E., Murdolo, A., Chen, J., Murray, L., Block, K., Quiazon, R., & Warr, D. (2016). *Promoting community-led responses to violence against immigrant and refugee women in metropolitan and regional Australia: The ASPIRE Project: Key findings and future directions.* Australia's National Research Organisation for Women's Safety Limited (ANROWS).

VicHealth. (2004). *The health costs of violence: measuring the burden of disease caused by intimate partner violence: a summary of findings.* Carlton: VicHealth.

Victoria Police. (2009). *Crime Statistics 2008–09.* Corporate Statistics, Corporate Strategy and Performance, Victoria Police.

Walker, L. E. (1980). *The battered woman.* New York: Harper & Row.

Weiss, S. J., Ernst, A. A., Blanton, D., Sewell, D., & Nick, T. G. (2000). EMT domestic violence knowledge and the results of an educational intervention. *The American Journal of Emergency Medicine, 18,* 168–171.

Weiss, S., Garza, A., Casaletto, J., Stratton, M., Ernst, A., Blanton, D., & Nick, T. G. (2000). The out-of-hospital use of a domestic violence screen for assessing patient risk. *Prehospital Emergency Care, 4*, 24–27.

World Health Organization. (2008). *A global response to elder abuse and neglect: building primary health care capacity to deal with the problem worldwide: main report. WHO, Ageing and Life Course Unit & Université de Genève. Centre Interfacultaire de Gérontologie*. Geneva: WHO.

World Health Organization. (2011). *Elder maltreatment fact sheet*. Geneva: WHO.

World Health Organization. (2013a). *Global and regional estimates of violence against women: prevalence and health effects of intimate partner violence and non-partner sexual violence. WHO, Department of Reproductive Health and Research, London School of Hygiene and Tropical Medicine, South African Medical Research Council*. Geneva: WHO.

World Health Organization. (2013b). *Responding to intimate partner violence and sexual violence against women: WHO clinical and policy guidelines*. Geneva: WHO.

World Health Organization. (2014). *Health care for women subjected to intimate partner violence or sexual violence: a clinical handbook*. Geneva: WHO.

Wu, V., Huff, H., & Bhandari, M. (2010). Pattern of physical injury associated with intimate partner violence in women presenting to the emergency department: a systematic review and meta-analysis. *Trauma, Violence and Abuse, 11*, 71–82.

Yon, Y., Mikton, C. R., Gassoumis, Z. D., & Wilber, K. H. (2017). Elder abuse prevalence in community settings: a systematic review and meta-analysis. *The Lancet Global Health, 5*, e147–e156.

SECTION 15:
The Paramedic Approach to the Patient Displaying Changes in Behaviour: Mental Health and Mental Illness

Behaviour changes are not necessarily the result of mental illness: they can be caused by a number of physical diseases or by the effects of both prescribed and illicit drugs. When such behaviour is observed in the community, the public have few options other than to request attendance by paramedics and/or the police. An increasing proportion of paramedic cases involve mental illness and as such paramedic education needs to focus on this in addition to physical illnesses.

Chapters in this section outline a structured approach to assessing and managing the patient displaying changes in behaviour. Chapter 52 discusses how physical causes of behavioural changes must be eliminated prior to the diagnosis of common mental illnesses. Direct treatment of most acute mental illnesses is well beyond the scope of paramedic practice, but transporting these patients to centres where they can be treated requires gaining their consent and cooperation.

In rare circumstances, patients can be agitated and even suspicious of paramedics. The law carefully regulates the use of both chemical and physical restraints to transport patients with a mental illness as a last resort.

Chapter 53 describes principles and processes to de-escalate acute behavioural episodes and to gain the cooperation of patients being transported for assessment and treatment. This de-escalation process is effective for episodes of aggression regardless of the cause.

CHAPTER 52

Mental Health Conditions

By Louise Roberts

OVERVIEW

- Patients displaying changes in behaviour which are indicative of changes in mental health status and potential mental illness are common in the out-of-hospital setting and they present paramedics with unique clinical and management challenges.
- Changes in behaviour can be caused by alterations in the body's physiology due to organic causes such as infection or can be a result of mental illness.

- Patients presenting with altered behaviour require a specific approach to assessment, including the Mental State Assessment and Examination.
- These patients often have physical injuries as a result of their inability to adequately protect themselves from harm.
- Patients who are demonstrating that they are likely to come to harm can be involuntarily transported to hospital under legal provisions.

Introduction

According to the World Health Organization (WHO, 2013), mental health is a state of emotional and social wellbeing in which a person can fulfil their abilities, cope with the normal stressors of life, work productively and make a contribution to their community. Changes in mental health status and functioning may occur over the course of an individual's life. These changes fall across a spectrum of severity, from common mental health problems, which cause distress but are short-lived, to more severe mental illnesses. Mental illnesses are defined as those which cause significant 'disturbances in thinking, perception and behaviour' (Dogra et al., 2017). They are characterised by having a longer duration, impaired functioning in at least one area of the individual's life and have a detrimental impact on the person's ability to cope (Bloch et al., 2017; Mindframe National Media Initiative, 2012). It is widely recognised that defining mental illness and their associated characteristics (see Box 52.1) is often difficult, and struggles to separate psychopathology from normal variances in human behaviour such as sadness after a loss and shyness (Stein et al., 2010). In the past 10 years research is starting to shed light on the relationship between physiological changes in the body and their association with the development of mental illness. Research has been broadly focused on the effects of genetics, changes in neuroanatomy and physiology, neurotransmitters, the immune system, the endocrine system and the relationship with the gut microbiome, specifically in its effects on mood, in the development of mental illness (Bloch et al., 2017).

This chapter provides an assessment framework as part of the paramedics' tool box to understand and assess changes in behaviour and assist with differential diagnosis. The challenge for paramedics is to consider the broad causes of altered behaviour which can be due to a primary mental health problem, a non-mental health issue (e.g. a physical/organic cause such as hypoglycaemia) or an interaction of both. Paramedics need to ensure that the non-mental health causes of these presentations are considered, explored and treated, and a holistic assessment is done so as not to discount either mental or physical health issues.

It should be noted that within the mental health sector the term 'mental health consumer' or persons with 'lived experience' is used in preference to 'patient'. For the sake of consistency within this text, however, the collective term 'patient' is used.

Prevalence of out-of-hospital and emergency department mental health presentations

In any single year, 1 in 5 Australian adults will experience a mental illness: in 2014–15, 17.5% of Australians self-reported having a mental or behavioural condition (Australian Bureau of Statistics [ABS], 2015). Anxiety-related and mood (affective) disorders were the most frequently reported with 11.2% and 9.3% respectively of the population experiencing these conditions within a 12-month period (ABS, 2015).

Broadly, the most common presentations of mental illness in the out-of-hospital setting are anxiety and mood (or *affective*) disorders, presentations of

BOX 52.1 Characteristics of a mental/psychiatric disorder

Features

A mental/psychiatric disorder is a behavioural or psychological syndrome or pattern that occurs in an individual:

- the consequences of which must be clinically significant distress (e.g. a painful symptom) or disability (i.e. impairment in one or more important areas of functioning)—that is, they must not be merely an expected response to common stressors and losses (e.g. the loss of a loved one) or a culturally sanctioned response to a particular event (e.g. trance states in religious rituals)
- that reflects an underlying psychobiological dysfunction
- that is not solely a result of social deviance or conflicts with society.

Other considerations

It must have diagnostic validity using one or more sets of diagnostic validators (e.g. prognostic significance, psychobiological disruption, response to treatment). It must also have clinical utility (e.g. contribute to better conceptualisation of diagnoses or to better assessment and treatment).

Source: Stein et al. (2010).

self-harm, suicide ideations and suicide attempts, psychosis and schizophrenia, and drug and alcohol issues. Accurate statistics regarding the number of mental health presentations attended by Australian and New Zealand paramedics are difficult to obtain due to misleading categorisation of jobs at dispatch, uncertainty regarding the individual's diagnosis at the point of assessment (Roberts & Henderson, 2009) and difficulties linking out-of-hospital data with hospital patient care records. More recent data here in Australia has tried to address these issues by examining patient records directly. The data focused on paramedic attendance to self-harm and mental health-related presentations in Australia from 2013 and showed Ambulance Victoria attended over 15,000 cases related to anxiety and more than 6000 cases of depression, over 6000 suicide attempts and 2000 cases of self-injury in a 12-month period (Lloyd et al., 2015). Similar prevalence rates were found in other Australian states, which demonstrates the vital role paramedics play in providing care and

treatment for those in the community with mental health problems and illness.

To add to this picture emergency departments (EDs) nationally in Australia managed an estimated 273,439 presentations with a mental health-related principal diagnosis during 2015–16 (3.7% of all ED occasions of service, excluding the Australian Capital Territory) (AIHW, 2017). According to the AIHW 12.8% of presentations were classified as *emergency* (requiring care within 10 minutes), with 77.5% of mental health-related presentations classified on initial assessment as being either *urgent* (requiring care within 30 minutes) or *semi-urgent* (requiring care within 60 minutes) (AIHW, 2017).

Current reporting and trends recognised globally suggest that these figures are only likely to increase in the coming years, due to the mainstreaming of mental health services and a steadily increasing demand for services, which has not been met by increases in funding (Lowthian et al., 2011). As such, paramedics need to be well educated in the areas of mental health and risk assessments and have a working knowledge of the primary diagnoses likely to present to emergency services.

The mental health system: why the increase in the out-of-hospital attendance to those with mental health concerns

Since the early 1970s the human rights movement and the advent of medications to manage more severe mental illness such as antipsychotics underpinned the movement of people from institutionalised (inpatient) care to community mental health care (deinstitutionalisation). More recently there has been a significant push in public policy to reduce seclusion and restraint practices, promote and embed the principle of least-restrictive practice and move mental health services to the general health system and the community. The trend towards earlier-discharge inpatient units (short-stay units), hospital avoidance, significant losses in mental health beds and funding (Bradbury et al., 2017) and greater provision of community and primary mental health care has moved the demand for service to the out-of-hospital and primary healthcare settings (e.g. greater involvement of general practitioners, community mental health services, non-government organisations and emergency services) (Jespersen et al., 2016).

While community treatment is the preferred option when possible, there is still a need to transport patients whose mental illness has unexpectedly exacerbated to require ED or psychiatric inpatient unit care. Admission to the ED allows for further medical assessment to rule out other causes of changed behaviour as well as a specialist psychiatric assessment to determine the most appropriate treatment option for the patient at that time. Possible outcomes include admission to treat an organic cause, admission to a psychiatric inpatient unit or discharge back home with follow-up by community mental health services. In other instances paramedics, depending on their assessment and the circumstances, may use alternative referral pathways such as local mental health teams, mental health triage consultation, mental health liaisons in either the ambulance operation centres or the ED or transport the patient directly to an inpatient mental health facility. The referral pathways vary according to specific local guidelines, laws and collaborations between available services.

Concepts of recovery and the biopsychosocial model of care

Mental illness effects an individual's ability to function whether it is changes in the body's physiology, psychology or social and occupational functioning (see Box 52.2). Therefore, understanding the aetiology of the illness or identifying one clear causative factor becomes more difficult and often not as crucial as the context and the story from the

person themselves. To be able to provide context and understanding and build the effective therapeutic relationship paramedics need to understand the concepts of recovery and the biopsychosocial model of care.

Paramedics are in a unique position to observe patients in their home environment, to identify community and social supports, facilitate engagement and communication between health professional and patient, and act as an advocate during the clinical handover of vital information if further care is required. An exclusive focus on the patient's physiological signs and symptoms may result in the loss of meaningful and crucial information, which might prolong the patient's episode of care. While the biomedical model of illness and treatment has distinct advantages in the out-of-hospital field, where timely intervention is crucial and the linking of signs and symptoms to specific diagnostic criteria and treatment pathways is useful, it fails to account for broader factors which influence health outcomes. For example, depression is three times more likely after a patient suffers an acute myocardial infarction (AMI), despite there being no specific physical link that directly ties the damage of myocardial cells to decreased release of serotonin in the brain (Lichtman et al., 2008). Similarly, depressive symptoms after an AMI are predictors of increased mortality and worse health status, despite there being no direct physiological link between brain and cardiac function (Mallik et al., 2006).

The biomedical model also fails to account for the importance of the patient–practitioner relationship in terms of successful recovery (the therapeutic relationship).

The biopsychosocial model

> To provide a basis for understanding the determinants of disease and arriving at rational treatments and patterns of health care, a medical model must also take into account the patient, the social context in which he lives, and the complementary system devised by society to deal with the disruptive effects of illness, that is, the physician role and the health care system. This requires a biopsychosocial model.
>
> *Engel (1977)*

The biopsychosocial model on the other hand suggests that illness is the result of a complex interplay of psychological, social and biological factors, each of which should be considered in our assessment and treatment of the patient (Engel, 1977). While the biomedical model seeks to separate the biological factors from other factors, the biopsychosocial

---

BOX 52.2 Biological, psychological and social factors that may impact on mental health

Biological
Genetics, nutritional status, general state of health or, in more specific cases, structural abnormalities in the brain or variable levels of neurotransmitters such as dopamine, serotonin, noradrenaline, GABA.

Psychological
Early experiences (childhood), personality, intelligence, attitudes and values, self-image and self-esteem, temperament, coping skills, stress and others.

Social
Family relationships, social supports, social skills, cultural background, as well as other environmental factors such as employment and others.

Note: Some of the items identified can be considered within multiple categories.

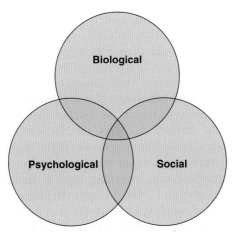

Figure 52.1
The integrated relationship between the biological, psychological and social domains identified by Engel.

approach asserts that no single factor can be considered in isolation. Rather, the biological, social and psychological aspects of an individual's life affect each other so that changes in one area will have an impact in another. This relationship is represented in Figure 52.1.

The advantage of the biopsychosocial model is that it allows us to view a person as a whole being and provides a framework to understand the wide range of factors which may affect health and individual variation. This ensures that important factors in the individual's health status are not missed. It also lends itself to multidisciplinary treatment models, with a combination of social, physical and psychological treatments being recognised and included in care provision. Unfortunately the model is not as prescriptive in terms of its assessment and treatment. Additionally, it has been argued that a further separation of biology and psychology can be arbitrary, if not misleading (Tavakoli, 2009).

Regardless of the theoretical debate, a basic understanding of the biopsychosocial model is important for paramedics, as it directs mental health assessment and treatment models and provides a framework for communication between mental health disciplines.

The recovery approach
'Recovery' is broadly defined as a 'deeply personal, unique process of changing one's attitudes, values, goals, skills and/or roles. It is a way of living a satisfying, hopeful and contributing life even within the limitations caused by illness' (Anthony, 1993, p. 14). The challenging question for paramedics is what does this actually mean and how do we understand and apply this concept to practice in the out-of-hospital setting?

The recovery approach focuses on the relationship between the clinician and the patient. A key principle is the ability to listen and support the person with the lived experience of mental illness. Their perspective and voice is fundamental to creating a therapeutic relationship which moves from a 'deficit' framework (the person is unable, incapable or lacks capacity) to one that acknowledges the person has abilities and strengths and can contribute to their own care planning, and should be supported in doing so as much as possible (Leonhardt et al., 2017). The idea of recovery acknowledges that every individual is different and due to illness may have challenges in making their own decisions and looking after themselves, but should be treated with respect, dignity and in the least-restrictive and most-inclusive manner possible (Isaacs et al., 2017).

Recovery also strongly points to the social systems and environmental factors which shape a person's life. Recovery suggests you can aim towards creating a positive and contributing life even though you have or are experiencing changes in mental health, social and family circumstances, work or personal environments, or trauma and stress. This leads us to consider the holistic nature of care, 'person-centred' care and the biopsychosocial model of health.

Pathophysiology
As mentioned, the causes of mental illness are complex and involve biological, social and psychological factors which interrelate to create changes in behaviour that are disruptive and distressing for the person. Biological factors involve genetic, neurochemical, neuroendocrine, immunology and inflammation basis for mental illness as well as changes in brain function and structure. Gene studies, for example, have shown hereditability and the role of multiple genes is significant in the development of mental illness. These studies have shown roughly half the risk of developing addiction and depression is hereditary. Genes and their interaction with the environment play an important role in the development of schizophrenia with the general population lifetime risk at around 1% compared to 10% in those with a family history (Bloch et al., 2017).

Recently more research has been done into the role of the neurotransmitters dopamine, serotonin, norepinephrine (noradrenaline) and their post-synapsis receptors and their association with depression and its development. Neurotransmitters such as serotonin and gamma-aminobutyric acid (GABA), the chief inhibitory neurotransmitter in the brain, interact with the emotional centres in the brain such as the amygdala, pre-frontal cortex, hippocampus, thalamus and hypothalamus and play a major role in how anxiety develops (Nuss, 2015).

Advances in scanning techniques such as functional magnetic resonance imaging (fMRI) have allowed researchers to map and record brain function and structure in those with mental illness. Changes in volume and function of the pre-frontal cortex (e.g. in schizophrenia) are thought to be significant and contribute to the development of psychosis (Bloch et al., 2017).

The relationship between the endocrine system and the brain and the role of the immune system and inflammation are two areas currently creating a lot of interest in the quest to understand the development of mental illness. The hypothalamic–pituitary–adrenal (HPA) axis particularly plays a large role in regulating the body's stress response and is thought to be integral to the development and presentation of anxiety (Graeff, 2017). Recent evidence investigating immune cells and their signalling indicates they also play a crucial role in the pathophysiology of major depressive disorder (MDD) and bipolar disorder (BD). The release of neuroactive cytokines, particularly interleukins, is altered in these disorders and creates neuroinflammation within the microglia cells within the central nervous system (Bhattacharya et al., 2016).

Psychological factors relate to those factors which are central to the person's personality, early life experiences and coping mechanisms, and how they view themselves and their world (see Box 52.2). Social factors are those which explore how the person interacts and engages with others such as their relationships, support networks, employment and cultural background

Definitions

In the mental health arena the classification of mental illness is based in the *International Classification of Diseases (ICD)* or the *Diagnostic and Statistical Manual of Mental Health Disorders Fifth edition (DSM-5)* (American Psychiatric Association, 2013). Both provide a guide to how mental health is identified and its characteristics. The following outlines the common presentations seen in the community and out-of-hospital environment.

Table 52.1 provides symptoms, common medications and recommendations for out-of-hospital management of all the following conditions.

Anxiety disorders are one of the most common mental health issues seen in the community with approximately 14% of Australian adults experiencing an anxiety disorder over a 12-month period (AIHW, 2017). There are a number of different types of anxiety disorders (panic attacks and panic disorders, generalised anxiety disorder, phobias, substance/medication-induced anxiety disorder) but all involve the person experiencing fear (the emotional response to a perceived or real imminent threat) and/or anxiety (anticipation of future threat) with associated behaviours that are prolonged and do not appear to match the level of threat or the situation. Anxiety disorders are characterised by the body's autonomic responses (flight, fight and freeze) such as increased heart rate (palpitations) and breathing rate, sweating, nausea, trembling, widened eyes and dilated pupils, feeling dizzy or lightheaded, tingling and numbness in extremities, and a feeling of being outside yourself (depersonalisation). A patient may also demonstrate or describe avoidance behaviours associated with the situation or objects which trigger their anxiety (DSM-5).

Mood disorders are very common, with more than 1 million Australians reporting a past depressive episode. MDD is characterised by disturbances in mood and behaviour. Typical symptoms of a depressive episode include lowered mood, changes in appetite (significant increase or decrease) and sleep (insomnia or hypersomnia), loss of interest or pleasure in usual activities, lowered motivation and energy, social withdrawal and difficulty concentrating. Suicidal thoughts may also be present. To meet the diagnostic criteria for MDD, symptoms must occur over a 2-week period and impact on the person's ability to perform everyday tasks. Understanding and identifying MDD is extremely important, as it can be a debilitating disorder that has strong links to suicidal ideation (thoughts of suicide) and attempted suicide (DSM-5).

Bipolar disorder is the name used to describe a set of conditions that involve prolonged 'mood swings' that impair functioning, the most severe of which is bipolar I (Black Dog Institute, 2010). Individuals with bipolar I experience long periods of high mood or mania, followed in most cases by periods of depression. First onset of the disorder typically occurs either in the late teens or in middle to late adulthood, and like many mental illnesses it is more likely to occur at times of heightened stress.

> ### PRACTICE TIP
>
> **Ask!**
> - What is the reason for the call-out today? How long has X been an issue for you? What changes or symptoms have you noticed? Can you identify anything that may have triggered this change?
> - What have you tried so far to manage X?
> - Has anything been useful in the treatment of X?
> - Are you on any medications?
> - What support do you have?

Table 52.1: Common mental illnesses encountered by paramedics

Disorder	Symptoms	Common medications	Management
Schizophrenia	*Positive symptoms* Delusions Hallucinations Disorganised speech Grossly disorganised behaviour *Negative symptoms* Affective flattening Alogia Avolition Anhedonia Thought disorder	*Atypical antipsychotics* Fluanxol depot (flupenthixol) Serenace, Haldol decanoate (haloperidol) Neulactil (pericyazine) *Typical antipsychotics* Abilify (aripiprazole) Risperdal (risperidone) Seroquel (quetiapine) Clopine (clozapine) Olanzapine (particularly useful in that it can be given in wafer form)	• Obtain a history from family or loved ones if available. When acutely unwell, many psychotic patients have limited insight into their condition. Obtaining information from an observer may therefore allow for a more accurate and thorough history. • If the patient is experiencing a perceptual or thought disturbance it is important to give them adequate time to respond to questions, make questions brief and clear and, if necessary, draw their attention back to you. • Warn the patient before undertaking an exam or approaching them closely. In the case of psychosis, the presence of hallucinations or paranoid delusions may mean that they are easily startled or concerned about your actions, so this simple preventative measure may ensure safety. • Treat the patient with dignity and respect. While patients with psychosis may experience a loss of contact with reality at the time of their encounter with emergency services, most recall the manner in which they were treated when they become lucid. • Limit external stimuli. If necessary turn off any televisions or radios and limit any competing sounds as stimulus overload may increase the likelihood of agitation and confusion. • Do not dispute delusions. These beliefs are generally fixed and when challenged may result in the patient disengaging. • Do not actively support delusions, which may be detrimental to the patient's long-term progress. Sidestep the issue instead; for example, 'That sounds very distressing for you. Perhaps we should have that checked out at hospital'. • Patients may not openly report hallucinations. Look for other observable signs that the person is experiencing a perceptual disturbance; for example, long delays in responses or very quick responses, appearing distracted, appearing to respond to a stimulus that you cannot see/hear, inappropriate responses such as laughing out of context. While you may not be able to confirm that the patient is experiencing a perceptual disturbance, documenting your observations and outlining them at handover is essential. • Avoid whispering or talking about the patient nearby as it may encourage paranoia.
Depression	Lowered mood Loss of energy Lowered motivation Loss of interest in usual activities Feelings of worthlessness Sleep disturbance (i.e. insomnia or hypersomnia) Poor concentration Recurrent thoughts of suicide	*Selective serotonin re-uptake inhibitors (SSRIs)* Prozac or Lovan (fluoxetine) Zoloft (sertraline) Aropax (paroxetine) Cipramil (citalopram) Luvox (fluvoxamine) *Tricyclics* Tryptanol, Endep (amitriptyline)	• If you have concerns regarding someone's mental state, sharing your observations with the patient and expressing your concerns may facilitate further discussion. • Psychomotor retardation or a slowing of cognitive processing may occur in individuals during a major depressive episode. It is important to limit external stimuli during assessment, which may be taxing on concentration. It is also important to make questions clear and concise, allowing time for the individual to respond and be patient.

Table 52.1: Common mental illnesses encountered by paramedics—cont'd

Disorder	Symptoms	Common medications	Management
		Tofranil melipramine (imipramine) Prothiaden, Dothep (dothiepin) Allegron (nortriptyline) Surmontil (trimipramine) Anafranil (clomipramine) Sinequan, Deptran (doxepin) *Monoamine oxidase inhibitors (MAOIs)* Parnate (tranylcypromine) Nardil (phenelzine)	• Present yourself in a warm and empathetic manner. Patients are often sensitive to perceived criticism and comments such as 'Why didn't you call earlier?' come across as critical, even if it isn't the intention. • Complete a risk assessment where appropriate.
Bipolar I	Significant mood variations ranging from depressed mood to mania Depression as per above Mania Inflated self-esteem or grandiosity Decreased need for sleep Pressured speech Flight of ideas Distractibility Excessive involvement in pleasurable activities	*Mood stabilisers* Lithium (lithium carbonate) *Anticonvulsants that act as mood stabilisers* Epilim (sodium valproate) Lamictal (XR lamotrigine)	• Interviewing patients during a manic episode may be difficult, as they are easily distracted. Use the patient's name to draw their attention, maintain eye contact and, if necessary, draw the patient's attention back to any unanswered questions. • Communication may appear one-sided due to the patient's pressured speech patterns. If the patient is engaging in a monologue, be firm and clear and interrupt the patient if necessary. • If the patient presents with psychomotor agitation and wishes to pace, tap or jiggle their legs, allow them to do so (if practicable). Attempting to control the patient by making them take a seat or requesting that they cease any additional movement may result in unnecessary agitation. • If pacing is getting in the way of engagement, be flexible and consider pacing alongside the patient. • Encourage eye contact and breaths between bursts of speech, which will allow you time to speak and may assist the patient to calm their body. • Maintain clear professional boundaries, as highly sexualised behaviour may occur during a manic episode.
Panic disorder	Intense fear or discomfort that develops abruptly and reaches a peak within 10 minutes Palpitations Sweating Trembling or shaking Feeling of choking Fear of losing control or going crazy Fear of dying Paraesthesia Chest pain or discomfort Shortness of breath	*Anxiolytics* Xanax (alprazolam) Lexotan (bromazepam) Rivotril (clonazepam) Rohypnol (flunitrazepam) Ativan (lorazepam) Serepax (oxazepam) Normison (temazepam) Valium (diazepam)	• Provide clear, direct and limited education; for example 'You are breathing very quickly right now, which is making you feel lightheaded. I need you to calm your body for me ...' • Have one paramedic approach and manage the patient. • Focus on behavioural techniques such as deep breathing to decrease activation of the sympathetic nervous system. While talking-based treatments can be helpful after an episode, the patient's ability to engage will be limited at the peak of the panic attack. • Deep-breathing techniques focus on taking slow, deep breaths through the diaphragm. Direct the patient to breathe in through their nose and out through their mouth, blocking out any external stimuli. You may also wish to use your hand as a visual guide to indicate when to inhale and exhale. • Decrease distracting external stimuli. If this is not possible, encourage the patient to maintain their gaze on a fixed point or to close their eyes and focus only on their breath. • Use a slow, calm tone of voice and provide positive feedback to the patient as appropriate.

Table 52.1: Common mental illnesses encountered by paramedics—cont'd

Disorder	Symptoms	Common medications	Management
Substance abuse	Substance use resulting in failure to fulfil major role obligations (e.g. work) Substance use in situations in which it is physically dangerous Substance-related legal issues	Agonists that produce similar addiction states to the substance (e.g. methadone) Antagonists that competitively block receptor sites (e.g. ReVia [naltrexone]) Anti-craving medications Medications that block drug metabolism (e.g. Antabuse)	• Refer to Chapter 27 for management details.
Borderline personality disorder (BPD)	Instability in mood, relationships, behaviour and self-image Fear of abandonment Chronic feelings of isolation and emptiness Impulsiveness		• Individuals exhibiting the challenging behaviours associated with BPD often elicit strong responses from healthcare workers and may be negatively labelled (Muir-Cochrane et al., 2010). It is important to be familiar with your own attitudes as patients often sense when they are not being valued and are likely to disengage as a result. • Respond to the person not the person's diagnosis or label (Muir-Cochrane et al., 2010). • When treating individuals with chronic feelings of emptiness and frequent self-harm it can be easy to feel disheartened. Try to remember that while self-harm may be an unhelpful attempt to engage healthcare workers, patients do the best they can with the emotional and other resources they possess. Treatment is likely to be long term, so patience and a longitudinal perspective are required. • Set clear boundaries with the patient about acceptable and unacceptable behaviour. While setting boundaries in Case study 1 led the patient to disengage for a period of time, it would have been unprofessional and ultimately unhelpful for the paramedic to discuss his marital status and family life with the patient. • When in an appropriate setting consider debriefing with your colleague about the case so that any residual issues or concerns can be processed. Debriefing should allow you to approach each new situation with professionalism and a positive outlook, which is important when patients re-present often (Campbell & Farrell, 2009).
Posttraumatic stress disorder	Traumatic event is re-experienced (e.g. nightmares) Persistent avoidance of stimuli associated with the trauma Increased arousal (e.g. hypervigilance)	*Antidepressants* Zoloft (sertraline)	• While PTSD may not occur routinely in the field, paramedics should be aware of the signs of this disorder as the prevalence rate among emergency workers is thought to be 5–20% (Bennett et al., 2004). • If concerned about a colleague do not be afraid to approach them and air your concerns. The success of many PTSD treatments decreases over time, so early intervention is best.

continued

Table 52.1: Common mental illnesses encountered by paramedics—cont'd

Disorder	Symptoms	Common medications	Management
Dementia	Progressive decline over months to years Memory impairment Cognitive disturbances (e.g. aphasia)	*Cholinesterase inhibitors* Aricept (donepezil) Exelon (rivastigmine) Reminyl (galantamine)	• Promote a trusting and supportive relationship. This includes introducing yourself by name and identifying your role, establishing and maintaining eye contact, being respectful and empathetic, and using encouragement and praise where appropriate. • Minimise risk to the patient, self and carer. If a patient with dementia becomes aggressive, try to identify the trigger in their environment and separate the patient from the trigger. If the agitation has occurred in response to requests to do something, give them time and allow them to cool off before continuing. • Minimise disruption and dissipate stress or emotion. Wherever possible, avoid putting the patient in unfamiliar situations or situations where they have no control, as this may increase anxiety and therefore the likelihood of aggression. • Promote a person-centred model of care. Explain why you are there and your intentions, actions and motives. As an illustration, explain procedures before conducting them and ask for permission before you touch the patient, if possible. Actions such as the patient moving their arm to enable you to apply a blood pressure cuff provide implied consent. • Keep questions short and simple and identify with the emotions and actions being expressed. Even if the patient's words are garbled, their expressions of emotion should be easily read. • Ensure the patient's needs are met and the service outcome is person-led. Observe the patient's current needs and their environment, as this may provide information related to future case management. • Ensure the patient is left with a supportive and caring person. Encourage continuity of care by providing a thorough handover to hospital staff or caregivers and ensure that any handover is explained to the patient (CSHISC, 2011).

Delirium	Rapid onset over hours to days Decreased attention Altered conscious state Disorientation Rambling or nonsense speech Reversed sleep–wake cycle Hallucinations	Treatment as per underlying condition	• Identify medical condition associated with the delirium. Conditions include:
			  › central nervous system (e.g. head trauma, infection)
			  › metabolic causes (e.g. kidney failure, low blood sugar)
			  › cardiac and respiratory system (e.g. myocardial infarction, respiratory failure)
			  › systemic illness (e.g. tumour, postoperative state; Compton & Kotwicki, 2007).

In order to synthesise the available material common medications encountered by paramedics have been identified.

Key symptoms of a manic episode include high energy levels, irritability, grandiosity, racing thoughts, decreased sleep and increased engagement in pleasurable or risky activities (e.g. indiscriminate spending or sexual activity).

Psychosis is an umbrella term used to describe a group of conditions that are characterised by disturbances in thoughts, sensory perception, beliefs and understanding of the world around you and the associated behaviour. Psychosis involves a loss of contact with reality (Kuipers et al., 2014). The majority of patients with psychosis experience their first episode in adolescence or early adulthood. The lifetime risk of developing a psychotic disorder is difficult to calculate as it relies on individuals presenting to centres where the diagnosis can be made and, as with many mental illnesses, sufferers may actively avoid such services or be unable to access them for significant periods of time although unwell. While classed as a low-prevalence mental illness, accounting for around 3% of cases presenting to Australian specialised mental health services (Department of Health, 2010a), the severity and impact of psychotic disorders means that sufferers are likely to come into contact with the hospital sector when they are acutely unwell (Frost et al., 2002). Psychosis may be caused by illness such as schizophrenia, organic causes such as drug intoxication or metabolic causes such as diabetes (Queensland Ambulance Service, 2008). When someone is experiencing a psychotic episode for the first time, a definitive diagnosis may be difficult to identify, as diagnoses require observation and in some symptoms need to be prevalent for at least 1 month during a 6-month period (DSM-5).

Common symptoms of a psychotic disorder include hallucinations, delusions and formal thought disorder. A hallucination is defined as a sensory experience that occurs in the absence of any external stimuli (Davidson et al., 2004). Hallucinations may occur in one or more of the five senses (i.e. they may be visual, auditory, tactile, gustatory or olfactory in nature). Auditory hallucinations tend to be the most common followed by visual hallucinations. Delusions are firmly held beliefs despite evidence to the contrary. Formal thought disorder refers to problems in the organisation and interpretation of ideas, which can affect communication and make it challenging for others to understand. Other symptoms that may occur during a psychotic episode include flat or blunted affect, social withdrawal, changes in sleeping and eating patterns, and an absence of hygiene or personal grooming (Davidson et al., 2004)

Checking for adherence to medications is important in patients with psychosis, as non-adherence has been estimated to occur in between 40% and 50% of cases in those living with schizophrenia. The non-adherence to medications contributes to relapse and increases the need for and number of hospital admissions (Tessier et al., 2017; Awad, 2004; Battaglia, 2001), with symptom relapse being more severe compared with patients who maintain their medications as directed (Saba et al., 2007). Changes in routine and stresses such as job changes can precipitate non-compliance or trigger symptoms.

Borderline personality disorder (BPD) refers to a pervasive instability in mood, relationships, behaviour and self-image with a primary difficulty in regulating and understanding emotions. Individuals with this disorder fear abandonment and often experience chronic feelings of isolation and emptiness. Impulsiveness is commonly seen in this condition and may contribute to destructive behaviours such as self-harm and addictions (Polk & Mitchell, 2009). As a personality disorder, BPD is not formally diagnosed until the patient is 18 years of age or older, when personality is considered to be a more stable and developed entity. These traits and symptoms may, however, occur in younger individuals.

All patients with a diagnosed mental illness can have a relationship with health services in which they frequently access care on a crisis basis with little ongoing support. This is especially the case for patients with BPD and for this reason most patients will have an established multidisciplinary plan that outlines the expected response for all of the clinicians involved in their care. There is also a perception that the changes in behaviour associated with BPD can be interpreted as patients using the ambulance response to seek attention and that their presentation is not equivalent to those suffering a physical illness (see Box 52.3).

As our population grows older and a greater emphasis is placed on maintaining people in their own homes and providing care within the residential environment, paramedics are increasingly dealing with presentations involving dementia, delirium and older persons with complex care needs.

The term **delirium** refers to a change in cognition and consciousness that develops over a short period of time. Possible symptoms include an altered conscious state, decreased attention, a reversed sleep–wake cycle, disorientation, rambling or illogical speech, agitation and seeing things that do not exist (hallucinations). Delirium often has a clear cause which, if treated, can result in a reversal of symptoms (e.g. the classic urinary tract infection).

The term **dementia** describes the symptoms of a large group of illnesses that cause a progressive decline in a person's cognition, memory and general functioning (Community Services and Health Industry

BOX 52.3 Mental illness and ambulance misuse

The question of misuse of ambulance services by patients with mental illness has been raised (Roberts & Henderson, 2009). Local and international literature, however, suggests that ambulances are not being misused by these patients (Fry & Brunero, 2004; Larkin et al., 2006). An Australian study by Fry and Brunero (2004) reported that 42% of patients with a mental illness who presented to ED were brought in by ambulance, while 39% were transported by police. They also noted that this group had higher triage codes on average than other attending patients, suggesting a higher urgency for patients with mental illness.

An international study by Larkin and colleagues (2006) supports these findings, with mental health patients deemed as higher urgency and more likely to result in admission than the general patient population, suggesting that ambulance services were not misused by this group. The transport of patients with a mental illness is indeed an appropriate use of ambulance resources and ambulance paramedics are well-placed to support the needs of patients, their families and the community during a mental health crisis.

Skills Council [CSHISC], 2009). There are many different forms of dementia, each with its own cause. Alzheimer's disease is by far the most common cause of dementia, accounting for 50–70% of all cases (CSHISC, 2009). Dementia can occur at any age but is more common after the age of 65.

Law and mental health

Identifying the legal requirements for out-of-hospital treatment of mental health patients can be a challenging task. While mental health legislation exists in all states and territories within Australia and in New Zealand, the jurisdictions differ in terms of the criteria for involuntary treatment, recognised practitioners and requirements. For this reason it is important to understand the agreed universal principles of mental health treatment.

Universal requirements

The fundamental aim of mental health legislation is to protect, promote and improve the lives and mental wellbeing of citizens.

WHO (2005, p. 1)

Key rights outlined by the WHO include quality in treatment delivery, non-discrimination, the rights

to privacy and individual autonomy, freedom from inhumane and degrading treatment, the principle of the least-restrictive environment and the rights to information and participation in the treatment process (WHO, 2005). The World Medical Association (2006) states that compulsory treatment should be used only when medically necessary and for the shortest possible duration.

Australia and New Zealand

Mental health legislation differs across jurisdictions, but each is informed by the universal requirements described above and the Convention on the Rights of Persons with Disabilities (CRPD). In Australia, there has been a move towards uniformity with the creation of the National Mental Health Reform Strategy (Department of Health, 2011).

Voluntary versus involuntary

Our aim is to provide care in the least-restrictive manner possible and therefore our goal should be to facilitate mental health care on a 'voluntary' basis where the patient agrees to further assessment and treatment for their mental illness ('voluntary' or 'informal' patients) (Forrester & Griffiths, 2001). However, other individuals who are experiencing mental ill health and are not able to safely be left at home and have diminished capacity to be able to make decisions may require 'involuntary' treatment and transport by the ambulance service and the implementation of the relevant Mental Health Act. Such patients require admission for treatment of their mental illness to ensure their own safety or the safety of others but for whatever reason cannot or will not consent. Although specific guidelines for involuntary treatment differ, some common criteria include that the person appears to have a mental illness and immediate treatment is required and the person presents a risk of harm to self or others and the person requires admission to a mental health facility for treatment (Forrester & Griffiths, 2001).

The decision to enact an involuntary treatment order is clearly a serious one, as it involves the revocation of a person's right to consent. For this reason a number of checks are included within mental health legislation to ensure a fair and just process. These include a request for admission from a friend, carer or authorised person; review from a psychiatrist following admission; limitations to detention periods; an appeals process; and, in most jurisdictions, a formal review board to monitor cases and ensure compliance with relevant legislation.

Exclusions

According to the United Nations (2002), there are a number of exclusions to involuntary treatment. Grounds for which someone cannot be held include:

political, economic or social status; membership of a cultural, racial or religious group; family or professional conflict; non-conformity with moral, social, cultural or political values or religious beliefs prevailing in the person's community; or any other reason not directly related to mental health status.

Confidentiality

Maintaining patient confidentiality is of paramount importance. However, the legal system recognises that there are times when the directive to keep a patient's information confidential comes into direct conflict with the directive to maintain their safety. As an illustration, consider the case of an 88-year-old female who has attempted suicide following the death of her husband by taking a substantial overdose. Her daughter finds her in time and calls for an ambulance. During the assessment phase the patient confides that she intends to carry out her suicide plan once she is discharged home.

She forbids the health professional from disclosing the information to her daughter or anyone else, fearing that her daughter will be distressed and that doctors may attempt to intervene in her plan. Although this information might ordinarily be considered confidential, the risk the patient poses to herself is clear and immediate and therefore outweighs her rights to confidentiality. In this case, the health professional is likely to be permitted to disclose her plan to her doctors to ensure that she remains safe. Thus, rights to confidentiality may be mitigated by risk. For more specific information regarding confidentiality and consent in the case of mental illness and risk-specific behaviour, refer to the mental health legislation and/or health records legislation in your relevant jurisdiction.

The Mental State Assessment

The patient who presents with changes in behaviour poses a number of challenges with assessment and management in the out-of-hospital setting. Mental health assessment and treatment in the out-of-hospital setting is complex due to the broad nature of mental illness and the close association between mental health problems/mental illness and physical illness.

For patients with changes in behaviour it is impossible to completely separate assessment from management: from the moment paramedics commence communicating with these patients they will be simultaneously assessing, managing and even treating. In almost every case, however, paramedic management will include communication as a tool for intervention and verbal de-escalation.

The initial aim of assessment is to establish clinician and patient safety. This includes a scene assessment, observing the body language and interactions of those on the scene and, if circumstances allow, to obtain the patient's vital signs to systematically eliminate other physical (organic) causes for the changes in behaviour. Organic causes such as diabetes and other metabolic syndromes, hypoxia, hypotension, head injury, sepsis, intoxication, poisoning and cerebrovascular accident (CVA) can all present with changes in behaviour and should be considered and addressed if possible in the assessment and treatment of the patient. Diabetes, metabolic syndromes, cardiac issues and lowered life expectancy are all well documented co-occurring challenges for those living with mental illness. The physical effects from social isolation and/or the breakdown of support networks and relationships (e.g. malnutrition, dehydration and substance use) and the high incidence of homelessness often associated with mental illness are important when assessing the patient in the out-of-hospital setting. Assessment relies on careful history taking, skilful communication and the gathering of information from the person and others if the situation allows.

Faced with a patient who may not be able to provide an accurate history or the changes in behaviour are too discrete and not obvious the challenge for paramedics is to safely identify the symptoms of concern, differentiate between the various causes of changes in behaviour, facilitate person-centred care and provide immediate support and treatment. To do this the paramedic needs to actively listen, observe and communicate with empathy. Techniques such as emotion recognition and acknowledgment, paraphrasing and summarising and open and non-threatening speech and body language are all vital in the development of the therapeutic relationship.

Mental State Examination

The Mental State Examination (MSE) or Mental State Assessment is a systematic assessment of a patient's mental health or state of mind at any given point in time (Victorian Government Department of Health, 2008). This formalised process of observation and questioning ensures that clinicians do not miss symptoms of concern. While the MSE provides a vital clinical picture and handover information it is important to note that it should never be the sole basis for a diagnosis. Different versions of the MSE exist but cover the following domains: behaviour and appearance, affect and mood, perception, thought flow and thought content, conversation and speech, orientation and cognition, insight and judgment with particular interest in how the person is interacting with you and their environment (Table 52.2).

Table 52.2: Mental State Examination categories and features

Category	Features
Appearance	Age (reference to what extent the person appears stated age) Gender Mode of dress (Appropriate for weather and context?) Level of hygiene and self-care Build, physical condition and nutritional status Physical changes and abnormalities Posture and gait Facial expressions Piercings and tattoos
Behaviour	Eye contact (Is it maintained, do they engage and does It match circumstance?) Activity level or psychomotor retardation or agitation (e.g. decreased or increased movement, pacing, disorganised or aimless movements, repetitive movements and mannerisms) Posture and gait Mannerisms and expressive gestures (e.g. hand wringing, grimacing, tics) Engagement with interviewer and how they are interacting with their environment and others Extrapyramidal symptoms
Speech	Rate (rapid or slowed?) Volume and pitch Quantity (How much speech is being produced? Does it seem inappropriate or pressured?) and cadence and tone
Mood	Patient's self-reported emotional state
Affect	Patient's observed emotional state Congruence (any incongruence between the patient's affect and their reported mood should be noted; e.g. patient reports feeling 'great' but presents as extremely depressed)
Thought form	Logical (Are the patient's responses logical?) Goal-directed (Does the patient answer the questions asked?) If not, there may be a disruption of logical connections between ideas including circumstantiality (talking around the point) and tangentiality (going off the point, but links between ideas are evident) In more severe cases patients may present with a formal thought disorder (e.g. flight of ideas, perseveration, word salad, echolalia, clang associations)
Thought content	Delusions are firmly held beliefs despite evidence to the contrary; commonly encountered delusions include: • paranoid delusions (e.g. thoughts that others are watching them) • grandiose delusions (e.g. belief that patient is invincible) • delusions of reference (e.g. thoughts that the newsreader is speaking directly to them) • thought insertion (e.g. concerns that the paramedic or others are putting ideas into their head) • thought withdrawal (e.g. concerns that paramedic is taking away their thoughts) Obsessions (thoughts) or compulsions (actions) Suicidal ideation or deliberate self-harm is included in this section but also forms an integral part of risk assessment
Perception	Hallucinations (changes in sensory perception and may be auditory, visual, tactile, olfactory or gustatory)
Concentration	Organised (i.e. focused) or easily distracted Memory (if concerns with short- or long-term memory are apparent in the basic assessment, note this down) Insight (Does the patient have insight into their condition and their current environment and situation?) Orientation (identifying orientation to time, who they are and where they are is a good start) Concentration (Can the patient concentrate during the assessment?) Judgment (Is the patient able to make sensible decisions regarding their own mental health, safety and other daily events?)

It is important to note that the MSE is a standard assessment tool useful for patients with varying presentations, not just those presenting with a mental illness. While the MSE focuses exclusively on the patient's mental state, it is a part of an overall clinical assessment which include the person's physical observations, broader social and personal support networks, help-seeking behaviours, living environment (e.g. cleanliness, order, indication of ability to attend to daily living skills), sleeping patterns and appetite and should be included as a part of the clinical handover.

While paramedics do not engage in formal mental health diagnoses they do engage in the development of a clinical formulation to allow for a working diagnosis so that out-of-hospital treatment and service can be initiated. To make a clinical decision, even if it is to transport, paramedics must be able to perform a basic differential diagnostic process in order to identify the most appropriate treatment for the patient. You should therefore be able to identify whether the likely cause is a mental illness and, if so, what group of disorders is most likely (e.g. psychotic disorder versus anxiety disorder). The term 'diagnosis' is used within this context as a working hypothesis with the understanding that it is in no way final or definitive.

Ask!
- What is bothering you the most today?
- What is your previous medical history?
- [To bystanders] Exactly what behaviour did you observe?

Look for!
- Signs of an organic cause for abnormal behaviour
- An elevated temperature
- Abnormalities in pulse, blood pressure and respiratory rate
- Blood glucose level
- Sympathetic response giving pale, clammy skin and dilated pupils
- Signs of drug use

CASE STUDY 1

Case 14934, 0954 hrs.

Dispatch details: A 19-year-old female short of breath and in an altered conscious state in a stairway at her university.

Initial presentation: The paramedics arrive to find a frail, young-looking woman who is visibly distressed and hyperventilating.

1 ASSESS

The approach to this patient, a young female university student, should take into account her current vulnerability, social circumstance and age. Assuming no direct danger from the scene, the paramedics must ensure the patient feels safe for them to approach and take into account that this could be an assault or other trauma-related circumstance. Therefore, communication needs to be tailored accordingly. Approaching with relaxed body language, non-threatening position, tone of voice and empathy is vital to creating an effective patient rapport and therapeutic relationship, which often creates a feeling of safety in the patient allowing more effective history taking and sharing of their story. It is possible to maintain a relaxed posture while still keeping an eye on the safety of the situation. Patients with disturbed behaviour are rarely a threat to paramedic safety if they are handled with respect and sympathy. If preliminary observations of the scene and the patient suggest the presence of agitation or aggression that could threaten paramedic safety, modifications to the approach, assessment and treatment of the patient will need to be made to ensure everyone's safety (see Chapter 53). In this case, the observed behaviour is not threatening which allows paramedics to establish a set of baseline vital sign observations

Gaining baseline observations (vital sign observations and initial observations of her behaviour, posture and interaction) will assist in differentiating between physical concerns which may be related to her current presentation, such as infection or injury, an acute stress response and/or mental illness such as anxiety or posttraumatic stress. Adequately setting up rapport with the patient and gaining baseline observations aids paramedics in formulating a diagnosis and management pathway, but also meet the expectations of the patient and can quickly gain their confidence and trust. This can be extremely useful when it comes time to ask more delicate details regarding the patient's social and mental health history, such as if there is a history of panic attacks or family history of anxiety or depression. It may also serve to distract the patient, resulting in a decline of her sympathetic nervous response.

Vital signs

Provided it is safe to do so and meets clinical assessment needs, obtaining the patient's vital signs and your initial observations of behaviour, scene and social context is a good starting point. While obtaining a full set of respiratory and perfusion observations, closely observe the patient's behaviour and start to include these factors in the assessment. Questions at this stage can focus on excluding physical causes such as a recent fall, illness or history of metabolic disorders such as thyroid disease or diabetes.

Mental State Examination

Table 52.3 provides an overview of the systematic way the Mental State Examination can describe and outline the patient's mental state from Case study 1.

Table 52.3: Example Mental State Examination

	Presentation	Interpretation
Appearance	This patient is of slim build and is dressed in neat casual clothing. Her hair is slightly dishevelled and with very pale appearance around her face and arms. Facial expression is distressed with tears running down her cheeks and widened eyes. Her self-care and grooming appear to be well attended to.	Her appearance suggests that being overweight is not a factor in her breathing difficulties. As her dress and hygiene are well attended to, the dishevelled nature of her appearance provides a contrast of note. Distress may occur in many instances when an ambulance is called, providing little input for differential diagnosis.
Behaviour	The patient's body appears to be heaving as if she is struggling for breath and she is visibly trembling. Her breathing rate slows during assessment and her trembling diminishes. Her eye contact is initially very limited but this also improves as rapport develops. No tics or unusual motor movements are observed. She is engaged throughout.	Note heaving breaths despite clear breath sounds. As she does not have a temperature, the trembling may provide a clue suggestive of anxiety or adrenaline release. This is consistent with limited eye contact on first meeting, which may or may not be present in patients with asthma, but is very common in those with anxiety.
Speech	The patient's voice is barely audible at times during the assessment. She shows no signs of pressured speech and her conversation is limited but coherent. Her quantity of speech is limited when she feels short of breath, but improves during assessment.	The improvement in speech and breathing rate is important, as no formal physiological treatment has yet been offered, suggesting that the physiological difficulty has resolved itself. The soft tone may be due to lack of breath but is also common in patients with anxiety.
Mood	She self-reports that she feels 'stressed out' and 'worried'.	This report is likely to be consistent for most patients who call an ambulance and thus offers few diagnostic clues. It would be worthwhile noting whether her response appears exaggerated compared with other patients or is consistent with current external stressors.

Table 52.3: Example Mental State Examination—cont'd

	Presentation	Interpretation
Affect	She appears to be visibly distressed and anxious during the assessment. Her mood and affect are congruent.	This patient's distress makes some psychiatric conditions, such as mania, less likely, but increases the likelihood of anxiety or depression.
Thought form	When able to respond, her answers are logical, with no disruptions to thought flow and content. She can follow a train of thought and remains on topic.	Clarity in thought form makes head injury, intoxication and more specific psychiatric conditions such as psychosis less likely. It is, however, consistent with anxiety.
Thought content	She identifies a number of stressors, including her final law exams, uncertainty regarding future career choices and whether she actually wants to pursue law, and a relationship breakdown. She denies any suicidal ideation or deliberate self-harm. While she is concerned about the possibility of a heart attack, her ideas are not fixed and are not of a delusional quality. Nil obsessions or compulsions noted.	This information is vital for treatment as it speaks to her risk of harm. To adequately assess for risk, seek further information about help-seeking, whether she has experienced these feelings before, what internal and external resources she has and can she access them. She also identifies a number of psychosocial stressors that are current, appear overwhelming and are likely to be enhanced when she is on campus. These stressors could have precipitated an anxiety-related event.
Perception	Nil perceptual disturbance reported. No mannerisms consistent with perceptual disturbance. She recognises that although she may consider leaving study that this is not the end of her ability to find a career and she has other skills.	The absence of perceptual disturbance makes some forms of trauma, intoxication and more specific psychiatric conditions such as psychosis less likely. It is, however, consistent with anxiety. Her recognition of her own strengths is also crucial to understanding her view of herself and the current circumstances. The ability to have a more positive perception of self tends to suggest depression and risk of harm is less likely.
Concentration	She is easily distracted by onlookers during the assessment. While she is oriented to time, person and place, she has limited insight into the cause of her presentation, believing that she is having a heart attack.	This aspect of the assessment provides vital clues for this patient's treatment. As she appears distracted by onlookers (and distressed as per affect), all efforts should be made to remove the crowd or the patient. Her belief that she is having a serious medical event may also heighten her distress and thus should be addressed via education; for example, 'Our assessment indicates that you are not having a heart attack but may be experiencing X, Y, Z …'

Risk assessment

Initially the risk assessment aims to identify the risk the patient poses to the paramedic (harm to others) and to themselves (deliberate or accidental self-harm), which suggests paramedics need to be capable of performing a basic risk assessment to ensure their own safety and that of their patients. Although a basic risk assessment focuses on the physical risk of harm, other important considerations add to our understanding and clinical decisions regarding risk. The patient's level of engagement, presence of alcohol or drug use, personal and external resources, access to those resources, support networks and help-seeking behaviour, past medical history of mental illness, and individual capacity are also key areas to history taking and risk assessment.

It may be argued that paramedics are not mental health professionals and as such should not have to perform a risk assessment. To counter this argument increasingly paramedics are being asked to make clinical decisions around referral pathways and whether the person needs hospital management (hospital avoidance); therefore, they are expected to be able to assess and make clinical judgments which includes when attending those with mental illness. Recent data also shows that paramedics are attending cases that are more primary mental healthcare focused and so they may not transport the patient to hospital and should be familiar with a basic risk assessment. In some circumstances the patient may well meet the criteria for involuntary admission on the grounds of their risk. If a risk assessment is not completed, this option will not be available and the patient may have a poorer outcome than if a good assessment had been done. Follow-up, transport and access to some form of definitive assessment and care is the best option to ensure patient safety and fulfil the paramedic's duty of care.

Types of risk

Harm to others

In the out-of-hospital environment it is essential for paramedics to check for dangers prior to and when entering any scene. Being able to assess the potential for harm from the environment, patient or a third party is crucial to maintaining your own safety and the safety of others. Key to assessing risk is the ability to recognise changes in body language, speech and tone of voice and the interaction between yourself and the patient and others at the scene.

Accidental self-harm

Accidental self-harm refers to unintended harm that may come to a patient as a result of their mental state. Individuals with thought disturbance, perceptual disturbance(s) and/or active delusions may be considered to be at greater risk of accidental self-harm. Accidental self-harm can be assessed as a part of a formal MSE, most notably in the areas of judgment and insight.

Deliberate self-harm

Deliberate self-harm encompasses a spectrum of behaviour from minor self-inflicted injury to more serious suicide attempts. If adequate rapport has been established between patient and paramedic, acts of deliberate self-harm or intent will generally be disclosed in step 1 in the model below. In some instances, however, previous self-harm or intent may not be as overt. In these instances the paramedic may need to ask the patient directly.

The four-stage model

The different forms of risk can be assessed using the following four-stage model (see Fig 52.2). To illustrate application of the model, a patient with suicidal intent is considered here (see also Case study 2 in this chapter).

- *Step 1: Plan.* When considering this aspect of the risk assessment you are interested in whether the patient has plans to complete suicide. This is best identified by asking the question directly. If the patient does identify a desire to commit harm, you need to ask further information about their plan, as a more defined plan may be suggestive of a higher degree of risk of actually going through with the intention. Here it is also important to understand the person's perception and if they view suicide as the only solution to their current situation, what supports they have and do they feel they can use those supports, and to consider and ask what has changed or precipitated these feelings. Depending on the answers to these, the risk of suicide may be higher and protective factors may be limited.
- *Step 2: Means and lethality.* Once the patient's plan has been identified, you need to establish whether the patient has access to the means required

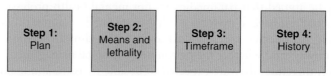

Figure 52.2
The four stages of risk assessment.

to carry out their plan and how likely those means are to be lethal. For example, a patient may have a clearly defined plan to shoot themselves but may not own a gun or have access to any firearms, whereas a patient who has access to the means is likely to be at increased risk. This element of the assessment may also be important to ensure your own safety.

- *Step 3: Timeframe.* Establishing the intended timing of the attempt is also important. A clear and in many cases shorter timeframe may increase the risk or indicate how long you have to manage the situation. Some patients make plans to self-harm or commit suicide on the anniversary of a significant event (e.g. the death of a partner). It is important to identify these patients and ensure the details are clearly documented and communicated at handover, because although the patient's immediate risk may be lower, their future risk may be increased and they may need additional support at that time.
- *Step 4: History.* The patient's history may reflect other risk factors that are important in determining your immediate treatment plan. Other factors may be important in determining a patient's risk of harm or suicide and research suggests that the risk factors in Box 52.4 should be considered.

Legal status

Assessing the patient's legal status is important at this point, as it may determine specific treatment options. The paramedic should determine whether the patient is being treated involuntarily (under a form of community treatment order) for a mental illness or, if they are not, whether they require and are eligible for this form of treatment. This patient does not appear to be a risk to herself or others, she has no clear history of mental illness and does not appear to require inpatient treatment for a mental illness. As such, the paramedics need to (and should be able to) treat her as a voluntary patient.

BOX 52.4 Risk factors for suicide

History
A history of past suicide attempts or having a loved one who has completed suicide may increase risk (Hirschfeld & Davidson, 1998).

Age
The ABS indicates that 30–34 year olds are statistically more likely to complete suicide (ABS, 2002). While the rate of suicide completion among adolescents aged 15–19 years is not as high as for other groups, suicide is the second highest cause of death in this age group after motor vehicle crashes (ABS, 2002).

Gender
Males are more likely to complete suicide, while females have a higher recorded rate of suicide attempts (Hirschfeld & Davidson, 1998). This difference is not necessarily due to the intent of the patient, but rather the means selected.

Depression
Depression has been linked to suicide. Paramedics should take note of patients who have been severely depressed and recently experienced an improvement in their mood. In some individuals this mood shift can be attributed to feelings of relief as they have made a decision to end their life, thus in their mind addressing their concerns. Severely depressed individuals may lack the energy and planning required to action suicidal feelings, but an improvement in their symptoms provides room for them to consider the idea further (Cheng et al., 2000; Hirschfeld & Davidson, 1998).

Alcohol/drug use
Substance use lowers inhibitions and may therefore increase risk (Cheng et al., 2000; Hirschfeld & Davidson, 1998).

Social support
Social support may be viewed as a protective feature in the person's history, whereas a lack thereof may increase risk (Australian Government, 2012).

Chronic illness
Patients with a chronic illness are more likely to commit suicide (Hirschfeld & Davidson, 1998).

Initial assessment summary

Problem	Chest pain and short of breath
Conscious state	GCS = 15 (despite reports of an altered conscious state)
Position	Sitting
Heart rate	112 bpm
Blood pressure	110/80 mmHg
Skin appearance	Pink, warm, dry
Speech pattern	Speaks in short sentences
Respiratory rate	28 bpm
Respiratory rhythm	Even cycles
Chest auscultation	Clear air entry
Pulse oximetry	99% on room air
Temperature	37.1°C
Pain	4/10
History	She was climbing the stairs when she began to feel dizzy and faint. Her hands began to shake and she became increasingly nauseated. She felt that her heart was going to burst from her chest and was worried something was 'seriously wrong' with her. She tried to finish climbing the stairs to remove herself from public view but she almost collapsed trying and so remained on the stairwell. She says that this is the first time she has had these symptoms. She cannot identify any medical issues that might have contributed to her presentation. She has a past history of asthma.

If we consider this case with regard to both the biomedical and the biopsychosocial models, even in the absence of a significant underlying cause such as supraventricular tachycardia, the biomedical model can explain some of this patient's symptoms (e.g. tetany in the hands and palpitations), but it cannot explain why her emotional state ultimately produced these physical symptoms. In this case study social stressors (recent exams and limited social support) brought on biological changes (increased heart rate, increased respiration rate). Her psychological interpretation of the events (thoughts that she was seriously ill and that her symptoms were harmful) increased her anxiety, resulting in a progression of her physiological symptoms. This case illustrates the manner in which social, biological and psychological factors can interact, resulting in mental health concerns.

② CONFIRM

The essential part of the clinical reasoning process is to seek to confirm your initial hypothesis by finding clinical signs that should occur with your provisional diagnosis. You should also seek to challenge your diagnosis by exploring findings that do not fit your hypothesis: don't just ignore them because they don't fit.

What else could it be?
Organic

Assessment of the patient's perfusion status, including an electrocardiograph (ECG), should rule out hypotension as a cause of an altered conscious state. Accurate assessment of the ECG will exclude paroxysmal supraventricular tachycardia (see Chapter 23) as an underlying cause of her elevated heart rate. Chest auscultation which indicates equal and adequate air entry to the lungs will tend to exclude a respiratory cause such as hypoxia and asthma for her presentation and this should correlate with normal oxygen saturation (SpO_2) readings. In this context the signs of hypocarbia (tetany) are consistent with the elevated respiratory rate. A neurological exam should rule out CVA and seizure.

DIFFERENTIAL DIAGNOSIS

Mental illness
Or
- Organic (e.g. cerebral hypoxia, hypotension, head injury, CVA, infection [especially encephalitis, meningitis], arrhythmias leading to hypotension)
- Metabolic (e.g. hypoglycaemia, hyperglycaemia, electrolyte imbalances, renal failure, liver failure)
- Intoxicants (e.g. alcohol, stimulants, hallucinogenics)
- Other cause (e.g. reactive anger/aggression, exposure to a traumatic scene)

Metabolic

A blood glucose reading (BGL) greater than 3.5–4 mmol and an enquiry as to a history of diabetes or other metabolic disorders should exclude this group of physical causes. Although infection can cause changes in behaviour, the infection needs to be severe and it is not likely to occur with normal vital signs and without a significant fever. A normal tympanic temperature will exclude an infectious cause severe enough to lead to altered behaviour in a young person. Similarly, disorders causing electrolyte imbalances sufficient to cause abnormal behaviour may also create abnormal vital signs. In this case the pulse is elevated but the blood pressure, temperature and BGL are within normal limits. The ECG reveals no arrhythmia.

Intoxicants

By now the patient has seen the paramedics perform a number of tests that have produced objective (and within normal range) results and should be gaining a degree of trust in their assessment. This is an opportune time to enquire if they could be suffering from alcohol or drug effects. But rather than ask these confronting (and accusational) questions directly, explore the more normal aspects of the patient's dietary intake first. 'Have you had breakfast today?' is an innocent question that opens the line of enquiry. 'Have you taken any medication today?' followed by 'Are there any medications you have missed taking today?' can add to the information gathered. At this point enquiries about alcohol can seem routine and far less judgmental. The patient denies any drug or alcohol use.

Other cause

After all of these factors have been ruled out, the paramedic can begin to enquire about events immediately prior to the onset of symptoms. Remember, effective patient care uses the patient to assist. Ask the patient whether they can identify anything that may have triggered this change. If sufficient rapport has been built with the patient by this time and a thorough physical assessment has reassured the patient that the illness is not physical, you may be surprised by the honesty of their answer. The patient cannot offer a trigger for the current episode.

Given the above has excluded physical causes of this patient's presentation, it leaves a working diagnosis of anxiety with links to either panic attacks or panic disorder to generalised anxiety disorder.

③ TREAT

Despite the frequency and severity of cases of mental illness, these conditions do not fit easily into the minds or practice of many paramedics. This may be because mental illness rarely requires the administration of medication by paramedics. Like most other conditions, however, there is a well-structured treatment plan that will suit most situations (see Fig 52.3).

Emergency management

Communicate

Establishing good rapport is essential from the outset of treatment. Rapport is facilitated by the warmth of your approach, attempts to understand the patient's position and maintaining respect for the patient. The use of active listening, paraphrasing, emotion recognition and summarising are essential skills during communication. These skills are particularly important for patients displaying changes in behaviour who may have been laughed at, stared at or dismissed in the past. These experiences often make the patient more sensitive to perceived criticism, making appropriate communication a vital part of treatment and an intervention in itself.

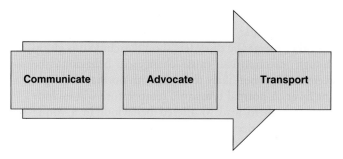

Figure 52.3
For paramedics, managing mental illness is challenging because it does not fit the normal clinical approach. Instead, these cases can be sequenced as communicate, advocate and transport.

Out-of-hospital care is filled with significant pressures, the most obvious being quick and efficient treatment and transport of patients. As a paramedic you must balance these pressures with the need to engage patients for not only the patient's benefit but for clinical management. A loss of engagement may result in treatment refusal or an escalation in emotional and physical distress, which result in poorer patient outcomes and are often more time-consuming. Patients will feel dismissed and disempowered and recognise and react to a rushed or disorganised assessment; remember you are there to provide a service and excellent clinical care.

In this patient's case, the treating paramedic should keep their voice low, their tone reassuring and their manner calm. It may be helpful to coach the patient through some deep-breathing exercises, which will serve the dual purpose of distraction and symptom management.

Advocate

In some instances the paramedic may be required to advocate for a patient, ensuring that they receive the best possible treatment in the least-restrictive manner. Individuals presenting with changes in behaviour often attract an audience and you may be required to clear the scene to ensure that the patient's privacy and dignity are maintained. If the patient has close support networks present such as friends and family which are providing a sense of safety you will want to maximise their presence and support. Paramedics may also need to advocate to other professionals, such as the police, to ensure that the patient's needs are adequately met. In this case the paramedics may need to clear the scene to minimise distress caused by bystanders.

Transport

Transportation not only enables access to mental health care but also can be considered a point of care provision itself (Department of Health, 2011). While the transport protocols between police, mental health services and ambulance services may vary across jurisdictions, ambulance services are generally considered to hold primary responsibility for the transport of people with a mental illness. Paramedics have a vital role if the person is too ill to be transported by mental health clinical staff alone (Department of Health, 2011), have other medical illness or other physical conditions which require management or require sedation or restraint. If they are agitated or have engaged in criminal activity, the police may be the most appropriate form of transport (Department of Health, 2010b; Health Department of Western Australia, 2012; Queensland Ambulance Service, 2012). Patients may favour an ambulance over a police vehicle as it could be viewed as less stigmatising and in many cases more appropriate, as paramedics have more training in mental health care compared with their police counterparts. As this patient has agreed to transport, is not an involuntary patient and is not aggressive, the primary transport choice is an ambulance. If other referral pathways are available such as follow-up with mental health teams, GP or through consultation with mental health triage, this patient may be able to be provided care by other means.

Sedation

The question of sedation to facilitate transport of patients with mental illness is often raised. In the vast majority of cases sedation is not necessary. With effective communication most patients will feel listened to and engage with paramedics and agree to transport if required, although the length of time to gain their consent may vary. In some cases, however, paramedics will be faced with agitated patients (who may or may not have a mental illness) who require a different approach. The sedation guidelines used in Australia and New Zealand were devised with this group in mind. Primary considerations for these patients include the availability and appropriateness of less-restrictive options such as verbal de-escalation: the need for early backup or support from other agencies (e.g. police or mental health teams), the provisions under local mental health legislation and the scope of practice of the clinician which vary across jurisdictions. Guidelines for safe sedation are described in local jurisdictional guidelines.

④ EVALUATE

The aim of the evaluation phase is to ensure that the selected intervention is appropriate. This may be assessed by considering the following.

- *Is the intervention working?* The treatment outcomes in the case of mental illness are as varied as the illnesses themselves. In some cases you will see a decrease in concerning symptoms, while in others there may be no apparent change in symptom severity. At the very least, you can assist the patient by building strong rapport and a collaborative and therapeutic relationship.
- *Is the patient safe?* Ensuring your safety and the patient's is of paramount importance. Safety should be considered from the outset, but you should also re-evaluate the scene and the patient's status throughout the intervention period.
- *Has the patient consented to transport or appropriate follow-up?* With appropriate communication and support most patients consent to transport or connection with further services. If the patient refuses transport but requires an urgent psychiatric assessment, you may need to reconsider your choice and communicate in a more direct but respectful manner. Highlight the need for transport and your concerns for the patient and consider offering limited options; for example, 'I am quite worried about the possibility of your harming yourself and, as such, I cannot leave you at home. I have a duty of care to ensure that you are transported to hospital but you do have a choice regarding your transport. You can travel in the ambulance or I can call the (police/community mental health team, etc.) and ask them to transport you. Which would you prefer?' If the patient continues to deteriorate, you may need to reconsider your initial diagnosis or communication strategies. Have you effectively eliminated physical causes? Can you approach the patient in a different manner or can your partner approach the patient?

In this patient's case, the paramedics would expect to see a change in her sympathetic activation (e.g. decrease in heart rate, improved respiratory rate) as a result of their intervention.

Specific treatment guidelines

Table 52.1 earlier in this chapter provides an overview of common mental illnesses encountered in paramedic practice and their associated symptoms, medications and specific management strategies.

Investigations

Hospital staff will again screen for and eliminate organic causes. Once this screening has been completed and a psychiatric cause is considered more likely, a psychiatric consultant will be called and a determination made regarding the next course of treatment.

Hospital admission

Modern psychiatric inpatient treatment is considered to be short-term and intensive intervention to minimise risk and manage symptoms. Care is provided 24 hours a day by a multidisciplinary team of professionals including psychiatrists, psychologists, mental health nurses, social workers and occupational therapists. Treatment is tailored to the needs of the individual, but is likely to include a medication review, short-term psychological treatment and family support. Inpatient wards also run comprehensive activity programs such as cooking, problem-solving groups and art therapy. Occasionally, treatment will be delayed in favour of observation if the patient's diagnosis or symptom profile is unclear. Admission to a short-stay ward may be required for some intensive treatments, such as electroconvulsive therapy.

Long-term treatment and impacts

Patients are generally discharged to a community mental health service for follow-up. A case manager will be allocated and a longer-term treatment plan devised. The case manager links the patient's mental health supports together, ensuring continuity of care, to monitor the patient's mental state on an ongoing basis and to evaluate their progress over time (Victorian Government Department of Health, 2008). The course of a mental illness varies according to the individual, their diagnosis and the supports available. While some patients require only one hospital admission, others will have regular involvement with mental health and emergency services. With support and appropriate intervention, recovery from a mental illness is possible.

CASE STUDY 2

Case 09755, 1423 hrs.

Dispatch details: A 29-year-old male complaining of back pain.

Initial presentation: The paramedics arrive at a farm that is relatively isolated. A dishevelled male walks slowly to the door to allow them to enter.

 ASSESS

1434 hrs Primary survey: The patient is conscious and talking.

1435 hrs Chief complaint: He has lower back pain.

1437 hrs Vital signs survey: Perfusion status: HR 68 bpm, BP 120/70 mmHg, skin pink and dry.
Respiratory status: RR 16 bpm, good clear air entry bilaterally.
Conscious state: GCS = 15.

1441 hrs Pertinent hx: The patient says he has had lower back pain for the past 3 months but it has become so bad that it is almost impossible to sleep. As a result he is constantly lethargic, which is a concern given the physically taxing nature of farm work. He is not maintaining and only engaging in limited eye contact and his voice is flat and sounds detached. He appears drawn, tired and has obviously lost weight, based on his loose clothing.

The paramedics are aware that flooding 8 months ago had a significant impact on local farmers, resulting in a loss of stock and, for many, significant financial strain. When asked if he has people to assist him with heavy lifting on the farm, the patient says that he had to let most of his farm hands go, though one remains. This placed a significant burden on him and the stress led to conflict with his wife and a subsequent separation almost 4 months ago.

1444 hrs Secondary survey: There is no specific tenderness to his lower back and his range of movement does not appear particularly limited.

Although this patient presents with a clear physical complaint (back pain), strict adherence to this complaint during the assessment period without consideration of his flat affect, monotone speech and limited eye contact may limit the history taking solely to his pain and possible mechanisms of injury. Without prompting he may not disclose his stressors or his risk. It is also worth considering at this point that often chronic pain or disability result in or occur in conjunction with anxiety and depression.

② CONFIRM

In many cases paramedics are presented with a collection of signs and symptoms that do not appear to describe a particular condition. A critical step in determining a treatment plan in this situation is to consider what other conditions could explain the patient's presentation.

What else could it be?
Chronic musculoskeletal back pain
The lack of any tender areas in the patient's back and the relatively normal range of movement would seem to exclude chronic musculoskeletal back pain and a range of inflammatory arthritis and myositis conditions.

Occult malignancy
Weight loss could be a sign of occult malignancy or diabetes. Lack of any symptoms associated with malignancy makes this less likely but this is still a diagnosis that has to be considered in the background during his hospital investigation.

Hyperglycaemia (diabetes)
The weight loss could be caused by prolonged hyperglycaemia but little else fits this clinical picture. The normal blood sugar and lack of any history of urinary frequency and excessive thirst effectively exclude diabetes.

Hypothyroidism
The early symptoms of hypothyroidism include fatigue, joint pain and depression but the disease is generally associated with weight gain, not loss. The patient does not report any increased sensitivity to cold or change to his hair and nails. This does not fit the clinical picture but it should be investigated at hospital.

Intracranial tumour
Intracranial tumour can present with a mood disorder although it would be unusual to have no other focal signs or symptoms evident. This diagnosis cannot be excluded at this stage.

Undisclosed problem with alcohol/drugs of addiction
An undisclosed problem with alcohol or drugs of addiction could present with a depressed mood and weight loss, although it is likely that history or evidence of the problem would have occurred in the evaluation thus far. When asked

---

PRACTICE TIP

Psychomotor retardation or a slowing of cognitive processing may occur in individuals during a major depressive episode. In such individuals it is important to limit external stimuli during assessment, which may be taxing on concentration. It is also important to make questions clear and concise, and allow time for the individual to respond. Be patient.

DIFFERENTIAL DIAGNOSIS

Clinical depression
Or
- Chronic musculoskeletal back pain
- Occult malignancy
- Hyperglycaemia (diabetes)
- Hypothyroidism
- Intracranial tumour
- Undisclosed problem with alcohol/drugs of addiction

direct (but not threatening) questions regarding his alcohol/drug use, the patient denies any issues. It should be noted that admission to drug and alcohol use or an addiction doesn't actually preclude depression and mood disorders as a diagnosis in the field and should not change the management of this patient.

In the absence of any physical factors and applying the patient's history and presentation to the MSE, clinical depression appears as a strong factor in his decision to request help for his back pain. Further assessment by health specialists will be needed to exclude other possibilities.

③ TREAT

With a provisional diagnosis of depression and considering this patient's setting of isolation and ongoing stress it is essential that this patient is engaged with the wider health system and paramedics are perfectly placed to do this. Recognising the need for support and further assessment any discussion around mental health and depression should be done openly and honestly with the patient. A frank acknowledgment that his current circumstances are difficult and challenging and having difficulty coping would not be unexpected opens the line of communication for him to talk and discuss what is occurring for him and how he feels about it. An inexperienced paramedic might use the 'need to investigate' his back pain as a way to encourage the patient to agree to transport to hospital. However, during his hospital assessment it will quickly become obvious that the paramedics have lied and this may make him less likely to seek treatment in the future. Open, honest and empathetic exploration of his condition will not only align the patient and crew's expectations of what should occur, but will also provide more information for the paramedics to make an informed decision regarding treatment options. At this point a risk assessment should be conducted, and this can be done using the four-stage model presented earlier in the chapter.

1447 hrs: The paramedics complete a risk assessment for the patient as follows:

Plan: The patient indicates that he has contemplated suicide. The paramedics ask for further information regarding his plan. He details the plan, noting that he has gone so far as to write a goodbye note to his family.

Means: The patient admits that he has access to firearms, his chosen method, indicating a high degree of risk.

Timeframe: He indicates that he will wait until after his daughter's birthday next week, as he does not want her to be sad on her birthday.

History: He denies any past suicide attempts, but advises that his paternal grandfather committed suicide when he was 45.

Based on the risk assessment, this patient is a very high risk of suicide. He is actively depressed, with a number of current social and personal stressors; he also has a clearly defined plan, access to the means and a timeframe; as well as a family link to suicide. Broader considerations which also identify high risk are that he appears to have diminished resources (both internal and external) with reduced capacity to cope plus physical, social and family isolation. It is key to note, however, that he has a clear protective factor regarding his daughter and that relationship might be able to be used as a recognition of strength and life purpose (e.g. 'Tell me about your daughter. You said her birthday is next week and you want her to enjoy the day.'). This provides an opening to understand his current circumstances, the nature of his relationships and what support he sees as possible and existing.

He clearly needs urgent assessment, care and safety within the mental health and hospital system. From an out-of-hospital perspective, the objectives of care are to provide: a safe space for the patient to feel listened to and not

BOX 52.5 General advice in cases of suicide risk

- Secure the environment and remove any unwanted distractions or stressors (this may include loved ones). Remove any accessible means of harm.
- Do not leave the person alone.
- Listen to the person's story and try to identify the factors that led to an increase in risk at that specific point in time.
- Many suicidal patients feel ambivalent about their desire to die or feel that they have no other option. Acknowledge the patient's feelings and identify protective factors (i.e. reasons they have not acted on their plans or reasons to live). Do not try to talk the patient out of their feelings as they will feel ignored and possibly more helpless.
- Be empathetic. While some clinicians may view suicide as pointless or selfish, expressing these views is unprofessional and unlikely to be helpful to the patient.
- Encourage access to definitive treatment. If the patient is reluctant, explore legal options such as an involuntary status. The specifics of this option will vary depending on the local jurisdiction.
- If all attempts fail and the person acts on their plans, seek immediate support and debriefing. Suicide can be very distressing and it is important that you take care of yourself.

judged; therapeutic communication which acknowledges his emotions and also his strengths; and transport in a safe and supportive manner (see Box 52.5). As his risk of self-harm is quite high, it is essential that he is informed and understands that this information will be handed over at hospital so that he can receive the most appropriate support possible.

As he contacted the ambulance service, provided he is supported sensitively and with empathy, it is likely that he will agree to further support and mental health care which begins with his transport. The main aim is to facilitate this transport in the most dignified and least-restrictive way while continuing to communicate with and assess him. If the paramedics have established a therapeutic rapport they will be well-placed to deliver a comprehensive handover, including the patient in the process to ensure that they feel empowered and in line with person-centred care.

As a last resort, if the patient is reluctant to be transported and unwilling to receive further care the paramedics may need to use their legal powers under mental health legislation to force transport. They may need to consider administering a chemical restraint to help reduce the level of distress and trauma for the patient, but this should only be used if absolutely necessary and all other means have been exhausted. If paramedics need to apply physical restraint to transport safely or obtain an intravenous line (IV), they must take extreme care not to compress his chest or diaphragm and continually monitor the patient for any changes in respiratory, cardiac or perfusion status. Mental illness should not preclude pain relief and managing this patient's pain with carefully titrated doses is strongly encouraged.

4 EVALUATE

Effective out-of-hospital management of mental illness rarely requires the administration of medications and as such there is unlikely to be any significant change in the patient's presentation during transport. Maintaining the patient's dignity is likely to lead to an uneventful journey to hospital.

PRACTICE TIP

Small quantities of IV midazolam repeated to effect are safer than large quantities delivered intramuscularly.

CASE STUDY 3

Case 09157, 1207 hrs.

Dispatch details: A 25-year-old male with uncontrolled haemorrhage to his left arm. The caller states that the patient inflicted the wound intentionally.

Initial presentation: When the paramedics arrive they find the patient pacing around the room. His wound has been bandaged by his mother and is no longer bleeding. The patient presents as dishevelled, irritable and suspicious, and asks the paramedics to show their credentials before submitting to a physical examination.

 ASSESS

1215 hrs Primary survey: The patient is conscious and talking.

1216 hrs Chief complaint: He reports that he lacerated his arm while searching for a tracking device that 'they' had implanted under his skin.

1218 hrs Vital signs survey: The patient eventually sits at the request of the paramedics, although his legs move restlessly throughout the examination.

Perfusion status: HR 90 bpm; unable to obtain BP due to the patient's agitation; skin pale and dry.

Respiratory status: RR 24 bpm, no increase in respiratory effort and no apparent respiratory disturbance evident on visual inspection while questioning the patient.

Conscious state: GCS = 14, confused to time.

1220 hrs Pertinent hx: The patient denies a history of mental illness, although his mother reports that he was diagnosed with schizophrenia 5 years ago. She says that he has been well for the past 4 years, but became irritable and withdrawn after losing his job 5 weeks ago. She has noticed a decline in his sleep and appetite since then.

1223 hrs Further mental health questioning: While the patient is able to answer most questions, paramedics note long pauses in his responses and diminished concentration and focus. He engages only in limited eye contact and is unable to identify who 'they' are, except to say that 'they' watch him and always seem to know where he is. He also articulates concerns that his mother is trying to poison him and that his friends are talking about him. It is important for paramedics to understand the nature of the delusions and the hallucinations, whether there is any suggestion that voices or beliefs are commanding the patient to hurt themselves or others and the likelihood of the patient acting on those commands. The comment from the patient that he believes his mother is trying to poison him is significant and should be considered in your risk assessment.

1228 hrs Secondary survey: There is no loss of sensation, movement and circulation to his left hand. Unless there is an indication of arterial bleeding, visualising any wound before transport is usually recommended as it may require a specific hospital for treatment, but in this case the crew leave the bandage in place to reduce distress and stimulus to the patient.

This case is challenging in that the patient is presenting with both psychosis (clear evidence of delusions—fixed false beliefs, increased psychomotor movement, changes in sleep and appetite patterns) and a physical injury that requires treatment. His behaviour is likely to make the paramedics wary and may affect their ability to communicate effectively. His discussion provides insight into his thought processes, revealing a paranoid delusion and lack of insight into his previous medical history and his current state. The clinical picture is consistent with psychosis, although the precipitating cause could be primary schizophrenia alone, an exacerbation due to drug use or possibly a combination of both.

2 CONFIRM

In many cases paramedics are presented with a collection of signs and symptoms that do not appear to describe a particular condition. A critical step in determining a treatment plan in this situation is to consider what other conditions could explain the patient's presentation.

What else could it be?
Acute drug reaction
A psychotic reaction to drugs, particularly stimulant drugs such as amphetamines, is not unusual and should be managed in a similar way to a primary psychotic state related to schizophrenia. Anecdotally, drug-induced psychosis may be associated with more dramatic delusions resulting in more intense and violent responses from the patient. A psychotic reaction to prescribed medications (including steroids) will occasionally occur: this can be either a direct effect of the drug or an interaction with an underlying psychotic condition. Unfortunately, excluding drug use without the use of toxicology relies on the history, which in this case may be unreliable.

Encephalitis
An acute psychotic state can be the first presentation of encephalitis and no other signs of infection may be obvious in the early stages. Although this is very unusual it is not impossible and should be considered, particularly if there is no previous history or obvious precipitating cause of the psychosis. This cannot be effectively excluded in the out-of-hospital setting and even without an arm wound this factor would necessitate transport to hospital to determine.

Focal epilepsy
Focal epilepsy can give rise to acute episodes of changes in behaviour, but this is not usually psychotic and should have a definite onset and offset associated with the epileptic activity. This is not consistent with this patient's presentation.

Hyponatraemia or other electrolyte imbalance
An electrolyte imbalance can precipitate disturbed behaviour that may be psychotic in nature. Hyponatraemia associated with excessive drinking of water or adrenal gland failure can present with delusional psychotic behaviour before progressing to cause seizures. An absence of suggestive history is helpful but a normal set of blood tests is necessary to exclude this hypothesis. It is worth considering in previously undiagnosed patients who are at risk of hyponatraemia (i.e. those attending dance parties or raves where the combination of excessive activity and drug use increases the risk). The patient's history does not include these activities.

Thyrotoxicosis
Endocrine abnormalities such as thyrotoxicosis can produce a hyperactive state with some paranoid component, especially if the patient has an underlying mental illness. The absence of excessive tachycardia, tremors and signs of a

DIFFERENTIAL DIAGNOSIS
Psychosis
Or
- Acute drug reaction
- Encephalitis
- Focal epilepsy
- Hyponatraemia or other electrolyte imbalance
- Thyrotoxicosis
- Hypoglycaemia

hypermetabolic state would make this diagnosis unlikely but formal thyroid function tests would exclude it completely.

Hypoglycaemia

The presence of a normal blood sugar excludes hypoglycaemia as a possible cause of the abnormal behaviour.

<table>
<tr><td>

PRACTICE TIP

If using physical restraint:
- place no pressure on the patient's chest or abdomen; the patient should be face up to allow good observation of ventilation
- ensure that it is possible to rapidly roll the patient onto their side if they vomit.

</td></tr>
</table>

③ TREAT

Further assessment and treatment in hospital is needed for this patient where the full range of possible alternative diagnoses can be excluded and he can be offered antipsychotic medication and stabilisation in a controlled environment. He is considered a high risk of accidental self-harm (as noted by his laceration) and could be a risk of harm to others should his paranoid delusions escalate given his current state of agitation.

The patient is able to engage to some extent with paramedics so he may voluntarily agree to transport, in which case the treatment will be aimed at making the experience as stress-free as possible for him while gaining further insight into his current state of mind and possible precipitating causes. Unusually, his paranoia may preclude the paramedics from treating his wound with pain relief. Always offer patients with physical injuries the option of receiving pain relief, but do not try to force the administration of medications.

④ EVALUATE

Should he not have enough insight or the capacity to make a decision regarding his own care, legal options may have to be pursued. This patient appears to be suffering from a mental illness, is considered a high risk of accidental self-harm due to his delusions (e.g. laceration to his arm) and thus cannot remain at home, and requires assessment and management in hospital. This would fulfil the legislative requirements for involuntary treatment and transport in most states. To achieve safe transport, chemical restraint may be considered and is the preferred option over physical restraint, the aim being to use the least-restrictive form of restraint that is compatible with both the patient's and the crew's safety.

Effective out-of-hospital management of mental illness rarely requires the administration of medications or restraints and as such there is unlikely to be any significant change in the patient's presentation during transport.

If physical or chemical restraint is used either temporarily or during transfer, several risks should be considered: 1. the risk of positional asphyxia, in which the victim is unable to breathe properly because of restrictions to chest movement caused by the restraint; and 2. the risk that a sedated patient becomes unconscious and vomits and the physical restraint prevents the paramedics from turning the patient quickly onto their side to clear the airway. While mechanically restraining the patient may be needed to ensure safety, it can prove fatal if the patient cannot be rolled quickly should they vomit.

CASE STUDY 4

Case 10020, 0831 hrs.

Dispatch details: A 25-year-old female in a gaming lounge with abnormal behaviour.

Initial presentation: Casino staff direct the paramedics to the patient in the gaming lounge where she has been for the past 40 hours and refuses to leave. They called the ambulance when they noticed that she was behaving unusually and had difficulty talking to her. The paramedics notice that she is extremely slim and dressed in bright, vibrant clothing.

1 ASSESS

In response to the paramedics' greeting the patient reports that she is a university student studying for her final exams. She goes on to discuss the last movies she has seen. When one of the paramedics firmly redirects her towards her behaviour she reports that in the last 4 weeks she has stopped eating as she has not been hungry. Her sleeping patterns have also altered dramatically: she has had a maximum of 2 hours sleep per night in the last few days. She says that she has been far too busy to sleep as she has significant study commitments and a professional tennis career to prepare for. Without appearing to draw breath, she acknowledges that she has never had formal tennis lessons or played regularly, but remains certain that she will be wildly successful. She is very flirtatious with bystanders and the treating paramedic.

0847 hrs Vital signs survey: Perfusion status: HR 98 bpm, weak and irregular, BP 140/100 mmHg, skin flushed and dry.

Respiratory status: RR 18 bpm, good clear air entry, L = R, normal work of breathing, no complaint of dyspnoea.

Conscious state: GCS = 15.

The treating paramedic notes that the patient presents with grandiose and disorganised thought patterns and pressured speech (a rapid, constant stream of speech which tends to be disorganised and difficult to interrupt). She speaks in a loud voice with little connection between ideas and it appears not in context to the situation. She admits to using amphetamines in the past 48 hours but denies any sustained or long-term use. Her symptoms are typical of a bipolar I manic episode.

2 CONFIRM

In many cases paramedics are presented with a collection of signs and symptoms that do not appear to describe a particular condition. A critical step in determining a treatment plan in this situation is to consider what other conditions could explain the patient's presentation.

What else could it be?
Amphetamine or stimulant use
Hypomania describes a state of euphoria and disinhibition that is often associated with excessive confidence and hypersexuality. It can be distinguished from

mania by an absence of psychotic symptoms but the two should be considered as part of a continuum as opposed to separate conditions. The most likely alternative diagnosis for hypomania is amphetamine or other stimulant use. Differentiation will depend on whether there is a history of drug use, a history of bipolar cycles and a previous diagnosis. Without drug screening it can be very difficult to differentiate between pure bipolar hypomania and drug-induced hypomanic behaviour—or, as in this case, a combination of both. The diagnosis is difficult to determine in the field but it could be relevant to immediate management.

Other organic brain syndrome

There are relatively few organic brain syndromes that mimic this degree of hypomanic behaviour. Possibly hyperstimulation associated with excessive amounts of circulating adrenaline or other catecholamines might present like this. Her pulse and blood pressure are not excessively elevated which suggests a systemic adrenaline-like syndrome is not likely. Serotonin syndrome is a potentially life-threatening condition caused by the interaction of serotonin re-uptake inhibitors with other drugs that results in the release of too much serotonin. It can produce a hyperactive state but it does not normally have the disordered ideas that are typical of a bipolar hypomanic phase. In addition, serotonin syndrome is always associated with physiological changes such as increases to temperature, heart rate and blood pressure. This does not fit the clinical picture in this case.

(3) TREAT

This patient's use of amphetamines will have exaggerated her hypomanic/manic state and allowed her to remain conscious for long periods of time without sleep. If someone who knows her well can be found they may be aware of a formal diagnosis of bipolar disorder or at least be aware of what medications she has been taking or is supposed to take.

The patient has no insight into her behaviour and so will be challenging to interact with and convince that she needs help. A slow, steady approach will allow her more opportunity to process information. This interaction should be handled by one member of the crew, who should concentrate on slowing down in response to her hypomanic speech patterns. The paramedics should consider discussing her physical symptoms (i.e. her lack of sleep, drug use and limited food intake) with her to see whether she will engage in treatment for these issues. Wherever possible, she should be encouraged to access treatment voluntarily.

The treating paramedics' risk assessment suggests that this patient is at risk of accidental self-harm and possible harm to others if left untreated. Given this assessment, the enacting of legislative powers needs to be considered. This patient meets the criteria for involuntary treatment for most jurisdictions. The paramedics have a duty of care to provide access to definitive mental health treatment. In this case since she has altered insight and capacity she cannot be left and requires transport to hospital or inpatient mental health care. Paramedics can provide her with as much choice as possible with the understanding that she will be transported to further care (e.g. comfort) without mechanical restraints. Police may need to intervene if the safety of the clinicians, public or person is at risk. Involving the police has advantages in terms of extra assistance and an authoritative presence but it can sometimes inflame the situation. The benefits and risks of police involvement need to be considered before escalating to this level.

The clinical decisions are further complicated by the patient's amphetamine use, which can mimic many of the symptoms of mania. When making a

---

DIFFERENTIAL DIAGNOSIS

Bipolar
Or
- Amphetamine or stimulant use
- Other organic brain syndrome

differential diagnosis, clinicians at the receiving hospital will construct a careful timeline to identify the presence of symptoms in relation to her substance use. They may also wish to monitor her for an extended period to determine whether her symptoms remain after the amphetamines have been metabolised and excreted from her system.

A number of ambulance services support the administration of benzodiazepines such as midazolam to manage amphetamine overdose. This guideline was mostly developed for the small cohort of patients who present with painful bruxism, twitching, scratching and hypertension, but it can also be used as a last resort in aggressive patients. There are very strict guidelines regarding the use of sedatives to facilitate the transport of involuntary patients who are mentally ill. It is perceivable that the paramedics could misinterpret this patient's history and find themselves administering a sedative against their local Mental Health Act. Consultation to support this decision would be recommended.

4 EVALUATE

Effective out-of-hospital management of mental illness rarely requires the administration of medications and as such there is unlikely to be any significant change in the patient's presentation during transport. Maintaining the patient's dignity and not engaging or challenging her delusions is likely to lead to an uneventful journey to hospital.

Summary

Patients presenting with changes in behaviour require a different approach from those presenting with physiological abnormalities. Much more care must be taken in all forms of communication with these patients and a slower, less intimidating approach is often required. These patients are extremely vulnerable and need to be protected from harm. In addition to the changes in behaviour, any physiological issues must be addressed in an effort to either reverse the changes in behaviour evident at presentation or manage any trauma that has occurred as a result.

References

American Psychiatric Association. (2013). Diagnostic and statistical manual of mental disorders (5th ed.). Washington, DC: APA.

Anthony, W. A. (1993). Recovery from mental illness: the guiding vision of the mental health service system in the 1990s. *Psychosocial Rehabilitation Journal, 16*(4), 11–23.

Australian Bureau of Statistics (ABS). (2002). *Year Book Australia, 2001.* Retrieved from www.abs.gov.au/ausstats/abs. (Accessed 30 January 2012).

Australian Bureau of Statistics. (2015). *National Health Survey: First Results, 2014-15.* https://www.abs.gov.au/ausstats/abs@.nsf/Lookup/by%20Subject/4364.0.55.001–2014-15–Main%20Features–Mental%20and%20behavioural%20conditions–32.

Australian Government. (2012). *National Suicide Prevention Strategy.* Retrieved from www.health.gov.au/internet/mentalhealth/publishing.nsf/content/national-suicide-prevention-strategy-1. (Accessed 30 January 2012).

Australian Institute of Health and Welfare. (2017). *Mental health services—in brief 2017.* Cat. no. HSE 192. Canberra: AIHW.

Awad, G. A. (2004). Antipsychotic medications: compliance and attitudes toward treatment. *Current Opinion in Psychiatry, 17*(2), 75–80.

Battaglia, J. (2001). *Compliance with treatment in schizophrenia.* American Psychiatric Association: 53rd Institute on Psychiatric Services. Retrieved from www.medscape.com/viewarticle/418612. (Accessed 17 January 2012).

Bennett, P., Williams, Y., Page, N., Hood, K., & Woollard, M. (2004). Levels of mental health problems among UK emergency ambulance workers. *Emergency Medicine Journal, 21*, 235–236. doi:10.1136/emj.2003.005645.

Bhattacharya, A., Derecki, N. C., Lovenberg, T. W., & Drevets, W. C. (2016). Role of neuro-immunological factors in the pathophysiology of mood disorders. *Psychopharmacology, 233*(9), 1623–1636.

Black Dog Institute. (2010). *Bipolar disorder explained.* Retrieved from www.blackdoginstitute.org.au/public/bipolardisorder/bipolardisorderexplained/index.cfm. (Accessed 14 January 2012).

Bloch, S., Green, S., Janca, A., Mitchell, P., & Robertson, M. (2017). *Foundations of clinical psychiatry*. Melbourne University Publishing.

Bradbury, J., Hutchinson, M., Hurley, J., & Stasa, H. (2017). Lived experience of involuntary transport under mental health legislation. *International Journal of Mental Health Nursing, 26*(6), 580–592.

Campbell, C., & Farrell, G. (2009). Personality disorders. In R. Elder, K. Evans & D. Nizette (Eds.), *Psychiatric and mental health nursing* (2nd ed.). Sydney: Elsevier.

Cheng, A. T. A., Chen, T. H. H., Chen, C., & Jenkins, R. (2000). Psychosocial and psychiatric risk factors for suicide: case-control psychological autopsy study. *The British Journal of Psychiatry, 177*, 360–365.

Community Services and Health Industry Skills Council (CSHISC). (2009). *Dementia training for ambulance workers: Learner's guide*. Strawberry Hills: Department of Health and Ageing.

Community Services and Health Industry Skills Council (CSHISC). (2011). *Key Principles: Skills for Ambulance Workers in Responding to People with Dementia*. Retrieved from www.psychology.org.au/publications/tip_sheets/dementia/#s5. (Accessed 24 November 2011).

Compton, M. T., & Kotwicki, R. J. (2007). *Responding to individuals with mental illnesses*. Sudbury, MA: Jones & Bartlett.

Davidson, G. C., Neale, J. M., & Kring, A. M. (2004). *Abnormal psychology* (9th ed.). Boston: John Wiley & Sons.

Department of Health. (2010a). *People living with psychotic illness*. Canberra: Department of Health.

Department of Health. (2010b). *Ambulance transport of people with a mental illness protocol 2010*. Melbourne: Mental Health, Drugs and Regions Division.

Department of Health. (2011). *Safe Transport of People with a Mental Illness: Chief Psychiatrists Guideline*. Retrieved from www.health.vic.gov.au/mentalhealth/cpg/safetransport.pdf. (Accessed 31 January 2012).

Dogra, N., Lunn, B., & Cooper, S. (Eds.), (2017). *Psychiatry by ten teachers*. CRC Press.

Engel, G. L. (1977). The need for a new medical model: a challenge for biomedicine. *Science, 196*(4286), 129–136.

Forrester, K., & Griffiths, D. (2001). *Essentials of Law for health professionals*. Australia: Harcourt.

Frost, B., Carr, V., & Halpin, S. (2002). *Employment and psychosis: low prevalence disorder component of the national study of mental health and wellbeing, Bulletin 3*. Canberra: Department of Health and Ageing.

Fry, M., & Brunero, S. (2004). The characteristics and outcomes of mental health patients presenting to an emergency department over a twelve-month period. *Australian Emergency Nursing Journal, 7*(2), 21–25.

Graeff, F. G. (2017). Translational approach to the pathophysiology of panic disorder: focus on serotonin and endogenous opioids. *Neuroscience and Biobehavioral Reviews, 76*, 48–55.

Health Department of Western Australia. (2012). *Protocol between the Western Australia Police Service and the Mental Health Division of the Health Department of Western Australia*. Retrieved from www.chiefpsychiatrist.health.wa.gov.au/docs/guides/Protocol_Between_WA_Police_Mental_Health_Division.pdf. (Accessed 4 February 2012).

Hirschfeld, R. M. A., & Davidson, L. (1998). Risk factors for suicide. In A. J. Frances & R. E. Hales (Eds.), *Review of Psychiatry* (Vol. 7). Washington DC: American Psychiatric Association.

Isaacs, A. N., Sutton, K., Dalziel, K., & Maybery, D. (2017). Outcomes of a care coordinated service model for persons with severe and persistent mental illness: a qualitative study. *The International Journal of Social Psychiatry, 63*(1), 40–47.

Jespersen, S., Lawman, B., Reed, F., Hawke, K., Plummer, V., & Gaskin, C. J. (2016). The impact of integrating crisis teams into community mental health services on emergency department and inpatient demand. *The Psychiatric Quarterly, 87*(4), 703–712.

Kuipers, E., Yesufu-Udechuku, A., Taylor, C., & Kendall, T. (2014). Management of psychosis and schizophrenia in adults: summary of updated NICE guidance. *BMJ: British Medical Journal, 348*.

Larkin, G. L., Claassen, C. A., Pelletier, A. J., & Camargo, C. A. (2006). National study of ambulance transports to United States emergency departments: importance of mental health problems. *Prehospital and Disaster Medicine, 21*(2), 82–90.

Leonhardt, B. L., Huling, K., Hamm, J. A., Roe, D., Hasson-Ohayon, I., McLeod, H. J., & Lysaker, P. H. (2017). Recovery and serious mental illness: a review of current clinical and research paradigms and future directions. *Expert Review of Neurotherapeutics, 17*(11), 1117–1130.

Lichtman, J., Bigger, J. T., Blumenthal, J. A., Frasure-Smith, N., Kaufmann, P. G., Lesperance, F., Mark, D. B., Sheps, D. S., Taylor, C. B., & Froelicher, E. S. (2008). Depression and coronary heart disease. *Circulation, 118*, 1768–1775.

Lloyd, B., Gao, C. X., Helibronn, C., & Lubman, D. I. (2015). *Self-harm and mental health-related ambulance attendances in Australia: 2013 data*. Fitzroy, Victoria: Turning Point.

Lowthian, J. A., Jolley, D. J., Curtis, A. J., Currell, A., Cameron, P. A., Stoelwinder, J. U., & McNeil, J. J. (2011). The challenges of population ageing: accelerating demand for emergency ambulance services by older patients, 1995–2015. *The Medical Journal of Australia, 194*, 574–578.

Mallik, S., Spertus, J. A., Reid, K. J., Krumholz, H. M., Rumsfeld, J. S., Weintraub, W. S., Agarwal, P., Santra, M., Bidyasar, S., Lichtman, J. H., Wenger, N. K., & Vaccarino, V. (2006). Depressive symptoms after acute myocardial infarction. *Archives of Internal Medicine, 166*, 876–883.

Mindframe National Media Initiative. (2012). *Mental illness and suicide in the media: a mindframe for police*. Retrieved from www.mindframe-media.info/site/index.cfm?display =105553. (Accessed 30 January 2012).

Muir-Cochrane, E., Barkway, P., & Nizette, D. (2010). *Mosby's pocketbook of mental health*. Sydney: Elsevier.

Nuss, P. (2015). Anxiety disorders and GABA neurotransmission: a disturbance of modulation. *Neuropsychiatric Disease and Treatment*, *11*, 165.

Polk, D. A., & Mitchell, J. T. (2009). *Prehospital behavioural emergencies and crisis response*. Sudbury, MA: Jones & Bartlett.

Queensland Ambulance Service. (2008). *Mental health intervention project: mental state assessment*. Brisbane: Queensland Government.

Queensland Ambulance Service. (2012). *Transport of Patients with a Mental Illness in Queensland*. Retrieved from www.ambulance.qld.gov.au/about/pdf/qems_mental_ health_transport.pdf. (Accessed 4 February 2012).

Roberts, L., & Henderson, J. (2009). Paramedic perceptions of their role, education, training and working relationships when attending cases of mental illness. *Journal of Emergency Primary Health Care*, *7*(3).

Saba, G., Mekaoui, L., Leboyer, M., & Schuhoff, F. (2007). Patient's health literacy in psychotic disorders. *Neuropsychiatric Disease and Treatment*, *3*(4), 511–517.

Stein, D. J., Phillips, K. A., Bolton, B., Fulford, K. W. M., Sadler, J. Z., & Kendler, K. S. (2010). What is a mental/psychiatric disorder? From DSM-IV to DSM-V. *Psychological Medicine*, *40*(11), 1759–1765.

Tavakoli, H. R. (2009). A closer evaluation of current methods in psychiatric assessments: a challenge for the biopsychosocial model. *Psychiatry*, *6*(2), 25–30.

Tessier, A., Boyer, L., Husky, M., Baylé, F., Llorca, P. M., & Misdrahi, D. (2017). Medication adherence in schizophrenia: the role of insight, therapeutic alliance and perceived trauma associated with psychiatric care. *Psychiatry Research*, *257*, 315–321.

United Nations. (2002). *Principles for the protection of persons with mental illness and the improvement of mental health care*. Retrieved from www.who.int/ mental_health/policy/en/UN_Resolution_on_protection _of_persons_with_mental_illness.pdf. (Accessed 4 February 2012).

Victorian Government Department of Health. (2008). *A guide to mental health terminology*. Retrieved from www.health.vic.gov.au/mentalhealth/termnlgy.htm. (Accessed 30 January 2012).

World Health Organization (WHO). (2005). *WHO resource book on mental health, human rights and legislation*. Geneva: WHO.

World Health Organization (WHO). (2013). *Mental health: strengthening our response. Fact sheet N220*. Retrieved from www.who.int/mediacentre/factsheets/fs220/en. (Accessed 12 January 2013).

World Medical Association. (2006). *WMA statement on ethical issues concerning patients with mental illness*. Retrieved from www.wma.net/en/30publications/ 10policies/e11. (Accessed 4 February 2012).

De-Escalation Strategies

By Ashley Denham and Joelene Gott

OVERVIEW

- Managing patients with mental illness in the community can be stressful for both patients and those that care for them.
- Managing aggressive patients with physical or chemical restraint increases the chance of harm to both the patient and the paramedics.
- De-escalation techniques are paramount in the safe and respectful management of patients with mental illness.

Introduction

The out-of-hospital environment is one that can be exciting and challenging for paramedics; however, this uncontrolled environment also brings an element of risk. While the majority of patients and their families are grateful when paramedics arrive, literature shows that healthcare workers, especially paramedics who work in uncontrolled environments, are at greater risk of experiencing patient aggression and violence. Verbal assault has been shown to be the most common form of aggression, although many paramedics report that they have experienced many incidents of violent or aggressive acts towards them (Wongtongkam, 2017).

The ability to verbally de-escalate agitated and aggressive patients has been identified as one of the most important and effective tools that paramedics can use. However, the response to aggression continues to be reactive, rather than preventative. Aggression continues to be viewed as something that paramedics need to 'manage' rather than addressing the issue early on and preventing the aggression from occurring (Baby et al., 2018). The situation should be quickly contained and preventative de-escalation techniques should be utilised prior to interventional, or pharmacological, measures for managing aggression (Du et al., 2017).

Aggression

Aggression can be a result of a number of conditions, such as medical conditions, substance abuse, mental health issues or preexisting traits of aggression and violence (Wongtongkam, 2017). Aggression and violence can result in short- and long-term physical and psychological harm for victims. It can result in burnout, exhaustion, decreased productivity, increased absenteeism and poor patient care. The financial costs are also significant (Hallett & Dickens, 2017).

Aggression is behaviour that is directed at another individual with the intent to cause harm, whether that be verbally, psychologically or physically. The cause of aggression can be intrinsic (such as mental health, substance misuse, intellectual disability) or extrinsic (such as social and environmental conditions) (see Table 53.1). Some conditions can also increase the risk that a patient will experience aggression, such as head injury, Huntington's Disease, learning disability and alcohol or substance misuse. Due to the multiple possible causes of aggression, a wide variety of people in the population are at risk of displaying aggressive behaviour (Spencer & Johnson, 2016).

De-escalation

Spencer and Johnson (2016) describe de-escalation as talking with an agitated or aggressive patient/bystander in a particular way that is able to avoid violence and escalation of the behaviour. De-escalation allows the perpetrator to regain some sense of self and calm down.

De-escalation comprises a set of techniques and skills that include verbal and nonverbal communication with the patient and others around specific to the setting and situation (Spencer & Johnson, 2016). It is important to understand that de-escalation is about communication and negotiation, not command and control (Cowin et al., 2003).

Bowers (2014) described a de-escalation model to assist healthcare providers manage aggressive and agitated patients/bystanders (see Fig 53.1).

1. Delimiting the situation. Immediately make the situation safe for you and others around you. In this step you may press a duress alarm or contact security or police. You should also keep a safe distance from the patient so you are not putting yourself in immediate danger.

Table 53.1 Differential diagnoses for the cause of aggression or agitation

System	Conditions
Metabolic/endocrine	• Electrolyte abnormalities (sodium, calcium, magnesium, potassium, phosphate) • Hypoglycaemia • Hyperglycaemia (e.g. diabetic ketoacidosis/hyperosmolar hyperglycaemic non-ketoacidosis) • Hypoxia • Hypercarbia • Renal or liver failure • Thyrotoxicosis • Myxoedema coma • Nutritional deficiency (e.g. Wernicke's encephalopathy, vitamin B12 deficiency)
Infection	• Sepsis • Systemic infections • Fever-related delirium
Neurological	• Head injury • Stroke • Intracranial mass • Intracranial haemorrhage • Central nervous system infection (e.g. meningitis, encephalitis, abscess) • Seizure • Dementia
Toxicological	• Anticholinergic intoxication • Stimulant intoxication • Steroid psychosis • Antibiotic reaction • Other drug reaction • Carbon monoxide toxicity • Alcohol intoxication or withdrawal • Toxic alcohols • Serotonin syndrome • Neuroleptic malignant syndrome
Other conditions	• Shock (e.g. hypovolaemic, cardiogenic, distributive, obstructive) • Burn • Hypothermia • Hyperthermia
Psychiatric	• Psychosis • Schizophrenia • Paranoid delusions • Personality disorder

Source: Gottlieb et al. (2018).

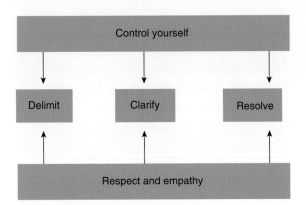

Figure 53.1
De-escalation model.
Source: Bowers (2014).

2. Clarify. Clarify the problem with the patient and find out what the patient is angry or agitated about or why. Make sure you speak clearly and try to sort out any confusion the patient may have. Ask open-ended questions and offer help to the patient. Keep the patient oriented by reminding them where they are, who you are and that you are there to help. If applicable, leverage any existing relationship you may have with the patient or some common ground you have established.

3. Resolve. Find a way of dealing with the complaint that satisfies the patient and your duty of care. Try and be polite and avoid being inflexible or authoritarian. Be apologetic

and flexible and, if not always possible, explain to the patient the reasons behind the rules/decisions. Take your time and really listen to what the patient is saying. If they are engaging in conversation with you, that is a success.

The above model only works if the person conducting the de-escalation is in control of themselves and their emotions at every stage, and they're expressing respect and empathy for the patient (see Fig 53.1).

Try and control yourself and stay calm. During an intense, highly volatile situation you may feel anxiety or frustration at what is occurring. It is very important that this is not communicated to the patient at any point. The following are some strategies that can assist with this.

- Try to understand the patient's point of view and the context.
- Have confidence in your own de-escalation skills, and have a backup plan if the de-escalation is unsuccessful.
- Know your restraint protocols and techniques in case they are required.
- Maintain a professional, calm and confident manner.

- Use open non-defensive body language, a relaxed facial expression and a calm tone.
- Don't take the situation personally as the aggression is rarely caused by or directed at paramedics but instead at events leading up to their attendance.
- Avoid getting into an argument by trying to defend or justify yourself.

Endeavour to display empathy and respect to the patient at all times. Respect can be shown by actions, such as tone of voice, eye contact, patience and facial expressions throughout the encounter. It can also be evident in what you say, along with how you listen and try and understand their point of view. It is important to ensure you don't make light of what they are saying or how they are feeling, nor should you try and tell the patient how they should feel.

DIFFERENTIAL DIAGNOSES

What are some of the differential diagnoses you are considering with this type of presentation?

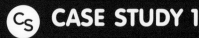

CASE STUDY 1

Case 12555, 1645 hrs.

Dispatch details: A 48-year-old female displaying abnormal behaviour. Call made by concerned neighbours.

Initial presentation: The patient is sitting on the couch in her neighbour's house. She is rocking back and forth on the couch, not making eye contact with paramedics. The patient abruptly yells out that she has no underwear on and can't go anywhere. She allows vital signs to be taken, all of which are within normal limits. The patient states that she had a pain in her ear and her behaviour has continued to become more and more abnormal. The patient agrees to go to the hospital and walks to ambulance. Once in the ambulance, she begins to have visual and auditory hallucinations, with outbursts of aggression and violence to paramedics.

CASE STUDY 2

Case 13971, 0815 hrs.

Dispatch details: A 54-year-old male, generally unwell with agitated behaviour. Call made by family member.

Initial presentation: The patient is lying on the couch with his wife and daughter on scene. Initially patient seems to be sleeping; however, when spoken to he became verbally aggressive. The patient yells at the paramedics to leave his home, and proceeds to spit on one officer's face. Police are called and the patient is physically restrained. Basic vital signs are taken, which shows a decrease in BP (90/50) and BGL (2.5 mmol/L). The patient does not agree to attend hospital and continues with his verbal aggression, becoming physically violent. The patient is escorted into the ambulance by police, and continues with his aggressive behaviour en route to hospital.

DIFFERENTIAL DIAGNOSES

What are some of the differential diagnoses you are considering with this type of presentation?

Summary

Agitation and aggression are becoming a more common patient presentation in the out-of-hospital environment. Identification of the aggressive patient and early intervention is a required skill for all paramedics. De-escalation should be the first line of intervention to calm an aggressive patient before attempting pharmacological or physical restraint. The most important part of the de-escalation process is the paramedics' personal self-control and ability to show respect and empathy in a calm and non-judgmental way. It is important to remember that not all agitation and aggression is caused by mental illness, but there are many differential diagnoses, some of which paramedics can treat. Many successful de-escalation cases are a result of the paramedics' approach to the situation and ability to calm the situation and gain a patient's trust.

If the de-escalation techniques are not successful, and the agitation and aggression continue and the situation becomes uncontrollable or unsafe, chemical or physical restraint should be considered. Chemical, or pharmacological, restraint involves medications such as droperidol, midazolam or other similar drugs. Each state and territory in Australia uses a different pharmacological option for the use of sedation of aggressive patients, and these medications all have different mechanisms of action. Consideration and preparation should always be taken when deciding to use pharmacological intervention, as many of the medications have side effects that affect the patient's conscious state and their respiratory drive. The aim of all interventions to treat and calm an aggressive patient should be the safety of the paramedics, the patient and bystanders, and allowing the patient to be transported to definitive care in the safest possible way.

References

Baby, M., Gale, C., & Swain, N. (2018). Communication skills training in the management of patient aggression and violence in healthcare. *Aggression and Violent Behavior, 39*, 67–82.

Bowers, L. (2014). A model of de-escalation. *Mental Health Practice, 17*, n.9.

Cowin, L., Davies, R., Estall, G., Berlin, T., Fitzgerald, M., & Hoot, S. (2003). De-escalating aggression & violence in the mental health setting. *International Journal of Mental Health Nursing, 12*, 64–73.

Du, M., Wang, X., Yin, S., Shu, W., Hao, R., Zhao, S., Rao, H., Yeung, W., Jayaram, M. B., & Xia, J. (2017). De-escalation techniques for psychosis-induced aggression or agitation. *The Cochrane Database of Systematic Reviews,* (4), CD009922, 1–24.

Gottlieb, M., Long, B., & Koyfman, A. (2018). Approach to the agitated emergency department patient. *The Journal of Emergency Medicine*, 1–11.

Hallett, N., & Dickens, G. L. (2017). De-escalation of aggressive behaviour in healthcare settings: concept analysis. *International Journal of Nursing Studies, 75*, 10–20.

Spencer, S., & Johnson, P. (2016). De-escalation techniques for managing aggression (protocol). *The Cochrane Database of Systematic Reviews,* (1), CD012034, 1–13.

Wongtongkam, N. (2017). An exploration of violence against paramedics, burnout and posttraumatic symptoms in two Australian ambulance services. *International Journal of Emergency Services, 6*(2), 134–146.

SECTION 16:
The Paramedic Approach to Obstetric, Neonatal and Paediatric Patients

In this section

Birth is a normal event and only rarely should it be considered as a medical emergency: for the most part mother and infant do well without the clinician having to face complex clinical decisions. Relatively few babies are born before the mother arrives at hospital, although paramedics may occasionally be required to assist in a normal delivery and very rarely they may be required to attend a complex birth or to assist in the resuscitation of a neonate who has been delivered without adequate ventilation or perfusion.

Birth and neonatal resuscitation are examples of situations that are relatively rare in paramedic experience and require a clear systematic approach. If the delivery is normal and resuscitation of the infant is unnecessary, there are essentially no elements of clinical reasoning to apply and an algorithmic approach to management is both safe and sufficient. The paramedic role is to provide clinical and caring support. Even when complications arise with either the mother or the infant, emergency management tends to follow predictable pathways involving well-specified algorithms, and the need for clinical reasoning and problem-solving beyond that associated with resuscitation principles is limited.

However, this is also a time when the emotional aspect of the scene places further pressure on the paramedic facing an unfamiliar task. As such, a prescriptive and directive approach to managing birth and neonatal resuscitation makes sense. Unlike previous chapters, which explore the 'what else could it be' approach to assessment and decision-making, the chapters in this section focus on clear and detailed procedural instructions. The information is intended to give paramedics a systematic approach that minimises clinical challenges and maximises the transfer of clinical responsibility for definitive care. One of the most useful pieces of advice in this setting is to share the problem with those who work with obstetrics and neonatal resuscitation. Paramedics are part of a larger multidisciplinary team, and as team players are not expected to manage all situations alone when expertise and advice is available.

CHAPTER 54

Imminent Birth

By Gayle McLelland

OVERVIEW

- In 2017 in Australia, 1974 women or 0.7% of all births were unplanned births before arrival (BBAs) at hospital, for which paramedics could potentially have been the initial primary health provider (Australian Institute of Health and Welfare 2019). While the number of BBAs remains low, since 1991 it has almost doubled in some areas (McLelland et al., 2011).
- Most of the births encountered by paramedics are normal vertex presentations and require minimal intervention (McLelland et al., 2013; McLelland et al., 2018).
- Close to two-thirds of BBAs happen prior to arrival of paramedics, with 66% of women identified to be in the second stage of labour delivering prior to arrival at hospital. Most were clinically uncomplicated (McLelland et al., 2018).
- Although rare, paramedics may encounter potentially life-threatening obstetric emergencies including breech birth, shoulder dystocia and cord prolapse (McLelland et al., 2013; McLelland et al., 2018).
- The most frequent maternal complication at an unplanned birth is postpartum haemorrhage occurring in 6.2–6.5% of all BBAs (McLelland et al., 2013).
- Admissions to special care units are 2 (Beeram et al., 1995) to 6.25 (Rodie et al., 2002) times greater for BBAs than for in-hospital births.

Introduction

Labour is the process that enables expulsion of the fetus, placenta and membranes through the birth canal. Normal labour is the spontaneous onset of contractions that occurs between 37 and 42 weeks' gestation and is completed within 18 hours with the presentation of the baby in a head-first or cephalic presentation. Labour, and the eventual birth of a baby, is a harmonious balance between correct anatomy, precise physiology and the mechanics of the baby travelling through the pelvis. Often referred to as the '5Ps'—passage, passenger, powers, psychology and problems (White et al., 2011)—a successful birth requires the right combination of all of these factors.

Physiology

Although labour is physiologically a continuous process, for educational and clinical purposes it is divided into three stages (Pairman et al., 2014). The first stage involves the onset of painful contractions causing effacement and dilation of the cervix; the second stage starts after the cervix has fully opened and lasts until the birth of the baby; and the third stage involves delivery of the placenta (Pairman et al., 2014; Rankin, 2017; see Tables 54.1 and 54.2). The factors that initiate labour are not fully understood but it is widely accepted that it commences due to a combination of fetal, placental and maternal factors (Coad & Dunstall, 2011; Fraser & Cooper, 2009; Rankin, 2017).

The female pelvis or passageway

The human pelvis consists of four bones. The posterior wall comprises the sacrum and the coccyx bone; and the lateral and anterior walls consist of three fused bones: the ilium, the ischium and the pubis. These bones join to form a border around an empty space, which in females allows the passage of the baby through the pelvis (Pairman et al., 2014; Rankin, 2017). This passage can be divided into three zones: the pelvic brim, the pelvic cavity and the pelvic outlet. The pelvic brim separates the upper flare of the iliac fossa, or false pelvis, from the lower basin-shaped true pelvis. The pelvic cavity is the area of the pelvis between the pelvic brim and the outlet. It is bordered anteriorly by the symphysis pubis and pubic bones; laterally by the interior of ilium and the body of the ischium; and posteriorly by the sacrum. The obstetric pelvic outlet is the lower portion of the pelvis and is bordered by the lower edges of the symphysis pubis anteriorly, the sacrum posteriorly and the ischial tuberosities laterally. The female pelvis is generally wider and shallower than the male pelvis and is categorised into one of four different shapes: gynaecoid, android, platypelloid and anthropoid (see Fig 54.1) (Rankin, 2017). While the gynaecoid pelvis is thought to be ideal for childbirth, a woman may have any one of the four shapes or a combination of two or more shapes (Coad & Dunstall, 2011). The dimensions of each type of pelvis vary greatly, but the gynaecoid pelvis is the widest (see Table 54.3).

Table 54.1: The three stages of labour

Stage 1
Commences with the onset of painful regular contractions until full dilation, or 10 cm dilation, of the cervix. Or clinically until the woman experiences the uncontrollable urge to push. The first stage is further divided into three phases. **Latent:** The cervix thins and effaces but there is very little dilation. The contractions can often be irregular at the start and be more than 10 minutes apart and lasting for 30 secs. As labour becomes more established they become more regular as they get closer together. With the progression of labour, contractions become regular, closer together and longer, often lasting up to a minute. Can take 6–8 hours in a primigravida. **Active:** The cervix rapidly dilates at an approximate rate of 1 cm/hour in primigravidas and 1.5 cm/hour in multigravidas from 4 cm up to 9 cm. During this stage contractions are regular, often less than 5 minutes apart, and can last up to a minute. **Transitional:** Occurs when the cervix is ≥ 9 cm until full dilation and the rate of dilation often slows at this stage. Full dilation is when the cervix is 10 cm and labour moves into the second stage.

Stage 2
Commences when the cervix is fully dilated or 10 cm dilated until the expulsion of the fetus. The woman often experiences an uncontrollable urge to open her bowels or push. As the second stage continues the urge to push becomes increasingly stronger, there is often anal pouting and perineal bulging until the presenting part becomes visible.

Stage 3
Commences with the birth of the baby and is completed when the placenta and membranes are expelled and the associated bleeding has been controlled.

Source: Coad & Dunstall (2011); Fraser & Cooper (2009); Pairman et al. (2014); and Rankin (2017).

Table 54.2: Length of stage of labour

	Nulliparous (first birth)	Parous (has previously given birth)
Active first stage	Average 8 hours Up to 18 hours	Average 5 hours Up to 12 hours
Second stage	Within 2 hours	Within 1 hour
Physiological third stage	Up to 1 hour	Up to 1 hour
Active third stage	Up to 30 minutes	Up to 30 minutes

Source: National Institute for Health and Care Excellence (2017).

Table 54.3: Pelvic measurements of gynaecoid pelvis

	Anteroposterior	Oblique	Transverse
Brim	11 cm	12 cm	13 cm
Cavity	12 cm	12 cm	12 cm
Outlet	13 cm	12 cm	11 cm

Source: Rankin (2017).

The fetal head or passenger

Equally important in the passage of the baby through the pelvis is the size, shape and position of the baby's head. Due to the large brain, the fetal head is comparatively large for the human pelvis but with the skull flexed on the neck the smallest diameter presents to the pelvis (Rankin, 2017). The passage is optimised further by the pliable nature of the baby's skull. While the facial and base of skull regions are almost completely ossified by birth, the cranium bones are not completely joined. The five large bones (two frontal, two parietal and one occipital) and two smaller bones (two temporal) that form the cranium (or vault) are connected with membranous sutures with fontanels where two or more bones meet (Rankin, 2017). The sutures and fontanels facilitate small movements between the bones, which enable them to overlap: the change in the shape of the skull assists with the baby's journey through the pelvis (Coad & Dunstall, 2011).

Labour

First stage

The release of prostaglandins and the hormone oestradiol allows the cervix to soften and stretch, or dilate. The cervix will eventually form part of the birth canal. As the cervix changes, there are also changes in the muscle of the uterus, the myometrium. The tone of the myometrium changes to allow coordinated contractions from the top, or fundus, increasing uterine pressure (Coad & Dunstall, 2011; Rankin, 2017). Once labour is initiated, a positive feedback loop known as Ferguson's reflex commences and will not finish until the birth of the baby (see Fig 54.2). Ferguson's reflex describes the increase in the production of oxytocins caused by the pressure of the presenting part of the baby on the cervix. This increase in oxytocins stimulates the myometrium to contract more strongly, longer and

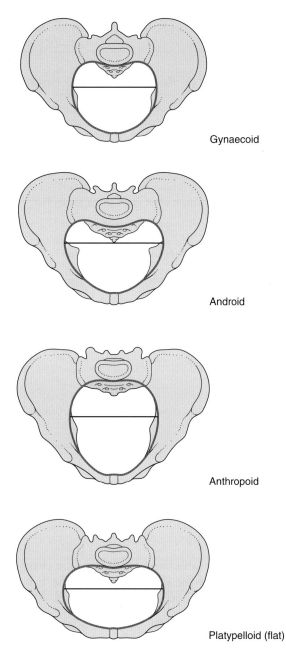

Figure 54.1
The four types of female pelvis.
Source: Pairman et al. (2014).

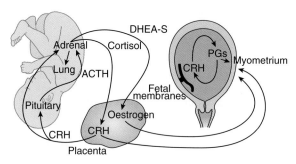

Figure 54.2
Positive feedback loop during labour. ACTH = adrenocorticotrophic hormone; CRH = corticotrophin-releasing hormone; DHEA-S = dehydroepiandrosterone sulfate; PGs = prostaglandins.
Source: McLean & Smith (2001).

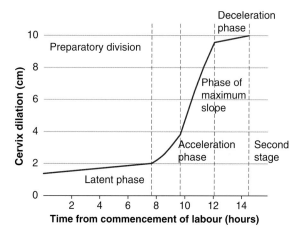

Figure 54.3
Friedman's curve, a typical graph depicting the progress of labour where cervical dilation is plotted against time. The curve is divided into latent and active phases, with the active phase further divided into acceleration, maximum slope and deceleration.
Source: Pairman et al. (2014).

with more frequency, which in turn causes thinning and dilation of the cervix (see Fig 54.3).

The upper and lower segments of the uterus work together during contractions. With each contraction the myometrium constricts, causing the upper segment of the uterus to descend as the baby moves through the birth canal, further strengthening Ferguson's reflex. During the first stage contractions occur somewhat irregularly up to 20 minutes apart, becoming more frequent until they are 3 minutes apart. The duration of contractions is typically brief at the start (10–15 seconds) but will increase up to 1 minute by the end of this stage (Coad & Dunstall, 2011; Rankin, 2017).

As the labour progresses the lower segment of the uterus stretches and the cervix continues to thin or efface until there is full dilation. During the stretching of the lower segment, a membrane (the chorion) separating the baby from the mother detaches from the surface of the uterus and traps a small sack of amniotic fluid between the baby's head and the cervix. This is called the forewaters. The hindwaters is the remainder of the fluid behind the baby. As the cervix dilates, the pressure in the forewaters increases until they burst into the birth canal. While the membranes can rupture at any time during or even before labour, the physiological moment is when the cervix is fully dilated and entering the second stage. Towards the end of the first stage, as the cervix dilates quickly, the woman may have a bloody mucosal vaginal loss or a

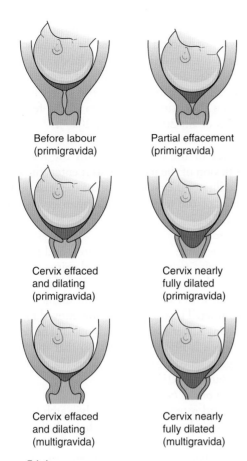

Before labour
(primigravida)

Partial effacement
(primigravida)

Cervix effaced
and dilating
(primigravida)

Cervix nearly
fully dilated
(primigravida)

Cervix effaced
and dilating
(multigravida)

Cervix nearly
fully dilated
(multigravida)

Figure 54.4
Cervical dilation for primigravida and multigravida.
Source: Pairman et al. (2014).

'show'. During pregnancy the cervix forms a mucus plug called the operculum, which assists in protecting the uterus from ascending infection (Rankin, 2017). Expulsion of the operculum at the end of pregnancy is known as a 'show' and often signifies changes to the cervix. The mucus plug or 'show' often continues to be expelled during labour as the cervix is dilating. Unfortunately, a 'show' is not a reliable indicator of time to birth, as a woman can have a 'show' at any stage during or prior to labour. Although the woman's body is preparing for labour in the final weeks of pregnancy and she may experience some discomfort, the actual definition of labour is the onset of painful regular contractions until full dilation of the cervix. The process of effacement is illustrated in Figure 54.4 and the cervix usually effaces and dilates faster in women who have previously had a baby.

The first stage of labour can be divided into three phases: latent (early), active and transitional. The latent phase is the period from the commencement of cervical effacement (thinning) and dilation until it is 3 cm dilated. The contractions commence irregularly at 15–20 minutes apart and may last up to 30 seconds but they become more coordinated and closer together. Once the cervix is more than 3 cm dilated, the active phase starts and continues until the cervix is 8–9 cm dilated. Dilation is much more rapid in the active phase, with the cervix dilating at an average of 1.5 cm per hour (Rankin, 2017). In addition, the contractions become more regular: three occurring in 10 minutes and lasting up to 60 seconds. When the cervix is 8–9 cm dilated, the woman enters the transitional phase. During this period the rate of dilation often slows and there may be a brief lull in uterine activity (Fraser & Cooper, 2009). During transition the woman often experiences restlessness and may become distressed, demanding pain relief.

Second stage
The second stage of labour is much shorter than the first; it begins at full dilation of the cervix and lasts until the birth of the baby. It can last up to 2 hours in a primigravida and 1 hour in a multigravida but can be as short as 5 minutes (Rankin, 2017). Since the length of this stage varies between women the best practice is to allow each woman to follow her own urges. The woman may have short 5–6-second pushes during one contraction or she may have the desire to bear down for longer (Coad & Dunstall, 2011; Rankin, 2017). Forcing her to push without the desire or stopping her from pushing when she needs to may cause hypoxia to the baby or exhaustion in the mother (Coad & Dunstall, 2011; Rankin, 2017).

At the commencement of the second stage the contractions become less intense as the mother experiences a quiet period or lull as the baby's head descends into the vagina. This can last between 10 and 30 minutes. During this important period there is no need to force the mother to push until she has the desire to do so herself (Rankin, 2017). As the baby descends further and the head becomes visible, the second stage progresses to an active period when the woman has an increasing urge to push or possibly defecate (Rankin, 2017). With each contraction the woman will bear down and the baby moves forwards and rotates in accordance with the pelvic floor. When the contractions subside it is possible that the baby may retreat back up the vagina until the next contraction (Coad & Dunstall, 2011). As the baby descends further, the perineum starts to stretch to allow passage of the baby's head (refer to the mechanism of labour below). When the widest part of the baby's head stretches the vulva to its maximum, the head often remains stationary or is said to be crowning. At this point the severity of the pain can cause the woman instinctively to stop pushing as she takes a quick breath or pants. This natural reflex prevents rapid delivery of the head, which could cause trauma to the perineum (Coad & Dunstall, 2011).

The baby is born facing the maternal anus but will rotate as its head realigns with the rest of the body in the pelvis (restitution). After restitution, the baby continues to turn a complete 90° until its head is perpendicular with the maternal midline as the anterior shoulder rotates in the pelvis. Rotation of the anterior shoulder continues as it follows the curve of the pelvis until it exits the vagina and the posterior shoulder immediately follows. With the birth of the comparatively large head and shoulders, the baby's body is instantly born with a gush of the amniotic fluid of the hindwaters (Coad & Dunstall, 2011).

Mechanism of labour

The journey of the baby into and through the pelvis is often referred to as the **mechanism of labour**. The successful completion of the mechanism of labour relies on two independent factors: the shape and the size of the presenting part of the fetus (Pairman et al., 2014; Rankin, 2017). Regardless of the orientation of the fetus in the uterus prior to delivery, there are three common principles to the mechanism: 1. the fetus will descend; 2. the leading part of the fetus will meet resistance against the pelvis floor and then rotate forwards; and 3. the last emerging part of the fetus will rotate around the pubic bone. Normal labour requires that the baby is in a longitudinal lie and that the attitude is one of good flexion so that the occiput is the presenting part, as detailed in Figure 54.5.

The stages of delivery are outlined below and in Figure 54.6.

Descent

Often the descent of the fetal head into the inlet of the pelvis occurs in the final weeks of pregnancy, especially for a primigravida. It is possible that the head will not descend until after the commencement of labour for a multigravida. As labour progresses the fetal head descends into the pelvis in transverse diameter but ease of entering the pelvis is largely reliant on the attitude or flexion of the fetal head (Pairman et al., 2014; Rankin, 2017).

Flexion

The force of the contractions on the fetal spine forces flexion of the fetal head as it enters the pelvis. This facilitates the presentation of the least possible diameter of the fetal head (Pairman et al., 2014; Rankin, 2017).

internal rotation

Due to the force of the contractions and the shape of the pelvis, including the ischial spines, once the fetal head has completely entered it rotates so that it lines up with the anteroposterior diameter of the pelvic outlet. The occiput has now moved forwards and is lying under the symphysis pubis. The position of the neck is slightly changed so that the head is no longer aligned with the shoulders (Pairman et al., 2014; Rankin, 2017).

Extension of the head

As the head moves under the pelvic arch it swivels on the pubic bone and pushes through the vagina, causing it to extend upwards. The forehead, face and chin then pass across the perineum (Pairman et al., 2014; Rankin, 2017), as illustrated in Figure 54.7.

Restitution

With the birth of the head, the shoulders enter the pelvis. The head appears to turn slightly externally as it realigns itself with the shoulders.

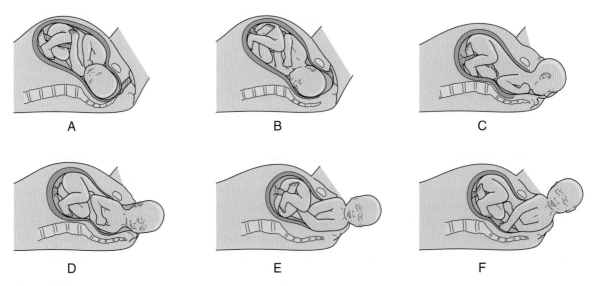

Figure 54.5
Mechanism of labour.
Source: Pairman et al. (2014).

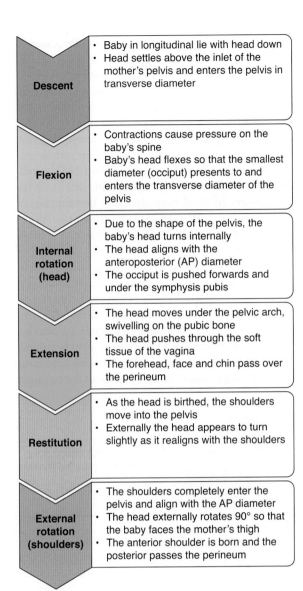

Descent	• Baby in longitudinal lie with head down • Head settles above the inlet of the mother's pelvis and enters the pelvis in transverse diameter
Flexion	• Contractions cause pressure on the baby's spine • Baby's head flexes so that the smallest diameter (occiput) presents to and enters the transverse diameter of the pelvis
Internal rotation (head)	• Due to the shape of the pelvis, the baby's head turns internally • The head aligns with the anteroposterior (AP) diameter • The occiput is pushed forwards and under the symphysis pubis
Extension	• The head moves under the pelvic arch, swivelling on the pubic bone • The head pushes through the soft tissue of the vagina • The forehead, face and chin pass over the perineum
Restitution	• As the head is birthed, the shoulders move into the pelvis • Externally the head appears to turn slightly as it realigns with the shoulders
External rotation (shoulders)	• The shoulders completely enter the pelvis and align with the AP diameter • The head externally rotates 90° so that the baby faces the mother's thigh • The anterior shoulder is born and the posterior passes the perineum

Figure 54.6
The stages of delivery.

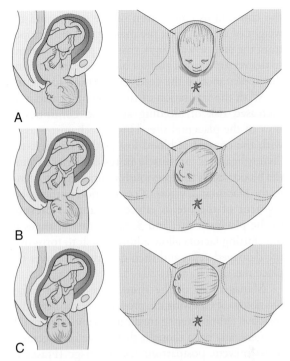

Figure 54.7
The head rotating and descending in the second stage.
Source: Marshall & Raynor (2014).

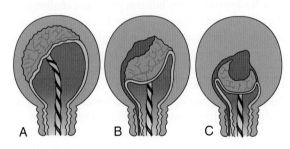

Figure 54.8
The third stage of labour commences after delivery,
A. The uterus contracts and the placenta separates,
B, and eventually passes down the birth canal, C.
Source: Marshall & Raynor (2014).

External rotation (shoulders)

As the shoulders continue to enter the pelvis, they align themselves with the anteroposterior diameter. The anterior shoulder hits the pelvic floor and moves under the symphysis pubis. This causes the head to continue to rotate so that the baby faces either the woman's left thigh or her right thigh. After the birth of the anterior shoulder, the posterior follows as it passes the perineum.

Third stage

The birth of the baby marks the commencement of the third stage. The contractions change and the rate slows (Pairman et al., 2014; Rankin, 2017). This stage can last between 5 and 60 minutes and is a vulnerable time for the mother as she has an increased risk of haemorrhage during this period

(Coad & Dunstall, 2011). After the birth of the baby the uterus contracts down upon itself; this reduction in size reduces the surface area of the placental site. The veins become more congested and rupture, causing the firm placenta to buckle and detach from the more flexible myometrium. The continuing contraction of the uterus causes the oblique muscle fibres to constrict around the blood vessels supplying the placenta, preventing drainage of blood back into the maternal system (see Fig 54.8). The increasingly congested placenta usually detaches from a central point and its escalating weight forces the separation of the edges followed by the membranes (Coad & Dunstall, 2011; Pairman et al., 2014; Rankin, 2017). Thus with the continuous contraction of the uterus and the weight of the placenta, the membranes are stripped from the uterine wall. Signs that the placenta is about to deliver are a small gush of blood (separation) and the appearance of the cord lengthening (descent).

With the separation of the placenta, there is an increased risk of bleeding as blood continues to flow to the placental site. Three mechanisms assist with the control of blood loss at this stage: 1. the 'living ligatures' or muscle fibres constrict around the blood vessels that previously connected the uterus to the placenta; 2. vigorous contraction of the upper segment of the uterus effectively applies pressure to the placental site; and 3. temporary changes in the clotting factors allow a fibrin mesh to form over the damaged veins and then quickly form over the placental site (Rankin, 2017).

Management of the third stage can be either physiological (allowing the process to occur naturally) or active (administering medications and therapy). It has generally been thought that active management helps prevent postpartum haemorrhage (Fraser & Cooper, 2009; Rankin, 2017) but recent research has questioned this belief (Pairman et al., 2014). At present, physiological management is recommended only for low-risk births but this presents a challenge in the pre-hospital setting as—purely by definition—out-of-hospital births are considered high risk in that they always occur in an unplanned setting, without the expected continuity of care, and often are precipitated births. However, most births that occur in the out-of-hospital setting are in fact normal vertex presentations and require little or no intervention (McLelland et al., 2018; Moscovitz et al., 2000; Verdile et al., 1995). As such, paramedics should be confident that physiological management should be adequate in most cases. In fact, in practical terms there are no in-field options for management of the third stage except allowing the placenta to separate and deliver naturally. The gush of blood that accompanies this may seem dramatic but if palpation reveals a firm uterus (a little bigger than a cricket ball), paramedics can be reassured that there should be no further bleeding from the placental bed.

Maternal physiological adaptation during labour

Cardiovascular system

A progressive rise in cardiac output with each contraction adds 300–500 mL of blood to the circulating volume and increases the woman's heart rate (Coad & Dunstall, 2011; Pairman et al., 2014; Rankin, 2017). There are also increases in diastolic and systolic blood pressure: increasing 5 seconds before a contraction and returning to baseline after the contraction. In the first stage, there may be a rise of 35 mmHg systolic and 25 mmHg diastolic; and in the second stage the diastolic can rise up to 55 mmHg and the systolic can rise higher than in the first stage (Coad & Dunstall, 2011; Pairman et al., 2014; Rankin, 2017). With the delivery of third-stage dramatic haematological changes occur and parameters return to pre-labour levels (Coad & Dunstall, 2011; Pairman et al., 2014; Rankin, 2017).

Supine hypotension remains a risk during labour, with the pregnant uterus pressing on the inferior vena cava and causing a reduction in cardiac return (Coad & Dunstall, 2011; Pairman et al., 2014; Rankin, 2017; see Fig 54.9). As a guiding principle, paramedics should avoid allowing a pregnant woman to lie supine. In transit this means using either the left lateral position or a wedge under the right hip to tilt the pregnant

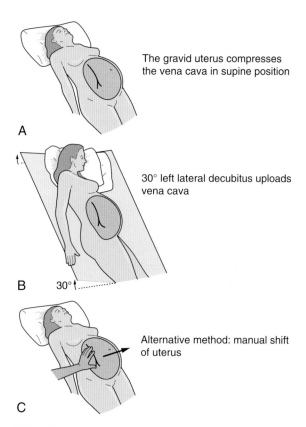

The gravid uterus compresses the vena cava in supine position

A

30° left lateral decubitus uploads vena cava

B   30°

Alternative method: manual shift of uterus

C

Figure 54.9
Supine hypotension. The weight of the gravid uterus can compress the inferior vena cava when the patient is supine, A. This can be managed by tilting the patient at least 30° to the left, B, or manually displacing the uterus to the left, C.
Source: Pairman et al. (2014).

uterus away from the vena cava. Unfortunately, most ambulances have a stretcher mounted on the right side of the vehicle so the paramedics have to turn the patient away from them, making observations that much harder. Loading the woman feet first is a possible solution but it removes the paramedic's ability to sit at her head and manage her airway or to secure her using the appropriate safety restraints.

Haematological system

To keep blood loss during delivery to a minimum, changes occur in the haematological system, including a state of increased coagulation (this precedes and follows delivery by several weeks) and physiological anaemia as a result of the increase in blood volume (increased plasma volume) but not in the amount of red blood cells. During labour, however, haemoconcentration can occur as a result of dehydration from exertion. Stress and muscular activity can also precipitate an increase in the formation of red blood cells (erythropoiesis). During labour and immediately postpartum, there is an increase in neutrophils and the white cell count may increase up to $25–30 \times 10^9/L$ (Coad & Dunstall, 2011; Pairman et al., 2014; Rankin, 2017).

Respiratory system

In active labour, hyperventilation from pain or anxiety can lead to a temporary respiratory alkalosis with the typical signs of hyperventilation (peripheral paraesthesia). A respiratory acidosis can occur if contractions are too close together (unlikely in spontaneous-onset labour) or if the woman holds her breath too long when pushing during the second stage (Coad & Dunstall, 2011; Rankin, 2017). Both conditions are generally self-resolving and do not require any intervention. However, both may indicate inadequate pain relief.

Renal system

Increased aldosterone secretion stimulates an increase in sodium loss (and potassium retention). There is a chance of dehydration so fluid intake should be maintained, particularly in prolonged labour or in labour occurring in hot conditions (Coad & Dunstall, 2011; Rankin, 2017).

 CASE STUDY 1

Case 10923, 1036 hrs.

Dispatch details: A 37-year-old woman, 39 weeks' gestation; membranes have ruptured; in labour.

Initial presentation: On arrival at the scene the paramedics find the patient leaning over the couch in her lounge room. She is able to answer questions in between contractions. Her neighbour is in attendance as they are unable to contact the patient's husband, who has gone to a country town for work. He is out on site, so is unreachable at the moment. The woman's 3-year-old daughter is also present.

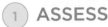 **ASSESS**

Patient history

On questioning the patient tells the crew that her membranes ruptured an hour ago and the amniotic fluid was clear. She is having contractions every 6–8 minutes but at this stage can breathe through them. She does not report an urge to push. This is her fifth pregnancy: three of her children are at school and one is with her.

In order to prepare a treatment plan the crew need to know:
- the history of this labour
- the history of this pregnancy

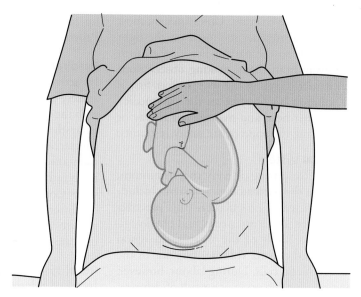

Figure 54.10
Feeling for a contraction.
Source: Pairman et al. (2014).

- the history of previous pregnancies and births
- a general medical history.

This labour

- *When did the contractions start? How often are they coming?* It is possible in this situation that a woman may be so distressed that she may state she is feeling contractions long after they finish, so the paramedics should try to feel the contractions if they can (see Fig 54.10).
- *Have the membranes ruptured?* The membranes can rupture at any point before or during labour, even when the head is crowning. If the membranes are still intact when the head delivers, they need to be ruptured manually by tearing them. The membranes must not be ruptured manually if they cannot be visualised. Once the membranes have ruptured, the amniotic fluid should be clear to slightly pink in colour. Any other colour is significant: green to brown could indicate a distressed baby and any shade of red could indicate bleeding.
- *Is there any other vaginal discharge?* Mucus mixed with a small amount of blood, or a 'show', indicates normal detachment of the membranes as the cervix is dilated. If the mucus becomes more heavily blood-stained, it may indicate that the cervix is nearing full dilation. Any amount of frank bleeding should be considered abnormal.
- *When did the mother feel the baby move last?* Paramedics have no ability to monitor the baby's wellbeing or health and asking about movements provides only an indication about the baby's health. Babies do not continually move in utero and often have 'sleep periods' where they are very quiet, so a lack of movement does not necessarily indicate a problem. If the mother has had a trouble-free pregnancy and is at term, and the labour is spontaneous and trouble-free, there is no reason to think there is a problem.
- *Are there any signs of the second stage or imminent delivery?* For example, uncontrollable urge to push, anal pouting, perineal bulging or presenting part on view.
- *When did the mother last void?* It is important to ask when the woman last urinated to assess fluid status, as dehydration can slow the progress of labour

and a full bladder can become an obstruction during the second stage of labour (Pairman et al., 2014).

This pregnancy

- *What is the mother's gravida and parity?* Generally, if a woman is a nullipara, the labour will take longer than if she is a multigravida (Pairman et al., 2014). However, there are exceptions to any rule so paramedics should always assess the woman's physical and clinical signs.
- *What is the gestation in weeks?* Rather than asking the baby's due date, it is better to ask the gestation in weeks. Determining the gestation of the baby allows the paramedics to assess the risk associated with a premature infant (see Ch 55).
- *Have there been any obstetric complications during the pregnancy?* Complications such as pre-eclampsia, gestational diabetes or antepartum haemorrhage can assist in gauging the risk of associated intrapartum or postpartum complications (Coad & Dunstall, 2011; Fraser & Cooper, 2009; Pairman et al., 2014; Rankin, 2017).

Previous pregnancies and births

- *Has the mother had any previous pregnancies and births? Were there any complications?* Women who have pregnancy and birth complications may be at greater risk of similar complications with subsequent pregnancies. Paramedics should assess the potential risk for this birth by obtaining a thorough history of previous births and pregnancies, such as shoulder dystocia, breech presentation and postpartum haemorrhage.

Past or present medical history

- *Does the woman have any chronic medical conditions?* For example, asthma, cardiac conditions.
- *Is there any acute exacerbation of chronic medical conditions?*
- *Has the patient had any recent acute medical conditions?* For example, upper respiratory tract infection, urinary tract infection.
- *Does the patient have any allergies?*

Initial assessment summary

Problem	Labour
Conscious state	GCS = 15
Position	Standing
Heart rate	92 bpm
Blood pressure	125/70 mmHg
Skin appearance	Pink, warm, dry
Speech pattern	Normal between contractions
Respiratory rate	18 bpm, becomes more erratic during contractions
Respiratory rhythm	Even cycles
Chest auscultation	Good breath sounds bilaterally
Pulse oximetry	99%
Temperature	37.4°C
Pain	Little to no pain between contractions; 8/10 during contractions
History	Gravida 5, para 4. Her membranes ruptured an hour ago and the amniotic fluid is clear. She is having contractions every 6–8 minutes but at this stage is able to breathe through them. She does not report an urge to push. Her last labour was over in less than 4 hours.
Physical assessment	No signs of the second stage of labour.

D: There are no immediate dangers.
A: The airway is not compromised.
B: Breathing is normal.
C: The patient is well perfused and there is no obvious haemorrhage.

The patient is a multigravida presenting in the first stage of labour of a near full-term uncomplicated pregnancy. Previous vaginal deliveries were uneventful and she has no complicating medical conditions. There does not appear to be any sign of fetal distress.

<table>
<tr><td>

DIFFERENTIAL DIAGNOSIS

First stage of labour
Or
- Second stage of labour and imminent delivery likely

</td></tr>
</table>

② CONFIRM

The challenge facing the crew is this situation is to decide whether there is time to transport the patient to hospital for the birth or whether the birth is imminent and they should prepare to deliver the baby prior to transport. Such are the uncertainties with the progression of labour that this judgment has to be made on a case-by-case basis considering the resources available, the distance to hospital and the patient's presentation. Although it is possible to deliver a baby in the ambulance it is not well-suited to the procedure and should be avoided if possible.

The following criteria should be assessed prior to making a decision about transport:
- contractions
- vaginal discharge
- signs of imminent delivery
- wellbeing of the baby
- signs of the second stage of labour and an imminent delivery.

Contractions

Definitive diagnosis of labour can be made only by performing a vaginal examination to assess cervical effacement and dilation. This skill is not commonly within the scope of practice for paramedics, so they need to rely on clinical assessment of contractions (see Box 54.1). The onset of early labour is often signified by the commencement of irregular contractions occurring 15–20 minutely that may last up to 30 seconds. During this period paramedics may discuss options with the patient and her family regarding staying home longer or travelling independently to hospital versus being transported in an ambulance. They can explain that labour is not fully established and she has time to organise herself further.

> ## BOX 54.1 Contractions
>
> Contractions are often described as intermittent waves of pain reaching a crescendo and then tapering, with a period of little or no pain in between. The frequency of contractions is measured from the beginning of one contraction until the beginning of the next and is described in one of two ways: 1. by how often they come (i.e. 3 minutely, 5 minutely, 10 minutely); and 2. by how often they occur in a 10-minute period (i.e. 3 in 10 minutes, 2 in 10 minutes or 1 in 10 minutes). The length of a contraction is measured from the beginning of that contraction until the end (i.e. 20 seconds, 30 seconds, 45 seconds and 60 seconds). In normal labour contractions rarely last longer than a minute or the baby would be compromised (Rankin, 2017). With the mother's permission to feel for a contraction, the paramedic should place one hand on the uterine fundus. The abdomen will become increasingly tenser for a period of time, usually no longer than 60 seconds, and then it will relax for a period of time before becoming tense again.

Each labour will have unique characteristics depending on several factors, including the number of previous babies the woman has had, the position and presentation of this baby, the gestation in weeks and whether there are other obstetric or medical complications. Labour is a dynamic process during which the contractions increase in strength, duration and frequency. A patient may describe the frequency of contractions by how many minutes apart they are but it is important that the paramedic is also aware of the length. Assessing the contractions accurately will assist in determining the appropriate form of pain relief. As the labour progresses, the contractions may come three times in 10 minutes and last up to 60 seconds. This often signifies that the woman is in active labour. Even so, the birth could still be several hours away. If the patient is very distressed and demanding, it is likely that she has entered the transitional phase but that does not always rule out the opportunity to transport.

In this case the patient's calm presentation, the timing of the contractions and the lack of an urge to push during the contractions suggest that birth is not imminent.

Vaginal discharge

Assessing the vaginal discharge during labour will assist paramedics to gauge the wellbeing of both the mother and the baby as well as assisting in decision-making. Vaginal discharge can include the expelled mucus plug as the cervix dilates, amniotic fluid and any vaginal bleeding. In this case, the discharge appears normal and does not indicate any urgency.

Signs of imminent delivery

As the second stage can take up to an hour to complete, there is often enough time to transport the patient to hospital but paramedics should consider the circumstances in which they have been requested. Most mothers have a plan for the birth and requesting an ambulance may suggest that events are occurring faster than anticipated, which could indicate a rapid progression of labour. An uncontrollable urge to push or bear down, uncontrollable grunting and an urge to defecate should all be considered as imminent signs of birth. As the baby descends through the pelvis, this will progress to anal pouting or puckering, perineal bulging and the presenting part becoming visible. It is worth noting that the rate of progression can slow or even halt and concurrent preparation for transport is always advisable. More often than not, the births that paramedics attend progress quickly and may require the paramedics to support the mother through the birth. In this case there are no signs of imminent delivery.

The baby's wellbeing

One of the key assessments of fetal wellbeing is to monitor the fetal heart rate (FHR) through labour and especially in relation to the contractions. Paramedics do not commonly have the equipment to monitor the FHR, however, so assessing fetal wellbeing is difficult in this setting. Enquiring about the last fetal movements provides a small amount of information about the baby's wellbeing, but babies do not continually move in utero so a lack of movement does not necessarily indicate a problem. This patient says she felt her baby kick 15 minutes before she called for the ambulance. As her membranes have ruptured and the fluid appears clear, there is no suggestion that the baby is distressed.

Signs of the second stage of labour and an imminent delivery

While this patient's heart rate may be higher than that of a non-pregnant woman of her age, it is not unexpected in pregnancy and especially during labour. Her respiratory rate is within normal limits but respiratory hyperventilation is common in the first stage of labour. The patient is having two strong contractions every 10 minutes and they are lasting for 50 seconds. She is panting through the contractions and is relatively pain-free between them.

The crew make the sound decision that the patient is in the active phase of the first stage of labour and can be transported the estimated 20 minutes to hospital.

TREAT

Emergency management

Safety

While the patient is in her own home, she should be allowed to remain in a position of comfort until the initial assessments and evaluations have been completed. For safety reasons, she should be transported in either a semi-recumbent or a lateral position to avoid supine hypotensive syndrome. If her membranes ruptured on the floor, check that there are no slip hazards.

Last micturition

As the baby descends into the pelvis, the bladder is vulnerable to traumatic damage (Fraser & Cooper, 2009). In addition, a full bladder can delay the progress of the baby's head as it descends during the second stage (Rankin, 2017). Prior to transport, the paramedics should encourage the woman to pass urine, as there will be little chance until they arrive at the hospital.

Vaginal discharge

A maternity pad placed at the labia will enable the crew and the receiving hospital to accurately describe and measure vaginal loss.

Analgesia

Regular contractions can be very painful. The possibility of not giving birth in the intended place, with the expected carers, can be extremely stressful and exacerbate the patient's discomfort (Pairman et al., 2014). If the patient requires analgesia, the use of numerical scores as an assessment tool for pain is not recommended for a woman in labour (National Institute for Health and Care Excellence, 2007). The intermittent nature of contraction pain makes it difficult to manage and fast-acting inhaled analgesics are better suited than long-lasting IV agents such as opioids, which can have a sedative effect between contractions. Opiates also cross the placental barrier and so their use in late labour risks producing respiratory depression in a newborn infant and even drowsiness for several days after birth, which can affect the baby's breastfeeding (National Institute for Health and Care Excellence, 2017).

When paramedics have no option but to administer an opioid analgesic, it is important that they assess the mother completely to ensure that they are satisfied she is not near the second stage. Philosophically, the management of pain for a woman in labour is very different from many of the other cases paramedics manage. The woman in labour should be treated as a 'normal' or 'well' event not an 'emergency' or 'ill' event. Certainly as the out-of-hospital context is unplanned and the usual in-hospital or home birth resources are unavailable, there is some risk. But most unplanned births are uncomplicated and occur without undue incident.

While paramedics cannot provide the continuity of care that has been shown to be a key element of successful progress in labour, they can provide a calm and reassuring environment for the mother. Building rapport and trust with the mother will reassure her that she is safe and is essential for delivering safe but adequate pain relief.

Oxygen

Physiological anaemia is commonly experienced in late pregnancy, but labour is a normal process so oxygen is not required in this situation. Although oxygen may be administered during obstetric emergencies, it is important to note that there is no recent quality evidence to support the effectiveness or not of this practice (Pairman et al., 2014). Although the flow of oxygen to the placenta is reduced in normal labour, the normal-term fetus adapts well by redistributing the flow of blood to protect vital organs such as the heart and brain, so overall the fetal circulation is unaffected by the pressure of the contractions (Steer & Flint, 1999).

Preparation for an emergency birth

Although many of the women in labour attended to and transported by paramedics do not actually give birth prior to arrival at hospital, it is wise for the crew to prepare for emergency birth. This includes arranging to rendezvous with another crew en route or preferably at the scene, as it can take more than two crew members to manage both the mother and the infant if problems arise. The majority of babies are born without incident, but crews should also routinely prepare the scene for neonatal resuscitation (see Ch 55).

1116 hrs: After travelling for 12 minutes, the patient becomes very distressed and commences a guttural groaning. She tells the paramedics that she needs to push. Upon visual inspection, the paramedics notice anal pouting and perineal bulging.

The decision to pull over for delivery is difficult. However, the paramedics have to set up not only for delivery but also for potential resuscitation of the newborn in a very tight environment.

Comfort/analgesia

Often a woman feels relief when she pushes according to her own natural urges during the second stage (Fraser & Cooper, 2009; Pairman et al., 2014; Rankin, 2017). As well as assessing the frequency, length and intensity of the contractions, the paramedics should assess how the woman pushes during the contractions. It can be normal for a woman to have several short 5-second pushes in one contraction.

The imminent signs of delivery

Once the baby has descended, the bobbing of the presenting part on the perineum should be visible to the paramedics. If the rate of progression appears to halt or slow, the paramedics will need to consider recommencing transport, as this could be a sign that there may be an unexpected problem. They also need to ensure that the mother does not progress too rapidly and have an explosive birth. They can prevent this by coaching her on her breathing throughout the contractions. Provided the baby does not become stuck, the head should be delivered within a few minutes of it being visible between the labia. The paramedics want the baby's head to be delivered, but not so rapidly that it causes damage to the baby and to the perineum, hence this is the phase where they will instruct the patient to pant in an effort to control the rate of delivery.

Vaginal discharge

The paramedics should continue to assess the colour and amount of vaginal discharge. Often, as the cervix dilates fully, a more heavily blood-stained 'show' will be discharged. While this is normal, any frank bleeding should be considered abnormal (Fraser & Cooper, 2009; Pairman et al., 2014; Rankin, 2017). If the membranes have not already ruptured, they will usually rupture at the commencement of the second stage but this cannot be guaranteed (Fraser & Cooper, 2009).

Fetal wellbeing

As the baby descends, fetal oxygenation is threatened due to cord or head compression, so the paramedics need to continue to monitor the amniotic fluid, looking for meconium staining. It is not unusual for fetal movements to be reduced or difficult to detect during the second stage.

Position

Usually during the second stage a woman should be able to assume any position where she feels the most comfortable. Squatting, kneeling on all fours or standing positions all produce a 28% increase in the outlet compared to supine or semi-recumbent positions. However, the back of the ambulance can be restrictive and may limit the amount of freedom the woman has, especially when moving.

The birth process

The paramedics should allow the mother to follow her instincts and push as she wants. There is no evidence to support the practice of instructing the mother to push (Valsalva manoeuvre) and it has been suggested that this could cause problems for both mother (Rankin, 2017) and baby (Pairman et al., 2014).

Initially, with contractions the baby's head will advance and recede: this slowly stretches the perineum to allow it to accommodate the baby's head (see Fig 54.7). Once the baby's head remains on the perineum and does not recede (crowning), the mother may complain of a burning sensation as the perineum stretches. During this time, the paramedics can encourage the mother to pant to minimise the possibility of perineal damage associated with a rapid birth. While the mother is pushing, she may defecate. This is quite normal. Placing a pad over the rectum will enable the paramedics to keep the area clean.

Most babies will birth spontaneously with minimal or no hands-on assistance. However, rapid descent of the head has been associated with an increase in maternal perineal tears. Lightly placing fingers on the descending head can provide support in a rapid birth and prevent perineal tears (Pairman et al., 2014). However, it is important not to place too much pressure on the head so that its progress is hindered.

Once the baby's head is born, there is a rest period between contractions. Traditionally at this time the baby is checked to see whether the cord is wrapped around the neck and to identify whether it needs to be cut to relieve pressure. For the mother this is an awkward procedure and many women find it uncomfortable or even painful. Most babies birth through the cord, so cutting the cord at this stage needs careful consideration as it will remove the only source of oxygen the baby receives and could cause further distress (Pairman et al., 2014). Paramedics should avoid cutting the cord unless it is obstructing the descent of the baby through the pelvis. As the baby is born the paramedics should still be assessing the amniotic fluid for any change in colour.

With the next contraction the baby's shoulders enter the pelvis and rotate into the anterior-posterior diameter of the outlet position. This rotation of the shoulder is observed externally as the baby's head restitutes to come into alignment with the shoulders. This is a natural movement and should not be forced. With the next contraction the woman may need to be encouraged to give another push and the anterior shoulder should deliver. If it does not deliver spontaneously, the paramedic may need to apply some gentle upward traction if she is on all fours. Following the birth of the anterior shoulder, some gentle downward traction will deliver the posterior shoulder. Immediately the rest of the baby will follow.

The time of birth should be noted.

Care of the baby

1132 hrs: Immediate care of the baby commences (see Ch 55). One paramedic takes responsibility for the baby and the other cares for the mother. They assist the patient to roll over so that she can hold her baby. With the patient's permission, the paramedics place the baby skin-to-skin on her abdomen and they wrap both mother and baby in a blanket to keep them warm.

While paramedics should not force breastfeeding, it often occurs naturally with mother and baby in this position. This will stimulate the release of oxytocin, which aids in the completion of the third stage.

Many ambulance services have operating instructions requiring all patients to be secured appropriately in a moving vehicle that would (taken literally) include a newborn baby. Paramedics have to balance the very real risk of hypothermia that is easily prevented with skin-to-skin contact (in the absence of a heated cot in the ambulance) with the risk of injury associated with an ambulance crash.

The birth of the baby signals the end of second stage of labour and the commencement of the third stage.

The third stage

Contractions/pain

The uterus continues to contract after the birth of the baby, but usually this does not cause any undue distress. Rarely, a woman may experience painful 'after pains' and require analgesia. Increasing pain could be a sign of trauma (uterine rupture, for instance) and while reassuring the patient the paramedics should be re-evaluating for any signs of peritonism.

Vaginal discharge

The paramedics need to check for any vaginal discharge at the end of the second stage and the beginning of the third stage. While there is a slight possibility that signs of meconium as the baby is born could indicate that the baby was stressed, it is more likely to be a normal bowel action (see Ch 55). A gush of blood can be a sign of normal placental separation, but other causes should be considered. If there is continual bleeding, especially greater than 500 mL, the paramedics should manage this postpartum haemorrhage by controlling obvious sources of haemorrhage with direct pressure and instituting volume replacement as usual.

Perineal damage

The perineum should be assessed for tearing or trauma and managed if required. Applying a combined dressing or maternity pad has two benefits: 1. it provides pressure to arrest bleeding; and 2. it aids assessment of any further bleeding.

Position

For transport during the third stage the mother can assume a position of comfort. But the paramedics need to continually assess for signs of separation and descent, as they may need to stop the ambulance to deliver the placenta. The best position for delivery of the placenta is an upright position (Coad & Dunstall, 2011), which is not optimum in a moving vehicle.

Last void

The paramedics should document the last time the patient voided as a full bladder can delay completion of the third stage and contribute to postpartum haemorrhage (Coad & Dunstall, 2011; Pairman et al., 2014). This information will be useful to pass on to the midwifery staff.

Management

The third stage is a vulnerable period in the out-of-hospital setting with an increased risk of postpartum haemorrhage (Coad & Dunstall, 2011; Rankin, 2017). Crews need to weigh the benefits of the physiological third stage against the possible need to manage complications. As the physiological third stage can take up to an hour, the paramedics should resume transport while continually assessing for signs of separation and descent. There is no need to pull the cord or manipulate the uterus at any time.

Unless neonatal resuscitation is required or transferring the mother to the stretcher proves problematic, the cord should remain intact during transport to facilitate the physiological third stage (Fraser & Cooper, 2009; Pairman et al., 2014; Rankin, 2017). If the cord has been clamped or cut during the birth or before it stops pulsating, the physiology of the third stage is altered and active management is required (Pairman et al., 2014).

In the out-of-hospital setting physiological management of the third stage must be considered the most appropriate option but it depends on the circumstances. For a birth at term, leaving the cord intact until it ceases pulsation is sensible. Unfortunately, unplanned births before arrival (BBAs) at hospital have a greater risk of maternal and neonatal complications (McLelland et al., 2013) so it may not always be possible to physiologically manage the third stage. That said, true active management of the third stage can prove difficult in the out-of-hospital setting.

Use of out-of-hospital pharmacology depends on the availability of the drugs and the ambulance service guidelines but may include intramuscular Syntocinon or oral/rectal misoprostol. If the ambulance service guidelines recommend pharmacology only with postpartum haemorrhage, the paramedics should be alert to the increased risk of bleeding once the umbilical cord has been cut. With good reason, many out-of-hospital guidelines (Woollard et al., 2008) advise against paramedics practising controlled cord traction, but this technique may be necessary if there is a postpartum haemorrhage (see Case study 5 and Box 54.3 later in this chapter).

Unless the third stage is complicated by excessive bleeding, there is no rush to deliver the placenta in the out-of-hospital setting and so active management is not often necessary. Sometimes the mother may have a desire to push again and will spontaneously deliver the placenta. Otherwise, it is wisest to allow the placenta to remain in situ and leave management of third stage to the maternity staff. If the placenta is delivered during transport, it should be placed in a plastic bag and taken to hospital. The paramedics can check that the placenta is complete but this will be done again in the maternity unit.

Hospital admission

Ideally, the paramedics should transport the patient to the hospital that she has booked into as it will have a record of her obstetric history and medical history, including her blood group. A common exception to this is if the baby is premature and requires a special care nursery (SCN) or neonatal intensive care unit (NICU). Other possible exceptions include that the hospital is too far away.

There are a variety of models of care available to pregnant women. The patient could be under the care of a midwife or a medical practitioner such as an obstetrician. Even if the baby was born outside the hospital, the primary carer will oversee the overall management. On admission to the hospital, management will depend on the patient's condition. If the placenta has not been delivered, she will be admitted to the birthing suite; if it has been delivered, she will be admitted into postnatal care. Any perineal or vaginal lacerations will be repaired; and twice per day the involution of the uterus will be checked to ensure that it is descending as required and her vaginal loss (lochia) and any sutures will be checked for signs of infection.

As much as possible mother and baby will remain together unless the baby needs to be admitted to SCN or NICU. A normal, healthy term baby will room in with the mother and she will be encouraged to breastfeed as soon as possible. The length of hospital stay varies from 2 to 5 days for a normal birth. Even if the baby is in SCN or NICU, most women will be discharged within this timeframe.

Investigations

Any required investigations depend on the woman's condition; often, for a normal birth no investigations are required. If the mother is a negative blood group, the baby's blood group will be checked; if the baby is a positive blood group, the mother will receive anti-D within 72 hours of the birth. This will prevent the mother forming antibodies against the blood type of any subsequent babies she may carry. If the woman has suffered excessive bleeding, her haemoglobin and blood group will be checked.

Follow-up

Discharge follow-up for a normal birth is largely dependent on the model of care chosen by the woman. In the caseload model, the woman will continue to be cared for by the midwife or midwives of that team. Women not in the caseload model will be visited by the hospital domiciliary midwife for up to a week after the birth. The number of visits made depends on the length of the woman's stay in hospital: the shorter the stay, the more visits. Women in the medical model will visit their medical practitioner approximately 6 weeks after discharge.

Once the woman has been discharged from the services provided by the hospital, the maternal child and health nurse will usually make at least one visit to the woman's home. Thereafter, the woman will usually go to the maternal child and health centre to have her baby's health monitored.

CASE STUDY 2

Case 11121, 2245 hrs.

Dispatch details: A 25-year-old female, who is 34 weeks' pregnant, is in labour with her second child.

Initial presentation: The ambulance crew find the patient lying in a left lateral position on her bed. She tells them that she thought the contractions would stop but they have got stronger since her membranes ruptured.

---

(1) ASSESS

2258 hrs History: She says that her contractions started at 6 tonight and she is now having three contractions in 10 minutes. Her membranes ruptured an hour ago and the amniotic fluid has been clear. She also had a show earlier in the day. Her husband does not have a driver's licence and they have no-one to drive her to hospital. She has had the urge to push during the last few contractions. This is her second pregnancy and she has had one live birth.

2300 hrs Examination: The patient has anal pouting and perineal bulging. As the paramedics prepare to assist with the birth, they observe fresh meconium when she pushes. With the next push, they realise that the presenting part is the baby's buttocks.

Breech presentation

In a **breech presentation** the presenting part of the baby is the sacrum, foot or knee. There are four types of breech presentation (see also Fig 54.11).

- *Extended, frank or incomplete breech* occurs in 45–50% of breech presentations, usually in women who are having their first baby. The baby's thighs are flexed with the legs extended at the knees so the feet lie adjacent to the baby's head.
- *Complete or flexed breech* occurs in 10–15% of breech presentations, usually in women who have previously had babies. The baby's thighs are flexed and crossed, with the feet close to the buttocks.
- *Footling breech* is rare and occurs more commonly in premature births, usually before 34 weeks (Fraser & Cooper, 2009). One or both of the hips and knees are extended and the feet present below the buttocks.
- *Knee breech* is the rarest breech presentation with one or both hips extended and the knees flexed, presenting below the buttocks.

The proportion of breech presentations decreases as the gestational age of the baby increases, from 25% at < 28 weeks' gestation to no more than 10% at 34 weeks' and 1–3% at term (Pairman et al., 2014).

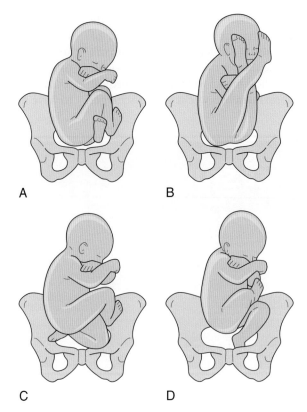

Figure 54.11
Types of breech presentation. A Complete. B Frank or extended. C Footling (kneeling). D Footling (single).
Source: Pairman et al. (2014).

Risk factors for a breech presentation include:
- extended legs in utero
- multiple pregnancy
- preterm labour
- polyhydramnios
- hydrocephaly
- uterine abnormality
- placenta praevia (Pairman et al., 2014).

There are no definite warning signs to diagnose a breech but often breech births are preceded by fresh or thick meconium after the membranes rupture (Royal Women's Hospital, 2006). Due to compression of the abdomen as it passes into the pelvis the baby often passes meconium. This is not a sign of fetal distress unless it occurs in early labour (Fraser & Cooper, 2009). In early labour the meconium will be blended more with the amniotic fluid to give it a brown- or green-stained appearance that occurs with fetal distress.

3 TREAT

Breech delivery has its own specific problems associated with the timely delivery of the baby before hypoxia causes damage. Because the widest part of the baby is following and not leading, there is a concern that the baby may become stuck. However, a minimalistic hands-off approach is best unless the progress of the birth is impeded: intervention is rarely required (Pairman et al., 2014). All other aspects of the delivery and at the resuscitation are similar to the normal situation.

When the perineum is distended by the buttocks, the paramedics should place the woman in the lithotomy position with her buttocks at the edge of the bed or couch and her legs pulled back at a 90° angle by either herself or two bystanders. Consider using dining chairs or other furniture for her to rest her legs (Woollard et al., 2008).

The paramedics should observe the buttocks as they progress through the perineum. The breech should rotate spontaneously to the sacroanterior position (the baby's back should be anterior to the mother). If the baby's back is not anterior to the mother, it may be necessary to gently rotate the baby to achieve this position. To rotate the baby, hold the baby's buttocks over the iliac crests and gently rotate so the baby's back is towards the midline of the mother's abdomen. It is important not to squeeze the baby's abdomen or pull on the baby's legs.

The paramedics should continue to observe the descent of the baby's buttocks through the perineum. As the buttocks continue to descend, the knees will pass through the introitus and the legs should spontaneously deliver. If the legs are extended, they may not deliver until the chest is born (Pairman et al., 2014). If progress is halted at this point, it may be necessary to assist delivery of the legs using two fingers to apply gentle flexion at the popliteal fossa or behind the knee joint and two fingers of the same hand over the baby's shin to bring the legs down, one at a time. Once the baby's legs are delivered, they should allow the baby to descend to its shoulders. At this stage it is possible to gently palpate the cord to check the fetal heart rate, but overhandling the cord can cause it to spasm (Pairman et al., 2014). Do not pull down on the cord (ALSO, 2004; Woollard et al., 2008).

Usually the baby's shoulders will spontaneously deliver without any interference. If this does not occur, it may be because the arms are extended over the baby's head, thus stopping progress of the baby's head through the pelvis due to the added bulk of the arms. To enable the head to enter the pelvis, it will be necessary to assist by using Løvset's manoeuvre (see Fig 54.12). This involves a series of rotations and downward traction of the baby. Keeping the back uppermost, the paramedic rotates the baby's body as much as 180° so that the posterior shoulder is lying under the symphysis pubis, then sweeps the first arm across in front of the baby's face (like a cat licking its face) and down beside the baby's chest. Then, keeping the baby's back uppermost, the paramedic rotates the baby back in the opposite direction at least 180° and using the same manoeuvre brings the second arm down and delivers the shoulders.

Once the shoulders are visible the baby's head will enter the mother's pelvis and the baby must be born within 6 minutes (Pairman et al., 2014). While it is important to be cognisant of this timeframe, it is also necessary to avoid a rapid birth as sudden decompression can lead to intracranial haemorrhage. The paramedic should allow the baby to hang and be hands off. If the back starts to rotate off centre, the baby can be gently rotated back by encircling the pelvic girdle with two hands. Wrapping a warm towel around the baby's bottom can help avoid hypothermia. Once the nape of the baby's neck and hairline are visible, the mother should be encouraged to lean forwards at the waist to tilt her pelvis, aiding clearance of the baby's mouth and nose. Do not tug or pull the baby at any stage during this process.

Sometimes it is necessary to provide assistance for the birth of the baby's head using the modified Maurice-Smellie-Viet manoeuvre (see Fig 54.13). To ensure favourable diameters, the head must be birthed by flexion. One paramedic should apply suprapubic pressure to encourage flexion of the occiput while the other second paramedic kneels in front of but lower than the woman. The second paramedic straddles the baby's body over one arm with the ring and index finger on the baby's cheeks (maxillae) and the middle finger on the baby's

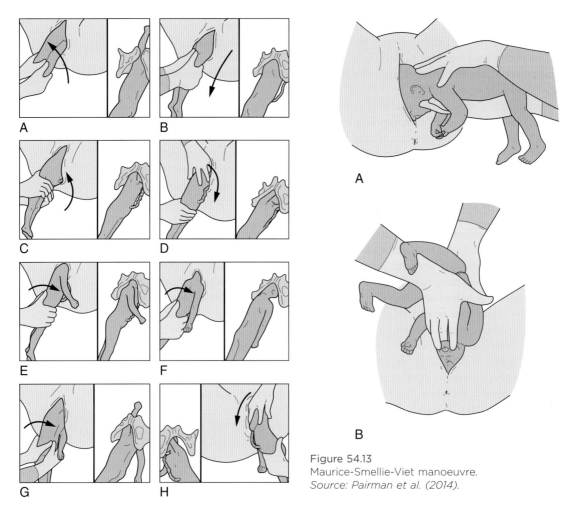

Figure 54.12
Løvset's manoeuvre.
Source: Pairman et al. (2014).

Figure 54.13
Maurice-Smellie-Viet manoeuvre.
Source: Pairman et al. (2014).

chin. The other hand is on the baby's back with the middle finger pushing down on the baby's head to keep it in the flexed position, but some traction on the shoulders may be required with the other fingers. The second paramedic slowly brings the head downwards keeping the body in a neutral position and brings the baby in a large arch to lie on the mother's stomach.

If there is continued difficulty with the birth of the baby's head, the paramedics should place the mother in the McRobert's position (see Fig 54.14). One paramedic should apply suprapubic pressure to assist with flexion of the baby's head. If the head still does not deliver, the mother should be maintained in this position and transported as quickly as possible to the nearest obstetric facility (Pairman et al., 2014; Woollard et al., 2008).

Once the baby has been born, the paramedics should manage the baby as per neonatal resuscitation and manage the third stage as per normal vaginal birth. When the baby and mother are stable, they should be transported to hospital.

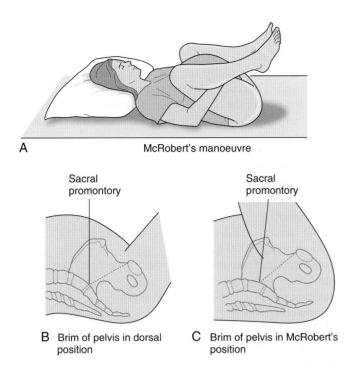

A   McRobert's manoeuvre

B   Brim of pelvis in dorsal position

C   Brim of pelvis in McRobert's position

Figure 54.14
McRobert's position.
Source: Pairman et al. (2014).

CS CASE STUDY 3

Case 13157, 0700 hrs.

Dispatch details: A 38-year-old female, who is 42 weeks pregnant, is in labour.

Initial presentation: The paramedics find the patient semi-recumbent on the couch. She tried to get in the car but was unable to.

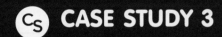

1 ASSESS

0710 hrs History: The patient says her contractions commenced at 5 this morning. They have been unbearable for about an hour and she has been pushing for half an hour. She also says that her previous two children were large and she has been diagnosed with gestational diabetes during this pregnancy.

0715 hrs Examination: On examination the paramedics notice anal pouting and perineal bulging. As they prepare to assist with the birth her membranes spontaneously rupture and they observe that the amniotic fluid has a greenish colour. With each contraction the patient pushes but the progress is slow, so the paramedics decide to transport her. However, as they prepare to transfer her to the stretcher, the baby's head becomes visible, so they decide to stay. The baby's head crowns after the patient pushes for five more contractions. The head is birthed but it fails to restitute.

Shoulder dystocia

The simplest definition of **shoulder dystocia** is when the baby's head is delivered but the progression of the shoulders into the maternal pelvis fails because the anterior shoulder, or occasionally the posterior shoulder, is impacted under the pubis symphysis. However, a more accurate definition is that when the usual downward traction of the head fails during normal vaginal birth, additional manoeuvres are required to assist the progression of the shoulders into the pelvis to facilitate the birth.

An incidence rate of 0.6% for shoulder dystocia has been reported in North America and the UK (Alhadi et al., 2001). Around 48% of all cases occur in infants < 4000 g (Baskett & Allen, 1995). There is an increased occurrence in women with a prolonged active first stage and a prolonged second stage (Alhadi et al., 2001).

Predisposing factors include:

- macrosomic baby (> 4000 g)
- maternal diabetes mellitus, including type 1, type 2 and gestational diabetes, leading to a large baby
- small maternal pelvis (e.g. platypelloid pelvis)
- increasing maternal age > 35 years old
- maternal BMI > 30
- short maternal stature
- post-maturity
- previous history of shoulder dystocia
- prolonged active first and second stages of labour.

However, it is often unpredictable with no predisposing factors.

Warning signs of shoulder dystocia

In the out-of-hospital setting early recognition of probable shoulder dystocia is the most effective management. Given that shoulder dystocia has been shown to be associated with a prolonged second stage (Alhadi et al., 2001), if the woman is not progressing well in the second stage the paramedics should transport her to the nearest obstetric facility.

If transport is not an immediate option (due to location or distance to hospital), shoulder dystocia presenting with an obstructed second stage may respond to a manoeuvre that changes the angle of the pelvis relative to the spine, creating a little more room for the anterior shoulder to slip under the symphysis pubis at the front of the pelvis. There are a number of positions, all of them with esteemed individuals' names, but they are all a combination of changing the angle of the pelvis and applying a little downward traction to help the shoulder slip under the symphysis pubis. If these techniques do not work, the patient needs to be in expert hands as soon as possible.

Recognition of shoulder dystocia

Signs of shoulder dystocia as the head is birthing include:

- difficulty with progress of the head and chin
- the head burrows into the perineum ('turtle neck' sign)
- restitution of the head does not occur, a sign that the shoulders have not entered the pelvis.

Do not confuse 'bed' dystocia or 'snug shoulders' with 'mild' dystocia (Pairman et al., 2014). 'Bed' dystocia occurs when a woman lies in the semi-Fowler's or semi-recumbent position and the baby's head is born into the mattress of the bed. The shoulders are not impacted behind the pubis symphysis. While progress of the head may be slow, the 'turtle neck' sign does not occur. This is easily managed by changing the woman's position to all fours, standing or rolling to the left lateral (Pairman et al., 2014).

3 TREAT

As shoulder dystocia is often unexpected, paramedics should know the basic manoeuvres used to manage this obstetric emergency. It is advisable to request a second ambulance, especially as there is an increased likelihood of the baby requiring supportive measures after this type of delivery. Management requires at least two paramedics and may even need the assistance of any available bystanders to employ the following manoeuvres.

- Continue to use downward traction to deliver the baby's head but do not twist the head or use excessive force.
- As quickly as possible the mother should be placed in a semi-recumbent position on one pillow. Her knees should be pulled to her chest, slightly abducting, in the McRobert's manoeuvre (see Fig 54.14 and Box 54.2). If the mother is very tired she may need some assistance with this. Attempt to birth the baby again by applying gentle downward traction to the baby.
- If the McRobert's manoeuvre is unsuccessful, the mother should continue to remain in that position. The second paramedic should apply suprapubic pressure to the anterior shoulder and perform the Rubin 1 manoeuvre (see Box 54.2). Initial continuous pressure should be applied for 30 seconds but if this is not successful, the second paramedic should rock back and forth on the heel of the hand for a further 30 seconds. During this procedure the paramedic assisting should continue to apply gentle downward traction.
- If the above manoeuvres are unsuccessful, the mother should be placed on all fours or in the Gaskin position with her head as low as possible, her pelvis as high as possible and her hips well flexed (see Box 54.2). Apply gentle downward traction to the posterior shoulder (i.e. nearest to the mother's back).
- If this is not successful, the mother should be placed in the ambulance and transported to the nearest obstetric facility. The receiving hospital should be notified of the problem and the impending arrival.

BOX 54.2 Limitations in the out-of-hospital setting

In a hospital or home birth, procedures such as episiotomy and internal manoeuvres are used for shoulder dystocia. However, the value of an episiotomy in shoulder dystocia is often debated (Baston, 2006) and internal manoeuvres can be complicated. While paramedics are limited by the procedures they can perform in the out-of-hospital setting, 58% (Gherman et al., 2006) to 90% (Carlin & Alfirevic, 2006) will be successfully managed by using the McRobert's, Rubin 1 or Gaskin manoeuvre.

The McRobert's manoeuvre has benefits for both the mother and the baby. This position rotates the sacrum backwards, straightening it relative to the lumbar vertebrae and allowing the pelvic inlets to open to the maximum diameter possible. This enables the symphysis pubis to rotate over the top of the anterior shoulder. Simultaneously the fetal spine straightens, facilitating the posterior shoulder passing over the sacral promontory into the hollow of the sacrum (Carlin & Alfirevic, 2006; Pairman et al., 2014; Rankin, 2017).

In the Rubin 1 manoeuvre the second paramedic should attempt to identify the baby's back by checking which way the baby is trying to face. Remember, although restitution will not have occurred completely at this stage, the baby will be trying to turn one way rather than the other. Once the back is identified, the second paramedic should stand on that side of the mother. With both hands interlocked but using the heel of one hand (external compression style), the second paramedic with moderate pressure should push down and away on the anterior shoulder (Carlin & Alfirevic, 2006; Pairman et al., 2014; Rankin, 2017).

In the Gaskin manoeuvre the woman is placed in the 'all fours' position. In reality, this is an upside-down McRobert's manoeuvre. The flexible sacroiliac joint opens, increasing the anteroposterior diameter by a further 1–2 cm and allowing sufficient room to deliver the posterior shoulder (Carlin & Alfirevic, 2006; Pairman et al., 2014; Rankin, 2017).

- En route apply oxygen to the mother and if able insert an intravenous therapy line. Do not stay on scene to do this as this is a true emergency.
- If the baby is born during any of this procedure the neonate should be managed as per the neonatal resuscitation guidelines (see Ch 55). The mother should be managed as per the third stage. She will be at greater risk of postpartum haemorrhage due to perineal trauma and an atonic uterus.

 CASE STUDY 4

Case 11834, 1420 hrs.

Dispatch details: A 34-year-old woman, who is 35 weeks' pregnant, in labour, membranes broken.

Initial presentation: The ambulance crew find the patient sitting in a chair in the manager's office of the local supermarket, in labour with her sixth child.

 ASSESS

1435 hrs History: The patient says was doing the weekly shopping when she felt a gush of clear fluid from her vagina. She has been having slight pains all morning but they have become more frequent since her membranes ruptured. She says that she can feel something in her pants but has been too scared to look.

1438 hrs Examination: On inspection the paramedics see part of the umbilical cord hanging from her vagina. There are no signs of the second stage.

Cord prolapse

In **cord presentation** the baby's umbilical cord lies in front of the presenting part but the membranes have not ruptured. When the membranes have ruptured this becomes **cord prolapse** (see Fig 54.15). An occult cord prolapse lies adjacent to the presenting part and an overt cord prolapse lies below the

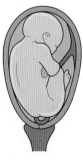
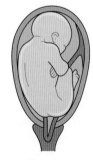

Presentation   Prolapse

Figure 54.15
In cord presentation the baby's umbilical cord lies in front of the presenting part and the membranes have not ruptured. When the membranes rupture this becomes cord prolapse.
Source: Pairman et al. (2014); Henderson & Macdonald (2004).

presenting part. Cord prolapse may occur if a woman is not in labour, or is in the first stage or third stage. As paramedics do not have the equipment to monitor the fetal heart it is not possible for them to diagnose and therefore manage either a cord presentation or an occult cord prolapse. The incidence of cord prolapse is around 0.2–0.4% of all births (Carlin & Alfirevic, 2006).

Predisposing factors include:

- a high presenting part
- multigravida
- malpresentation (e.g. breech, shoulder, face or brow; transverse or oblique lie)
- prematurity or birth weight < 2.5 kg
- multiple birth (e.g. twins, triplets)
- excessive amniotic fluid (polyhydramnios)
- mother of Afro-Caribbean descent with high assimilation pelvis
- after external cephalic version (for breech).

③ TREAT

Without the equipment to diagnose an occult cord prolapse, paramedics can only manage the condition when they visualise the cord external to the vagina. It is generally outside the scope of practice for paramedics to perform a vaginal examination and the mother could still be in the first stage of labour. Even if they suspect that the mother is in the second stage of labour, the paramedics should deliver the baby *only* if the presenting part is in view, as the second stage can take as up to an hour or more to complete. If the presenting part is in view, the birth of the baby is the fastest way to remove the cord compression.

The aim of managing an overt prolapse is to prevent or minimise cord compression by the presenting part by elevating the pelvis as high as possible. Because cord compression effectively cuts off the oxygen supply to the fetus the key is to take the pressure off the presenting part as it engages with the pelvis. This will cause transport difficulties, as it is hard to maintain a high pelvis position in a moving environment. Direct communication with the receiving facility will not only allow them preparation time but will also provide the paramedics with advice, particularly with reference to manual disimpaction of the presenting part from the pelvis.

If the mother is not in labour

- Place her in the 'all fours' position, knees to chest, with the pelvis as high as possible in the air (Curran, 2003; Pairman et al., 2014; Rankin, 2017; Woollard et al., 2008).
- While there is little evidence supporting the effectiveness of oxygen to assist fetal distress, providing supplemental oxygen to the mother remains a common and acceptable practice (Curran, 2003; Rankin, 2017).
- If the cord is external to the vagina it may be in danger of cooling and drying out. However, overhandling the cord can cause spasming and vasoconstriction. Paramedics need to be aware of these dangers but it may be necessary to gently place the cord in the vagina to prevent it drying out (Woollard et al., 2008). If the cord continually falls out, it may be necessary to cover it with saline-soaked gauze.
- One paramedic should insert a hand into the woman's vagina and manually push the presenting part off the cord with at least two fingers. This can be very difficult, particularly if the presenting part is very high (Curran, 2003; Pairman et al., 2014; Rankin, 2017; Woollard et al., 2008).
- Transport as quickly as possible to the nearest obstetric facility. The safest position during transport is the exaggerated Sims or left lateral position. The woman's pelvis must remain higher than her shoulders to keep the presenting part off the cord.

If the mother is in labour
- Perform all of the above.
- Provide the mother with pain relief—usually inhaled, unless contraindicated.
- Encourage the mother to pant during contractions and avoid pushing down unless the presenting part is in view.

If the presenting part is in view
- Prepare to assist with the birth of the baby.
- Coach the mother to push hard when she has a contraction.
- Prepare neonatal resuscitation equipment (see Ch 55).

 CASE STUDY 5

Case 11268, 0345 hrs.

Dispatch details: A 29-year-old woman who is 38 weeks' pregnant is in labour and pushing.

Initial assessment: The ambulance crew find the patient in the bathroom lying against the wall, with her baby, still attached to the umbilical cord, in her arms.

 ASSESS

0358 hrs History: The baby was born 10 minutes ago.

0406 hrs Examination: Following a vital signs survey, the paramedics transfer the patient to the bedroom. They note some blood loss on the floor. The bleeding continues substantially after delivery of the placenta, so they check her uterus and notice that it is boggy (not contracted).

Postpartum haemorrhage
A **postpartum haemorrhage (PPH)** can be defined as blood loss of greater than 500 mL from the time of the birth of the baby, including the third stage, until 24 hours later. A very severe primary PPH involves a blood loss greater than 1000 mL. However, sometimes blood loss is difficult to quantify during birth as it is often mixed with amniotic fluid. PPH can also be defined as any amount of postpartum bleeding that causes haemodynamic compromise (Coad & Dunstall, 2011; Royal College of Obstetricians and Gynaecologists, 2011; Rankin, 2017; Woollard et al., 2008).

The incidence of primary PPH ranges from 5% to 15% of all births (Rankin, 2017). PPH has been reported in Australia at a rate of 6.2–6.5% of all BBAs (Flanagan et al., 2017; McLelland et al., 2018). It was the leading cause of maternal death in the UK between 2003 and 2005 (Royal College of Obstetricians and Gynaecologists, 2011). Two-thirds of women who have a primary PPH have no identifiable risk factors (Pairman et al., 2014).

For causes of PPH, think of the '4 Ts'.
- **T**one: causes 90% of PPH (Pairman et al., 2014)
  - Atonic uterus includes precipitate births, prolonged labour, multiple birth, grand parity, prolonged third stage
- **T**rauma
  - Perineal tears includes precipitous birth, malposition

- **T**issue
    - › Retained products includes either whole or partial placenta or membranes
- **T**hrombin: causes < 1% of PPH (ALSO, 2004)
    - › Clotting disorders due to pre-eclampsia or haemolysis elevated liver enzymes low platelets (HELLP) syndrome, pyrexia, deep vein thrombosis (DVT)

Signs of primary PPH

Visible blood loss is often the first sign, so any visible loss must be assessed. Due to changes in the cardiovascular system at term (Coad & Dunstall, 2011; Dundas, 2003; Rankin, 2017) early signs of shock can be masked until the woman has lost up to one-third of her blood volume (Pairman et al., 2014) and is very compromised, so paramedics should be alerted to:

- an increase in heart rate by 20 bpm
- any decrease in blood pressure
- any signs of pallor.

Although unlikely, if clots are retained in an atonic uterus the first signs of a primary PPH would be:

- cold, clammy and pale skin
- an enlarged and boggy uterus
- altered conscious state (Rankin, 2017).

③ TREAT

Although postpartum haemorrhage can be very dramatic and is definitely life-threatening, a massive haemorrhage is much nearer to the paramedic's usual emergency management than emergencies associated with delivery. Life-threatening postpartum haemorrhage is thankfully relatively rare in paramedic practice so it is recommended that paramedics consult with the receiving facility for advice and support as they attempt to control the haemorrhage with compression.

Paramedic management

The aim of paramedic management is to recognise bleeding early and to stop or minimise blood loss to prevent a severe postpartum haemorrhage (> 1000 mL).

Specific management

Paramedics should request support from a second crew to allow them to concentrate on the mother's condition while ensuring that the baby is supported.

If the placenta has not yet delivered

- Any vaginal bleeding after birth indicates the placenta has separated. Ask the mother to push the placenta out. If unable to cut the cord, use controlled traction to deliver the placenta (see Box 54.3). This is not usually recommended in the out-of-hospital setting but in an emergency may be necessary (Woollard et al., 2008).
- Check the uterine fundus for a contracted uterus. An empty contracted uterus does not bleed. If the uterus has contracted:
    - › Do not 'fiddle' with it as it may cause it to relax. Do not 'rub up' or massage it.

BOX 54.3 Controlled cord traction

In the out-of-hospital setting controlled cord traction should be undertaken only if absolutely necessary for postpartum haemorrhage and if oxytocic medication has been administered.

› Check for any visible laceration and apply direct pressure (Fraser & Cooper, 2009; Pairman et al., 2014; Rankin, 2017).
› Manage as below.

If the placenta has delivered but the uterus has not contracted

- Using a circular motion with a cupped hand massage or rub up the uterine fundus until it is firm. Warn the woman first, as this is painful (Fraser & Cooper, 2009; Pairman et al., 2014; Rankin, 2017).
- Manage as below.

Postpartum haemorrhage management

After delivery of the placenta and contraction of the uterus, the following management is required.

- Have the woman lie down. Her legs can be elevated on a pillow (Fraser & Cooper, 2009) but her pelvis should not be tilted.
- Commence oxygen at 8 L/min via mask (Mathai et al., 2007; Pairman et al., 2014; Woollard et al., 2008).
- Insert two large-bore (16 gauge or as wide as available) intravenous cannula and commence 1–2 litres of crystalloid solution (e.g. Hartmann's, normal saline) (World Health Organization, 2017; Pairman et al., 2014; Woollard et al., 2008). While crystalloid fluids may prove successful in restoring volume in mild or moderate PPH, consideration must be given to haemodilution and coagulopathy if large volumes of fluids are administered (Schorn & Phillippi, 2014).
- Give oxytocic drugs if available (e.g. IM Syntocinon 10 IU/s; Misoprostol 800 microgram oral/rectal).
- Ask the woman to empty her bladder if she is able to (Fraser & Cooper, 2009; Pairman et al., 2014; Rankin, 2017; Woollard et al., 2008).
- Encourage the baby to breastfeed if possible.
- Notify the receiving hospital and transport as quickly as possible.
- If available, consider administration of tranexamic acid (TXA) 1 g IV. While still relatively uncommon in the out-of-hospital setting, TXA has been shown to reduce mortality in women suffering a PPH (WOMAN Trial Collaborators, 2017).
- Other manoeuvres that can be used if bleeding continues are bimanual compression and aortic compression. The use of these is governed by local guidelines and procedures and should be undertaken only as a last resort by paramedics in the field.

Procedure for delivering the placenta

- Guard the uterus with one hand to prevent inversion by placing the hand over the symphysis pubis and applying gentle pressure downwards and backwards. Do not move this hand until the placenta is visible in the introitus.
- Apply gentle downwards traction on the cord with the other hand until the placenta is visible at the opening of the vagina.
- Do not pull or tug. If the cord does not descend, stop traction and wait for the cord to descend.
- Once the placenta can be seen at the introitus, grasp the cord where it joins the placenta.
- Remove the hand on the symphysis pubis and use this hand to hold the emerging placenta.
- With a twisting motion aid complete delivery of the placenta and membranes. The twisting action assists in removing as much of the membranes as possible.
- Massage the fundus until it is firmly contracted.

If the uterus is not contracting and bleeding still continues after fundal massage and the administration of oxytocic drugs, more invasive measures

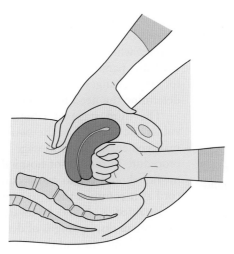

Figure 54.16
Bimanual compression.
Source: Pairman et al. (2014).

may be required. Bimanual compression is preferred in the hospital setting as it is effectively direct pressure on the placental site. However, in the pre-hospital setting without long gloves this may put paramedics at risk of blood-borne diseases. Aortic compression, which temporarily stops the flow to the uterus and thus prevents bleeding, is often preferred. Both methods are very painful, so if the woman does not have an altered conscious state, she should be offered pain relief.

For bimanual compression:
- Wear long, preferably sterile gloves.
- Insert one hand into the vagina and remove any obvious clots.
- Form a fist and place it in the anterior fornix of the vagina, applying pressure against the anterior wall of the uterus.
- Using the other hand, apply pressure deep in the abdomen behind the uterus on the posterior wall (see Fig 54.16).

For aortic compression:
- Form a fist and push it into the woman's abdomen slightly above the umbilicus and to the left.
- Push firmly through the abdominal wall, causing compression of the aorta supplying the uterus. The pulsation of the aorta is easy to feel through the abdominal wall.
- Effectiveness can be assessed by checking cessation of the femoral pulse. If the femoral pulse cannot be felt, compressions are adequate. If the pulse is felt, compressions are inadequate. Check extremities for anoxia.

Both methods are only temporary and immediate transport to the nearest maternity service is required.

Further research

Research continues to look at how Australian paramedics respond to and manage out-of-hospital obstetric emergencies. Further research is required to validate in the out-of-hospital setting recent advances in obstetric and midwifery care such as the findings of the WOMAN trial into tranexamic acid use for postpartum haemorrhage (WOMAN Trial Collaborators, 2017).

A Delphi study of ambulance managers revealed that obstetrics is one of the few clinical areas where paramedics want further continuing education (Snooks et al., 2009). In the United Kingdom, a Prehospital Obstetric Emergency Training (POETs) course is now available for qualified paramedics (Woollard et al., 2008). The course is held over 2 days and focuses on training paramedics to manage obstetric emergencies. An improvement in the outcomes of out-of-hospital deliveries would suggest that specialised training would be useful in other areas.

Summary

Most out-of-hospital births are full term and uncomplicated. Although minimal intervention will be required, paramedics still need a basic understanding of the physiology of labour to enable clinical decision-making. Obtaining a thorough obstetric and medical history will enable them to make appropriate clinical decisions regarding out-of-hospital management of the patient. Paramedics will rarely encounter obstetric complications but they do need an understanding of the basic manoeuvres in order to manage them.

It is important to be able to recognise the difference between the first and the second stage of labour: when to 'stay' or 'go'. Since labour is dynamic, paramedics need to continually monitor for any changes in the woman's condition to determine the need to stop en route to hospital.

The third stage of labour is often the most vulnerable time for the woman. Physiological management of the third stage is the recommended procedure in the out-of-hospital setting and paramedics should try to avoid cutting the umbilical cord as it commits them to active management.

Paramedics should be aware that by the time the woman displays signs of deterioration or shock during labour, she and the baby are already haemodynamically compromised.

Unless there is a medical reason for separation, mother and baby should remain together, skin-to-skin, during transport.

References

Alhadi, M. G., Byrne, P., & McKenna, M. (2001). Shoulder dystocia: risk factors and maternal and perinatal outcome. *Journal of Obstetrics and Gynaecology: The Journal of the Institute of Obstetrics and Gynaecology, 21*(4), 352–354. doi:10.1080/01443610120059860.

ALSO. (2004). *Advanced life support in obstetrics provider manual* (4th ed.). Kansas: American Academy of Family Physicians.

Australian Institute of Health and Welfare. (2019.) Australia's mothers and babies 2017—in brief. Perinatal statistics series no. 35. Cat. no. PER 100. Canberra: AIHW.

Baskett, T., & Allen, A. (1995). Perinatal implications of shoulder dystocia. *Obstetrics and Gynecology, 86*(1), 14–17.

Baston, H. (2006). Midwifery basics: complications (5). Shoulder dystocia. *The Practising Midwife, 9*(2), 36–39.

Beeram, M., Solarin, K., Young, M., & Abedin, M. (1995). Morbidity and mortality of infants born before arrival at the hospital. *Clinical Pediatrics, 34*(6), 313–316.

Carlin, A., & Alfirevic, Z. (2006). Intrapartum fetal emergencies. *Seminars in Fetal & Neonatal Medicine, 11*(3), 150–157. [Review].

Coad, J., & Dunstall, M. (2011). *Anatomy and physiology for midwives* (3rd ed.). Edinburgh: Churchill Livingstone.

Curran, C. A. (2003). Intrapartum emergencies. *Journal of Obstetric, Gynecologic, and Neonatal Nursing, 32*(6), 802–813. doi:10.1177/0884217503258425.

Dundas, K. (2003). Obstetrics: the physiological changes. *Hospital Pharmacist, 10*(6), 242, 245–247, 251–254.

Flanagan, B., Lord, B., & Barnes, M. (2017). Is unplanned out-of-hospital birth managed by paramedics 'infrequent', 'normal' and 'uncomplicated'? *BMC Pregnancy and Childbirth, 17*(1), 436.

Fraser, D. M., & Cooper, M. A. (Eds.), (2009). *Myles textbook for midwives* (15th ed.). London: Elsevier.

Gherman, R. B., Chauhan, S., Ouzounian, J. G., Lerner, H., Gonik, B., & Goodwin, T. M. (2006). Shoulder dystocia: the unpreventable obstetric emergency with empiric management guidelines. *American Journal of Obstetrics and Gynecology, 195*(3), 657–672. [Review].

Henderson, C., & Macdonald, S. (2004). *Mayes midwifery: a textbook for midwives* (13th ed.). London: Baillière Tindall.

Marshall, J., & Raynor, M. (2014). *Myles textbook for midwives* (16th ed.). London: Elsevier.

Mathai, M., Sanghvi, H., & Guidotti, R. (2007). Integrated management of pregnancy and childbirth. In M. McCormick (Ed.), *Managing complications in pregnancy and childbirth: a guide for midwives and doctors*. Geneva: World Health Organization.

McLean, M., & Smith, R. (2001). Corticotrophin-releasing hormone and human parturition. *Reproduction (Cambridge, England), 121*, 496.

McLelland, G., McKenna, L., & Archer, F. (2011). No fixed place of birth: unplanned BBAs in Victoria, Australia. *Midwifery, 29*(2), e19–e25. doi:10.1016/j.midw.2011.12.002.

McLelland, G., Morgans, A., Archer, F., & McKenna, L. (2013). Incidence of unplanned births before arrival to hospital and the involvement of emergency medical services: a structured literature review. *Journal of Emergency Primary Health Care, 9*(2), 414–418.

McLelland, G., McKenna, L., Morgans, A., & Smith, K. (2018). Epidemiology of unplanned out-of-hospital births attended by paramedics. *BMC Pregnancy and Childbirth*, *18*(1), 15.

Moscovitz, H. C., Magriples, U., Keissling, M., & Schriver, J. A. (2000). Care and outcome of out-of-hospital deliveries. *Academic Emergency Medicine: Official Journal of the Society for Academic Emergency Medicine*, *7*(7), 757–761.

National Institute for Health and Care Excellence. (2007). *Intrapartum Care of Healthy Women and their Babies during Childbirth: Clinical Guideline 55*. London: National Collaborating Centre for Women's and Children's Health, National Health Service. Retrieved from http://publications.nice.org.uk/intrapartum-care-cg55.

National Institute for Health and Care Excellence. (2017). *Intrapartum care for healthy women and babies: Clinical Guideline 190*. London: National Health Service. Retrieved from https://www.nice.org.uk/guidance/cg190/chapter/recommendations.

Pairman, S., Pincombe, J., Thorogood, C., & Tracy, S. (Eds.), (2014). *Midwifery preparation for practice* (3rd ed.). Sydney: Elsevier.

Rankin, J. (2017). *Physiology in Childbearing: With Anatomy and Related Bioscience* (4th ed.). London: Elsevier Health Sciences.

Rodie, V. A., Thomson, A. J., & Norman, J. E. (2002). Accidental out-of-hospital deliveries: an obstetric and neonatal case control study. *Acta Obstetricia et Gynecologica Scandinavica*, *81*(1), 50–54.

Royal College of Obstetricians and Gynaecologists. (2011). *Prevention and Management of Postpartum Haemorrhage*. Retrieved from www.rcog.org.uk/womens-health/clinical-guidance/prevention-and-management-postpartum-haemorrhage-green-top-52. (Accessed 2 May 2012).

Royal Women's Hospital. (2006). *Breech: Management of Breech Presentation. Clinical Guidelines*. Retrieved from www.thewomens.org.au/BreechManagementofBreechPresentation?printView=true. (Accessed 1 May 2012).

Schorn, M. N., & Phillippi, J. C. (2014). Volume replacement following severe postpartum hemorrhage. *Journal of Midwifery & Women's Health*, *59*(3), 336–343. https://doi.org/10.1111/jmwh.12186.

Snooks, H., Evans, A., Wells, B., Peconi, J., Thomas, M., Woollard, M., Guly, H., Jenkinson, E., Turner, J., Hartley-Sharpe, C., & 999 EMS Research Forum Board. (2009). What are the highest priorities for research in emergency prehospital care? *Emergency Medicine Journal*, *26*(8), 549–550.

Steer, P., & Flint, C. (1999). ABC of labour care: physiology and management of normal labour. *BMJ*, *318*(7186), 793–796. doi:10.1136/bmj.318.7186.793.

Verdile, V. P., Tutsock, G., Paris, P. M., & Kennedy, R. A. (1995). Out-of-hospital deliveries: a five-year experience. *Prehospital and Disaster Medicine*, *10*(1), 10–13.

White, L., Duncan, G., & Baumle, W. (Eds.), (2011). *Foundations of maternal and paediatric nursing* (3rd ed.). Clifton Park: Thomson Delmar Learning.

WOMAN Trial Collaborators. (2017). Effect of early tranexamic acid administration on mortality, hysterectomy, and other morbidities in women with post-partum haemorrhage (WOMAN): an international, randomised, double-blind, placebo-controlled trial. *The Lancet*, *389*(10084), 2105–2116.

Woollard, M., Simpson, H., Hinshaw, K., & Wieteska, S. (2008). Training for prehospital obstetric emergencies. *Emergency Medicine Journal*, *25*(7), 392–393.

World Health Organization. (2017). *Managing Complications in Pregnancy and Childbirth: A guide for midwives and doctors* 2nd Edition. Geneva: World Health Organization.

CHAPTER 55

Neonatal Resuscitation

By Rosemarie Boland

OVERVIEW

- The vast majority of newborn babies undergo a successful transition to extrauterine life without the need for any intervention other than drying, provision of warmth and ensuring a clear airway.
- Fewer than 6% of all newborn babies in Australia require assistance to establish effective respirations with positive pressure ventilation. Less than 0.2% require advanced resuscitation interventions (external cardiac compressions, intubation and drug administration).
- Newborn babies are cyanosed or 'dusky' when they are born. This is normal and does not require any intervention if the baby is breathing or crying and has a heart rate above 100 bpm.
- The key to successful resuscitation in newborn babies is effective ventilation. When performed correctly, positive pressure ventilation results in a rapid improvement in heart rate, usually without the administration of supplementary oxygen.

- If positive pressure ventilation is required, room air (21% oxygen) should be used initially, as it has been shown to result in a significantly lower mortality rate compared with using 100% oxygen.
- High-flow 100% oxygen is indicated only if the newborn has a heart rate less than 60 bpm after at least 30 seconds of effective positive pressure ventilation in air.
- Preterm birth (before 37 completed weeks' gestation) is associated with a higher risk of stillbirth and infant mortality and morbidity.
- In 2017, there were 806 planned home births reported nationally in Australia, representing 0.3% of all births. Unintentional home births are rare.
- The lack of exposure to neonates requiring resuscitation suggests that paramedics should use an algorithmic approach to these cases to ensure all basic care is delivered.

Introduction

Live birth is defined as the complete expulsion or extraction from its mother of a product of conception, irrespective of the duration of pregnancy, which, after such separation, breathes or shows any other evidence of life, such as beating of the heart, pulsation of the umbilical cord or definite movement of voluntary muscles, whether or not the umbilical cord has been cut or the placenta is attached (Australian Institute of Health and Welfare [AIHW], 2019). A **stillbirth** (fetal death) is defined as a death occurring prior to the complete expulsion or extraction from the mother of a product of conception of 20 or more completed weeks' gestation or 400 g or more birth weight. The stillbirth rate remains constant in Australia at 7.1 per 1000 births (AIHW, 2019).

Babies are considered **full term** between 37 and 42 completed weeks' gestation. **Post-term birth** is birth that occurs after 42 or more completed weeks' gestation. **Preterm birth** is defined as birth before 37 completed weeks' gestation (AIHW, 2019). In 2017, 8.7% of babies born in Australia were preterm, with most preterm births occurring between 32

and 36 weeks' gestation (AIHW, 2019). Preterm birth is associated with a higher risk of mortality and morbidity. These risks are even higher when preterm birth occurs in an out-of-hospital setting (Boland et al., 2018).

Viability is the earliest gestational age at which a newborn baby can survive outside the mother's womb. This is currently 22–23 weeks' gestation for live born babies admitted to a neonatal intensive care unit (NICU) in Australia or New Zealand (Chow et al., 2019). Of the 101 babies born < 24 weeks' gestation in Australia and New Zealand who were offered neonatal intensive care in 2017, 55 (55%) survived to discharge home (Chow et al., 2019). By 24 weeks' gestation, 68% of babies offered intensive care survived to hospital discharge.

It is important to note that a 'viable' baby born at 22–24 weeks' gestation may not necessarily be resuscitated and offered intensive care. At periviable gestational ages (22–24 weeks), many parents decide neonatal intensive care is not in the best interests of their baby and opt for comfort (palliative) care at birth. These decisions are based on the risks of neurosensory impairment (deafness, blindness) and disability (cerebral palsy) in surviving children and their predicted quality of life. Between 2009 and 2016 in Victoria, 5% of babies born at 22 weeks and 40% of babies born at 23 weeks were offered intensive care. All those not offered intensive care died at their birth hospital (Boland & Doyle, 2019). By 24 weeks' gestation, 85% were offered intensive care. In Western Australia, 8% of 22-week babies, 81% of 23-week babies and 95% of 24-week babies were offered intensive care between 2004 and 2010 (Sharp et al., 2018). Hence, when interpreting survival data for periviable babies, it is critical to determine if the denominator is all live births or only babies offered neonatal intensive care and to be aware that the provision of active versus palliative care will influence survival data.

Survival rates are significantly lower for babies born very preterm (28–31 weeks) and extremely preterm (22–27 weeks) in the out-of-hospital environment (Boland et al., 2016; Stewart et al., 2017; Boland et al., 2018). In Victoria, only 5 babies born before 27 weeks' gestation have survived following out-of-hospital birth over a 20-year period from 1990–2009 (Boland et al., 2018). Babies born in the out-of-hospital environment are also twice as likely to be stillborn compared with babies born in a hospital at 22–27 weeks' gestation and four times as likely to be stillborn at 28–31 weeks' gestation (Boland et al., 2018). Spontaneous preterm labour will often occur within days of fetal death in utero. If equipment to monitor fetal heart rate in transit to hospital is not available, paramedics will not know if the baby has already died in utero or will be live born. Paramedics need to be aware that babies born in a residential home or in an ambulance before 28 weeks' gestation do not have similar survival rates compared with hospital-birth infants, even if resuscitated and transferred to a hospital with a NICU after birth. Paramedics attending the birth of an extremely preterm baby should consult with a neonatologist from the neonatal emergency retrieval team in their state or area, preferably via the ambulance clinician, to discuss appropriate management of the baby. The difficult ethical decisions about ongoing resuscitation can then be made from a position of more information and in a more controlled environment.

Extremely preterm babies have better prospects for survival and improved quality of survival if they are born at a tertiary perinatal centre with a NICU (Marlow et al., 2014; Boland et al., 2016; Boland et al., 2018). Where possible, women in preterm labour at less than 32 weeks' gestation should be preferentially transferred to a perinatal centre by the paramedic crew, even if this means bypassing

a maternity hospital on route. In most states of Australia and in some areas of New Zealand, this directive is written into ambulance service clinical practice guidelines (Stewart et al., 2017).

Pathophysiology

In the transition from intrauterine life to extrauterine life the fetus undergoes complex physiological, hormonal and cardiovascular changes to survive outside the womb. Most newborns undergo this transition with minimal assistance. Less than 6% of all newborn babies in Australia require assistance to establish effective ventilation at birth and fewer than 0.2% require advanced resuscitation measures to survive (AIHW, 2019).

During fetal life, the placenta acts as the gas exchange organ. Oxygen diffuses across the placental membrane from the mother's blood to the fetus' blood. The fetal alveoli are expanded, but are liquid-filled. Blood flow to the fetal lungs is minimal and the blood vessels perfusing the fetal lungs are constricted. Pulmonary blood flow is low because pulmonary vascular resistance (PVR) is high. Almost 90% of right ventricular output bypasses the lungs and enters the systemic circulation via the ductus arteriosus (see Fig 55.1). The ductus arteriosus connects the main pulmonary artery with the descending aorta, acting as a low-resistance right-to-left shunt between the fetal pulmonary circulation and the systemic circulation (Crossley et al., 2009). Systemic vascular resistance (SVR) is low, primarily because resistance in the placental circulation is low.

Blood from the umbilical vein flows to the inferior vena cava (IVC), across the right atrium to the left atrium via the foramen ovale and from the pulmonary artery into the aorta across the ductus arteriosus. This maintains the brain and myocardium with the most highly oxygenated blood within the fetal circulation. During intrauterine life the fetus is relatively hypoxaemic with a PO_2 of 20–25 mmHg (Merrill & Ballard, 2005). Fetal oxygen saturations are approximately 50–60%, but fall to a mean of 40–50% during labour (East et al., 2002). Fetal haemoglobin has a higher affinity for oxygen compared with adult haemoglobin and the fetus has a greater tissue resistance to acidosis. This allows the fetus to compensate for the changes in oxygen consumption and interruption to gas exchange during labour (Merrill & Ballard, 2005).

While the fetal circulation is dependent on the placenta for gas exchange, postnatal circulation is reliant on pulmonary gas exchange. The successful transition to pulmonary gas exchange after birth

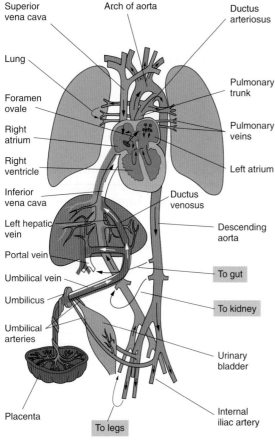

Oxygen saturation of blood

▓ High oxygen content   ▓ Medium oxygen content
▓ Poor oxygen content

Figure 55.1
Fetal circulation.
The fetal circulation includes the normal circulatory structures plus the umbilical vein, umbilical arteries, ductus venosus (DV), foramen ovale (FO) and ductus arteriosus (DA). Oxygenated blood travels from the placenta via the umbilical vein, through the DV to the right atrium, where it supplies the heart and brain. Blood is diverted from the high-resistant pulmonary circuit to the low-resistant systemic circuit via the FO and DA. Deoxygenated blood returns to the placenta via the umbilical arteries, which receive 55% of fetal cardiac output.
Source: Pairman et al. (2014).

requires clearance of airway liquid and a large decrease in PVR to prevent right ventricular output bypassing the lungs (Crossley et al., 2009). Most newborns will make vigorous efforts to breathe at birth. The pressure created during inspiration causes fetal lung liquid to move out of the alveoli and into the surrounding lung tissue. This can occur in as few as 5–10 breaths. Lung liquid is cleared from the tissue via the blood vessels and lymphatics. The first breaths for a newborn require a much greater

negative pressure difference within the thorax than all subsequent respirations.

With the onset of ventilation, oxygen tension rises. There is an eight- to ten-fold increase in blood flow to the lungs due to a large decrease in PVR. The decrease in PVR is mostly due to pulmonary capillary recruitment and relaxation of blood vessels caused by lung aeration and increased oxygen content of the blood. SVR increases in response to loss of the placental circulation, constriction of the umbilical arteries and vein and clamping of the umbilical cord. By 1 minute after birth, with effective breathing and an adequate circulation, the newborn's oxygen saturation of haemoglobin (SpO$_2$) will reach a mean of 66%. By 7–10 minutes after birth, SpO$_2$ will have reached a mean of 90% when measured by pulse oximetry (Dawson et al., 2010a).

As PVR decreases and SVR increases, the pressure gradient across the ductus arteriosus reverses, resulting in reverse shunting of blood from left to right into the pulmonary circulation. The foramen ovale (which prior to birth allowed shunting of blood from the right atrium to the left atrium) closes because the pressure gradient reverses. With increased pulmonary blood flow the left atrial pressure rises, effectively closing the foramen ovale. These combined changes, along with biochemical factors (prostaglandins) that control constriction of the smooth muscle of the ductus arteriosus, eventually lead to closure of the fetal cardiovascular shunts. In healthy term infants, functional closure of the ductus arteriosus begins within hours of birth and is complete by 96 hours after birth. The transition from fetal to extrauterine life is then complete. Anatomical closure of the ductus arteriosus usually occurs by 1–2 weeks of postnatal age. In the fullness of time, most people will undergo fibrosis around the valve, effectively sealing it.

It is important to note that during the functional stage of ductal closure, any condition causing hypoxia and acidosis in the newborn can result in the ductus reopening (Weisz & McNamara, 2017). This return to a 'fetal-type' circulation, but without the placental circuit for oxygenation, can lead to life-threatening hypoxia and is not compatible with postnatal life. Infants who are born with critical congenital heart disease (cCHD) are sometimes able to use this patent ductus to allow mixing of oxygenated and deoxygenated blood at the level of the ductus to survive for a short period after birth. They will deteriorate when the duct begins to constrict. This problem may present as an infant who is severely compromised immediately after birth or within hours of birth, or the first week of life, depending on

Table 55.1 Comparison of vascular and pulmonary functions before and after birth

Body structure	Fetal function	Extrauterine function
Aorta	Carries oxygenated blood from left ventricle and deoxygenated blood from the pulmonary arteries to fetal organs and placenta	Carries oxygenated blood from left ventricle into systemic circulation
Ductus venosus (DV)	Shunts most of the oxygenated blood from the placenta to the inferior vena cava	Disappears within 2 weeks of birth: becomes the ligamentum venosum
Foramen ovale (FO)	Connects the right and left atria: permits oxygenated blood from the right atrium to bypass the right ventricle and pulmonary circuit and go directly into the left atrium	Functionally closes soon after birth: anatomically seals during childhood
Ductus arteriosus (DA)	Shunts blood from the pulmonary artery directly into the aorta	Functionally closes soon after birth: eventually becomes the ligamentum arteriosum
Umbilical arteries and veins	Carry blood to and from placenta: the organ of respiration before birth	Clamped at birth, obliterating placental connections; become ligaments
Lungs	Distended with fluid, minimal pulmonary circulation, fetal respiratory movements	Expanded and aerated; pulmonary circulation allows CO_2 and O_2 exchange; organ of respiration

Source: Niermeyer et al. in Gardner et al. (2016).

whether the anomaly is a cCHD with duct-dependent systemic flow, duct-dependent pulmonary flow or transposition of the great arteries (Khalil et al., 2019).

Table 55.1 summarises the differences in vascular and pulmonary functions in fetal life compared with extrauterine (postnatal) life.

Identifying the newborn at risk of disorders during transition

Failure of the newborn to undergo a successful transition to extrauterine life may result from fetal compromise during pregnancy, labour or at the time of birth, or as a consequence of any congenital anomaly that compromises oxygenation. During pregnancy, there are a number of factors associated with a higher risk of problems during transition that potentially require resuscitation intervention at birth (see Box 55.1).

Prior to birth and/or during labour, any event that compromises placental function or blood flow through the umbilical cord can lead to fetal hypoxia. The fetus compensates in response to hypoxia by initiating the 'diving reflex' (similar to that seen in diving mammals) to preferentially redistribute blood to the brain, adrenal glands and heart and away from the lungs, liver, spleen, intestines and kidneys (Merrill & Ballard, 2005). The fetus is also capable of switching to anaerobic metabolism, using the glycogen stores in the liver for glycolysis. As most glycogen stores are laid down in the third trimester of pregnancy, preterm babies and growth-restricted babies may not have sufficient glycogen stores to maintain anaerobic metabolism for a prolonged

period of time. Events that can compromise uterine, placental or umbilical blood flow before and during labour include:

- antepartum haemorrhage
- placental abruption
- cord prolapse
- cord compression
- a true knot or a nuchal cord (cord wrapped tightly around the baby's neck)
- maternal pre-eclampsia or eclampsia.

At birth, lung aeration is central to the transition to extrauterine life. If breathing is not established, PVR will remain high and the ductus arteriosus will remain open. Deoxygenated blood will continue to bypass the pulmonary circulation and enter the systemic circulation. The failure of PVR to decrease is known as persistent pulmonary hypertension of the newborn (PPHN). Conditions associated with PPHN include meconium aspiration syndrome, sepsis, pneumonia, asphyxia and respiratory distress syndrome (Weisz & McNamara, 2017). This can progress to a vicious cycle of worsening tissue hypoxia, ischaemia and metabolic acidosis, ultimately causing irreversible organ damage or death.

Failure to breathe effectively at birth

There are various reasons why a newborn baby may not breathe at birth or fail to breathe effectively despite efforts to do so. These include:

- respiratory depression secondary to hypoxia (before or during birth)
- failure to generate sufficient pressure during inspiration to force lung liquid from the

BOX 55.1 Factors associated with a higher risk of problems during transition

Maternal risk factors

- Maternal age < 16 or > 35 years
- No antenatal care
- Substance abuse
- Drug therapy (lithium, adrenergic blocking agents, narcotics)
- Chronic maternal illness (anaemia, congenital heart disease)
- Diabetes mellitus
- Maternal infection
- Prolonged rupture of membranes > 18 hours before birth of the baby
- Chorioamnionitis (a bacterial infection of the membranes surrounding the fetus: associated with preterm labour)
- Bleeding during the second trimester of pregnancy
- Previous stillbirth or neonatal death

Fetal risk factors

- Twins, triplets or higher order multiples
- Preterm labour (especially less than 35 weeks' gestation)
- Post-term birth (after 42 weeks' gestation)
- Large for dates (birth weight > 90th centile)
- Fetal growth restriction (fetal weight < 3rd centile for gestational age)
- Fetal anaemia or Rh isoimmunisation
- Polyhydramnios (excessive amniotic fluid)
- Oligohydramnios (deficiency of amniotic fluid)
- Breech or any other presentation other than cephalic (head down)
- Reduced fetal movement before the onset of labour
- Thick meconium in the amniotic fluid

CAUTION!

Never administer naloxone to the baby of a mother suspected of using opiates. Naloxone can cause an acute withdrawal and seizures in the newborn.

---

alveoli and allow air to enter the alveoli: this is more common in very premature babies who have weaker respiratory muscles, a possible lack of surfactant and reduced drive to breathe (Australian and New Zealand Committee on Resuscitation [ANZCOR], 2016)

- the effects of maternal drugs, especially narcotics used within 4 hours of giving birth (including opiates given therapeutically by clinicians)
- meconium (or blood) blocking the airway
- structural anomaly affecting the airways (rare).

Meconium obstructing the airway

Meconium is the first faeces passed by the baby and contains amniotic fluid, mucus, lanugo (hair shed from the fetal skin), epithelial cells, bile and water. It is odorous, black or dark green and viscous. If the fetus becomes distressed in utero, it can pass meconium into the amniotic fluid. Placental insufficiency (especially in post-term babies), maternal hypertension, pre-eclampsia or maternal drug use can all cause fetal distress in utero. As the fetus becomes more hypoxic, the anal sphincter relaxes and meconium is passed into the amniotic fluid. In response to continued hypoxia, the fetus begins to gasp, leading to inhalation of the meconium into the fetal lungs before birth. This can cause meconium aspiration syndrome after birth—a complex interplay of chemical pneumonitis, surfactant dysfunction and partial or complete obstruction of the airway leading to gas trapping, alveoli collapse and atelectasis (see Fig 55.2). As the disease progresses, the baby becomes increasingly acidotic, hypoxic and hypercapnic and may develop PPHN. Clinically, the baby may have meconium staining (especially of the umbilical cord, skin and fingers) and develop early-onset respiratory distress.

The incidence of meconium aspiration syndrome is 1.5 per 1000 births in Australia (Safer Care Victoria, 2018a). Meconium aspiration syndrome is rare in newborns before 34 weeks' gestation and is more common in term and post-term infants. In a baby who is breech, meconium in the amniotic fluid can be a normal occurrence and does not necessarily indicate fetal distress.

Look for!

- Hyperinflated (barrel-shaped) chest
- Nasal flaring
- Retraction and recession (in-drawing) of the lower ribs and sternum
- Respiratory rate > 60 bpm
- Worsening cyanosis

Listen for!

- Widespread 'wet' inspiratory crackles

Structural anomalies affecting the airways

Newborn babies are obligatory nose breathers up to 8 weeks of age. If there is a structural blockage of the airway, a baby will not be able to establish effective breathing. Structural malformations of the airway are very rare. If diagnosed during pregnancy,

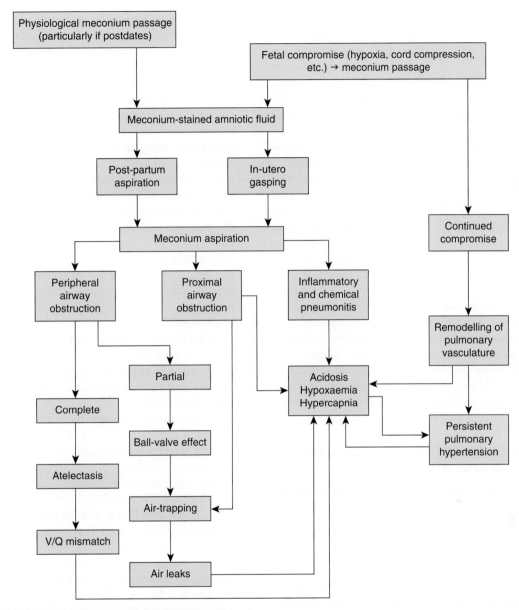

Figure 55.2
The pathophysiology of meconium aspiration syndrome.
Source: Kliegman et al. (2011).

any plans for a home birth should be abandoned. Although rare, it is important to consider a structural anomaly as a differential diagnosis in a newborn baby who is making efforts to breathe but remains cyanosed and has limited, unilateral or no chest wall movement. Some of the structural airway anomalies in newborn babies include the following.

- *Choanal atresia.* A narrowing or blockage of the nasal airway by tissue or bony cartilage. May be unilateral or bilateral. Incidence: 0.8 per 10,000 births in Australia (Abeywardana & Sullivan, 2008).

- *A pharyngeal airway malformation* (e.g. Pierre Robin sequence). Small mandible, cleft palate and a large tongue that falls back into the pharynx obstructing the airway when the baby is lying supine. Incidence: 1.6 per 10,000 births (Consultative Council on Obstetric and Paediatric Mortality and Morbidity, 2017).

- *Diaphragmatic hernia.* The abdominal contents (intestines ± the liver) have herniated through a hole in the diaphragm, causing a hypoplastic lung on the affected side. Incidence: 2.5 per 10,000 births in Australia (Abeywardana & Sullivan, 2008).

• *Pneumothorax.* May occur spontaneously at birth with the pressures exerted during the first breaths of life (incidence: 1–2 per 100 births) or as a result of use of excessive pressure during bag-valve-mask (BVM) ventilation.

The newborn with an airway malformation will usually try to make vigorous efforts to inhale air into the lungs, but will become bradycardic and cyanosed as they become increasingly hypoxic. These babies usually have other signs of respiratory distress, such as nasal flaring, intercostal or sub-costal retraction and recession (in-drawing of the ribs) and a respiratory rate above 60 bpm.

Providing effective positive pressure ventilation with a BVM may prove challenging in the presence of an airway malformation, even for a paramedic with advanced airway management skills.

Failure to establish effective ventilation after birth

If a newborn fails to establish effective ventilation after birth, the following will occur:

- bradycardia (HR < 100 bpm) resulting from lack of oxygen to the myocardium
- apnoea/further depression of the respiratory drive resulting from lack of oxygen to the brainstem
- hypotension as a result of hypoxia, bradycardia and poor cardiac contractility; this can be further exacerbated in the presence of hypovolaemia following fetal blood loss and/or shock
- poor muscle tone secondary to insufficient oxygen delivery to the muscles, brain and other organs
- central cyanosis (persisting beyond 10 minutes of postnatal age) resulting from hypoxaemia.

Unlike adults requiring resuscitation, asystole is extremely rare in newborns. Newborns usually have a healthy myocardium, which is depressed by hypoxaemia rather than vascular disease. Therefore, the key to successful resuscitation of a newborn is effective positive pressure ventilation.

Preparing for the birth of a baby

Although the need for resuscitation can be anticipated in some instances, there are many times when it is not. Paramedics transporting women in labour and attending births must have the necessary equipment ready to resuscitate every baby, no matter how 'low risk' the mother. Essential equipment for basic newborn resuscitation includes:

- a warm environment, including warm towels (in a patient's home, towels can be warmed in a tumble dryer, time permitting; in an ambulance, turn the heating up to 'high' and close all the doors)
- a 50 × 50 cm sheet of bubble wrap to place over the newborn after drying (this is extremely effective at maintaining warmth while allowing the paramedic to visualise the baby's breathing efforts)
- a 28 × 38 cm polyethylene 'zip-lock' (Glad™) bag with a square hole cut in the end opposite the zip-lock big enough for the baby's head (for newborns < 32 weeks' gestation or < 1500 g birth weight)
- a digital thermometer to measure per axilla or rectal temperature
- a 240-mL self-inflating bag (preferably with a positive end expiratory pressure [PEEP] valve, set at 5 cm H_2O)
- face masks: small enough for a preterm baby (35 mm) and a term baby (50 mm)
- a small oxygen mask (Hudson™) and green Argyle oxygen tubing
- nasal oxygen cannulae: neonatal size
- a stethoscope (preferably neonatal size)
- 8-Fg, 10-Fg and 12-Fg suction catheters
- a portable suction unit (be aware that most ambulances do not have low-flow suction; the recommended negative suction pressure for clearing the airway of a newborn is 100 mmHg [13 kPa or 133 cm H_2O])
- a portable oxygen cylinder with a flow meter and tubing, able to deliver a flow of 8–10 L/min
- oropharyngeal (Guedel™) airways: sizes 00 and 0 (not used routinely in newborns unless there is an airway malformation)
- two umbilical cord clamps
- a firm surface on which to lay the baby supine (in the home, place a warm towel on top of two folded blankets on the floor near the mother)
- newborn size 3-lead ECG electrodes ('dots').

Also desirable are:
- a pulse oximeter with a neonatal sensor, able to be applied to the baby's right hand or right wrist
- a woollen hat (in the home environment, ask the mother if she has a hat for the baby; if not, a corner of a warm towel will suffice).

Paramedics with advanced training in airway management (intensive care paramedics) should also carry:

- endotracheal tubes (ETTs): sizes 2.5 mm, 3.0 mm, 3.5 mm (uncuffed)
- laryngoscope with a straight blade: sizes 0 and 1
- end-tidal colorimetric CO_2 detector (Pedi-Cap™ is recommended for newborns)
- laryngeal mask airway: size 1 (for newborns > 2000 g or > 34 weeks' gestation)
- intraosseous (IO) needle or IO gun (0.5 mm)
- tapes for securing endotracheal tube and intraosseous needle
- adrenaline, 1 : 10,000
- 0.9% sodium chloride
- 10% glucose
- needles and syringes for drawing up and administering medications.

Stress-reliever 'liquorice sticks' are not recommended as they add significant dead space to the ETT and increase the risk of accidental extubation. Cuffed ETTs are not recommended for newborns as they can cause serious damage to the airway mucosa (Kezler & Chatburn, 2017). Oropharyngeal (Guedel™) airways are not routinely recommended in newborns as they can cause vagal reactions. An oropharyngeal airway may be useful in a baby with an airway malformation such as Pierre Robin sequence to prevent the baby's large tongue from occluding the airway.

 CASE STUDY 1

Case 10805, 1435 hrs.

Dispatch details: A 29-year-old female who is 39 weeks' pregnant with her third child is in labour.

Initial presentation: The ambulance crew find the patient leaning over her kitchen bench having a strong contraction. She appears to be quite distressed and says she has been having contractions every 2 minutes since she called the ambulance. A neighbour is present and is caring for the patient's other two children. With the next contraction, the patient exhales loudly and groans 'The baby is coming!' Her membranes rupture and the amniotic fluid is clear. As she kneels on all fours on the floor, the baby's head is visible between her legs. With the next contraction, the baby is born. The baby girl cries immediately and is moving all her limbs vigorously, but she appears cyanosed.

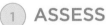 **ASSESS**

Evaluating a newborn's need for assistance during transition begins within seconds of the birth and continues until the transition to extrauterine life is complete. Most newborn babies respond to the stimulation of being born and the cool air of the birth environment by crying lustily. They will move all four limbs and assume a posture of flexion. As they establish regular respirations, their heart rate will rise above 100 bpm within a minute of birth. Newborn babies who are breathing or crying, are flexed or moving their limbs immediately after birth and who have a heart rate above 100 bpm within a minute of birth do not require resuscitation. If these responses are weak, stimulate the baby to breathe by rubbing the baby gently, but briskly, with a towel. Shaking, slapping, spanking or holding a newborn upside-down is potentially dangerous and should **never** be used as a means of stimulation.

PRACTICE TIP

- A newborn who is flexed and moving their limbs is unlikely to be severely compromised.
- A newborn who is floppy, not moving and has an extended posture is likely to require resuscitation.

A newborn who is bradycardic at birth with absent or gasping respirations and poor muscle tone (floppy posture) and who is not moving is more likely to have experienced a significant hypoxic ischaemic event before or around the time of birth. This baby will require more than stimulation to establish effective breathing. Dry this baby quickly and prepare to initiate resuscitation.

Initial assessment of *every* newborn baby to determine whether the baby requires more than routine care at birth is based on the following four questions.

1. Is the baby term gestation?
2. Is the amniotic fluid clear of meconium?
3. Is the baby breathing or crying?
4. Is the baby flexed or moving their limbs?

If the answer to any of these questions is 'no', the newborn requires further assessment and initiation of basic life support interventions. These follow a standardised clinical approach. Follow the principles of ensuring that the patient has a clear airway, is breathing and has a circulation, but initiate specific interventions that are unique to the newborn baby.

Patient history

At 39 weeks' gestation, this baby is considered term gestation. The amniotic fluid was clear when the mother's membranes ruptured just prior to the baby being born. Although the paramedics do not have a maternal history other than knowing this is the mother's third baby, the baby's condition at birth will dictate what actions need to be taken to assist the baby during the transition to extrauterine life. Any preexisting medical conditions or complications during pregnancy should still be ascertained, but assessing the baby should be the first priority.

At birth the baby was crying and moving all four limbs. There was no meconium in the amniotic fluid. Based on this assessment, the paramedics determine she does not require resuscitation. They can treat her as a vigorous (normal) newborn, applying the principles of routine care:

- ensuring a clear airway
- providing warmth
- maintaining ongoing assessment and documentation of the baby's vital signs.

Airway

A baby's airway is anatomically different from that of an adult or older child. Babies have a large head, a short neck and a large tongue. Their tracheal diameter is narrower and their trachea is shorter. The cricoid is the narrowest part of the airway and the larynx is higher and more anterior than that of an adult, at C2–C3 (see Fig 55.3).

To open the airway, position the baby with the head in a neutral or slightly extended position. Avoid both flexion and hyperextension of the head as this can occlude the airway. Most newborn babies will clear their own airway at birth and do not require suctioning.

Breathing

Uncompromised newborns will normally make vigorous efforts to inhale air into the lungs. Healthy term newborns can exert negative pressures of −80 cm H_2O for the first breaths to expand the lungs and clear fetal lung fluid (ANZCOR, 2016). After the initial breaths, the pressures exerted are much lower. It is common for newborn babies to pause for a few seconds after these first large breaths and then to establish a regular breathing pattern. A normal respiratory rate in a newborn baby is 40–60 bpm. In the first hours after birth, a higher respiratory rate is common, as fetal lung liquid is being cleared.

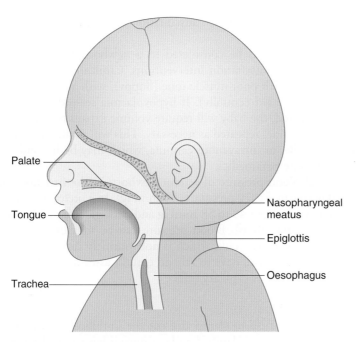

Figure 55.3
The anatomy of the newborn infant.
The sagittal sections of the neck of a newborn shortly after birth. Note that in newborns and infants, the neck is shorter and the larynx is located more cephalad.
Source: Snell & Smith (1993).

Recession or retraction (in-drawing) of the lower ribs and sternum, or the onset of persistent expiratory grunting, is a sign that the baby is experiencing difficulties keeping the lungs expanded. This is most commonly seen in premature babies who lack pulmonary surfactant. It may also be observed in babies with meconium aspiration syndrome and newborns with early-onset sepsis (e.g. Group B streptococcus infection, acquired in utero).

Persistent apnoea or gasping respirations, especially in a newborn with poor muscle tone and a heart rate below 100 bpm, is a serious sign. This indicates significant compromise. Positive pressure ventilation should be initiated without delay.

Cardiovascular

With the onset of regular breathing, the newborn's heart rate should rise quickly and should be consistently above 100 bpm within a minute of birth. Some babies will take up to 90 seconds to achieve a heart rate above 100 bpm (Dawson et al., 2010b). Thereafter, the baby's heart rate will vary between 110 and 160 bpm. A heart rate less than 100 bpm in a baby who is not breathing or is breathing inadequately is an indication for positive pressure ventilation.

Listening over the apex of the heart with a stethoscope is the best method of assessing the newborn's heart rate at birth. Peripheral and carotid pulses are extremely difficult to feel in newborns. An alternative method is to palpate the base of the umbilical cord while it is still pulsating. However, palpation of the cord is inferior to auscultation as the heart rate tends to be underestimated (Kamlin et al., 2006), potentially resulting in newborn babies receiving interventions they do not require. In paramedic practice, an ECG can be used to continuously measure heart rate if newborn-size 3-lead ECG electrodes are available. Placement of ECG leads in extremely preterm (EP) babies may result in damage to their friable skin. In the absence of a neonatal sensor to monitor heart rate and oxygen saturations, auscultation of the heart rate in EP babies is recommended.

Hypovolaemia should be considered in a newborn infant who remains bradycardic despite resuscitation interventions. Clinically, the newborn may be extremely pale, with poor muscle tone (floppy), with a capillary refill time of > 3 seconds (assessed centrally). If hypovolaemia secondary to blood loss or shock is suspected, the baby will require volume expansion with 10 mL/kg 0.9% sodium chloride, repeated as necessary. This will require insertion of an intraosseous needle, or intravenous cannula, which may be beyond the scope of practice of some paramedics.

The normal blood pressure of a term newborn in the first hour of life is 70/44 mmHg (mean arterial pressure = 53 mmHg). In a preterm infant, systolic blood pressure varies from 48 to 58 mmHg and diastolic from 24 to 36 mmHg (Safer Care Victoria, 2016). Blood pressure can be measured only with an appropriate-sized newborn cuff, which is not routinely carried by ambulance personnel. Paramedics will have to rely on clinical assessment of perfusion by nonspecific signs such as capillary refill.

Cutting the umbilical cord

There is no need to rush to clamp and cut the umbilical cord in a vigorous newborn. The cord can be clamped and cut once it has stopped pulsating (see Ch 54 for more details). Delaying cord clamping for up to 3 minutes after birth is beneficial to babies as it increases their blood pressure and improves iron status during infancy (ANZCOR, 2016).

Currently, there is insufficient evidence from human trials to support or refute delaying clamping in a non-vigorous newborn. Immediately after birth the uterine arteries begin to constrict, so gas exchange via the placental circulation cannot be relied upon in a newborn who has failed to establish effective ventilation at birth. In addition, placental function and gas exchange may well have been impaired before birth. In this situation, prompt initiation of resuscitation interventions should take priority over delayed cord clamping (ANZCOR, 2016).

Separating the mother and the baby by cutting the umbilical cord will make it easier for each paramedic to treat one patient, considering there are now two patients.

Colour

Assessment of colour is a poor proxy for tissue oxygenation in the first few minutes after birth in newborn babies (O'Donnell et al., 2007). At 1 minute of postnatal age, a healthy uncompromised newborn will have a mean oxygen saturation of haemoglobin of 60%, hence their cyanosed or 'dusky' appearance. The oxygen saturations of a healthy newborn will reach a mean of 73% by 2 minutes after birth and can take up to 7–10 minutes to reach a mean of 90% when measured by pulse oximetry (Dawson et al., 2010a). For this reason, colour is not used as part of the initial assessment to identify the newborn requiring more than routine care at birth.

It is very common for newborn babies to have acrocyanosis: a blue/purplish discolouration of the hands and feet. This is completely normal in the first 24 hours after birth and does not indicate systemic desaturation. No intervention is required. Acrocyanosis is not an indication for oxygen therapy.

Persistent central cyanosis, with or without other signs of respiratory distress in a newborn, will require out-of-hospital treatment with oxygen therapy. Extreme pallor that does not resolve with BVM ventilation is a very concerning sign in a newborn. It can indicate severe acidosis and hypotension due to poor cardiac output, with or without hypovolaemia (ANZCOR, 2016).

Initial assessment summary

Problem	Post-birth management of newborn
Appearance	Initially cyanosed
Pulse	> 100 bpm
Grimace	Crying
Activity	Moving all limbs
Respiratory effort	Crying and breathing

D: There is no environmental danger to the mother, baby or the crew.

R: Crying.

A: The baby's airway appears clear and there are no visible secretions (blood or meconium).

B: The baby is breathing and crying

C: The baby's heart rate is > 100 bpm.

Although the baby initially appears cyanosed the heart rate and muscle tone are good. While central cyanosis is a critical sign in adults, it is common in newborns in the first few minutes after birth. The entire clinical picture needs to be considered.

2 CONFIRM

The mother has told the paramedics that she is 39 weeks' gestation and expecting one baby. Twins would confound this clinical scene. The paramedics would need to call for immediate backup if this mother was giving birth to twins, as then there would be three patients to stabilise and transport.

The paramedics have seen that the amniotic fluid is clear of meconium. The baby is crying and has good tone, which would indicate that her heart rate is likely to be above 100 bpm. Although the baby appeared cyanosed at birth, this is a normal finding in the first minute after birth and does not require intervention if the baby is breathing, moving and has a heart rate above 100 bpm.

The paramedics perform a set of initial observations on the baby to confirm:

- Is the baby's heart rate above 100 bpm when auscultated with a stethoscope over the apex?
- Is the baby continuing to breathe at a rate of 40–60 bpm?
- Are there any signs of increased work of breathing (nasal flaring, chest recession or expiratory grunting)?
- Is the baby becoming centrally pink over the first minutes after birth (pink gums, mucous membranes and chest)?

As they make their initial assessment of the baby, the paramedics need to reassure the mother that her baby looks healthy. She will want to know (or confirm) what sex her baby is and that her baby has no obvious abnormalities. The paramedics should look for any other obvious congenital anomalies of the head, neck, face, limbs, spine and genitalia.

The paramedics should note and document the time of birth. They also need to allocate the baby a 1- and a 5-minute Apgar score (see Table 55.2). The Apgar score is *not* used to guide the resuscitation process: rather, it is assigned retrospectively to summarise the newborn's transition to extrauterine life and to quantify the newborn's response to any resuscitation interventions. Bear in mind that a non-vigorous newborn requires immediate intervention at birth, well before the 1-minute Apgar score is assigned. Conversely, a vigorous newborn can score '0' for colour at 1 minute, but not require resuscitation. Heart rate is the most important of the five signs and colour is the least useful (Australian Resuscitation Council, 2016). Initial assessment of the baby is therefore based on assessment of breathing, muscle tone and heart rate. Subsequent assessment

Table 55.2 Apgar score

Apgar score	0 points	1 point	2 points
Appearance (colour)	Cyanosed	Partially pink	Pink
Pulse (heart rate)	Absent	< 100 bpm	> 100 bpm
Grimace: response to stimulation	No response	Some response	Crying
Activity (muscle tone)	Limp	Some flexion	Flexed arms and legs that resist extension
Respiratory effort	Apnoea	All other types of respiratory effort	Breathing and crying lustily

is based on breathing, heart rate, muscle tone and colour. Assessment of the baby's temperature is also important before and during transport to hospital to detect hypothermia. (Aim for normothermia: a rectal or per axilla temperature of 36.5–37.5°C.) Use a digital thermometer to assess the baby's temperature. A newborn baby's external auditory canal is usually too small to obtain an accurate temperature using a tympanic membrane thermometer.

 TREAT

Emergency management

Safety

This baby has been born in her mother's kitchen. If there had been time, it would have been ideal to move the mother to her bed for the birth, then an area on the floor beside the bed could have been set up with warm blankets and towels to receive the baby. The paramedics needed to be ready to 'catch' this baby, ideally with warm towels ready, to prevent her from being born onto the cold hard floor of the kitchen. As a minimum, the crew should have the obstetric kit and newborn BVM ventilation device on hand.

Warmth

As this baby is vigorous, she should be dried quickly and placed on her mother's chest, skin-to-skin to maintain warmth. A warm blanket should be placed over both of them and a woollen hat (or the corner of a warm towel) placed on the baby's head. This is important as newborn babies can lose heat quickly due to the large surface area of their head.

If a baby is not vigorous at birth, they should be placed supine onto warm towels and blankets on the floor beside the mother (or on the end of the stretcher if in the ambulance). The baby should be dried quickly, especially the head, and the wet towel removed and replaced with a clean warm one. A hat should be placed on the baby's head and a piece of bubble wrap placed over the baby's body, up to the neck, leaving the head exposed. This will allow the paramedics to continue to assess and treat the baby, while maintaining warmth.

 EVALUATE

Continue to assess the newborn.

- Is the baby breathing effectively?
- Is the baby's heart rate > 100 bpm?
- Does the baby have good muscle tone?
- Is the baby pinking up over the first few minutes after birth?
  If yes, the baby should be nursed skin-to-skin with the mother.
  If not, the baby will require the next steps of resuscitation: ensuring a clear airway and initiation of positive pressure ventilation if the heart rate is < 100 bpm or the baby is not breathing.

Newborn airway management
Position to open the airway
Position the baby supine with the head in a neutral or slightly extended position. Avoid both flexion and hyperextension of the head as this can occlude the airway. Check if there is obvious blood or secretions in the airway (mouth and nares). Remember that babies are nose breathers, so need clear nares to breathe. Placing a rolled towel or blanket (~5 cm thick) underneath the baby's shoulders can help maintain the baby's head in the neutral position to open the airway.

Clear the airway only if necessary
Newborns normally do not require suctioning of their mouth, oropharynx or nose at birth: they are able to clear their own airway very effectively. Suctioning can cause more harm than benefit to a newborn and adverse effects include a vagal reaction, resulting in laryngeal spasm, bradycardia and delaying the time to onset of spontaneous breathing (ANZCOR, 2016). Suctioning can also cause damage to soft tissues. If it is required, it should be brief (no more than 5 seconds) and the suction catheter should be passed no more than 5 cm in a term infant. The negative pressure should not exceed 100 mmHg (13 kPa, 133 cm H_2O). Most standard suction units in Australian ambulances are not capable of delivering such low negative pressures. The corner of a towel can be used to wipe any secretions from the corner of the mouth and nose in the majority of newborns.

Visible blood in the oropharynx or nasopharynx may need to be removed by gently suctioning the mouth, followed by the nose. The mouth is suctioned first so that any blood in the pharynx is cleared and cannot be inhaled once the baby's nares are clear and the baby gasps and takes their first breath. (Remember that newborn babies are nose breathers.)

The baby born through meconium-stained amniotic fluid
If the baby is born though meconium-stained amniotic fluid or there is obvious meconium in the mouth or nose, management at birth differs slightly. Ideally, these babies need their airway cleared before being dried and stimulated to breathe. Management of meconium in the airway is dictated by the condition of the baby at birth.
- If the newborn is vigorous (breathing or crying, good muscle tone and HR > 100 bpm) and there is no obvious meconium in the mouth, suctioning is not indicated.
- If there is meconium visible in the mouth, suction the oropharynx, followed by the nares (only if necessary).

- If the baby is not vigorous (not breathing, flaccid and HR < 100 bpm), the aim is to clear the airway before drying and stimulating the baby to breathe. Suction the oropharynx, followed by the nasopharynx (only if necessary).
- If a paramedic is present at the birth of a non-vigorous baby born through thick meconium-stained fluid, the paramedic may suction the oropharynx under direct vision with a laryngoscope to clear meconium from around the vocal cords.

Current evidence regarding suctioning of non-vigorous meconium-exposed infants does not either support or refute the practice. Suction under direct vision should *not* be performed if the baby has already cried or has established ventilation, as this can further compromise the baby and does not alter the outcome in terms of developing meconium aspiration syndrome (ANZCOR, 2016).

Having cleared the airway and positioned the baby to open the airway, reassess the baby.

Positive pressure ventilation
Positive pressure ventilation with a BVM is indicated if:
- the baby is not breathing
- the baby has gasping respirations (a serious sign indicating neurological compromise secondary to asphyxia)
- the heart rate is less than 100 bpm *after* drying and stimulating the baby to breathe.

Face-mask placement
The face mask should be large enough to cover the baby's nose and mouth without covering the eyes or overlapping the chin. Paramedics need to carry a range of sizes of face masks for term (50 mm) and preterm (35 mm) babies. A face mask with a cushioned rim is preferable to a mask without a rim (ANZCOR, 2016). Face-mask leaks up to 60% are common and can impede effective BVM ventilation (Wood et al., 2008). Just because the mask fits does not mean the seal is adequate. Improvement in the baby's heart rate is the most important indication that BVM ventilation is effective. If the heart rate is not improving, ensure the airway is clear, then reapply the mask and try to improve the seal.

240-mL bag vs 600-mL bag
A 240-mL BVM should ideally be used to ventilate a newborn baby of any birth weight. (See the infant self-inflating bag in Fig 55.4.) This is because the tidal volume of a newborn is approximately 5–10 mL/kg body weight (ANZCOR, 2016). If chest rise is not achieved with a 240-mL bag, it is most likely because there is a large leak between the face and the mask. Ensure the airway is clear:

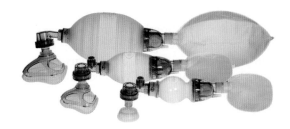

Figure 55.4
Comparison of disposable self-inflating bags with PEEP valve for BVM ventilation: adult: 1500 mL; paediatric: 600 mL; infant: 240 mL (recommended size for newborn babies).
Source: Image provided courtesy of Laerdal.

briefly suction the oropharynx to clear any secretions and reposition the head in a neutral position. Try reapplying the mask to improve the seal.

The technique for mask ventilation

The paramedic should position themselves directly behind the baby's head. With the baby's head in a neutral or slightly extended ('sniffing') position, roll the mask onto the baby's face from the chin upwards and over the mouth and nose. Using the thumb and index finger, hold the mask by the outer rim, applying equal downward pressure on the mask. Using the third finger of the same hand, apply an equal amount of jaw lift upwards. Do not hyperextend the head, as this will occlude the airway. Commence BVM ventilation at a rate of 40–60 breaths per minute. Count 'breathe two three, breathe two three, breathe two three' as you squeeze and release the bag.

Peak inflating pressures required for initial breaths to open the lungs and for subsequent breaths are variable and influenced by gestational age, mode of birth and underlying lung disease. If available, it is ideal to use a device that allows the peak inspiratory pressure (PIP) and positive end expiratory pressure (PEEP) to pre-set (e.g. a T-piece device—NeoPuff™ or similar). T-piece devices are usually only available in hospital settings and are routinely carried by dedicated neonatal retrieval teams. In term newborns, start with an initial PIP of 30 cm H_2O. In very preterm babies born < 32 weeks' gestation, start with an initial PIP of 20–25 cm H_2O. If you are in an ambulance setting and unable to measure the PIP, squeeze the bag just hard enough so that the chest and upper abdomen move slightly. The chest wall movement should be equal to that seen in normal quiet breathing (ANZCOR, 2016). Avoid delivering excessive pressures and volumes, especially if using a 600-mL paediatric bag. This may lead to overdistension of the alveoli, causing a pneumothorax. Immature preterm lungs can also

be damaged from delivery of high tidal volumes, even with a 240-mL bag (Björklund et al., 1997). If a PEEP valve is attached to the bag, set it to 5 cm H_2O. PEEP assists preterm newborn babies to establish and maintain functional residual capacity; it also helps improve their oxygenation (Siew et al., 2009).

Most newborn babies respond very quickly to effective positive pressure ventilation. When performed correctly, this will result in a rapid improvement in heart rate, usually without the administration of supplementary oxygen (ANZCOR, 2016). Once it is clear the baby is responding to BVM ventilation, as evidenced by an improvement in heart rate, the PIP and ventilation rate can and should be reduced (ANZCOR, 2016).

Mouth-to-mouth-and-nose resuscitation

If a 240-mL or 600-mL bag is not available, rescue breathing by mouth-to-mouth-and-nose ventilation should be used. The paramedic should apply their mouth over the baby's mouth and nose and give small inflations at a rate of 40–60 breaths per minute (~1 breath per second). Aim to achieve a visible rise and fall of the chest. Continue until the baby's heart rate increases to above 100 bpm and the baby is breathing spontaneously.

Air or oxygen for resuscitation

Newborn babies requiring BVM ventilation should initially be resuscitated with air (21% oxygen). High-flow 100% oxygen should be reserved for those severely compromised newborns who do not respond to resuscitation efforts within the first minutes of life. Level 1 evidence from randomised controlled trials comparing initiating resuscitation with air (21% oxygen) versus 100% oxygen in newborns consistently demonstrates a significant reduction in mortality when air is used (Davis et al., 2004). In term newborns, the use of 100% oxygen has also been shown to delay the time taken by the newborn to initiate breathing or crying (Vento et al., 2001).

Newborn babies, especially premature babies, can become rapidly and dangerously hyperoxic when exposed to 100% oxygen. There is increasing evidence that even brief exposure to excessive oxygenation can be harmful to the newborn baby, both during and after resuscitation. Use of 100% oxygen reduces cerebral perfusion in newborn babies (Davis et al., 2004) and enhances oxidative stress for up to 4 weeks after birth (Vento et al., 2001, 2002; Perlman et al., 2010).

Pulse oximetry is used routinely at in-hospital births to guide supplemental oxygen administration. To avoid hyperoxia, the oxygen concentration is reduced once the newborn's SpO_2 is above 90%.

Table 55.3 Target pre-ductal* saturations for newborn babies during resuscitation

Time from birth (in minutes)	Target pre-ductal saturations for newborn babies during resuscitation
1 minute	60–70%
2 minutes	65–85%
3 minutes	70–90%
4 minutes	75–90%
5 minutes	80–90%
10 minutes	85–90%

Source: ANZCOR (2016).

*Pre-ductal saturations are obtained by placement of the pulse oximeter probe on the infant's right hand or right wrist. All other limbs are post-ductal.

The aim of supplemental oxygen administration is to achieve the normal rise of SpO_2 over the first minutes of life seen in healthy term infants. The pre-ductal target saturations for newborn babies during the first minutes after birth are shown in Table 55.3. A neonatal sensor is required to measure oxygen saturations. The sensor should be placed onto the baby's right hand or right wrist to obtain pre-ductal readings of SpO_2. The pre-ductal saturations reflect brainstem oxygen delivery and have better perfusion and oxygenation than post-ductal saturations from the left hand, left foot or right foot (Mariani et al., 2007). As long as there is adequate cardiac output and peripheral blood flow for the oximeter to detect a pulse, the oximeter will display a continual measurement of heart rate and SpO_2, both of which are extremely useful during resuscitation of a newborn baby.

If paramedics do not have access to a neonatal sensor and therefore cannot measure the baby's SpO_2, the following principles apply with regard to the use of supplemental oxygen for newborn resuscitation.

- Normal healthy newborns are cyanosed or dusky at birth and take several minutes to 'pink up'. If they are breathing or crying, with a heart rate above 100 bpm, they do not require supplemental oxygen.
- Visual assessment of the presence or absence of cyanosis has poor correlation to the baby's PaO_2 and SpO_2.
- The only absolute indication for the administration of 100% high-flow oxygen during resuscitation is if the newborn has a heart rate less than 60 bpm after *at least* 30 seconds of effective BVM ventilation in air.
- If the heart rate is between 60 and 100 bpm and the baby is breathing ineffectively, 100%

oxygen can be used briefly until the heart rate improves to above 100 bpm.

- If the baby remains persistently centrally cyanosed and/or has signs of respiratory distress (respiratory rate greater than 60 bpm, nasal flaring, retraction or recession, cyanosis), the paramedics should consult with the neonatal emergency retrieval service via the ambulance clinician regarding management. Some babies will require intubation and positive pressure ventilation, while others may be safe to transport self-ventilating with 2 L of oxygen delivered by nasal cannulae or a Hudson™ face mask.

Chest compressions

A newborn baby who has suffered significant peripartum hypoxic ischaemia, with or without an associated acute sentinel event (e.g. placental abruption or antepartum haemorrhage), may present in circulatory collapse with poor cardiac output and may not respond to positive pressure ventilation. Asystole at birth or after birth is rare. Remember: fewer than 2 per 1000 live born babies in Australia require chest compressions at birth (AIHW, 2019).

Even if the heart rate is less than 60 bpm at birth, at least 30 seconds of effective BVM ventilation should be performed before chest compressions are initiated. This differs from adults, where compressions are commenced as soon as possible in the absence of a palpable pulse. A heart rate less than 60 bpm and performing chest compressions are an absolute indication for the use of 100% high-flow oxygen via the BVM.

PRACTICE TIP

Newborn babies usually have a healthy myocardium, which is depressed by hypoxaemia. Effective ventilation is the key to resuscitation.

Technique

In newborns, the two-thumb, hand-encircling technique (see Fig 55.5A) is the preferred option. Using this technique, both thumbs are superimposed on one another or placed side by side on the lower third of the sternum (just below the nipples), with the hands encircling the newborn's torso. The chest should be compressed one-third of the anterior–posterior diameter. This technique has been shown

PRACTICE TIP

Signs of effective BVM ventilation include:
- improvement in the heart rate above 100 bpm
- a slight rise of the chest and upper abdomen
- improvement in oxygenation (SpO_2 and/or colour).

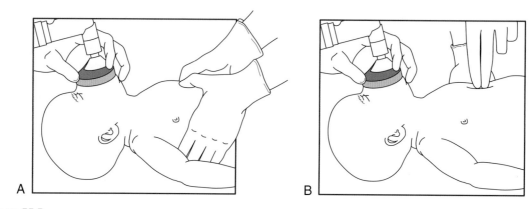

Figure 55.5
A The two-thumb, hand-encircling technique (recommended). **B** The two-finger technique.
Source: Niermeyer et al. (2016).

to have advantages over the two-finger technique (see Fig 55.5B) because it:

- improves peak systolic and coronary perfusion pressure
- results in more consistent depth of compressions over prolonged periods of time
- is easier to perform and less tiring compared with the two-finger technique (ANZCOR, 2016).

The ratio of compressions to inflation

In the newborn, the ratio of compressions to BVM inflation is 3:1, providing a higher rate of inflation than a 15:2 ratio (ANZCOR, 2016). This ratio is used for both one- and two-person resuscitation teams. The aim is to achieve 90 compressions and 30 inflations per minute (2 events per second, 120 events per minute). Count 'One two three breathe, one two three breathe' as you compress, compress, compress, inflate; compress, compress, compress, inflate. The compressions should be paused while the positive pressure inflation is delivered (unless the baby has been intubated, in which case there is no need to pause compressions to deliver the positive pressure inflation via the ETT). The baby's chest should fully expand between compressions, but the paramedic's hands should not move from their position around the baby's torso. Chest compressions should be delivered for at least 30 seconds with minimal interruption before checking the heart rate again. If a pulse oximeter is providing a continuous reading of heart rate and oxygen saturations, this is evidence of effective output.

Ongoing management

Paramedics with appropriate training may perform these procedures in the out-of-hospital environment:

- insertion of a laryngeal mask airway (LMA) in babies > 2000 g or > 34 weeks' gestation

- intravenous or intraosseous (IO) access
- medication and fluid administration.

Intubation

Intubation is appropriate in the following out-of-hospital situations:

- the baby's heart rate is not improving with BVM ventilation
- the baby is born through meconium and is not vigorous at birth
- the baby is extremely premature (< 28 weeks' gestation, < 1000 g birth weight)
- the baby is born without a detectable heart rate.

The heart rate should improve following intubation with effective delivery of positive pressure ventilation. See Table 55.4 for the appropriate endotracheal tube sizes.

Insertion of an LMA

If intubation is impossible or not feasible, or the provider is not trained in neonatal intubation, a size 1 LMA may be used to secure an airway in a newborn > 2000 g or > 34 weeks' gestation. The ANZCOR guidelines (2016) state an LMA should be considered as an alternative to tracheal intubation if face-mask ventilation is unsuccessful and tracheal intubation is unsuccessful or not feasible (ANZCOR, 2016).

Intravenous or IO access

Since so few babies require the administration of drugs following birth, paramedics will most likely be unfamiliar with gaining access to the intravascular space. Compared with adults, using IO devices may be faster and more reliable.

The IO route is quickly becoming the preferred method of establishing access in the out-of-hospital environment. The preferred site is the proximal tibia. Aim to enter a few centimetres below the

Table 55.4 Selecting the correct size endotracheal tube

Gestational age (weeks)	Endotracheal tube size (uncuffed ETT)	Estimated birth weight	Actual birth weight in grams	Depth of insertion from upper lip*
23–24	2.5 mm	<1 kg	500–699 g	5.5 cm
25–26			700–899 g	6.0 cm
27–29			900–999 g	6.5 cm
30–32	3.0 mm	1–2 kg	1000 g	7.0 cm
33–34			1500 g	7.5 cm
			2000 g	8.0 cm
35–37	3.5 mm	3 kg (or greater)	2500 g	8.5 cm
38–40			3000 g	9.0 cm
41–43			4000 g	10.0 cm

*Weight in kg + 6 cm can be used to estimate the depth of insertion for babies > 1 kg birth weight.

tibial tuberosity at the centre of the flat anteromedial surface. Direct the needle caudally away from the upper tibial epiphysis (Safer Care Victoria, 2018b). The distal anterolateral surface of the tibia is an alternative site. The distal femur and sternum should not be used in babies (Safer Care Victoria, 2018b). An 18-gauge IO needle is preferable to using an IO gun in a premature baby (ANZCOR, 2016). An IO gun should be used with extreme caution in a premature baby, especially one weighing less than 1500 g due to the fragility of the baby's small bones and the small IO space.

Umbilical venous catheterisation (UVC) is *not* a supported procedure in paramedic practice. There is a risk of cannulating the umbilical artery and inadvertently administering vasoactive drugs into the artery (e.g. adrenaline). Complications include bleeding, infection, perforation, clot formation, cardiac arrhythmias, hepatic necrosis and portal hypertension (Safer Care Victoria, 2018c). Peripheral cannulation (IV) is extremely difficult in a newborn who is shocked or collapsed. Since it is also time-consuming it is better to proceed with patient transport.

Medications and fluid administration

The priority during advanced resuscitation of a newborn baby is to ensure that the continuity and technique of external chest compressions and positive pressure ventilation is not compromised. However, if external chest compressions with positive pressure ventilation in 100% oxygen fail to restore the heart rate and circulation, then adrenaline may be required. Adrenaline is indicated if the heart rate is below 60 bpm after at least 30 seconds of external chest compressions with BVM ventilation in 100% oxygen (and at least 30 seconds of effective BVM

ventilation in air before external cardiac compressions are commenced). Adrenaline should preferably be administered intravenously (ANZCOR, 2016). Inserting a peripheral line in a shocked or collapsed newborn is extremely difficult. An IO needle can be used as an alternative if there is no IV access (ANZCOR, 2016). There is insufficient evidence for use of the endotracheal adrenaline, as the safety and efficacy of the endotracheal dose has not been studied in human neonates. If the endotracheal route is used, ANZCOR state that it is likely that a higher dose will be required to achieve the desired effect. If the tracheal route is used, up to 10 times the IV dose (50–100 microgram/kg) should be used (ANZCOR, 2016).

Volume expanders may be indicated in a baby in whom hypovolaemia secondary to fetal blood loss or septic shock is suspected. Normal saline is the volume expander of choice in the out-of-hospital setting—0.9% sodium chloride for volume expansion is indicated if:

- blood loss is suspected and the baby appears shocked
- the baby appears very pale,
- capillary refill > 4 seconds,
- perfusion is poor
- femoral pulses are weak
- the baby is not responding to resuscitation measures with an improvement in heart rate.

Consideration should be given to preventing and treating hypoglycaemia in all babies, especially those who have required resuscitation at birth. Adverse neurological outcomes have been demonstrated in newborns with hypoglycaemia following a hypoxic ischaemic insult (Salhab et al., 2004). Although the optimal range of blood glucose concentration to minimise brain injury is still to be defined, aim to maintain the baby's blood glucose level ≥ 2.5 mmol/L (ANZCOR, 2016). IM glucagon can be administered if IV or IO access is not available for a continuous 10% glucose infusion. Glucagon acts by mobilising glycogen from the liver. If the baby has inadequate stores of glycogen (e.g. extremely preterm baby or growth-restricted baby), glucagon treatment may not be as effective.

The following drugs are not indicated in newborn resuscitation.

- *Lignocaine, atropine, calcium, magnesium, potassium, vasopressin* and *amiodarone* are not indicated in the resuscitation of a newborn baby at any time.
- *Sodium bicarbonate.* Level 1 evidence from two human trials has failed to demonstrate a beneficial impact on survival, neurological outcome or acid–base balance in asphyxiated babies (Lokesh et al., 2004; Murki et al., 2004). The known side effects include depressed myocardial function, exacerbation of intracellular hypercarbia, paradoxical intracellular acidosis, reduced cerebral blood flow and increased risk of intraventricular haemorrhage in preterm babies.
- *Naloxone.* This is not indicated in initial newborn resuscitation as there is no evidence of benefit and substantial evidence of risk (myocardial depression, cardiac arrhythmias, exacerbation of cerebral white-matter neuro-histological injury; Van Woerkom et al., 2004). The first priority is to provide BVM ventilation if the baby is not breathing. If there is any suspicion that the mother is an intravenous drug user, naloxone is absolutely contraindicated in the baby, as it can cause an acute withdrawal and seizures.

Documentation

The paramedics should document the following whenever a birth occurs in the out-of-hospital setting:

- time of birth (this is not always possible if the birth occurred prior to the paramedics' arrival)
- time of first spontaneous breath
- resuscitation interventions, timing and response (including BVM ventilation, use of 100% oxygen, external chest compressions, adrenaline or sodium chloride administration)
- heart rate, respiratory rate, respiratory effort, perfusion, tone and colour every 15 minutes during transport
- temperature (per axilla or rectal)
- blood glucose level (if possible)
- Apgar score at 1 and 5 minutes (and assessed every 5 minutes until the score is 7 or greater).

Birth during transport

Delivering a baby during transport adds a layer of complexity to the care of both mother and baby. Space (or lack thereof) is a significant issue. This will be a highly emotional and potentially chaotic situation, even if the baby is born in a healthy condition. If the baby requires resuscitation, this will have to be performed on the end of the stretcher at the mother's feet, in her full view. Even if the mother has a support person with her in the ambulance, that person will need to sit in the front passenger seat to give the paramedics room to work in the rear of the ambulance. All aspects of resuscitation and subsequent care of the baby are further complicated by the limitations of suitable equipment for sick newborns in the out-of-hospital environment, including monitoring equipment, umbilical catheters for intravenous access, an incubator for thermoregulation and assisted ventilation devices.

If the mother experiences complications during the birth (e.g. shoulder dystocia) or following the birth (e.g. postpartum haemorrhage), the paramedics will be further stretched. Backup assistance from a second crew is highly desirable if the birth is complicated or the baby is premature or compromised. Where possible, mother and baby should not be separated and each should have their own paramedic, but this may not be possible in some rural and remote areas. Ideally, a paramedic from the second crew can drive the ambulance while the two paramedics from the first crew care for the mother and her baby.

Paramedics are strongly advised to consult with a neonatologist from their local Newborn and Paediatric Emergency Transport Service or equivalent regarding ongoing emergency management of any baby requiring resuscitation and for all premature babies. The consultant can direct the paramedic crew to the most appropriate receiving hospital, which may not necessarily be the closest hospital, en route. The consultant may also activate a neonatal team to proceed to the receiving hospital to continue management of the baby and to transfer the baby to a tertiary hospital with a NICU.

There will be times when a baby is too premature or too severely asphyxiated to survive, despite the best efforts of the paramedics. If a baby has been stillborn or has died despite resuscitation efforts, the paramedics will find themselves in one of the most difficult situations they will face in their career. The death of a baby is devastating for all involved. Encourage the mother (and father, if he is present) to see their baby and allow one of the parents to hold the baby during transport to hospital if they wish. The hospital will arrange for SANDS (the

Stillbirth and Neonatal Death Support Association) to contact the parents and offer counselling to the family. It is equally important that the paramedics are provided with an opportunity to debrief and receive counselling following the death of a baby in their care.

Discontinuing resuscitation

The Australian Resuscitation Council guidelines and international guidelines state that it is reasonable to discontinue resuscitation of a newborn baby if there is no measurable heart rate after 10 minutes of maximal resuscitation (ANZCOR, 2016). Both survival and quality of survival deteriorate rapidly beyond this time and there is a very high risk of severe neurological disability if the baby does survive (Casalaz et al., 1998; Haddad et al., 2000). Where early death is inevitable, resuscitation is not indicated. This may be the case in babies born at the limits of viability (22–23 weeks' gestation) and those with known congenital anomalies that are incompatible with life (Lantos et al., 1988). The decision to withdraw or not to initiate resuscitation efforts is not an easy one. Where possible, this should be made in a hospital environment in consultation with the parents, who may have strong views on an acceptable risk of morbidity.

Hospital admission

On admission to the neonatal intensive or special care nursery, the following procedures are standard care for sick and/or premature babies:

- continuous cardiorespiratory, blood pressure, temperature and SpO_2 monitoring
- intubation and mechanical ventilation (or nasal continuous positive airway pressure [CPAP])
- intratracheal surfactant administration (to treat respiratory distress syndrome)
- frequent blood gas analysis during the acute stage of illness
- umbilical venous catheterisation (UVC) and umbilical arterial catheterisation (UAC)
- IV penicillin and gentamicin (for all babies with respiratory distress until blood cultures show no growth); aciclovir may be added if a viral herpes simplex virus infection is suspected (e.g. the mother has an active herpes lesion)
- IV therapy with 10% glucose at 60 mL/kg/day (day 1)
- volume expansion with 0.9% sodium chloride to treat hypovolaemia and metabolic acidosis
- inotropes (dopamine or dobutamine) to treat hypotension
- incubator care for thermoregulation

- therapeutic hypothermia (for babies with grade 2 or grade 3 hypoxic ischaemic encephalopathy [HIE])
- other imaging (head ultrasound to detect intraventricular haemorrhage in preterm babies; magnetic resonance imaging [MRI] to detect brain injury in babies with HIE).

Investigations

The following investigations and monitoring may be performed at the receiving hospital to diagnose and treat the underlying condition that has contributed to abnormal transition to extrauterine life:

- chest x-ray to diagnose respiratory distress syndrome, pneumonia, pneumothorax or meconium aspiration syndrome
- blood gas analysis including lactate to diagnose respiratory failure and/or metabolic acidosis
- urea and electrolytes to guide IV fluid replacement therapy
- full blood count, C-reactive protein, IT ratio and blood cultures to rule out infection
- blood glucose level to diagnose and treat hypoglycaemia
- continuous blood pressure monitoring via the UAC or peripheral arterial line to detect hypotension and guide the concentration of inotrope infusions
- continuous cardiorespiratory, SpO_2 and temperature monitoring to monitor cardiorespiratory stability and to guide supplemental oxygen therapy.

Follow-up

The baby's length of stay in hospital will vary according to gestational age and severity of illness. A healthy term infant born before arrival at hospital who was vigorous at birth would normally room in with their mother in the postnatal ward after a short period of observation in the special care nursery. The average length of stay for these babies is 2–4 days. The baby will receive a routine follow-up visit from the local maternal child health nurse within a week of discharge.

A preterm baby born at 24 weeks' gestation will be in hospital for 12–16 weeks on average. Those who develop chronic lung disease may be hospitalised for many weeks or even months beyond the term-corrected age. Extremely premature babies may be discharged home from hospital on low-flow oxygen therapy. Many require readmission for respiratory illnesses such as bronchiolitis during the first 6–12 months of life.

A term baby whose birth is complicated by meconium aspiration syndrome will usually require mechanical ventilation for a period of 4–12 days with high peak inspiratory pressures (30–35 cm H_2O).

These babies often require deep sedation, muscle relaxation and inhaled nitric oxide (iNO) while ventilated. PPHN often complicates severe cases of meconium aspiration syndrome (Safer Care Victoria, 2018a; Weisz & McNamara, 2017). Length of stay will vary according to the severity of the disease.

A baby with HIE secondary to peripartum hypoxia may or may not require mechanical ventilation. Babies with grade 1 (mild) HIE do not usually require ventilation, whereas a baby with grade 2 (moderate) or grade 3 (severe) HIE who is experiencing seizure activity is likely to be intubated and ventilated to protect the airway. As these babies do not usually have parenchymal lung disease (unless complicated by meconium aspiration syndrome) they usually require low ventilation pressures and slow rates. They may require inotropes to support cardiac output and blood pressure. Therapeutic hypothermia (deep body cooling to 33–34°C) is commenced for neuroprotection for babies ≥ 35 weeks' gestation with grade 2 or 3 HIE (Safer Care Victoria, 2018d). Length of stay varies according to the severity of HIE and ischaemic effects on other organs (brain, kidneys and myocardium). Treatment may be redirected to palliative care for babies with grade 3 HIE if MRI reveals extensive and irreversible brain damage.

 CASE STUDY 2

Case 10407, 1755 hrs.

Dispatch details: A 25-year-old female who is 26 weeks' pregnant has ruptured her membranes and is having contractions.

Initial presentation: The paramedics are met in the front drive of the house by the woman's partner. He is yelling, 'Quick, quick, she's had the baby!' He takes them to the bathroom where the woman is sitting on the floor holding a tiny newborn baby in her arms wrapped in a bath towel.

The preterm baby

All preterm babies, but especially those born before 28 weeks' gestation or weighing less than 1500 g at birth, become hypothermic very easily. Heat loss will be further exacerbated when birth occurs in an out-of-hospital setting, as paramedics have limited control over the temperature of the birth and transport environment.

The Australian and New Zealand Committee on Resuscitation (2016) neonatal resuscitation guidelines recommend using a polyethylene (food-grade, heat-resistant) zip-lock bag as a means of preventing extreme heat loss in very premature babies. The use of a polyethylene bag to prevent hypothermia is an evidence-based practice, used in hospitals routinely since 2006 for babies born before 32 weeks' gestation or weighing less than 1500 g at birth. To prepare the bag, cut a square hole just large enough for the baby's head to pass through the bag at the opposite end to the zip-lock. At birth, place the baby immediately, without drying (i.e. wet and warm) into the bag with the body completely covered and just the head exposed through the hole at the top. Then lock the bag under the baby's feet. Dry the baby's head and place a hat on it.

If the baby is breathing and has a heart rate above 100 bpm, the baby can be placed onto the mother's chest (skin-to-skin) and a warm blanket placed over the top of the two of them. If the baby requires resuscitation interventions, place the baby into a bag and cover with a warm towel and warm blankets next to the mother. Leave the baby in the bag with just their head out and cover the baby with a space blanket or warm towels. Ensure the baby has a hat or warm towels covering their head.

If the baby has already been born when the paramedics arrive on the scene, the baby will inevitably be hypothermic. The baby should be dried well and a hat placed on their head. A polyethylene bag can still be used as long as the paramedics are able to provide a radiant heat source directly onto the bag or warm blankets around the bag. During transport to hospital, if no incubator is available and if safe to do so, baby can be placed skin-to-skin with the mother, as her body temperature will maintain the baby's temperature far more effectively than using space blankets or warm blankets.

Hypothermia increases both mortality and morbidity, especially in very preterm babies. Preventing hypothermia is one of the most difficult challenges faced by paramedics in the out-of-hospital setting, for both term and preterm babies.

1 ASSESS

It might seem logical to ask the mother 'When was your baby due?' However, if the mother responds with a date that is several months away, it is somewhat challenging to calculate how preterm the baby is. When assessing any pregnant woman or her newborn baby, it is better to ask, 'How many weeks pregnant are you?' The crew may also ask the woman or her partner the following.
- How long ago was the baby born?
- Did the baby cry and move immediately after birth?
- Are you expecting more than one baby?
- Have you been well during your pregnancy?

1809 hrs Primary survey: The baby is wet and is still attached to the umbilical cord. She looks to be approximately 600–800 g. She is making some weak crying noises and moving her arms and legs.

1810 hrs Pertinent hx: The mother informs the crew that the baby cried as soon as she was born and was moving all her limbs. This is the mother's third baby. Her previous baby was also born preterm at 31 weeks' gestation.

1811 hrs Assessment: The baby is breathing rapidly but has marked intercostal chest recession. Her head is still wet. Her colour is pale. The umbilical cord is no longer pulsating.

1812 hrs Vital signs survey: Perfusion status: HR 150 bpm (auscultation), skin slightly centrally cyanosed, capillary refill > 4 seconds, temperature 34.6°C (per axilla).

Respiratory status: 88 bpm, equal air entry bilaterally, nasal flaring and grunting with each breath, marked intercostal and substernal retraction.

Conscious state: The baby has her eyes closed. She is lying in an extended posture.

2 CONFIRM

In many cases paramedics are presented with a complex situation involving more than one patient. A critical step in the treatment plan is to determine who should receive priority in this situation. The mother is conscious with no obvious haemorrhage but the newborn is clearly extremely preterm and is unable to breathe effectively. The paramedics' visual assessment confirms that the baby is experiencing the problems associated with preterm birth that they anticipated.

Assess!
- Is the newborn crying or breathing?
- Is the heart rate above 100 bpm?
- Does the newborn have good muscle tone?
- Are there obvious secretions in the mouth or nose?

TREAT

Emergency management

The first priority for the paramedics is to move this mother and her baby to a safer, warmer place than a cold bathroom floor. Simultaneously, they need to rapidly assess the baby's heart rate, work of breathing, tone and oxygenation (if possible). They also need to call for backup from an intensive care paramedic crew, as it is highly likely that this baby will require respiratory support before transport to hospital. At 26 weeks' gestation, early-onset respiratory distress and respiratory failure are inevitable. Preterm babies have the following anatomical and functional problems that result in an inability to support ventilation and oxygenation:

- underdeveloped alveolar saccules with limited surface area for gas exchange
- lack of pulmonary surfactant so alveoli collapse on expiration and functional residual capacity (FRC) is not established
- low compliance in the lung (small changes in volume in response to application of high pressures).

The lack of surfactant and decreased lung compliance lead to increased work of breathing, fatigue, atelectasis and a ventilation/perfusion (V/Q) mismatch (Gardner et al., 2016). Clinically the baby will be tachypnoeic (respiratory rate > 60 bpm), with grunting, nasal flaring and chest recession, and may be centrally cyanosed.

One paramedic clamps and cuts the umbilical cord while the other prepares an area in the bedroom to treat the baby. Having laid down a warm towel on top of two blankets, the paramedic cuts a hole in a 28 × 38 cm zip-lock bag. The baby is quickly carried into the bedroom and laid supine on the warm towel, dried and then placed with her body completely in the bag and her head outside of the bag. The paramedic zip locks the bag at the bottom and places a warm blanket over the bag. He dries the baby's head and uses a corner of a second towel to cover the top of her head.

1822 hrs: Perfusion status: HR 90 bpm (auscultation), skin slightly centrally cyanosed.

Respiratory status: No respiratory effort.

Conscious state: The baby has her eyes closed and has poor muscle tone (floppy).

1826 hrs: The paramedics commence BVM ventilation at a rate of 60 bpm. This rate is appropriate for a baby of 26 weeks' gestation with respiratory distress as she is likely to be hypercapnic. Her heart rate improves quickly with BVM ventilation to 130 bpm, but she remains cyanosed. As her colour is not improving and she has signs of marked respiratory distress, the paramedics BVM ventilate her using 100% oxygen.

If the respiratory distress remains severe, intubation should be considered according to local guidelines and the baby ventilated at 60 bpm, aiming for a tidal volume of 4–6 mL/kg.

The insertion of a UVC is not supported in paramedic practice. The risk of haemorrhage, inadvertent cannulation of the umbilical artery, drug or fluid administration into the artery, air embolism and infection are too great. While insertion of an IO needle is easier and quicker than peripheral venous cannulation of a newborn baby in the out-of-hospital setting, there is no IO needle small enough to safely cannulate a baby of 26 weeks' gestation (Safer Care Victoria, 2018b). The crew will not be able to gain IV access on this baby. Furthermore, such a procedure would only delay transport to hospital, which is a priority in this case.

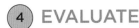 **EVALUATE**

Umbilical venous and arterial lines were inserted in hospital. A chest x-ray revealed respiratory distress syndrome. Surfactant replacement therapy was given intra-tracheally, maintenance fluids of 10% glucose were commenced, and IV penicillin and gentamicin were given for 7 days. A dobutamine infusion was also required to treat hypotension. The baby required high-frequency ventilation for 14 days and then extubation to nasal CPAP and then to high-flow nasal canulae (HFNC). She remained on HFNC for a further few weeks. She was discharged home after 14 weeks on low-flow oxygen of 100 mL/min.

Long-term role

Complications of prematurity and peripartum asphyxia can have lifelong effects. Extremely low birth weight babies (500–999 g birth weight) have increased rates of adverse neurodevelopmental outcomes such as cerebral palsy, deafness, blindness and severe developmental delay (Doyle et al., 2011). The rates of disability increase with decreasing gestational age.

 CASE STUDY 3

Case 10306, 0430 hrs.

Dispatch details: A 26-year-old female who is 41 weeks' pregnant is in labour for a planned home birth. There is thick meconium in the amniotic fluid. The midwife assisting with the home birth has requested transport to hospital.

Initial presentation: The paramedics are met by the woman's husband. He takes them into the lounge room where they find the woman on all fours over a fit ball. The midwife is listening to the fetal heart rate with a fetal Doppler monitor.

1 ASSESS

0444 hrs Primary survey: The woman is alert. She has just had a strong contraction lasting 1 minute. The fetal heart rate was 80 bpm during and for 30 seconds after the contraction.

0445 hrs Chief complaint: The midwife shows the crew a sanitary pad covered in thick meconium.

0446 hrs Pertinent hx: The midwife informs the crew that the woman was 8 cm dilated when she performed a vaginal examination (VE) 15 minutes ago. During the VE, the membranes ruptured and meconium was seen in the amniotic fluid. The woman is 41 weeks and two days pregnant. This is her first pregnancy. The woman has been in labour for 12 hours.

If this baby is breech, this could explain the meconium in the amniotic fluid. Meconium in a breech baby can be a normal finding that is not necessarily indicative of fetal distress. However, the fetal heart rate dropping to 80 bpm during and after a contraction is a sign that the fetus is distressed in utero.

PATIENT HISTORY

Ask!
- Is this your first baby?
- Are you expecting more than one baby?
- How long ago did your membranes ('waters') rupture?
- When did you first notice the meconium in the amniotic fluid?
- Is your baby positioned head down or breech?

989

0447 hrs Reassessment: The mother has another strong contraction and grunts, 'I need to push!'

0448 hrs Management: With the next three contractions, the midwife delivers the baby. He is floppy, not moving and not making any effort to breathe. His umbilical cord, fingers and toes are meconium stained.

The paramedics quickly suction the baby's oropharynx of meconium and then suction the nares. They dry the baby and stimulate him to breathe by rubbing his back and head with the towel. Then they remove the wet towel and replace it with a warm, dry towel.

0451 hrs Vital signs survey: Perfusion status: HR 78 bpm (auscultation), regular; skin warm, cyanosed.

Respiratory status: No respiratory effort following airway clearance.

Conscious state: Not moving and floppy.

② CONFIRM

In this case, the fact that the baby is not breathing is not in dispute. The first priority is to ventilate the baby.

The baby should be resuscitated in room air initially. Using 100% oxygen may further delay the time taken for him to take his first breath. The crew may need to provide supplementary oxygen if his heart rate does not improve with BVM ventilation. The first step is to provide BVM ventilation at a rate of 40–60 bpm in air (21%) for at least 30 seconds, then reassess the baby's heart rate and breathing effort. If the heart rate is 60–100 bpm, BVM ventilation should be continued and supplemental oxygen provided until the heart rate is above 100 bpm and the baby is breathing effectively. If the heart rate is below 60 bpm, chest compressions and 100% oxygen are now indicated.

③ TREAT

0452 hrs: The paramedics provide BVM ventilation at a rate of 30 bpm. This slower rate of ventilation is recommended because meconium aspiration is associated with gas trapping. Slowing the BVM rate enables a longer expiratory time. The paramedics aim for 0.5 seconds for inflation and 1.5 seconds for exhalation (2 seconds per inflation = 30 bpm). After 30 seconds of effective BVM ventilation, the baby starts to move and opens his eyes. He also takes some breaths on his own.

0453 hrs: Perfusion status: HR 110 bpm (auscultation), skin cyanosed but becoming pink.

Respiratory status: 20 bpm, equal air entry bilaterally.

Conscious state: The baby has opened his eyes and is moving his legs. His arms remain extended.

0454 hrs: The paramedics stop BVM ventilation as the baby is breathing spontaneously and his heart rate is > 100 bpm. However, the baby develops signs of respiratory distress over the next few minutes.

0456 hrs: Perfusion status: HR 140 (auscultation), skin centrally cyanosed.

Respiratory status: 60 bpm, equal air entry bilaterally, barrel-shaped chest, nasal flaring and grunting with each breath.

Conscious state: The baby is lying with his eyes closed. He is flexed but does not resist extension of his limbs.

0457 hrs: The paramedics commence oxygen at 2 L/minute via nasal cannula.

0500 hrs: The paramedics prepare to load the mother and baby for transport to hospital and document the events to date. The mother is assisted to the patient stretcher for transport. The baby is placed skin-to-skin with her.

④ EVALUATE

From the labour and birth history, the paramedics were anticipating this baby was at high risk of compromise at birth. They determine this baby is at risk of respiratory failure secondary to peripartum hypoxia-ischaemia, meconium aspiration. It is therefore anticipated this baby may not respond to initial resuscitation interventions and may continue to deteriorate in response to worsening hypoxia, acidosis, hypercapnia and PPHN. Consideration should be given to securing an airway in this baby for transport to hospital. The paramedics should consult with the neonatal emergency transport team to discuss the need for intubation and for an appropriate destination hospital. Backup from an intensive care ambulance team should be considered.

The baby required intubation shortly after arrival at the receiving hospital for worsening respiratory distress. His chest x-ray was consistent with meconium aspiration syndrome. He required ventilation for 48 hours and oxygen therapy for a further 4 days. He received IV antibiotics for 7 days. He was discharged home fully breastfeeding on day 9.

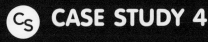

CASE STUDY 4

Case 11008, 0500 hrs.

Dispatch details: A 31-year-old female who is 38 weeks' pregnant has ruptured her membranes and is having regular contractions. She has gestational diabetes.

Initial presentation: The paramedics are met at the front door by the patient. They estimate her weight to be 120 kg. She tells them she has been having regular contractions since midnight. She is home alone as her husband is working a night shift and is due home at 7. She phoned for an ambulance when her membranes ruptured.

① ASSESS

0517 hrs Pertinent hx: The woman informs the paramedics that she was diagnosed with gestational diabetes mellitus (GDM) at 28 weeks' gestation. Her GDM has been diet controlled. She was booked for a planned induction in 2 days' time as the baby is large for dates on ultrasound. This is her first baby. She has a strong contraction lasting 1 minute and becomes distressed with the pain.

The paramedics need to determine whether there are any additional factors placing this baby at risk of requiring resuscitation. They establish that this is a term fetus and that the amniotic fluid was clear of meconium. They ascertain that her membranes ruptured less than 18 hours ago.

0524 hrs Treatment: The paramedics decide to assist the mother into the ambulance and proceed to the nearest maternity hospital, which is 35 km away. On the way, her contractions become closer and last longer.

0545 hrs Treatment: Approximately 30 km into the journey, she becomes extremely distressed with the pain and tells the paramedics she has a strong urge to push. They pull over to the side of the road in a truck stop. With the next four contractions, the baby's head is delivered, but the baby's shoulders are stuck. The baby's head is on the perineum for 6 minutes. They perform the McRobert's manoeuvre (see Ch 54) and the baby's body is born. The baby boy is floppy. He is not moving or making any effort to breathe. There is no blood or meconium in the amniotic fluid.

0600 hrs Vital signs survey: Perfusion status: HR 40 bpm (auscultation), skin cyanosed.
Respiratory status: No respiratory effort.
Conscious state: The baby is floppy.

2 CONFIRM

From the birth history, it was anticipated that this baby would be born in poor condition and likely to require resuscitation.

At birth, the baby is clearly compromised—not breathing or crying and with poor muscle tone. Given the baby's head was on the perineum for 6 minutes, the most likely problem is a hypoxic ischaemic insult.

3 TREAT

Emergency management

The paramedics quickly dry the baby and stimulate him to breathe by rubbing his back and head with a towel. They wipe the secretions from the corner of his mouth and nose with a corner of the towel. They remove the wet towel and replace it with a warm, dry towel, and cover the baby's head with a corner of the clean towel. They position him supine on the end of the stretcher with his head in a neutral position and place a small rolled towel under his shoulders to help maintain his head in a neutral position.

0602 hrs: The paramedics provide BVM ventilation at a rate of 60 bpm in air. They are achieving good chest wall rise with each BVM inflation. After 30 seconds of effective BVM ventilation, they re-evaluate the baby's heart rate, respiratory effort and muscle tone. A 3-lead ECG is applied to accurately monitor hear rate. There is no change.

0603 hrs: They connect the BVM to 100% oxygen. While one paramedic ventilates at 60 inflations per minute, the second auscultates the baby's heart rate again. There is still no change.

It is not routine practice to assess for a shockable arrhythmia in a newborn baby. Bradycardia occurs secondary to hypoxaemia, not because of cardiac arrhythmias such as ventricular fibrillation.

0604 hrs: The paramedics commence external chest compressions using the hand-encircling technique with BVM ventilation at a ratio of 3:1, using 100% oxygen. After 30 seconds of external chest compressions and BVM ventilation in 100% oxygen, the baby's heart rate is still 50 bpm. They contact the clinician and continue CPR. If the baby's heart rate is > 60 bpm but < 100 bpm, the paramedics should cease chest compressions but continue BVM ventilation, increasing the BVM ventilation rate to 40–60 bpm. They should continue BVM ventilation until the baby's heart rate is > 100 bpm and the baby is breathing spontaneously.

If the baby's heart rate is < 60 bpm, the paramedics should continue chest compressions and BVM ventilation at a ratio of 3:1 and ensure that they are using 100% oxygen via the BVM. They should reassess the baby after another

30 seconds of chest compressions and BVM ventilation with 100% oxygen. If the baby's heart rate is still < 60 bpm, advanced resuscitation interventions are indicated. The paramedics should call for backup from an intensive care paramedic crew if they have not already done so.

0605 hrs: Perfusion status: HR 70 bpm (auscultation), skin cyanosed, capillary refill > 4 seconds.

Respiratory status: RR 15, occasional gasping respirations, good air entry bilaterally with BVM ventilation.

Conscious state: The baby has opened his eyes but he remains very floppy. BGL: 1.1 mmol/L.

0606 hrs: The paramedics proceed to the receiving hospital. They have ceased chest compressions as the baby's heart rate is above 60 bpm but continue BVM ventilation in 100% oxygen at a rate of 40 bpm. They slow down the rate of BVM ventilation to avoid iatrogenic hypocapnia. The baby starts to move and opens his eyes, then takes some breaths on his own. The paramedics administer 1 mg of glucagon IM to treat the baby's low BGL.

4 EVALUATE

From the birth history, condition of the baby at birth and initial response to resuscitation interventions, it is clear this baby has experienced significant compromise.

In this case, the baby may continue to deteriorate. Establishing and maintaining an airway en route to the destination hospital is a priority. The neonatal transport team should be consulted regarding out-of-hospital management of his airway, ventilation and circulation and the most appropriate destination hospital.

The baby required intubation and ventilation shortly after arrival at the receiving hospital. Umbilical venous and arterial lines were inserted and maintenance fluids of 10% glucose were commenced and increased at 6 hours of age to 12.5% to treat hypoglycaemia. No abnormalities were detected on chest x-ray, and the full blood count, C-reactive protein and blood cultures were unremarkable. A dopamine infusion was required for 36 hours to treat hypotension. He was treated with therapeutic hypothermia for 72 hours. His MRI on day 4 was essentially normal and he was discharged home on day 10.

Hospital management

Paramedics need to be aware that a newborn infant of a diabetic mother is at risk of hypoglycaemia secondary to fetal hyperinsulinaemia after birth (Rozance et al., 2016). Babies of diabetic mothers are also at risk of being macrosomic (> 4000 g birth weight) and/or large for gestational age (> 90th percentile). This increases their risk of shoulder dystocia, birth injury, brachial nerve plexus and perinatal asphyxia. Surfactant synthesis can be delayed or inhibited in the fetus because of elevated fetal serum insulin levels, placing the newborn at increased risk of developing respiratory distress (Rozance et al., 2016).

Babies with moderate or severe HIE are also at risk of developing adverse neurodevelopmental outcomes as a result of hypoxic ischaemic damage to their brain such as cerebral palsy, cognitive delay and memory difficulties. At least 25% of survivors will have significant long-term major neurosensory problems (Jacobs & Tarnow-Mordi, 2010).

Future research

The survival rate for extremely preterm babies plateaued in the middle of the first decade after 2000 (Doyle et al., 2011). As it is unlikely that the lower limits of survival will be reduced beyond 22 weeks' gestation, the focus is on improving the long-term outcomes of extremely premature babies. For example, since 2010 magnesium sulfate has been routinely given to mothers at risk of preterm birth before 30 weeks' gestation because of its neuroprotective effects for the fetus (Doyle et al., 2009).

Therapeutic hypothermia is offering hope to parents whose babies have moderate or severe HIE. If commenced within 6 hours of birth, therapeutic hypothermia can reduce rates of cerebral palsy and cognitive impairment (Jacobs & Tarnow-Mordi, 2010). However, babies must meet strict criteria before this therapy is considered. Paramedics should not commence therapeutic hypothermia in the out-of-hospital environment because of its side effects of deep brain and body hypothermia. Current research is focusing on hypothermia in combination with various therapies, including the use of erythropoietin (Levene, 2010), xenon (a noble anaesthetic gas), cannabinoids and topiramate (an anticonvulsant).

Summary

Newborn babies rarely require resuscitation at the time of their birth: most newborns make vigorous efforts to inhale air into their lungs at birth and clear their own airway very effectively. Cyanosis is common immediately after birth and heart rate, breathing and muscle tone are the three criteria that should be used to assess the newborn at birth to determine the need for ongoing resuscitation interventions.

If the newborn does not start breathing or has a heart rate below 100 bpm after being dried and stimulated, BVM ventilation is indicated. When performed correctly, BVM ventilation will reliably result in a rapid improvement in heart rate, usually without the administration of supplementary oxygen. Air (21% oxygen) should be used initially, with 100% oxygen reserved for those babies who do not respond to BMV ventilation in the first few minutes of life.

Newborn babies lose heat very quickly and out-of-hospital interventions to manage hypothermia should be instigated as part of the resuscitation process.

Prematurity is associated with an increased risk of mortality and morbidity. Transferring the woman with threatened preterm labour to a tertiary perinatal centre before the birth of her baby increases the baby's chance of survival and quality of life.

References

Abeywardana, S., & Sullivan, E. A. (2008). *Congenital anomalies in Australia 2002–2003. Birth anomalies series no. 3 Cat. no. PER 41.* Sydney: AIHW National Perinatal Statistics Unit.

Australian and New Zealand Committee on Resuscitation (2016). *Section 12—Neonatal guidelines.* Retrieved from: https://resus.org.au/guidelines/ [Accessed 28 May 2018].

Australian Institute of Health and Welfare. (2019). *Australia's mothers and babies 2017—in brief. Perinatal statistics series no 35. Cat. no. PER 100.* Canberra: AIHW.

Australian Resuscitation Council. 2016. *ANZCOR Guideline 13.3—Assessment of the Newborn Infant.* https://resus.org.au/guidelines/index/.

Boland, R. A., & Doyle, L. W. (2019). Active management of periviable births at 22–24 weeks' gestation. *Journal of Paediatrics and Child Health, 55*(S1), 3–55.

Boland, R. A., Davis, P. G., Dawson, J. A., & Doyle, L. W. (2016). Outcomes of infants born at 22-27 weeks' gestation in Victoria according to outborn/inborn birth status. *Archives of Disease in Childhood. Fetal and Neonatal Edition, 0,* F1–F8.

Boland, R. A., Davis, P. G., Dawson, J. A., Stewart, M. J., Smith, J., & Doyle, L. W. (2018). Very preterm birth before arrival at hospital. *The Australian and New Zealand Journal of Obstetrics and Gynaecology, 58,* 197–203.

Björklund, L. J., Ingimarsson, J., Curstedt, T., John, J., Robertson, B., Werner, O., & Vilstrup, C. T. (1997). Manual ventilation with a few large breaths at birth compromises the therapeutic effect of subsequent surfactant replacement in immature lambs. *Pediatric Research, 42*(3), 348–355.

Casalaz, D. M., Marlow, N., & Speidel, B. (1998). Outcome of resuscitation following unexpected stillbirth. *Archives of Disease in Childhood. Fetal and Neonatal Edition, 78,* F112–F115.

Chow, S., Le Marsney, R., Creighton, P., Chambers, G. M., & Lui, K. (2019). *2017 Report of the Australian and New Zealand Neonatal Network.* Retrieved from: https://anznn.net/annualreports [Accessed 29 August 2019].

Consultative Council on Obstetric and Paediatric Mortality and Morbidity (2017). *Congenital anomalies in Victoria: 2007-2009. Melbourne, Victorian State Government.* Retrieved from https://www2.health.vic.gov.au/about/publications/researchandreports/congenital-anomalies-2007-09. Accessed 29 August 2019.

Crossley, K. J., Allison, B. J., Polglase, G. R., Morley, C. J., Davis, P. G., & Hooper, S. B. (2009). Dynamic changes in the direction of blood flow through the ductus arteriosus at birth. *The Journal of Physiology, 587*(19), 4695–4704.

Davis, P. G., Tan, A., O'Donnell, C. P. F., & Schulze, A. (2004). Resuscitation of newborn infants with 100% oxygen or air: a systematic review and meta-analysis. *The Lancet, 364*(9442), 1329–1333.

Dawson, J., Kamlin, C., Vento, M., Wong, C., Cole, T. J., Donath, S. M., & Morley, C. J. (2010a). Defining the reference range for oxygen saturation for infants after birth. *Pediatrics, 125*(6), e1340–e1347. doi:10.1542/peds.2009–1510.

Dawson, J., Kamlin, C., Wong, C., te Pas, A., Vento, M., Cole, T., Donath, S. M., Hooper, S. B., Davis, P. G., & Morley, C. J. (2010b). Changes in heart rate in the first minutes after birth. *Archives of Disease in Childhood. Fetal and Neonatal Edition*, *95*(3), F177–F181. doi:10.1136/adc.2009.169102.

Doyle, L. W., Crowther, C. A., & Middleton, P. (2009). Antenatal magnesium sulphate and neurologic outcome in preterm infants: a systematic review. *Obstetrics and Gynecology*, *113*, 1327–1333.

Doyle, L. W., Roberts, G., & Anderson, P. J., for the Victorian Infant Collaborative Study Group. (2011). Changing long-term outcomes for infants 500–999 g birth weight in Victoria, 1979–2005. *Archives of Disease in Childhood. Fetal and Neonatal Edition*, *96*(6), F443–F447. doi:10.1136/adc.2010.200576.

East, C. E., Colditz, P. B., Begg, L. M., & Brennecke, S. P. (2002). Update on intrapartum fetal pulse oximetry. *The Australian and New Zealand Journal of Obstetrics and Gynaecology*, *42*(1), 23–28. doi:10.1111/j.0004-8666.2002.00023.x.

Gardner, S. L., Enzman-Hines, M., & Nyp, M. (2016). Respiratory diseases. In S. L. Gardner, B. S. Carter, M. Enzman-Hines & J. A. Hernandez (Eds.), *Merenstein and Gardner's handbook of neonatal intensive care* (8th ed., pp. 565–643). St Louis: Mosby.

Haddad, B., Mercer, B. M., Livingston, J. C., Talati, A., & Sibai, B. M. (2000). Outcome after successful resuscitation of babies born with Apgar scores of 0 at both 1 and 5 minutes. *American Journal of Obstetrics and Gynecology*, *182*, 1210–1214.

Jacobs, S. E., & Tarnow-Mordi, W. O. (2010). Therapeutic hypothermia for newborn infants with hypoxic–ischaemic encephalopathy. *Journal of Paediatrics and Child Health*, *46*(10), 568–576. doi:10.1111/j.1440-1754.2010.01880.x.

Kamlin, C. O. F., O'Donnell, C. P. F., Everest, N. J., Davis, P. G., & Morley, C. J. (2006). Accuracy of clinical assessment of infant heart rate in the delivery room. *Resuscitation*, *71*(3), 319–321. doi:10.1016/j.resuscitation.2006.04.015.

Khalil, M., Jux, C., Rueblinger, L., Behrje, J., Esmaeili, A., & Schranz, D. (2019). Acute therapy for newborns with critical congenital heart disease. *Translational Pediatrics*, *8*(2), 114–126.

Kezler, M., & Chatburn, R. L. (2017). Overview of assisted ventilation. In J. P. Goldsmith, E. G. Karotkin, W. Alpert & G. K. Suresh (Eds.), *Assisted ventilation of the neonate* (6th ed., pp. 140–152). Philadelphia: Elsevier.

Kliegman, R. M., Stanton, B. F., Schor, N. F., St. Geme, J. W., III, & Behrman, R. E. (2011). *Nelson textbook of pediatrics* (19th ed.). Philadelphia: Saunders.

Lantos, J. D., Miles, S. H., Silverstein, M. D., & Stocking, C. B. (1988). Survival after cardiopulmonary resuscitation in babies of very low birth weight. Is CPR futile therapy? *The New England Journal of Medicine*, *318*, 91–95.

Levene, M. I. (2010). Cool treatment for birth asphyxia, but what's next? *Archives of Disease in Childhood. Fetal and Neonatal Edition*, *95*(3), F154–F157. doi:10.1136/adc.2009.165738.

Lokesh, L., Kumar, P., Murki, S., & Narang, A. (2004). A randomized controlled trial of sodium bicarbonate in neonatal resuscitation—effect on immediate outcome. *Resuscitation*, *60*(2), 219–223. doi:10.1016/j.resuscitation.2003.10.004.

Mariani, G., Dik, P. B., Ezquer, A., Aguirre, A., Esteban, M. L., Perez, C., & Fustiñana, C. (2007). Pre-ductal and post-ductal O2 saturation in healthy term neonates after birth. *The Journal of Pediatrics*, *150*(4), 418–421. doi:10.1016/j.jpeds.2006.12.015.

Marlow, N., Bennett, C., Draper, E., Hennessy, E., Morgan, A., & Costeloe, K. (2014). Perinatal outcomes for extremely preterm babies in relation to place of birth in England: the EPICure 2 study. *Archives of Disease in Childhood. Fetal and Neonatal Edition*, *99*(3), F181–F188.

Rozance, P. J., Mcgowan, J. E., Price-Douglas, W., & Hay, W. W. (2016). Glucose homeostasis. In S. L. Gardner, B. S. Carter, M. Enzman-Hines & J. A. Hernandez (Eds.), *Merenstein and Gardner's handbook of neonatal intensive care* (8th ed., pp. 337–359). St Louis: Mosby.

Merrill, J. D., & Ballard, R. A. (2005). Care of the high-risk infant. In G. B. Avery (Ed.), *Avery's diseases of the newborn*. Philadelphia: Saunders.

Murki, S., Kumar, P., Lingappa, L., & Narang, A. (2004). Effect of a single dose of sodium bicarbonate given during neonatal resuscitation at birth on the acid–base status on first day of life. *Journal of Perinatology*, *24*(11), 696–699.

Niermeyer, S., Clarke, S. B., & Hernandez, J. A. (2016). Delivery room care. In S. L. Gardner, B. S. Carter, M. Enzman-Hines & J. A. Hernandez (Eds.), *Merenstein and Gardner's handbook of neonatal intensive care* (8th ed., pp. 47–70). St Louis: Mosby.

O'Donnell, C. P. F., Kamlin, C. O. F., Davis, P. G., Carlin, J. B., & Morley, C. J. (2007). Clinical assessment of infant colour at delivery. *Archives of Disease in Childhood. Fetal and Neonatal Edition*, *92*(6), F465–F467. doi:10.1136/adc.2007.120634.

Pairman, S., Pincombe, J., Thorogood, C., & Tracy, S. (Eds.), (2014). *Midwifery preparation for practice* (3rd ed.). Sydney: Elsevier.

Perlman, J. M., Wyllie, J., Kattwinkel, J., Atkins, D. L., Chameides, L., & Goldsmith, J. P., on behalf of the Neonatal Resuscitation Chapter Collaborators. (2010). Special report: neonatal resuscitation. 2010 international consensus on cardiopulmonary resuscitation and emergency cardiovascular care science with treatment recommendations. *Pediatrics*, *126*(5), e1319–e1344. doi:10.1542/peds.2010-2972B.

Safer Care Victoria: Maternity and Newborn Clinical Network. (2016). *Blood pressure disorders (Online)*. Retrieved from https://www.bettersafercare.vic.gov.au/resources/clinical-guidance/maternity-and-newborn-clinical

-network/blood-pressure-disorders. Accessed 29 August 2019.

Safer Care Victoria: Maternity and Newborn Clinical Network. (2018a). *Meconium aspiration syndrome (Online).* https://www.bettersafercare.vic.gov.au/resources/clinical-guidance/maternity-and-newborn-clinical-network/meconium-aspiration-syndrome. Accessed 29 August 2019.

Safer Care Victoria: Maternity and Newborn Clinical Network. (2018b). *Intraosseous needle insertion for neonates (Online).* https://www.bettersafercare.vic.gov.au/resources/clinical-guidance/maternity-and-newborn-clinical-network/intraosseus-needle-insertion-for-neonates. Accessed 29 August 2019.

Safer Care Victoria: Maternity and Newborn Clinical Network. (2018c). *Umbilical vein catheterisation (Online).* https://www.bettersafercare.vic.gov.au/resources/clinical-guidance/maternity-and-newborn-clinical-network/umbilical-vein-catheterisation-for-neonates. Accessed 29 August 2019.

Safer Care Victoria: Maternity and Newborn Clinical Network. (2018d). *Encephalopathy in newborns. (Online).* https://www.bettersafercare.vic.gov.au/resources/clinical-guidance/maternity-and-newborn-clinica l-network/encephalopathy-in-neonates. Accessed 30 August 2019.

Salhab, W. A., Wyckoff, M. H., Laptook, A. R., & Perlman, J. M. (2004). Initial hypoglycemia and neonatal brain injury in term infants with severe fetal acidemia. *Pediatrics, 114*(2), 361–366.

Sharp, M., French, N., McMichael, J., & Campbell, C. (2018). Survival and neurodevelopmental outcomes in extremely preterm infants: 22-24 weeks of gestation born in Western Australia. *Journal of Paediatrics and Child Health, 54,* 194–199.

Siew, M. L., te Pas, A. B., Wallace, M. J., Kitchen, M. J., Lewis, R. A., Fouras, A., Morley, C. J., Davis, P. G., Yagi, N., Uesugi, K., & Hooper, S. B. (2009). Positive

end-expiratory pressure enhances development of a functional residual capacity in preterm rabbits ventilated from birth. *Journal of Applied Physiology, 106*(5), 1487–1493. doi:10.1152/japplphysiol.91591.2008.

Snell, R. S., & Smith, M. S. (Eds.), (1993). *Clinical anatomy for emergency medicine.* St Louis: Mosby.

Stewart, M. J., Smith, J., & Boland, R. A. (2017). Optimizing outcomes in regionalized perinatal care: integrating maternal and neonatal emergency referral, triage and transport. *Current Treatment Options in Pediatrics, 3*(4), 313–326.

Van Woerkom, R., Beharry, K. D., Modanlou, H. D., Parker, J., Rajan, V., Akmal, Y., & Aranda, J. V. (2004). Influence of morphine and naloxone on endothelin and its receptors in newborn piglet brain vascular endothelial cells: clinical implications in neonatal care. *Pediatric Research, 55,* 147–151.

Vento, M., Asensi, M., Sastre, J., García-Sala, F., Pallardó, F. V., & Viña, J. (2001). Resuscitation with room air instead of 100% oxygen prevents oxidative stress in moderately asphyxiated term neonates. *Pediatrics, 107*(4), 642–647.

Vento, M., Asensi, M., Sastre, J., Lloret, A., García-Sala, F., & Minana, J. (2002). Hyperoxemia caused by resuscitation with pure oxygen may alter intracellular redox status by increasing oxidized glutathione in asphyxiated newly born infants. *Seminars in Perinatology, 26*(6), 406–410.

Weisz, D. E., & McNamara, P. J. (2017). Cardiovascular assessment. In J. P. Goldsmith, E. G. Karotkin, W. Alpert & G. K. Suresh (Eds.), *Assisted ventilation of the neonate* (6th ed., pp. 124–139). Philadelphia: Elsevier.

Wood, F. E., Morley, C. J., Dawson, J. A., Kamlin, C. O. F., Owen, L. S., Donath, S., & Davis, P. G. (2008). Improved techniques reduce face mask leak during simulated neonatal resuscitation: study 2. *Archives of Disease in Childhood. Fetal and Neonatal Edition, 93*(3), F230–F234. doi:10.1136/adc.2007.117788.

CHAPTER 56

Paediatric Patients

By John Craven

OVERVIEW

- Paediatric patients can be challenging for paramedics as they may respond to illness and injury differently to adults.
- Parents and carers need to be engaged in the assessment and treatment of children as they can reference what is normal for the child and provide emotional support.
- Respiratory distress is one of the most common acute paediatric issues and respiratory failure is a leading cause of cardiac arrest in children.

Introduction

Paediatric patients represent a challenge to paramedics. Research suggests that cases involving children evoke anxiety and discomfort, and lack of confidence leads to a reluctance to initiate timely and appropriate treatment, possibly contributing to patient morbidity and mortality (Fowler et al., 2017). Training is often sparse and paramedics often feel underprepared and stressed. This is exacerbated by the fact that paediatric interactions are relatively infrequent, making up an estimated 4–8% of call outs (Miller et al., 2014).

Although only a small proportion of paediatric cases require emergency intervention due to a life-threatening condition (Drayna et al., 2015), children still present unique challenges as they are anatomically, physiologically and developmentally different to adults. They suffer from a range of conditions that are either not found in adults or present in different ways. The infrequency of interaction may impede the development of familiarity with both conditions and children themselves.

One of the common fallacies with children is that they sicken and die quickly. The reality is that children have a more responsive and compensative physiology than older people, in particular a dynamic cardiovascular system, and can compensate from disease insult more effectively. Accordingly, children will often not overtly appear unwell until the later stages of a critical illness, or they may display more subtle signs than adults. What is notable is that once a child's ability to compensate is overcome, they may rapidly deteriorate to deleterious result, hence the emphasis in paediatrics on the early detection of severe illness.

The ability to recognise that a child is seriously unwell is a key skill in the field of acute paediatrics; one of the major tasks of clinicians dealing with children is to identify the 'sick child' from a large undifferentiated group of children who may be potentially sick. Many children who have suffered poor outcomes in the healthcare system have long periods where the severity of their condition has not been recognised or has been significantly underestimated. Observation charts with normal reference ranges are now in common use and have been successful in aiding healthcare practitioners (see Fig 56.1).

When approaching all children, a rapid assessment can help differentiate the critically unwell child who needs immediate resuscitation and/or treatment from the less unwell child who can be assessed using the patient-centred interview. In addition to identifying potential diagnoses, the severity of illness should be assessed. Differentiating illness severity using terms such as 'mild', 'moderate', 'severe' and 'life-threatening' is a more sophisticated form of clinical assessment: an evaluation of the risk, clinical needs and extent of required intervention is made in addition to disease diagnosis. This aids treatment of the condition and aids communication of clinical urgency to other treating clinicians. There is a significant difference between the management of mild asthma and life-threatening asthma, for example.

While there are numerous diseases that may cause a child to become critically unwell, all fulminant pathological processes if untreated eventually result in either respiratory failure or circulatory collapse, which will progress to cardiac arrest (see Fig 56.2). Respiratory failure is generally due to obstruction of the respiratory system or failure of respiratory drive. Respiratory obstruction can occur in the upper or lower airways at the level of alveolar gas exchange. Shock, or circulatory collapse, is due to failure of the cardiac pump or intravascular depletion, either through fluid volume loss or maldistribution of fluid outside the central circulation.

SAAS MEDSTAR KIDS RDR CHARTS

Age		<3mths	3mths-1yr	1-4yrs	5-11yrs	12+yrs
Respiratory rate	≥80					
	65–79					
	60–64					
	55–59					
	50–54					
	45–49					
	40–44					
	35–39					
	30–34					
	25–29					
	20–24					
	17–19					
	15–16					
	12–14					
	10–11					
	8–9					
	≤7					
Resp distress	Severe					
	Moderate					
	Mild					
	Nil					
SaO$_2$	≥95%					
	92–94					
	90–91					
	≤89					
O$_2$ required	≥6L/min					
	2–6L/min					
	≤2L/min					
Heart rate	≥180					
	170s					
	160s					
	150s					
	140s					
	130s					
	120s					
	110s					
	100s					
	90s					
	80s					
	70s					
	60s					
	50s					
	40s					
	≤39					
Systolic BP	≥170s					
	160s					
	150s					
	140s					
	130s					
	120s					
	110s					
	100s					
	90s					
	80s					
	70s					
	60s					
	50s					
	≤49					
Central cap refill	>2sec					
	≤2sec					
Temperature	≥38.6°C					
	38.1–38.5					
	35.6–38					
	35.1–35.5					
	≤35					
Consciousness (AVPU)	P.U					
	V<10secs					
	awake					
	A. V					
Weight estimation		Age(mths)/2 + 4	Age(mths)/2 + 4	2 × Age(yrs) + 8	3 × Age(yrs) + 7	3 × Age(yrs) + 7
ETT size		3–3.5	3.5–4	Age/4 + 4	Age/4 + 4	Age/4 + 4
ETT depth (oral)		~10cm	10–12cm	Age/2 + 12	Age/2 + 12	~18cm
Gastric tube size (tr)		5–8	8	8–10	10	12

Figure 56.1
Early warning observation chart from SAAS MedSTAR.

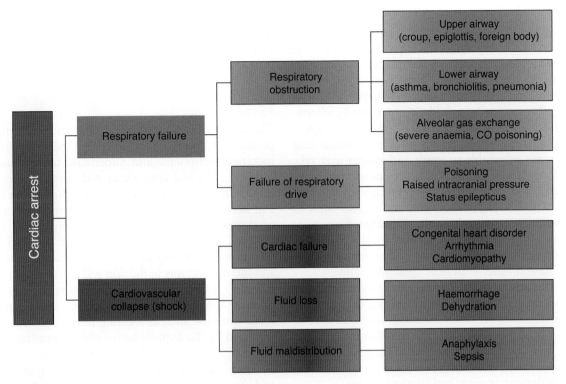

Figure 56.2
Progression of serious illness.

Identifying these underlying pathophysiological processes allows paramedics to treat severe illness urgently, effectively and somewhat empirically without necessarily identifying the specific underlying cause, which may take time and further diagnostic tests to ascertain.

Important differences in children

Children represent a diverse group of patients. In addition to having a unique range of diseases, they vary enormously in size, shape, weight, emotional response, intelligence and ability to socially interact. Knowledge of anatomical and physiological differences is required across this range to allow paramedics to competently manage a seriously ill or injured child.

Weight

The most rapid change in weight occurs in the first year of life. Term newborn babies have an average weight of 3.5 kg which increases to 10–12 kg by 1 year of age. Weight then increases by approximately 2 kg per year until the pubertal growth spurt begins at 10–12 years of age. As most medications and IV fluids are dosed per kilogram of body weight, it is important to establish a child's weight as soon as possible. A parent or carer will often be aware of a recent weight, especially with infants. As a guide, most medication dosing is calculated using 40 kg as a base for maximal adult dosing. This can often be used as a quick method of double-checking drug doses to prevent errors of overdosing.

Airway

The size, shape and proportions of the body change with growth. A number of these are clinically important in managing an acutely ill child.

The airway is influenced by the shape of the mouth and neck. In a baby, the head is proportionally large, the neck short and the shoulders thin, which influences a more flexed neck position when lying supine, resulting in airway narrowing. The tongue is relatively large, the floor of the mouth easily compressible and the larynx more acutely angled, all of which may impede the view during laryngoscopy. Infants are primarily nasal breathers up to approximately 6 months of age, and while a child below this age can breathe through their mouth when there is nasal obstruction, they do so only under duress and with increased effort.

Breathing

At birth, the lungs are developmentally immature. Over the first 2 years of life, there is a significant growth and development of the small airways and expansion of the surface area available for oxygen exchange. The result of this is that small children have less respiratory reserve and an increased likelihood of developing severe respiratory illness. The smaller size of the upper and lower airways increases the chance of airway obstruction from mucus production and airway inflammation, partly explaining the propensity of children in developing wheeze, stridor or respiratory distress in conditions such as croup, bronchiolitis and asthma. The immature lung is more vulnerable to insult and infants may take a long time to recover from periods of respiratory support or even simple chest infections.

The compliant chest wall and weaker muscles mean that infants rely on the diaphragm for respiratory effort, and in trauma this means that force may be transmitted easily to deeper organs such as heart and lungs with little chest wall damage.

Infants have a relatively greater metabolic rate and oxygen consumption; however, tidal volume remains proportionally constant across all ages at 5–7 mL/kg to adulthood. The combination of higher oxygen consumption with small lung volumes and limited respiratory reserve means that small children will desaturate more rapidly than adults.

Circulation

A newborn's circulating blood volume is estimated at 80 mL/kg, which is higher than in adults, although the actual volume is tiny. Relatively small blood losses can be critical.

In utero and at birth the ventricles of the heart are roughly equal. By 6 months of age, the altered pressures of the systemic and pulmonary circulations have caused the left ventricle to dynamically hypertrophy and become dominant. The rise in systemic vascular resistance from low levels as a newborn is reflected in the changing normal values of blood pressure until maturity.

Despite the small stroke volume of the newborn heart (approx. 1.5 mL/kg), the cardiac index is at the highest point of any stage of life. However, the relatively fixed stroke volume means that cardiac output is mostly related to heart rate. The infant vascular system is also more dynamic and the peripheral vascular system can quickly constrict to divert blood flow into the central circulation, resulting in improved circulation and reduced heat loss. This clinically appears as mottling of the skin and cool peripheries.

Infants have very high body surface area to weight ratios, which decrease as they grow. As such, they are prone to rapid heat loss and struggle to regulate their body temperature. Hypothermia is a significant issue if infants are stripped and exposed, such as in a resuscitation situation.

Fever

The human body actively regulates its own temperature. Cooling is achieved by perspiration, increased peripheral and superficial blood flow (causing a flushed appearance and warming thermoreceptors in the skin to give a sensation of 'hot'), and behavioural changes such as to remove layers of clothing. An increase in body temperature is achieved through vasoconstriction of superficial blood vessels (causing a pale or mottled appearance and thermoreceptors in the skin will give a sensation of 'cold'), piloerection of hair, shivering or rigors to create heat through muscle activity, and behavioural changes, such as wanting to rug up. This is regulated by the hypothalamus which lies adjacent to the pituitary in the limbic system of the brain.

Fever is a regulated part of the immune response and should be distinguished from heat stroke and malignant hyperthermia, which are unregulated and dangerous conditions. The process of developing a fever begins with white blood cells activating in the face of an infection and releasing endogenous pyrogens, which include cytokines such as interleukin 1 (IL-1), interleukin 6 (IL-6) and tumour necrosis factor (El-Radhi, 2012). These cytokines stimulate the hypothalamus to raise the body temperature set point and set in motion the process by which the body increases temperature. Fever is theorised to aid the immune system by improving blood flow and immune system activity, and inhibiting the activity or replication of many viruses and bacteria. A fever is generally considered when the temperature is greater than 38°C and is believed to not naturally exceed 42°C. Babies (0–3 months old) and immunosuppressed children may become hypothermic in response to infection instead of developing a fever. In these situations a temperature of less than 36°C is considered a sign of potential sepsis.

'Fever phobia' is a term coined during research in the 1980s when it was identified that health professionals and lay people had unreasonable fears that fever was an illness or could damage a person (Schmitt, 1980). While fever makes a child uncomfortable and the underlying cytokine release is associated with febrile convulsions, there are few other ill effects. Trying to cool a febrile child externally will cause them significant discomfort and is likely to induce shivering and rigors as the body attempts to maintain warmth. Medications

> ## PRACTICE TIP
>
> For a rapid cardiovascular assessment:
> - heart rate
> - pulse volume
> - central capillary refill time
> - blood pressure

with antipyretic actions, such as paracetamol and ibuprofen, are more successful and act directly upon cytokine production and will generally reduce a fever by approximately 1°C. However, the question needs to be asked as to why there is a need to bring down a fever. If temperature is regulated by the body with fever an active part of the immune response and there is little consequence of fever, it would seem counterproductive to the activity of the immune system to attempt this, other than to bring comfort to a patient. Thus, current recommendations are to not externally cool children with tepid baths or sponging, to keep them dressed comfortably and to use ibuprofen and paracetamol for their analgesic effect rather than as antipyretics (Chiappini et al., 2009).

Dehydration

Evaluation of dehydration (or hydration status) is a key element of paediatric assessment. Severe dehydration is far less common in developed countries such as New Zealand and Australia but does occur and can lead to death if unrecognised or untreated. Children can become rapidly dehydrated through acute vomiting or diarrhoeal disease or more insidiously with conditions such as diabetic ketoacidosis, and hydration status is an important clinical assessment in respiratory illnesses, such as bronchiolitis, where respiratory distress compromises the ability to feed or drink. A head-down examination for signs of dehydration is the best approach (see Box 56.1), starting with the anterior fontanelle, which should be palpable in most children up to 12 months of age. While decreased urine output is a good marker of dehydration when accurately measured, it is extremely hard to estimate in an acute setting as it progressively occurs from an early stage due to release of antidiuretic hormone (ADH). A clinical judgment of the severity of dehydration should be made which correlates roughly with a concept of the amount of body water that has been lost as a percentage of the total body weight, with mild dehydration being 1–2%, moderate being 5% and severe 10% or greater (see Fig 56.3). This allows for a rough estimate of fluid replacement that needs to occur. Rehydration may occur with oral fluids, via nasogastric route or intravenous (IV) (including intraosseous [IO]) route. Isotonic fluids (such as normal [0.9%] saline) should always be used for IV rehydration (Santillanes & Rose, 2018).

Cognition, behaviour and development

Children vary enormously in their development, which dictates their degree of responsiveness, interaction with strangers, intellectual ability and

---

BOX 56.1 Systematic dehydration assessment

- Anterior fontanelle (if present)
- Mental state
- Eyes
  - › Sunken
  - › Tears
- Mouth
  - › Dry cracked lips
  - › Dry mouth/decreased salivation
- Pulse and respiratory rate
- Blood pressure
- Skin turgor

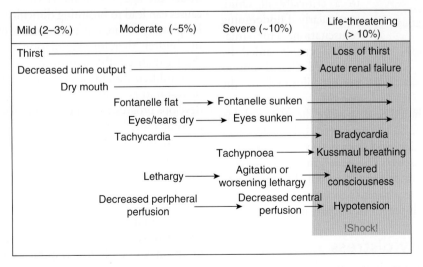

Figure 56.3
Severity of dehydration, with clinical signs.

emotional response. The assessment of children in an acute setting can be challenging but success is rewarding. The challenge is to modify the clinical approach appropriately for each child's development and emotional needs. No single technique is universally effective, and the experienced clinician employs a multitude of different approaches depending on the age and responses of the child. In general, an unrushed and gentle manner will be effective, particularly when parents are engaged and distraction techniques employed. Despite best efforts, however, some children will always remain difficult. With critically unwell children, a slow approach may need to be sacrificed to timely intervention.

The degree of activity and interaction of a child varies enormously with age, particularly in the first few years of life. The normal behaviour of an infant mostly consists of sleeping, waking, crying to feed, feeding and then sleeping again. Disruption or variation in this process may be the initial indicator of significant illness, as is a child who is not attentive and interested in their environment.

Parents and carers

Health professionals often misguidedly complain about how parents and carers complicate the paediatric interaction. In fact, they are the greatest ally in approaching a child. Parents and carers need to be engaged in the assessment and treatment process, and generally should be encouraged to remain by the child to provide emotional, and sometimes physical, support. Parents should always be allowed the opportunity to remain by the bedside of or next to a critically ill child, particularly if undergoing resuscitation. This situation is greatly aided by having a dedicated support person allocated to the parents.

Provision should be allowed for the effect a child's illness may have on parents or carers. They are often affected by anxiety and sleep deprivation, and may be unwell themselves. The term 'just a virus' is rarely appreciated by a concerned parent. Dismissing or failing to address a parent's concerns will adversely affect the development of rapport and trust.

PRACTICE TIP

Unwell children are often described as being 'flat'. This can be more objectively broken down into:
- level of alertness
- degree of spontaneous activity
- resting muscle tone/floppiness.

Respiratory distress

Respiratory distress is one of the most common acute paediatric issues, particularly among children

---

BOX 56.2 Causes of breathing difficulty in children

Upper airway obstruction	Croup
	Epiglottitis
	Foreign body
Lower airway obstruction	Asthma
	Bronchiolitis
	Foreign body
	Inhalational injury
	Pneumonia
	Pulmonary oedema
Disorders outside the lungs	Pleural effusion
	Empyema
	Rib fractures/flail chest
Abdominal causes	Peritonitis
	Abdominal distension/masses
Dysfunction of respiratory muscles	Neuromuscular diseases
Decreased respiratory drive	Seizures
	Poisoning
	Raised intracranial pressure
	Loss of consciousness
Increased respiratory drive	Diabetic ketoacidosis
	Anaemia
	Poisoning (causing metabolic acidosis)

---

under the age of 6 years. A variety of underlying causes can lead to breathing difficulty (see Box 56.2). Respiratory failure is a leading cause of cardiac arrest in children therefore ventilation is a vital part of the paediatric CPR algorithm.

Children should be evaluated as to their degree of respiratory distress (see Box 56.3). As a child develops progressively more respiratory distress, they become more lethargic, listless and non-interactive. Even if the diagnosis is unclear, effort should be made to localise the underlying pathological cause to upper respiratory tract, lower respiratory tract or an alternative cause such as cardiovascular, neurological or metabolic disease. Children who have respiratory distress due to a non-respiratory system disease tend to have effortless tachypnoea or an unexpectedly low respiratory rate.

Oxygen is the immediate primary treatment of all respiratory compromise. A mask should be

BOX 56.3 A rapid respiratory assessment

- Effort of breathing
  - › Respiratory rate
  - › Respiratory noises
  - › Recession
  - › Head bobbing/nasal flaring
- Efficacy of breathing
  - › Air entry (chest auscultation)
  - › Pulse oximetry
- Effects of respiratory inadequacy
  - › Heart rate
  - › Skin colour
  - › Mental status

applied to a self-ventilating patient, whereas assisted bag-valve-mask ventilation should be commenced should the child not be breathing or when respiration is inadequate. The delivery of oxygen takes priority until pulse oximetry is available when oxygen delivery can be titrated to achieve saturations of 94–98% in the previously normal child.

Out-of-hospital advanced airway management (endotracheal intubation) in children is difficult and significantly more challenging than in the controlled environment of the hospital resuscitation room. Paramedics will not be exposed to many paediatric cases requiring intubation, making lack of practice a further complicating factor. Regardless of cause, children rarely need intubation and the risk of exacerbating the child's condition must be balanced against clinical need for an endotracheal tube in the out-of-hospital environment.

Upper respiratory tract

Croup, or viral laryngotracheobronchitis, is by far the most common cause of acute upper respiratory tract obstruction in young children. However, there are many other causes that need to be considered such as inhaled foreign body, epiglottitis or bacterial tracheitis. The assessment and management of paediatric patients with upper respiratory tract conditions is discussed in Section 9.

Lower respiratory tract

Lower respiratory tract disease is also very common in children. In children under the age of 2 years, bronchiolitis predominates. Over the age of 2, asthma and viral chest infections are extremely common. Less common are other causes such as pneumonia, pneumothorax, pleural effusion and pulmonary embolus.

Bronchiolitis

Bronchiolitis is a viral lower respiratory tract infection that occurs in children under 2 years of age. Most cases are due to infection with either respiratory syncytial virus (RSV) or parainfluenza or human metapneumovirus (HMPV).

Significant development of the lungs occurs from the first inhalation at birth and continues for a number of years. During the first 2 years of life, there is rapid growth of alveoli (alveolarisation), development of microvasculature and proliferation of ciliated epithelial cells in the terminal airways, or bronchioles (Burri, 2006; Lewin & Hurtt, 2017). This last is important in bronchiolitis as it is the site of viral infection. Older children and adults regularly suffer chest infections caused by the same viruses but do not suffer the same severity of illness, apparently due to greater functional maturity of the lung.

Bronchiolitis tends to run a predictable course, with the child developing progressively worsening respiratory distress, cough and wheeze, which usually peaks on the fourth or fifth night from onset of symptoms (or third night from onset of wheeze). From this point the child usually slowly and progressively recovers with improving respiratory distress, but often with worsening and moistening of the cough as ciliated epithelial cells recover and begin to move debris and mucus from the lower airways.

Bronchiolitis is clinically characterised by initially dry 'wheezy' cough, symmetrical signs of respiratory distress, generalised wheeze and crackles on auscultation of the chest with progressive decrease in air entry with increasing severity.

Management is supportive: effective treatments have proven elusive (Ricci et al., 2015). Oxygen is applied to keep O_2 saturations > 94% and hydration is maintained through either IV or nasogastric route. Poor feeding, due to inability to suck and breathe at the same time, is usually a good marker of moderate to severe bronchiolitis and a sign that supplemental oxygen and fluids may be needed. Children at high risk of more severe disease include those with chronic lung disease, prematurity or age under 6 weeks.

Asthma

Asthma is a hyperreactive inflammatory response causing airway obstruction, which leads to respiratory distress, cough and wheeze. In children under 2 years of age, a viral exacerbation of asthma can be difficult to differentiate from bronchiolitis, as both demonstrate symptoms of inflammation of the lungs. The underlying process that causes asthma only occurs as the lung matures: it is common over 2 years of age, uncommon between 1 and 2 years of age and extraordinarily rare under 12 months.

The assessment and management of patients with asthma is discussed in Chapter 17.

Pneumonia

Pneumonia is defined as an infection of the lung parenchyma with alveolar infiltration leading to consolidation, which is where the spongy air-filled spaces of the lung becomes solid with mucus and inflammatory cells (Mackenzie, 2016). Pneumonia can be due to either bacterial or viral infection, and traditionally the most common bacterial organism isolated was *Streptococcus pneumoniae*, although this has become less common following development of a specific vaccine and mass vaccination of the early 2000s. Bacterial pneumonia will generally present with high fevers, breathlessness and a 'toxic'-looking child: listless, lethargic and flushed. The classic clinical signs of dull percussion, bronchial breath sounds and cough usually take several days to develop.

By contrast, viral pneumonia, and that caused by *Mycoplasma pneumoniae*, tend to present as a severe form of viral chest infection, with breathlessness, cough and generalised chest signs of wheeze and crackles.

Oxygen is the immediate primary treatment for respiratory compromise and should be delivered to keep SaO$_2$ > 92%. Appropriate antibiotics are the treatment for bacterial pneumonia: untreated bacterial pneumonia may disseminate into sepsis. Viral infections are generally self-limiting although in rare severe cases may cause acute respiratory distress syndrome (ARDS) and respiratory arrest.

Cardiovascular impairment and shock

Cardiac causes of cardiovascular impairment are relatively uncommon outside the neonatal period, when most congenital cardiac abnormalities appear. The remainder of children generally have an impairment due to loss of vascular tone (sepsis, anaphylaxis) or loss of intravascular volume (haemorrhage, dehydration).

> ### PRACTICE TIP
> The following features suggest an underlying cardiac abnormality:
> - cyanosis not responding to oxygen therapy
> - unexplained tachycardia
> - gallop rhythm (third heart sound) or murmur
> - enlarged liver
> - absent femoral pulses.

 CASE STUDY 1

Case 13885, 0920 hrs.

Dispatch details: A 16-day-old girl is distressed and has been feeding poorly since last night. She is now looking mottled and unwell.

Initial presentation: The paramedics enter the house and find the mother holding the child in her arms. The baby has a weak cry. The mother is visibly upset and has been crying. A small boy is also in the room.

 ASSESS

Patient history

Small babies can be difficult to assess. Babies primarily sleep, wake, feed, cry and fill their nappies. Uncovering symptoms specific to an illness can be difficult; however, some clues may be elicited by looking for changes in a baby's basic behaviour and appearance.

The baby's mother tells you that her daughter was born at term via normal vaginal delivery and had no postnatal problems. She went home on day 2 and was breastfeeding well until the previous day when she became fussy and was less interested in her evening breastfeed. She did not wake for a feed overnight and when her mother tried to feed her this morning, she just cried irritably.

She has been crying intermittently since and refuses to settle. She is breathing faster than usual and looks pale.

Initial assessment summary

Problem	Generally unwell
Conscious state	Alert
Position	In mother's arms
Heart rate	180 bpm, regular
Blood pressure	85/40 mmHg (right arm)
Skin appearance	Cool, mottled
Speech pattern	Short, irritable cry
Respiratory rate	63 bpm, shallow panting breaths
Respiratory rhythm	Panting breaths
Chest auscultation	Bilateral air entry; no crackles or wheeze
Temperature	35.8°C
Pulse oximetry	Unable to obtain trace
History	Poor feeding, irritable cry, respiratory distress

D: There are no dangers.
A: The airway is patent. No stridor.
B: There is increased respiratory rate with mild effort.
C: Heart rate is 180 bpm. Colour is mottled. Capillary refill time is 3 seconds.

2 CONFIRM

The essential part of the clinical reasoning process is to seek to confirm your initial hypothesis by finding clinical signs that should occur with your provisional diagnosis. You should also seek to challenge your diagnosis by exploring findings that do not fit your hypothesis: don't just ignore them because they don't fit.

This case demonstrates the difficulty of assessing a small baby. The most important assessment question—'Is this child sick?'—needs to be answered. Once this has occurred, a list of possible differentials should be composed. In the out-of-hospital setting, it is often better to target bodily systems initially rather than specific diagnoses; many diagnoses will require diagnostic testing that occurs in a hospital setting but treatment may need to be empirically initiated in the meantime. Seeking out specific symptoms and signs may help refute potential diagnosis or make them more likely.

What could it be?
Infective cause
The 'big four' serious bacterial infections in the neonatal period are pneumonia, sepsis, meningitis and urinary tract infection. Causative organisms are mostly the organisms that newborns are becoming colonised with as a part of normal life: *E. coli*, *Staphylococcus* and *Streptococcus* (especially group B). It can be difficult in the out-of-hospital setting to clinically differentiate these infections in a baby. This baby has signs of irritability, poor feeding, respiratory and cardiovascular distress, and a low temperature, all of which fit the criteria for potential serious bacterial infection. Further assessment for infection (urine screen, chest x-ray, blood count and culture, and lumbar puncture) needs to occur, with empirical treatment with IV antibiotics until infection is confirmed or excluded (usually at 48 hours).

Cardiac cause
Congenital cardiac defects occur in approximately 1% of newborns. Some of the more serious defects rely on a patent ductus arteriosus (PDA) to maintain adequate oxygenated blood flow around the body and are known as

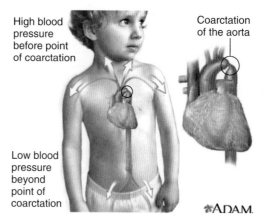

High blood
pressure
before point
of coarctation

Coarctation
of the aorta

Low blood
pressure
beyond
point of
coarctation

✷ADAM.

Figure 56.4
Coarctation of the aorta.

'duct-dependent circulations'. While most of these serious defects are detected with antenatal ultrasound, some of them, particularly coarctation of the aorta, can be difficult to diagnose. A child with a coarctation of the aorta relies on blood flow from the pulmonary arteries through the PDA to supply the left arm and lower body with blood (see Fig 56.4). In these situations, the PDA usually closes within the first month of life (rather than within the first few days) and the subsequent poor perfusion of oxygenated blood to the lower body leads to metabolic acidosis and progressive organ failure. Children appear 'toxic' in a similar way to children with sepsis, and it can be hard to differentiate initially. The absence of palpable femoral pulses is a diagnostic sign. Treatment is IV prostaglandin to reopen the ductus arteriosus and careful IV fluids to maintain good perfusion (Park, 2014).

Arrythmias are generally rare in the neonatal period but persistent supraventricular tachycardias (SVT) may occur. The newborn heart initially tolerates the increased cardiac work well, with heart rates 250–300 bpm, but over days to weeks the child progressively develops cardiac failure. As cardiac failure develops, poor feeding, breathlessness and poor perfusion occur.

Other rare causes of cardiac failure in this age group would be infective myocarditis or congenital cardiomyopathy.

Metabolic cause

Congenital adrenal hyperplasia is an uncommon condition where steroidogenesis cannot occur properly in the adrenals due to an absence of mediating enzymes. The resulting excess or deficit in mineralocorticoid, glucocorticoid and sex hormones results in a group of clinical conditions. Most commonly females develop virilisation of primary or secondary sex characteristics. Salt wasting due to absence of mineralocorticoids is also a common problem. In a male child (in whom virilisation is not apparent) and salt-wasting crisis may be the initial presentation, with shock due to profound hyponatraemia and the subsequent dehydration and vomiting. Treatment is acute rehydration, normalisation of electrolytes and replacement of hormones (Trapp et al., 2011).

Inflicted injury (NAI)

Inflicted injury, or non-accidental injury (NAI), should be considered in all cases where the diagnosis is unclear. See below for further information. Significant abdominal or chest injuries may present with an irritable child with poor feeding and potentially respiratory or circulatory compromise.

While loading the child for transport, the paramedic checks, but is unable to feel femoral pulses, making the likely diagnosis a congenital cardiac defect with a duct-dependent circulation.

③ TREAT

The patient is indeed unwell and should be transported to hospital. The child is self-ventilating and has adequate perfusion. The decision to transport the child without delay is a good one in this situation, as most of the necessary diagnostics and treatments are not accessible in the out-of-hospital setting.

A blood sugar level should be checked in all unwell children—the younger the child, the more important it becomes. Until it is demonstrated that oxygen is not required, oxygen should be provided at 4–6 L/minute via face mask.

If the child had been in an unstable or compromised condition, IV/IO access should be urgently obtained, IV fluid bolus of normal saline 10–20 mL/kg (or if BSL <2.5, 10% dextrose 2 mL/kg) given and antibiotics commenced. Intubation of the unwell neonate can be difficult, fraught with complications and may worsen the situation, particularly if the child is self-ventilating with no difficulties.

Infective cause

Bacterial infection needs to be treated with IV antibiotics, with the preferred empirical antibiotics in this age group being amoxicillin or cefotaxime with gentamicin. In most paramedic systems this will require urgent transfer to hospital. Shock should be initially treated with IV fluid boluses. Inotropes such as adrenaline and dopamine, or intubation and ventilation, may be required in extreme cases. Once again, the ideal place is the resuscitation room in hospital.

Cardiac cause

IV fluid boluses may be initially required to correct dehydration or perfusion deficiency. The mainstay of treatment is IV prostaglandin (PGE_1) to reopen the ductus arteriosus. A cardiac ultrasound is required to make the diagnosis and direct further treatment.

Supraventricular tachycardia (SVT) in the neonatal period is treated with vagal manoeuvres, medications such as adenosine or electro cardioversion. The treatment choice depends on the degree of compromise of the child. The most common vagal manoeuvre performed in this age group is to place the child or the child's head in a bucket of ice water, stimulating a diving reflex and a significant vagal response.

Metabolic cause

Congenital adrenal hyperplasia is diagnosed by a combination of physical signs and biochemical and hormonal abnormalities. Initial treatment is rehydration and normalisation of electrolytes, particularly sodium and potassium. Hydrocortisone and fludrocortisone are generally the drugs used to replace the absent mineralocorticoids and glucocorticoids.

Inflicted injury (NAI)

If inflicted, or non-accidental, injury cannot be ruled out or no alternative diagnosis found, a skeletal survey x-ray may be performed to find bony injuries. Child protection services should be contacted to assist in examining the child and interviewing the carers.

④ EVALUATE

The response to any management should be assessed and the child should be closely monitored during transport for deterioration.

Further evaluation may include a more complete examination looking for specific signs of disease. This may involve four limb blood pressures, checking for enlarged liver and femoral pulses for cardiac disease; bulging fontanelle or rash for sepsis/meningitis; or unexplained bruising for inflicted injury.

CASE STUDY 2

Case 14588, 1732 hrs.

Dispatch details: A 3-year-old boy is suffering a seizure following recent illness. His mother heard him make strange noises and found him on the lounge room floor. He had jerking movements of his limbs and panting respirations. As he was still breathing, she was advised to place him on his side and monitor his breathing and pulse. His mother was kept on the phone line and the seizure resolved after 7 minutes.

Initial presentation: The paramedics enter the house and find the boy lying on his side on the lounge room floor. There is the smell of vomit in the air. The boy is taking deep breaths but is not otherwise moving. A woman who identifies herself as his mother is kneeling near him.

 ASSESS

1744 hrs Chief complaint: Generalised seizure activity.

1745 hrs Vital signs survey: Airway is clear. There is some vomit around his mouth and on the floor but no audible respiratory noises.

RR: 24 with minimal work of breathing, SpO$_2$ 98%, air entry: L = R, no wheeze or crackles.

Perfusion status: HR 136, BP 98/56 mmHg, skin cool and pale, capillary refill 2 seconds.

Conscious state: GCS = 13 (E2 V2 M4). Eyes open briefly; he cries and localises painful stimulus.

1750 hrs Pertinent hx: The child is previously well and fully vaccinated. He was born term with no neonatal issues. He was unwell the last few days with viral symptoms (cough, runny nose). He was playing in the house while his mother made dinner. He has never suffered a convulsion before.

1801 hrs Assessment: Without fully regaining consciousness, another seizure occurs. His eyes are closed, his back arches and his limbs symmetrically tense and jerk. His breathing becomes shallow and panting, with oxygen saturations dropping to 93%. His mother turns to the paramedics with tears in her eyes. 'Do something!' she cries.

 CONFIRM

The essential part of the clinical reasoning process is to seek to confirm your initial hypothesis by finding clinical signs that should occur with your provisional diagnosis. You should also seek to challenge your diagnosis by exploring findings that do not fit your hypothesis: don't just ignore them because they don't fit.

The complaint of seizure may appear, and may be, a straightforward diagnosis in the case of idiopathic epilepsy. However, an underlying precipitant should always be sought, particularly if there is no previous history of seizures (see Fig 56.5). Posturing, asymmetry of movement, pupillary abnormality or presence of other signs such as fever or rash may give some indication of underlying pathology.

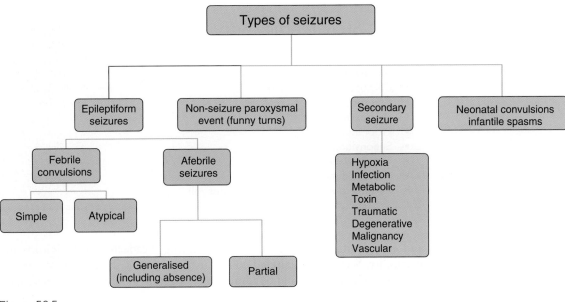

Figure 56.5
Types of seizures.

BOX 56.4 Criteria for simple febrile convulsion

- Presence of fever
- Age 9 months to 5 years
- Generalised tonic/clonic seizure
- Duration < 15 mins
- Post ictal period (usually 10–30 mins)
- Full recovery with no neurological deficits

What else could it be?
Febrile convulsion
Febrile convulsions are relatively common between 9 months and 5 years of age. It is estimated that approximately 4% of children (1 in 25) suffer at least one. Simple febrile convulsions, despite being unpleasant for parents to witness, are generally devoid of ill effects and the clinical impetus is to exclude serious causes of fever, such as sepsis and meningitis (Mastrangelo et al., 2014). Attempting to control fever has not been shown to prevent febrile convulsions (El-Radhi, 2012). It is currently thought that the immune system-mediated interleukin release that precipitates the febrile response is more likely to be causative in provoking febrile convulsions than fever (Pavlidou et al., 2013). In order to diagnose a simple febrile convulsion, a number of criteria need to be met in addition to the presence of a fever (see Box 56.4). If the criteria are not all met, it is called an atypical febrile convulsion, which is associated with a much higher rate of significant underlying disease. From an acute management perspective, simple febrile convulsions are generally of short duration (95% less than 5 minutes) and self-limiting. Children should be placed in a safe position on their side and observed once a blood sugar level is checked. Medication is not recommended unless status epilepticus occurs.

Intracranial infection
Meningitis has become rarer due to vaccination against some of the main causative bacterial agents, *H. influenza* and *S. pneumonia*. Both meningitis

PRACTICE TIP

- Has the midazolam been effective?
- Is the patient's ventilation/oxygenation adequate?
- Are there underlying causes that need to be identified and addressed?
- Has blood sugar been checked?
- Have the pupils been examined?

BOX 56.5 Medications with potential for severe toxicity in small doses

- Amphetamines
- Calcium channel blockers
- Chloroquine
- Hydroxychloroquine
- Propranolol
- Sulfonylureas
- Theophylline
- Tricyclic antidepressants
- Hydrocarbons (solvents, eucalyptus oil)

and encephalitis present with fevers, vomiting, headache, neck rigidity and irritability. Seizures and altered consciousness occur as the disease progresses. Empirical antibiotics should be administered urgently should bacterial meningitis be considered likely.

Intracranial mass
Solid brain tumours, abscesses and intracranial bleeds due to vascular malformation are uncommon but do occur in childhood. Tumours will generally present subtly with gradual onset of symptoms such as weight loss, vomiting and coordination loss but may present catastrophically once intracranial pressure reaches a critical point or if there is bleeding into the necrotic core of the tumour. If raised intracranial pressure is suspected as a cause for seizure or change in consciousness, the child should be nursed at an angle of 35° with their head up. In consultation with neurosurgeons an osmotic solution (mannitol or 3% saline) may be administered, vomiting, cough and seizures suppressed and then a move made to intubate the child safely with moderate hyperventilation (target pCO_2 30–35 mmHg).

Toxins/drugs
Young active children will explore and ingest toxins and medicines accidentally, particularly in the 1–3-year age range, when it is normal behaviour to ingest small objects discovered during exploration or in mimicking of parents. Self-harming is highly unusual pre-adolescence. The majority of medicines and environmental toxins require a significant ingestion to cause harm and most children will generally not ingest more than 2–3 tablets. However, there are a small number of drugs in which this can cause significant deleterious effects, particularly cardiac, antidepressant and anti-diabetic medications (see Box 56.5). An ECG and blood sugar level can aid diagnosis and are considered a mandatory part of poisoning assessment (Daly et al., 2011).

Trauma/inflicted injury
A head injury with significant intracranial injury may present with change of consciousness and/or seizure. This may be either accidental or inflicted; either way the acute impairment needs to be managed as a priority. Skull x-rays are no longer performed acutely as they add little to the clinical management of the patient. A CT of the brain provides more useful information as to intracranial pathology.

DIFFERENTIAL DIAGNOSIS
- Idiopathic seizure
- Febrile convulsion
- Hypoxia
- Head trauma
- Drugs/toxins
- Electrolyte abnormality
- Meningitis/encephalitis
- Hypoglycaemia/metabolic disorder
- Intracranial mass (tumour, abscess or bleed)

3 TREAT
Midazolam via the intramuscular route is effective and quickly absorbed, reaching peak effectiveness at around 10 minutes. It is much easier and faster than trying to obtain IV access in a patient that is actively seizing. IV, IO, intranasal or buccal routes may be used according to local guidelines.

1802 hrs: The child is kept in the lateral position. Oxygen is applied via mask at 10 L/minute. Midazolam is drawn up: a weight of 14 kg estimated (confirmed with his mother) and a dose of 1.4 mg calculated (at 0.1 mg/kg). Midazolam is administered intramuscularly to the left lateral thigh. A portable suction unit is brought near should further vomiting occur. His temperature is 36.7°C.

1805 hrs: He continues to seize. IV access is considered and prepared. A finger prick blood glucose is performed: 0.8 mmol. IV access is obtained without delay and he is administered 28 mL of 10% dextrose (2 mL/kg) without delay. His mother is informed of the result and she says that her mother, who is staying with them, is a diabetic and takes tablets for her sugar. She goes off to look for the tablets.

1810 hrs: He continues to seize. The blood glucose is rechecked and found to be 1.1 mmol. A second bolus of 2 mL/kg 10% dextrose is administered. His mother returns and hands over a box of gliclazide with an empty blister pack. 'There were lots of tablets lying on the floor', she says tearfully. 'Is he going to be okay?'

1812 hrs: A radio message for toxicology advice is placed and the paramedics prepare a third bolus of 10% dextrose. Preparation is made for urgent departure. A further dose of midazolam is considered but as the seizure is due to hypoglycaemia, correcting the blood glucose level is the primary treatment.

1815 hrs: He continues to seize. The blood glucose is rechecked and found to be 1.5 mmol. A third bolus of 2 mL/kg 10% dextrose is administered. The seizure stops. He is rapidly loaded into the ambulance. The toxicology advice is radioed back and advises an ongoing dextrose infusion and a priority transfer to the nearby hospital.

(4) ## EVALUATE

Evaluating the effect of any clinical management intervention should be performed in a timely manner and can provide clues to the accuracy of the initial diagnosis. Some conditions respond rapidly to treatment, so patients should be expected to improve if the diagnosis and treatment were appropriate. A failure to improve in this situation should trigger the clinician to reconsider the diagnosis.

In this case, the underlying cause of the seizures—hypoglycaemia—needs to be identified and addressed. Hypoglycaemia due to sulfonylureas can be profound and prolonged. For glucose replacement, 10% dextrose is used in preference to 50% glucose due to the sclerosing effect high-concentration glucose has on veins, which can rapidly cause them to obstruct. Octreotide is the specific antidote in this situation and should be administered as early as possible.

> **PRACTICE TIP**
> - Has the midazolam been effective?
> - Is the patient's ventilation/oxygenation adequate?
> - Are there underlying causes that need to be identified and addressed?
> - Has blood sugar been checked?
> - Have the pupils been examined?

CASE STUDY 3

Case 15868, 1943 hrs.

Dispatch details: A 10-year-old girl fell in the playground today and hurt her left arm and head. Her mother is concerned that she may have a serious injury. The girl has a background history of cerebral palsy.

Initial presentation: Paramedics have trouble finding the house: it is a dark and wet day in a built-up area. They are let into the house by the girl's mother who appears anxious and ushers them into the lounge, where the girl is sitting in a chair. She appears tall for her age and lean, with thin arms and legs. She has bruising visible on the left side of her face. She appears otherwise undistressed.

 ASSESS

As the girl is not requiring urgent management, a history is taken from her mother. She is an only child and lives with her mother. She has mild to moderate cerebral palsy which mostly affects her strength and coordination, but she is able to walk without aid. She attends the local primary school and is in Year 6.

Her mother says that she was at the playground this afternoon and fell off the monkey bars, which she often does, due to her clumsiness.

The girl is very quiet when approached to examine. Aside from flinching and looking nervous, she holds still. She is wearing a school dress with a light cardigan. She is thin with a fine build and although her long brown hair is pulled back into pony tail, it has come loose. She has several bruises on the left side of her face with some scattered skin tears and looks like she has been crying. Her lip is swollen and is split on the left. She holds out her left arm and circumferential bruising of the forearm is evident. No other abnormalities are found. Her observations are all in the normal range.

 CONFIRM

The essential part of the clinical reasoning process is to seek to confirm your initial hypothesis by finding clinical signs that should occur with your provisional diagnosis. You should also seek to challenge your diagnosis by exploring findings that do not fit your hypothesis: don't just ignore them because they don't fit.

What could it be?
Fracture
Fractures are very common in children: bones are weaker than ligaments and tendons in childhood but become progressively stronger and thicker with age. Thus, a child is more likely to break a bone than sprain or strain a ligament or dislocate a joint, and the force required to do so is much less. On the positive side, bone cells (osteoblasts and osteoclasts) are very active in childhood and most fractures heal very quickly, particularly when compared to an equivalent ligamentous injury.

Visibly deformed or painful limbs should be splinted for analgesia and ease of transport. Pain severity should be assessed and treated appropriately.

> ## BOX 56.6 Potential warning signs of inflicted or neglectful injuries
>
> - Delay in seeking medical attention
> - Story of the accident is vague or varies on retelling
> - Account of the accident is not compatible with the injury observed
> - The injury is not compatible with the child's level of development
> - The parent's affect is abnormal
> - The parent's behaviour gives cause for concern
> - The child's appearance and interaction with the parents is abnormal

Soft tissue injury

Bruises, abrasions and lacerations are common in childhood. More complex injuries, especially deep or complicated lacerations which may require exploration and washout, are less common. All limb injuries should be examined to exclude neurological or vascular impairment. In cases where the mechanism of injury is significant or when pain is out of proportion to the evident injury, underlying deep injuries, particularly of the abdomen, should be suspected. Abdominal injuries can be subtle and often take time to become clinically evident. Repeated examination over time is recommended.

Non-accidental or inflicted injury

Identification of children suffering abuse will not occur unless inflicted or neglectful causes of injuries are considered as part of the diagnostic process. In most cases, injuries can easily be explained on history and by presentation as being accidental or due to misadventure, but there are a number of factors that should alert the clinician to the possibility of an inflicted injury (see Box 56.6).

③ TREAT

The principles of musculoskeletal injury management are covered in Chapter 36, whereas pain management is covered in Chapter 30.

④ EVALUATE

If suspicion of abuse is roused, it is best to assume a non-judgmental attitude, ensure safety of the child and convey those concerns when handing over the patient. Intense interrogation of the parents/carers is unhelpful as it creates a combative environment which makes it more difficult for later investigation.

In this case the paramedics note that the child's bruising is mostly on the left side of the face and the mother had bruising on her right hand. Circumferential bruising of the wrist is not explained by a fall. No allegations were made and the child was taken to the nearby Children's Hospital Emergency Department for assessment. The paramedics quietly passed on their concerns to the emergency department staff. The child was admitted to hospital, and Child Protection Services were notified.

Australia and New Zealand have mandatory reporting of suspected child abuse, which places a legal obligation on certain groups of professions when presented with suspected abuse (Townsend & Luck, 2013). Each jurisdiction has a slightly different listing of mandated notifiers and paramedics should be aware of the legal obligations in their area.

Paramedics should take a pragmatic approach to reporting. As previously mentioned, they should not make accusations or ask direct questions that may arose suspicion in the carers connected with the child. After all, the parents or carers may be innocent and untrue allegations can be harmful to both the child and the parents or carers. Any report made should be factually correct, objective and without judgment. Take into consideration other possible causes of injuries or disease manifestations and focus on describing the situation rather than drawing conclusions. It is vitally important to avoid exaggeration in the hope of ensuring a successful outcome for the child. The report should be written as early as possible to the time when events become apparent.

Sudden unexplained death in infancy (SUDI)

The term 'sudden unexplained death in infancy' (SUDI) is superseding the well-known term 'cot death' or 'SIDS' (sudden infant death syndrome) as an attempt to discriminate cases where a cause of death can be found from those where a cause of death cannot. Public health campaigns in New Zealand and Australia over the last 25 years have dramatically reduced the risk of children dying in infancy. The main messages across both countries were encouraging supine sleep position, reducing exposure to tobacco smoke, encouraging breast feeding and providing a safe sleeping environment for the baby (Mitchell & Blair, 2012; Mitchell et al., 2012).

Unfortunately, unexplained deaths still occur and it is likely that paramedics will be called to attend when the child is discovered. If no CPR is being performed on attendance, and the child has no signs of life, death may be pronounced in accordance with local guidelines. Should CPR be performed, it should be continued until the situation and the condition of the child can be assessed. At this point a decision should be made to either cease CPR and pronounce death, or continue with advanced life support until the child can be transported to an emergency facility where they can be further assessed. It is recommended that parents be present during resuscitation efforts and, if staff numbers permit, have a senior staff member stand with them to provide comfort and explain what is happening. If the parents are interfering with resuscitation efforts, they should be gently escorted back from the scene.

Summary

Children present a challenge in paramedic practice due to unfamiliarity, and the variations in size, development and range of illnesses. Provided that a systematic and sensible approach is adopted, most children can be effectively assessed and treated or stabilised for transfer.

References

Burri, P. H. (2006). Structural aspects of postnatal lung development – alveolar formation and growth. *Neonatology*, *89*(4), 313–322.

Chiappini, E., Principi, P., Longhi, R., Tovo, P.-A., Becherucci, P., Bonsignori, F., Esposito, S., Festini, F., Galli, L., Lucchesi, B., Mugelli, A., de Martino, M., & Writing Committee of the Italian Pediatric Society Panel for the Management of Fever in Children. (2009). Management of fever in children: summary of the Italian pediatric society guidelines. *Clinical Therapeutics*, *31*(8), 1826–1843.

Daly, F., Little, M., Cadogan, M., & Murray, L. (2011). *Toxicology handbook*. Churchill Livingstone.

Drayna, P. C., Browne, L., Guse, C. E., Brousseau, D. C., & Lerner, E. B. (2015). Prehospital pediatric care: opportunities for training, treatment, and research. *Prehospital Emergency Care*, *19*, 441–447.

El-Radhi, A. (2012). Fever management: evidence vs current practice. *World Journal of Clinical Pediatrics*, *1*(4), 29–33.

Fowler, J., Beovich, B., & Williams, B. (2017). Improving paramedic confidence with paediatric patients: a scoping review. *Australasian Journal of Paramedicine*, *15*(1), 1–12.

Lewin, G., & Hurtt, M. E. (2017). Pre- and postnatal lung development: an updated species comparison. *Birth Defects Research*, *109*, 1519–1539.

Mackenzie, G. (2016). The definition and classification of pneumonia. *Pneumonia*, *8*, 14.

Mastrangelo, M., Midulla, F., & Moretti, C. (2014). Actual insights into the clinical management of febrile seizures. *European Journal of Pediatrics*, *173*(8), 977–982.

Miller, R., Eriksson, L., Fleisher, L., Wiener-Kronish, J., Cohen, N., & Young, W. (2014). *Miller's anaesthesia E-book*. Elsevier Health Services.

Mitchell, E. A., & Blair, P. S. (2012). SIDS prevention: 3000 lives saved but we can do better. *The New Zealand Medical Journal, 125*(1359), 50.

Mitchell, E. A., Freemantle, J., Young, J., & Byard, R. W. (2012). Scientific consensus forum to review the evidence underpinning the recommendations of the Australian SIDS and Kids Safe Sleeping Health Promotion Programme. *Journal of Paediatrics and Child Health, 48*(8), 626–633.

Pavlidou, E., Hagel, C., & Panteliadis, C. (2013). Febrile seizures: recent developments and unanswered questions. *Childs Nervous System, 29*(11), 2011–2017.

Ricci, V., Nunes, V. D., Murphy, M. S., & Cunningham, S. (2015). Bronchiolitis in children: summary of NICE guidance. *British Medical Journal, 350*.

Santillanes, G., & Rose, E. (2018). Evaluation and management of dehydration in children. *Emergency Medicine Clinics of North America, 36*(2), 259–273.

Schmitt, B. D. (1980). Fever phobia: misconceptions of parents about fevers. *JAMA Pediatrics, 134*(2), 176–181.

Townsend, R., & Luck, M. (2013). *Applied paramedic Law and ethics Australia and New Zealand*. Sydney: Elsevier.

Trapp, C. M., Speiser, P. W., & Oberfield, S. E. (2011). Congenital adrenal hyperplasia: an update in children. *Current Opinion in Endocrinology, Diabetes, and Obesity, 18*(3), 166–170.

Medications Commonly Encountered in Community Emergency Health

By Boyd Furmston

A lack of time, resources and diagnostic tools characterises the environment in which paramedics are required to operate. In this setting, much of the diagnostic load falls onto collecting and understanding the patient's history. Complexity such as poor cognition, language difficulties, illness and anxiety can limit the patient's ability to portray an accurate and concise narrative. In many cases, objective clues to the patient's past medical history can be used to assist in the clinical reasoning process behind the patients prescribed medications. Medications can be prescribed for a broad range of conditions while others are very specific and their prescription for a patient can identify conditions that the patient may not be able to articulate. Table A1.1 lists cardiac medications that paramedics will commonly encounter and identifies the conditions for which they are usually prescribed. Table A1.2 provides a broader list of common drugs and their primary uses.

Table A1.1 Cardiac medications

	Classification/action	Generic name	Common trade names	Clinical use (indicates diagnosed history)
	Cardiovascular agents/cardiac therapy/antihypertensives			
Vasodilators used to manage ischaemic chest pain	Nitrates	Glyceryl trinitrate	Nitro-Dur 5, 10 and 15; Anginine	History of: • Angina Increasing recent use may indicate shift from angina to ACS.
	Nitrates	Isosorbide mononitrate	Monodur, Imdur	History of: • Angina Longer-acting oral nitrates; indicate advanced CAD and recalcitrant angina. Patients on these drugs usually have a long CAD history.
	Potassium channel activators	Nicorandil	Ikorel	History of: • Angina Longer-acting oral nitrates; indicate advanced CAD and recalcitrant angina. Patients on these drugs usually have a long CAD history. These patients have often been identified as not being suitable for invasive therapies such as CABG and PCI.

Table A1.1 Cardiac medications—cont'd

	Classification/action	Generic name	Common trade names	Clinical use (indicates diagnosed history)
Antiarrhythmics	Class 1c	Flecainide	Flecatab, Tambocor	History of: • Atrial tachycardia • SVT (AF and SVT including WPW) Usually administered after other agents have proved ineffective.
	Class II	Atenolol Metoprolol tartrate Metoprolol succinate Propranolol Carvedilol	Noten Tenormin Tensig Lopresor Toprol XL Inderal Dilatrend	Routinely administered post-AMI. Primarily given during this period as antiarrhythmics, but they also reduce blood pressure. Can be prescribed for SVT. Can produce sense of lethargy/fatigue in weeks after commencing. Can also produce profound bradycardia. Some patients are particularly dose-dependent and may experience arrhythmias, hypertension and chest pain after missing just a single dose. Non-selective, therefore not often prescribed as can cause bronchospasm. Have little antiarrhythmic or antihypertensive effects. Prescribed to manage CCF, so indicate poor LVF.
	Class III	Amiodarone Sotalol	Aratac Cordarone Cardol Sotacor	History of: • Atrial tachycardia • SVT • Ventricular tachycardia Although amiodarone is used primarily as a ventricular antiarrhythmic in emergency medicine, it is effective in the treatment of AF and other SVTs when administered orally. Sotacor is usually administered as treatment for AF rather than hypertension.
	Class IV	Verapamil Diltiazem Amlodipine Nifedipine	Veracaps Isoptin Cardizem Nordip Adalat	History of: • Hypertension Selective calcium channel blockers with mainly vascular effects. Mild overdose can cause profound hypotension and bradycardia. Presence of these drugs usually indicates long-standing hypertension resistant to other treatments.
	Cardiac glycosides	Digoxin	Lanoxin	History of: • AF Used for rate control of AF. Narrow therapeutic range and pro-arrhythmic side effects have seen it replaced by amiodarone.
	Antiadrenergic agents, centrally acting	Methyldopa Clonidine	Hydopa Aldomet Clonidine hydrochloride Catapres	Hydopa may be considered a first-line antihypertensive agent in pregnancy. Clonidine can also be prescribed for dysmenorrhoea, ADHD and drug withdrawal.

continued

1017

Table A1.1 Cardiac medications—cont'd

	Classification/action	Generic name	Common trade names	Clinical use (indicates diagnosed history)
Antihypertensives	Antiadrenergic agents, peripherally acting	Prazosin	Minipress	Primarily an antihypertensive but commonly prescribed for benign prostatic hyperplasia.
	Arteriolar smooth muscle	Hydralazine	Alphapress	Causes a reflex increase in heart rate so rarely administered without other medications and not considered a first-line agent in pregnancy.
	Angiotensin-converting enzyme (ACE) inhibitors	Perindopril Enalapril Captopril Ramipril Lisonopril	Coversyl Renitec Capoten Ramace Zestril	History of: • Hypertension • CCF Effective and popular anti-hypertensives. Will produce profound hypotension (collapse) in small number of patients shortly after starting therapy.
	Angiotensin II receptor antagonists	Candesartan Irbesartan Losartan	Atacand Avapro Karvea Cozavan	History of: • Hypertension • CCF

Lipid-modifying agents

	Bile acid sequestrants	Cholestyramine Colestipol	Questran Lite Colestid	History of: • Hyperlipidaemia despite dietary modification Administered routinely post-AMI.
	HMG-CoA reductase inhibitors (statins)	Simvastatin Pravastatin Atorvastatin	Zocor APO-Pravastatin Pravachol Lipitor	
	Fibrates	Gemfibrozil	Lopid	

Antithrombotic agents

	Vitamin K antagonists Heparins	Warfarin sodium Enoxaparin sodium Dalteparin sodium	Coumadin Marevan Clexane Fragmin	History of: • AF • Heart valve replacement • DVT • PE
	Platelet aggregation inhibitors	Clopidogrel Abciximab Dipyridamole Aspirin	Clovix ReoPro Persantin Astrix Solprin Cardiprin	History of: • CAD/AMI • CVA/TIA (especially Persantin)
	Novel (New) Oral Anticoagulant (NOAC) Thrombin inhibitors & factor Xa inhibitors	Dabigatran Rivaroxaban Apixaban	Pradaxa Xarelto Eliquis	History of: • AF • Heart valve replacement • DVT • PE

Diuretics

	Loop diuretics	Frusemide	Lasix, Urex	History of: • Hypertension • CCF
	Thilazide diuretics	Hydrochloro-thiazide	Dithiazide	
	Potassium-sparing agents	Spironolactone	Aldactone Spiractin	

ACS = acute coronary syndrome; CAD = coronary artery disease; CABG = coronary artery bypass grafting; PCI = percutaneous coronary intervention; AMI = acute myocardial infarction; SVT = supraventricular tachycardia; AF = atrial fibrillation; WPW = Wolff-Parkinson-White; CCF = congestive cardiac failure; LVF = left ventricular failure; ADHD = attention deficit hyperactivity disorder; DVT = deep vein thrombosis; PE = pulmonary embolism; TIA = transient ischaemic attack.

Table A1.2 Non-cardiac medications

	Classification/action	Generic name	Common trade names
Ophthalmologicals (eye)			
Anti-glaucoma preparations and miotics	Beta-blocking agents	Timolol Betaxolol	Timopt, Tenopt Betoptic
	Sympathomimetics in glaucoma therapy	Brimonidine	Alphagan
	Carbonic anhydrase inhibitors	Acetazolamide Dorzolamide	Diamox Trusopt
	Prostaglandin agonists	Latanoprost	Xalatan
	Parasympathomimetics	Pilocarpine	Isopto Carpine
Decongestants and anti-allergics	Alpha-agonists	Naphazoline	Albalon
	Ophthalmic antihistamines	Levocabastine	Livostin
Ophthalmic antibiotics	Antibacterials	Chloramphenicol Tobramycin	Chlorsig Tobrex
Systemic hormonal preparations			
Hormone replacement therapies		Thyroxine Oestradiol	Oroxine, Eutrosig Zumenon
Corticosteroids for systemic use		Hydrocortisone Betamethasone Dexamethasone Cortisone Prednisolone Triamcinolone Methylprednisolone	Hysone 4, Hysone 20 Celestone Dexmethsone Cortate Panafcortelone Predsone Tricortone Aristocort Advantan Depo-Medrol
Contraceptives		Levonorgestrel with ethinyloestradiol	Microgynon 50 ED
Drugs for the treatment of osteoporosis		Alendronate Raloxifene	Fosamax Evista
Respiratory agents/drugs for obstructive airway disease			
Adrenergics	Short-acting selective β2 agonists	Salbutamol Terbutaline	Ventolin, Asmol Bricanyl
	Long-acting β2 agonists	Salmeterol Eformoterol	Serevent Oxis turbohaler
Other systemic drugs for obstructive airways disease			
	Anticholinergics	Ipratropium bromide Tiotropium	Atrovent Spiriva
Anti-allergic agents, excluding corticosteroids	Cromolyn/mast cell stabilisers	Cromolyn sodium	Intal
Glucocorticoids	Corticosteroids	Budesonide Fluticasone Beclomethasone	Pulmicort Flixotide Qvar
	Xanthines	Theophylline	Nuelin SR
	Leukotriene receptor antagonists	Montelukast	Singulair
Antihistamines for systemic use			
	Sedating antihistamines	Promethazine	Phenergan
	Non-sedating antihistamines	Loratadine Cetirizine Fexofenadine	Claratyne Zyrtec Telfast

continued

Table A1.2 Non-cardiac medications—cont'd

	Classification/action	Generic name	Common trade names
	Cough and cold preparations		
	Decongestants	Oxymetazoline Pseudoephedrine	Drixine Logicin sinus
	Cough suppressants	Pholcodine	Duro-Tuss
	Drugs used in diabetes		
Oral hypoglycaemic agents	Sulfonamides	Gliclazide Glibenclamide Glipizide Glimepiride	Diamicron Glimel Melizide Amaryl
	Alpha-glucosidase inhibitors	Acarbose	Glucobay 50, 100
	Biguanides	Metformin	Diaformin
	Thiazolidinediones	Rosiglitazone Pioglitazone	Avandia Actos
Insulin and analogues	Insulin, fast-acting	Insulin lispro, Insulin aspart and glulisine	Humalog NovoRapid Apidra
	Insulin, intermediate-acting	Insulin isophane Insulin isophane bovine	Humulin Hypurin isophane
Antidotes to insulin overdose	Glucagon	Glucagon	GlucaGen
	Dopaminergic agents	Apomorphine	Apomine
	DOPA and DOPA derivatives	Carbidopa/Levodopa Levodopa with benserazide	Sinemet Madopar 125
	Anticholinergics	Benxhexol Benztropine	Artane Cogentin
	Drugs for CNS disorders/anti-epileptics		
	Enhancement of inhibition by GABA	Clonazepam Phenobarbitone Vigabatrin Tiagabine Topiramate	Paxam, Rivotril Phenobarbitone Sabril Gabitril Epirimax, Topamax, Tamate
	Blockade of sodium channels	Phenytoin Sodium valproate Carbamazepine Lamotrigine Gabapentin Ethosuximide	Dilantin Epilim Tegretol Lamogine APO-Gabapentin, Neurontin Zarontin
	CNS disorders/antipsychotics/neuroleptics/psycholeptics		
Typical		Lithium	Lithicarb
Atypical	Dopamine receptor antagonists	Chlorpromazine Flupenthixol Pericyazine Clozapine Risperidol Haloperidol Olanzapine Aripiprazole Quetiapine	Largactil Fluanxol Neulactil Clopine Risperdal Serenace Zyprexa Abilify Seroquel

Table A1.2 Non-cardiac medications—cont'd

	Classification/action	Generic name	Common trade names
CNS disorders/anti-anxiety, sedative and hypnotic drugs (panic disorders etc)			
	Benzodiazepines	Diazepam Nitrazepam Temazepam Alprazolam Clonazepam Flunitrazepam Oxazepam	Valium Mogadon Temaze, Normison Xanax Rivotril Rohypnol Serepax
	Other anxiolytics	Zopiclone Buspirone	Imrest Buspar
CNS disorders/antidepressants/stress disorders			
	Tricyclic antidepressants	Amitriptyline Imipramine Nortriptyline Dothiepin Trimipramine Clomipramine Doxepin	Endep Tofranil, Melipramine Allegron Dothep Surmontil Anafranil Deptran, Sinequan
	Monoamine oxidase inhibitors (MAOIs)	Phenelzine Tranylcypromine Moclobemide	Nardil Parnate Aurorox
	Selective serotonin reuptake inhibitors (SSRIs)	Fluoxetine Paroxetine Sertraline Citalopram	Prozac Aropax, Paxil Zoloft Cipramil
CNS disorders/antidepressants/stress disorders			
	Serotonin/noradrenaline reuptake inhibitors (SNRIs)	Venlafaxine	Effexor-XR
Mood stabilisers		Lithium carbonate	Lithicarb
Anti-dementia drugs	Cholinesterase inhibitors	Donepezil Rivastigmine Galantamine	Aricept Exelon Reminyl
Antibiotics for systemic and topical use			
Antibacterials for systemic use	Cephalosporins	Cephalexin Cefaclor Ceftriaxone Clindamycin	Cefaclor GH Ceftriaxone ICP APO Clindamycin
	Tetracyclines	Doxycycline	Doryx
	Penicillins	Amoxycillin Ampicillin	Alphamox
	Macrolides	Azithromycin Roxithromycin Erythromycin	APO azithromycin Rulide Eryc
Antibiotics for topical use	Gram-negative aerobes	Mupirocin	Bactroban
Antifungals	Azole antifungals	Clotrimazole Fluconazole Ketoconazole Nystatin	Canesten Diflucan Nizoral Nilstat oral suspension
	Allylamine antifungal	Terbinafine	Lamisil
	Polyene macrolide	Amphotericin B Amorolfine	Fungilin Loceryl
Antivirals		Aciclovir	Acyclo-V, Zovirax

continued

1021

Table A1.2 Non-cardiac medications—cont'd

	Classification/action	Generic name	Common trade names
Drugs for the treatment of gastrointestinal system disorders			
Antiemetics	5HT3 receptor antagonist Dopamine antagonist	Ondansetron Prochlorperazine Metoclopramide	Onsetron, Zofran Stemetil Maxolon
Motion sickness	Anticholinergics	Hyoscine	Travacalm
Antidiarrhoeals	Opioid agonists	Loperamide	Imodium
Drugs for acid-related disorders	H2 receptor antagonists	Ranitidine	Zantac
Drugs for gastro-oesophageal reflux disease	Proton pump inhibitors	Esomeprazole Omeprazole Rabeprazole	Nexium Maxor Pariet
Cathartics and laxatives		Lactulose Psyllium husk powder	Actilax Metamucil orange smooth
Antacids		Aluminium hydroxide, magnesium hydroxide Magnesium bicarbonate	Mylanta Gaviscon
Analgesics			
Narcotic analgesics		Hydromorphone Codeine Oxycodone Morphine Tramadol	Dilaudid Various/codeine Endone/oxycontin Various/morphine Tramol
Non-narcotic analgesics, antipyretics	Salicylates	Aspirin	Solprin
	Antipyretic analgesics	Paracetamol	Panadol
Drugs for the treatment of neuropathic pain		Amitriptyline Pregabalin Gabapentin	Endep Lyrica Neurontin
Drugs for the treatment of inflammatory disorders	Non-steroidal anti-inflammatories	Aspirin Ibuprofen Indomethacin Naproxen Piroxicam	Solprin Nurofen Indocid Naprosyn Feldene
	Steroidal anti-inflammatories	Dexamethasone Prednisolone	Dexmethsone Panafcortelone
Anti-migraine preparations	Ergot alkaloids Selective serotonin 5HT-1 agonists	Methysergide Sumatriptan Cyproheptadine	Deseril Imigran Periactin

Glossary

aberrancy Departing from normal or the usual course.

abdominal compartment syndrome Describes the pathophysiological consequences of raised intraabdominal pressure; may be associated with any clinical condition that increases such pressure, including massive intraabdominal or retroperitoneal haemorrhage, intestinal obstruction or severe gut oedema.

ablation Therapy designed to destroy tissues that generate or sustain arrhythmias.

access catheter A plastic tubing device with two central lumens placed percutaneously in a large vein for the purpose of drawing blood into a renal replacement therapy circuit and enabling blood from the circuit to be returned to the patient.

access catheter site The position where the skin and large vein are punctured in order to place a vascular access catheter.

actigraph Used for measuring movement, in particular with regards to the quantity of sleep.

acute coronary syndrome (ACS) A broad spectrum of clinical presentations, spanning ST-segment elevation myocardial infarction through to an accelerated pattern of angina without evidence of myonecrosis.

acute kidney injury (AKI) Formerly known as acute renal failure (ARF), this describes the spectrum of illness including pathophysiological and clinical changes and causative factors associated with an abrupt loss of urine production.

acute liver failure (ALF) Liver cell injury occurring over a short period of time to a critical mass of liver cells; as a result, the liver is unable to maintain homeostasis.

acute lung injury (ALI) A distinct form of acute respiratory failure characterised by progressive hypoxaemia, reduced lung compliance and diffuse pulmonary infiltrates on chest x-ray.

acute-on-chronic liver failure (AoCLF) Results from an acute decompensation of chronic liver disease; can be precipitated by infection, bleeding or intoxication.

acute-phase proteins Proteins (also known as acute-phase reactants) that are synthesised in the liver in response to inflammation; include C-reactive protein, alpha-1-antitrypsin, coagulation factors (e.g. fibrinogen, prothrombin, factor VIII, plasminogen) and complement factors.

acute pulmonary oedema Sudden collection of fluid in the interstitial spaces and terminal airways of the lungs.

acute respiratory distress syndrome (ARDS) A life-threatening condition of the lungs whereby insufficient oxygen is drawn into the lungs, resulting in insufficient gas exchange.

acute tubular necrosis (ATN) A collective term reflecting pathological renal changes from various renal insults of a nephrotoxic or ischaemic origin.

adenosine triphosphate (ATP) A naturally occurring compound in the body that is converted to adenosine diphosphate, releasing energy for use within the body.

adult guardian An officer who is appointed to protect the interests and rights of adults with impaired decision-making capacity, no matter the type or cause of impairment. The adult guardian is an independent statutory officer.

advance directive A document that expresses a patient's preferences regarding end-of-life issues.

advanced life support (ALS) The provision of effective airway management, ventilation of the lungs and production of circulation using techniques additional to those used for basic life support.

afterload The load imposed on the muscle during contraction; translates to systolic myocardial wall tension.

allergen An antigen that causes an allergic response.

allograft Transplanted organ and tissue.

amylase An enzyme that breaks down starch, glycogen and dextrin to form glucose, maltose and the limit dextrins.

amyloid angiopathy Deposition of β-amyloid in the vessel walls of arteries within the brain; a morphological hallmark of Alzheimer's disease.

anabolism The phase of metabolism in which simple substances (e.g. amino acids) are synthesised into complex materials (e.g. proteins).

anaphylaxis A life-threatening allergic reaction.

angiodysplasia Swollen blood vessels in the colon prone to rupture and haemorrhage.

angio-oedema Leakage of fluid into the layers of the skin due to alterations in capillary permeability.

anosognosia A lack of knowledge or insight into one's disease.

antepartum haemorrhage Any bleeding from the genital tract after 20 weeks' gestation and before the birth of the baby.

anticoagulation The effect of a drug aimed at stopping blood from clotting.

anxiety A disorder characterised by excessive concern or worry, resulting in irritability, restlessness and disturbed sleep.

antigen Any substance that causes an immune response.

anxiolytic An intervention that inhibits anxiety.

antivenom A biological substance used to treat symptoms associated with envenomation.

APACHE score Abbreviation for Acute Physiology and Chronic Health Evaluation; a numerical value determined from a collection of predetermined criteria that enables the severity of an illness to be classified. The score provides a risk-of-death calculation and enables patients with critical illness to be compared in an objective manner.

aphasia Inability to speak.

apnoea No ventilatory effort.

apoptosis Normal physiologically programmed cell death; the main mechanism used to eliminate dysfunctional cells.

arrhythmia A broad term used to describe any rhythm other than sinus rhythm.

arterial blood gas An arterial blood sample taken to assess pH, bicarbonate, oxygen and carbon dioxide levels, and other electrolytes.

arteriovenous (AV) circuit The arterial and venous vascular access cannula or shunt and associated tubing necessary to carry blood in and out of a haemofilter and the circulation.

ascites An abnormal accumulation of fluid in the abdomen; commonly caused by liver dysfunction.

aspiration Movement of water or liquid into the lungs with resultant pulmonary damage.

asterixis A clinical sign indicating a lapse of posture, usually manifest in a bilateral flapping tremor at the wrist. Tremors are not symmetrical.

ataxia A lack of voluntary coordination of muscle movement.

atelectasis Collapse of part of the lung; caused by blockage of the air passage or external pressure on the lung.

atopy A genetic predisposition for hypersensitivity reactions to common environmental antigens.

Australasian Transplant Coordinators Association (ATCA) Formed to promote communication and collaboration among organ and tissue donor and transplant coordinators and to promote research, education and discussion of professional and ethical issues in the field in Australasia.

autonomy Ethical principle of self-determination and independence.

azotaemia Accumulation of excessive amounts of nitrogenous waste in the blood.

bacteraemia The presence of viable bacteria in the blood.

barotrauma Injury to the body due to changes in barometric or water pressure.

basic life support (BLS) The support of life by the initial establishment of and/or maintenance of airway, breathing and circulation and related emergency care.

benefit–cost The relative merits of an action based on the benefit that will be achieved and the possible cost (financial or other) that might result from such an action.

benefit–risk The relative merits of an action based on the benefit that will be achieved and the possible risk or adverse outcome that might occur from such an action.

berry aneurysm A saccular aneurysm that forms as an outpouching in a blood vessel; most often found at the base of the brain.

biopsy A medical procedure whereby a sample of tissue is taken for further analysis.

biphasic A pattern of electrical flow where the current reverses direction in the middle of the waveform, flowing first from one electrode pad through the heart to the second electrode pad and then from the second pad through the heart to the first pad.

bleb A blister-like pocket filled with air on the surface of the lungs.

brain death Death from confirmed irreversible cessation of all functions of the person's brain and/or absent intracranial blood flow.

bulla An air-filled cavity within the lung tissue.

cachexia Wasting of muscle; muscle atrophy associated with weakness, fatigue and a loss of appetite.

cadaveric donor Donor of tissue and solid organs after death.

capnography The monitoring of expired carbon dioxide.

cardiac arrest The cessation of cardiac mechanical activity, with the absence of a detectable pulse, and unresponsiveness and apnoea (or agonal respirations).

cardiac pacing The delivery of an electrical impulse to either or both of the atria and ventricles to initiate or maintain normal cardiac electrical activity.

cardiomyopathy A condition whereby the heart muscle becomes enlarged, dilated or stiff.

cardiopulmonary resuscitation (CPR) A technique of heart compression and inflation of the lungs used in an attempt to revive a person who has suffered a cardiac arrest.

care bundle A small collection of evidence-based activities applied to selected patients.

carina The junction of the left and right main bronchi.

carotid siphon The twisted segment of the internal carotid artery that extends from the point where the artery enters the skull through the carotid canal or foramen in the temporal bone and bifurcates into the anterior and middle cerebral arteries that form part of the cerebral artery circle: the circle of Willis.

catabolism The phase of metabolism in which complex materials (e.g. polysaccharides) are broken down into simple substances (e.g. monosaccharides) and release energy in the process.

catamenial pneumothorax A spontaneous pneumothorax occurring in women with a history of endometriosis; usually occurs shortly after the onset of menses.

catatonic A state of apparent unresponsiveness to external stimuli despite appearing awake.

cellulitis Bacterial infection of the skin, particularly the dermis and subcutaneous fascia.

chemoreceptor A sensor that responds to changes in the chemical composition of the blood.

chronic liver failure (CLF) Liver cell injury occurring over a prolonged period; the function of the residual liver cell mass is sufficient to maintain homeostasis.

chronic obstructive pulmonary disease (COPD) A progressive and irreversible condition that reduces inspiratory and expiratory lung capacity: this increases airway resistance and leads to loss of lung recoil.

chronic renal failure (CRF) A failure of normal kidney function with slow insidious onset, often related to degenerative diseases such as diabetes or chronic heart failure.

chronotrope An agent that increases the contraction rate.

clinical practice guidelines Statements about appropriate healthcare for specific clinical circumstances that assist practitioners in their day-to-day practice.

clinical reasoning The cognitive processes and strategies that clinicians use to make clinical decisions regarding patient assessment and care; synonymous with clinical decision-making.

clotting indices Blood tests that indicate the potential for blood to clot; usually time-based or expressed as a ratio of normal time taken for blood to clot.

coagulation factors Elements of the blood responsible for the formation of a blood clot (e.g. platelet count).

coagulopathy A disorder of the clotting mechanism of the blood that can be caused by preexisting disease, medications, pathophysiological conditions such as hypothermia and acidosis, or current treatments such as a massive blood transfusion.

cognitive impairment A deficiency in the ability to think, perceive, reason or remember that may result in loss of ability to attend to one's daily living needs.

cold ischaemic time The time from cross-clamp to when blood supply is re-established to an organ during transplant surgery.

colloid Large molecules that do not precipitate in solution.

colloid osmotic pressure Also known as oncotic pressure; the osmotic pressure of a colloid in solution.

complementary therapies Treatments that have not been considered part of standard Western medicine but that are increasingly being used in combination with standard medical treatments; may include therapies for pain, such as massage and relaxation techniques, and some nutritional therapies.

concept analysis A systematic process involving identification of all uses of a term, verification of common attributes and identification of manifestations of the term.

confidentiality The obligation of persons to whom private information has been given not to use that information for anything other than the primary purpose for which it was given.

consent The voluntary agreement of a person or a group, based on adequate knowledge and understanding of relevant material, to participate in research; informed consent is one possible result of the informed choice process—the other possible result is refusal.

continuous arteriovenous haemofiltration (CAVH) A technique of continuous renal replacement therapy whereby blood is driven by the patient's blood pressure through a filter containing a highly permeable membrane via an extracorporeal circuit originating in an artery and terminating in a vein.

continuous arteriovenous techniques All techniques of continuous renal replacement therapy (haemofiltration, haemodialysis and haemodiafiltration) whereby the patient's blood pressure (instead of a blood pump) drives blood through a filter containing a highly permeable membrane.

continuous positive airway pressure (CPAP) A treatment that uses a specific level of pressure applied to the airways in both the inspiratory and the expiratory phases of ventilation.

continuous renal replacement therapy (CRRT) A treatment applied continuously to replace renal function, including continuous veno-venous haemofiltration and continuous veno-venous haemodiafiltration.

controlled mechanical ventilation A ventilation mode that requires the patient to receive a neuromuscular blockade and sedation so that a fixed, non-triggered tidal volume and rate can be delivered.

contusion A bruise; an area where blood vessels have broken under the skin resulting in the blood moving into the surrounding tissue.

convection A process whereby dissolved solutes are removed with blood plasma water as it is filtered through the haemofilter membrane.

convulsion Seizure activity that is seen to cause the body to shake as a result of random muscular contractions.

cor pulmonale Alteration in the structure and function of the right ventricle caused by a respiratory disorder.

costochondritis Chest wall pain resulting from inflammation in the cartilaginous joints between the ribs and the sternum.

counterpulsation Rapid inflation of an intraaortic balloon catheter at the onset of diastole of each cardiac cycle and then deflation immediately before the onset of the next systole.

crepitation (crepitus) Crackling noise heard within the lungs during respiratory conditions such as pneumonia and acute pulmonary oedema.

cricothyroidotomy The establishment of an airway by making an incision through the cricothyroid membrane, enabling access to the trachea.

critical care nursing Specialised nursing care of critically ill patients who have an immediate life-threatening or potentially life-threatening illness or injury.

critical illness A state or disease process whereby life-support techniques and/or machines are required to sustain life until the patient recovers.

critically ill patients Patients who have an immediate life-threatening or potentially life-threatening illness or injury causing compromise to the function of one or more organs.

cross-clamp The act of clamping the aorta to achieve a controlled arrest of the heart, ceasing blood flow to all organs, and commencing infusion of cold perfusion fluid during organ retrieval surgery; marks the beginning of cold ischaemic time.

cryoanalgesia A method of analgesia aimed at disrupting neurosensory perception of pain using extreme cold.

cytokines Glycoproteins of low molecular weight that have immune function activity and are elevated as a result of bacterial multiplication and/or inflammation; high levels of cytokines can suppress immune function.

cytotoxin A substance that has a toxic effect on cells.

damage-control surgery A surgical approach that uses simple procedures for haemorrhage and contamination control prior to intensive medical management and partial recovery before an operation for definitive repair and reconstruction.

death The final cessation of the integrated functioning of the body; death is observed to have occurred when there is irreversible loss of brain function or irreversible cessation of circulation.

deep vein thrombosis (DVT) A thrombus (blood clot) formed in the deep veins, predominantly of the legs.

defibrillation The application of a controlled electrical shock to the victim's chest in order to terminate a life-threatening cardiac rhythm.

delusion A fixed, false belief despite logic suggesting otherwise.

denervation Loss of direct autonomic nervous system innervation.

deontological A philosophical view reflecting duty or a moral obligation to behave or act in a particular way.

depolarisation The electrical state in an excitable cell whereby the inside of the cell becomes less negative relative to the outside.

dermonecrotic Causing necrosis of the skin.

designated officer According to Australian law, a person appointed by the governing body of a health institution to authorise consent for non-coronial postmortems and organ and tissue retrieval for transplant and research.

designated specialist According to Australian law, a person appointed by the governing body of a health institution with authority to confirm brain death.

diabetic ketoacidosis (DKA) A metabolic derangement resulting from a relative or absolute insulin deficiency; characterised by hyperglycaemia, cellular dehydration and intravascular volume depletion, ketosis and electrolyte abnormalities.

diagnosis-related group (DRG) A method to standardise the diagnoses used to classify patients into uniform groups; it allows for weighting/comparison of one DRG with another so that relative resource use for each can be analysed.

dialysate The solution administered into the ultra-filtrate-dialysate compartment of the haemofilter of a haemodialyser in order to achieve solute clearance by diffusion.

dialysis Purification of blood by diffusion of waste substances through a membrane.

diaphoresis Sweating.

diathesis Predisposition to a particular disorder or disease.

diastole The phase of relaxation pertaining to the heart.

diffusion A process whereby solutes are transported across a semipermeable membrane.

diplopia Double vision.

disseminate intravascular coagulation (DIC) Widespread formation of fibrin clots, platelet and coagulation protein consumption and occlusion of microvasculature, resulting in impaired cellular tissue oxygen delivery.

DonateLife Organ Donor Coordinator Also referred to as an Organ Donor Coordinator, State Organ Donor Coordinator or State Donor Nurse Consultant in various jurisdictions.

donation Refers to organ and tissue donation; an organ donor may also be a tissue donor and some donors are tissue donors only.

donation after cardiac death Also known as non-heart-beating donation; donor of selective solid organs and tissues after cardiac death rather than brain death.

dose intensity How much renal replacement therapy is applied or prescribed for a given time.

drowning The process of experiencing respiratory impairment from submersion or immersion in a liquid.

dry drowning A submersion incident where no significant water (liquid) is aspirated into the lungs.

dysarthria Speech disorder as a result of motor incompetence.

dysphagia Difficulty swallowing.

dyspnoea The sensation of breathlessness or shortness-of-breath; can occur in the absence of any physiological evidence.

ecchymosis Blood in the tissues causing a blue or purplish patch.

eclampsia A severe variant of preeclampsia characterised by tonic–clonic seizures which are not caused by any preexisting disease or other identifiable causes (e.g. epilepsy, cerebral haemorrhage).

effacement The shortening and thinning of a tissue, most commonly the cervix during labour.

Ehlers-Danlos syndrome A group of hereditary disorders that affect connective tissue, primarily the joints, skin and blood vessel walls.

emancipatory practice development A continuous process used to improve an aspect of patient care through fostering empowerment of others and creating a transformational culture.

embolus A mass travelling freely within the intravascular space that can be gaseous, such as air, or solid, such as a blood clot or fatty mass. It has the potential to block the smaller vessels, depriving the tissues distal to this site of circulation.

endogenous Having an internal origin or cause.

endotracheal tube An artificial airway used in critical care settings to enable delivery of mechanical ventilation and clearance of airway secretions.

envenomation The injection of venom from a venomous animal.

erythema Redness of the skin or mucous membranes.

eschar A section of dead tissue that sheds off; most often occurs as a result of burns.

ethical Right or morally acceptable.

ethics The study of morals and values.

evidence-based nursing The deliberate and judicious use of practices, procedures and medications that are supported by rigorous evidence gained from research.

excitotoxicity A pathological process whereby nerve cells are damaged or die as a result of excessive neurotransmitter stimulation.

exogenous Having an external origin or cause.

exsanguinate To drain the blood; to bleed out to the point of death.

extracorporeal circuit (EC) The path for blood flow outside the body; includes the plastic tubing carrying the blood to a filter (or haemofilter or dialyser) from the vascular access catheter and from the filter back to the body via the access catheter again.

extracorporeal membrane oxygenation (ECMO) Circulation of blood outside the body to provide total artificial support of cardiac and pulmonary function.

eye care Cleansing of the eyes and the prevention of dry eyes and corneal abrasions by the use of artificial tears and measures to maintain eyelid closure.

faecalith A small segment of impacted faecal matter found in a small sac in the wall of the intestine.

family Those closest to a person in knowledge, care and affection, including the immediate biological family, the family of acquisition (related by marriage or contract) and the family of choice and friends (not related biologically or by marriage or contract).

fascia Connective tissue.

fibrosis The formation of excessive fibrous connective tissue in an organ or tissue.

filter (dialyser) A tubular-shaped device made up of plastic casing and the capillary fibres of the semipermeable membrane within it.

filter life (or functional life) of the extracorporeal circuit The passage of blood through the extracorporeal circuit, particularly if the haemofilter initiates blood clotting.

fulminant hepatic failure The definition of acute liver failure when associated with hepatic encephalopathy.

gestation The estimated gestational age of the baby in completed weeks using all available obstetric information (clinical estimation, ultrasound, cycle length, etc.), counting from the first day of the woman's last menstrual period. Commonly recorded as 35 + 2/40, indicating that the gestation is 35 weeks and 2 days.

glycogenolysis The breakdown of glycogen molecules to release glucose for energy.

glyconeogenesis The production of glucose from non-carbohydrate carbon substrates.

glycosuria Excretion of glucose in the urine.

haematemesis Vomiting blood.

haematochezia The passage of fresh blood from the anus.

haematuria Blood in the urine.

haemodiafiltration A process that uses both convection and diffusion as mechanisms for removal of waste solutes in the application of artificial kidney techniques.

haemodialyser A haemofilter designed principally to facilitate diffusion of plasma solutes from the blood.

haemodynamic monitoring The measurement of pressure, flow and oxygenation within the cardiovascular system.

haemofilter (blood filter) The primary functional component of the renal replacement therapy system, responsible for separating plasma water from the blood and/or allowing the exchange of solutes across the filter membrane by diffusion.

haemoptysis Coughing up blood.

haemorrhagic A tendency to bleed.

haemotympanum Blood in the tympanic cavity of the ear.

hallucination Perception without stimuli; can be visual, auditory, olfactory or a physical sensation.

heat exhaustion A severe form of heat illness that produces hyperpyrexia and collapse due to the inability to sweat.

heat–moisture exchanger A disposable humidification device that traps the water vapour from expired breath within the filter and moisturises subsequent inhaled breaths.

heat stroke Form of heat illness associated with severe water or salt depletion due to excessive sweating and a temperature lower than 40°C.

HELLP syndrome A severe variant of preeclampsia characterised by haemolysis, elevated liver enzymes and low platelets.

hemianaesthesia Loss of sensation on one side of the body.

hemiparesis Weakness on one side of the body.

hemiplegia Paralysis on one side of the body.

heparin A drug used to prevent blood clotting; administered to prevent clot formation following surgery and to prevent clotting when extracorporeal blood flow is required for dialysis or heart bypass operations.

hepatic encephalopathy (HE) The cerebral effects of liver failure, which may range from mild confusion to high risk of death from severe cerebral oedema and raised intracranial pressure.

hepatorenal syndrome (HRS) The development of renal failure in the setting of severe liver disease. It probably results from a reduction in renal perfusion caused by splanchnic vasodilation, which is a consequence of the production of the vasodilator substance nitric oxide by inflamed liver cells.

heterotopic Implantation of an organ into an abnormal anatomical position.

homonymous hemianopsia Loss of visual field on either the left or right of the vertical plane in both eyes. The loss of visual field is on the same side in both eyes.

Horner's syndrome Interruption of sympathetic nervous innovation to the eye resulting in the classic triad of miosis (pupil constriction), loss of hemifacial sweating and drooping eyelid.

hybrid A cross between two species; a mixture of approaches or techniques to provide renal replacement therapy (e.g. intermittent haemodialysis and haemofiltration).

hydrostatic pressure The pressure exerted by a fluid.

hyperaemia A process whereby the body adjusts the flow of blood to an area of tissue to meet its metabolic needs.

hyperglycaemic hyperosmolar non-ketotic state A metabolic derangement characterised by hyperglycaemia, cellular dehydration and intravascular volume depletion, and electrolyte abnormalities. Insulin excretion is maintained in this condition, so ketosis is not seen.

hypoglycaemia A blood sugar or glucose concentration generally below 4 mmol/L.

hypokinesis Reduced or slow movement.

hypothalamic–pituitary–adrenal (HPA) axis A system, the activation of which can lead to a host defence response and the release of catecholamines.

hypothalamus A portion of the brain controlling, among other things, behavioural and emotional responses.

hypothesis A proposition to explain a phenomenon.

hypoxaemia Inadequate oxygen within the blood to meet the demands of the body.

hypoxia Inadequate oxygen at a cellular level to meet cellular metabolic demands.

iatrogenic Illness or injury caused by a medical procedure.

immunoglobulin An antibody.

immunoneuroendocrine axis The nexus between the immune response and the hypothalamic–pituitary–adrenal axis and the response to stress.

immunosuppression Drug therapies to suppress the body's natural response to reject non-self organs.

Indigenous person Aboriginal or Torres Strait Islander person in Australia or Māori in New Zealand.

induction of labour A procedure performed for the purpose of initiating and stimulating the process of labour. This may include the artificial rupture of the membranes and/or the use of uterine-stimulating medication.

infant A child under 1 year of age.

infarction Death of tissue (necrosis) due to inadequate oxygen supply.

infection An inflammatory response to the presence of microorganisms or the invasion of normally sterile host tissue by those organisms.

infection control A series of policies and procedures aimed at reducing the risk of hospital-acquired infection and limiting the spread of infection.

innate immune system A natural immune system.

inoconstrictor An inotrope with vasoconstrictor properties.

inodilator An inotrope with vasodilator properties.

inotrope An agent that increases myocardial contractility.

insomnia An inability to fall asleep or remain asleep.

intensivist A medical specialist who diagnoses and prescribes treatment for a variety of life-threatening illnesses managed within the intensive care unit.

intermittent haemodialysis (IHD) Diffusive treatment during which blood and dialysate are circulated on the opposite sides (within the tubes/fibres and outside the fibres) of a semipermeable membrane in a counter-current direction in order to achieve diffusive solute removal.

intraaortic balloon pump (IABP) Mechanical assistance for a failing heart based on the principles of diastolic augmentation and systolic unloading by counterpulsation of a balloon in the aorta.

Introductory Donation Awareness Training (IDAT) The IDAT is a multidisciplinary workshop which provides introductory training and education to a range of health professionals working in organ, eye and tissue donation.

introitus The entrance to a hollow organ or canal, such as the vagina.

ischaemia The restriction of blood supply to a tissue resulting in hypoxia of the tissue distal to the restriction.

justice That which concerns fairness or equity, often divided into three parts: procedural justice, concerned with fair methods of making decisions and settling disputes; distributive justice, concerned with the fair distribution of the benefits and burdens of society; and corrective justice, concerned with correcting wrongs and harms through compensation or retribution.

lacrimation Secretion of tears.

legislation Laws that have been enacted by government (e.g. to define death and all aspects of organ and tissue donation).

limbic system The areas of the brain involved with emotions and memory.

lipase Any enzyme that is capable of degrading lipid molecules. Lipase breaks down lipids into simple fatty acids and glycerol that can be absorbed across the mucosa of the stomach and small intestine.

lipohyalinosis Disease of the small vessel of the brain characterised by vessel wall thickening.

living donor A living person who donates serum, tissue or solid organs.

living will An advance directive expressing an individual's wishes regarding healthcare if they become terminally ill and lose the ability to make decisions.

lumen The inside space of a tubular structure such as a blood vessel.

lysis Cellular destruction.

malaise A general feeling of discomfort or being unwell.

malignancy Cancerous cells that are able to spread to other sites within the body and invade and destroy tissues.

Mallory-Weiss tear A tear in the mucous membrane at the junction of the oesophagus and the stomach.

Marfan's syndrome A genetic disorder that affects the connective tissue, including bones, joints and blood vessels.

margination Adhesion to endothelium.

masticate To chew (food).

mechanical circulatory support Partial or total cardiovascular support devices such as an intraaortic balloon pump and ventricular assist devices.

melaena Black, tarry stools containing large amounts of blood, indicating blood loss in the upper digestive tract.

meninges The three layers of tissue that surround the brain and the spinal cord: the dura mater, the arachnoid mater and the pia mater.

metabolites Substances that are used or produced by enzyme reactions or other metabolic processes.

monophasic Pattern of electrical flow whereby the current flows in one direction throughout the pulse, from one electrode pad through the heart to the other electrode pad.

multigravida A woman's second (or third or fourth etc.) pregnancy.

multi-organ donor Donor of solid organs (i.e. kidneys, pancreas, heart, lungs, liver) and tissue.

multi-organ dysfunction syndrome (MODS) The presence of altered organ function in an acutely ill patient where homeostasis cannot be maintained without intervention.

Münchausen's syndrome by proxy A behaviour pattern whereby a carer misleads others into thinking that a person they are caring for has an illness in order to draw attention to themselves.

mydriasis Pupil dilation as a result of drugs, disease or other cause.

myoglobin Iron- and oxygen-binding protein found in the muscle.

myoglobinuria The presence of myoglobin in the urine.

myolysis The breakdown or lysis of muscle tissue.

myotoxins Toxins that cause muscle damage; predominantly found in snake venom.

near-drowning Survival for at least 24 hours after a submersion incident.

necrosis A form of cell death characterised by cellular swelling and loss of membrane integrity as a result of hypoxia or trauma.

negligence A legal term defined as causing damage unintentionally but carelessly. A court will determine negligence based on reasonable foreseeability that damage might have been possible, a duty of care existed to the person damaged, a breach in that duty could be demonstrated and that damages were indeed experienced by the victim.

neoplasm An abnormal mass of tissue resulting from the abnormal proliferation of cells.

nephrolithiasis Renal stones or calculi.

nephrologist A medical specialist who diagnoses and prescribes treatment, including dialysis, for kidney disease and failure.

neurotoxin A toxin that interrupts nervous system signalling.

neurotransmitter A chemical that transmits a signal across the synapse between nerve cells, or between a nerve cell and an effector tissue.

nitric oxide (NO) A gas used as an endothelium-derived relaxant factor via inhalation to produce selective pulmonary vasodilation.

nociceptors Unspecialised nerve cell endings that initiate the sensation of pain.

non-invasive ventilation Positive pressure ventilation delivered via a nasal or facial mask (i.e. not via an endotracheal tube or tracheostomy).

nystagmus Involuntary rapid eye movement.

objective assessment Assessment that is able to be measured.

older child A child between 9 and 14 years of age.

oliguria Low or minimal urine output.

oliguric renal failure Renal failure with the additional characteristic of urine output less than 0.5 mL/kg/h in adults and less than 1 mL/kg/h in infants.

operculum Mucus plug that forms in the cervix during pregnancy.

ophthalmoplegia Paralysis or weakness of an eye muscle.

'opt-in' donation Specific consent for donation required from the potential donor's next of kin.

'opt-out' donation A presumed consent system, where eligible persons are considered for organ retrieval at the time of their death if they have not previously indicated their explicit objection.

oral hygiene The prevention of plaque-related disease by the use of tooth brushing and other oral hygiene aids.

organ A part of the body that performs vital function(s) to maintain life; includes the kidneys, heart, lungs, liver and pancreas.

Organ and Tissue Authority The peak body that works with all jurisdictions and sectors to provide a nationally coordinated approach to organ and tissue donation for transplantation to maximise rates of donation.

orthotopic Implantation of an organ into a normal anatomical position.

osmosis The movement of a pure fluid through a semipermeable membrane from a region of low solute concentration to a region of high solute concentration.

osmotic pressure The pressure exerted on a semipermeable membrane by a solution containing solutes that cannot pass through the membrane.

palliative A field of healthcare focused on making terminally ill patients comfortable in the period between cessation of interventions aimed at recovery and the patient's death.

paraesthesia Altered sensation (e.g. pins and needles).

paranoia Irrational and persistent feeling that one is the subject of intrusive attention from others.

parenchyma The essential or functional element or tissue of an organ.

parity The number of viable offspring a woman has had.

partogram Birth suite chart that records maternal and fetal monitoring during labour and the progress of labour (e.g. strength and frequency of contractions, fetal descent).

percutaneous coronary intervention (PCI) A group of technologies used to treat coronary artery disease, including percutaneous transluminal coronary angioplasty; rotational, directional and extraction atherectomy; laser angioplasty; and implantation of intracoronary stents.

peristalsis Coordinated muscle contractions along a muscular tube (e.g. contractions along the bowel move food through the intestines).

personal information Information by which individuals can be identified. This is defined in the *Privacy Act 1988* (Cwlth) as information or an opinion, whether true or not, and whether recorded in a material form or not, about an individual whose identity is apparent, or can reasonably be ascertained, from the information or opinion.

personal protective equipment (PPE) Equipment such as gloves, eye protection and masks used to protect healthcare staff from infectious diseases.

phaeochromocytoma A cholinergic-secreting tumour on the adrenal gland.

phagocytosis Ingestion and destruction of microorganisms and cellular debris by capable cells.

pharmacogenetics The study of differences in drug responses based on genetic differences in metabolic pathways.

photophobia An inability to visually tolerate light.

piloerection The involuntary erection of body hair.

pneumothorax An abnormal accumulation of air in the pleural space around the lungs.

polycystic kidney disease (PKD) A genetic condition characterised by the growth of cysts on the kidneys.

polycythaemia High red blood cell count in the blood.

polymyositis A disease of the connective tissue causing muscle inflammation and weakness.

polysomnography The continuous recording of various physiological variables during sleep, including brain-wave activity, eye movement and muscle tone.

portocaval shunt A connection between the portal vein and the inferior vena cava to reduce blood flow to the liver in order to reduce hepatic hypertension. This will reduce the chance of rupture and haemorrhage of veins in the oesophagus and stomach.

positive end expiratory pressure (PEEP) Positive pressure at the end of the expiratory phase.

post-dilution Administration of replacement fluid into a patient's blood via the extracorporeal circuit after it exits the haemofilter (post-filter delivery).

postpartum haemorrhage More than 500 mL blood loss from the genital tract following birth; it is categorised as primary, within the first 24 hours following birth, or secondary, from 24 hours to 6 weeks postpartum.

practice development A continuous process of improvement designed to promote increased effectiveness in patient-centred care; enables healthcare teams to develop their knowledge and skills, transforming the culture and context of care.

pre-dilution Administration of replacement fluid into a patient's blood via the extracorporeal circuit prior to its entry into the haemofilter (pre-filter delivery).

preeclampsia A serious condition affecting some pregnant women from around 20 weeks' gestation characterised by hypertension, proteinuria and fluid retention.

preload The load imposed by the initial fibre length of the cardiac muscle before contraction (i.e. at the end of diastole).

pressure ulcer Any injury caused by unrelieved pressure that damages the skin and underlying tissue, usually over a bony prominence.

pressure-controlled ventilation A ventilatory mode used to minimise pulmonary volutrauma, where each breath is delivered to a pre-set level of inspiratory pressure; tidal volumes may therefore vary.

pressure-regulated volume control A ventilation mode in which a mandatory rate and target tidal volume are set and the ventilator delivers breaths using the lowest achievable pressure and a decelerating flow pattern.

primigravida First pregnancy.

privacy Having control over the extent, timing and circumstances of sharing oneself (physically, behaviourally or intellectually) with others. Implies a zone of exclusivity, where individuals are free from the scrutiny of others.

prophylactic Intended to prevent disease or symptoms.

proteolysis The breakdown of proteins into smaller polypeptides or amino acids.

protocol A document that provides the background, rationale and objectives of research and describes its design, methodology, organisation, conduct and the conditions under which it is to be performed and managed.

propagate To disperse or spread.

pruritus Itching.

ptosis Drooping of the eyelid.

pulmonary dynamic hyperinflation Hyperinflation of a native lung with an obstructive lung disease and concurrent compression of the single lung allograft leading to respiratory failure and cardiac tamponade.

pulse oximetry A method used to monitor peripheral arterial oxygen saturation.

pulsus paradoxus A drop in systolic blood pressure by > 10 mmHg during inspiration, resulting in a loss of radial pulse detection for the affected beats.

purulent Containing, causing or discharging pus.

pyrexia Fever or elevated temperature.

pyrogen A fever-inducing substance.

rapid sequence intubation (RSI) The rapid induction of a patient using a combination of anaesthetic and paralysing agents given in quick succession to allow for the intubation of the airway.

recipient A person who receives organs and/or tissues from another person (the donor).

refeeding syndrome May occur in patients who have not received nutritional support for some time; involves life-threatening fluid and electrolyte shifts after initiation of aggressive nutritional support therapies.

rejection Destruction of the allograft due to the body's ability to identify self from non-self.

renal replacement therapy (RRT) Any treatment that replaces renal function; includes intermittent haemodialysis and peritoneal dialysis.

research Systematic, rigorous investigation to establish facts, principles and new knowledge.

research participant Individual about whom a researcher obtains data through intervention or interaction with that person or their identifiable private information.

respect for person Has two fundamental aspects: 1. respect for the autonomy of those individuals who are capable of making informed choices and respect for their capacity for self-determination; and 2. protection of persons with impaired or diminished autonomy—that is, those individuals who are incompetent or whose voluntary capacity is compromised.

resuscitation The preservation or restoration of life by establishing and/or maintaining airway, breathing and circulation and related emergency care.

retrieval The removal of organs and/or tissues from a donor for the purposes of transplantation into another person.

return of spontaneous circulation (ROSC) The resumption of sustained cardiac activity; signs include breathing (more than a few gasps), coughing, a palpable pulse or a measurable blood pressure.

rhabdomyolysis The breakdown of muscle tissue due to a direct or an indirect muscle injury that results in the release of the contents of muscle fibres and cells.

rhinorrhoea Discharge of mucus through the nose (i.e. a runny nose).

risk The function of the magnitude of a harm and the probability of its occurrence.

root cause analysis A structured process of analysing each step in a chain of events that led to a mistake or an error. Commonly applied to the health setting, where a team of unbiased experts are called on to dispassionately investigate how and why an error might have been caused by looking more at the system problems that emerged than at individual negligence.

scavenger system A system that removes gas following exhalation from the patient or a device close to the patient through which medication is being delivered; its function is to avoid the environment and those other than the patient receiving the medication.

sensory overload A prolonged overstimulus of the senses that can result from excessive or prolonged periods of noise, light, odours and touch from both equipment and personnel.

sepsis A systemic inflammatory response to infection.

sepsis-induced hypotension A systolic blood pressure < 90 mmHg or a reduction ≥ 40 mmHg from baseline in the absence of other causes of hypotension.

septic shock A subset of severe sepsis, defined as sepsis-induced hypotension in the presence of perfusion abnormalities despite adequate fluid resuscitation.

severe acute respiratory syndrome (SARS) The term given to a new virulent respiratory infection.

severe sepsis Sepsis associated with organ dysfunction, hypoperfusion or hypotension.

skill mix The relative mix of skilled and experienced staff in a team; for instance, in intensive care there may be very experienced and qualified registered nurses, some not-so-experienced nurses with and without critical care qualifications, and some non-nursing personnel who provide basic care.

slow, low, efficient dialysis A dialysis-based treatment similar to intermittent haemodialysis but where dialysate and blood flow rates are reduced to provide a slower clearance rate with an extended time of treatment (e.g. 8–10 hours instead of 3–4 hours).

somatic nervous system Part of the peripheral nervous system that carries motor and sensory information to and from skeletal muscles.

Starling's law (mechanism) of the heart This states that the strength of a contraction is a product of the stretch of the myocardial fibres just prior to the contraction.

stress A state of mental or emotional strain or suspense.

subarachnoid space The space between the arachnoid mater and the pia mater in the meningeal layers surrounding the brain and the spinal cord.

subcutaneous emphysema The presence of air in the subcutaneous tissues, usually felt as crackling bubbles underneath the skin; occurs in the upper chest, neck and face.

submersion incident Encompasses both drowning and near-drowning events without the implication of time or prognosis.

sudden cardiac arrest (SCA) Unexpected natural death from a cardiac event reflected by an abrupt loss of consciousness and generally less than 1 hour after the onset of symptoms.

surfactant A substance that lowers surface tension. In the lungs this makes the alveoli more stable, ensuring that they do not collapse during the increased intrathoracic pressure of exhalation.

sympathetic nervous system A part of the autonomic nervous system or involuntary nervous system; it regulates tissues not under voluntary control (e.g. glands, heart, blood vessels and smooth muscle).

sympathomimetic Mimicking the sympathetic nervous system responses.

synchronised intermittent mandatory ventilation A ventilator mode that enables synchronisation of mandatory breaths controlled by the ventilator with patient-initiated spontaneous breaths.

systematic inflammatory response syndrome (SIRS) A nonspecific syndrome that occurs as a result of a wide variety of severe clinical insults.

systole The phase of contraction pertaining to the heart.

tachyphylaxis A decrease in the responsiveness to a substance following repeated administration.

tachypnoeic Having an increased ventilation rate.

technical practice development A continuous process used to improve an aspect of patient care.

tension pneumothorax A life-threatening dynamic condition whereby a pneumothorax expands to the point that it causes alterations to perfusion.

tetany Involuntary muscle contraction.

thalamus Midbrain structure with a significant role in relaying information from the various sensory receptors to other brain areas.

thrombosis The formation of a clot inside a blood vessel.

thrombotic microangiopathy Formation of microvascular platelet aggregates and occasionally fibrin formation typically in the setting of microvascular endothelium injury.

thoracentesis A procedure to remove fluid from the intrapleural space.

tidal volume The volume of air that is moved into or out of the lungs with each breath.

tissue A group of specialised cells (e.g. cornea, heart valves, bone, skin) that perform defined functions.

tissue-only donor A donor of musculoskeletal tissue (i.e. femur, tibia, humerus, pelvis, ligaments, tendons, fascia, meniscus), cardiac tissue (i.e. bicuspid, tricuspid valves, aortic and pulmonary tissue), eye tissue (i.e. cornea and sclera) and/or skin tissue.

tissue typing The process of laboratory testing to identify the human leucocyte antigen (HLA) phenotype from the genes on chromosome 6, which will determine the tissue groups of a potential donor.

transformational leadership A style of leadership characterised by developing a shared vision, inspiring and communicating, valuing others, challenging and stimulating, developing trust and enabling others.

transplant The surgical implantation of one or more organs and tissues from one human being to another.

Transplant Nurses' Association (TNA) Formed to advance the education of nurses and other health professionals involved in the transplant process.

Transplantation Society of Australia and New Zealand (TSANZ) A body whose members (scientists, doctors, transplant coordinators and research students) have an interest in all forms of transplantation.

transpulmonary gradient (TPG) Mean pulmonary artery pressure minus pulmonary artery wedge pressure.

transtentorial herniation Herniation of the brain through the tentorial notch.

transudate Fluid that has shifted through a membrane into the interstitial spaces; it is low in proteins.

trismus Clenching of the jaw, resulting in an inability to open the mouth.

trypsin An enzyme that acts to degrade protein; also referred to as a proteolytic enzyme or proteinase.

ultrafiltrate The fluid produced during ultrafiltration.

ultrafiltration A process whereby plasma water is removed from the circulation through a haemofilter, achieving body fluid or water loss.

unconsciousness A condition where a victim fails to respond to verbal or tactile stimuli.

unethical Wrong or morally unacceptable.

urticaria Transient raised and reddened itchy areas of skin; often referred to as hives.

utilitarian Ethical theory that presupposes that an action is right if it achieves the greatest good for the greatest number of people.

varices Abnormal, enlarged, dilated veins prone to rupture and haemorrhage.

vascular access catheter A device inserted into a central vein to allow blood to be pumped into and out of a filter.

vasoactive Causing vasoconstriction or dilation.

vasopressor A substance that promotes vasoconstriction.

veno-venous (VV) circuit The vascular access cannula or shunt and associated tubing necessary to carry blood into and out of the haemofilter and the circulation.

venous air trap A device preventing inadvertent pumping of air via the pump into a patient, causing air embolism.

ventilator-associated pneumonia (VAP) A nosocomial pneumonia that develops in a patient mechanically ventilated for 48 hours or more.

ventricular assist device (VAD) Full or partial ventricular assistance provided by implantation of an artificial heart.

vertex Head-down presentation; the normal presentation of a baby during delivery.

vesicular breath sounds The normal breath sounds heard over the lung fields at a distance from the larger airways.

Virchow's triad Three broad categories of factors that contribute to thrombosis: hypercoagulability, endothelial injury and stasis of blood flow.

vital capacity The maximum amount of air that can be expelled forcibly following full inhalation.

volume-controlled ventilation A procedure where the tidal volume and rate of ventilation are set and controlled.

voluntary Free of coercion, duress or undue inducement.

warm ischaemia The time taken from the withdrawal of ventilation and treatment to the confirmation of the death of a donation-after-cardiac-death donor and the commencement of infusion of cold perfusion fluid and/or organ retrieval.

wet drowning Aspiration of water or liquid into the lungs with resultant pulmonary damage during a submersion incident.

work of breathing The physical effort exerted to achieve spontaneous breathing. It is affected by lung compliance, chest wall resistance, muscle wasting (intercostals and diaphragm) and/or fatigue and the use of secondary muscles to aid breathing.

younger child A child from 1 to 8 years of age.

Index

Page numbers followed by 'f' indicate figures, 't' indicate tables, and 'b' indicate boxes.

A

Index